Behavioral and Emotional Disorders in Adolescents

Behavioral and Emotional Disorders in **Adolescents**

Nature, Assessment, and Treatment

Edited by
David A. Wolfe
Eric J. Mash

THE GUILFORD PRESS
New York   London

© 2006 The Guilford Press
A Division of Guilford Publications, Inc.
72 Spring Street, New York, NY 10012
www.guilford.com

Printed in the United States of America

This book is printed on acid-free paper.

Last digit is print number: 9   8   7   6   5   4   3   2   1

Library of Congress Cataloging-in-Publication Data

Behavioral and emotional disorders in adolescents : nature, assessment, and treatment /
edited by David A. Wolfe, Eric J. Mash.
    p. cm.
  Includes bibliographical references and index.
  ISBN 1-59385-225-8 (hardcover)
  1. Mental illness—Diagnosis.   2. Behavioral assessment of
children.   3. Psychodiagnostics.   I. Wolfe, David A.   II. Mash, Eric J.
  RJ503.5.B436 2006
  618.92′89—dc22

                                     2005012856

To our wives, Barb and Heather

About the Editors

David A. Wolfe, PhD, holds the RBC Chair in Children's Mental Health at the Centre for Addiction and Mental Health (CAMH), and is a Professor of Psychology and Psychiatry at the University of Toronto. He is a fellow of the American Psychological Association and past president of Division 37 (Child, Youth, and Family Services). Dr. Wolfe has broad research and clinical interests in abnormal child and adolescent psychology, with a special focus on child abuse, domestic violence, and developmental psychopathology. He has authored numerous articles and books on these topics, especially in relation to the impact of early childhood trauma on later development in childhood, adolescence, and early adulthood. Dr. Wolfe is the 2005 recipient of the Donald O. Hebb award for Distinguished Contributions to Psychology from the Canadian Psychological Association.

Eric J. Mash, PhD, is a Professor of Psychology in the Department of Psychology and Program in Clinical Psychology at the University of Calgary. He is a fellow of the American and Canadian Psychological Associations; has served as an editor, editorial board member, and editorial consultant for many scientific and professional journals; and has written or edited numerous books and journal articles related to children's mental health, child and adolescent psychopathology, child and adolescent psychotherapy, and child and family assessment. Dr. Mash's research has focused on family relationships across a variety of child and family disorders, including attention-deficit/hyperactivity disorder, conduct problems, internalizing disorders, and maltreatment. He is a recipient of the Leadership Education in Neurodevelopmental Disabilities Distinguished Alumnus Award from the Oregon Health & Science University.

Contributors

Mona Abad, MA, Graduate Clinical Psychology Program, Loyola University, Chicago, Illinois

Ana M. Abrantes, PhD, Addictions Research, Butler Hospital, Brown University, Providence, Rhode Island

Lisa Armistead, PhD, Department of Psychology, Georgia State University, Atlanta, Georgia

Elizabeth Mayfield Arnold, PhD, Department of Psychiatry and Behavioral Medicine, Wake Forest University, Winston-Salem, North Carolina

Sasha G. Aschenbrand, MA, Child and Adolescent Anxiety Disorders Clinic, Department of Psychology, Temple University, Philadelphia, Pennsylvania

Howard E. Barbaree, PhD, Law and Mental Health Program, Centre for Addiction and Mental Health, Toronto, Ontario, Canada; Department of Psychiatry, University of Toronto, Toronto, Ontario, Canada

Russell A. Barkley, PhD, Department of Psychiatry, State University of New York Upstate Medical University at Syracuse, Syracuse, New York

Alexandra Boeving, PhD, Department of Psychiatry, Medical University of South Carolina, Charleston, South Carolina

Robert F. Bornstein, PhD, Department of Psychology, Gettysburg College, Gettysburg, Pennsylvania

Elizabeth Bromley, MD, New York State Psychiatric Institute, New York, New York

Ronald T. Brown, PhD, Department of Public Health, Temple University, Philadelphia, Pennsylvania

Sandra A. Brown, PhD, Department of Psychology, University of California at San Diego, La Jolla, California; Veterans Affairs San Diego Healthcare System, San Diego, California

Laura Arnstein Carpenter, PhD, Department of Pediatrics, Medical University of South Carolina, Charleston, South Carolina

Debbie Chiodo, MA, MEd, Centre for Prevention Science, Centre for Addiction and Mental Health, London, Ontario, Canada

Shannon E. Daley, PhD, Department of Psychology, University of Southern California, Los Angeles, California

Stephanie Sergent Daniel, PhD, Department of Psychiatry and Behavioral Medicine, Wake Forest University, Winston-Salem, North Carolina

Elisabeth M. Dykens, PhD, Department of Psychology and Human Development and Kennedy Center Institute, Vanderbilt University, Nashville, Tennessee; Neuropsychiatric Institute, University of California, Los Angeles, California

Rex L. Forehand, PhD, Department of Psychology, University of Vermont, Burlington, Vermont

Deborah Friedman, PhD, Graduate Clinical Psychology Program, Loyola University, Chicago, Illinois

Edward Garrido, PhD, Department of Psychology, Southern Methodist University, Dallas, Texas

David B. Goldston, PhD, Duke Child and Family Study Center and Department of Psychiatry and Behavioral Sciences, Duke University School of Medicine, Durham, North Carolina

Deborah Gorman-Smith, PhD, Department of Psychiatry, University of Illinois at Chicago, Chicago, Illinois

Constance Hammen, PhD, Department of Psychology, University of California, Los Angeles, California

Kristina A. Hedtke, MA, Child and Adolescent Anxiety Disorders Clinic, Department of Psychology, Temple University, Philadelphia, Pennsylvania

Robert M. Hodapp, PhD, Department of Special Education, Vanderbilt University, Nashville, Tennessee

Grayson N. Holmbeck, PhD, Department of Psychology, Loyola University, Chicago, Illinois

Barbara Jandasek, MA, Graduate Clinical Psychology Program, Loyola University, Chicago, Illinois

Jeffrey G. Johnson, PhD, Department of Psychiatry, College of Physicians and Surgeons, Columbia University, New York, New York; New York State Psychiatric Institute, New York, New York

Ernest N. Jouriles, PhD, Department of Psychology, Southern Methodist University, Dallas, Texas

Jody Kamon, PhD, Treatment Research Center, University of Vermont, Burlington, Vermont

Ellie Kazemi, MA, Graduate School of Education and Information Studies, University of California, Los Angeles, California

Philip C. Kendall, PhD, Child and Adolescent Anxiety Disorders Clinic, Department of Psychology, Temple University, Philadelphia, Pennsylvania

Beth A. Kotchick, PhD, Department of Psychology, Loyola College in Maryland, Baltimore, Maryland

Julie S. Kotler, MS, Department of Psychology, University of Washington, Seattle, Washington

Calvin M. Langton, PhD, Department of Psychiatry, University of Toronto, Toronto, Ontario, Canada

Angela LaRosa, MD, College of Health Professions, Medical University of South Carolina, Charleston, South Carolina

Daniel le Grange, PhD, Department of Psychiatry, University of Chicago, Chicago, Illinois

Orly Lipka, PhD, Department of Educational and Counseling Psychology and Special Education, University of British Columbia, Vancouver, British Columbia, Canada

James Lock, MD, PhD, Department of Psychiatry and Behavioral Sciences, Stanford University School of Medicine, Stanford, California

Eric J. Mash, PhD, Department of Psychology, University of Calgary, Calgary, Alberta, Canada

Anna McCarthy, MA, Department of Psychology, University of Houston, Houston, Texas

Robert J. McMahon, PhD, Department of Psychology, University of Washington, Seattle, Washington

Jennine S. Rawana, PhD, Centre for Prevention Science, Centre for Addiction and Mental Health, London, Ontario, Canada

Beth A. Rosner, PhD, Neuropsychiatric Institute, University of California, Los Angeles, California

Karen D. Rudolph, PhD, Department of Psychology, University of Illinois at Urbana–Champaign, Champaign, Illinois

Linda S. Siegel, PhD, Department of Educational and Counseling Psychology and Special Education, University of British Columbia, Vancouver, British Columbia, Canada

Joel R. Sneed, PhD, Department of Psychology, New York University, New York, New York

Steven G. Spector, MD, Child Study Center, Yale University, New Haven, Connecticut

Patrick H. Tolan, PhD, Department of Psychiatry and Institute for Juvenile Research, University of Illinois at Chicago, Chicago, Illinois

Fred R. Volkmar, PhD, Child Study Center, Yale University, New Haven, Connecticut

David A. Wolfe, PhD, Centre for Prevention Science, Centre for Addiction and Mental Health, London, Ontario, Canada; Departments of Psychology and Psychiatry, University of Toronto, Toronto, Ontario, Canada; Faculty of Education, University of Western Ontario, London, Ontario, Canada

Kenneth J. Zucker, PhD, Child, Youth, and Family Program, Clarke Institute of Psychiatry, Centre for Addiction and Mental Health, Toronto, Ontario, Canada

Preface

After years of neglect, research and clinical practice in regard to problems of adolescence have been expanding at a rapid pace. In the past decade, theories on development and psychopathology of adolescents have been advanced, along with improved research tools that allow us to examine more closely unique features of this period of development. Nonetheless, it is easy to overlook the many ways that adolescent development and disorders differ from those affecting children and adults. Much of the research on disorders of childhood and adolescence has been based primarily on samples of children. There has been inadequate representation of adolescents in many of these samples, sometimes leading to unsupported assumptions that the disorders are similar across development. We now know that adolescence is a period in which the central nervous system, especially brain functions, continues to unfold. This ongoing development is sometimes associated with emotional and behavioral changes that would be considered normal during this particular age period. However, some of this rapid change in physical and psychological development is associated with new adjustment problems and disorders that represent a shift in developmental course from earlier childhood.

The challenge facing editors of a book on adolescence is to capture the current status of this field, which is expanding rapidly and changing constantly. We began by deciding which disorders were most important and needed greater detail and expansion in relation to their expression during adolescence. We then identified experts who dedicated their professional careers to each of the disorders and asked them to address the specific issues pertaining to this age period. We provided them with a framework of the type of information that we wanted our readers to have and then let them tell us the current state of knowledge and the direction the field was taking for each of the disorders. We wanted the authors to capture current developments in the field and provide comprehensive and up-to-date summaries of each disorder. They were asked to focus their discussion on what is known about the disorders but also to give attention to the implications of assessment and treatment issues as they relate to adolescents. Each author or group of authors was asked to provide basic information about a particular disorder and to address questions such as the following: What do we know about this disorder? What is its course and outcome? What are the known theories and empirical findings? What is the current knowledge that deserves future attention? In addressing these questions, experts were directed to cover the nature of the behavior, symptoms, and/or cognitive and emotional deficits that define the core of each disorder; any criteria that exist to establish the presence of the disorder in adolescents or to form a diagnosis; an epidemiological description of the prevalence, gender distribution, and ethnic and cultural factors that may be known about the disorder in adolescents; developmental course and different pathways shown to be associated with the disorder, and which link the disorder during adolescence with prior development and later outcomes; the psychiatric, psychological, and social disorders or problems that may coexist with the disorder; and an overview of known and suspected causes of the disorder (etiology). As in our books on the theory, assessment, and treatment of childhood disorders (Mash & Barkley, 2003, 2006; Mash & Terdal, 1997), the authors have done a terrific job of assembling current information about adolescent disorders and problems and making this readily available to our readers.

The book begins with an introductory section that includes chapters covering general issues associated with understanding and intervention with adolescents. These chapters address developmental issues of adolescence and special issues associated with treatment/prevention. These chapters are followed by sections that include chapters on specific adolescent disorders and problems. The text provides comprehensive coverage of most forms of adolescent psychopathology, including attention-deficit and disruptive behavior disorders, mood disorders, anxiety disorders, developmental and learning disorders, eating disorders, abuse and trauma, health-related problems, and other common problems. The intent is to create an integrative state-of-the-art account of what is currently known about behavioral and emotional disorders in adolescents. For some problems, particularly those that were first identified in childhood (e.g., autism), very little was known about the adolescent manifestations of the disorder. For other disorders first manifested in childhood (e.g., attention-deficit/hyperactivity disorder), there was a larger knowledge base but not one that suggested unique differences between the basic features of the disorder in children versus adolescents. Finally, for other disorders with a later age of onset (e.g., depression and eating disorders), there was a substantial amount of information about these disorders in adolescents. However, in most cases, it was evident that an understanding of the causes, assessment, and treatment of the disorder in adolescents was evolving.

We wish to extend our sincere appreciation to the many professionals who took the time to share their knowledge and help us to prepare this comprehensive volume on disorders of adolescence. We are indebted to them for their substantial time commitment in researching the background materials and writing these chapters. We recognize as well the considerable effort it sometimes took to separate findings on adolescents from those studies that included adolescents and children together in their samples. Many others deserve our gratitude as well. Kitty Moore, Executive Editor at The Guilford Press, supported the project from its outset to completion, and the staff at Guilford—Sarah Lavender Smith, Carolyn Graham, Judith Grauman, and Laura Specht Patchkofsky—guided the manuscript through the production process. The administrative and secretarial talents of Shannon Burns in London and Alison Wiigs in Calgary were essential to the completion of this book. We also want to thank Seymour Weingarten (Editor-in-Chief) and Bob Matloff (President) at The Guilford Press for their unwavering support of this and our other books. Finally, we thank our families for giving up the family time needed to complete a book such as this and for their patience, support, and encouragement of our work in the field.

DAVID A. WOLFE, PhD
ERIC J. MASH, PhD

REFERENCES

Mash, E. J., & Barkley, R. A. (Eds.). (2003). *Child psychopathology* (2nd ed.). New York: Guilford Press.

Mash, E. J., & Barkley, R. A. (Eds.). (2006). *Treatment of childhood disorders* (3rd ed.). New York: Guilford Press.

Mash, E. J., & Terdal, L. G. (Eds.). (1997). *Assessment of childhood disorders* (3rd ed.). New York: Guilford Press.

Contents

I

INTRODUCTION

1

Behavioral and Emotional Problems in Adolescents
Overview and Issues

David A. Wolfe
Eric J. Mash

Behavioral and emotional problems in adolescents affect a significant number of young people, with considerable personal and societal costs. Estimates of mental health treatment expenditures for adolescents in the United States are substantial, and considerably more than for younger children (Ringel & Sturm, 2001). Because these estimates do not include costs associated with the educational, child welfare, and juvenile justice systems, or indirect costs of adolescent mental illness such as future lost wages due to lower educational attainment, they likely underestimate the overall costs associated with behavioral and emotional problems in adolescents.

Recent research into such adolescent disorders as conduct disorder, substance abuse, mood disorders, suicide, eating disorders, anxiety disorders, relational violence, attention-deficit/hyperactivity disorder (ADHD), and other problems indicates that adolescence presents unique challenges as compared with other developmental periods (American Psychological Association, 2002; Cicchetti & Rogosch,

2002). The epidemiology, expression, gender differences, comorbidities, developmental pathways, contexts, and causes of these disorders in adolescents are different than for other ages. These differences derive in part from the fact that adolescence is a transitional period of rapid developmental change, characterized by multiple interacting influences (United Nations, 2002). These changes and influences include physical maturation, emerging sexuality, need for autonomy, growing peer influence, new sources of stress associated with physical appearance and relationships, and exposure to a variety of stressors that may place adolescents at risk for concurrent and later problems (Kazdin, 2000). Paradoxically, adolescents show improvements in strength, speed, reaction time, mental reasoning abilities, immune function, among others; yet, their overall morbidity and mortality rates *increase* 200–300% from childhood to late adolescence (Burt, 2002).

Disorders that occur during the period from the onset of puberty (at about age 11 or 12)

and ending with independence and entry into early adulthood (around 18–24 years) have not received the attention given to disorders of childhood or adulthood (Irwin, Burg, & Cart, 2002). However, this situation is changing as developmental psychopathologists and clinical practitioners from a wide range of disciplines are increasingly recognizing the special aspects of development, behavior, and adjustment needed to understand, assess, and treat adolescents with behavioral and emotional disorders (Cicchetti & Rogosch, 2002; Holmbeck & Kendall, 2002).

An integrative conceptual framework for understanding the different forms of behavioral and emotional problems in adolescents has been lacking, and knowledge is new and has not been presented in a single source (Holmbeck & Kendall, 2002). Students, researchers, and practitioners who are interested in adolescent psychopathology and its assessment and treatment must currently sift through numerous articles and texts on developmental psychopathology, looking for, and trying to separate, specific mention of adolescent problems from broader discussions that focus on both child and adolescent disorders combined (e.g., Mash & Barkley, 2003, in press).

The current volume compiles the best and most up-to-date theory and research on understanding, assessing, and treating adolescents with behavioral and emotional problems, with a special sensitivity to the changes in physical, intellectual, psychosocial, and emotional development that occur during adolescence. The presentation focuses on the malleability of adolescents as a function of peer, family, school, community, and other influences while recognizing that it is during this period that distinct developmental pathways may also become well established (Davis, Banks, Fisher, & Grudzinskas, 2004; Steinberg & Morris, 2001). Although the focus of this volume is on disorders in adolescents, we recognize that it is necessary to link these problems with previous and future time periods as contexts for understanding, assessing, and treating these disorders.

WHY A SPECIAL FOCUS ON ADOLESCENT DISORDERS?

Adolescence represents an important developmental link between childhood or environmental circumstances and adult outcomes, in which previous adaptational patterns or difficulties may decrease, continue, intensify, or change (Steinberg, 2004). It involves rapid changes in emotional, social, physical, and intellectual development, resulting in an extremely diverse group of young people. At the early stages of adolescence an individual is beginning to form an identity separate from parents and family members, while turning to peers as one's source of personal support and social information. A mere 7–10 years later they are expected to be capable of self-sufficiency and independence. Not surprisingly, there are also significant changes in the types and frequency of mental disorders and problem behaviors that accompany these rapid changes in adolescent (Holmbeck & Kendall, 2002). Eccles and colleagues (1993) emphasize that problems in adolescence have an early beginning involving issues of autonomy and control with family members, particularly concerning family decisionmaking processes. Self-esteem plays a role in how well each adolescent negotiates these developmental tasks, and he or she needs to be a part of the solution to problems related to family decision making. In general, positive family relationships, including being able to discuss problems with parent(s), have been found to have a protective association for engaging in high-risk behaviors during adolescence (Resnick, Ireland, & Borowsky, 2004).

"Adolescence" is typically defined by chronological age (11–18 years), although physical, social, and cognitive development is often taken into account as well (American Psychological Association, 2002). Based on this age range, adolescents represent the fastest growing age group in the United States, particularly in urban areas (Annie E. Casey Foundation, 2002). Proportionately, the number of children ages 13–17 in the United States has increased by 12% over the past 8 years, compared to only a 4% increase among children under age 18 (Annie E. Casey Foundation, 2002). In addition, the population of adolescents in the United States is becoming increasingly racially and ethnically diverse. Nearly 40% of youngsters ages 10–19 identify as Hispanic or nonwhite, and ethnic and racial diversity among adolescents is projected to increase even further in the coming years (U.S. Census Bureau, 2005). From a global perspective, adolescents comprise 20% of the world's population and 85% reside in developing countries (Blum & Nelson-Mmari, 2004). It has been estimated by the World Health Organization (WHO, 1997) that over the 50-year period from 1970 to 2025 the number of urban youth will increase worldwide by 600%.

Researchers in adolescent development have long maintained that more meaningful distinctions within this broad developmental category are necessary for genuine insights into these rapid changes. These distinctions break down into three age ranges, although the exact boundaries are somewhat arbitrary: early (ages 11–13), mid (ages 14–16), and late adolescence (ages 17–20). Of course, there are no established rules for being an adolescent. Some preteens appear to enter this stage well in advance of their biological age, while others have difficulty leaving childhood behind. There is a similar discrepancy in maturity at the older end of adolescence, affecting the rate at which individuals emerge into adult responsibility and personal autonomy.

Historically, society has been largely concerned about the negative aspects of adolescent development, such as behavior problems and risk behaviors, with little attention paid to factors promoting healthy youth development (Burt, Resnick, & Novick, 1998). Consequently, with the exception of education, services for youth have traditionally existed to address or prevent youth problems, with little corresponding attention given to promoting youth development (Catalano, Hawkins, Berglund, Pollard, & Arthur, 2002). This emphasis has resulted in an assortment of youth services focused on "fixing" adolescents with emotional or behavioral problems, including those who engage in experimental risk behaviors. Similarly, many interventions are restricted to single issues such as substance use or early pregnancy, with inadequate consideration given to the shared underlying causes of such visible concerns (Burt, 2002). Other factors influencing youth's decisions and choices, such as their families, their environments, and the developmental context in which emotional and behavioral problems occur, have similarly received insufficient attention and integration (Biglan, Brennan, Foster, & Holder, 2004).

Today's shift in thinking about adolescent emotional and behavioral problems is leading to major advances in accepting and supporting adolescents as valuable members of society, gradually rejecting the negative viewpoint based on fear and poor understanding. Although adolescence is a period of greater risk than any other in terms of academic failure, violence, and health-compromising behaviors (Wolfe, Jaffe, & Crooks, 2006), it is recognized more and more as a period of tremendous opportunity for establishing the skills and values needed for adult life. This period of development has always been challenging and fraught with ups and downs, as teens seek independence from their families and establish their own identities. Yet, the last two decades have seen considerable effort expended to understand adolescent development and psychopathology, and efforts are underway to address some of the large gaps in education and services. Most important, studies examining adolescent behavior in its ecological context and in light of its special vulnerabilities and opportunities have led to greater awareness of normal and abnormal adolescent behavior (Cicchetti & Rogosch, 2002).

As a result of this increased focus, major transformations have begun in how adolescent behaviors are understood and how healthy and adaptive behaviors can be promoted. These transformations began, in large part, with concerted efforts by governmental and nongovernmental agencies to target the high rates of health-compromising behaviors among adolescents (U.S. Department of Health and Human Services [USDHHS], 2000). These efforts have been matched with increased funding for research on various aspects of adolescent development and disorders, along with ways to assist youth facing the difficult challenges of this period. What is emerging is a more youth-friendly and inclusive approach to emotional and behavior disorders of adolescence and problems associated with health-compromising behaviors (e.g., substance use and precocious or unsafe sexual behavior). This shift has also brought positive and innovative strategies to promote healthy, safe choices and lifestyles during this critical period of development (Irwin, 2003).

THE SIGNIFICANCE OF ADOLESCENT MENTAL HEALTH PROBLEMS

Adolescents with emotional and behavioral disorders, or some lesser degree of impairment, must also navigate the many challenges of this tumultuous period, and they may face greater obstacles in adapting to these rapid changes and demands. Consequently, there has also been increasing attention to adolescent mental health problems over the past decade, which derives from a number of sources. First, many young people experience significant mental health problems that interfere with normal development and functioning, with as many as 1 in 5 children and adolescents experiencing significant difficulties (Costello et al., 1996; Roberts, Attkisson, & Rosenblatt, 1998), and 1 in 10 having a diagnosable disorder that causes some level of impairment (Burns et al., 1995; Roberts et al., 1998; Shaffer et al., 1996). In one community sample of adolescents ages 14–17 years, it was found that 15.5% of females and 8.5% of males reported a diagnosable mental disorder (Romano, Tremblay, Vitaro, Zoccolillo, & Pagnani, 2001). Females had significantly higher rates of internalizing, anxiety, and depressive disorders than males, whereas externalizing disorders were significantly higher among males. These figures likely underestimate the magnitude of the problem for several reasons. Notably, community surveys do not include a substantial number of youth who do not meet diagnostic criteria for a mental disorder but who may manifest subclinical or undiagnosed disturbances that place them at high risk for the later development of more severe clinical problems (McDermott & Weiss, 1995). In fact, specific mental health symptoms and impairments in functioning at school and home may be stronger predictors of adolescents' later academic and social adjustment than a mental health diagnosis per se (Vander Stoep, Weiss, McKnight, Beresford, & Cohen, 2002). In addition, cultural and contextual factors may influence how adolescents express their symptoms or seek help, from problem identification to choice of treatment providers (Cauce et al., 2002).

Demographic Factors

Whereas sex differences in problem behaviors are negligible in children under the age of 3 (Gadow, Sprafkin, & Nolan, 2001), they become increasingly evident with age. Boys show higher rates of early-onset disorders that involve some form of neurodevelopmental impairment, and girls show more emotional disorders with a peak age of onset in adolescence (Rutter, Caspi, & Moffitt, 2003). For example, boys generally have higher rates of reading disorders, autism spectrum disorders, attention-deficit disorder, and early-onset persistent conduct problems, whereas girls have higher rates of depression and eating disorders (Rutter et al., 2003).

The normal developmental trajectories for girls and boys across the two major dimensions of Internalizing and Externalizing behaviors were examined by Dutch researchers to determine how these major problem areas change from childhood to adolescence (Bongers, Koot, van der Ende, & Verhulst, 2004). Boys' externalizing problems start out higher than girls in preschool and early elementary years; however, these problems decrease gradually for both boys and girls until they almost converge by age 18. The opposite pattern emerges for internalizing problems. Parents report similar rates of internalizing problems for boys and girls in early childhood, but girls outpace boys in these problems during the transition to adolescence (Bongers et al., 2003).

There is also some evidence and concern that the frequency of certain adolescent disorders such as conduct and oppositional disorders and some types of depression are showing an earlier age of onset and increasing in prevalence as a result of societal changes and conditions that create growing risks for young people (Kovacs, 1997). Researchers in the United Kingdom, for example, examined conduct, hyperactive, and emotional problems among three population samples of 15- to 16-year-olds over 25 years and found that rates of conduct problems, in particular, are increasing (Collishaw, Maughan, Goodman, & Pickles, 2004). They found a substantial rise in adolescent conduct problems for both boys and girls, which did not differ by social class or family type. They also found evidence for a recent rise in emotional problems but mixed evidence in relation to hyperactive behavior. Other community surveys have also identified increases in oppositional defiant behaviors but not in other youth problems (Achenbach, Dumenci, & Rescorla, 2003). Some of the social conditions affecting rates of these disorders include multigenerational adversity in inner cities, chronic poverty in women and children, pressures of family breakup, teenage pregnancy and parenting, physical abuse and neglect, sexual abuse (including victimization via the Internet), homelessness, problems of the rural poor, difficulties of North American Native adolescents, adjustment problems of adolescents in immigrant families, and conditions associated with the impact of prematurity, HIV (human immunodeficiency virus), cocaine, and alcohol on young people's growth and development (McCall & Groark, 2000).

Ethnicity

Racial and ethnic minority persons comprise a substantial and vibrant segment of many countries, enriching each society with many unique strengths, cultural traditions, and important contributions. In the United States these groups are growing rapidly, with current projections showing that by 2025 they will account for more than 40% of all Americans (President's New Freedom Commission, 2003). Minority children in the United States are overrepresented in rates of some disorders, such as substance abuse, delinquency, and teen suicide (McLoyd, 1998). However, once the effects of socioeconomic status (SES), sex, age, and referral status are controlled, very few differences in the rate of children's psychological disorders emerge in relation to race or ethnicity (Achenbach, Howell, Quay, & Conners, 1991). Some minority groups, in fact, show even less psychopathology after controlling for SES (Samaan, 2000).

Even though rates of problems are similar, significant barriers remain in access, quality, and outcomes of care for minority children. As a result, American Indians, Alaska Natives, African Americans, Asian Americans, Pacific Islanders, and Hispanic Americans bear a disproportionately high burden of disability from mental disorders (Morreale, Kapphahn, Elster, Juszczak, & Klein, 2004), and areas in which disability is manifested may also differ depending on race and ethnicity (Ezpeleta, Keeler, Alaatin, Costello, & Angold, 2001). Specifically, the system has neglected to incorporate respect or understanding of the histories, traditions, beliefs, languages, and value systems of culturally diverse groups. Misunderstanding and misinterpreting behaviors have led to tragic consequences, including inappropriately placing minorities in the criminal and juvenile justice systems (President's New Freedom Commission, 2003).

Despite the growing ethnic diversity of the North American population, ethnic representation in research studies and the study of ethnicity-related issues more generally have received relatively little attention in studies of child and adolescent psychopathology (García Coll, Akerman, & Cicchetti, 2000). Research has generally been insensitive to possible differences in prevalence, age of onset, developmental course, and risk factors related to ethnicity (Kazdin & Kagan, 1994), and to the considerable heterogeneity that exists within specific ethnic and racial groups (Murry, Bynum, Brody, Willert, & Stephens, 2001). Consequently, a critical gap exists in many areas of normal and abnormal adolescent development for minority youth (Ohye & Daniel, 1999). Although global comparisons of the prevalence of different types of problems for different ethnic groups are not likely to be very revealing, studies into the processes affecting the form, associated factors, and outcomes of different disorders for various ethnic groups hold promise for increasing our understanding of the relationship between ethnicity and emotional and behavioral problems of adolescence (Bradley, Corwyn, Burchinal, McAdoo, & Garcia Coll, 2001).

Evidence gathered by the WHO (2001) suggests that by the year 2020, child and adolescent neuropsychiatric disorders will rise proportionally by over 50%, internationally, to become one of the five most common causes of morbidity, mortality, and disability among children. Unfortunately, youth who are not identified as having mental health problems and who do not receive appropriate services often end up in the criminal justice or mental health systems as young adults. In fact, about three-quarters of 21-year-olds with mental disorders have experienced problems at a younger age (Offord, 2000). Youth with mental disorders are at a much greater risk for school underachievement, school failure, and dropout and of not being fully functional members of society in adulthood (Ezpeleta et al., 2001; Vander Stoep, Weiss, Kuo, Cheney, & Cohen, 2003).

In 1998, total mental health utlization costs for youth with problems were estimated to be more than $11 billion (Ringel & Sturm, 2001). Nonetheless, 70% or more of youth who experience serious difficulties neither seek nor receive help for their problems (Achenbach et al., 2003; Sheffield, Fiorenza, & Sofronoff, 2004; Sourander et al., 2004). The costs of adolescent disorders include not only human suffering of both the afflicted youth and the family and community members with whom they come into contact but also economic and social costs. Using estimates of economic loss, medical costs, and quality-of-life indicators, Miller (2004) estimates the cost of problem behaviors among *all* youth in the United States at $435 billion in 1998. This breaks down to $12,300 per youth ages 12–20 each year ($1,500 in resources, $3,400 in future work losses, and $7,400 in quality of life). The costs incurred by *multiproblem* youth (i.e., those who have more than one mental health disorder or engage in multiple risk behaviors) is even more startling: These individuals account for 77–80% of the total cost of youth behavior problems, estimated at $2.5 million per multiproblem youth.

Experimental Risk Behaviors

Early to midadolescence is a particularly important transitional period for healthy versus problematic adjustment (Cicchetti & Rogosch, 2002). The greatest categories of risk behaviors during adolescence include drug and alcohol abuse, unsafe sexual behavior, school failure and dropout, and delinquency/crime/violence (Lerner & Castellino, 2002). Not surprisingly, the leading causes of death among youth stem from accidents and violence resulting from high-risk behaviors (Blum & Nelson-Mmari, 2004; Irwin et al., 2002).

Between the ages of 11 and 16, adolescents rapidly start to experiment with alcohol, drugs, smoking, sex, and violence in their peer and dating relationships. Substance use, risky sexual behavior, violence, accidental injuries, and mental health problems are prominent concerns that make adolescence a particularly vulnerable period (Kilpatrick et al., 2000; Leitenberg & Saltzman, 2000). Risk-taking behaviors account for 70% of adolescent mortality, which more than doubles between early (ages 10–14) and later (15–19) adolescence (Irwin et al., 2002). Whether or not they get involved with these potential risks directly, it is happening around them and they often find themselves in situations in which they have to make choices. For some, their role may become one of crisis counselor or bystander, and they may even encourage their peers to make safer choices. For others, the escalating experimentation of their peers may influence them to make harmful or premature choices. More likely, most adolescents will find themselves in both roles during their teen years. Regardless of their role, youth are desperate for information and guidance to help them handle the choices, pressures, and consequences associated with this tumultuous stage.

One of the first major contemporary advances in understanding adolescence and risk behaviors began with the recognition that many of these experimental risk behaviors are interconnected. Rather than studying youth risk behaviors as if they were separate and independent problems, researchers and clinicians noted that factors that increased the risk of one behavior, such as substance use, were highly similar to those that increased other behaviors, such as unsafe sexual behavior. A good example of this convergence comes from the substance abuse literature, in which alcohol and drug abuse were seen as related cousins, largely connected to (and sometimes responsible for) the youth's other problem behaviors. Similarly, researchers and clinicians involved with other youth problems, such as risky sexual behavior, violence, or crime, likewise began to see the overlap in predictors of these behaviors, challenging past assumptions that each outcome had a unique or independent pathway (Jessor, Donovan, & Costa, 1991).

Not only are risk behaviors related to one another and often occur in the same individual, these behaviors are important in terms of the goals of adolescence. Jessor, who conducted much of the pioneering work in this area and formulated problem behavior theory around the concept of co-occurrence and common causal factors, points out how some behaviors seen as problems are "functional, purposive, instrumental, and goal-directed, and that the goals involved are often those that are central in normal adolescent development" (Jessor et al., 1991, p. 378). Many of these goals are typical of ordinary adolescent development and not signs of disorder, which explains why risk behaviors that play an adaptive role during adolescence can be difficult to change, much less eliminate. Smoking, drinking, drug use, and early sexual activity, for example, can be instrumental in gaining peer acceptance and respect, establishing autonomy from parents, repudiating norms and values of conventional authority, coping with anxiety or failure, or affirming one's maturity. These activities can also be physically and psychologically dangerous or can compromise short- and long-term health.

Because adolescence must prepare an individual to manage adult roles and privileges, developmentalists generally accept that some amount of experimentation and transition is necessary. The issue becomes when, how, and with what they will experiment, as well as what role adults should play in ensuring they make safe and responsible choices. About 80% of high school students have tried alcohol, 60% have tried cigarette smoking, and 50% have tried marijuana (Johnston, O'Malley, & Bachman, 2003); it is equally telling that very few adolescents (about 6%) refrain entirely from such behaviors (Moffitt, Caspi, Dickson, Silva, & Stanton, 1996). The challenge faced by parents, teachers, and professionals is how to keep teens safe, given that the majority (but not all) will experiment with adult privileges such as smoking, sex, and alcohol use, as well as with known illegal or unsafe activities (Wolfe et al., 2006).

Youths' relationships and their peer culture also play a significant role in understanding many of the motives and beliefs underlying their healthy or harmful choices. These relationships include past and present interactions with parents and family members, which shape many of their current attitudes and provide the foundation for making safe versus risky choices. These relationships also include their peer group and peer culture, which set the context for new opportunities to experiment with adult privileges, challenge rules, or define their own boundaries and choices. Rather than viewing youth behaviors primarily in terms of their degree of risk or harm, it is worthwhile to consider that risk behaviors almost always occur in the context of a relationship. As noted by Jessor and colleagues (1991), this relationship context reflects developmental circumstances, such as resolving disputes with parents or peers, seeking status or acceptance, or seeking new pleasures. Thus, it often comes down to the individual's skill at negotiating relationship issues, particularly with parents, peers, and romantic partners, which determines his or her degree of risk during this experimental period.

Getting a grasp on the myriad explanations for youth problem behaviors and disorders is daunting, as such behavior is clearly multidetermined (Mash & Dozois, 2003). Although numerous theories attempt to explain why some youth engage in particular risk behaviors, especially substance use and delinquency, few consider multiple risk behaviors and their underlying connections. A narrow, single-problem focus made sense when researchers were attempting to identify the vast number of variables needed to explain a single problem behavior. Today, it is necessary to consider how similar factors, such as poor parent-

ing or role models, can lead to diverse outcomes, such as substance abuse or unsafe sex. Equally important is the need to consider how different factors can lead to similar adolescent outcomes, such as loss of a parent or abuse in childhood and adolescent depression. Identifying the common theoretical constructs and processes provides a more complete picture of an adolescent's experience and best informs universal efforts at education and prevention (Catalano et al., 2002).

Researchers have proposed many theories for why adolescents engage in risk behaviors. Some of these theories focus more narrowly on specific cognitive or behavioral processes that precede such behavior, while others involve processes rooted in childhood, early family interactions, and wide-ranging cultural factors. Although no one particular theory or conceptual model can fully accommodate all the likely processes contributing to adolescent risk behaviors, each has added pieces to the puzzle that permit a more complete picture. Researchers also determined that risk and problem behaviors are correlated, implying that the same individuals often show a number of risk behaviors beyond the one or two that may have initially been of concern (Dryfoos, 1990; Jessor et al., 1991). Such discoveries had an important bearing on theoretical explanations for risk and problem behaviors and have spawned a growing movement toward a more comprehensive, integrated study of adolescent risk and problem behaviors. Current theories use a developmental systems perspective that emphasizes the importance of adolescent-context relationships for understanding and enhancing the trajectory of change through adolescence into adulthood (Lerner & Castellino, 2002). Fortunately, theories stemming from the various fields of sociology, psychology, criminology, and many others have become less isolated from one another, allowing their important contributions to be integrated and more readily applied (Biglan et al., 2004).

Behavioral and Emotional Problems

The chapters in this volume provide comprehensive coverage of a wide range of behavioral and emotional problems of adolescents. These problems generally fall into two broad categories: (1) diagnosable disorders such as anxiety and depression, and (2) difficulties that do not fit neatly into current diagnostic categories but are significant problems nonetheless (e.g., dating violence and risky sexual behaviors). Although we consider problems in both of these categories in separate chapters, most adolescents are known to experience multiple symptoms and problems, and there is much overlap among categories (Hoffmann, Bride, McMaster, Abrantes, & Estroff, 2004). For example, using semistructured diagnostic interviews, more than 50% of referred adolescents have been found to meet criteria for two or more DSM-IV Axis I diagnoses (Youngstrom, Findling, & Calabrese, 2003).

The DSM-IV-TR (American Psychiatric Association [APA], 2000) makes few developmental allowances for disorders of adolescents, with most diagnostic criteria for adolescents being the same as those for children or adults. The large section of DSM that is labeled "Disorders Usually First Diagnosed in Infancy, Childhood, or Adolescence" consists almost exclusively of disorders that first occur during infancy and childhood (e.g., attention-deficit and disruptive behavior disorders and pervasive developmental disorders) rather than ones with a predominantly adolescent onset. On the other hand, many disorders with a predominantly adolescent onset (e.g., depression and eating disorders) are diagnosed using the same criteria as for adults, with minor age-related adjustments. In most cases, DSM age-related adjustments are not differentiated based on developmental period. For example, in the case of a major depressive episode, irritability can substitute for depressed mood for both children *and* adolescents. Although there is much evidence to indicate that the same criteria used to diagnose many adult disorders can also be used to diagnose adolescents, current diagnostic systems are generally insensitive to the developmental concerns of adolescents. For example, although older adolescents have been found to report more depressive symptoms than adults and similar symptom persistence (Wight, Sepúlveda, & Aneshensel, 2004), it is not known whether the greater number of symptoms represents a higher actual risk for depression in adolescents or whether certain symptom criteria are generally more likely to occur during adolescence (e.g., sleep disturbances or suicidal ideation).

The most common disorders of adolescents are conduct disorder, substance abuse, and anxiety and depression. In addition, there are also several other disorders and problems (e.g.,

eating disorder, bipolar disorder, personality disorder, suicidal behavior, and self-harm) that are most likely to first occur during adolescence but occur far less often than conduct problems, substance abuse, and anxiety and depression. Because of their common occurrence or relatedness to adolescence, our knowledge base about both of these types of disorders and problems in adolescents is substantial. On the other hand, there are many disorders that first occur during childhood, such as learning disorders, pervasive developmental disorders, mental retardation, and ADHD, that typically continue into adolescence and adulthood. Because these disorders have traditionally been viewed as "disorders of children," they have not been extensively studied in adolescents. Until recently, the main features and associated characteristics of these disorders during adolescence were viewed as changing in expression but essentially the same as for children. As a result, the chapters on these topics that follow tell as much about what we do not yet know about these disorders in adolescents as what we do, and they outline important areas in which further research is needed.

Finally, a number of chapters in this volume are devoted to important problems of youth that, although not disorders per se, are serious concerns in their own right. These include adolescent health and chronic illness, adolescent sexual risk behavior, problems related to sex role development and gender identity disturbances, deviant sexual behavior, violence in adolescent dating relationships, and abuse and trauma. Many of these difficulties may be related to mental disorders and other problems in adolescents in ways that are only beginning to be investigated and understood. For example, in a community sample of adolescents, Goodwin, Lewinsohn, and Seely (2004) found that respiratory symptoms were associated with an increased risk of any mental disorder, particularly depression, substance use disorder, panic attacks, and ADHD. Although this relationship was partly accounted for by demographic differences, hypochondriasis, functional impairment, and cigarette smoking, these factors did not completely explain the association. These and other findings highlight the importance of examining mechanisms to account for the possible relationships between adolescent health-related problems and mental disorders (e.g., environmental risk factors or family vulnerability).

DEVELOPMENTALLY INFORMED PERSPECTIVES ON ADOLESCENT PSYCHOPATHOLOGY

The field of developmental psychopathology in adolescence has shifted dramatically with the increasing recognition that many of the same risk and protective factors predict diverse outcomes, including substance abuse, delinquency, school dropout, and mental disorders (Catalano et al., 2002). Furthermore, from a developmental perspective, there are many interesting parallels between the milestones and behaviors of young children and those of young adolescents, with some important differences. Both age groups have the highest level of problem behaviors of any other age period (Mash & Wolfe, 2005), especially in terms of noncompliant, disruptive, or difficult behaviors. Both age periods are also marked by rapid physical and emotional development. Perhaps most telling is how both age groups have difficulty controlling or regulating their emotions, usually under particular circumstances such as paying attention in class or sharing with peers or siblings.

An important difference between the developmental processes of young children and those of adolescents is connected to the fundamental goals demanded of each of them by their environment and biology. Whereas the young child's "job" is to form a secure, close relationship to his or her caregivers, the adolescent's role is to expand his or her attachments to peers and romantic partners. Under nonstressful circumstances, most adolescents accomplish this step by continuing to use their relationship with parents as a secure base to explore their autonomy and independence (Allen, McElhaney, Kupermine, & Jodl, 2004). Traditional folklore maintains that adolescents are *expected* to be troublesome and aggravating as they plot a course from their childhood connections to their adolescent peer group and struggle with rapid hormonal and environmental changes. Although this simplified and negativistic view has some truth to it, it overattributes adolescent emotional and behavior problems to their stage of development. Accordingly, insufficient consideration may be given to the *true* warning signs of problems, assuming they would grow out of it or there was little that could be done.

Today's view of adolescence focuses more on developmental issues and challenges accompanying the transition from childhood to adulthood (Holmbeck, Friedman, Abad, & Jandasek, Chapter 2, this volume). During adolescence, individuals often "try on" different characteristics and roles and are therefore more open to experimenting with new ways of relating to others. Adolescents start to make their own decisions about important issues affecting their lives. Self-reliance, self-control, and independent decision making all increase during the teen years, with a shift away from the family and onto the peer group. To the frustration of many parents, conformity to parental opinions gradually decreases while the tendency to be swayed by peers increases in early adolescence before it declines (Crockett & Petersen, 1993). Thus, by providing adolescents with growth opportunities that emphasize a more positive mode of relating to others, this natural inclination to try new patterns can be used to strengthen their interpersonal capacities. Conversely, if adolescents are not provided with helpful messages about ways to adapt to their ever-changing personal and interpersonal demands, they will be more vulnerable to the bombardment of other, less healthy messages and expectations.

Adolescence is a time of tremendous reorganization and transformations of the body, the mind, and one's responsibilities. Along with biological changes, more advanced thinking abilities develop in concert with social changes and the transition into new roles and expectations. The rate at which these changes take place is uneven, leaving a gap between physiological changes on the one hand, and cognitive and emotional maturity on the other. This gap may account for some of the observed risk-taking behaviors characteristic of adolescents. For example, pubertal changes are accompanied by increased novelty and sensation seeking, yet one's emotional self-regulation often does not fully mature until adulthood (American Psychological Association, 2002). As a result, it has been argued that interventions should begin with the premise that adolescents are inherently more likely than adults to take risks and should focus on reducing the harm associated with risk-taking behavior (Steinberg, 2004). An understanding of all the different changes taking place during adolescence provides the foundation for understanding the observed rise in risk behaviors and changes in emotional and behavioral problems.

Biological Influences

Navigating puberty is one of the major challenges faced by adolescents (Silbereisen & Kracke, 1997). Adolescents undergo significant psychological and emotional changes, in conjunction with physical changes, which are often related to gender (Graber, 2003). For example, they face transformations in physical appearance, such as breast development in females and growth of facial hair for males, and a dramatic increase in height. During this period, most youth will physically mature from children into adults, although males continue to grow into their early 20s. Self-image may be temporarily threatened as teens come to terms with all the physical changes, including bodily maturations and facial changes, each influencing the way they feel about themselves. The impact of puberty differs across the board: Some youth feel attractive, grown up, and confident, while others feel self-conscious, ugly, and afraid. These physical changes are intertwined with psychological and emotional transitions. Physical changes affect self-image and behavior while also prompting changes and reactions in others. Changes in a child's physical appearance may, for instance, elicit different types of behavior from parents, peers, and others. In addition to these types of challenges, adolescent moods tend to fluctuate more frequently over the day as compared to the disposition constancy of adults.

The extent to which early or late onset of puberty may affect emotional and behavioral problems is worthy of consideration. Early onset of puberty in girls has been found to be associated with a number of risk behaviors, including cigarette smoking and consumption of alcohol (Stattin & Magnusson, 1990). Furthermore, girls who mature younger tend to start dating earlier and often choose older partners (Silbereisen & Kracke, 1997). Involvement with older partners has been identified as a link in the observed relationship between premature physical maturation and earlier onset of sexual activity for girls (Stattin & Magnusson, 1990). In addition, early pubertal development relates to a younger age of sexual debut for both males and females (Capaldi, Crosby, & Stoolmiller, 1996). Self-report of appearing older or more mature than peers tends to coincide with earlier sexual involvement (Resnick et al., 1997). Earlier age at menarche has also been found to correlate with riskier sexual practices, most likely by increasing the likelihood of affiliating with older boyfriends, which, in turn, increases the chance of engaging in sexual risk behavior (Mezzich et al., 1997). Moreover, Baumeister, Flores, and Marin (1995) found that, among Latina adolescents, later age at menarche was associated with *not* becoming pregnant in adolescence.

Early as well as late onset of puberty, particularly early-maturing girls and late-maturing boys, is also associated with increased risk for emotional and behavioral problems. For example, early-maturing girls have been found to be at higher risk for depression, substance abuse, disruptive behaviors, and eating disorders (Ge, Conger, & Elder, 2001; Graber, Lewinsohn, Seeley, & Brooks-Gunn, 1997; Striegel-Moore & Cachelin, 2001). Similarly, early-maturing boys are more likely to be involved in high-risk behaviors such as sexual activity, smoking, or delinquency (Flannery, Rowe, & Gulley, 1993; Harrell, Bangdiwala, Deng, Webb, & Bradley, 1998). In contrast to girls, late maturation for boys is associated with greater risk for depression, conflict with parents, and school problems (Graber et al., 1997). Moreover, late-maturing boys are at greater risk of harassment and bullying due in part to their smaller physical stature (Pollack & Shuster, 2000).

In addition to outward pubertal changes taking place during adolescence, hormonal and nerve-related changes occur in the brain, which have been shown to affect teens' behavior. One significant hormonal change is the increased activity of the hypothalamic–pituitary–adrenal (HPA) axis, which plays a central role in the biological response to stress (Walker, 2002; Walker & Bollini, 2002). Heightened stress levels during adolescence have been attributed in large part to this more active HPA axis. The prefrontal cortex, where emotional control, impulse restraint, and rational decision making take place, grows quickly during adolescence. However, because this part continues to mature and grow throughout puberty and into early adulthood, it logically follows that most teens have not yet fully developed any of the aforementioned abilities, particularly during early and midadolescence (Durston et al., 2001). To a certain extent, this finding explains why many teenagers engage in high-risk and impulsive behavior: They simply lack the cognitive and self-regulatory skills to consistently make positive, well-considered decisions.

Cognitive and Emotional Influences

Adolescence is also a time of important cognitive and social development in which individuals learn to think more rationally and become capable of thinking hypothetically. Adolescents can consider extended time perspectives, not just the here and now, and adjust their goals and behavior accordingly; however, processing of information is still less systematic than formal and will depend on their prior knowledge and understanding. It is emblematic that their ability to consider and understand emotionally arousing topics is less sophisticated than that of adults. At the same time they must develop and use effective decision-making skills involving complex interpersonal relationships. These skills include an awareness of possible risks and considerations of future consequences, balancing their own interests with those of their peers, family members, and dating partners. Thus, cognitive-developmental changes in adolescence, such as increases in abstract thinking and changes in how self-evaluations are made (via social comparison rather than in terms of absolute standards) may affect both the type and strength of cognitive vulnerabilities for particular disorders (e.g., body image and eating disorders, self-appraisal and depression, hostile attributional bias, and conduct disorders).

Many of the cognitive and emotional changes that occur in adolescence are gender-related (Maccoby, 1998). For example, adolescent girls are more likely to initiate verbal exchanges and show greater responsiveness to the verbalizations of others than boys, and they are also more likely to think and talk about the emotional aspects of relationships than boys (Crick & Zahn-Waxler, 2003). As a result of these and other gender differences, the ways in which males and females think about social situations, regulate their emotions, and express their behavior and the types of mental health problems they develop during adolescence can vary considerably (Bell, Foster, & Mash, 2005a, 2005b). For example, with respect to body change strategies, adolescent boys attempt to become more muscular, whereas adolescent girls attempt to lose weight, and these differences are related to biological, psychological, and sociocultural influences (Muris, Meesters, van de Blom, & Mayer, 2005).

Self-identity and self-esteem also change dramatically during adolescence. Self-esteem reflects the person's judgment of his or her personal competence across such domains as attractiveness, acceptance by others, and academic, athletic, and interpersonal success. Self-identity, in turn, becomes more solidified as young adults develop a coherent picture of their capabilities and limitations and select and commit to their personal choices related to sexual, occupational, and social roles. In parallel, teens develop greater capability for abstract thought, which enables them to formulate a more complex view of themselves, coupled with greater self-reflection, social comparison, and autonomous decision making (Crockett & Peterson, 1993). However, Harter (1990) points out that these important changes are accompanied by certain vulnerabilities. Teens' overestimates of their confidence may lead to failure, while underestimates of their own confidence may lead to the avoidance of challenge and a diminished opportunity for growth. Optimally, teens should have the opportunity to explore a wide range of possible options in these domains before having to make commitments to one's identity. For example, even though their abilities are roughly the same, adolescent girls tend to feel more confident about their reading and social skills than boys, whereas adolescent boys tend to feel more confident about their athletic and math skills (Eccles, Barber, Jozefowicz, Malenchuk, & Vida, 1999).

As a result of the aforementioned neurological processes and experience in general, adolescents' intellectual and cognitive abilities become more sophisticated, their expectations about relationships become more realistic, and their ability to regulate emotions becomes more finely tuned. In addition, more advanced cognitive skills such as reasoning and problem solving emerge and are consolidated. More advanced thinking abilities also imply an increased propensity to consider hypothetical situations and abstract concepts, skills that affect how one thinks about the self, relationships, and the world. Along with this comes the ability to think from more than one perspective or angle—to consider what is being observed versus what is possible. As adolescents mature, they also gain the ability to plan ahead, anticipate the response of others, and become better debaters and arguers, all of which contribute to and are affected by increased problem solving in class and the ability to reflect on moral dilemmas.

This increased ability to think about possibilities may also lead to becoming lost in thoughts and worries. Adolescents first become capable of metacognition, or "thinking about thinking." As a result, they experience an increased propensity to monitor thoughts, more intense self-absorption, and often a belief that their own behavior is the focus of everyone else's concern and attention (the latter is known as the false audience consensus). Social cognition—thinking about people, relationships, human behavior, and social conventions such as social norms, guidelines for social interaction, and justice—is also an important part of adolescent growth. Adolescents are starting to make their own decisions about important issues affecting their lives. Self-reliance, self-control, and independent decision making all increase during the teen years, with a shift away from the family and onto the peer group. To the frustration of many parents, conformity to parental opinions gradually decreases while the tendency to be swayed by peers increases in early adolescence before it declines (Crockett & Peterson, 1993).

Social and Behavioral Influences

As cognitive and emotional development continues, adolescents begin to comprehend their own emotions and develop the ability to understand or analyze why they feel a certain way, which facilitates the formation of more long-lasting, mutual, and healthy relationships. Two distinguishing features of adolescence are the importance of peers and the development of romantic relationships. Most teens shift their focus of interest from parents to peer relations and develop the capacity for intimacy with other youth. Along with this new found type of relationship follows the sense of a greater need for privacy from family, which almost without fail leads to a change in family relationships. Although this shift to greater independence leads to less exclusive and intense relationships between parents and children, it does not necessarily mean a decrease in the importance of the parent–child relationship. Indeed, some research has shown that while youth turn to their peers for more superficial decisions (e.g., clothes and beliefs about curfews), parents are more influential than peers in more serious matters of religious beliefs, moral values, and political ideas (Steinberg & Morris, 2001).

Relationships are of central importance in adolescence, to the extent that some researchers have coined them the "organizing principle" of adolescence and teenage peer networks (Collins & Sroufe, 1999). The development of romantic relationships in particular encourages independence, assists with identity formation, and fosters skills for intimacy. These fledgling romances also provide a training ground for the development and refinement of interpersonal skills such as negotiation, reciprocity, emotional closeness, and disclosure. Romantic relationships also serve a function within the peer group and may be a way to gain status and acceptance.

While all these adjustments to family and peer relations are taking place, social status and social roles also transform. Newfound rights, privileges, and responsibilities are acquired during the latter phases of this developmental stage, such as the permission to drive, marry, vote, drink, and smoke. These changes in social status allow teens to take on fresh roles and try new activities. Social positioning also changes as adolescents begin training for adult roles, such as work, family roles, and responsibilities in their community. It is also the time in life when individuals generally attain adult status and training, with the completion of formal schooling and/or job training.

While simultaneously attempting to cope with all of the physical, cognitive, and emotional changes, adolescents must also deal with the challenge of developing an identity. As mentioned earlier, teens establish an identity beyond their family role by developing relationships with others and becoming more emotionally detached from their parents. Healthy same-sex relationships play a key role in the growth of an individual and a sense of self in relation to others. It is also a period of role experimentation—trying on different roles until the "true self" is found. Adolescents may even change their identity from context to context, particularly around the ages of 14–16. For example, an individual might be typically shy at school but behave in an outgoing manner at summer camp (Steinberg & Morris, 2001). At the same time, the need to be seen as a unique person while also fitting in with others poses an inner struggle for most teens. These challenges are all part of the changes in identity, self-esteem, and self-conceptions that occur during the teenage years, as new activities and roles trigger a new evaluation of self. Cultural identity is another critical part of this process, especially for adolescents who are not part of the white–Anglo majority (Phinney, 1990).

Along with these changes comes the need to establish a sense of autonomy and a healthy sense of independence. Teens strive to assert their own independence and to be seen as self-sufficient by others. To do so, they must become less emotionally dependent on parents; therefore, the ability to make independent decisions and establish a personal core set of values and morals is vital during these years. Attempts to achieve a balance between autonomy and connectedness lead to the push–pull behavior some parents observe in their adolescents: Youth may be childlike and affectionate one moment, and aloof strangers the next.

Intimacy takes on an important role as well, as adolescence is a time of forming close and caring relationships with others. Most teenagers experience a change in their capacity for intimacy with others, especially as far as their peers are concerned. They move from sharing activities and interests to relationships that involve openness, honesty, loyalty, and keeping confidences. Adolescence is a time for forming trusting and loving relationships, and expressing sexual feelings and enjoying physical contact with others represents one manifestation of this intimacy. Changes in emotions, motivations, behaviors, and relationships with others are also common. Teenagers often attempt to incorporate sexuality into a sense of self. In other words, they develop sexual values and morals and try to come to terms with relationships. Developing a sexual identity is a major component of developing intimacy, although the development of sexual identity may be a largely unconscious process for nonsexual minority youth (Savin-Williams, 1998).

Another developmental task of adolescence is the desire for a sense of achievement. Being successful and competent members of society and making decisions with long-term consequences are integral parts of attaining this sense of accomplishment. An evaluation of one's own competencies, capabilities, aspirations, and expectations for the future take on a major role in decision making during this period. However, as noted earlier, this process can be unduly influenced by gender stereotypes and expectations, that is, despite similar abilities, adolescent girls tend to feel more confident about their reading and social skills than boys, and adolescent boys tend to feel more confident about their athletic and math skills (Eccles

et al., 1999). Males also value control and perceive themselves as more willing to take on leadership roles and responsibilities, whereas females tend to value relationship involvement, social relationships, and a desire of more affection, of intimate personal relationships, and for others to initiate more positive personal relationships with them (Bakken & Romig, 1992).

TREATMENT AND PREVENTION CHALLENGES

Although significant, given proper understanding, resources, and priorities, behavioral and emotional problems of adolescence can be significantly attenuated. In response to these mounting concerns, adolescents' special needs and problems are receiving greater attention, especially because efficacious treatments are available for many adolescent behavioral and emotional problems and serious consequences are largely preventable. For example, with respect to treatment, meta-analytic reviews have found medium to large effect sizes for adolescent interventions that are comparable to those reported for children and adults (Weisz & Hawley, 2002). However, far fewer treatment outcome studies have been conducted with adolescents than children and few psychosocial treatments have been developed *specifically* for adolescents. For example, nearly all the treatments for adolescents that were evaluated in the meta-analysis by Weisz and Hawley (2002) were either upward adaptations of treatments developed for children or downward adaptations of treatments developed for adults.

For youth to make healthy and adaptive choices, their home, community, and societal structures must be supportive. Understanding what interventions are most appropriate, however, requires understanding of the timing and nature of investments over the course of a lifetime and the factors and constraints that affect decisions to invest in children and youth by parents, family members, and young people themselves. Investing in youth preserves the benefits of prior investments in children, helps to recover some of the benefits for those who may not have had earlier assistance, and addresses new risks that arise during this period (Catalano et al., 2002). Only through more concerted efforts to assist youth will society complete the chain of education and services beginning in infancy and childhood that will lead to lasting changes in health and productivity across the lifespan.

Furthermore, contemporary views of youth are predicated on the grounds that efforts to assist others must be *inclusive* rather than *exclusive*. Such a model builds on strengths rather than attempting to treat known weaknesses alone. Within the framework of a health promotion model, it is often more useful to look for the "at-risk" indicators and reduce their potency rather than wait for the person to show the undesired behavior. For example, because most forms of violence occur within the context of a close or intimate relationship, we have progressed considerably in terms of identifying preexisting risk factors that are amenable to change or elimination. Yet, policies and actions still remain overly focused on the discovery of individual deviancy and problem behaviors that will account for the tremendous expected differences between "problem" and "nonproblem" youth.

From the standpoint of prevention, health promotion efforts to reduce harm from normal risk taking and experimentation in adolescence are being implemented in primary health care settings, schools, and community programs (Irwin et al., 2002). The most effective prevention programs strive for ways to involve youth in education and prevention efforts rather than deliver programs that lack youth input and commitment, as such efforts are rewarding through the promotion of cooperation and mutual support (Wolfe et al., in press). To foster healthy adolescent development, efforts to reduce or prevent risk behaviors are needed, along with an equal commitment to helping young people understand life's challenges and responsibilities and to developing the necessary skills to succeed as adults. Youths need developmentally appropriate knowledge and education, delivered in a nonjudgmental and highly salient format, which emphasizes their choices, responsibilities, and consequences. In effect, they need to be prepared, not scared. Youth, especially high-risk youth, need education and skills to promote healthy relationships, to develop peer support, and to establish social action aimed at ending violence in relationships. They need to feel connected not only to their peers, which is relatively easy, but also to their school, family, and community. Such connection requires a commitment to building capacity in each community to be inclusive of all youth; to see each adolescent as a person rather than a potential problem. The ultimate act of inclusion is to empower youth to identify the critical issues they face and the solutions that are most meaningful to the reality of their lives and circumstances.

As a result of efforts targeting infants and children in the first few years of life, major progress in prevention science has occurred. These initiatives have built on the growing body of literature related to infant brain development and the crucial attachment process that sets the foundation for subsequent development, future relationships, and the ways in which attachments disturbances are related to various forms of adolescent psychopathology (Cicchetti & Toth, 1996; Hilburn-Cobb, 2004). However, adolescence remains a poor second cousin when it comes to empirically supported treatment and prevention initiatives (Weisz & Hawley, 2002). At the extreme, there is a belief that investing in adolescence has fewer dividends than investing in earlier stages of development. That is, much of the die has been cast in attitudes and behavior, and intervention is targeted to those who are readily identifiable because of their acting-out behavior. There may some truth to the view that the cost/benefit ratio of interventions is higher during adolescence. This fact should not lead to abandoning the full potential of this stage of development for meaningful prevention efforts. Because adolescent problems have been neglected relative to those of children, throughout the volume we look at the expression and treatment of various disorders in both childhood and adolescence when information about adolescents is lacking.

CONCLUSIONS

Although we have always known that adolescence is a unique and important period of development, research documenting its significance had lagged far behind research on children and adults. Throughout the 1990s this picture began to change dramatically, due in large part to expanding techniques for studying neurodevelopmental processes in the brain. As neuroimaging techniques advanced our understanding of areas of the brain that are immature relative to other areas of growth, theories of adolescent risk behaviors and mental disorders likewise expanded to accommodate knowledge of biological processes and their interaction with social/environmental factors. Knowledge of adolescent development across cognitive, social, and biological dimensions likewise informed theories of the interplay between normal and abnormal adolescent behavior throughout this turbulent growth period. Simultaneously, we have seen a major shift in moving from the view of "fixing" adolescent problems and risk behaviors toward engaging youth in health promotion and positive solutions. More and more efforts are underway today to involve adolescents in learning healthy alternatives to risk behaviors and to tailor the delivery of knowledge and assistance to their developmental level and needs.

At the same time, there remains a lack of sensitivity to identifying adolescent emotional and behavioral disorders as unique from those presenting in child- or adulthood, and balancing knowledge of adolescent development with that of psychopathology. To address this need, the following chapters examine carefully how child-based disorders are often expressed during adolescence, noting similarities and differences that may be crucial to the choice of prevention or intervention. To this end, authors of each chapter discuss the increasing attention directed to understanding, assessing, and treating behavioral and emotional problems of adolescents. What emerges is a more balanced view of the special needs of this age group in relation to their ongoing physical, social, and cognitive development.

REFERENCES

Achenbach, T. M., Dumenci, T. M., & Rescorla, L. A. (2003). Are American children's problems still getting worse? A 23–Year comparison. *Journal of Abnormal Child Psychology, 31*, 1–11.

Achenbach, T. M., Howell, C. T., Quay, H. C., & Conners, C. K. (1991). National survey of problems and competencies among four- to sixteen-year-olds: Parents' reports for normative and clinical samples. *Monographs of the Society for Research in Child Development, 56*(3, Serial No. 225).

Allen, J. P., McElhaney, K. B., Kupermine, G. P., & Jodl, K. M. (2004). Stability and change in attachment security across adolescence. *Child Development, 75*, 1792–1805.

American Psychiatric Association. (2000). *Diagnostic and statistical manual of mental disorders* (4th ed., text rev.). Washington, DC: Author.

American Psychological Association. (2002). *Developing adolescents: A reference for professionals.* Washington, DC: Author.

Annie E. Casey Foundation. (2002). *Kids count data book.* Baltimore: Author.

Bakken, L., & Romig, C. (1992). Interpersonal needs in middle adolescence: Companionship, leadership and intimacy. *Journal of Adolescence, 15*(3), 301–316.

Baumeister, L. M., Flores, E., & Marin, B. V. (1995). Sex information given to Latina adolescents by parents. *Health Education Research, 10*(2), 233–239.

Bell, D. J., Foster, S. L., & Mash, E. J. (2005a). *Handbook of behavioral and emotional problems in girls.* New York: Kluwer/Plenum Press.

Bell, D. J., Foster, S. L., & Mash, E. J. (2005b). Understanding behavioral and emotional problems in girls. In D. J. Bell, S. L. Foster, & E. J. Mash (Eds.), *Handbook of behavioral and emotional problems in girls* (pp. 1–24). New York: Kluwer/Plenum Press.

Biglan, A., Brennan, P. A., Foster, S. L., & Holder, H. D. (2004). *Helping adolescents at risk: Prevention of multiple problem behaviors.* New York: Guilford Press.

Blum, R. W., & Nelson-Mmari, K. (2004). The health of young people in a global context. *Journal of Adolescent Health, 35*, 402–418.

Bongers, I. L., Koot, H. M., van der Ende, J., & Verhulst, F. C. (2004). Developmental trajectories of externalizing behaviors in childhood and adolescence. *Child Development, 75*(5), 1523–1537.

Bradley, R. H., Corwyn, R. F., Burchinal, M., Pipes McAdoo, H., & García Coll, C. (2001). The home environments of children in the United States. Part II: Relations with behavioral development through age thirteen. *Child Development, 72*(6), 1868–1886.

Burns, B. J., Costello, E. J., Angold, A., Tweed, D., Stangl, D., Farmer, E. M. Z., & Erkanli, A. (1995). Data watch: Children's mental health service use across service sectors. *Health Affair, 14*, 147–159.

Burt, M. R. (2002). Reasons to invest in adolescents. *Journal of Adolescent Health, 31*(6, Suppl. 1), 136–152.

Burt, M. R., Resnick, G., & Novick, E. R. (1998). *Building supportive communities for at-risk adolescents: It takes more than services.* Washington, DC: American Psychological Association.

Capaldi, D. M., Crosby, L., & Stoolmiller, M. (1996). Predicting the timing of first sexual intercourse for at-risk adolescent males. *Child Development, 67*(2), 344–359.

Catalano, R. F., Hawkins, J. D., Berglund, M. L., Pollard, J. A., & Arthur, M. W. (2002). Prevention science and positive youth development: Competitive or cooperative frameworks? *Journal of Adolescent Health, 31*(6, Suppl. 1), 230–239.

Cauce, A. M., Domenech-Rodriguez, M., Paradise, M., Cochran, B. N., Shea, J. M., Srebnik, D., & Baydar, N. (2002). Cultural and contextual influences in mental health help seeking: A focus on ethnic minority youth. *Journal of Consulting and Clinical Psychology, 70*, 44–55.

Cicchetti, D., & Rogosch, F. A. (2002). A developmental psychopathology perspective on adolescence.

Journal of Consulting and Clinical Psychology, 70, 6–20.

Cicchetti, D., & Toth, S. L. (Eds.). (1996). *Adolescence: Opportunities and challenges.* Rochester, NY: University of Rochester Press.

Collins, W. A., & Sroufe, L. A. (1999). Capacity for intimate relationships: A developmental construction. In W. Furman, B. B. Brown, & C. Feiring (Eds.), *The development of romantic relationships in adolescence* (pp. 125–147). New York: Cambridge University Press.

Collishaw, S., Maughan, B., Goodman, R., & Pickles, A. (2004). Time trends in adolescent mental health. *Journal of Child Psychology and Psychiatry, 45,* 1350–1362.

Costello, E. J., Angold, A., Burns, B. J., Erkanli, A., Stangl, D. K., & Tweed, D. L. (1996). The Great Smoky Mountains Study of youth: Functional impairment and serious emotional disturbance. *Archives of General Psychiatry, 53,* 1137–1143.

Crick, N. R., & Zahn-Waxler, C. (2003). The development of psychopathology in males and females: Current progress and future challenges. *Development and Psychopathology, 15,* 719–742.

Crockett, L. J., & Petersen, A. C. (1993). Adolescent development: Health risks and opportunities for health promotion. In S. G. Millstein & A. C. Petersen (Eds.), *Promoting the health of adolescents: New directions for the twenty-first century* (pp. 13–37). London: London University Press.

Davis, M., Banks, S., Fisher, W., & Grudzinskas, A. (2004). Longitudinal patterns of offending during the transition to adulthood in youth from the mental health system. *Journal of Behavioral Health Services and Research, 31,* 351–366.

Dryfoos, J. G. (1990). *Adolescents at risk: Prevalence and prevention* (Vol. 9). New York: Oxford University Press.

Durston, S., Hulshoff Pol, H. E., Casey, B. J., Giedd, J. N., Buitelaar, J. K., & van Engeland, H. (2001). Anatomical MRI of the developing human brain: What have we learned? *Journal of the American Academy of Child and Adolescent Psychiatry, 40*(9), 1012–1020.

Eccles, J., Barber, B., Jozefowicz, D., Malenchuk, O., & Vida, M. (1999). Self-evaluations of competence, task values, and self-esteem. In N. G. Johnson & M. C. Roberts (Eds.), *Beyond appearance: A new look at adolescent girls* (pp. 53–83). Washington, DC: American Psychological Association.

Eccles, J. S., Midgley, C., Wigfield, A., Buchanan, C. M., Reuman, D., Flanagan, C., & MacIver, D. (1993). Development during adolescence: The impact of stage-environment fit on young adolescents' experiences in the schools and in families. *American Psychologist, 48,* 90–101.

Ezpeleta, L, Keeler, G., Alaatin, E., Costello, E. J., & Angold, A. (2001). Epidemiology of psychiatric disability in childhood and adolescence. *Journal of Child Psychology and Psychiatry, 42,* 901–914.

Flannery, D. J., Rowe, D. C., & Gulley, B. L. (1993). Impact of pubertal status, timing, and age on adolescent sexual experience and delinquency. *Journal of Adolescent Research, 8*(1), 21–40.

Gadow, K. D., Sprafkin, J., & Nolan, E. E. (2001). DSM-IV symptoms in community and clinic preschool children. *Journal of the American Academy of Child and Adolescent Psychiatry, 40*(12), 1383–1392.

Garcia Coll, C., Akerman, A., & Cicchetti, D. (2000). Cultural influences on developmental processes and outcomes: Implications for the study of development and psychopathology. *Development and Psychopathology, 12,* 333–356.

Ge, X., Conger, R. D., & Elder, G. H., Jr. (2001). Pubertal transition, stressful life events, and the emergence of gender differences in adolescent depressive symptoms. *Developmental Psychology, 37,* 404–417.

Goodwin, R. D., Lewinsohn, P. M., & Seely, J. R. (2004). Respiratory symptoms and mental disorders among youth: Results from a prospective, longitudinal study. *Psychosomatic Medicine, 66,* 943–949.

Graber, J. A., Lewinsohn, P. M., & Seeley, J. R., & Brooks-Gunn, J. (1997). Is psychopathology associated with the timing of pubertal development? *Journal of the American Academy of Child and Adolescent Psychiatry, 36*(12), 1768–1776.

Graber, J. S. (2003). Puberty in context. In C. Hayward (Ed.), *Gender differences at puberty* (pp. 307–325). New York: University Press.

Harrell, J. S., Bangdiwala, S. I., Deng, S., Webb, J. P., & Bradley, C. (1998). Smoking initiation in youth: The roles of gender, race, socioeconomics, and developmental status. *Journal of Adolescent Health, 23*(5), 271–279.

Harter, S. (1990). Self and identity development. In S. S. Feldman & G. R. Elliott (Eds.), *At the threshold: The developing adolescent* (pp. 352–387). Cambridge, MA: Harvard University Press.

Hillburn-Cobb, C. (2004). Adolescent psychopathology in terms of multiple behavioral systems: The role of attachment and controlling strategies and frankly disorganized behavior. In L. Atkinson & S. Goldberg (Eds.), *Attachment issues in psychopathology and intervention* (pp. 95–135). Mahwah, NJ: Erlbaum.

Hoffmann, N. G., Bride, B. E., MacMaster, S. A., Abrantes, A. M., & Estroff, T. W. (2004). Identifying co-occuring disorders in adolescent populations. *Journal of Addictive Behaviors, 23,* 41–53.

Holmbeck, G. N., & Kendall, P. C. (2002). Introduction to the special section on clinical adolescent psychology. Developmental psychopathology and treatment. *Journal of Consulting and Clinical Psychology, 70.* 3–5.

Irwin, C. E. (2003). Adolescent health at the crossroads: Where do we go from here? *Journal of Adolescent Health, 33,* 51–56.

Irwin, C. E., Burg, S. J., & Cart, C. U. (2002). America's adolescents: Where have we been, where are we going? *Journal of Adolescent Health, 31*(6, Suppl. 1), 91–121.

Jessor, R., Donovan, J. E., & Costa, F. M. (1991). *Beyond adolescence: Problem behavior and young adult development.* New York: Cambridge University Press.

Johnston, L. D., O'Malley, P. M., & Bachman, J., G. (2003). *Monitoring the future, national results on adolescent drug use. Overview of key findings.* Bethesda, MD: National Institute on Drug Abuse, U.S. Department of Health and Human Services, Public Health Service, National Institutes of Health.

Kazdin, A. E. (2000). Adolescent development, mental disorders, and decision making of delinquent youths. In T. Grisso & R. G. Schwartz (Eds.), *Youth on trial: A developmental perspective on juvenile justice* (pp. 33–65). Chicago: University of Chicago Press.

Kazdin, A. E., & Kagan, J. (1994). Models of dysfunction in developmental psychopathology. *Clinical Psychology: Science and Practice, 1,* 35–52.

Kilpatrick, D. G., Acierno, R., Saunders, B., Resnick, H. S., Best, C. L., & Schnurr, P. P. (2000). Risk factors for adolescent substance abuse and dependence: Data from a national sample. *Journal of Consulting and Clinical Psychology, 68*(1), 19–30.

Kovacs, M. (1997). Depressive disorders in childhood: An impressionistic landscape. *Journal of Child Psychology and Psychiatry, 38,* 287298.

Leitenberg, H., & Saltzman, H. (2000). A statewide survey of age at first intercourse for adolescent females and age of their male partners: Relation to other risk behaviors and statutory rape implications. *Archives of Sexual Behavior,* 203–215.

Lerner, R. M., & Castellino, D. R. (2002). Contemporary developmental theory and adolescence: Developmental systems and applied developmental science. *Journal of Adolescent Health, 31*(6, Suppl. 1), 122–135.

Maccoby, E. E. (1998). *The two sexes: Growing up apart, coming together.* Cambridge, MA: Harvard University Press.

Mash, E. J., & Barkley, R. A. (Eds.). (2003). *Child psychopathology* (2nd ed.). New York: Guilford Press.

Mash, E. J., & Barkley, R. A. (Eds.). (in press). *Treatment of childhood disorders* (3rd ed.). New York: Guilford Press.

Mash, E. J., & Dozois, D. J. A. (2003). Child psychopathology: A developmental–systems perspective. In E. J. Mash & R. A. Barkley (Eds.), *Child psychopathology* (2nd ed., pp. 3–71). New York: Guilford Press.

Mash, E. J., & Wolfe, D. A. (2005). *Abnormal child psychology* (3rd ed.). Belmont, CA: Wadsworth/ Thomson.

McCall, R. B., & Groark, C. J. (2000). The future of applied child development research and public policy. *Child Development, 71,* 197–204.

McDermott, P. A., & Weiss, R. V. (1995). A normative typology of healthy, subclinical, and clinical behavior styles among American children and adolescents. *Psychological Assessment, 7,* 162–170.

McLoyd, V. C. (1998). Socioeconomic disadvantage and child development. *American Psychologist, 53,* 185–204.

Mezzich, A. C., Tarter, R. E., Giancola, P. R., Lu, S., Kirisci, L., & Parks, S. (1997). Substance use and risky sexual behavior in female adolescents. *Drug and Alcohol Dependence, 44*(2–3), 157–166.

Miller, T. R. (2004). The social costs of adolescent problem behavior. In A. Biglan, P. A. Brennan, S. L. Foster, & H. D. Holder (Eds.), *Helping adolescents at risk: Prevention of multiple problem behaviors* (pp. 31–56). New York: Guilford Press.

Moffitt, T. E., Caspi, A., Dickson, N., Silva, P., & Stanton, W. (1996). Childhood-onset versus adolescent-onset antisocial conduct problems in males: Natural history from ages 3 to 18 years. *Development and Psychopathology, 8*(2), 399–424.

Morreale, M. C., Kapphahn, C. J., Elster, A. B., Juszczak, L., & Klein, J. D. (2004). Access to health care for adolescents and young adults. *Journal of Adolescent Health, 35,* 342–344.

Muris, P., Meesters, C., van de Blom, W., & Mayer, B. (2005). Biological, psychological, and sociocultural correlates of body change strategies and eating problems in adolescent boys and girls. *Eating Behaviors, 6,* 11–22.

Murry, V. M., Bynum, M. S., Brody, G. H., Willert, A., & Stephens, D. (2001). African American single mothers and children in context: A review of studies on risk and resilience. *Clinical Child and Family Psychology Review, 4*(2), 133–155.

Offord, D. R. (2000). Prevention of antisocial personality disorder. In J. L. Rapoport (Ed.), *Childhood onset of "adult" psychopathology: Clinical and research advances* (pp. 379–398). Washington, DC: USic.

Ohye, B. Y., & Daniel, J. H. (1999). The "other" adolescent girls: Who are they? In N. G. Johnson, M. C. Roberts, & J. Worell (Eds.), *Beyond appearance: A new look at adolescent girls* (pp. 115–129). Washington, DC: APA Books.

Phinney, J. (1990). Ethnic identity in adolescents and adults: A review of the research. *Psychological Bulletin, 108,* 499–514.

President's New Freedom Commission on Mental Health. (2003). *Achieving the promise: Transforming mental health care in America.* Retrieved February 16, 2004, from http://www.mentalhealthcommission.gov

Resnick, M. D., Bearman, P. S., Blum, R. W., Bauman, K. E., Harris, K. M., Jones, J., et al. (1997). Protecting adolescents from harm: Findings from the National Longitudinal Study on Adolescent Health. *Journal of the American Medical Association, 278*(10), 823–832.

Resnick, M. D., Ireland, M., & Borowsky, I. (2004). Youth violence perpetration: What protects? What predicts? Findings from the National Longitudinal Study of Adolescent Health. *Journal of Adolescent Health, 35,* 424.e1–424.e10

Ringel, J. S., & Sturm, R. (2001). National estimates of

mental health utilization and expenditures for children in 1998. *Journal of Behavioral Health Services and Research, 28,* 319–333.

Roberts,R., Attkisson, C., & Rosenblatt, A. (1998). Prevalence of psychopathology among children and adolescents. *American Journal of Psychiatry, 155,* 715–725.

Romano, E., Tremblay, R. E., Vitaro, F., Zoccolillo, M., & Pagani, L. (2001). Prevalence of psychiatric diagnoses and the role of perceived impairment: Findings from an adolescent community sample. *Journal of Child Psychology and Psychiatry, 42,* 451–461.

Rutter, M., Caspi, A., & Moffitt, T. E. (2003). Using sex differences in psychopathology to study causal mechanisms: Unifying issues and research strategies. *Journal of Child Psychology and Psychiatry, 44,* 1092–1115.

Samaan, R. A. (2000). The influences of race, ethnicity, and poverty on the mental health of children. *Journal of Health Care for the Poor and Underserved, 11,* 100–110.

Savin-Williams, R. C. (1998). " . . . *And then I became gay": Young men's stories.* New York: Routledge.

Shaffer, D., Fisher, P. Dulcan, M. K., Davies, M., Piacentini, J., Schwab-Stone, M. E., et al. (1996). The NIMH Diagnostic Interview Schedule for Children Version 2.3 (DISC-2.3): Description, acceptability, prevalence rates, and performance in the MECA study. *Journal of the American Academy of Child and Adolescent Psychiatry, 35,* 865–877.

Sheffield, J. K., Fiorenza, E., & Sofronoff, K. (2004). Adolescents willingness to seek psychological help: Promoting and preventing factors. *Journal of Youth and Adolescence, 33,* 495–507.

Silbereisen, R. K., & Kracke, B. (1997). Self-reported maturational timing and adaptation in adolescence. In J. Schulenberg & J. L. Maggs (Eds.), *Health risks and developmental transitions during adolescence* (pp. 85–109). Cambridge, UK: Cambridge University Press.

Sourander, A., Multimaki, P., Santalahti, P., Parkkola, K., Haavisto, A., Helenius, H., et al. (2004). Mental health service use among 18-year-old adolescent boys: A prospective 10-year follow-up study. *Journal of the American Academy of Child and Adolescent Psychiatry, 43,* 1250–1258.

Stattin, H., & Magnusson, D. (1990). *Pubertal maturation in female development.* Hillsdale, NJ: Erlbaum.

Steinberg, L. (2004). Risk taking in adolescence: What changes, and why? *Annals of the New York Academy of Sciences, 1021,* 51–58.

Steinberg, L., & Morris, A. S. (2001). Adolescent development. *Annual Review of Psychology, 52,* 83–110.

Striegel-Moore, R. H., & Cachelin, F. M. (2001). Etiology of eating disorders in women. *Counseling Psychologist, 29*(5), 635–661.

U.S. Census Bureau. (2005). Census 2000 PHC-T-9. Population by age, sex, race, and Hispanic or Latino origin for the United States: 2000. *Census 2000 Summary File 1.* Retrieved January 4, 2005, from http://factfinder.census.gov

U.S. Department of Health and Human Services. (2000). *Promoting better health for young people through physical activity and sports: A report to the President from the Secretary of Health and Human Services and the Secretary of Education.* Washington, DC: U.S. Government Printing Office.

United Nations. (2002). *Adolescence: A rite of passage.* New York: Author.

Vander Stoep, A., Weiss, N. S., Kuo, E. S., Cheney, D., & Cohen, P. (2003). What proportion of failure to complete secondary school in the US population is attributable to adolescent psychiatric disorder? *Journal of Behavioral Health Services and Research, 30,* 119–124.

Vander Stoep, A., Weiss, N. S., McKnight, B., Beresford, S. A. A., & Cohen, P. (2002). Which measure of adolescent psychiatric disorder diagnosis, number of symptoms, or adaptive functioning best predicts adverse young adult outcomes? *Journal of Epidemiology and Community Health 56,* 56–65.

Walker, E. (2002). Adolescent neurodevelopment and psychopathology. *Current Directions in Psychological Science, 11*(1), 24–28.

Walker, E., & Bollini, A. M. (2002). Pubertal neurodevelopment and the emergence of psychotic symptoms. *Schizophrenia Research, 54*(1–2), 17–23.

Weisz, J. R., & Hawley, K. M. (2002). Developmental factors in the treatment of adolescents. *Journal of Consulting and Clinical Psychology, 70.* 21–43.

Wight, R. G., Sepúlveda, J. E., & Aneshensel, C. S. (2004). Depressive symptoms: how do adolescents compare with adults? *Journal of Adolescent Health, 34,* 314–323.

Wolfe, D. A., Jaffe, P., & Crooks, C. (2006). *The Relationship Connection: Comprehensive strategies for reducing adolescent risk behaviors.* New Haven, CT: Yale University Press.

World Health Organization. (1997, December). *Fact sheet #186.* Geneva: Author.

World Health Organization. (2001). *Noncommunicable diseases and mental health.* Geneva: Author.

Youngstrom, E. A., Findling, R. L., & Calabrese, J. R. (2003). Who are the comorbid adolescents? Agreement between psychiatric diagnosis, youth, parent, and teacher report. *Journal of Abnormal Child Psychology, 31,* 231–245.

2

Development and Psychopathology in Adolescence

Grayson N. Holmbeck
Deborah Friedman
Mona Abad
Barbara Jandasek

Both the quantity and quality of research on adolescent development and adolescent psychopathology have increased rapidly over the past two decades. In 1986, the Society for Research on Adolescence held its first meetings. The first *Annual Review of Psychology* chapter focusing on adolescent development appeared in 1988 (Petersen, 1988), with three chapters on the topic appearing since 1995 (Compas, Hinden, & Gerhardt, 1995; Lerner & Galambos, 1998; Steinberg & Morris, 2001). Several journals devoted exclusively to research on adolescent development and adolescent mental health are available (*Journal of Research on Adolescence, Journal of Youth and Adolescence, Journal of Early Adolescence, Journal of Adolescent Research*). Moreover, several journals have devoted special issues or sections to various aspects of adolescent development: *American Psychologist* (Takanishi, 1993), *Developmental Psychology* (Zahn-Waxler, 1996), and the *Journal of Consulting and Clinical Psychology* (Holmbeck & Kendall, 2002). Recently, Division 53 (the Society

for Clinical Child Psychology) of the American Psychological Association added "Adolescent" to its name (the Society for Clinical Child and Adolescent Psychology), with its journal being renamed as well (*Journal of Clinical Child and Adolescent Psychology*). Finally, an informal review of journals in psychology (e.g., *Development and Psychopathology, Journal of Consulting and Clinical Psychology*) and psychiatry (e.g., *Journal of the American Academy of Child and Adolescent Psychiatry*) reveals that adolescent psychopathology continues to receive increasing attention.

Despite all this attention to the second decade of life, few papers have appeared that integrate across the developmental and psychopathology literatures. (One recent exception was the special section on Clinical Adolescent Psychology: Developmental Psychopathology and Treatment appearing in the *Journal of Consulting and Clinical Psychology* [Holmbeck & Kendall, 2002].) The potential for cross-fertilization between the fields of developmental psychology and clinical–child psychology is perhaps no more evident than in research focusing on adolescent psychopathology (Holmbeck et al., 2000; Holmbeck & Shapera, 1999; Holmbeck & Updegrove, 1995). Adolescence is a transitional developmental period between childhood and adulthood that is characterized by more biological, psychological, and social role changes than any other stage of life, except infancy (Feldman & Elliott, 1990; Holmbeck et al., 2000). Indeed, change is *the* defining feature of adolescence. Given the many changes that characterize adolescent development, it is not surprising that there are also significant changes in the types and frequency of psychological disorders and problem behaviors that are manifested during adolescence, as compared to childhood. Adolescence is a period of development when a maladaptive pathway may be altered in an adaptive direction by exposure to protective processes or intervention; similarly, maladaptive pathways may begin anew during this period. Moreover, distinctions between normal and abnormal are sometimes less clear during this developmental period than they are in earlier developmental periods (Cicchetti & Rogosch, 2002).

The influence of theories from the field of *developmental* psychopathology is evident in recent research on adolescent problem behaviors. Developmentally oriented research has documented the importance of the following for the psychosocial functioning of the child and adolescent (Graber & Brooks-Gunn, 1996; Schulenberg, Maggs, & Hurrelmann, 1997): the timing (early vs. late) of developmental events, the cumulative impact of multiple events that occur simultaneously, and the fit between the developmental needs of an adolescent and the adolescent's environmental context. Contextual perspectives on adolescent psychopathology also have their roots in developmental theory (Bronfenbrenner, 1979).

The field of *developmental psychopathology* has provided us with a vocabulary with which to explain the unfolding of psychopathology over the adolescent developmental period (e.g., developmental trajectories, resilience, risk and protective processes, continuity/discontinuity, hetero- and homotypic continuity, multifinality, equifinality; Cicchetti & Rogosch, 1999a, 2002). Moreover, research based on a developmental psychopathology perspective has advanced our understanding of the developmental precursors and correlates of adolescent psychopathology. On the other hand, those who develop treatment strategies for adolescents have been slow to incorporate developmental principles into their treatment approaches (Cicchetti & Rogosch, 2002; Holmbeck et al., 2000; Holmbeck, Greenley, & Franks, 2003; Weisz & Hawley, 2002). In fact, most treatments for adolescents were originally developed for other age groups (i.e., children or adults) and subsequently adapted for teenagers (Weisz & Hawley, 2002), although there are exceptions (e.g., Henggeler, Schoenwald, Borduin, Rowland, & Cunningham, 1998).

By adopting a developmental perspective on psychopathology during adolescence, we can begin to ask different kinds of questions. For example, one might pose the following:

1. How (and why) does age of onset vary across disorders?
2. Do prenatal and early childhood precursors differ for childhood-onset versus adolescent-onset versions of the same disorder?
3. How does the symptom presentation of a particular childhood-onset disorder change as the child negotiates the developmental tasks of adolescence?
4. How does mastery (or lack of mastery) of adolescent developmental tasks influence adolescents' ability to manage future adversities as well as their adaptational trajectory over time?
5. What developmental pathways manifested in childhood increase the probability that psychopathology will develop in adolescence?
6. What resilience processes make it less likely that certain symptoms will emerge in the future?
7. What types of developmental pathways lead to which types of psychopathologies and are multiple antecedent developmental pathways possible for the same psychopathology?
8. Are factors associated with the onset of a disorder similar or different from factors associated with the maintenance of a disorder?
9. What developmental and contextual processes moderate (e.g., cognitive development and neighborhood quality) and/or mediate (e.g., autonomy development) associations between socialization influences (e.g., parenting) and future adjustment outcomes?
10. What behaviors are typical for the age period (e.g., experimentation with drugs)

and which are indicative of more serious psychopathology?

The purpose of this chapter is to review the developmental changes and milestones of adolescence and their impact on adolescent psychopathology. First, we provide an overview of a framework for understanding adolescent development and adjustment. In reviewing the components of this framework, we discuss the implications that each component has for adolescent psychopathology. Second, we review the tenets of the field of developmental psychopathology and the implications that this field has for understanding psychopathology during adolescence. Finally, we review several concepts from this field and discuss how each is related to different forms of adolescent psychopathology. Specifically, we focus on the following: developmental trajectories (including multifinality and equifinality), the onset and maintenance of psychopathology, age-of-onset research, resilience, risk and protective factors, comorbidity, shared and nonshared environment effects, person–environment fit research, and research on culture and contextualism.

A FRAMEWORK FOR UNDERSTANDING ADOLESCENT DEVELOPMENT AND ADJUSTMENT

It is our contention that adolescent psychopathology is best understood within the context of the major tasks of this developmental period. We believe that an appreciation for the rapid developmental changes of adolescence and the contexts of such development will aid the clinician and researcher in considering such issues in their clinical and research endeavors. The framework presented here summarizes major constructs that have been studied by researchers in this field and is based on earlier models presented by Hill (1980), Holmbeck (Holmbeck et al., 2000; Holmbeck & Updegrove, 1995), Steinberg (2002), and Grotevant (1997). The model is biopsychosocial in nature, insofar as it emphasizes the biological, psychological, and social changes of the adolescent developmental period (see Figure 2.1). In addition to this focus on intraindividual development, we have also attempted to incorporate more recent discoveries from studies of contextual effects during adolescence. For example, recent research has gone

beyond asking whether family variables are associated with adolescent adjustment outcomes and now attempts to isolate those contexts or circumstances in which such associations are most pronounced. In short, this model is both developmental and contextual.

At the most general level, the framework presented in Figure 2.1 indicates that the primary developmental changes of adolescence have an impact on the developmental outcomes of adolescence *via* the interpersonal contexts in which adolescents develop. In other words, the developmental changes of adolescence have an impact on the behaviors of significant others, which, in turn, influence ways in which adolescents resolve the major issues of adolescence, namely, autonomy, sexuality, identity, and so on.

For example, suppose that a young preadolescent girl begins to mature physically much earlier than her age-mates. Such early maturity will likely have an impact on her peer relationships insofar as early-maturing girls are more likely to date and initiate sexual behaviors at an earlier age than are girls who mature on time (Magnusson, Stattin, & Allen, 1985). Such impacts on male peers may influence the girl's own self-perceptions in the areas of identity and sexuality. In this way, the behaviors of peers in response to the girl's early maturity could be said to *mediate* associations between pubertal change and outcomes such as identity and sexual behavior (and therefore account, at least in part, for these significant associations). We use the term "mediation" because of the proposed A → B → C relationship inherent in this example, whereby B is hypothesized to mediate associations between A and C (see Baron & Kenny, 1986, and Holmbeck, 1997, for a more thorough explanation of mediated effects).

Such causal and mediational influences may vary depending on the demographic and intrapersonal context in which they occur (see Figure 2.1: "Demographic and Intrapersonal Moderating Variables"). Specifically, associations between the primary developmental changes and the developmental outcomes may be *moderated* by demographic variables such as ethnicity, gender, socioeconomic status, and the like. We use the term "moderated" because it is expected that associations between the primary changes and developmental outcomes may differ depending on the demographic status of the individual (see Baron & Kenny, 1986, and Holmbeck, 1997, for a more thorough explanation of moderated effects). For

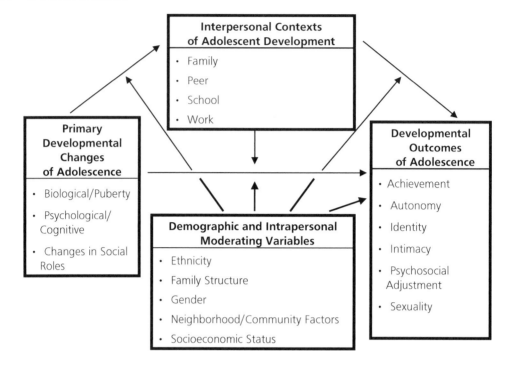

FIGURE 2.1. A framework for understanding adolescent development and adjustment. From Holmbeck and Shapera (1999). Copyright 1999 by John Wiley & Sons, Inc. Reprinted by permission.

example, if associations between pubertal change and certain sexual outcomes *only* held for girls, we could infer that gender moderates such associations. In addition to serving a mediational role as described previously, the interpersonal contexts (i.e., family, peer, school, and work contexts) can also serve a moderating role in the association between the primary changes and the developmental outcomes. For example, early maturity may lead to poor adjustment outcomes *only* when families react to early pubertal development in certain ways (e.g., with increased restriction and supervision); in this example, familial reactions to puberty moderate associations between pubertal development and adjustment.

Primary Developmental Changes of Adolescence

The framework in Figure 2.1 specifies three types of primary developmental changes that occur during adolescence: biological/pubertal, psychological/cognitive, and changes in social roles. They are viewed as "primary" because they are universal across cultures and because they often occur temporally prior to the devel-

opmental outcomes of adolescence (changes in autonomy, identity, sexuality, etc.). Despite the universality and intensity of these changes, there has unfortunately been a decided lack of attention to these developmental issues in the adolescent clinical literature, particularly the cognitive-developmental changes of adolescence. Such lack of attention to cognitive development (perhaps in favor of pubertal development) is likely a function of the difficulty in assessing the cognitive-developmental changes (and the relative ease with which puberty can be assessed, particularly those aspects of pubertal development that are observable). In this section, we provide a brief overview of each type of change as well as examples of research that has examined links between these developmental changes and adolescent psychopathology.

Biological/Pubertal Changes

Adolescence is a time of substantial physical growth and change (Brooks-Gunn & Reiter, 1990). Tanner (1962) charted most of the characteristics of these changes in males and females. Changes in body proportions, facial characteristics, voice, body hair, strength, and coordination are found in boys and changes in body proportions, body hair, breast growth, and menarcheal status are found in girls. Crucial to the understanding of this process is the knowledge that the peak of pubertal development occurs two years *earlier* in the modal female than in the modal male (e.g., the adolescent growth spurt peaks at age 12 in girls and at age 14 in boys; Steinberg, 2002). *Intra*individual variation is also evident with respect to the onset of different pubertal changes (e.g., breast development typically occurs prior to menarche for girls). Moreover, there is substantial variation between individuals in the time of onset, duration, and termination of the pubertal cycle (Brooks-Gunn & Reiter, 1990), and these differences have social consequences. Thus, it is possible, for example, that two 14-year-old boys may be at very different stages of pubertal development, such that one boy has not yet begun pubertal changes and the other boy has experienced nearly all pubertal events. Any of the following factors can have an influence on the timing of pubertal change: Genetic factors, ethnicity, environmental stress and social class, nutrition, health, the presence of certain chronic illnesses, and percentage of body fat (American Psychological Association, 2002).

Research also suggests that both *pubertal status* (an individual's placement in the sequence of predictable pubertal changes) and *pubertal timing* (timing of changes relative to one's age peers) have an impact on the quality of family relationships and certain indicators of psychosocial adaptation and psychopathology (Alsaker, 1995; Graber, Brooks-Gunn, Paikoff, & Warren, 1994; Holmbeck & Hill, 1991; Laursen, Coy, & Collins, 1998; Paikoff & Brooks-Gunn, 1991; Sagrestano, McCormick, Paikoff, & Holmbeck, 1999). With respect to pubertal timing, early-maturing girls, for example, are at risk for a variety of adaptational difficulties, including depression, substance use, early sexual risk behaviors, eating problems and disorders, and family conflicts (American Psychological Association, 2002). Early-developing boys, on the other hand, are favored over later-developing boys for involvement in athletic activities, dating, and social events (Richards, Abell, & Petersen, 1993), but late-maturing boys may be at risk for depression and school problems (American Psychological Association, 2002; Graber, Lewinsohn,

Seeley, & Brooks-Gunn, 1997). Gender differences also appear in the manner in which puberty is linked with adjustment outcomes. Whereas early-maturing girls appear to be at risk for depressive symptoms, boys are most at risk for such symptoms when they experience accelerated pubertal change (Ge et al., 2003). It is important to note that most of the psychological effects of pubertal changes are probably not direct but, rather, are moderated or mediated by responses of the individual or significant others to such changes (see Figure 2.1; Holmbeck, 1996; Paikoff & Brooks-Gunn, 1991). Finally, evidence has been found for links between hormonal changes associated with puberty and subsequent mood and behavioral changes (Angold, Costello, Erkanli, & Worthman, 1999; Buchanan, Eccles, & Becker, 1992).

Other links between physical development and psychopathology have been found in past research. For example, the rate of overweight adolescents has increased threefold since 1980 (to 14%; American Psychological Association, 2002), with such rates being even higher in some ethnic groups (e.g., African American girls). Such overweight adolescents are at risk for other health-related problems and social discrimination. Dissatisfaction with body weight and body preoccupation is normative during adolescence, but some adolescents also develop eating disorders, with most cases being females (90%; American Psychological Association, 2002).

At a more complex level of analysis, some researchers have found that the influence of puberty (e.g., early maturity) on psychopathology (e.g., depression) is moderated by other factors (e.g., cognitive development). For example, Rierdan and Koff (1993) found that early-maturing girls who were also functioning at low levels of ego development had higher levels of depression than other girls in their sample. Others have isolated similar interactive effects: (1) girls who are both postmenarcheal and involved in mixed-sex social activities are more likely to have symptoms of eating disorders (Cauffman & Steinberg, 1996), (2) in boys, relations between testosterone levels and risk behaviors and depression are moderated by quality of family relationships (Booth, Johnson, Granger, Crouter, & McHale, 2003), (3) early-maturing girls who also have experienced more recent stressful events are most likely to exhibit depressive symptomatology (Ge, Conger, & Elder, 2001), and (4) the effect of pubertal transition effects on externalizing problems and affiliation with deviant peers is moderated by family and neighborhood conditions (Ge, Brody, Conger, Simons, & Murry, 2002).

Finally, other biological variables (other than those related to puberty) have been linked with psychopathology. Research that has examined links between early temperament and adolescent problem behaviors has found that very young uninhibited children are more likely to score higher on problem behaviors during adolescence than inhibited children (Schwartz, Snidman, & Kagan, 1996). Similarly, measures of childhood temperament have also been linked with convictions for violent offenses in late adolescence (Henry, Caspi, Moffitt, & Silva, 1996). Prenatal and perinatal factors in early childhood are also implicated in both internalizing and externalizing problems (Allen, Lewinsohn, & Seeley, 1998) and associations between adrenocorticol activity and internalizing symptoms have been demonstrated (Klimes-Dougan, Hastings, Granger, Usher, & Zahn-Waxler, 2001). Recently, some have suggested the intriguing possibility that hormonal changes during puberty may have an impact on expression of genes that may, in turn, be associated with changes in risk for psychopathology (Walker, 2002).

Psychological/Cognitive Changes

Piaget (1970, 1972) provided a comprehensive stage theory of cognitive development, which, until recently, has dominated this field of study. He identified adolescence as the period in which formal operational thinking emerges and when adult-level reasoning can take place. Adolescents who have achieved such thinking abilities are able to think more complexly, abstractly, and hypothetically. They are able to think in terms of possibilities and many are able to think realistically about the future. Moreover, they are able to employ meta-cognition, or the ability to think about one's own thoughts.

Although there is general agreement that a shift in thinking occurs during the transition from childhood to adolescence, critics of the Piagetian approach have suggested alternatives (Moshman, 1998). Proponents of the information-processing perspective, for example, have attempted to identify specific changes in cognitive activity that may account for advances in thinking. They maintain that there are significant advances in the following areas during adolescence: (1) processing capacity or efficiency (e.g., memory and organization of information); (2) knowledge base; and (3) cognitive self-regulation (Keating, 1990). These factors together make it easier for adolescents to simultaneously process multiple symbolic representations (e.g., they are better able to generate a complete list of solutions for a problem). It is important to note that the information-processing and Piagetian perspectives are not necessarily mutually exclusive. Piaget's theory describes a qualitative shift in adolescent thinking that appears to begin around age 11 or 12, and the information-processing perspective complements this theory because it suggests possible cognitive features that underlie this shift.

In addition to the Piagetian and information-processing perspectives, a third approach to cognitive development during adolescence is the contextualist perspective. Vygotsky (1978) has suggested that psychological processes have a social basis. According to this approach, social interactions, particularly verbal communication, have an important influence on cognitive development. Lochman, White, and Wayland (1991) have applied a contextual approach to the development of problem solving. They note that caregivers structure their child's environment and resolve their child's problems, and through dialogue and observation, children internalize "idiographic" ways of perceiving the world and solving problems. This perspective on cognitive development is unique because it emphasizes the role of the cognitive "environment." Indeed, cognitive development does not occur in a vacuum but, rather, is fostered or hindered via interactions with the social world (Higgins, Ruble, & Hartup, 1983). Of interest here are the child's socially relevant cognitions such as one's understanding of significant others and their behaviors. The development of roletaking and empathy skills, increases in the sophistication of attributional processes in social situations, and the development of prosocial behavior are a few of the important social cognitive-developmental tasks (Guerra, 1993; Nelson & Crick, 1999).

Overall, it appears that a fairly sophisticated way of thinking develops during adolescence, which is characterized by abstraction, consequential thinking, and hypothetical reasoning. Although the processes that underlie the shift in adolescent thinking are not well understood, it appears that increases in efficiency, capacity, and attentional control are important factors. In addition, from a contextual point of view, environmental factors seem to be of importance. We now turn to a discussion of associations between cognitive developmental processes and adolescent psychopathology.

One aspect of cognitive development that has been examined in relation to psychopathology is moral development (i.e., the development of an individual's values and sense of ethics; American Psychological Association, 2002). In studies of delinquent adolescents, scores on measures of moral development are usually higher in nondelinquent adolescents versus delinquent adolescents and such measures are also able to discriminate between delinquent adolescents who are high versus low on psychopathy (Chandler & Moran, 1990; Trevethan & Walker, 1989). Analogous findings have emerged in studies of ego development. For example, those with affective disorders are more likely to have higher ego development scores than those with conduct disorders (Noam, Paget, Valiant, Borst, & Bartok, 1994; Noam, Recklitis, & Paget, 1991). Problem-solving ability has also been linked with symptomatology. For example, Lenhart and Rabiner (1995) found that social problem solving (e.g., the ability to integrate multiple perspectives in a social conflict) was linked with social competence in a sample of adolescents (e.g., lower levels of behavioral and emotional problems, less aggression in the classroom, and more competence in social interactions).

Finally, in a series of studies on the effects of IQ on adjustment, Luthar and colleagues have shown that IQ serves a protective function for adolescents, although IQ also appears to moderate associations between adjustment variables (Luthar & Ripple, 1994; Luthar & Zigler, 1992). With respect to the latter, those adolescents with high IQs and high levels of distress were more likely to show decreases in social competence over time. No association between distress and social competence was found for those with low IQs. Luthar and Ripple (1994) speculated that those with higher IQs are more aware of their own levels of internal distress than those with low IQs.

Clinically, the techniques of some psychotherapies (such as cognitive-behavioral therapy; CBT) emphasize self-reflection (thinking about how one thinks), consequential thinking (reflecting on the impact of a particular pattern of thinking or behaving), and consideration of future possibilities (thinking about how change in thinking or behaving might, in turn, impact on one's life in the future). Thus, the techniques of such therapies rely on complex symbolic processes, which typically require a high level of cognitive development. Of course, some adolescent clients may not be capable of advanced symbolic processing, particularly in the domain of their problem. Although adolescence is often a time of dramatic cognitive development, there is also considerable interindividual variability in the degree to which such development has taken place. It follows, then, that an adolescent's level of cognitive development is likely to impinge on or facilitate the success of some psychotherapeutic techniques (Holmbeck et al., 2000, 2003; Shirk, 1999). Indeed, a meta-analysis by Durlak, Fuhrman, and Lampman (1991) revealed that CBT is more likely to be effective with older (and more cognitively mature) adolescents. Adolescents who do not have such higher-level cognitive abilities may benefit from treatment that initially focuses on changing/accelerating cognitive-developmental processes (e.g., means–ends thinking and perspective taking; Shirk, 1999; Temple, 1997). That is, the therapist may find it necessary to promote the developmental changes that are necessary for the child to benefit from subsequent therapeutic interactions (provided, of course, that the child is developmentally ready to experience such changes and that there is adequate environmental support to maintain the changes).

Social Redefinition

A variety of changes in the social status of children occur during adolescence (Steinberg, 2002). Although such social redefinition is universal, the specific changes vary greatly across different cultures. In some nonindustrial societies, public rituals (i.e., rites of passage) take place soon after the onset of pubertal change. In Western industrialized societies, the transition is less clear, but analogous changes in social status do take place. Steinberg (2002) cites changes across four domains: *interpersonal* (e.g., changes in familial status), *political* (e.g., late adolescents are eligible to vote), *economic* (e.g., adolescents are allowed to work), and *legal* (e.g., late adolescents can be tried in adult court systems). In addition, adolescents are able to obtain a driver's permit and they can get married. Leaving home in late adolescence also serves to redefine one's social role. Finally, research suggests that stereotypical gender role expectations are intensified during the adolescent period (Galambos, Almeida, & Petersen, 1990).

Such changes in social role have clinical implications. Adolescents' abilities to adapt to changing societal expectations for acceptable behavior will vary. In fact, some adolescents engage in risky behavior as a way of identifying with adult role models (American Psychological Association, 2002). Expected roles are less clear in this culture than is the case in less industrialized societies; there is little consensus about what constitutes "normal" behavior for adolescents in Western culture (e.g., conflicting messages concerning sexuality and substance abuse are frequently presented in the media). Future research should examine whether psychopathology is a possible outcome of failure to sort through conflicting expectations.

Interpersonal Contexts of Adolescence

Figure 2.1 specifies four interpersonal contexts: (1) family, (2) peer, (3) school, and (4) work. Adolescents are embedded within multiple systems; clearly, these systems are implicated in various types of adolescent psychopathology and all are appropriate targets for interventions.

Family Context

Adolescence is a time of transformation in family relationships (Collins, 1990; Holmbeck, 1996; Paikoff & Brooks-Gunn, 1991; Steinberg, 1990). As noted earlier, recent research involving large representative samples of adolescents (see Arnett, 1999) has *not* supported the extreme version of the early storm and stress perspective (Freud, 1958; Hall, 1904). Despite such disconfirming evidence, it appears that public policy and the public's beliefs are still in line with this out-of-date perspective (Buchanan et al., 1990; Holmbeck & Hill, 1988). For example, those who write for mass media publications will often invoke concepts such as rebelliousness and parent–adolescent conflict to make points about the negative nature of adolescence. In a recent national survey of adults, 71% provided negative labels for the typical American teenager (e.g., "rude" and "irresponsible"; Public Agenda, 1999).

Although serious parent–child relationship problems are not typical during early adolescence (Holmbeck, Paikoff, & Brooks-Gunn, 1995), a period of increased emotional distance in the parent–adolescent relationship appears at the peak of pubertal change (Holmbeck & Hill, 1991; Laursen et al., 1998; Paikoff & Brooks-Gunn, 1991). For example, amount of time spent with family members decreases from 35% to 14% from 5th grade to 12th grade; however, connections between adolescents and other family members continue to be present for the large majority of adolescents (Larson, Richards, Moneta, Holmbeck, & Duckett, 1996). Although there also may be an increase in conflict and negative affect, most adolescents negotiate this period *without* severing ties with parents or developing serious disorders (Collins & Laursen, 1992). Also, families with adolescents are more likely to experience conflict over mundane issues rather than basic values (Montemayor, 1983). Any discontinuities in the parent–child relationship during the transition to adolescence tend to occur against a backdrop of relational continuity (Holmbeck, 1996). Moreover, some have argued that the conflicts that arise during the transition to adolescence may serve an adaptive role; indeed, increases in conflicts may indicate that adjustments are needed in parenting and the manner in which decisions are made in the family (Cooper, 1988; Holmbeck, 1996).

One of the major tasks for parents during this developmental period is to be responsive to adolescents' needs for increasing responsibility and decision making power in the family while at the same time maintaining a high level of cohesiveness in the family environment, monitoring their offspring's behavior, and having clear developmental expectations (American Psychological Association, 2002). Parents who lack flexibility and adaptability during this developmental period, particularly in areas of strictness and decision making, tend to have offspring with less adaptive outcomes (Fuligni & Eccles, 1993; Holmbeck et al., 1995).

It also appears that parent–adolescent relationships are altered by the cognitive changes discussed earlier. For example, adolescents are increasingly able and willing to discuss (and argue about) issues with their parents in more complex ways, to see the flaws in their parents' arguments, to imagine what it would be like to have different parents, and to think about their parents' marital relationship separate from their own relationships with their parents (American Psychological Association, 2002). Interestingly, parent–adolescent conflicts over day-to-day issues may be more distressing for the parent than for the child (Robin & Foster, 1989; Steinberg, 2001).

With respect to adolescent psychopathology, many family variables have been implicated in past work (see Fiese, Wilder, & Bickham, 2000, for a review). Parent–child interactions characterized by dysfunctional levels of anger (Kobak, Sudler, & Gamble, 1991) have been associated with depressive symptoms during adolescence. Coercive family interactions during childhood and adolescence (i.e., reciprocation of aversive behaviors between parent and child) have been found to increase risk for antisocial behavior in adolescence (Compton, Snyder, Schrepferman, Bank, & Shortt, 2003). Numerous parenting variables (e.g., positive parenting, psychological control, overprotectiveness, monitoring, involvement, and consistency of discipline) have been linked with outcomes such as externalizing symptoms (Holmbeck et al., 2002), internalizing symptoms (Barber & Harmon, 2002), and substance use (Colder & Chassin, 1999). Finally, adolescent attachment organization has also been found to be associated with future levels of delinquency (Allen et al., 2002). Current research is beginning to move beyond such "main effects" findings and is beginning to examine factors that moderate (Allen et al., 2002; Allen, Moore, & Kuperminc, 1997) and mediate (Holmbeck et al., 2002) effects of family and parent variables on adolescent psychopathology.

Peer Context

One of the most robust predictors of adult difficulties (e.g., dropping out of school and criminality) is poor peer relationships during childhood and adolescence (Parker & Asher, 1987). Most now agree that child–child relationships are necessities and not luxuries and that these relationships have positive effects on cognitive, socialcognitive, linguistic, sex role, and moral development (American Psychological Association, 2002; Berndt & Savin-Williams, 1993; Parker & Asher, 1987). Although controversial, some have argued that peers have a more substantial impact on social development than do parents (Harris, 1998).

Peer relationships during childhood and adolescence appear to evolve through a series of developmental stages (e.g., Brown, 1990; La Greca & Prinstein, 1999; Selman, 1980). Selman (1980), for example, presented a theory of the growth of interpersonal understanding, the stages of which correspond to developmental levels of social perspective taking. Many adolescents are increasingly able to employ advanced levels of role-taking skills, which serve to enhance the maturity of their relationships. Sullivan (1953) also provided a stage theory for the development of peer relationships where he stressed the importance of interpersonal relationships and the differences between child–child and parent–child relationships (Youniss, 1980). With respect to adolescence, Sullivan described his notion of "chumship" and maintained that this (typically) same-sex friendship is a critical developmental accomplishment. It is with this relationship that the child presumably learns about intimacy, and this friendship serves as a basis for later close relationships. Young adolescents also often associate with a peer group; in fact, it is normative to do so. Concerns about conformity to peer norms reach a peak during this period (American Psychological Association, 2002), which may produce stress and intense concerns about belonging to a particular peer group. Adolescents tend to become involved in mixed-sex groups in midadolescence and gradually move toward dyadic intimate relationships in later adolescence. Peers tend to select as friends individuals like themselves (selection effects), and they tend to subsequently influence each other over time (socialization effects; Dodge & Pettit, 2003).

Although families and peers each provide unique contributions to development and adjustment, it is also true that the family can provide a secure base for a child's exploration into the world of peers. Hartup (1992) suggests that healthy family relationships are a necessary basis for the development of healthy peer relationships, especially in light of the following findings: (1) children and adolescents usually adhere to their parents' values even during increases in peer involvement; (2) parent and peer values are typically quite similar, especially with regard to important issues; and (3) differences between parent and peer values are more likely when adolescents have distant relationships with their parents and when they associate with peers who endorse antisocial behaviors.

Those who fall off the normative developmental peer relationship trajectory as described earlier are at risk for developing problems such as aggression, delinquency, and substance use (American Psychological Association, 2002; Brown, Dolcini, & Leventhal, 1997). For example, association with deviant peers in early childhood is associated with early-onset conduct problems that continue into adolescence (Dodge & Pettit, 2003). Specifically, such a pathway may be from disruptive behavior in kindergarten to aggression in middle childhood to delinquency in early adolescence (Tremblay, Masse, Vitaro, & Dobkin, 1995). Tolan, Gorman-Smith, and Henry (2003) proposed a similar multilink model for youth violence that begins with community and neighborhood factors; such factors are hypothesized to disrupt parenting practice that, in turn, would lead to higher levels of gang membership and peer violence.

Like the research on family factors, research on peer relationships has matured to the point where mediational and moderational models have been proposed (Brown et al., 1997). For example, Dishion, Capaldi, Spracklen, and Li (1995) have found that association with deviant peers mediated associations between family factors and drug use. This research by Dishion and colleagues also suggests that there are interactions across peer and family domains such that similarity between best friend and target child drug use is higher when parental monitoring is low. Similarly, unilateral forms of family decision making (i.e., parents are solely responsible for making decisions) are more highly associated with externalizing behavior problems when a child affiliates with antisocial peers. Links have also been found between early childhood maltreatment and dating violence as mediated by posttraumatic stress disorder symptoms, particularly for girls (Wekerle et al., 2001).

School Context

Another context of adolescent development is the school environment. Scholars have maintained that not only should we be interested in the school's impact on cognition and achievement, but that we should also examine how the school is an important environment for the development of one's personality, values, and social relationships (Entwisle, 1990; Trickett & Schmid, 1993). With increasing age, children are exposed to more complex school environments (Minuchin & Shapiro, 1983). Movement between schools (such as between an elementary school and a junior high school) can be viewed as a stressor, with multiple school transitions producing more deleterious effects (Petersen & Hamburg, 1986; Simmons & Blyth, 1987). Simmons and Blyth (1987) found, for example, that children (and particularly girls) who switch from an elementary school into a junior high school (as opposed to staying in a K–8 school) will show significant self-esteem decrements and that recovery in self-esteem is not likely for a sizable number of these young adolescents. Presumably, these decreases in self-esteem are due, at least in part, to movement from a protected environment (i.e., elementary school) to an impersonal environment (junior and senior high school).

As is the case with school transitions, the school environment also has an impact on adolescent development. Physical setting, limitations in resources, philosophies of education, teacher expectations, curriculum characteristics, and interactions between teacher and student have been found to be related to a variety of child and adolescent outcomes (Minuchin & Shapiro, 1983; Rutter, Maughan, Mortimore, & Ouston, 1979). High school students, for example, appear to profit from nonauthoritarian teaching approaches (Rutter et al., 1979). Also, the high rates of dropouts in some school districts indicate that the school environment and the needs of the students have not been well matched (Eccles et al., 1993). On a positive note, larger schools provide a larger number and variety of peers with whom the adolescent can interact.

With respect to psychopathology, Roeser, Eccles, and Sameroff (1998) have found links between the school learning environment (e.g., support for competence and autonomy and relationships with teachers) and subsequent emotional functioning and achievement. More generally, Eccles and colleagues (Eccles, Lord, Roeser, Barber, & Hernandez Jozefowicz, 1997; see also Roeser & Eccles, 2000) have proposed a stage–environment fit theory to explain variability in school-related outcomes (see section below on person–environment fit). Among African American high school students, level of school motivation is linked with subsequent drug use that is linked, in turn, with graduation status (Zimmerman & Schmeelk-Cone, 2003). With respect to school dropouts during adolescence, it appears that dropping out is a process that has its origins in early childhood, with the following serving as significant predictors: early home environment, quality of early caregiving, socioeconomic status, IQ, and other mental health variables (Jimerson, Egeland, Sroufe, & Carlson, 2000).

Work Context

The last context that we consider is the work environment (Greenberger & Steinberg, 1986; Lewko, 1987). Although more than 80% of all high school students in this country work before they graduate (Steinberg, 2002) and many government agencies have recommended that adolescents work, little research has been done on the effects of such work on adolescent development and the adolescents' relationships with significant others.

Based on the research done to date (e.g., Greenberger & Steinberg, 1986), however, it seems clear that the work environment has both positive *and* negative effects on adolescent development. Although adolescent work tends to be associated with an increased sense of self-reliance, it is also associated with (1) cynical attitudes toward future work, (2) less time with families and peers, (3) less involvement in school, (4) a greater likelihood of drug abuse and delinquent acts (Finch, Mortimer, & Ryu, 1997), and (5) less time for self-exploration and identity development. It is important to note that the causal direction of such associations has not yet been clarified. Although the number of hours that an adolescent works is important to consider (American Psychological Association, 2002), the primary problem with many adolescent jobs seems to be their monotonous and stressful nature. Clearly, the quality of the position and the context or meaning of the position for the adolescent (rather than merely the number of hours) are important factors to consider in examining adjustment outcomes (Finch et al., 1997).

Developmental Outcomes of Adolescence

As can be seen in Figure 2.1, the developmental changes of adolescence impact on the interpersonal contexts of adolescent development that, in turn, impact on the developmental outcomes of adolescence. In this section, we discuss the following developmental outcomes of adolescence: achievement, autonomy, identity, intimacy, and sexuality (see Figure 2.1). Psychosocial adjustment is not reviewed in this section because it is a more general focus of this chapter and is discussed throughout.

Achievement

For the first time in one's life, decisions made during one's adolescence can have serious consequences for one's future education, career, and choice of extracurricular activities (Henderson & Dweck, 1990). Some adolescents decide to drop out of school whereas others complete their education and graduate from high school. Some decide to continue on to college or graduate school. For those who remain in school, it is during high school that most adolescents are, for the first time, given the opportunity to decide which classes they want to take. Such decisions present the adolescent with new opportunities but also limit the range of possible employment and educational options available to the adolescent. After graduation from high school, adolescents typically decide whether they want to pursue more education or whether they wish to seek full-time employment—a decision that is certainly affected by one's socioeconomic status. Finally, adolescence is a time of preparation for adult work roles, a time when vocational training begins. Given the increase in choices, one might expect to see an increase in anxiety around "life decisions." Those who have developed higher-order cognitive abilities are likely at an advantage when they begin to make education and career-related decisions (see aforementioned section on the school context for examples of psychopathology research on achievement-related constructs).

Autonomy

Autonomy is a multidimensional construct in the sense that there is more than one type of adolescent autonomy (Hill & Holmbeck, 1986; Steinberg, 1990). Emotional autonomy is the capacity to relinquish childlike dependencies on parents (Fuhrman & Holmbeck, 1995; Steinberg & Silverberg, 1986). Adolescents increasingly come to deidealize their parents, to see them as "people" rather than simply as parenting figures, and to be less dependent on them for immediate emotional support. When adolescents are behaviorally autonomous, they have the capacity to make their own decisions and to be self-governing. Being behaviorally autonomous does not mean that adolescents never rely on the help of others. Instead, they become increasingly able to recognize those situations in which they have the ability to make their own decisions versus those situations in which they will need to consult with a peer or parent for advice.

All the following are important to consider regarding the autonomy of an individual adolescent: (1) the degree to which the adolescent is responsible in managing the level of autonomy he or she has been granted, (2) whether parent and child have realistic expectations for the level of autonomy that should be granted in the future, (3) the degree to which there is a discrepancy between how much autonomy the parent is willing to grant and the amount of autonomy the adolescent is able to manage (Holmbeck & O'Donnell, 1991), (4) the parents' responses to their child's attempts to be autonomous (i.e., do they have the ability to foster healthy levels of autonomy in their offspring?), (5) the degree of flexibility demonstrated by parents in changing their parenting around autonomy issues (Holmbeck et al., 1995), and (6) the degree to which the child is susceptible to peer pressure, which typically increases to a peak in early adolescence, due in part to an increase in peer pressure prior to early adolescence and an accompanying decrease in susceptibility to parental pressure (Steinberg, 2002). Moreover, treatments that are applied to adolescents "must be reconceptualized in terms of mutual rather than unilateral interventions" (Shirk, 1999, p.64).

Allen and colleagues (1997) have examined adolescent problem behaviors such as delinquency in relation to deviations in normative autonomy development. Specifically, they were interested in providing a possible explanation for the curvilinear trend during adolescence in the frequency of problem behaviors (i.e., the sharp increase in such behaviors at the beginning of adolescence followed by a sharp decrease in late adolescence). They argue that adolescents become increasingly interested in exploring behaviors that are different than those expected by parents, including involvement in behaviors that signal increasing maturity (e.g., alcohol use). Moreover, it may be that adolescents who acquire such autonomy in the context of problematic attachments with parents are most at risk for developing problem behaviors. When the process is adaptive, adolescents exhibit increasing levels of autonomy in areas of personal choice (e.g., hair style) within a context of connected relationships with parents while accepting parental authority in areas of more importance (e.g., school performance). Although most adolescents are likely to experiment with some deviant behavior, they are less likely to become engaged in highly deviant behaviors with deviant peers when adaptive familial protective factors are in place (see the section "Risk, Resource, Protective, and Vulnerability Factors").

Allen and colleagues (1997) draw on their own work to argue that autonomy development is more likely to be adaptive if it is achieved via negotiation where family members consider the reasoning of each others' positions rather than through hostile interactions involving unilateral parental decision making. With respect to the latter, Allen's research suggests that when behaviors that undermine an adolescent's autonomy are present in a family, hostility increases. Moreover, such familial hostility is likely to spill over into their relations with peers as well. When this occurs, such adolescents may be in a pattern of seeking autonomy at the expense of relationships, thus placing them at risk for associations with deviant peers.

Identity

A major psychological task of adolescence is the development of an identity (Erikson, 1968; Harter, 1990). Adolescents develop an identity through role explorations and role commitments. One's identity is multidimensional and includes self-perceptions and commitments across a number of domains, including occupational, academic, religious, interpersonal, sexual, and political. Although the notion that all adolescents experience identity crises appears to be a myth, identity development is recognized as an important adolescent issue (Harter, 1990).

Research in the area of identity development has isolated at least four identity statuses that are defined with respect to two dimensions: commitment and exploration. These identity statuses are identity moratorium (exploration with no commitment), identity foreclosure (commitment with no exploration), identity diffusion (no commitment and no systematic exploration), and identity achievement (commitment after extensive exploration). A given adolescent's status can change over time, reflecting increased maturation and development or, alternatively, regression to some less mature identity status. Perhaps most important, an adolescent's identity status can also vary depending on the domain under consideration (e.g., academic vs. interpersonal). The process of identity formation appears to be different for males and females. Identity development in males appears to involve struggles with autonomy and themes of separation whereas identity development in females is more likely to be intertwined with the development and maintenance of intimate relationships (although both genders may experience either or both processes; Gilligan, Lyons, & Hanmer, 1990; Harter, 1990).

As an alternative to traditional identity theories, Nurmi (1997) provided a stage model for the self-definition process. Rather than being a process that is linked specifically with the adolescent stage of development, Nurmi maintains that the self-definitional process becomes salient during any major developmental transition throughout the lifespan. Nurmi also describes mental health outcomes of the various stages of self-definition. For example, past research suggests that a lack of commitment to school and family is linked with suicide attempts during adolescence. A lack of problem solving and planning ability with respect to life goals is associated with a variety of mental health outcomes (e.g., dropping out of school, substance use, and depression; Nurmi, 1997). Moreover, the degree to which there is a fit between an adolescent's goals and the available options in the environment also has an impact on subsequent mental health. Finally, those with high personal standards coupled with repeated failures are more likely to exhibit both internalizing (e.g., suicidal behavior) and externalizing (e.g., delinquency) behavior.

Intimacy

It is not until adolescence that one's friendships have the potential to become intimate (Savin-Williams & Berndt, 1990). An intimate relationship is characterized by trust, mutual self-disclosure, a sense of loyalty, and helpfulness. Intimate sharing between friends increases during adolescence as do adolescents' intimate knowledge of their friends. All relationships become more emotionally charged during the

adolescent period and adolescents are more likely to engage in friendships with opposite sex peers than are children. Girls' same sex relationships are described as more intimate than are boys' same sex relationships. Having intimate friendships is adaptive; adolescents with such friendships are more likely to have high self-esteem. Some scholars have proposed that friendships change during the adolescent period because of accompanying social-cognitive changes. The capacity to exhibit empathy and take multiple perspectives in social encounters makes it more likely that friendships will become similarly more mature, complex, and intimate.

Sexuality

Most children have mixed reactions to becoming a sexually mature adolescent. Parents also have conflicting reactions to such increasing maturity. Despite the high rates of sexual activity during adolescence (nearly 70% of adolescents have had sexual intercourse by age 18; Steinberg, 2002), we know very little about normal adolescent sexuality (whether heterosexual or homosexual), primarily due to the difficulty in conducting studies on this topic (Katchadourian, 1990). A host of factors are associated with the onset and maintenance of sexual behaviors. Pubertal changes of adolescence have both direct (hormonal) and indirect (social stimulus) effects on sexual behaviors. Ethnic and religious differences in the onset of sexuality also exist. Finally, personality characteristics (e.g., the development of a sexual identity) and social factors (e.g., parent and peer influences) also serve as antecedents to the early onset of adolescent sexual behaviors. For example, McBride, Paikoff, and Holmbeck (2003) found that family conflict was associated with earlier sexual debut in African American adolescents. Moreover, those with more advanced pubertal development, higher levels of family conflict, and lower levels of positive affect in observed family interactions were more likely to debut early.

The increasing rates of sexually transmitted diseases among adolescents and the fact that many young adults with AIDS (acquired immune deficiency syndrome) probably became infected as adolescents would suggest that adolescent sexuality is deserving of considerable attention from researchers and mental health practitioners working with adolescents. Also, as discussed later in the section "Comorbidity during Adolescence," early onset of adolescent sexuality is often viewed as part of a more general adolescent problem behavior syndrome.

DEVELOPMENTAL PSYCHOPATHOLOGY OF ADOLESCENCE

Given this overview of the biopsychosocial framework for the study of adolescent psychopathology, we now turn to a discussion of the developmental psychopathology perspective on adolescence (Cicchetti & Rogosch, 2002). In the first section, we discuss the major assumptions and tenets of the developmental psychopathology perspective. Following this, sections on issues relevant to a developmental psychopathology perspective on adolescence are provided: developmental trajectories (including multifinality and equifinality), the onset and maintenance of psychopathology, age-of-onset research, resilience, risk and protective factors, comorbidity, shared and nonshared environment effects, person–environment fit research, and research on culture and contextualism.

Assumptions, Tenets, and Research Objectives of Developmental Psychopathology

Developmental psychopathology is a multidisciplinary "macro-paradigm" that combines knowledge from psychology, psychiatry, epidemiology, medicine, neurobiology, and other fields (Cicchetti & Rogosch, 2002). The goal of the discipline is to understand the unfolding of psychopathology over the lifespan and how the processes that lead to psychopathology are affected by normative developmental milestones and contextual factors (Cicchetti & Rogosch, 2002; Mash & Dozois, 2003). Developmental psychopathologists are concerned with the full range of typical and atypical behavior. Of particular interest with respect to adolescence is how a particular symptom or cluster of symptoms can be understood in relation to the previously discussed developmental challenges of the adolescent period (Cicchetti & Rogosch, 2002).

Some of the assumptions, tenets, and research objectives of this field (particularly in relation to the study of adolescent psychopathology) are as follows (Cicchetti & Rogosch, 2002; Mash & Dozois, 2003):

1. A given type of adolescent psychopathology is best understood via a complete examination of experiences and trajectories leading up to the problem behavior as well as trajectories that occur subsequent to the problem behavior.

2. It is assumed that *multifinality* (i.e., two children with the same symptoms or experiences at one point in time may have different outcomes during adolescence) and *equifinality* (i.e., two adolescents with the same symptoms at one point in time may have developed those symptoms along different pathways) are more the rule rather than the exception; relatedly, a single factor is usually not necessary or sufficient to produce a given psychopathology (Kazdin, Kraemer, Kessler, Kupfer, & Offord, 1997).

3. Knowledge is enhanced when our understanding of normative child and adolescent development is used to further our understanding of adolescent psychopathology (see example above in the section "Autonomy").

4. Similarly, knowledge of normal adolescent development can be enhanced by the study of atypical adolescent development (Sroufe, 1990).

5. It is of interest to understand the full range of adolescent functioning (including clinical, subclinical, and normative forms of behavioral functioning) across multiple domains. Distinctions between normal and abnormal are particularly likely to become blurred during the adolescent developmental period (e.g., boundaries between problem drinking and normative experimentation have not been clearly delineated).

6. It is of interest to understand why some adolescents who are at risk for disorder or who have been exposed to adversity do not show symptoms (i.e., resilient adolescents).

7. Relations between antecedent events/adaptations and subsequent psychopathology are assumed to be probabilistic (Kazdin et al., 1997). One corollary of this assumption is that early historical adaptations (e.g., anxious attachment) may not themselves be psychopathological or even a sufficient condition for subsequent psychopathology (Sroufe, 1997; Sroufe, Carlson, Levy, & Egeland, 1999). Rather, such earlier adaptations and pathways are probabilistically associated with the quality of later functioning (i.e., continuity), but discontinuity is also possible (a process that Cicchetti & Rogosch, 2002, refer to as probabilistic

epigenesis). For example, those children with compromised development from earlier stages (e.g., early aggressiveness in kindergarten) are probabilistically more at risk (than their noncompromised counterparts) for continuing on maladaptive pathways as they navigate the challenges of adolescence (e.g., the development of advanced social skills and close, intimate friendships). With respect to early attachment difficulties, such early experiences may have an impact on the child's neurophysiology and ability to regulate emotions, which may, in turn, be predictive of later social and individual pathology (Sroufe et al., 1999), but such outcomes clearly do not occur in all cases.

8. Development occurs via continuous and multiple reorganizations across all domains of child and adolescent functioning (e.g., physical, social, cognitive, neurological, and emotional).

9. It is assumed that adolescents play an important role in determining their own development and outcomes of development (e.g., by the environments in which they choose to engage and by changing these environments over time) via transactional processes between individual and environment.

10. The large number of transitions during adolescence (as compared with other stages of development across the lifespan) provide many opportunities for a redirection of prior maladaptive trajectories (Graber & Brooks-Gunn, 1996) as well as more possibilities for movement onto maladaptive pathways.

11. Factors associated with the onset of a disorder may be distinct from those associated with the maintenance of a disorder (Mash & Dozois, 2003; Steinberg & Avenevoli, 2000).

Given this broad coverage of the developmental psychopathology perspective, we now provide more specific reviews of some of the major constructs from this field including their relevance to adolescent psychopathology.

Developmental Trajectories during Adolescence: Multifinality and Equifinality

As implied previously, proponents of the developmental psychopathology perspective attempt to understand how pathology unfolds over time rather than examining symptoms at a single time point. As a consequence, developmental psychopathologists have found the notion of "developmental trajectories" very useful

(Cicchetti & Rogosch, 2002). For example, one could examine alcohol use in adolescence and isolate different developmental trajectories of such use over time (e.g., some adolescents may show rapid increases in alcohol use over time, some may show gradual increases, while others may show increases followed by decreases; Schulenberg, Wadsworth, O'Malley, Bachman, & Johnston, 1996). It is also assumed that some developmental trajectories are indicative of a developmental failure that probabilistically increases the chances that a psychopathological disorder will develop at a later point in time (Cicchetti & Rogosch, 2002). Thus, there is an interest in isolating early-onset trajectories that portend later problems. As an example, Dodge and Pettit (2003) point out that children who have early difficult temperaments (i.e., an early trajectory) who are also rejected by their peers for 2 or more years by grade 2 have a 60% chance of developing a serious conduct problem during adolescence. Again, this confluence of trajectory (i.e., difficult temperament) and risk factor (i.e., chronic peer rejection) does not automatically produce an adolescent with conduct disorder; rather, it merely increases the odds that the adolescent will develop such a disorder.

Given the vast individual differences in trajectories in any given domain of functioning, developmental psychopathologists have also been interested in the concepts of multifinality and equifinality (Cicchetti & Rogosch, 1996). Multifinality occurs when there are multiple outcomes in those who have been exposed to the same antecedent risk factor (e.g., maternal depression). Given equivalent exposure to a parent who is depressed, not all adolescents so exposed will develop along identical pathways. For example, Marsh, McFarland, Allen, McElhaney, and Land (2003) examined outcomes of adolescents with insecure preoccupied attachment orientations. Those with mothers who displayed low levels of autonomy in observed interactions were more likely to display internalizing symptoms. Conversely, those with mothers who displayed very high levels of autonomy were more likely to exhibit risky behaviors. Thus, we see multiple outcomes (i.e., multifinality) in adolescents who all have the same initial risk factor (i.e., insecure preoccupied attachment orientation). It is important to note, however, that these conclusions were based on cross-sectional data; thus a preoccupied attachment could also be an outcome of symptomatology.

Equifinality occurs when individuals with the same level of psychopathology achieved such pathology via different pathways. Evidence for equifinality has emerged in recent research. For example, Harrington, Rutter, and Fombonne (1996) found that suicidal behavior can be reached via different paths, one involving depression and another involving conduct disorder. Similarly, in girls, it appears that several of the same outcomes (e.g., anxiety disorders, substance use, school dropout, and pregnancy) emerge in those with depression *or* conduct disorder (Bardone, Moffitt, Caspi, Dickson, & Silva, 1996). Finally, Gjerde and Block (1996) suggested that depressed adult women and men progress along very different adolescent developmental pathways prior to developing depression. It is worth noting, from an intervention perspective, that the presence of equifinality would suggest that different versions of a given treatment for a given problem may be needed depending on the pathway by which an individual progressed toward psychopathology (Holmbeck et al., 2003).

In a study that sought to examine the prevalence of both multifinality and equifinality across internalizing and externalizing symptoms, Egeland, Pianta, and Ogawa (1996) found support for both processes. For early internalizing symptoms, multifinality was likely such that early internalizing pathways could lead to variety of diagnoses in adolescence. Equifinality was also found for later diagnoses of depression and anxiety, such that a variety of paths preceded such diagnoses. The findings for early externalizing symptoms were similar, although there was more continuity over time (i.e., early externalizing symptoms leading to antisocial outcomes) as would be expected based on prior research.

When one recognizes the notion that multiple trajectories are possible, even when the starting point is the same (i.e., multifinality), one may be interested in devising a typology of such trajectories. For example, Lacourse, Nagin, Tremblay, Vitaro, and Claes (2003) were able to isolate different trajectories of delinquent group membership in boys and their association with subsequent violent behaviors (see Zucker, Ellis, Fitzgerald, Bingham, & Sanford, 1996, for a similar example involving a typology of alcoholics, or Broidy et al., 2003, for an example involving adolescent outcomes of typologies of childhood aggression). Such approaches have been termed "person-oriented" approaches (as opposed to "variable-oriented") insofar as people are clustered into groups based on the similarity of their characteristics or patterns of trajectories over time (Bergman & Magnusson, 1997). Groups are differentiated based on their patterning or profile of scores on antecedent or outcome variables of interest. With respect to typologies of trajectories, Chassin, Pitts, and Prost (2002) were able to identify three trajectory groups of binge drinkers and then went on to isolate antecedent predictors of trajectory memberships as well as subsequent outcomes. As noted earlier, such trajectories can assume quadratic forms (i.e., U-shaped or inverted U-shaped functions; Garber, Keiley, & Martin, 2002).

The Onset and Maintenance of Psychopathology during Adolescence

It appears that factors that lead to the *onset* or initiation of a developmental trajectory are often different than those that *maintain* an individual on a developmental trajectory (Steinberg & Avenevoli, 2000). With respect to the latter, an individual who has begun on a particular pathway may continue on the pathway or may be deflected from the pathway (Sroufe, 1997). Factors that deflect an individual from a maladaptive trajectory may be chance events, developmental successes, or protective processes that serve an adaptive function (Mash & Dozois, 2003). In an analogous fashion, other factors may deflect individuals from adaptive trajectories onto maladaptive trajectories. It is an assumption of developmental psychopathology that maintenance on a pathway is more likely than deflection, particularly when an individual has moved through several developmental transitions on the same pathway (Steinberg & Avenevoli, 2000).

What do we know about factors that lead to the onset of maladaptive paths versus those that serve to maintain individuals on such pathways? Steinberg and Avenevoli (2000) argue that researchers have tended to confuse factors that lead to the onset versus those that lead to the maintenance of psychopathology and that this confusion has hampered progress in the field of developmental psychopathology. With respect to "onset," Steinberg and Avenevoli argue (from a "diathesis–stress" perspective) that biological predispositions (e.g., temperament and nature of autonomic arousal) can exacerbate or decrease the degree to which individuals are vulnerable to the impact of subsequent environmental stressors. Thus, two individuals exposed to the same stressor may begin on different pathways (e.g., anxiety vs. depression vs. aggression vs. no pathology) depending on the specific nature of each individual's biological predispositions. Put another way, stressors appear to have *nonspecific effects* on the onset of pathology due to the moderating effect of particular biological vulnerabilities (Steinberg & Avenevoli, 2000). These authors argue that future research on the elicitation of psychopathology needs to begin to isolate particular combinations of biological vulnerabilities and environmental threats that precede engagement with maladaptive developmental pathways. Indeed, such evidence is beginning to emerge; Brennan, Hall, Bor, Najman, and Williams (2003) found that early-onset and persistent aggression is predicted by interactions of biological and social risks (see discussion of early- vs. late-onset psychopathology below). Similarly, Caspi and colleagues (2003) found support for a gene × environmental stress interaction effect in predicting depressive symptoms.

With respect to "maintenance," Steinberg and Avenevoli (2000) argue that environmental stressors have *specific effects* on the course of psychopathology. Thus, it is possible that two individuals can begin on the same pathway (due to having the same biological predispositions and same level of exposure to early stressors) but may have very different long-term outcomes if their environments differ. For example, two young children who have started on an early aggression pathway may diverge from each other over time because one of them is exposed to incompetent parenting, lack of structure, and deviant peers and the other is not (also see Dodge & Pettit, 2003). Those who begin on an "early aggression" trajectory are probabilistically more likely to associate with deviant peers and "choose" maladaptive environments, but this is clearly not always the case for every affected child. Steinberg and Avenevoli also provide evidence that those who continue on certain paths and select certain environments are also more likely to strengthen the synaptic weights or connections of the original biological predisposition (e.g., the nature of the child's arousal regulation capacities), making it even less likely that the individual will desist from this behavior or be deflected from the maladaptive developmental trajec-

tory. Put another way, psychopathology is likely to be maintained in individuals when the symptoms or the antecedents of the symptoms are repeated (Steinberg & Avenevoli, 2000). Returning to the example above, "lack of structure" in the family environment may not be a factor in the onset of conduct problems, but it may help to maintain these problems because it permits more exposure to deviant peers and permits the pathology to become more ingrained and entrenched (Steinberg & Avenevoli, 2000).

Given this theoretical background, we turn to a review of the research in the area of onset and maintenance of adolescent psychopathology. Researchers in several areas have begun to distinguish between onset and maintenance in their research designs (e.g., see Brook, Kessler, & Cohen, 1999, in the area of substance use; see Patterson, Forgatch, Yoerger, & Stoolmiller, 1998, in the area of antisocial behavior). For example, Dodge and Petit (2003) provided a model of chronic conduct problems that is consistent with the notions advanced by Steinberg and Avenevoli (2000; see above). These authors argue that the bulk of research on conduct problems in childhood and adolescence suggests that children with certain neural or psychophysiological predispositions are more likely to begin a trajectory leading to conduct problems in adolescence. Such children are more likely to be parented harshly or neglected, given their early difficult temperament. Outside the family, such children are more likely to be aggressive and to engage in conflict with peers during early childhood. According to Dodge and Pettit, such children enter elementary school in an at-risk state (although this transition is also an opportunity for deflection). Most often, such children experience peer rejection and have difficult relations with teachers. This combination of harsh parenting and peer rejection serves to crystalize the trajectory, making it less likely that deflection will occur. Although adolescence is another transitional opportunity, such children are at risk for affiliation with deviant peers. In fact, Dodge and Pettit provide evidence that such children react psychophysiologically in ways that make it uncomfortable for them to interact with typical peers. At this point, other cognitive strategies also play a role (e.g., the greater likelihood of hostile attributions). Movement toward a diagnosis of conduct disorder is overdetermined in such adolescents, with the probability of such an outcome increasing rapidly with age because of a confluence of multiple contributing factors.

In describing a developmental psychopathology model of depression, Hammen (1992) argues that cognitive vulnerabilities (e.g., negative view of self and negative self-schema) may be developed over time as a consequence of problematic relations and attachments with parents. Such cognitions make these individuals more vulnerable to subsequent stressors, with depression being the eventual outcome. Interestingly, Hammen provides evidence that depression-prone individuals are also more likely to generate new stressors or exacerbate existing ones, thus fueling the cycle (see Petersen et al., 1993, for a similar perspective on adolescent depression).

Although we have argued thus far that factors associated with the onset of psychopathology may differ from those associated with its maintenance, this is not always the case. For example, Patterson and colleagues (1998) found that early-onset antisocial behavior (during preadolescence) is linked with early arrests (before age 14) which are, in turn, linked with chronic offending in later adolescence (at age 18). Most relevant to this discussion, they also found that the factors that were associated with the onset of the trajectory (i.e., problematic parental discipline and monitoring, marital transitions, social disadvantage, and deviant peer involvement) were the same factors that were associated with the maintenance of this "chronic offending" trajectory.

Age-of-Onset Research

A related line of research focuses on the age of the child or adolescent when symptoms of psychopathology begin. Interestingly, it appears that both the antecedents and long-term outcomes for "early-onset" children and adolescents differ significantly from those who are "late onset" (Aguilar, Sroufe, Egeland, & Carlson, 2000). This is important because it suggests that studies of adolescents that do not take "age of onset" into account in sampling procedures will likely combine across multiple subgroups of adolescents who vary significantly in severity and chronicity (Cicchetti & Rogosch, 2002).

Perhaps the most widely cited example of such age-of-onset differences is Moffitt's (1993) distinction between "life-course-persis-

tent" and "adolescence-limited" delinquents. The former exhibit earlier conduct problems than the latter and they are more likely to have neuropsychological problems, difficult early temperament, inadequate parenting and family dysfunction, hyperactivity, and psychopathic personality traits (Moffitt, Caspi, Dickson, Silva, & Stanton, 1996; although there is some debate about whether the neuropsychological difficulties predate the conduct problems; Aguilar, Sroufe, England, & Carlson, 2000).

The outcomes for the life-course-persistent delinquents tend to be worse than for their adolescence-limited counterparts, with higher rates of adult criminality and violence, substance dependence, and adult work-related problems (Cicchetti & Rogosch, 2002; Moffitt, Caspi, Harrington, & Milne, 2002). The conduct problems of adolescence-limited delinquents are more likely to abate over time than is the case for the life-course-persistent delinquents (although the former are not without problems, as they are also at risk for mental health problems and high levels of life stress; Aguilar et al., 2000; Moffitt et al., 2002). Clearly, these are very different pathways with different antecedents and outcomes. On the other hand, if they were studied together at only one point in time (e.g., mid to late adolescence), their behaviors may appear similar (Moffitt, Caspi, Dickson, Silva, & Stanton, 1996). Finally, Moffitt and colleagues (2002) recently suggested that there is a third group of boys who are aggressive as children but with low levels of conduct problems in adolescence (in earlier work, these boys were referred to as "recoveries"). These individuals are also at risk for problems in adulthood, but at lower levels than the other two groups just described. Moreover, their problems are more likely to be of the internalizing type (depression, anxiety, etc.). An analogous distinction has been made in the literature on adolescent alcohol use. Zucker, Fitzgerald, and Moses (1995) described three types of adolescent and young adult "alcoholisms," each with different ages of onset, antecedents, and long-term consequences (see Schulenberg et al., 1996, for a similar approach to adolescent alcohol use).

Interestingly, it appears that Moffitt's (1993) distinction between the two types of delinquent adolescents (i.e., child onset vs. adolescence limited) applies only to boys. Silverthorn and Frick (1999) propose that the childhood-onset form may be the only one that applies to girls, but with one important difference. Delinquent adolescent girls appear to have the same antecedents as life-course-persistent boys, but their conduct problems emerge later than in boys. Thus, it appears that adolescent girls are more likely to fit a delayed-onset, life-course-persistent subtype.

With respect to internalizing symptoms, there is some suggestion that the antecedents of childhood symptoms of depression differ from those of adolescent symptoms (Duggal, Carlson, Sroufe, & Egeland, 2001). Whereas variables indexing the overall family context are associated with symptoms in childhood, factors such as maternal depression (in girls) and lack of supportiveness in the early rearing environment (in boys) were more highly associated with symptoms during adolescence. On the other hand, it is difficult to determine whether such differences in findings relate more to the question of onset versus maintenance (see above) or early versus late onset. In the literature on depression, distinctions have also been made between adolescent-onset and adult-onset depression. Those with the former differ from those with the latter insofar as the former are more likely to have perinatal problems, psychopathology in their family background, caretaker instability, and other mental health problems (Jaffee et al., 2002).

Resilience

As noted earlier, developmental psychopathologists are interested in understanding the full range of normative and atypical functioning. In fact, researchers have examined a subset of individuals in the normative range, namely, those who function adaptively despite exposure to significant levels of risk and/or adversity (e.g., trauma, social disadvantage, marital transitions, difficult temperament, and high genetic loading for psychopathology). Rather than moving along a maladaptive developmental trajectory (as would be expected, given their prior history), these "resilient" adolescents manage to defy their at-risk status. From a prevention and intervention perspective, adolescents who exhibit resilience are of interest because they can provide much needed information to researchers and interventionists regarding factors that protect at-risk individuals from developing later problems. The issue of resilience is also relevant to the study of multifinality; adolescents with a particular risk

factor (e.g., a substance-abusing parent) are likely to vary in outcome (e.g., substance use vs. normal functioning), with one of these paths being a resilience pathway (Cicchetti & Rogosch, 1999b). Moreover, an adolescent may display resilience with respect to one outcome (e.g., academic achievement) but not necessarily with respect to another (e.g., peer relations). Indeed, researchers have found that some inner-city adolescents who have experienced high levels of uncontrollable stress may be resilient in some areas (e.g., school performance and behavioral conduct) but not in others (e.g., they may exhibit high levels of internalizing symptoms; Luthar, Doernberger, & Zigler, 1993).

How does resilience develop? Researchers and theorists agree that resilience is best viewed as a dynamic process that unfolds over time based on transactions between the individual and the environment rather than as a single variable operating at a single point in time within an adolescent (Mash & Dozois, 2003; Sroufe, 1997). Interestingly, past research suggests that individual and environmental factors that characterize resilient adolescents are similar to those that provide developmental advantages to any child. Superior intellectual functioning, easy temperament, and close relations with caring adults are characteristics that can protect a child exposed to adversity (Masten & Coatsworth, 1998) but they also provide advantages for other children as well. Also, research by Stouthamer-Loeber and colleagues (1993) suggests that protective and risk effects often occur within the same variables, such that scores on one end of a continuum may be protective (e.g., superior intellectual functioning) whereas scores on the other end of the continuum produce higher risk status (e.g., low intellectual functioning). Also, a variable may be protective by increasing adaptation or by decreasing maladaptation (Stouthamer-Loeber et al., 1993; see more detailed discussion in the next section).

Risk, Resource, Protective, and Vulnerability Factors

Generally, research on risk and protective factors is focused on understanding the adjustment of youth who are exposed to varying levels of adversity. A protective factor either ameliorates negative outcomes or promotes adaptive functioning. To isolate a true "protective factor," however, there must be a particular stressor that influences the sample under investigation. The protective factor serves its protective role only in the context of adversity; a protective factor does not operate in low adversity conditions.

Protective factors are contrasted with resource factors (sometimes referred to as "promotive factors"; Stouthamer-Loeber, Loeber, Wei, Farrington, & Wikstrom, 2002). Specifically, a factor that has a positive impact on the sample *regardless* of the presence or absence of a stressor is a "resource factor" (Rutter, 1990). For example, if a positive father–child relationship reduces behavior problems only in children of depressed mothers but has no impact for children of nondepressed mothers, then the father–child relationship would be conceptualized as a "protective factor" (see Figure 2.2). However, if the positive father–child relationship reduces behavior problems in all children, regardless of mothers' level of depression, then it would be conceptualized as a "resource factor" (Rutter, 1990; Figure 2.2). A model may also identify a positive father–child relationship as both a "protective" and "resource" factor if it reduces behavior problems in children who have depressed mothers *more* than in children who have nondepressed mothers, but if it also produces a

significant reduction in behavior problems for all children, regardless of level of maternal depression. It is also important to note that a protective factor represents a moderational effect (Holmbeck, 1997; see the statistically significant interaction effect in Figure 2.2), whereas a resource factor represents an additive effect. Statistically, a resource factor emerges as two main effects.

"Risk" and "vulnerability" factors operate in the much same way as "resource" and "protective" factors but in the opposite direction (see Figure 2.3). A "vulnerability" factor is a moderator that increases the chances for maladaptive outcomes in the presence of adversity (Rutter, 1990). Similar to a "protective factor," a "vulnerability factor" only operates in the context of adversity. By contrast, a variable that negatively influences outcome regardless of the presence or absence of adversity is a "risk factor" (Rutter, 1990). For example, witnessing violence in the home environment is conceptualized as a "vulnerability" factor if it only increases behavior problems in children who are also exposed to a stressor, such as viewing extensive violence on television (Figure 2.3). A vulnerability factor is a moderator and is demonstrated statistically with a significant interaction effect. Witnessing violence in the

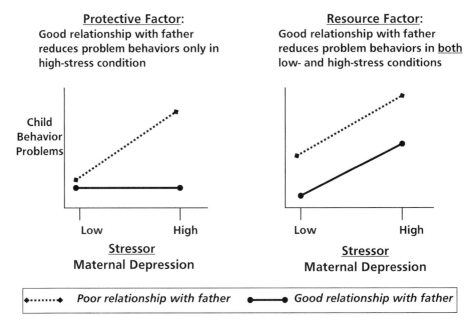

FIGURE 2.2. Protective and resource factors. From Rose, Holmbeck, Coakley, and Franks (2004). Copyright 2004 by Lippincott Williams & Wilkins. Reprinted by permission.

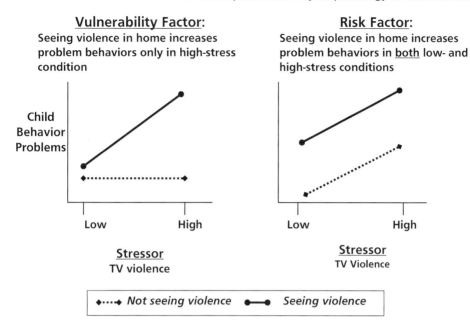

FIGURE 2.3. Vulnerability and risk factors. From Rose, Holmbeck, Coakley, and Franks (2004). Copyright 2004 by Lippincott Williams & Wilkins. Reprinted by permission.

home can be conceptualized as a "risk" factor if it results in an increase in child behavior problems for all children, regardless of the amount of TV violence witnessed. As with resource factors, a risk factor represents an additive effect (i.e., two main effects). A model may also identify a factor as being both a "risk" and "vulnerability" factor if it increases the chance of a maladaptive outcome in samples with and without exposure to a stressor, but increases the chances for maladaptive functioning significantly more in the sample with the stressor.

To summarize, if a factor significantly promotes or impairs the chances of attaining adaptive outcomes in the face of a stressor then it operates via "protective" or "vulnerability" mechanisms, respectively. In these cases, the factor serves a moderational role. However, if a factor significantly promotes or impairs the chance of attaining adaptive outcomes without differentiating between the presence or absence of a stressor, then it is conceptualized as operating via "resource" or "risk" mechanisms, respectively.

Many examples of these types of effects have appeared in the literature. For example, in their study of maltreatment and adolescent behavior problems, McGee, Wolfe, and Wilson (1997) found that the association between severity of

physical abuse and internalizing symptoms was moderated by gender. Specifically, the association was positive and significant for girls but not for boys. In other words, being "male" could be considered a protective factor for the development of internalizing symptoms when exposed to high levels of physical abuse. Gorman-Smith and Tolan (1998) found that associations between exposure to violence and young adolescent anxiety/depression symptoms was moderated by level of family cohesion. The effect was only significant (and positive) at low levels of cohesion. At high levels of cohesion, the effect was nonsignificant, suggesting that family cohesion buffers (or protects against) the negative effects of exposure to violence on adolescent mental health.

Some investigators have sought to examine risk factors as causal chains over time (i.e., mediation; Holmbeck, 1997). For example, Tolan and colleagues (2003) examined a causal chain as a predictor of violent behaviors in adolescence, which included the following variables (in temporal order): community structure characteristics, neighborliness, parenting practices, gang membership, and peer violence. Woodward and Fergusson (1999) examined predictors of increased rates of teen pregnancy and found a causal chain that began with early conduct problems; such problems were associated with subsequent risk-taking behaviors in adolescence, which placed girls at risk for teen pregnancy.

Comorbidity during Adolescence

Comorbidity involves the presence of two or more disorders within a single individual; one typically uses the term "comorbidity" when disorders co-occur at rates greater than expected from each disorder's base rate (e.g., attention-deficit/hyperactivity disorder and conduct disorder; Hinshaw, Lahey, & Hart, 1993; Mash & Dozois, 2003). Although some comorbidities may be the result of definitional ambiguities or methodological artifacts (see Mash & Dozois, 2003), comorbidity does seem to occur with regularity in adolescence. For example, the various problem behaviors of adolescence tend to be intercorrelated, insofar as they tend to co-occur within the same individuals. One well-known clustering scheme suggests that there are two broadband categories of psychopathology (Achenbach, 1985): *internalizing* problems (i.e., disorders that represent problems within the self such as depression, anxiety, somatic complaints, and social withdrawal) and *externalizing* problems (i.e., disorders that represent conflicts with the external environment such as delinquency, aggression, and other self-control difficulties). Alternatively, Jessor and colleagues (Jessor, Donovan, & Costa, 1991; Jessor & Jessor, 1977) have proposed that a "problem behavior syndrome" characterizes some adolescents, such that there tend to be high intercorrelations among several types of problem behavior (e.g., drug use, sexual intercourse, drinking, and aggression). According to problem behavior theory, such behaviors develop as a function of the same etiological factors and, therefore, tend to co-occur in the same individuals (findings that have been replicated in other laboratories; e.g., Bingham & Crockett, 1996; Farrell, Danish, & Howard, 1992; although see Loeber, Farrington, Stouthamer-Loeber, & Van Kammen, 1998, for an alternative perspective).

Some studies have shown evidence for comorbidity that combines across the internalizing and externalizing dimensions. For example, Capaldi (1991) studied four groups of boys: those with depressed mood only, those with conduct problem only, those with both problems, and those with neither. Findings suggested that the poorest adjustment occurred for those in the comorbid group. Like many who study comorbidity, Capaldi (1991) was also interested in whether there was a temporal relationship between the two disorders. Specifically, she found that once a conduct disorder is in place, multiple failures across multiple contexts (i.e., family and peer) place such young adolescents at risk for subsequent depressive symptoms. Similarly, Aseltine, Gore, and Colten (1998) examined four groups of participants with presence versus absence of depression and substance use. They found distinctive risk factors for depression, substance use, and their comorbidity.

Shared and Nonshared Environment Effects

The field of behavior genetics has attempted to shed light on how the behavioral variation observed among adolescents can be ascribed to genetic and environmental processes. Recent research in this area has contributed to the field of developmental psychopathology by investigating how both "nature" and "nurture" are the sources of abnormal as well as normal development (O'Connor & Plomin, 2000; Rende & Plomin, 1995). Before summarizing behavioral genetics research findings that apply to the developmental psychopathology of adolescence, we follow with a brief review of the methodology of this field of research.

Classic behavior genetics research methods include family, twin, and adoption study designs. Adoption and twin studies, which are quasi-experimental designs in which the family members of varying genetic relatedness are compared, are needed to disaggregate genetic and environmental sources of variance. For example, if heredity affects a behavioral trait, it follows that identical twins will be more similar to each other on that trait than will fraternal twins. A stepfamily design is also sometimes used in which monozygotic (MZ) twins and dizygotic (DZ) twins are compared, along with full siblings, half siblings, and unrelated siblings living in the same household (O'Connor & Plomin, 2000; Pike & Plomin, 1996; Rende & Plomin, 1995).

Most of the work in behavior genetics has employed an additive statistical model. One basic assumption of the additive model is that genetic and environmental influences are independent factors that sum to account for the total amount of individual variation. This model partitions the variance of the characteristic being studied among three components: genetic factors, shared environmental influences, and nonshared environmental influences. In these studies, genetic factors are considered to be all characteristics that are inherited. A heritability estimate, which ascribes an effect size to genetic influence, is calculated. The variance left over is then ascribed to environmental influences (Collins, Maccoby, Steinberg, Hetherington, & Bornstein, 2000; O'Connor & Plomin, 2000; Pike & Plomin, 1996; Rende & Plomin, 1995).

Environmental influences are then further subdivided into shared and nonshared types. The term "shared environment" refers to those environmental factors that produce similarities in developmental outcomes among siblings in the same family. If siblings are more similar than would be expected from their shared genetics alone, it implies an effect of the environment that is shared by both siblings, such as being exposed to marital conflict or poverty, or being parented in a similar manner. In the foregoing example, shared environmental influence is estimated indirectly from correlations among twins by subtracting the heritability estimate from the MZ twin correlation. Nonshared environment, which refers to those environmental factors that produce behavioral differences among siblings in the same family, can then be estimated. Nonshared environmental influence is calculated by then subtracting the MZ twin correlation from 1.0 (O'Connor & Plomin, 2000; Pike & Plomin, 1996; Rende & Plomin, 1995).

In the stepfamily design described previously, shared environmental influence is implicated when correlations among siblings are large across all types of sibling pairs including those that are not related. On the other hand, nonshared environmental influence is implicated when siblings correlations are low across all pairs of siblings of varying genetic relatedness including monozygotic twins, as variation among monozygotic twins, being 100% genetically similar, must be attributable to differences in environment (O'Connor, McGuire, Reiss, Hetherington, & Plomin, 1998).

Results of multiple studies with genetically sensitive designs suggest that most aspects of child and adolescent psychopathology show evidence of genetic influence (O'Connor & Plomin, 2000; Pike & Plomin, 1996; Rende & Plomin, 1995). Autism and Tourette's disorder

in particular have been demonstrated to be mostly genetically determined (Pike & Plomin, 1996; Rende & Plomin, 1995). Genetic factors have also been found to strongly influence externalizing behaviors, including aggression (Deater-Deckard & Plomin, 1999). While the results are less clear, genetic influence has also been associated with the development of internalizing problems as well (Rende, Plomin, Reiss & Hetherington, 1993; Thapar & McGuffin, 1994). However, genetic influence does not account for all the variance in psychopathological disorders (O'Connor & Plomin, 2000; Pike & Plomin, 1996; Rende & Plomin, 1995). The environmental conditions under which adolescents are socialized have also been proven to play an important role. Interestingly, however, it is those environmental factors that are nonshared, those that create differences among siblings, and not shared environmental factors, that seem to contribute to a large portion of the variation. Environmental factors that have been postulated to be nonshared include differential treatment by parents, peer influences, and school environment (O'Connor & Plomin, 2000; Pike & Plomin, 1996; Rende & Plomin, 1995).

Nonshared environmental factors have been implicated in hyperactivity, anorexia nervosa, aggression, and internalizing symptoms (Pike & Plomin, 1996). In addition, the combination of nonshared and genetic influences may influence the adolescent's choice of peer group (Iervolino et al., 2002). Juvenile delinquency appears to be one exception to the rule in that shared environmental factors have been shown to be more influential than nonshared environmental or genetic factors (Pike & Plomin, 1996).

Behavior genetics research has more recently gone beyond the partitioning of variance into genetic and environmental components toward investigating questions that are increasingly pertinent to the study of developmental psychopathology. Recent research has examined how differential parenting practices may produce differing developmental outcomes among siblings. One study found that over 50% of the variance in antisocial behavior and 37% of the variance in depressive symptoms were associated with conflictive and negative parenting behavior that was directed specifically at the adolescent (Reiss et al., 1995). However, research has also suggested that longitudinal associations between both parenting behavior and adolescent adjustment may be partly explained by genetic factors (Neiderhiser, Reiss, Hetherington & Plomin, 1999), suggesting that genetically influenced characteristics of the child may elicit specific types of parenting behavior. In this way, nonshared experiences of siblings may in fact reflect genetic differences such as differences in temperament (Plomin, Reiss, Hetherington, Howe, & George, 1994). One adoption study found that adolescents who were at genetic risk for the development of antisocial behavior by virtue of having a biological parent with a disorder were more likely than adolescents without this risk to be exposed to coercive parenting by their adoptive parents. It is important to note, however, that negative parenting behaviors still contributed to adolescent externalizing behavior over and above the effect of genetic predisposition (O'Connor, Deater-Deckard, Fulker, Rutter, & Plomin, 1998).

Another important question examined in behavioral genetics research is whether genetic influences are more prominent at the extreme range of a psychopathological condition. By examining the full range of symptomatology rather than specific diagnoses, behavior genetics research may highlight the continuity or discontinuity between normal and abnormal development (Rende & Plomin, 1995). One study shows that, while variation in subclinical depressive symptoms is mostly influenced by genetics, adolescent depressive disorder appears to be influenced mostly by shared environmental factors (Rende et al., 1993). Behavior genetic research has also demonstrated that genetic influences may partly explain comorbidity among disorders (O'Connor & Plomin, 2000). One study has found that half of the correlation between externalizing and internalizing behaviors in adolescence can be explained by common genetic liability (O'Connor, McGuire, et al., 1998).

Researchers have pointed to the many limitations of behavior genetics research that need to be considered when evaluating these findings (Collins et al., 2000; Jackson, 1993; Maccoby, 2000; Rutter, Pickles, Murray, & Eaves, 2001). In particular, the additive statistical model, the assumption that lies at the heart of behavior genetics methodology, has been criticized as neglecting to consider the potentially important contribution of gene–environment interactions. In addition, genetic and environmental influences may be correlated (Collins et al., 2000; Jackson, 1993; Maccoby, 2000; Rutter et al., 2001; Steinberg & Morris, 2001). Stable heritability estimates are also difficult to calculate. These estimates are highly influenced by the range of genetic and environmental variation within the sample and also tend to be influenced by reporter. For example, parent reports of child characteristics tend to show lower heritability estimates than when children or teachers report on the same characteristics, or when observational measures are used (Maccoby, 2000). If heritability estimates are unstable, then estimates of environmental influences, derived from heritability estimates, are also unstable (Maccoby, 2000). Critics have suggested that environmental influences cannot be estimated without being measured directly. However, the methodology used in studies examining environmental factors, such as differential parenting, may also be difficult to interpret. Sibling pairs in these samples are assumed to vary only according to genetic similarity. However, genetic similarity may be confounded with family structure in that full siblings are likely to have more congruent parenting experiences than half-siblings or stepsiblings (Jackson, 1993; Maccoby, 2000). Also, shared events, such as those found in similar family environments, may contribute to nonshared variance in that different siblings may be affected differently by the same experiences (O'Connor & Plomin, 2000).

Person–Environment Fit Research

Person–environment fit theory focuses on the interaction between characteristics of the individual and the environment, such that not only does the individual influence his or her environment, but the environment also has an impact on the individual. The adequacy of this fit between a person and the environment can affect one's motivation, behavior, and overall mental and physical health (Eccles et al., 1993). That is, if the fit is optimal, the individual's functioning may be facilitated; if it is unsuitable, the individual may experience maladaptation.

Traditionally, research on person–environment fit has focused on vocational issues. Specifically, such research examines how individual satisfaction and adjustment within certain careers vary as a function of career/personality match (Swanson & Chu, 2000). Research in this field has suggested that individuals will seek out environments that complement their personality, which in turn leads to increased satisfaction and motivation. However, when individuals find themselves in a work environment that is not congruent with their personality, they will work to change the environment or their perceptions of the environment (Swanson & Chu, 2000).

The person–environment fit paradigm has also been successfully integrated within a developmental framework. Within this developmental perspective, person–environment fit theory or, more specifically, stage–environment fit theory postulates that the combination of an individual's developmental stage and the surrounding environment produce change within the individual (Eccles & Midgley, 1989). Proponents of this perspective maintain that synchronizing the trajectory of development to the characteristics and changes in the surrounding environment will encourage positive growth and maturity (Eccles et al., 1993). As noted earlier, the magnitude and variety of changes occurring during the adolescent period distinguishes adolescence as an especially sensitive developmental period. According to stage–environment fit theory, adaptation is more likely if changes within the individual are matched with supportive change within the adolescent's three main environments: school, home, and peer.

One environmental change that marks early adolescence is the transition from elementary school to junior high school. Several negative changes within the individual have been associated with this transition, such as decreases in motivation, self-concept, and self-confidence, as well as increased academic failure (Eccles et al., 1993). This phenomenon may be due to several differences between elementary schools and junior high schools that make the latter less developmentally appropriate for students in this age range. In fact, the Michigan Study of Adolescent Life Transitions (MSALT) found that, as compared to elementary schools, junior high schools were characterized by a greater emphasis on discipline and control, less opportunities for the students to participate in decision making, less personal and positive teacher–student relationships, and lower cognitive requirements for assigned tasks (Eccles et al., 1993). Thus, a stage–environment mismatch within the school environment may be associated with negative changes within the adolescent that often occur at this time.

Patterns of change in the adolescent's home environment are also supportive of the stage–environment hypothesis. During adolescence, the process of establishing greater independence from parents results in greater conflict and modification of roles between the child and parents (Fuligni & Eccles, 1993). Collins (1990) postulated that maladaptive conflicts may occur when there is a poor fit between the child's desire for autonomy and opportunities for such independence. Consideration of pubertal development has provided further support for this theory. In general, early-maturing girls report that they are less satisfied with levels of autonomy and decision making provided at home and in school as compared to their less physically mature peers. In addition, these same girls also report lower self-esteem (Eccles et al., 1993). However, this effect did *not* hold for those girls who were afforded higher participation in decision making (Eccles et al., 1993).

Another notable aspect of stage–environment fit is how congruence, or lack thereof, in one environment may affect functioning in another environment. Current research suggests that compatibility of stage–environment match in one setting is associated with functioning in other settings. For example, a positive home environment characterized by involvement in decision making was directly associated with higher intrinsic school motivation (Eccles et al., 1991).

Person–environment fit theory has also been expanded to include the role of temperament. Individual differences in an adolescent's temperament and its fit to the environment are associated with both positive and negative developmental change. The Pennsylvania Early Adolescence Transitions Study (PEATS) found that a good fit between changing parental and peer demands and an adolescent's temperament was related to positive friendships, higher ratings of self-competence, and positive adjustment (East et al., 1992; Lerner & Lerner, 1994). On the other hand, a negative fit between adolescent temperament and parental demands was associated with lower academic and social competence, as well as peer and conduct problems (Talwar, Nitz, & Lerner, 1990). Thus, examining individual temperament in addition to environment and developmental stage may enrich the goodness-of-fit model.

Culture and Contextualism

Research on culture and contextual factors has become more common in the developmental psychology literature (Garcia Coll, Akerman, & Cicchetti, 2000). Such research has revealed that there may be individual pathways to psychopathology that vary depending on type of neighborhood, ethnicity, or sociocultural circumstances (Rutter, 1997). Also, norms for appropriate behavior as well as the type of processes that are protective may vary across culture (Cicchetti & Rogosch, 2002). Moreover, help-seeking behaviors (e.g., initial problem identification and choice of treatment provider) appear to vary across cultures (Cauce et al., 2002). A major question in the literature is, How do culture and context affect a child's development trajectory and the development of symptomatology?

Demographic changes in the United States have produced a steady increase of minority populations in the United States that underscores the need to study acculturation and other cultural issues (Garcia Coll et al., 2000). Although culture has been defined as the continual passing of socially transmitted patterns from one generation to another that govern the thoughts, values, and behaviors of individuals in all societies (Hallowell, 1934), the continually changing role of culture in the lives of adolescents makes it a difficult topic to investigate (Garcia Coll et al., 2000). On the other hand, taking culture into consideration in developmental psychopathology research can help to validate and extend current theories of normal development in a number of ways (Garcia Coll et al., 2000): (1) cultural research can reveal what developmental progressions or associations between predictors and outcomes are culture-specific versus which are universal (Greenberger & Chen, 1996), (2) such research can isolate pathways to adaptive and maladaptive outcomes that vary across cultural groups, and (3) research may suggest factors crucial for mental growth that are culture specific versus culturally invariant (e.g., parental warmth appears to be crucial across cultures [Greenberger & Chen, 1996]; but "kinship" may be particularly crucial for African American adolescents [Taylor, 1996]). Garcia Coll and Magnuson (1999) call for a paradigm shift in research whereby culture and context would be placed at the core rather than the periphery of understanding and investigating developmental processes.

Antisocial behavior, in particular, has been found to be influenced by a number of contextual variables. Numerous studies have also shown the strength of parental criminality as a predictor of antisocial behavior in the offspring (e.g., Farrington, 1995), but the extent to which this risk is genetically or environmentally mediated remains unclear. Antisocial behavior has also been found to result from a lack of social cohesion in the neighborhood (Sampson, Raudenbush, & Earls, 1997). School factors also seem to be influential during childhood and adolescence, but peer group effects are most evident with respect to adolescence-limited antisocial behavior (Rutter, Giller, & Hagell, 1998). Rutter (1997) examined the effects of extrafamilial or social variables such as schools, peer groups, community characteristics, and poverty on psychopathology, specifically antisocial personality disorder and conduct problems. Some evidence suggests that at least some of the influence of these variables on adolescent behavior is indirect, perhaps being mediated by parenting or family relationships (Conger, Conger, Elder, & Lorenz, 1993; Patterson, 1995).

A number of issues have yet to be addressed in investigating the role of contextualism in developmental psychopathology. First, we need to use more systematic and carefully crafted assessments of cultural context. Future research must "unpack culture" to gain a better understanding of its role in developmental psychopathology (e.g., Cooper, Jackson, Azmitia, & Lopez, 1998). Intervention is another area affected by the study of culture and context. Little work has been directed toward understanding and applying culturally sensitive modes of intervention, despite research showing that interventions that incorporate knowledge of cultural issues may be more effective (Sameroff & Fiese, 1990; Toth & Cicchetti, 1999).

CONCLUSIONS

The goal of this chapter was to demonstrate the utility of adopting developmental and developmental psychopathology perspectives for the advancement of knowledge on adolescent psychopathology. By discussing the components of a biopsychosocial framework, we were able to document ways in which our understanding of psychopathology has been facilitated by consideration of the primary developmental issues of the adolescent period. Indeed, there are multiple changes in the types and frequencies of psychopathological symptoms that are exhibited during adolescence. The implications of the timing of developmental change as well as the importance of fit between the needs of adolescents and their environmental contexts have been emphasized.

The remaining sections of the chapter were devoted to providing an overview of the field of developmental psychopathology and the relevance of its assumptions and tenets for adolescent psychopathology. Knowledge of research in this important field of study will be useful to the clinician who seeks to conceptualize and treat adolescent psychopathology. Developmental psychopathologists are concerned with how psychopathology develops and is maintained, how and why adolescents move along (or are deflected from) specific developmental trajectories, how resilience processes reduce the likelihood of psychopathology for some adolescents, how the ability to master certain developmental tasks affects the manner in which future adversities will be managed, and how certain types of childhood risk profiles increase the probability that other forms of maladaptive behavior will emerge during adolescence. Research on these issues has moved the field of clinical child and adolescent psychology beyond an interest in static diagnostic issues to a more complete understanding of how psychopathological process unfolds over time. We hope that this developmental perspective is useful to those who wish to conduct research or develop prevention or intervention programs for adolescents who are navigating the challenges of this important developmental period.

ACKNOWLEDGMENTS

Completion of this chapter was supported in part by research grants from the March of Dimes Birth Defects Foundation (No. 12-FY01-0098) and the National Institute of Mental Health (No. R01-MH50423).

REFERENCES

Achenbach, T. M. (1985). *Assessment and taxonomy of child and adolescent psychopathology.* Beverly Hills, CA: Sage.

Aguilar, B., Sroufe, L. A., Egeland, B., & Carlson, E. (2000). Distinguishing the early-onset/persistent and adolescence-onset antisocial behavior types: From birth to 16 years. *Development and Psychopathology, 12,* 109–132.

Allen, J. P., Marsh, P., McFarland, C., McElhaney, K. B., Land, D. J., Jodl, K. M., & Peck, S. (2002). Attachment and autonomy as predictors of the development of social skills and delinquency during midadolescence. *Journal of Consulting and Clinical Psychology, 70,* 56–66.

Allen, J. P., Moore, C. M., & Kuperminc, G. P. (1997). Developmental approaches to understanding adolescent deviance. In S. S. Luthar, J. A. Burack, D. Cicchetti, & J. R. Weisz (Eds.), *Developmental psychopathology: Perspectives on adjustment, risk, and disorder* (pp. 548–567). New York: Cambridge University Press.

Allen, N. B., Lewinsohn, P. M., & Seeley, J. R. (1998). Prenatal and perinatal influences on risk for psychopathology in childhood and adolescence. *Development and Psychopathology, 10,* 513–529.

Alsaker, F. D. (1995). Timing or puberty and reactions to pubertal changes. In M. Rutter (Ed.), *Psychosocial disturbances in young people: Challenges for prevention* (pp. 37–82). New York: Cambridge University Press.

American Psychological Association. (2002). *Developing adolescents: A reference for professionals.* Washington, DC: Author.

Angold, A., Costello, E. J., Erkanli, A., & Worthman, C. M. (1999). Pubertal changes in hormone levels and depression in girls. *Psychological Medicine, 29,* 1043–1053.

Arnett, J. J. (1999). Adolescent storm and stress, reconsidered. *American Psychologist, 54,* 317–326.

Aseltine, R. H., Gore, S., & Colten, M. E. (1998). The co-occurrence of depression and substance abuse in late adolescence. *Development and Psychopathology, 10,* 549–570.

Barber, B. K., & Harmon, E. L. (2002). Violating the self: Parental psychological control of children and adolescents. In B. K. Barber (Ed.), *Intrusive parenting: How psychological control affects children and adolescents* (pp. 15–52). Washington, DC: American Psychological Association.

Bardone, A. M., Moffitt, T. E., Caspi, A., Dickson, N., & Silva, P. A. (1996). Adult mental health and social outcomes of adolescent girls with depression and conduct disorder. *Development and Psychopathology, 8,* 811–829.

Baron, R. M., & Kenny, D. A. (1986). The moderator-mediator variable distinction in social psychological research: Conceptual, strategic, and statistical considerations. *Journal of Personality and Social Psychology, 51,* 1173–1182.

Bergman, L. R., & Magnusson, D. (1997). A person-oriented approach in research on developmental psychopathology. *Development and Psychopathology, 9,* 291–319.

Berndt, T. J., & Savin-Williams, R. C. (1993). Peer relations and friendships. In P. H. Tolan & B. J. Cohler (Eds.), *Handbook of clinical research and practice with adolescents* (pp. 203–220). New York: Wiley.

Bingham, C. R., & Crockett, L. J. (1996). Longitudinal adjustment patterns of boys and girls experiencing early, middle, and late sexual intercourse. *Developmental Psychology, 32,* 647–658.

Booth, A., Johnson, D. R., Granger, D. A., Crouter, A. C., & McHale, S. (2003). Testosterone and child and adolescent adjustment: The moderating role of parent–child relationships. *Developmental Psychology, 39,* 85–98.

Brennan, P. A., Hall, J., Bor, W., Najman, J. M., & Williams, G. (2003). Integrating biological and social processes in relation to early-onset persistent aggression in boys and girls. *Developmental Psychology, 39,* 309–323.

Broidy, L. M., Nagin, D. S., Tremblay, R. E., Bates, J. E., Brame, B., Dodge, K. A., et al. (2003). Developmental trajectories of childhood disruptive behaviors and adolescent delinquency: A six-site, cross-national study. *Developmental Psychology, 39, 222–245.*

Bronfenbrenner, U. (1979). *The ecology of human development.* Cambridge, MA: Harvard University Press.

Brook, J. S., Kessler, R. C., & Cohen, P. (1999). The onset of marijuana use from preadolescence and early adolescence to young adulthood. *Development and Psychopathology, 11,* 901–914.

Brooks-Gunn, J., & Reiter, E. O. (1990). The role of pubertal processes. In S. S. Feldman & G. R. Elliott (Eds.), *At the threshold: The developing adolescent* (pp. 16–53). Cambridge, MA: Harvard University Press.

Brown, B. B. (1990). Peer groups and peer cultures. In S. S. Feldman & G. R. Elliott (Eds.), *At the threshold: The developing adolescent* (pp. 171–196). Cambridge, MA: Harvard University Press.

Brown, B. B., Dolcini, M. M., & Leventhal, A. (1997). Transformations in peer relationships at adolescence: Implications for health-related behavior. In J. Schulenberg, J. L. Maggs, & K. Hurrelmann (Eds.), *Health risks and developmental transitions during adolescence* (pp. 161–189).Cambridge, UK: Cambridge University Press.

Buchanan, C. L., Eccles, J. E., Flanagan, C., Midgley, C., Feldlaufer, H., & Harold, R. (1990). Parents' and teachers' beliefs about adolescence: Effects of sex and experience. *Journal of Youth and Adolescence, 19,* 363–394.

Buchanan, C. M., Eccles, J. S., & Becker, J. B. (1992). Are adolescents the victims of raging hormones?: Evidence for activational effects of hormones on moods and behavior at adolescence. *Psychological Bulletin, 111,* 62–107.

Capaldi, D. M. (1991). Co-occurrence of conduct problems and depressive symptoms in early adolescent boys: I. Familial factors and general adjustment at grade 6. *Development and Psychopathology, 3,* 277–300.

Caspi, A., Sugden, K., Moffitt, T. E., Taylor, A., Craig, I. W., Harrington, H., et al. (2003). Influence of life stress on depression: Moderation by a polymorphism in the 5–HTT gene. *Science, 301,* 386–389.

Cauce, A. M., Domenech-Rodriguez, M., Paradise, M.,

Cochran, B. N., Shea, J. M., Srebnik, D., & Baydar, N. (2002). Cultural and contextual influences in mental health help-seeking: A focus on ethnic minority youth. *Journal of Consulting and Clinical Psychology, 70,* 44–45.

Cauffman, E., & Steinberg, L. (1996). Interactive effects of menarcheal status and dating on dieting and disordered eating among adolescent girls. *Developmental Psychology, 32,* 631–635.

Chandler, M., & Moran, T. (1990). Psychopathy and moral development: A comparative study of delinquent and nondelinquent youth. *Development and Psychopathology, 2,* 227–246.

Chassin, L., Pitts, S. C., & Prost, J. (2002). Binge drinking trajectories from adolescence to emerging adulthood in a high-risk sample: Predictors and substance abuse outcomes. *Journal of Consulting and Clinical Psychology, 70,* 67–78.

Cicchetti, D., & Rogosch, F. A. (1996). Equifinality and multifinality in developmental psychopathology. *Development and Psychopathology, 8,* 597–600.

Cicchetti, D., & Rogosch, F. A. (1999a). Conceptual and methodological issues in developmental psychopathology research. In P. C. Kendall, J. N. Butcher, & G. N. Holmbeck (Eds.), *Handbook of research methods in clinical psychology* (2nd ed., pp. 433–465). New York: Wiley.

Cicchetti, D., & Rogosch, F. A. (1999b). Psychopathology as risk for adolescent substance use disorders: A developmental psychopathology perspective. *Journal of Clinical Child Psychology, 28,* 355–365.

Cicchetti, D., & Rogosch, F. A. (2002). A developmental psychopathology perspective on adolescence. *Journal of Consulting and Clinical Psychology, 70,* 6–20.

Colder, C. R., & Chassin, L. (1999). The psychosocial characteristics of alcohol users versus problem users: Data from a study of adolescents at risk. *Development and Psychopathology, 11,* 321–348.

Collins, W. A. (1990). Parent–child relationships in the transition to adolescence: Continuity and change in interaction, affect, and cognition. In R. Montemayor, G. Adams, & T. Gullotta (Eds.), *Advances in adolescent development: From childhood to adolescence: A transitional period?* (Vol. 2, pp. 85–106). Beverly Hills, CA: Sage.

Collins, W. A., & Laursen, B. (1992). Conflict and relationships during adolescence. In C. U. Shantz & W. W. Hartup (Eds.), *Conflict in child and adolescent development* (pp. 216–241). New York: Cambridge University Press.

Collins, W. A., Maccoby, E. E., Steinberg, L., Hetherington, E. M., & Bornstein, M. H. (2000). Contemporary research on parenting: The case for nature and nurture. *American Psychologist, 55,* 218–232.

Compas, B. E., Hinden, B., & Gerhardt, C. (1995). Adolescent development: Pathways and processes of risk and resilience. *Annual Review of Psychology, 46,* 265–293.

Compton, K., Snyder, J., Schrepferman, L., Bank, L., &

Shortt, J. W. (2003). The contribution of parents and siblings to antisocial and depressive behavior in adolescents: A double jeopardy coercion model. *Development and Psychopathology, 15,* 163–182.

Conger, R. D., Conger, K. J., Elder, G. H., & Lorenz, F. O. (1993). Family economic stress and adjustment of early adolescent girls. *Developmental Psychology, 29,* 206–219.

Cooper, C. R. (1988). Commentary: The role of conflict in adolescent–parent relationships. In M. R. Gunnar & W. A. Collins (Eds.), *21st Minnesota Symposium on Child Psychology* (pp. 181–187). Hillsdale, NJ: Erlbaum.

Cooper, C. R., Jackson, J. F., Azmitia, M., & Lopez, E. M. (1998). Multiple selves, multiple worlds: Three useful strategies for research with ethnic minority youth on identity, relationships, and opportunity structures. In V. C. McLoyd & L. Steinberg (Eds.), *Studying minority adolescents: Conceptual, methodological, and theoretical issues* (pp. 111–125). Hillsdale, NJ: Erlbaum

Deater-Deckard, K., & Plomin, R. (1999). An adoption study of etiology of teacher and parent reports of externalizing behavior problems in middle childhood. *Child Development, 70,* 144–154.

Dishion, T. J., Capaldi, D., Spracklen, K. M., & Li, F. (1995). Peer ecology of male adolescent drug use. *Development and Psychopathology, 7,* 803–824.

Dodge, K. A., & Pettit, G. S. (2003). A biopsychosocial model of the development of chronic conduct problems in adolescence. *Developmental Psychology, 39,* 349–371.

Duggal, S., Carlson, E. A., Sroufe, L. A., & Egeland, B. (2001). Depressive symptomatology in childhood and adolescence. *Development and Psychopathology, 13,* 143–164.

Durlak, J. A., Fuhrman, T., & Lampman, C. (1991). Effectiveness of cognitive-behavior therapy for maladapting children: A meta-analysis. *Psychological Bulletin, 110,* 204–214.

East, P. L., Lerner, R. M., Lerner, J. V., Soni, R. T., Ohannessian, C. M., & Jacobson, L. P. (1992). Early adolescent–peer group fit, peer relations, and psychosocial competence: A short-term longitudinal study. *Journal of Early Adolescence, 12,* 132–152.

Eccles, J. S., Buchanan, C. M., Flanagan, C., Fuligni, A., Midgley, C., & Yee, D. (1991). Control versus autonomy during early adolescence. *Journal of Social Issues, 47,* 53–68.

Eccles, J. S., Lord, S. E., Roeser, R. W., Barber, B. L., & Hernandez Jozefowicz, D. M. (1997). The association of school transitions in early adolescence with developmental trajectories through high school. In J. Schulenberg, J. L. Maggs, & K. Hurrelmann (Eds.), *Health risks and developmental transitions during adolescence* (pp. 283–320). Cambridge, UK: Cambridge University Press.

Eccles, J. S., & Midgley, C. (1989). Stage-environment fit: Developmentally appropriate classrooms for young adolescents. In C. Ames & R. Ames (Eds.), *Research on motivation in education: Goals and cognitions* (Vol. 3, pp. 139–186). San Diego, CA: Academic Press.

Eccles, J. S., Midgley, C., Wigfield, A., Buchanan, C. M., Reuman, D., Flanagan, C., & MacIver, D. (1993). Development during adolescence: The impact of stage–environment fit in young adolescents' experiences in schools and in families. *American Psychologist, 48,* 90–101.

Egeland, B., Pianta, R., & Ogawa, J. (1996). Early behavior problems: Pathways to mental disorders in adolescence. *Development and Psychopathology, 8,* 735–749.

Entwisle, D. R. (1990). Schools and the adolescent. In S. S. Feldman & G. R. Elliott (Eds.), *At the threshold: The developing adolescent* (pp. 197–224). Cambridge, MA: Harvard University Press.

Erikson, E. (1968). *Identity: Youth and crisis.* New York: Norton.

Farrell, A. D., Danish, S. J., & Howard, C. W. (1992). Relationship between drug use and other problem behaviors in urban adolescents. *Journal of Consulting and Clinical Psychology, 60,* 705–712.

Farrington, D. P. (1995). The Twelfth Jack Tizard memorial lecture: The development of offending and antisocial behavior in childhood: Key findings from the Cambridge study in delinquent development. *Journal of Children Psychology and Psychiatry, 36,* 929–964.

Feldman, S. S., & Elliott, G. R. (Eds.). (1990). *At the threshold: The developing adolescent.* Cambridge, MA: Harvard University Press.

Fiese, B. H., Wilder, J., & Bickham, N. L. (2000). Family context in developmental psychopathology. In A. J. Sameroff, M. Lewis, & S. M. Miller (Eds.), *Handbook of developmental psychopathology* (2nd ed., pp. 115–134). New York: Kluwer.

Finch, M. D., Mortimer, J. T., & Ryu, S. (1997). Transition into part-time work: Health risks and opportunities. In J. Schulenberg, J. L. Maggs, & K. Hurrelmann (Eds.), *Health risks and developmental transitions during adolescence* (pp. 321–344). Cambridge, UK: Cambridge University Press.

Freud, A. (1958). Adolescence. *Psychoanalytic Study of the Child, 13,* 231–258.

Fuhrman, T., & Holmbeck, G. N. (1995). A contextual-moderator analysis of emotional autonomy and adjustment in adolescence. *Child Development, 66,* 793–811.

Fuligni, A. J., & Eccles, J. S. (1993). Perceived parent–child relationships and early adolescents' orientation toward peers. *Developmental Psychology, 29,* 622–632.

Galambos, N. L., Almeida, D. M., & Petersen, A. C. (1990). Masculinity, femininity, and sex role attitudes in early adolescence: Exploring gender intensification. *Child Development, 61,* 1905–1914.

Garber, J., Keiley, M. K., & Martin, N. C. (2002). Developmental trajectories of adolescents' depressive symptoms: Predictors of change. *Journal of Consulting and Clinical Psychology, 70,* 79–95.

Garcia Coll, C. T., Akerman, A., & Cicchetti, D. (2000). Cultural influences on developmental processes and outcomes: Implications for the study of development and psychopathology. *Development and Psychopathology, 12,* 333–356.

Garcia Coll, C. T., & Magnuson, K. (1999). Cultural influences on child development: Are we ready for a paradigm shift? In C. Nelson & A. Masten (Eds.), *Minnesota Symposium on Child Psychology* (Vol. 29, pp. 1–24). Mahwah, NJ: Erlbaum.

Ge, X., Brody, G. H., Conger, R. D., Simons, R. L., & Murry, V. M. (2002). Contextual amplification of pubertal transition effects on deviant peer affiliation and externalizing behavior among African American children. *Developmental Psychology, 38,* 42–54.

Ge, X., Conger, R. D., & Elder, G. H. (2001). Pubertal transition, stressful life events, and the emergence of gender differences in adolescent depressive symptoms. *Developmental Psychology, 37,* 404–417.

Ge, X., Kim, I. J., Brody, G. H., Conger, R. D., Simons, R. L., Gibbons, F. X., & Cutrona, C. E. (2003). It's about timing and change: Pubertal transition effects on symptoms of major depression among African American youths. *Developmental Psychology, 39,* 430–439.

Gilligan, C., Lyons, N. P., & Hanmer, T. J. (Eds.). (1990). *Making connections: The relational worlds of adolescent girls at Emma Willard School.* Cambridge, MA: Harvard University Press.

Gjerde, P. F., & Block, J. (1996). A developmental perspective on depressive symptoms in adolescence: Gender differences in autocentric–allocentric modes of impulse regulation. In D. Cicchetti & S. L. Toth (Eds.), *Adolescence: Opportunities and challenges* (Vol. 7, pp. 167–196). Rochester, NY: University of Rochester Press.

Gorman-Smith, D., & Tolan, P. (1998). The role of exposure to community violence and developmental problems among inner-city youth. *Development and Psychopathology, 10,* 101–116.

Graber, J. A., & Brooks-Gunn, J. (1996). Transitions and turning points: Navigating the passage from childhood through adolescence. *Developmental Psychology, 32,* 768–776.

Graber, J. A., Brooks-Gunn, J., Paikoff, R. L., & Warren, M. P. (1994). Prediction of eating problems: An 8-year study of adolescent girls. *Developmental Psychology, 30,* 823–834.

Graber, J. A., Lewinsohn, P. M., Seeley, J. R., & Brooks-Gunn, J. (1997). Is psychopathology associated with the timing of pubertal development?, *Journal of the American Academy of Child and Adolescent Psychiatry, 36,* 1768–1776.

Greenberger, E., & Chen, C. (1996). Perceived family relationships and depressed mood in early and late adolescence: A comparison of European and Asian Americans. *Developmental Psychology, 32,* 707–716.

Greenberger, E., & Steinberg, L. (1986). *When teenagers work: The psychological and social costs of adolescent employment.* New York: Basic Books.

Grotevant, H. D. (1997). Adolescent development in family contexts. In W. Damon (Ed.), *Handbook of child psychology* (Vol. 3, pp. 1097–1149). New York: Wiley.

Guerra, N. G. (1993). Cognitive development. In P. H. Tolan & B. J. Cohler (Eds.), *Handbook of clinical research and practice with adolescents* (pp. 45–62). New York: Wiley.

Hall, G. S. (1904). *Adolescence.* New York: Appleton.

Hammen, C. (1992). Cognitive, life stress, and interpersonal approaches to a developmental psychopathology model of depression. *Development and Psychopathology, 4,* 189–206.

Harrington, R., Rutter, M., & Fombonne, E. (1996). Developmental pathways in depression: Multiple meanings, antecedents, and endpoints. *Development and Psychopathology, 8,* 601–616.

Harris, J. R. (1998). *The nurture assumption: Why children turn out the way they do.* New York: Free Press.

Harter, S. (1990). Self and identity development. In S. S. Feldman & G. R. Elliott (Eds.), *At the threshold: The developing adolescent* (pp. 352–387). Cambridge, MA: Harvard University Press.

Hartup, W. W. (1992). Peer relations in early and middle childhood. In V. B. Van Hasselt & M Hersen (Eds.), *Handbook of social development: A lifespan perspective* (pp. 257–281). New York: Plenum Press.

Henderson, V. L., & Dweck, C. S. (1990). Motivation and achievement. In S. S. Feldman & G. R. Elliott (Eds.), *At the threshold: The developing adolescent* (pp. 308–329). Cambridge, MA: Harvard University Press.

Henggeler, S. W., Schoenwald, S. K., Borduin, C. M., Rowland, M. D., & Cunningham, P. B. (1998). *Multisystemic treatment of antisocial behavior in children and adolescents.* New York: Guilford Press.

Henry, B., Caspi, A., Moffitt, T. E., & Silva, P. A. (1996). Temperamental and familial predictors of violent and nonviolent criminal convictions: Age 3 to age 18. *Developmental Psychology, 32,* 614–623.

Higgins, E. T., Ruble, D. N., & Hartup, W. W. (Eds.). (1983). *Social cognition and social development: A sociocultural perspective.* New York: Cambridge University Press.

Hill, J. P. (1980). *Understanding early adolescence: A framework.* Carrboro, NC: Center for Early Adolescence.

Hill, J. P., & Holmbeck, G. N. (1986). Attachment and autonomy during adolescence. In G. J. Whitehurst (Ed.), *Annals of child development* (Vol. 3, pp. 145–189). Greenwich, CN: JAI Press.

Hinshaw, S. P., Lahey, B. B., & Hart, E. L. (1993). Issues of taxonomy and comorbidity in the development of conduct disorder. *Development and Psychopathology, 5,* 31–49.

Holmbeck, G. N. (1996). A model of family relational transformations during the transition to adolescence:

Parent–adolescent conflict and adaptation. In J. A. Graber, J. Brooks-Gunn, & A. C. Petersen (Eds.), *Transitions through adolescence: Interpersonal domains and context* (pp.167–199). Mahwah, NJ: Erlbaum.

Holmbeck, G. N. (1997). Toward terminological, conceptual, and statistical clarity in the study of mediators and moderators: Examples from the child–clinical and pediatric psychology literatures. *Journal of Consulting and Clinical Psychology, 65,* 599–610.

Holmbeck, G. N., Colder, C., Shapera, W., Westhoven, V., Kenealy, L., & Updegrove, A. (2000). Working with adolescents: Guides from developmental psychology. In P. C. Kendall (Ed.), *Child and adolescent therapy: Cognitive-behavioral procedures* (2nd ed., pp. 334–385). New York: Guilford Press.

Holmbeck, G. N., Greenley, R. N., & Franks, E. A. (2003). Developmental issues and considerations in research and practice. In A. E. Kazdin & J. R. Weisz (Eds.), *Evidence-based psychotherapies for children and adolescents* (pp. 21–41). New York: Guilford Press.

Holmbeck, G. N., & Hill, J. P. (1988). Storm and stress beliefs about adolescence: Prevalence, selfreported antecedents, and effects of an undergraduate course. *Journal of Youth and Adolescence, 17,* 285–306.

Holmbeck, G. N., & Hill, J. P. (1991). Conflictive engagement, positive affect, and menarche in families with seventh-grade girls. *Child Development, 62,* 1030–1048.

Holmbeck, G. N., Johnson, S. Z., Wills, K. E., McKernon, W., Rose, B., Erklin, S., & Kemper, T. (2002). Observed and perceived parental overprotection in relation to psychosocial adjustment in preadolescents with a physical disability: The mediational role of behavioral autonomy. *Journal of Consulting and Clinical Psychology, 70,* 96–110.

Holmbeck, G. N., & Kendall, P. C. (2002). Introduction to the special section on clinical adolescent psychology: Developmental psychopathology and treatment. *Journal of Consulting and Clinical Psychology, 70,* 3–5.

Holmbeck, G. N., & O'Donnell, K. (1991). Discrepancies between perceptions of decision-making and behavioral autonomy. In R. L. Paikoff (Ed.), *Shared views in the family during adolescence: New directions for development* (No. 51, pp. 51–69). San Francisco: Jossey-Bass.

Holmbeck, G. N., Paikoff, R. L., & Brooks-Gunn, J. (1995). Parenting adolescents. In M. Bornstein (Ed.), *Handbook of parenting* (Vol. 1, pp. 91–118). Mahwah, NJ: Erlbaum.

Holmbeck, G. N., & Shapera, W. F. A. (1999). Research methods with adolescents. In P. C. Kendall, J. N. Butcher, & G. N. Holmbeck (Eds.), *Handbook of research methods in clinical psychology* (2nd ed., pp. 634–661). New York: Wiley.

Holmbeck, G. N., & Updegrove, A. L. (1995). Clinical-developmental interface: Implications of developmental research for adolescent psychotherapy. *Psychotherapy, 32,* 16–33.

Iervolino, A. C., Pike, A., Manke, B., Reiss, D., Hetherington, E. M., & Plomin, R. (2002). Genetic and environmental influences in adolescent peer socialization: Evidence from two genetically sensitive designs. *Child Development, 73,* 162–174.

Jackson, F. J. (1993). Human behavioral genetics, Scarr's theory, and her views on interventions: A critical review and commentary on their implications for African-American children. *Child Development, 64,* 1318–1332.

Jaffee, S. R., Moffitt, T. E., Caspi, A., Fombonne, E., Poulton, R., & Martin, J. (2002). Differences in early childhood risk factors for juvenile-onset and adult-onset depression. *Archives of General Psychiatry, 59,* 215–222.

Jessor, R., Donovan, J. E., & Costa, F. M. (1991). *Beyond adolescence: Problem behavior and young adult development.* New York: Cambridge University Press.

Jessor, R., & Jessor, S. L. (1977). *Problem behavior and psychosocial development: A longitudinal study of youth.* New York: Academic Press.

Jimerson, S., Egeland, B., Sroufe, L. A., & Carlson, B. (2000). A prospective longitudinal study of high school dropouts: Examining multiple predictors across development. *Journal of School Psychology, 38,* 525–549.

Katchadourian, H. (1990). Sexuality. In S. S. Feldman & G. R. Elliott (Eds.), *At the threshold: The developing adolescent* (pp. 330–351). Cambridge, MA: Harvard University Press.

Kazdin, A. E., Kraemer, H. C., Kessler, R. C., Kupfer, D. J., & Offord, D. R. (1997). Contributions of risk-factor research to developmental psychopathology. *Clinical Psychology Review, 17,* 375–406.

Keating, D. P. (1990). Adolescent thinking. In S. S. Feldman & G. R. Elliott (Eds.), *At the threshold: The developing adolescent* (pp. 54–89). Cambridge, MA: Harvard University Press.

Klimes-Dougan, B., Hastings, P. D., Granger, D. A., Usher, B. A., & Zahn-Waxler, C. (2001). Adrenocortical activity in at-risk and normally developing adolescents: Individual differences in salivary cortisol basal levels, diurnal variation, and responses to social challenges. *Development and Psychopathology, 13,* 695–719.

Kobak, R. R., Sudler, N., & Gamble, W. (1991). Attachment and depressive symptoms during adolescence: A developmental pathways analysis. *Development and Psychopathology, 3,* 461–474.

Lacourse, E., Nagin, D., Tremblay, R. E., Vitaro, F., & Claes, M. (2003). Developmental trajectories of boys' delinquent group membership and facilitation of violent behaviors during adolescence. *Development and Psychopathology, 15,* 183–197.

La Greca, A. M., & Prinstein, M. J. (1999). Peer group. In W. K. Silverman & T. H. Ollendick (Eds.), *Devel-*

opmental issues in the clinical treatment of children (pp. 171–198). Boston, MA: Allyn & Bacon.

Larson, R. W., Richards, M. H., Moneta, G., Holmbeck, G., & Duckett, E. (1996). Changes in adolescents' daily interactions with their families from ages 10 to 18: Disengagement and transformation. *Developmental Psychology, 32,* 744–754.

Laursen, B., Coy, K. C., & Collins, W. A. (1998). Reconsidering changes in parent–child conflict across adolescence: A meta-analysis. *Child Development, 69,* 817–832.

Lenhart, L. A., & Rabiner, D. L. (1995). An integrative approach to the study of social competence in adolescence. *Development and Psychopathology, 7,* 543–561.

Lerner, J. V., & Lerner, R. M. (1994). Explorations of the goodness-of-fit model in early adolescence. In W. B. Carey & S. C. McDevitt (Eds.), *Prevention and early intervention: Individual differences as risk factors for the mental health of children* (pp. 161–169). New York: Brunner/Mazel.

Lerner, R. M., & Galambos, N. L. (1998). Adolescent development: Challenges and opportunities for research, programs, and policies. *Annual Review of Psychology, 49,* 413–446.

Lewko, J. H. (Ed.). (1987). *How children and adolescents view the world of work* (No. 35). San Francisco: Jossey-Bass.

Lochman, J. E., White, K. J., & Wayland, K. K. (1991). Cognitive-behavioral assessment and treatment with aggressive children. In P. C. Kendall (Ed.), *Child and adolescent therapy: Cognitive-behavioral procedures* (pp. 25–65). New York: Guilford Press.

Loeber, R., Farrington, D. P., Stouthamer-Loeber, M., & Van Kammen, W. B. (1998). *Antisocial behavior and mental health problems: Explanatory factors in childhood and adolescence.* Mahwah, NJ: Erlbaum.

Luthar, S. S., Doernberger, C. H., & Zigler, E. (1993). Resilience is not a unidimensional construct: Insights from a prospective study of inner-city adolescents. *Development and Psychopathology, 5,* 703–717.

Luthar, S. S., & Ripple, C. H. (1994). Sensitivity to emotional distress among intelligent adolescents: A short-term prospective study. *Development and Psychopathology, 6,* 343–357.

Luthar, S. S., & Zigler, E. (1992). Intelligence and social competence among high-risk adolescents. *Development and Psychopathology, 4,* 287–299.

Maccoby, E. (2000). Parenting and its effects on children: On reading and misreading behavior genetics. *Annual Review of Psychology, 51,* 1–27.

Magnusson, D., Stattin, H., & Allen, V. L. (1985). A longitudinal study of some adjustment processes from mid-adolescence to adulthood. *Journal of Youth and Adolescence, 14,* 267–283.

Marsh, P., McFarland, F. C., Allen, J. P., McElhaney, K. B., & Land, D. J. (2003). Attachment, autonomy, and multifinality in adolescent internalizing and risky behavioral symptoms. *Development and Psychopathology, 15,* 451–467.

Mash, E. J., & Dozois, D. J. A. (2003). Child psychopathology: A developmental–systems perspective. In E. J. Mash & R. A. Barkley (Eds.), *Child psychopathology* (2nd ed., pp. 3–71). New York: Guilford Press.

Masten, A. S., & Coatsworth, J. D. (1998). The development of competence in favorable and unfavorable environments: Lessons from research on successful children. *American Psychologist, 53,* 205–220.

McBride, C. K., Paikoff, R. L., & Holmbeck, G. N. (2003). Individual and familial influences on the onset of sexual intercourse among urban African American adolescents. *Journal of Consulting and Clinical Psychology, 71,* 159–167.

McGee, R. A., Wolfe, D. A., & Wilson, S. K. (1997). Multiple maltreatment experiences and adolescent behavior problems: Adolescents' perspectives. *Development and Psychopathology, 9,* 131–149.

Minuchin, P. P., & Shapiro, E. K. (1983). The school as a context for social development. In P. H. Mussen (Ed.) & E. M. Hetherington (Vol. Ed.), *Handbook of child psychology* (Vol. IV, pp. 197274). New York: Wiley.

Moffitt, T. E. (1993). Adolescence-limited and life-course persistent anti-social behavior: A developmental taxonomy. *Psychological Review, 100,* 674–701.

Moffitt, T. E., Caspi, A., Dickson, N., Silva, P., & Stanton, W. (1996). Childhood-onset versus adolescent-onset antisocial conduct problems in males: Natural history from ages 3 to 18 years. *Development and Psychopathology, 8,* 399–424.

Moffitt, T. E., Caspi, A., Harrington, H., & Milne, B. J. (2002). Males on the life-course-persistent and adolescence-limited antisocial pathways: Follow-up at age 26 years. *Development and Psychopathology, 14,* 179–207.

Montemayor, E. (1983). Parents and adolescents in conflict: All families some of the time and some families most of the time. *Journal of Early Adolescence, 3,* 83–103.

Moshman, D. (1998). Cognitive development beyond childhood. In D. Kuhn & R. S. Siegler (Eds.), *Handbook of child psychology: Cognition, perception, and language* (Vol. 2, pp. 957–978). New York: Wiley.

Neiderhiser, J. M., Reiss, D., Hetherington, E. M., & Plomin, R. (1999). Relationships between parenting and adolescent adjustment over time: Genetic and environmental contributions. *Developmental Psychology, 35,* 680–692.

Nelson, D. A., & Crick, N. R. (1999). Rose-colored glasses: Examining the social information-processing of prosocial young adolescents. *Journal of Early Adolescence, 19,* 17–38.

Noam, G. G., Paget, K. F., Valiant, G., Borst, S., & Bartok, J. (1994). Conduct and affective disorders in developmental perspective: A systematic study of adolescent psychopathology. *Development and Psychopathology, 6,* 519–532.

Noam, G. G., Recklitis, C. J., & Paget, K. F. (1991). Pathways of ego development: Contributions to maladaptation and adjustment. *Development and Psychopathology, 3,* 311–328.

Nurmi, J. (1997). Self-definition and mental health during adolescence and young adulthood. In J. Schulenberg, J. L. Maggs, & K. Hurrelmann (Eds.), *Health risks and developmental transitions during adolescence* (pp. 395–419). Cambridge, UK: Cambridge University Press.

O'Connor, T. G., Deater-Deckard, K., Fulker, D., Rutter, M., & Plomin, R. (1998). Genotype-environment correlations in late childhood and early adolescence: Antisocial behavioural problems and coercive parenting. *Developmental Psychology, 34,* 970–981.

O'Connor, T. G., McGuire, S., Reiss, D., Hetherington, E. M., & Plomin, R. (1998). Co-occurrence of depressive symptoms and antisocial behavior in adolescence: A common genetic liability. *Journal of Abnormal Psychology, 107,* 27–37.

O'Connor, T. G., & Plomin, R. (2000). Developmental behavior genetics. In A. J. Sameroff & M. Lewis (Eds.), *Handbook of developmental psychopathology* (pp. 217–235). New York: Plenum Press.

Paikoff, R. L., & Brooks-Gunn, J. (1991). Do parent–child relationships change during puberty? *Psychological Bulletin, 110,* 47–66.

Parker, J. G., & Asher, S. R. (1987). Peer relations and later personal adjustment: Are lowaccepted children at risk? *Psychological Bulletin, 102,* 357–389.

Patterson, G. R. (1995). Coercion as a basis for early age of onset for arrest. In J. McCord (Ed.), *Coercion and punishment in long-term perspectives* (pp. 81–105). Cambridge, UK: Cambridge University Press.

Patterson, G. R., Forgatch, M. S., Yoerger, K. L., & Stoolmiller, M. (1998). Variables that initiate and maintain an early-onset trajectory for juvenile offending. *Development and Psychopathology, 10,* 531–547.

Petersen, A. C. (1988). Adolescent development. In M. R. Rosenzweig & L. W. Porter (Eds.), *Annual review of psychology* (Vol. 39, pp. 583–608). Palo Alto, CA: Annual Reviews.

Petersen, A. C., Compas, B. E, Brooks-Gunn, J., Stemmler, M., Ey, S., & Grant, K. E. (1993). Depression in adolescence. *American Psychologist, 48,* 155–168.

Petersen, A. C., & Hamburg, B. A. (1986). Adolescence: A developmental approach to problems and psychopathology. *Behavior Therapy, 17,* 480–499.

Piaget, J. (1970). Piaget's theory. In P. H. Mussen (Ed.), *Manual of child psychology* (3rd ed., pp. 703–732). New York: Wiley.

Piaget, J. (1972). Intellectual evolution from adolescence to adulthood. *Human Development, 15,* 112.

Pike, A., & Plomin, R. (1996). Importance of nonshared environmental factors for childhood and adolescent psychopathology. *Journal of the American Academy of Child and Adolescent Psychiatry, 35,* 560–570.

Plomin, R., Reiss, D., Hetherington, E. M., Howe, G. W., & George, W. (1994). Nature and nurture: Genetic contributions to measures of the family environment. *Developmental Psychology, 30,* 32–43.

Public Agenda. (1999). *Kids these days '99: What Americans really think about the next generation.* New York: Author.

Reiss, D., Hetherington, E. M., Plomin, R., Howe, G. W., Simmens, S. J., Henderson, S. H., et al. (1995). Genetic questions for environmental studies: Differential parenting of siblings and its association with depression and antisocial behavior in adolescence. *Archives of General Psychiatry, 52,* 925–936.

Rende, R., & Plomin, R. (1995). Nature, nurture, and the development of psychopathology. In D. Cicchetti & D. J. Cohen (Eds.), *Developmental psychopathology: Theory and methods* (Vol. 1, pp. 291–314). New York: Wiley.

Rende, R., Plomin, R., Reiss, D., & Hetherington, E. M. (1993). Genetic and environmental influences on depressive symptomatology in adolescence: Individual differences and extreme scores. *Journal of Child Psychology and Psychiatry and Allied Disciplines, 34,* 1387–1398.

Richards, M., Abell, S. N., & Petersen, A. C. (1993). Biological development. In P. H. Tolan & B. J. Cohler (Eds.), *Handbook of clinical research and practice with adolescents* (pp. 21–44). New York: Wiley.

Rierdan, J., & Koff, E. (1993). Developmental variables in relation to depressive symptoms in adolescent girls. *Development and Psychopathology, 5,* 485–496.

Robin, A. L., & Foster, S. L. (1989). *Negotiating parent–adolescent conflict: A behavioral–family systems approach.* New York: Guilford Press.

Roeser, R. W., & Eccles, J. S. (2000). Schooling and mental health. In A. J. Sameroff, M. Lewis, & S. M. Miller (Eds.), *Handbook of developmental psychopathology* (2nd ed., pp. 135–156). New York: Kluwer.

Roeser, R. W., Eccles, J. S., & Sameroff, A. J. (1998). Academic and emotional functioning in early adolescence: Longitudinal relations, patterns, and prediction by experience in middle school. *Development and Psychopathology, 10,* 321–352.

Rose, B. M., Holmbeck, G. N., Coakley, R. M., & Franks, E. A. (2004). Mediator and moderator effects in developmental and behavioral pediatric research. *Journal of Developmental and Behavioral Pediatrics, 25*(1), 1–10.

Rutter, M. (1990). Psychosocial resilience and protective mechanisms. In J. Rolf, A. S. Masten, D. Cicchetti, K. H. Nuechterlein, & S. Weintraub (1990). *Risk and protective factors in the development of psychopathology* (pp. 181–214). New York: Cambridge University Press.

Rutter, M. (1997). Antisocial behavior: developmental psychopathology perspectives. In D. M. Stoff & J. Breiling (Eds.), *Handbook of antisocial behavior* (pp. 115–124). New York: Wiley.

Rutter, M., Giller, H., & Hagell, A. (1998). *Antisocial behavior by young people.* New York: Cambridge University Press.

Rutter, M., Maughan, B., Mortimore, P., & Ouston, J. (1979). *Fifteen thousand hours: Secondary schools and their effects on children.* Cambridge, MA: Harvard University Press.

Rutter, M., Pickles, A., Murray, R., & Eaves, L. (2001). Testing hypotheses on specific environmental causal effects on behavior. *Psychological Bulletin, 127,* 291–324.

Sagrestano, L. McCormick, S. H., Paikoff, R. L., & Holmbeck, G. N. (1999). Pubertal development and parent–child conflict in low-income African-American adolescents. *Journal of Research on Adolescence, 9,* 85–107.

Sameroff, A., & Fiese, B. (1990). Transactional regulation and early interaction. In S. Meisels & J. Shonkoff (Eds.), *Handbook of early intervention* (pp. 119–149). New York: Cambridge University Press.

Sampson, R. J., Raudenbush, S. W., & Earls, F. (1997). Neighborhoods and violent crime: A multilevel study of collective efficacy. *Science, 277,* 918–924.

Savin-Williams, R. C., & Berndt, T. J. (1990). Friendship and peer relations. In S. S. Feldman & G. R. Elliott (Eds.), *At the threshold: The developing adolescent* (pp. 277–307). Cambridge, MA: Harvard University Press.

Schulenberg, J., Maggs, J. L., & Hurrelmann, K. (1997). Negotiating developmental transitions during adolescence and young adulthood: Health risks and opportunities. In J. Schulenberg, J. L. Maggs, & K. Hurrelmann (Eds.), *Health risks and developmental transitions during adolescence* (pp. 1–19). Cambridge, UK: Cambridge University Press.

Schulenberg, J., Wadsworth, K. N., O'Malley, P. M., Bachman, J. G., & Johnston, L. D. (1996). Adolescent risk factors for binge drinking during the transition to young adulthood: Variable- and pattern-centered approaches to change. *Developmental Psychology, 32,* 659–674.

Schwartz, C. E., Snidman, N., & Kagan, J. (1996). Early childhood temperament as a determinant of externalizing behavior in adolescence. *Development and Psychopathology, 8,* 527–537.

Selman, R. L. (1980). *The growth of interpersonal understanding: Developmental and clinical analyses.* New York: Academic Press.

Shirk, S. R. (1999). Developmental therapy. In W. K. Silverman & T. H. Ollendick (Eds.), *Developmental issues in the clinical treatment of children* (pp. 60–73). Boston: Allyn & Bacon.

Silverthorn, P., & Frick, P. J. (1999). Developmental pathways to antisocial behavior: The delayed-onset pathway in girls. *Development and Psychopathology, 11,* 101–126.

Simmons, R. G., & Blyth, D. A. (1987). *Moving into adolescence: The impact of pubertal change and school context.* New York: Aldine de Gruyter.

Sroufe, L. A. (1990). Considering normal and abnormal together: The essence of developmental psychopathology. *Development and Psychopathology, 2,* 335–347.

Sroufe, L. A. (1997). Psychopathology as an outcome of development. *Development and Psychopathology, 9,* 251–268.

Sroufe, L. A., Carlson, E. A., Levy, A. K., & Egeland, B. (1999). Implications of attachment theory for developmental psychopathology. *Development and Psychopathology, 11,* 1–13.

Steinberg, L. (1990). Interdependence in the family: Autonomy, conflict, and harmony in the parent–adolescent relationship. In S. S. Feldman & G. L. Elliott (Eds.), *At the threshold: The developing adolescent* (pp. 255–276). Cambridge, MA: Harvard University Press.

Steinberg, L. (2001). We know some things: Adolescent-parent relationships in retrospect and prospect. *Journal of Research on Adolescence, 11,* 1–20.

Steinberg, L. (2002). *Adolescence* (6th ed.). Boston: McGraw-Hill.

Steinberg, L., & Avenevoli, S. (2000). The role of context in the development of psychopathology: A conceptual framework and some speculative propositions. *Child Development, 71,* 66–74.

Steinberg, L., & Morris, A. S. (2001). Adolescent development. *Annual Review of Psychology, 52,* 83–110.

Steinberg, L., & Silverberg, S. (1986). The vicissitudes of autonomy in early adolescence. *Child Development, 57,* 841–851.

Stouthamer-Loeber, M., Loeber, R., Farrington, D. P., Zhang, Q., Van Kammen, W., & Maguin, E. (1993). The double edge of protective and risk factors for delinquency: Interrelations and developmental patterns. *Development and Psychopathology, 5,* 683–701.

Stouthamer-Loeber, M., Loeber, R., Wei, E., Farrington, D. P., & Wikstrom, P. H. (2002). Risk and promotive effects in the explanation of persistent serious delinquency in boys. *Journal of Consulting and Clinical Psychology, 70,* 111–123.

Sullivan, H. S. (1953). *The interpersonal theory of psychiatry.* New York: Norton.

Swanson, J. L., & Chu, S. P. (2000). Applications of person–environment psychology to the career development and vocational behavior of adolescents and adults. In W. E. Martin Jr. & J. L. Swartz-Kulstad (Eds.), *Person–environment psychology and mental health: Assessment and intervention* (pp. 143–168). Mahwah, NJ: Erlbaum.

Takanishi, R. (1993). The opportunities of adolescence—Research, interventions, and policy: Introduction to the special issue. *American Psychologist, 48,* 85–88.

Talwar, R., Nitz, K., & Lerner, R. M. (1990). Relations among early adolescent temperament, parent and peer demands, and adjustment: A test of the goodness of fit model. *Journal of Adolescence, 13,* 279–298.

Tanner, J. (1962). *Growth at adolescence* (2nd ed.). Springfield, IL: Charles C. Thomas.

Taylor, R. D. (1996). Adolescents' perceptions of kinship support and family management practices: Association with adolescent adjustment in African American families. *Developmental Psychology, 32,* 687–695.

Temple, S. (1997). *Brief therapy for adolescent depression.* Sarasota, FL: Professional Resource Press.

Thapar, A., & McGuffin, P. (1994). A twin study of depressive symptoms in childhood. *British Journal of Psychiatry, 165,* 259–265.

Tolan, P. H., Gorman-Smith, D., & Henry, D. B. (2003). The developmental ecology of urban males' youth violence. *Developmental Psychology, 39,* 274–291.

Toth, S. L., & Cicchetti, D. (1999). Developmental psychopathology and child psychotherapy. In S. Russ & T. Ollendick (Eds.), *Handbook of psychotherapies with children and families* (pp. 15–44). New York: Plenum Press.

Tremblay, R. E., Masse, L. C., Vitaro, F., & Dobkin, P. L. (1995). The impact of friends' deviant behavior on early onset of delinquency: Longitudinal data from 6 to 13 years of age. *Development and Psychopathology, 7,* 649–667.

Trevethan, S. D., & Walker, L. J. (1989). Hypothetical versus real-life moral reasoning among psychopathic and delinquent youth. *Development and Psychopathology, 1,* 91–103.

Trickett, E. J., & Schmid, J. D. (1993). The school as a social context. In P. H. Tolan & B. J. Cohler (Eds.), *Handbook of clinical research and practice with adolescents* (pp. 173–202). New York: Wiley.

Vygotsky, L. (1978). *Mind in society: The development of higher psychological processes.* Cambridge, MA: Harvard University Press.

Walker, E. F. (2002). Adolescent neurodevelopment and psychopathology. *Current Directions in Psychological Science, 11,* 24–28.

Weisz, J. R., & Hawley, K. M. (2002). Developmental factors in the treatment of adolescents. *Journal of Consulting and Clinical Psychology, 70,* 21–43.

Wekerle, C., Wolfe, D. A., Hawkins, D. L., Pittman, A., Glickman, A., & Lovald, B. E. (2001). Childhood maltreatment, posttraumatic stress symptomatology, and adolescent dating violence: Considering the value of adolescent perceptions of abuse and a trauma mediational model. *Development and Psychopathology, 13,* 847–871.

Woodward, L. J., & Fergusson, D. M. (1999). Early conduct problems and later risk of teenage pregnancy in girls. *Development and Psychopathology, 11,* 127–141.

Youniss, J. (1980). *Parents and peers in social development: A Sullivan–Piaget perspective.* Chicago: University of Chicago Press.

Zahn-Waxler, C. (1996). Environment, biology, and culture: Implications for adolescent development. *Developmental Psychology, 32,* 571–573.

Zimmerman, M. A., & Schmeelk-Cone, K. H. (2003). A longitudinal analysis of adolescent substance use and school motivation among African American youth. *Journal of Research on Adolescence, 13,* 185–210.

Zucker, R. A., Ellis, D. A., Fitzgerald, H. E., Bingham, C. R., & Sanford, K. (1996). Other evidence for at least two alcoholisms. II: Life course variation in antisociality and heterogeneity of alcoholic outcome. *Development and Psychopathology, 8,* 831–848.

Zucker, R. A., Fitzgerald, H. E., & Moses, H. D. (1995). Emergence of alcohol problems and the several alcoholisms: A developmental perspective on etiologic theory and life course trajectory. In D. Cicchetti & D. Cohen (Eds.), *Developmental psychopathology: Vol. 2. Risk, disorder, and adaptation* (pp. 677–711). New York: Wiley.

3

Interventions for Adolescent Psychopathology
Linking Treatment and Prevention

Jody Kamon
Patrick H. Tolan
Deborah Gorman-Smith

"What treatment, by whom, is most effective for this individual with that specific problem, under which set of circumstances?" (Paul, 1967, p. 111) This question posed by Gordon Paul, over 35 years ago, focused on what we need to know to have a solid approach for intervention for psychopathology. Today, the field of clinical adolescent psychology continues to struggle to meet the challenges in that question. There has been considerable scientific study of interventions for adolescent disorders since that time with the goal of providing science-based answers to each of the aspects of Paul's question. Over the past three decades, there has been a rapid growth in the knowledge base about interventions and in the sophistication of what is judged to be an intervention that works, whether treatment or prevention. The question implies that we need a compendium of knowledge about interventions across all areas of adolescent psychopathology and related problems. Acquiring this knowledge can be understood as consisting of two tasks: (1) determining whether a given intervention works; and (2) determining under what circumstances and for whom it has the intended effects. A third task, not explicit in Paul's question but equally important, involves determining how the intervention works.

Determining whether intervention programs work is typically differentiated into two parts. First, clinical researchers try to establish the *efficacy* of an intervention. Establishing efficacy involves the process of determining whether a proposed intervention can significantly eliminate, reduce, or prevent the identified problem (Lonigan, Elbert, & Bennett-Johnson, 1998). Usually, this stage of testing is characterized by careful control of the conditions of the study to maximize internal validity; emphasizing minimization of alternative explanations for effects found. Also, at this stage priority is placed on minimizing methodological impediments to scientific confidence that the intervention had positive effects. Once an intervention program is deemed efficacious, research progresses to the next step—attempting to demonstrate that the program is also *effective*, meaning it shows positive benefits under less artificial and less carefully controlled conditions. Effectiveness is defined as the process of establishing how well an intervention works, under the conditions it would most typically be delivered, usually a community or general clinical practice setting (Lonigan et al., 1998). Effectiveness studies place less emphasis on controlling conditions of program delivery and more on evaluating interventions under typical conditions.

Determining *for whom and under what* circumstances intervention effects occur can be considered an issue of moderation effects (Holmbeck, 1997). The emphasis is often twofold in developing a strong understanding of moderating effects. First is determining for what groups and subgroups the intervention is beneficial. Often the interest is in demographic groups or groups that may differ in level or types of symptoms or related risk factors prior to intervention. A second interest is how the circumstances of intervention provision may affect its impact. For example, can an intervention delivered in a clinic have the same impact if delivered in a school? Or, does a violence prevention effort have an effect in highly violent communities that correspond to effects in other communities?

Determining *how* an intervention works depends on measurement of the strategies and activities of the intervention and how their use relates to changes in the processes thought to mediate the problem of interest. The emphasis is on testing whether the intervention effect on symptoms and functioning can be explained by changes in theoretically emphasized characteristics and processes (Baron & Kenny, 1986). For instance, cognitive-behavioral interventions for adolescent depression focus on reducing depressive symptoms, in part by decreasing negative thoughts. However, if we see reductions in depressive symptoms posttreatment, we cannot assume that one of the mechanisms of action responsible for improvements in treatment is a decrease in negative thoughts. Before drawing such a conclusion, treatment research examining cognitive-behavioral interventions for adolescent depression needs to test whether reductions in negative thoughts mediate depressive symptomatology posttreatment.

This chapter focuses on prevention as well as treatment, viewing them as both complementary and closely related avenues for fostering adolescent mental health. While it is still common to consider treatment and prevention separately, this chapter takes the view that, in fact, they are components in a spectrum of approaches needed to address adolescent mental health needs. We first review what is known about the efficacy and effectiveness of treatment and prevention for the most prevalent disorders of adolescence. We follow with a discussion of some pertinent issues and illustrative findings about mediation and moderation effects, concluding with implications for moving toward evidenced-based practice in adolescent interventions. It is important to note that many prevention programs occur prior to adolescence or in early adolescence as they are intended to prevent problems that often first appear in adolescence. Thus, the prevention programs we review later in the chapter target children with the goal of preventing psychopathology in adolescence.

TREATMENT AND PREVENTION RATHER THAN TREATMENT VERSUS PREVENTION

Although treatment and prevention of mental health problems of youth have long coexisted as part of psychology and related mental health disciplines, there has been a boundary between these with little crossover of evaluation efforts, particularly summary and review efforts. Although many reasons might be cited, this disconnection seems to have limited the understanding of each area, emphasizing allegiance to either treatment or prevention at the cost of a broader intervention spectrum perspective incorporating both.

Originally, treatment was considered separately from prevention. Prevention efforts were classified into three types: primary, secondary, and tertiary (Commission on Chronic Illness, 1957). Primary prevention is defined as programs that attempt to decrease the incidence of a disorder or illness by intervening with normal populations (Durlak & Wells, 1998; Mrazek & Haggerty, 1994). Secondary prevention, on the other hand, attempts to lower prevalence rates of established cases of the disorder or illness (Mrazek & Haggerty, 1994). Finally, tertiary prevention is defined as intervention that attempts to decrease the degree of dysfunction or disability associated with an existing disorder or illness (Mrazek & Haggerty, 1994).

This classification system has been superseded by another classification system that operates from a risk–benefit perspective targeting specific portions of the general population (Gordon, 1983). The risk–benefit perspective is defined as weighing the risk of an individual acquiring a disease against the cost, risk, and discomfort of the prevention program. Similar to the previous system, Gordon's system includes three categories: universal, selective, and indicated. However, this system also relates prevention to treatment and, in subsequent form, is used to relate prevention and treatment as a spectrum of interventions intended to address mental health problems (Mrazek & Haggerty, 1994). Universal prevention interventions target all members of an eligible population (Mrazek & Haggerty, 1994). Thus, universal programs are typically designated for the general public or for all members of a specific group such as high school students or parents. Selective prevention programs focus on groups of individuals who are at risk for future problems but who are not currently dysfunctional. The chance of developing the identified problem for these individuals is elevated compared to the general population (Mrazek & Haggerty, 1994). One example of individuals targeted for selective interventions includes youth of depressed parents who are consequently at greater risk for experiencing depression. Indicated prevention is defined as interventions intended for individuals who display "risk factors" or "abnormalities" that place them at high risk for future development of the disorder or illness (Mrazek & Haggerty, 1994). By this definition, one might consider indicated prevention programs to be the same as treatment. However, Gordon (1983) distinguishes this last type of prevention from treatment by clarifying that those individuals receiving indicated prevention programs are not symptomatic of the actual disorder or illness (e.g., show subsyndromal levels of symptoms). In subsequent refinement, this continuum included differentiation of treatment that is meant to repair or ameliorate symptoms from treatment that is intended to help manage a more chronic condition.

This spectrum is illustrated in Figure 3.1. This classification system includes three broad sections: prevention, treatment, and maintenance. Prevention interventions include only those programs designed for individuals who have not experienced the initial onset of a disorder. Treatment interventions are defined as programs that are (1) therapeutic in nature and (2) designed for individuals who display diagnostic levels of a disorder or whose symptoms approach diagnostic levels. Maintenance interventions include programs that are (1) supportive, educational, and/or pharmacological in nature, and (2) designed for individuals who have met psychiatric diagnostic levels, whose illness continues, and who may need long-term support (Mrazek & Haggerty, 1994). While this

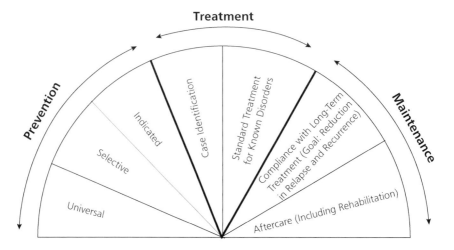

FIGURE 3.1. Interventions as a spectrum of related strategies. From Mrazek and Haggerty (1994). Copyright 1994 by National Academies Press. Reprinted by permission.

spectrum approach has often not been integrated into reviews of prevention and even less into reviews of treatment, we suggest that it provides a broad and useful perspective. While treatment and prevention can differ not only according to when they are implemented and how the population is targeted, the relative value of a given intervention seems more ascertainable if viewed within this spectrum (Tolan, 2002). The emphasis is on the relative level of risk of a person or group and the likely benefit of a given intervention rather than a presumption that one type of intervention is always preferable.

EVIDENCE OF EFFICACY

Treatment Efficacy

Over the past two decades we have made strides in testing the efficacy of many interventions for various types of adolescent psychopathology (Kazdin & Weisz, 2003). This has occurred for prevention as well as for treatment. Several years ago, a task force of the American Psychological Association's Division 12 on Clinical Child Psychology reviewed child and adolescent treatment outcome research and designated 25 interventions as empirically supported for use with children (Lonigan et al., 1998). Of those 25 interventions, 14 have been found to be efficacious with adolescent populations as well (Weisz & Hawley, 2002). Several of these interventions are summarized later in this chapter.

Research examining interventions for adolescent psychopathology has indicated that many interventions meant to have psychotherapeutic impact can be beneficial to the majority of adolescent clients if properly delivered (Kazdin, Bass, Ayers, & Rodgers, 1990; Weisz, Donenberg, Han, & Kauneckis; 1995; Weisz, Weiss, Alicke, & Klotz, 1987; Weisz, Weiss, Han, Granger, & Morton, 1995). Two of the meta-analyses cited previously assessed treatment outcome effects for adolescents specifically, separate from children. These two meta-analyses showed treatment effect sizes fall in the moderate to large range (e.g., median effect size of .58 standard deviation units in the review by Weisz et al., 1987, and of .82 in the study by Weisz, Weiss, et al., 1995). This range of effect sizes can be translated approximately to an average of 58–82% of adolescent clients receiving psychotherapy have better post-

treatment status than untreated comparisons. These effect sizes are on a par with those found for both children and adults and are as large, if not larger, than those found for many common medical procedures (Lipsey & Wilson, 1993; Weisz & Hawley, 2002). These effect sizes are based on a relatively equal number of studies of externalizing and internalizing problems, with a range of both genders well represented among the studies. In addition, therapist training levels have been fairly consistent across types of problems, suggesting that fidelity in intervention delivery is an important contributor to efficacy (Kazdin, Seigel, & Bass, 1992; Weisz et al., 1987).

These overall summary statistics demonstrate that basic efficacy exists for strongly conceptualized and carefully implemented treatments across disorders affecting adolescents. Meta-analyses have also suggested that effect size is not just dependent on intervention content but is also related to more structured interventions, more careful evaluation as part of the intervention, more careful and consistent training of providers, and provider fidelity to the protocol intervention (Lipsey & Wilson, 1993; Weisz et al., 1987). These findings suggest a strong advantage of research-based interventions for aiding adolescent mental health, including the type of organization and implementation approaches characterizing these interventions (e.g., structured, protocol-driven, careful training and supervision).

One implication is that a deliberate shift is needed toward using such evidence-based treatments as the interventions of choice for the disorder for which they are efficacious. There are examples of efficacious interventions for each of the most prevalent disorders affecting adolescents. Using such interventions seems preferable to using untested approaches or an eclectic mixing of techniques. However, knowing which programs produce benefits compared to no treatment or a less organized treatment-as-usual condition does not necessarily mean that the tested intervention is uniquely effective or that untested interventions are necessarily ineffective. Further, these tests do not, in general, provide information regarding under which circumstances such programs are most likely to work or how their effects might vary by populations and circumstances.

At the same time, there remains much room for improvement in the area of adolescent treatment. Often, interventions designed for use with adolescents are either downward adaptations of adult interventions or upward adaptations of child interventions. In fact, among the 14 interventions found to be efficacious with adolescents, only one was designed originally and specifically for adolescents (Weisz & Hawley, 2002). Adapting programs designed with older and younger populations for use with adolescents can neglect developmental issues specific to adolescence that might affect treatment success. Such developmental issues include biological (e.g., pubertal development), psychological (e.g., cognitive development), and social (e.g., peer and family relationships) changes. To date, adolescent treatment research has often failed to incorporate developmental theory or research into treatment models and/or when discussing research findings (Weisz & Hawley, 2002). Considering developmental theory in adolescent treatment research can better inform case conceptualization and risk appraisal, which can, in turn, affect treatment outcome.

In addition, while we have begun to identify efficacious interventions for adolescent populations, we have yet to substantially answer for whom, under what circumstances, and how most of these efficacious interventions work. Understanding interventions for adolescents thus rests on summarizing what is known and also noting important unresolved issues in advancing knowledge further. For instance, evidence suggests that rates of certain types of disorders increase in adolescence, such as depression, conduct problems, substance use, and specific types of anxiety disorders (e.g., social phobia and panic disorder) (Lerner, Villaruel, & Castellino, 1999; Reed & Wittchen, 1998). Comorbidity is also high, with some adolescents experiencing as many as three co-occurring psychological disorders (American Psychiatric Association, 1994). We discuss these issues about adolescent treatment and prevention within this chapter. The perspective throughout is that while some initial frameworks have been developed for disorders such as depression, anxiety, conduct, and attention-deficit/hyperactivity disorders (Weisz & Hawley, 2002), as well as substance use (Austin, Mcgowan, & Wagner, 2005), we are still in the early stages of developing a sophisticated and varied regime of intervention approaches for adolescent mental health problems.

Translating Treatment Efficacy to Effectiveness

The efficacy demonstrations that are the basis of the meta-analysis effect sizes differ from common clinical practices in several ways. They were more likely to (1) be behavioral or cognitive-behavioral than other approaches; (2) use specially trained therapists; (3) have carefully defined inclusion rules; (4) recruit participants; and (5) provide manualized or protocol-based interventions compared to common clinical practice (Weiss & Weisz, 1990; Weisz, Weiss, et al., 1995). Their generalization to common practice may be limited (Weisz, Weiss, & Donenberg, 1992). Also, as noted by Kazdin and colleagues (1992), most available studies do not include evaluations of most of the wide variety of psychotherapeutic methods being employed in the community with children and adolescents.

It may well be that many of the key concerns in determining effective practices are not easily addressed in most clinical trial research designs, rendering limited information about what works in a fashion that is considered informative from the perspective of practitioners and agencies (Chorpita, 2003). In other words, even though emotional state, behavior, and attitude change can be demonstrated under controlled field experimental conditions, empirical tests of clinical intervention services, as normally delivered, do not demonstrate benefits (Weisz, Donenberg, et al., 1995). For example, Weisz and Jensen (2001) reviewed 14 studies of treatment effectiveness for children and adolescents (ages 2–18) in which the following criteria needed to be present to be included in their analyses: (1) youth were clinic referred rather than recruited; (2) treatment was conducted in service-oriented clinics or agencies rather than nonclinical settings such as university labs; (3) therapy was delivered by practicing clinicians rather than researchers or trained research assistants; (4) therapy was an existing part of services offered by the clinic rather than a research-based treatment procedure within a larger clinical trial; and (5) studies needed to provide a comparison between the treated group and a control group that received either a placebo or no intervention. Results from their analyses found that the mean effect size across the 14 studies was –0.001. In other words, the average treated youth was no better after treatment than youngsters in the control group.

Such research suggests that adolescent treatment services provided in common clinical practice settings produce negligible effects compared to the efficacy research described earlier reporting effect sizes of up to .82 (Weisz, Weiss, et al., 1995). One conclusion that can be drawn is that intervention studies are of limited utility for guiding practice because they do not test the most common approaches or use common practices. An alternative interpretation is that common practices and approaches are not reliably beneficial and should be reorganized to follow the practices and use of the interventions found to have efficacy. This latter interpretation is supported by a recent study that showed that greater fidelity to a proven program designed to treat adolescent delinquency and related risk factors was related to effects (Henggeler, Schoenwald, Liao, Letourneau, & Edwards, 2002). Although there is a substantial and growing number of treatment efficacy studies, the status is still one of a thin strand of findings that is relatively limited in regard to defining the importance of implementation and service delivery characteristics, testing how efficacious interventions can be integrated into typical practices and procedures, or determining what service provider or client characteristics might constrain the benefits derivable from a given intervention. Extensive and concentrated efforts on developing a larger set of efficacious studies and empirical tests of training, supervision, and setting variations in intervention delivery and effects are key to moving beyond this promising but not assuring state of knowledge.

Prevention Efficacy

Similar to treatment, there has been a substantial production of empirical trials of prevention strategies for adolescent problems. However, unlike treatment, much of prevention of adolescent problems is based on interventions that occur during childhood years. Prevention also differs from treatment because often the focus is on either more general mental health issues or a particular social problem such as the prevention of drug abuse, teen pregnancy, academic failure, and aggression and violence rather than defined disorders or in preventing developmental risk related to multiple problematic outcomes (Durlak & Wells, 1997). There are also numerous prevention efforts that promote healthy development or have

nonspecific prevention effects (Cowen, 1997; Durlak & Wells, 1997). In addition, compared to treatment efforts, prevention efforts have focused more on organizing intervention trials around the portion of the population targeted and the stage of development of the problem at which prevention occurs (Price & Lorion, 1989). Universal programs, for example, work to prevent disorders and the incidence of problem behaviors among the general population, usually focusing on the whole population. Selective or high-risk preventive efforts focus on children and youth (or families) exhibiting or experiencing one or more risk factors empirically linked to the problem of interest. Indicated prevention efforts overlap with many treatment foci, as they target those evidencing early states of or a strong proclivity toward the problem to be prevented (Price & Lorion 1989; Tolan, 2002). For example, multisystemic treatment (MST) targets youth already involved in the juvenile justice system and works to prevent further incidents or greater seriousness of antisocial behavior. It could be viewed either as treatment or as an indicated prevention effort (Tolan & Guerra, 1994; Tolan & Gorman-Smith, 1997).

Meta-analyses of prevention programs support a judgment of efficacy for most mental health problems of children. However, this judgment is not based on the comprehensive reviews such as those found for treatment. For example, Durlak and Wells (1997), in perhaps the broadest meta-analysis of prevention for children to date, only considered primary or universal prevention efforts. Durlak and Wells note an average effect size of .30 for externalizing problems and .32 for internalizing problems. These effects are often sustained at follow-up (often about 1 year later). The effect sizes at follow-up for externalizing problems averaged .25 standard deviation units and for internalizing problems averaged .40 standard deviation units. Other meta-analyses and critical reviews have focused on specific areas of prevention, most often targeted/selective and indicated interventions. There is consistency across these reviews in identifying efficacy for a broad set of preventive interventions, with some examples for the major issues of youth mental health such as depression, anxiety, and conduct problems (Lipsey & Wilson, 1993; Tolan & Guerra, 1994; Tolan, 1996).

Although one can conclude that there are efficacious prevention efforts for most disorders and mental health problems of adolescence, it is less clear how specific the interventions are in which problems and disorders they affect. It is common for multiple problems and risk markers to be affected. An important notation in evaluating the research on prevention efficacy is that many prevention efforts have an implicit (and often explicit) emphasis on affecting developmental processes with an expectation of ensuring a general benefit for later adolescent behavior and mental health (Shure & Spivack, 1982). The view is that by altering important, more general processes one can divert developmental trajectories from problematic outcomes, reducing prevalence of later disorders and related problems. For example, one well-regarded prevention program, Promoting Alternative Thinking Strategies (PATHS), targets elementary-age children with the goal of preventing later emotional and behavioral problems by increasing overall emotional competence and management of emotions that might affect behavior. PATHS has been replicated in several instances; showing benefits for social problem solving and understanding of emotions, reductions in the number of youth who later experience internalizing and externalizing symptoms, and effects on conduct, social competence, and impulsivity (Greenberg & Kusche, 1998).

Thus, judging prevention efficacy has an additional complexity in that the focus may be on processes thought to protect and promote mental health and effective functioning generally. Similarly, interventions may affect many areas of mental health and indicators of functioning rather than a very specific disorder or single theorized etiological process. What is unclear is whether this is due to affecting shared risk processes, the comprehensiveness of the multicomponent interventions, or an interdependence of capability and risk (e.g., by aiding social competence and reducing susceptibility and exposure to social processes that might precipitate mental health problems in an at-risk youth). It is also not clear if the more general effects often found in prevention suggest some more general impact than often reported in treatment or simply more consideration of multiple impacts (Tolan & Gorman-Smith, 2003). Nevertheless, this does limit the extent to which a compendium can be compiled of prevention efforts for a given disorder or problem.

Similar to Weisz, Donenberg, and colleagues' (1995) consideration of what service organization methods were characteristic of efficacious treatment, Nation and colleagues (2003) reviewed previously published prevention studies targeting elementary-age children and early adolescents to identify common guiding principles of effective prevention programs. Results from their review highlighted nine principles that effective programs had in common. The first set of principles are related to program characteristics and, among other things, (1) are comprehensive in addressing a range of precursors or mediators relevant to the target problem; (2) utilize varied teaching methods to increase participants' skills; (3) expose participants to significant dosage in terms of contact hours, including follow-up booster sessions; (4) aid in the development of programs based on etiological and intervention theories; and (5) provide opportunities for participants to develop strong, positive relationships with a significant person in their lives. The second set of principles involves matching programs to the target group and includes the following: (1) delivery of intervention timed to have maximum impact; and (2) design of intervention that is culturally appropriate for participants. The last set of principles focuses on implementation and evaluation of prevention programs and includes the following: (1) outcome evaluations to determine programs' effectiveness; and (2) sufficient training, support, and supervision for staff members to enhance implementation of program. Not surprisingly, there is considerable overlap between these principles and those identified via meta-analyses of treatment (Weisz, Donenberg, et al., 1995).

Translating Prevention Efficacy to Effectiveness

There has not been the body of studies in application of prevention that there is in treatment to allow the meta-analytic examination of how effects might differ in practice from those found in basic efficacy studies. However, there are several efforts underway to test the impact of fidelity on the effects of prevention programs. For instance, in a recent effort to disseminate efficacious violence and drug use prevention, the Blueprints program (U.S. Department of Health and Human Services, 2001), evaluated the role of adherence on prevention program outcomes (Elliott & Mihalic, 2004). This effort emphasized two important trends among the attempts to disseminate ten Blueprint programs. First, many of the program developers were not prepared for translation of their programs to larger-scale implementation and several of the programs were difficult to disseminate without development to organize for application beyond efficacy trials. Second, although good adherence could be achieved with strong technical assistance (e.g., about 75–85% fidelity in most cases), this result required substantial effort. The authors note that adherence did relate to treatment outcome, with those user sites with less fidelity having limited impact. Similarly, a recent survey, focused on school-based violence prevention programming, found that most prevention programs being used had not been empirically tested (Gottfredson, 2001). Of the small proportion of schools using empirically tested programs, most were not implementing these as designed and had little or no technical assistance and management support. The few emerging results are consistent with those for treatment in suggesting that strong adherence and careful implementation as designed are likely to be key in achieving effectiveness.

GAP BETWEEN EFFICACY AND EFFECTIVENESS FINDINGS

Two conclusions can be drawn from the variance in effects demonstrated in efficacy studies and typical practice. One conclusion is that existing, non-research-based treatments used in general clinical practice and the tendency to mount prevention efforts without reliance on research-based programs leads to ineffective interventions. An alternative conclusion is that programs found to be efficacious within controlled research settings do not translate to the "real world." Limited research to date favors the first conclusion (Elliot & Tolan, 1999), and evidence addressing the second conclusion is virtually nonexistent. What little research exists examining the translation of efficacious programs into community settings suggests that such programs can be translated successfully through a careful merging of adherence to the intervention protocol and close collaboration between researchers developing and testing such programs and community-based

clinicians (Connor-Smith & Weisz, 2003; Henggeler et al., 2002). The translation problem then is how to ensure adequate fidelity and how to train community resources in the use of efficacious interventions, adherence to their protocols, and access to needed technical assistance.

If the goal is to implement efficacious interventions with fidelity, doing so is not just a technical exercise. It involves some thorny yet relatively unexplored problems of how to ensure adherence to intervention protocols and how to determine the essential characteristics of a given intervention to which adherence is sought. By adherence, we refer to the extent to which individuals and/or groups within general clinical practice settings include the prescribed components of efficacious interventions and omit proscribed components of such interventions (Yeaton & Sechrest, 1981). Unfortunately, there has not been much scientific study of what are the essential components of any of the efficacious interventions or how variation in adherence might affect impact. Adherence to treatment protocols has been measured in only 19% of child and adolescent outcome studies (Kazdin et al., 1990). Although some efforts have shown that adherence does affect impact, it remains unclear what is driving this effect (Henggeler et al., 2002). Is it completing the assigned tasks? Is it strong engagement and enthusiasm within a general framework provided by the intervention? Is it increasing structure and having a stable approach and strong regular supervision?

If the second conclusion is drawn—that efficacy research may be limited because it is often undertaken in unrealistic conditions—it leads to additional implications for translation other than treatment fidelity. From this perspective the inability to translate efficacious treatment programs into community settings relates to research designs that emphasize basic or main effects and therefore deemphasize how effects might depend on person and situation characteristics. They also rely on delivery organization and homogeneity among the clientele and settings of service delivery that are not typical of practice. In other words, perhaps the impact of empirically validated programs in "real-world" settings is drastically reduced because the circumstances of clients seeking treatment in general clinical practice or in how prevention efforts are organized are typically different from those of research-based interventions. If so, it is less a matter of adherence to fidelity of efficacious interventions undertaken with unrealistic levels of control over participant characteristics, conditions of implementation, and provider adherence. Instead, it is more a matter of undertaking strong scientific evaluations of promising approaches within more real-world settings (Tolan, 2004).

It is likely that both conclusions are warranted and each can inform progress in research and intervention practice. Research on two intervention programs provide some strong clues about issues of critical importance in translating research to practice and implementation of efficacious programs into practice in community settings. The Nurse–Family Partnership program, developed by David Olds, focuses on prevention of later child and adolescent problems through improving early health and development of low-income first-time mothers (including adolescent mothers) and their children through prenatal and infancy home visiting by nurses (Olds, 2002; Olds et al., 2002). The goal of this program is to change the future life-course trajectories of high-risk mothers and their children. The program is research and theory driven and has been tested in three separate randomized controlled research trials to determine the program's efficaciousness with different populations in different settings (Elmira, NY; Memphis, TN; and Denver, CO). Over time, results indicated that the program was successful in reducing dysfunctional care of children, improving maternal life course, and reducing not only child behavior problems but adolescent externalizing behaviors as well (Olds, 2002; Olds et al., 2002).

Since the success of this program, other similar types of programs have been attempted in community settings during the past 5 years. However, these programs have not been able to achieve the successful outcomes demonstrated by the Nurse–Family Partnership program (Olds, 2002). Thus, Olds and colleagues have attempted to collaborate with community and state agencies to ensure that the Nurse–Family Partnership program is implemented with fidelity. Olds argues that at least three conditions are necessary to ensure the fidelity of efficacious programs when implementing them in community settings. First, the communities and organizations that intend to adopt the program need to be fully knowledgeable about and sup-

portive of the program. Second, staff implementing the treatment program need to be well trained and supported to conduct the treatment program in the same manner in which it was conducted during the research trials. Third, data need to be collected as the program is being disseminated into communities to determine the effectiveness of the program within each individual community setting. Collecting such data helps to facilitate quality improvement efforts (Olds, 2002). Maintaining these conditions in an effort to ensure treatment fidelity can aid in translating this and other treatment and prevention programs into community settings.

The second program, MST, developed by Scott Henggeler and colleagues, is in a similar stage of development as the Nurse–Family Partnership program. The MST program is an intensive family-based treatment program used to treat violent juvenile offenders (Henggeler, Schoenwald, Borduin, Rowland, & Cunningham, 1998). Similar to the Nurse–Family Partnership program, the MST program has undergone multiple randomized controlled trials to determine the efficacy of this treatment program. Results from randomized controlled trials have consistently demonstrated MST's efficacy in reducing the number of arrests, drug use, and periods of incarceration. In addition the effort increases family cohesion and quality of peer relations. These results are sustained over time (Henggeler, Cunningham, Pickrel, Schoenwald, & Brondino, 1996).

As with the Nurse–Family Partnership program, the demand for MST in communities across the country grew as word of the program's success spread. Currently, MST programs are being implemented in thirty U.S. states and eight nations (Henggeler, 2003). When transporting MST into community settings, research has indicated through two separate studies of MST in community settings that adherence to the MST protocol is significantly related to better treatment outcomes for youth and their families (Schoenwald, Henggeler, Brondino, & Rowland, 2000). To increase the likelihood of maintaining the integrity of the MST program in community settings, several key variables have been identified (Brown et al., 1997). These variables are similar to those defined earlier by Olds in that they focus on the characteristics of the agency/organization and the therapist. In addition, Brown and colleagues argue that, because implementing MST is costly, it is important to establish a number of good funding resources.

The Nurse–Family Partnership program and the MST program provide two examples of ways in which research-based, efficacious intervention programs can be successfully translated into the real world. In addition, fidelity research on translating such interventions into practice settings provides information regarding key ingredients necessary to ensure fidelity is maintained. Such research suggests that when disseminating research-based programs into community practice, it is important that the treatment protocols are adhered to closely. However, these initial findings suggest that it is equally important that researchers and community providers continue to collaborate to better determine what conditions are necessary for effective interventions.

EVIDENCE-BASED INTERVENTIONS FOR ADOLESCENTS

Treatment Examples

As mentioned in the beginning of this chapter, the American Psychological Association's Division 12 (Clinical Psychology) Task Force on the Promotion and Dissemination of Psychological Procedures set out to identify empirically supported treatments for children and adolescents (Lonigan et al., 1998). To aid them in this endeavor, the Task Force established guidelines for categorizing treatment programs by level of evidence. Treatments categorized as "probably efficacious" needed to meet the following criteria: (1) conducted at least two, well-controlled, randomized, between-group studies demonstrating the intervention to be more effective than a no-treatment control group; (2) within these studies the sample characteristics were clearly described; and (3) the treatment used a treatment manual that clearly described the program and how to implement it (Lonigan et al., 1998). Treatments categorized as "well established" also had to have undergone two, well-controlled, randomized, between-group studies, conducted by different researchers, demonstrating the treatment program to be more effective than an alternative treatment programs (Lonigan et al., 1998). The Task Force identified 25 empirically supported treatments (Lonigan et al., 1998). As mentioned earlier, of those 25, 14 have been found to demonstrate positive outcomes with adolescents

(Weisz & Hawley, 2002). Similar efforts and compendiums of efficacious treatments can be found (e.g., Kazdin & Weisz, 2003). Examples of such efforts are reviewed here.

Treatment for Antisocial Behavior

MST, mentioned in the previous section of this chapter, is one of four treatment programs for adolescent antisocial behavior identified as probably efficacious under the criteria developed by the Division 12 Task Force (Brestan & Eyberg, 1998). The other three include anger control training with stress inoculation, assertiveness training, and rational-emotive therapy (Brestan & Eyberg, 1998). MST was initially developed with the goal of providing comprehensive mental health services to adolescents engaging in serious antisocial behavior and their families (Henggeler et al., 1998). In fact, the MST program is the only treatment program designed specifically for adolescents instead of evolving from a downward adaptation of adult programs or an upward adaptation of child programs (Weisz & Hawley, 2002).

MST operates from the belief that serious antisocial behavior is multidetermined by different systems surrounding the individual including youth characteristics and beliefs, family characteristics, peer relationships, school performance, and neighborhood characteristics (Henggeler et al., 1998). Because research suggests that there are multiple determinants of antisocial behavior, Henggeler and colleagues felt that a program designed to address the specific determinants within each family must be flexible as such determinants can vary significantly from family to family. Thus, each family that participates in the MST program collaborates with practitioners to establish family-specific treatment goals, as well as to develop and implement interventions to meet these goals. As Henggeler and colleagues have indicated, the capacity of MST to "address the multiple determinants of serious clinical problems in a comprehensive, intense, and individualized fashion . . . is one of the key components of the success of MST" (Henggeler et al., 1998, p. 8).

As the delivery of MST services needs to be flexible, the MST program does not provide practitioners with a session-by-session breakdown as one might typically see with other empirically supported manualized interventions. Rather, MST provides practitioners with nine guiding principles of the intervention and allows for flexibility within each principle. In addition, there is a strong belief that the interventions developed by the therapist, youth, and family will be most effective if implemented in the youths' natural environments. Often, this means that therapists provide intensive, home-based services. Duration of treatment is time limited, lasting 3 to 5 months depending on the intensity and number of problems and also on the effectiveness of the interventions.

Numerous studies have been conducted regarding the efficacy and effectiveness of MST for delinquent youth, as well as for other types of challenging clinical populations. Initial studies were university based, and involved doctoral-level students as the primary interventionists (Borduin, Henggeler, Blaske, & Stein, 1990; Borduin et al., 1995; Brunk, Henggeler, & Whelan, 1987; Henggeler et al., 1986). Findings from these studies indicated that MST improved family relations and reduced problematic behaviors such as adolescent antisocial behavior, adolescent sexual offending, and abusive or neglectful behavior by parents toward their children compared to other treatments such as individual outpatient counseling, behavior therapy, and typical community treatment offered to delinquent youth. In addition, results from a 4-year follow-up of one study demonstrated that only 26% of youth who received MST engaged in subsequent criminal behavior postintervention compared to 71% of youth who received individual therapy (Borduin et al., 1995). Such research suggested that MST was a promising intervention for youths with more severe types of psychopathology. However, it had not been tested within a general clinical practice setting at that point.

Consequently, a randomized controlled trial comparing the effectiveness of MST delivered through a community-based, state-run mental health center to regular services offered by the local juvenile justice department was conducted (Henggeler, Melton, & Smith, 1992). Results indicated that youth who received MST demonstrated a decrease in criminal activity and an increase in positive family relations and more prosocial peer relationships when compared to youth receiving services typically provided by the Department of Juvenile Justice (Henggeler et al., 1992). In addition, at the time of follow-up, nearly 2½ years later, the percentage of MST youth who had not been arrested postintervention was twice as high as the percentage rate for youth receiving regular juvenile justice services (Henggeler, Melton, Smith, Schoenwald, & Hanley, 1993).

Henggeler, Schoenwald, and Pickrel (1995) suggested that the success of MST in community settings is based on involving community therapists who resemble university-based therapists with regard to training and supervision, as well as the use of a treatment model that is structured, focused, and as ideally suited to meet the client's needs as possible. It has also been suggested that the flexible and individualized nature of MST enhances its transportability into community settings. Research examining the effectiveness of MST in community-based settings has found that poorer MST treatment outcomes, as compared to findings from previous efficacy/effectiveness studies, were associated with a lack of fidelity or adherence to the MST treatment principles (Henggeler, Melton, Brondino, Scherer, & Hanley, 1997).

Research on the MST program provides an excellent example of the transition from the development of an efficacious, university-based program to an effective, community-based program. As mentioned earlier, MST is being implemented worldwide. In addition, MST has been used with diverse samples of youth—males and females, Caucasian and African American, rural and urban, youth from single- and two-parent homes, and youth from a wide range of socioeconomic status. More recently, MST has begun to be used with other types of populations as well. It has been tested with substance-dependent youth, youth with severe psychiatric problems, and even youth with chronic medical conditions such as diabetes (Henggeler, 2003).

Finally, studies have examined potential mediators of MST outcomes (Huey, Henggeler, Brondino, & Pickrel, 2000). Huey and colleagues used path analysis to examine whether parental monitoring, family functioning, and deviant peer associations mediated MST adherence and youth delinquency. Changes in parental monitoring and family functioning were found to mediate MST adherence and youth delinquency. In addition, deviant peer associations served as a mediator between parental monitoring and treatment outcome, as well as for family functioning and treatment outcome (Huey et al., 2000). This research increases our understanding of how MST works. Based on these findings, we know, for instance, that adherence to MST produces increases in parental monitoring, which in turn produces decreases in deviant peer associations, resulting in an overall decrease in antisocial behavior. Understanding how a treatment affects change is important in order to maximize treatment efficiency. This concept is discussed in more detail later in the chapter.

Treatment for Anxiety Problems

To treat adolescent anxiety, Philip Kendall and colleagues developed the C.A.T. Project. The C.A.T. Project is a 16-session intervention specifically designed to treat adolescents with anxiety disorders or anxious problems (Kendall, Choudhury, Hudson, & Webb, 2002). The C.A.T. Project targets 14- to 17-year-old adolescents and is based on the empirically supported treatment the Coping Cat (Kendall et al., 2002). The Coping Cat was designed to treat anxiety in children ages 8–13. Both interventions use the theoretical principles of cognitive-behavioral therapy (CBT) and both treat adolescents with the C.A.T. Project targeting older adolescents and the Coping Cat targeting younger adolescents.

Drawing on CBT theory, which postulates that abnormal behaviors and faulty cognitions can be changed, the C.A.T. Project is divided into two sections. The first eight sessions are focused on identifying the adolescent's anxiety problems, increasing the adolescent's flexibility in thinking about these problems and developing strategies to change the adolescent's reactions, as well as his or her parents' reactions, when the adolescent becomes anxious. The cognitive-behavioral strategies are presented in a four-step plan, using the acronym FEAR. FEAR stands for the following four steps: **F**eeling frightened, **E**xpecting bad things to happen, **A**ttitudes and actions that will help, and **R**ewards and results (Kendall et al., 2002). These steps involve the adolescent identifying physical sensations related to anxious feelings, identifying anxious thoughts during anxious situations, developing positive ways of thinking and behaviors that will decrease anxiety in scary situations, and developing self-evaluation skills and self-rewards for success. The second section includes eight more sessions that focus solely on the application and practice of the strategies developed in the first eight sessions through exposure therapy to increasingly anxiety-provoking situations. The C.A.T. Project uses a leader manual and adolescent workbook that provide a session-by-session breakdown.

As mentioned earlier, the C.A.T. Project is based on and is consistent with the Coping Cat intervention. One of the main differences between the two interventions is that the C.A.T. Project provides more information to adolescents regarding the nature of anxiety, whereas the Coping Cat, designed for children and younger adolescents, does not. In addition, the C.A.T. Project includes more on using the FEAR plan, especially in diverse situations. Because adolescents are typically more developed in their cognitive ability, the C.A.T. Project also focuses more on "thinking traps" and the types of cognitive processes that can increase anxiety compared to the Coping Cat. Finally, the C.A.T. Project utilizes a more sophisticated reward system than the Coping Cat's sticker system to reinforce adolescents' successes.

It is important to note that the C.A.T. Project is not as well researched as the Coping Cat. However, we feel it is a promising treatment for older adolescents with anxiety disorders. The C.A.T. Project is based on the Coping Cat in theory and session content and, as described later, research using the Coping Cat intervention has demonstrated success in treating anxiety disorders in children and young adolescents and has been determined probably efficacious. In addition, Kendall and colleagues have accounted for some of the developmental differences between children and younger adolescents and older adolescents in the creation of the C.A.T. Project intervention such as increases in cognitive ability. Because the C.A.T. Project uses strategies found to be effective with younger adolescents and accounts for particular developmental needs among older adolescents, it is highly likely that the C.A.T. Project will demonstrate similar levels of success as the Coping Cat. However, it is important that the C.A.T. Project undergo the same rigorous research process as the Coping Cat to better determine its overall efficaciousness and efficacy.

While the C.A.T. Project is currently being evaluated for efficacy, the Coping Cat and other CBT interventions for anxiety disorders have been indicated as probably efficacious treatments by the Division 12 Task Force (Ollendick & King, 1998). In two separate randomized controlled trials, use of the Coping Cat intervention was found to significantly decrease anxiety disorders in both children and younger adolescents compared to a wait-list control group (Kendall, 1994; Kendall et al., 1997). Specifically, results indicated that 64–71% of those in the treatment group no longer met diagnostic criteria for their primary diagnosis of an anxiety disorder at the end of treatment, compared with 5–6% of the wait-list control group (Kendall, 1994; Kendall et al., 1997). Furthermore, a follow-up study of the first intervention trial published in 1994 revealed that gains made by the treatment group were sustained 1 year and 3 years posttreatment (Kendall & Southam-Gerow, 1996). In addition, of the youth in the second study, 1-year follow-up results revealed that 53% continued to not meet criteria for an anxiety disorder (Kendall et al., 1997) and 7.4-year follow-up results indicated that 90% continued to not meet criteria for their primary anxiety disorder (Kendall, Safford, Flannery-Schroeder, & Webb, 2004). In the 7.4-year follow-up, youth who responded positively upon initially receiving the Coping Cat intervention also had lower levels of substance use involvement and substance use–related problems (Kendall et al., 2004).

Research on the Coping Cat has also begun to examine for whom and under what circumstances this treatment for anxiety disorders is most effective. One study by Treadwell, Flannery-Schroeder, and Kendall (1995) examined differences in anxiety and treatment outcome based on sex and ethnicity. Youth diagnosed with an anxiety disorder, ages 8–13, participated in the Coping Cat treatment. Forty-one percent of the sample was female, 89% were Caucasian, and 11% of the sample of youth identified themselves as African American. Results demonstrated no significant differences in self-reported fears/anxieties and parent and teacher reports of fears/anxieties, or in diagnoses based on either sex or ethnicity. In addition, Treadwell and colleagues found no significant differences on treatment outcome by sex or ethnicity. These results suggest that boys and girls, as well as Caucasian and African American youth, experience similar fears and anxieties and respond similarly to the Coping Cat treatment. However, as this is only one study examining characteristic differences within the treatment populations, the findings are by no means conclusive. Future studies in this area need to be conducted to further address potential sex and ethnic differences with greater certainty.

Kendall and colleagues (2001) also examined comorbidity and its potential effect on treatment outcome. Seventy-nine percent of participating youth had at least one comorbid psychiatric diagnosis. Youths were randomly assigned to either a treatment group that received the Coping Cat intervention or a wait-list control group. Results indicated that while pretreatment comorbidity was not associated with differences in treatment outcome, treatment did appear to reduce comorbidity (Kendall, Brady, & Verduin, 2001). While 79% of youth met criteria for at least one additional disorder at intake, only 20% of youth continued to meet criteria for an additional disorder at follow-up (Kendall et al., 2001). This is an important finding as adolescents may sometimes experience as many as three or more co-occurring disorders. Thus, if the Coping Cat reduces incidence of comorbidity among younger adolescents, we are hopeful that the C.A.T. Project will likely have a similar impact on comorbid conditions among older adolescents experiencing anxiety disorders.

While studies examining the impact of sex, ethnicity, and even comorbidity on treatment outcome serve to increase our understanding of for whom the Coping Cat works, such research cannot tell us the mechanisms of action responsible for the program's efficacy. However, two such studies exist, one of which examined anxious and negative self-talk as a mediator between the Coping Cat intervention and treatment outcome (Treadwell & Kendall, 1996). More specifically, the authors hypothesized that youth participating in the Coping Cat intervention would experience decreases in anxious and negative self-talk, which, in turn, would result in decreases in symptoms of anxiety. Results indicated that based on youth reports, self-talk did serve as a mediator between treatment and treatment outcome (Treadwell & Kendall, 1996). A second study by Chu and Kendall (2004) looked at positive involvement at multiple points throughout treatment as a potential predictor of treatment outcome. Youth who displayed increased involvement midtreatment were significantly less likely to continue to meet criteria for their primary anxiety disorder at the end of treatment compared to youth who displayed less involvement (Chu & Kendall, 2004). Level of youth involvement at the beginning of treatment did not predict treatment outcome (Chu & Kendall, 2004). These results suggest that positive involvement by the midpoint of treatment may serve to produce more favorable outcomes. Such research provides important groundwork in helping us understand how the Coping Cat treatment works and hopefully encourages future research on mediators and moderators of treatment outcome.

Treatment for Depression

For adolescent depression, one of the only treatment programs to be determined as probably efficacious was developed by Gregory Clarke, Peter Lewinsohn, Hyman Hops and colleagues (Clarke, Lewinsohn, & Hops, 1990; Kaslow & Thompson, 1998; Lewinsohn, Clarke, Rhode, Hops, & Seeley, 1996). Adolescent Coping with Depression, like the C.A.T. Project, is based on principles from CBT and is also psychoeducational in that it teaches youth and their families about the etiology of depression, as well as skills they can use to alleviate depressive symptoms. Similar to the C.A.T. Project, Adolescent Coping with Depression is delivered with the use of a leader's manual, an adolescent workbook, and a parent workbook, which provide a session-by-session breakdown.

Adolescent Coping with Depression consists of 16 group sessions that last 2 hours each (Clarke et al., 1990; Lewinsohn et al., 1996). Sessions are held twice weekly for 8 weeks and typically include four to eight adolescents per group. Treatment sessions focus on helping adolescents develop relaxation skills; build a wide range of pleasant activities they can engage in; reduce negative thoughts; and increase social, communication, and problem-solving skills. The objective of developing these skills is that adolescents will improve their ability to regulate their moods and to manage situations that contribute to their depression. Parents of adolescents can participate in a separate but related program to support their adolescent in his or her treatment. The program for parents includes nine sessions, lasting 2 hours each, which are held once weekly. Parent groups provide parents with an overview of the skills their adolescent is learning so that they can better support their youth in utilizing these skills.

Two randomized controlled research trials have been conducted demonstrating the efficacy of Adolescent Coping with Depression (Clarke, Rohde, Lewinsohn, Hops & Seeley, 1999; Lewinsohn, Clark, Hops, & Andrews, 1990). Each study involved adolescents, ages 14–18, diagnosed with a depressive disorder. In both studies, youth were randomly assigned to one of three treatment conditions: the CBT component for the depressed adolescent only, the CBT component for the depressed adolescent and the parent component, or the wait-list control. The only difference between the first and second study was that the second study included follow-up conditions for adolescents assigned to either of the two treatment groups (CBT adolescent only or CBT adolescent and parent). Youths who participated in either of the two treatment groups were then randomly assigned to one of three follow-up conditions for the next 24 months: assessments every 4 months with booster sessions, assessments only every 4 months, or assessments only every 12 months (Clarke et al., 1999). Results from both studies indicated that significantly fewer youth in either treatment condition met criteria for a depressive disorder postintervention compared to the wait-list control groups (Clarke et al., 1999; Lewinsohn et al., 1990). In addition, youth in the two treatment conditions reported significantly greater reductions in depressive and anxious symptoms and maladaptive cognition and reported greater involvement in pleasant activities. These treatment gains were maintained at the 2-year follow-up. For the later study that compared assessments plus booster sessions to assessments only, there were no significant differences between groups assigned to one of the three different follow-up groups (Clarke et al., 1999).

Recently, Clarke and colleagues (2002) published a study in which they compared the effectiveness of Adolescent Coping with Depression to usual care in a health maintenance organization (HMO) setting for depressed adolescents whose parents were also depressed. Therapist compliance in delivering Adolescent Coping with Depression was rated at 90.8% based on review of audiotaped sessions. Interestingly, results comparing the two treatment conditions found no significant treatment differences between the groups posttreatment and at 12- and 24-month follow-up periods: Both treatment groups improved substantially with between 89% and 92% of youth recovered at the 24-month follow-up period. The authors suggested several possible reasons for the lack of between-group differences. First, the target population was different from efficacy studies examining Adolescent Coping with Depression. Perhaps there is a greater genetic component contributing to depression among adolescents who have depressed parents. Second, although the authors examined treatment fidelity, conditions in this study were less controlled than previous efficacy studies in that the authors did not control for comorbidity and other potential moderating variables in this effectiveness trial. A third possibility is that usual services used specifically to treat adolescent depression are equally as effective as empirically supported interventions. As the authors suggested, further research needs to be conducted to further evaluate the effectiveness of Adolescent Coping with Depression in general clinical practice setting.

Research examining Adolescent Coping with Depression has also focused on both potential mediators and moderators (Kaufman, Rohde, Seeley, Clarke, & Stice, 2005; Rohde, Clarke, Lewinsohn, Seeley, & Kaufman, 2001; Rohde, Clarke, Mace, Jorgensen, & Seeley, 2004). The first study looked at four potential mediators of treatment and posttreatment depressive symptoms among youth diagnosed with major depression and conduct disorder (Kaufman et al., 2005). The four mediators included negative cognitions, engagement in pleasant activities, therapeutic alliance, and group cohesion. Adolescents who received Adolescent Coping with Depression were significantly more likely to experience reductions in negative thoughts, which, in turn, were related to reductions in depressive symptoms at the end of treatment. On the other hand, engagement in pleasant activities, therapeutic alliance, and group cohesion did not serve as mediators for treatment and posttreatment outcomes.

Overall treatment outcomes were also assessed in this sample of youth with major depression and comorbid conduct disorder at the end of treatment, as well as 6-month and 12-month posttreatment (Rohde et al., 2004). Youth were recruited from the juvenile justice system and randomly assigned to either Adolescent Coping with Depression or a life skills/tutoring control condition. Immediately following treatment, youth who received Adolescent Coping with Depression reported greater reductions in depressive symptoms and improvements in social functioning compared to youth in the control condition. However, rates of conduct problems did not change and end-of-treatment differences were no longer distinguishable between groups at the 6- and 12-month follow-up periods. Rohde and col-

leagues (2001) examined potential moderators using data from combining the two samples used in the initial aforementioned efficacy studies. Of 151 adolescents participating in treatment for depression, 40% had a comorbid disorder. Results indicated that comorbidity did not have a significant impact on the efficacy of the two treatment conditions compared to the control wait-list condition. In addition, while comorbid youth reported greater severity of depressive symptoms at intake, they also reported greater decreases in depressive symptoms posttreatment compared to youth without a comorbid disorder. Interestingly, depressed youth with comorbid substance abuse/dependence disorders experienced a slower time to recovery and youth with comorbid externalizing disorders experienced greater recurrence of depression compared to other comorbid youth. The results of these two studies that looked at comorbidity are important in that they pose a question that can only be answered by future research: Does the Adolescent Coping with Depression course need to be modified in some way to maximize efficacy and, ultimately, effectiveness, for depressed adolescents with substance abuse and externalizing diagnoses? Future treatment outcome research on this program can shed light on the answers to these and potentially other related questions.

Prevention Examples

Prevention of Antisocial Behavior

In 1990, two programs of research aimed at preventing antisocial behavior were launched. While quite different in focus, each tested theoretically driven interventions for aggression and related antisocial behavior and yielded efficacy evidence. The first, FastTrack (Conduct Problems Prevention Research Group, 1999), focused on preventing onset and reducing the long-term problems of children at risk for experiencing conduct disorders in adolescence. The second, the Metropolitan Area Child Study (Metropolitan Area Child Study Research Group, 2002a), focused on reducing average levels of aggression and serious antisocial behavior among school-age children living in high-risk urban communities. Both programs (1) target children with the objective of preventing antisocial behavior in early and late adolescence; (2) were built on prior promising efforts to organize multicomponent programs meant to affect the child and proximal developmental influences; and (3) were tested in a random-assignment trial over several years and have yielded efficacy for aggression and related risk markers (Conduct Problems Prevention Research Group, 1999; Gorman-Smith, 2003; Metropolitan Area Child Study Research Group, 2002a, 2002b).

Effects of the FastTrack Program

FastTrack focused on children beginning in first grade. Children were screened based on teacher and parent behavior ratings to focus on children displaying the most aggressive behavior. The intervention combined a parent training program with a social-cognitive program designed to facilitate emotional understanding and self-control, tutoring in reading for those in need, and a consultation program for classroom teachers. Intervention began in 1st grade and continued in some form up through the 10th grade. While the intervention was ongoing, it was less intensive toward the end of elementary school and, after a second intensive intervention during middle school, is less intensive during high school. This approach was based on the view that conduct disorder is a chronic problem, that most of those in the high-risk group targeted had multiple risk factors and needed multiple intervention needs, and that risk was most affected during key developmental transitions (Conduct Problems Prevention Research Group, 2002).

The universal-level program was composed of a classroom curriculum that was taught by teachers. This curriculum adapted PATHS (Kusche & Greenberg, 1994) to focus on prosocial behavior and friendship skills, emotional understanding and self-control, communication and conflict resolution skills, and problem-solving skills. The curriculum was designed to progress developmentally across grades 1–5 and ranged in length per year from 9 to 22 sessions. The indicated intervention was applied to only the high-risk children and their families and addressed six areas of risk and protective factors: (1) parenting; (2) child social problem-solving and emotional coping skills; (3) peer relations; (4) classroom atmosphere and curriculum; (5) academic achievement; and (6) home–school relations. These were targeted through parent training, home visiting, peer-pairing social skills support, parent–child relationship enhancement, social skills training, and academic tutoring.

While all received parenting groups, social skills training, and parent–child relationship enhancement sessions throughout the elementary school years, beyond first grade, there was variation in the extent to which home visiting, peer pairing, and academic tutoring was provided depending on need. These were applied where poor adaptation in these areas was noted. Staff were carefully trained educational and mental health professionals, with pairs of staff responsible for three groups that consisted of 15–18 families (Conduct Problems Prevention Research Group, 2002). Implementation was carefully monitored and well supported through ensuring school and family commitment to the program and extensive outreach to the families and schools.

FastTrack was tested in four cities (Durham, Nashville, State College Pennsylvania, Seattle), with students randomly assigned to intervention or controls (defined as treatment as usual) by school within site. Effects were first tested for the end of second grade, 2 years postintervention. Results were reported for the high-risk group separately from the whole cohort of the targeted youth. The high-risk intervention group evidenced positive effects on academic achievement, parenting practices, and child behavior ratings. These initial results suggest a significant impact on behaviors thought to serve as risk factors for developing conduct disorder as well as symptoms often comprising conduct disorder (Conduct Problems Prevention Research Group, 1999). Results for the general cohort showed improved social-cognitive skills, better peer acceptance, and teacher-rated behavior. At third grade, lower rates of special education referral were noted for intervention participants compared to high-risk controls (Conduct Problems Prevention Research Group, 2002). Notably, these whole group results were consistent whether or not it included the high-risk subgroup in the universal intervention effects analyses (Conduct Problems Prevention Research Group, 1999).

The Conduct Problems Prevention Research Group has also reported on predictors of effects with a particular focus on predictors of outcome at the end of third grade (Conduct Problems Prevention Research Group, 1999, 2002). In the universal intervention group, demographic characteristics have not been important moderators, although some initial effects did not generalize across sexes (Conduct Problems Prevention Research Group, 1999). However, psychopathology and level of social support of the parent did moderate level of impact for several measures of child aggression and oppositional behavior. However, these moderators' strength varied some by outcome and source (Conduct Problems Prevention Research Group, 2002). These results suggest that a complex set of person and situation characteristics need to be considered to understand variation in impact based on timing of testing outcome and the aspect of functioning of interest.

Effects of the Metropolitan Area Child Study

The Metropolitan Area Child Study was intended to prevent adolescent violence, school failure, and other antisocial behavior. This intervention study combined a social-cognitive intervention for students with teacher training and consultation that was provided to all students in an intervention school (Guerra, Eron, Huesmann, Tolan, & Van Acker, 1997). High-risk students received small-group social-cognitive training and a family intervention. The interventions were delivered for 2 years to seven successive cohorts of students in two midwestern cities (Chicago and Aurora, IL). While the Chicago schools were in neighborhoods with some of the highest crime and poverty rates in the country (e.g., inner-city communities; Wilson, 1987), the Aurora schools served impoverished and crime-burdened (urban-poor) communities but had more social and economic resources. In other words, the Chicago communities typify those found in the inner city of very large cities, whereas Aurora communities typify those found in most American cities. This design permitted consideration of how the social ecology might affect impact of the intervention. A second design feature of this study was to compare the effects if the intervention was undertaken earlier (e.g., beginning in second grade) versus later (e.g., beginning in fifth grade). A third design feature was to compare the effects of less intensive intervention (e.g., the classroom intervention only, compared to the classroom plus the small group, compared to the classroom plus small group plus family intervention).

The interventions were meant to affect different contributors to risk for aggression, violence, and related problems such as school fail-

ure and substance abuse. For example, the teacher consultation and training was intended to improve teacher behavior management and instructional methods, which should reduce off-task time in classroom and misbehavior of high-risk youth. Teachers participated in a series of workshops that included information about effective instructional and behavior management techniques followed by opportunities to rehearse use of such skills under supervision of trainers. These workshops were followed up by monthly meetings with teams of teachers to review implementation of the strategies and issues they faced in their classrooms (Gorman-Smith, 2003). The social-cognitive classroom program was intended to aid children in developing skills such as mean–ends thinking, norms about aggression, and aggression-related cognitive rehearsal that were expected to reduce tendency to use aggression.

The program consisted of 20 sessions over 2 years and provided one class session per week. Research staff provided the training, which emphasized basic social-cognitive coping skills such as means–ends thinking, development of alternate responses in the face of frustration, and orientation of self-concept to personal goals and social responsibilities. Units teaching youth to apply these coping skills to different typical social conflicts and aggression-provoking situations followed the initial skill-building sessions. In these sessions, exercises and rehearsals of use of skills were emphasized (Guerra et al., 1997). The small-group program was intended to build on these social-cognitive skills and improve peer relationship skills and social skills. Thus, while covering the same topics as the classroom social-cognitive intervention, these groups (meeting once a week), focused on more practice of skills, self-control skills, and management of peer relationships. Like the classroom social-cognitive effort, these sessions were highly structured and included information, cognitive exercises, and behavioral practice (Letendre, Henry, & Tolan, 2003).

The family intervention was intended to improve or maintain strong parenting practices, aid family communication, and support effective family problem solving. The 22-week program emphasized development of clear and consistent parenting, use of positive parenting and strong monitoring, clear and direct communication among family members, organization of family rules and roles, and family problem solving for developmental and social setting problems. This intervention component only lasted over 1 school year (Tolan & McKay, 1996). Results from tests of proximal effects suggest that the impact depends to some extent on which outcome is of interest but overall such effects are limited to youth provided early intervention. In addition, some effects are related to community type. Effects did not evidence gender dependency, nor is there evidence of ethnic group differences beyond those associated with community type.

Initial tests of effects focused on aggression and academic functioning. Overall benefit for high-risk youth was found for aggression from the full intervention (all three components) in the urban-poor but not inner-city communities, if delivered early in the elementary school years. However, among the highest-risk portion of the sample, there were positive effects from the full intervention, if offered early, in both types of communities. This finding suggests that in high-risk communities a strong direct effect on aggression requires a multicomponent approach, particularly one with a strong family approach (Metropolitan Area Child Study Research Group, 2002a). Subsequent path analysis suggested that the program led to improved parenting, which related to more child compliance and less aggression (Tolan, Hanish, McKay, & Dickey, 2002). Further survival analyses suggest longer-term benefits in delaying onset of substance use (Tolan, 2001).

Initial tests of effects on academic functioning showed a positive effect across community types, even for the classroom intervention condition only, but only for those in the early intervention condition (Metropolitan Area Child Study Research Group, 2002b). Subsequent analyses showed that the program led to better use of teacher attention to manage child behavior and more on-task time during instruction, suggesting that the target of training led to improved achievement (Gorman-Smith, 2003).

Test of the impact on social cognition related to aggression showed that the social-cognitive interventions affected measured features such as perceived norms, cognitive scripts related to aggression, and social problem solving as expected. In addition, improvement in these social-cognitive features was related to decreased aggression subsequent to the initial intervention (Metropolitan Area Child Study Research Group, 2003).

Prevention of Anxiety

With regard to the prevention of anxiety, the Queensland Early Intervention and Prevention of Anxiety Project has developed an empirically supported prevention program for children and adolescents, ages 7–16, at risk for developing anxiety disorders in adolescence and adulthood (Barrett, Lowry-Webster, & Turner, 2000a, 2000b; Dadds, Spence, Holland, Barrett, & Laurens, 1997; Dadds et al., 1999). Their prevention program targets youth displaying mild anxious features to youth meeting criteria for an anxiety disorder but who are in the less severe range. Based on definitions of prevention discussed earlier, this prevention program falls in the range of indicated to targeted prevention. The prevention program was originally called The Coping Koala but was changed to the FRIENDS program in 1999. The FRIENDS program is presented in 10 group sessions and is an Australian modification of the Coping Cat anxiety intervention program developed by Kendall (reviewed earlier in this chapter). The FRIENDS prevention program utilizes the same principles and strategies as the Coping Cat, only it teaches them within a group format.

Dadds and colleagues (1997) have conducted one large-scale, randomized controlled trial comparing the efficacy of the Coping Koala Prevention Program to a no-intervention control group. Children and younger adolescents from eight different schools were screened for anxiety problems. Those displaying multiple symptoms of anxiety were selected to participate and randomly assigned to either the Coping Koala prevention intervention or a monitoring group. Posttreatment results indicated that youth in the intervention group displayed significantly reduced rates of anxiety compared to the monitoring group and that these results were maintained 6 and 24 months after the intervention was delivered (Dadds et al., 1997, 1999). Interestingly, girls in the intervention group who reported higher levels of anxiety pretreatment still displayed significant anxiety problems at the 24-month follow-up.

Since the program changed its name, there have been numerous evaluations attesting to its efficacy. The FRIENDS prevention program has been evaluated within a randomized controlled trial as a universal prevention program delivered in school settings (Lowry-Webster, Barrett, & Dadds, 2001; Lowry-Webster,

Barrett, & Lock, 2003). Results indicated that youth who received the FRIENDS program experienced significant reductions in anxious symptoms compared to youth in the comparison condition, even after controlling for preintervention levels of symptomatology. In addition, youth who reported higher levels of anxiety at the onset of the intervention also experienced greater reductions in depressive symptoms at the end of treatment. These gains were maintained at the 12-month follow-up.

The FRIENDS program has also been evaluated based on the type of staff delivering the intervention (teachers vs. psychologists; Barrett & Turner, 2001) and with youth of various racial and ethnic backgrounds (Barrett, Sonderegger, & Sonderegger, 2001; Barrett, Sonderegger, & Xenos, 2003). In comparing the effectiveness of the prevention program as delivered in a school setting by either teachers or psychologists, results indicated that youth in both the teacher-led and psychologist-led intervention groups experienced fewer symptoms of anxiety postintervention compared to youth in the usual condition, suggesting that the FRIENDS program can be effectively delivered within the school setting by school staff. The FRIENDS prevention program was also utilized with non-English-speaking immigrant youth in Australia (Barrett et al., 2001, 2003). Compared to the wait-list control condition, immigrant youth in the prevention condition displayed lower anxiety and a more positive future outlook and these gains remained present at the 6-month follow-up assessment. The authors suggest strategies for enhancing the FRIENDS prevention intervention to be more culturally sensitive.

Currently, the FRIENDS program has been adopted in over eight different countries and is endorsed by the World Health Organization. However, despite its success, future research is needed to examine whether the impact of the prevention program on anxiety is maintained over a longer period of time, more specifically, throughout the course of adolescence. In addition, it is important that future studies continue to examine the impact of sex, ethnicity, age, and other related variables on the efficacy and effectiveness of the FRIENDS program. The finding that the prevention program was not as effective for girls with more severe anxiety problems suggests that for these girls, perhaps a more intensive prevention program or one that includes additional components specific to

this population is needed. Another possibility for this difference may be that the timing of the prevention program needs to be examined.

Prevention of Depression

There are several empirically proven programs that can be considered prevention of depression. Some focus on youth based on elevated levels of depression (Clarke et al., 1995), while others target children at risk due to parental affective disorder (Beardslee et al., 1996). Beginning in 1990, Beardslee, Versage, Wright, and Salt (1997) have been evaluating an intervention for children and early adolescents, ages 8–15 whose parents have been diagnosed with an affective disorder. As these youth are far more likely to be diagnosed with an affective disorder and other mental health problems in adolescence and adulthood than youth of parents who do not have mood disorders, the intent was to target this high-risk group prior to the emergence of clinical-level mood disorder (Beardslee, Versage, & Galdstone, 1998). Beardslee and colleagues developed two short-term interventions that take different approaches to affecting risk. The first is a two-session psychoeducational lecture and the second is a four to eight session clinician-centered intervention designed to aid families in communication about depression and improve youth's ability to cope with stress and other depression risk factors.

The family-clinician-centered intervention focuses on enabling families to discuss the specific problems related to the affective disorder of the parent, which serves as a general model for family communication. In addition, the clinician acts as a family consultant through periodic check-ins from the family (Beardslee et al., 1997). Results have indicated increased resilience on the part of at-risk children as well as improved family communication overall. Children and adolescents in the study reported an increase in coping skills and an improved ability to make sense of their internal and external environments (Beardslee et al., 1997, 1998). As theorized, communication improved within the family and coping increased. It appears the clinician-centered approach leads to stronger and better sustained effects. However, there has not been a study reporting on the impact on rates of adolescent affective disorder at this point. One major limitation is that the rate of eventual disorder even among those with a family history of affective disorder may not be high enough to permit sensitive detection of effects in the sample.

RELATING INTERVENTION EFFECTS TO HOW AND FOR WHOM THEY WORK

As noted at the outset of this chapter, intervention research should aim to provide direction that not only indicates what the effective approaches are but also demonstrates how the interventions work as theorized and determines for whom a given intervention is advisable. As noted previously, some of the empirically based interventions have had tests of whether outcomes were attributable to the intervention targets (mediators) and to what extent results vary by demographic, risk, and developmental–ecological differences (moderators). However, treatment outcome research examining mediators and moderators is still, for the most part, a rarity, especially in the area of prevention. The remainder of this chapter highlights the importance of considering mediators and moderators in adolescent treatment and prevention research.

Tests for Mediator Effects

A mediator is defined as a variable that accounts for the relation between the independent or predictor variable and the dependent or outcome variable (Baron & Kenny, 1986). As applied to intervention evaluation, the interest is in how change in a target of the intervention can explain the difference in the level of an outcome variable attributed to intervention participation. Mediating variables attempt to explain why or how effects occur. For instance, perhaps we hypothesized that the impact of CBT on anxiety was due to the increase in coping skills developed during intervention. To determine this, the following four conditions would need to be met: (1) a significant relation between intervention participation and reduced anxiety symptoms posttreatment; (2) a significant relation between participation and improved coping skills; (3) a significant relation between improved coping skills and lower anxiety symptoms; and (4) a substantial reduction in the relation between participation and lower anxiety symptoms once the relation between change in coping skills and change in symptoms is considered (MacKinnon & Dwyer,

1993). It should be noted that as most interventions have several targets and emphasize multiple beneficial processes, it might be that tests of a single process might not fully explain mediation effects. In addition, there may be complex dependencies between processes and activities of a given intervention and between activities targeting theoretical mediators and nonspecific characteristics such as intervention provider experience that can affect outcomes (Letendre et al., 2003).

Weersing and Weisz (2002) recently reviewed treatment outcome studies for anxiety, depression, and disruptive behaviors among children and adolescents to assess the current state of clinical research in examining mediators. Their findings indicated that 30% of anxiety trials, 79% of depression trials, and 77% of disruptive behavior trials measured potential mediating variables. In addition, a majority of the studies examining potential mediating variables found that treatment significantly impacted these variables. Unfortunately, most of the treatment studies reviewed that included mediating variables failed to test for mediation. Rather, the potential mediators were often treated as outcome variables. Weersing and Weisz found this to be true even in studies whose primary objective was to seek mediation effects. The potential mediating variables were often measured simultaneously with the treatment outcome variables. Thus, even if the investigators of those studies wanted to reanalyze the data to assess for mediators, they are unable to do so because of when the data was collected temporally. To better understand mediators in adolescent treatment, additional studies are needed that focus solely on treatment with adolescents, consist of a research design conducive to examining mediators, and include measures that specifically target potential mediators.

Prevention efforts focusing on mediation are even more scarce (Greenberg et al., 2003). Prevention theories often include more complex and multidimensional theories of mediation compared to intervention theories. Many prevention efforts include a presumption that intervention can affect developmental trajectories, not just reduce symptoms (Tolan & Gorman-Smith, 2003). In addition, many extend this developmental view to consider transactions between risk and effects of intervention; it could be that intervention not only reduces risk susceptibility but also has an ensuing reduction of risk exposure and may catalyze protective factors (Cowen, 1997). Some theories suggest that the developmental impact of prevention is to change the interrelation of risk factors or promote competencies that may generalize (Kellam & Rebok, 1992). These theoretical formulations bring forth complexities about interventions within a developmental perspective that may not be as explicitly considered in treatment. They may require theoretical specificity in testing mediation that goes well beyond what can be firmly drawn from existing normal development, risk, and intervention effects literature (Tolan, 2002; Tolan & Gorman-Smith, 2003).

One example of an attempt to test mediation or how a prevention intervention works was reported by Tolan and colleagues (2002). Through repeated assessments across the family intervention of the Metropolitan Area Child Study, this study first documented that intervention participants changed in targeted parenting practices and child behavior over the course of the intervention. In addition, the analyses related change in parenting to a strong alliance with the intervention provider and showed that this change in parenting subsequently mediated change between pretest level of aggression and posttest level of aggression. The relation of change in parenting to change in aggression was partially mediated by increased child compliance and social competence. Within the pattern of overall effects, a subsequent study showed that there were some families that engaged quickly and improved substantially in a linear change pattern, while others showed initial resistance and dips in skills prior to improvement, yet others never improved in parenting and showed no change in child aggression (Hanish & Tolan, 2001). Other examples of tests of mediation can be found in the literature, and it is becoming more common for intervention trials to include explicit focus on measuring process and change in targets as mediators of outcomes. However, knowledge remains limited as to the number of programs that have empirically demonstrated desirable effects.

Tests for Moderator Effects

A moderator is defined as a variable that explains variations in strength and/or direction of the relation between two other variables: the independent or predictor variable and the dependent or outcome variable (Baron & Kenny, 1986). As applied in intervention research, the interest is in characteristics and conditions that might explain differences in intervention effect levels. Moderator variables attempt to describe under what conditions or when certain effects will occur. For instance, a recent test of the SAFEChildren program, a program designed to affect parenting skills of participants living within inner-city communities, found that the impact on parenting skills was moderated by preintervention parenting capability (Tolan, Gorman-Smith, & Henry, 2003). More specifically, the impact on parental monitoring was limited to those parents showing lower parenting skills prior to intervention.

Typical moderators of interest include demographic characteristics such as sex and age; provider characteristics such as experience, adherence to protocols, and interpersonal skills; and setting characteristics such as school climate and community characteristics. Moderator analyses can be challenging to typical intervention research designs because they depend on the natural variation within the sample and the intervention provision, thus requiring substantial variation and large sample sizes. In addition, it means sampling so that different subgroups and conditions are systematically represented. Typically, these relations are tested by including an interaction term in the analysis equation to represent expectation of differential effect due to some difference on another variable (e.g., intervention by sex term to test for sex moderation). Such tests can strain the sensitivity capabilities (power) of many designs because of the need to precisely differentiate intervention effects from sex differences from the interaction of these two. In general, this means many moderation effects are likely to be underestimated.

Several meta-analyses have been conducted to explore potential moderators of treatment outcomes. Weisz, Donenberg, Han, and Weiss (1995) conducted a meta-analysis examining eight potential moderators for child and adolescent treatment outcomes. Results indicated that severity of target problem, setting (research vs. general clinical practice), and type of intervention (behavioral vs. nonbehavioral in nature) moderated treatment outcomes. Holmbeck and colleagues (2000) examined 34 studies of CBT with adolescents for consideration of developmental timing of the intervention. Only one study examined age as a moderator, limiting the understanding of how adolescent development and intervention effects might relate (how age and related developmental differences might moderate impact). Durlak, Fuhrman, and Lampman (1991) noted that available studies that suggested treatment effect sizes for adolescents were almost twice the number found for children. This research suggests that currently, while data implies that treatment for adolescents may be more effective than treatment for children, there is a limited basis for understanding how moderators such as adolescence and the stage of adolescence might affect intervention impact.

Several prevention programs have shown that effects are moderated by initial risk level (e.g., Metropolitan Area Child Study Research Group, 2002a; Stoolmiller, Eddy, & Reid, 2000). In addition, in some cases sex and age differences have been found to moderate intervention outcome, although not with much consistency (Conduct Problems Prevention Research Group, 1999; Metropolitan Area Child Study Research Group, 2002a). However, there are too few studies to permit substantive conclusions regarding the key conditions under which prevention interventions are most effective. Although many classes of moderators can be identified that are relevant to understanding what works for whom, we highlight three of particular relevance: contextual factors, cultural and ethnicity differences, and co-occurrence or comorbidity of problems. Each, of course, is a very complex issue on multiple levels, from construct definition to measurement operationalization to theorizing just what role they might play in intervention effects. In fact, it is a reasonable critique that these factors cannot be presumptively considered moderators; some theories might argue these are mediators or need to be integral to the intervention and not to be considered apart from it (Holmbeck, 1997). However, we focus on these three topics here because they are among those moderators most likely to be useful in developing a regime of interventions.

Contextual Factors

The contention that the context of an intervention can affect its impact seems less controversial than specifying *how* it might affect impact. Most commonly, context refers to social ecology in relation to a school or neighborhood, for example (Tolan, Guerra, & Kendall, 1995).

Evidence that context matters is supported by the difficulty in replicating the relationship of predictors of developmental functioning to risk across contexts (Catalano, Hawkins, Krenz, & Gillmore, 1993; Sue, Kuraski, & Srinivasan, 1999), of differential risk across settings (Gorman-Smith, 2003), and of differential relation of intervention to risk (Stoolmiller et al., 2000). For instance, research has indicated that parenting practices and their influence on development are partially determined by the sociological characteristics of the community (Furstenberg, 1993). Young mothers living in the most dangerous and poor urban neighborhoods, for example, isolated their families from neighborhood social activities in an effort to increase their family's safety (Furstenberg, 1993). Although this parenting strategy increased mothers' sense of safety, it also cut them off from developmentally valuable interactions with peers and tests of individual autonomy. Also, it may reduce opportunities for social support within their neighborhood. Additional research has found that in inner-city communities where there are strong neighborhood social relations, children in families marked by poor parenting and family relationships were less likely to show serious and chronic patterns of delinquency than children from such families living in communities without this protective neighborhood characteristics (Gorman-Smith, Tolan, & Henry, 2000). These examples demonstrate that the context of neighborhood (e.g., poor, inner-city, and dangerous) can have an impact on parenting, as well as on child and family outcomes.

Similarly, it is likely that one can find intervention effects to differ by community and other contextual characteristics such as school and setting of intervention (Multisite Violence Prevention Project, 2004). At the very least, context deserves careful consideration to determine when and how it might affect interventions, and more specifically how its consideration should be integrated when implementing a given approach. There are two aspects of context that seem clearly of importance in understanding interventions for adolescents. First, we must consider how contextual factors impact various forms of adolescent psychopathology and interventions. Theoretical and subsequent operationalization for the testing of contextual characteristics seems likely to improve the level of effects as well as certainty about under what circumstances a given intervention is likely to be effective. This can refer to including impact of context in the intervention design. For example, the MST intervention program reviewed earlier focuses on multiple systems affecting families based on prior risk studies. The program recognizes that families live within social systems and that such systems are important areas of functioning and can affect the ability of the intervention to change child risk and family functioning and to maintain any gains made in treatment. Interestingly, although the MST program used prior research studies examining the impact of context on risk, we did not come across any studies that examined context as a moderator for treatment outcomes among adolescents participating in the MST program.

Context consideration can also mean intervention that is context sensitive in design. For example, a recent prevention effort, the SAFEChildren program, focused on helping families within the inner-city manage the transition to first grade as well as ecological challenges such as protecting children from community violence (Tolan, Gorman-Smith, & Henry, 2003). Considering context in this manner can also mean varying interventions depending on the ecology of risk. Consider the study by Gorman-Smith and colleagues (2000), which found that children whose families lived in inner-city communities with protective neighborhood processes were less likely to be involved in serious and chronic delinquency compared to children whose families lived in inner-city communities but had no neighborhood social organization. Families in both communities had strong parenting practices but low levels of the family relationship characteristics of cohesion and emotional support. If we use this information to design an intervention program for inner-city youth engaging in delinquent behavior, we might design differential approaches to support and promote strong family functioning in these different contexts.

Another way in which contextual factors merit more consideration is because efficacy and effectiveness of adolescent interventions may differ substantially in different contexts. For example, the Metropolitan Area Child Study (Gorman-Smith, 2003; Metropolitan Area Child Study Research Group, 2002b) had a stronger and more general effect on social cognition related to aggression in urban poor communities than the more impoverished and burdened inner-city communities. Similarly, a comparison of the impact of SAFEChildren

seems to have some dependency on inner-city versus urban-poor economic level and whether or not there are neighborhood social processes found protective of youth living in inner-cities (Gorman-Smith et al., 2000).

Thus, it may be that variations in community characteristics and other important contexts such as schools and health care systems can have important influences on intervention benefits. Although several treatment and prevention programs consider context implicitly in their design or focus on those residing within communities considered high risk, these examples highlight the value of more explicit and carefully articulated consideration of the role context plays in risk development and its remediation or prevention. By examining the impact of contextual factors, we can learn how the effectiveness of intervention and prevention programs varies based on familial, peer, school, and community factors. Understanding how such programs may differ by family type or community, for instance, aids in the development of more flexible adolescent intervention programs that allow for adaptation depending on the population. In other words, we are better able to address the question of under what circumstances specific adolescent intervention programs work.

Cultural and Ethnicity Factors

The diversity of cultural and ethnic groups within our society is a compelling argument for consideration of these as potentially important influences on risk, intervention development, and likely effects, including variation in effects. Unfortunately, to date although there has been much clinical writing about this issue and there is increasing availability of risk and developmental studies that consider multiple ethnic groups and/or focus on cultural and ethnicity issues, these factors have not been substantially influential on treatment and prevention efforts to date (Catalano et al., 1993). For example, in a recent review of child and adolescent treatment outcome studies, over 80% of treatment outcome studies failed even to report the ethnic composition of their samples let alone evaluate the role of ethnicity in treatment (Weisz & Hawley, 1998).

When cultural factors have been considered in relation to intervention outcomes, such variables are often conceptualized as moderators. Researchers have sought to answer the question whether intervention outcomes differ based on race, ethnicity, or sex, often with the interest in showing that they do not; that the intervention is generalizable across groups. Although this information is important, it may be limited particularly when diversity of sampling is limited and not purposeful. Further, cultural sensitivity and cultural competence, meaning the intervention is built on adequate consideration of cultural values, concepts, and interest, require more than testing for demographic differences in effects. In part, this is impeded because there are not well-developed conceptualizations of cultural sensitivity or cultural competence. Also, there is no consensus about how ethnicity and race should be considered in intervention design and evaluation. Therefore, critical questions remain unanswered. For example, is the intervention culturally sensitive or what are the underlying variables accounting for any cultural differences or lack of cultural differences?

Suggestions have been made for how clinical research can incorporate cultural issues more favorably. First, intervention development and evaluation should be undertaken with cultural appropriateness, sensitivity, and competence as considerations from the initiation. Second, it is important that consideration of these be extended to operationalization in intervention activities, intended targets, measurement, personnel hiring and training, and analyses (Catalano et al., 1993). Third, it is important to examine interventions to date not just for a lack of difference by ethnic or cultural group but also for how they might be improved if more culturally sensitive (Padilla & Lindholm, 1995). Thus, the development of intervention programs and research examining the efficacy and effectiveness of such programs should involve individuals who are culturally sensitive to the populations for which the intervention is being targeted and have expertise in applying that to interventions (Sue et al., 1999). Accomplishing these three improvements may require ethnography and other qualitative descriptive methods to adequately capture the important considerations regarding the experiences and viewpoints of the targeted populations (Sue et al., 1999).

For intervention outcome evaluation there are several important examples. Delivery of intervention by culturally competent providers with culturally competent supervision is one. A second is to be extremely clear regarding their definitions of race and ethnicity (Sue et al., 1999). Investigators should also include mea-surement of characteristics likely to be associated with or considered competing explanations to ethnic or cultural effects, such as social class, education levels, community and neighborhood characteristics, and level of life event and situational stressors (Sue et al., 1999). Measurement equivalence is another important consideration, as this could underestimate or misdirect ethnic and cultural patterns.

A further important consideration is that intervention research occurs within the context of an often tense relationship between science and academia and minority groups and communities. Often, minority groups may be reluctant to participate in research that is brought to their communities, already developed by white, middle-class researchers in academic settings. Adequate implementation and cooperation for strong evaluation requires careful and thoughtful collaboration. In addition to benefits with sensitivity and implementation strength, such collaboration will also aid in the quality and complexity of process, mediators, and outcome, with sounder integration of cultural and ethnicity issues. Most directly, such collaboration can facilitate and improve ability to understand soundly intervention variations or consistencies and differences in processes related to benefits across groups.

As these many suggestions suggest, we are only now just beginning to understand issues related to intervention efficacy and effectiveness with diverse populations. Utilizing such strategies as those suggested by Sue and colleagues, as well as others, can enhance our understanding of the ways in which cultural factors can impact intervention and prevention efforts among diverse groups of adolescents and their families. The process of implementing such strategies requires an emphasis on training researchers and interventionists to be culturally sensitive and competent, developing intervention outcome studies that consider cultural factors in every stage of the study's design, and building collaborative relationships with diverse communities to encourage participation in the research process and ultimately, greater utilization of mental health services over time.

Comorbidity

The impact of comorbidity on the effects of interventions for adolescent disorders and related mental health problems is only beginning to be examined. Historically, in controlled treatment efficacy trials, participants who met criteria for more than the primary target disorder were screened out. For prevention, the comorbidity, and more generally the heterogeneity within the included sample, has often been ignored. Inclusion in a prevention program, if not a universal prevention intervention, has usually been driven by interest in a specific risk factor or outcome. More recently, however, treatment researchers have begun to realize the increasing need to include individuals with multiple disorders into efficacy and effectiveness trials as it is quite common for youth referred for intervention in a general clinical practice setting to be experiencing more than one disorder.

For instance, in the intervention programs reviewed earlier, research indicated that 40% of youth with a primary diagnosis of a depressive disorder also met criteria for a second disorder such as anxiety, attention-deficit/hyperactivity disorder (ADHD) or substance abuse (Rohde et al., 2001), and 79% of youth who met criteria for an anxiety disorder also met criteria for another disorder including a second anxiety disorder, ADHD, oppositional defiant disorder (ODD), depression, or conduct disorder (CD; Kendall et al., 2001). Research conducted in community outpatient clinics suggests that adolescents typically meet criteria for as many as three psychological disorders based on diagnostic interviews using the *Diagnostic and Statistical Manual of Mental Disorders* (4th ed.; American Psychiatric Association, 1994; Weisz & Hawley, 2002). Prevention outcome studies have also begun to examine intervention impact on subgroups, defined by differences in risk at pretest and possessing different risk factors (Conduct Problems Prevention Research Group, 2002; Stoolmiller et al., 2000). In addition, there has been more consideration of how effects on multiple outcomes might be due to comorbidity (Hawkins, Catalano, Kosterman, Abbott, & Hill, 1999).

Because comorbidity is so common among youth, neglecting to include youth with multiple disorders or examine comorbidity as a moderator in clinical research trials may produce intervention outcome results that are applicable only to a small subset of the adolescent population experiencing psychopathology. Perhaps comorbidity complicates the intervention process, impacting intervention outcomes in important ways that have yet to be discovered. For instance, treating an adolescent with depression may become much more challenging if the youth also presents with a substance abuse disorder. Questions arise, such as which problem should be focused on first or whether both problems should be approached simultaneously? If the primary diagnosis is depression and the therapist was intending to use Adolescent Coping with Depression, a group curriculum, how does the therapist build in individual sessions to address the substance use or does the therapist refer the youth to another clinic specializing in substance abuse? If the therapist chooses to refer the youth to a second clinic, how might that impact the family's ability to meet the growing therapeutic commitments in an effort to help their child? Questions can multiply quickly depending on the problem and because most clinical research has yet to incorporate the issue of comorbidity into their intervention designs, there is no roadmap for how best to address such issues.

In recent years, intervention researchers have begun to recognize the importance of examining comorbidity in intervention efficacy and effectiveness research. Thus, some studies exist that demonstrate ways to assess for comorbidity and its potential impact on intervention outcome, several of which were reviewed earlier in this chapter. Such research suggests that comorbidity does not negatively affect the impact of interventions for disorders such as anxiety but may affect the rate of impact or recurrence for disorders such as depression (Clarke et al., 1992; Kendall et al., 2001; Rohde et al., 2001). In fact, research examining interventions for anxiety disorders suggest that CBT interventions may generalize and decrease symptoms in additional disorders. It has been argued that because manualized cognitive-behavioral interventions use many similar skills, it is not surprising that an intervention for one disorder might generalize to a second disorder (Connor-Smith & Weisz, 2003).

On the other hand, research by Rohde and colleagues (2001) suggests that manualized interventions might not generalize easily, depending on the disorders involved. Their results indicated that youth with a comorbid diagnosis of substance abuse experienced a slower time to recovery and youth with comorbid diagnoses of ADHD or disruptive behavior disorders such as ODD or CD were more likely to experience a recurrence of depression posttreatment. Such findings present a different picture compared to the findings by Kendall and colleagues. Specifically, results from Rohde and colleagues suggest that for youth experiencing depression, a second psychological disorder may complicate treatment. Such complications may require intervention manual modifications. For example, for youth participating in intervention for depression, perhaps it is important to include optional modules designed to address substance abuse problems thereby increasing adolescents' rate of recovery. Likewise, it may be important to provide booster sessions for those adolescents experiencing depression and ADHD or an externalizing disorder.

Future evaluations seem likely to be enhanced to the extent that comorbidity or subgroup compositions in general are considered in sample selection as well as outcome evaluation. However, there is need for methodological as well as theoretical focus to make this adequately considered in most designs. As with the other important moderators and the mediation topics highlighted, moving toward effective practice rests on integrating needed complexity in program development and implementation, evaluation design, and results interpretation.

MOVING TOWARD EFFECTIVE PRACTICE

As these examples illustrate, we have efficacious treatment and prevention programs for several of the most common and concerning adolescent mental health problems. In some cases, effectiveness trials have been undertaken. In others, some comparisons have been made that can suggest how interventions work and for whom and under what circumstances effects can be sustained. Clearly, reliance on these interventions is preferable to practice based on individual judgment, yet it is not a state that can confidently guide practice. There is a consistently growing need to develop scientific bases for services that are effective in general clinical practice settings. This need calls for clinical research on adolescent intervention to move beyond the typical university-based settings and to integrate the complexities identified earlier.

Efficacious intervention programs should be examined within the contexts in which they most often occur: clinics, schools, and community settings. In fact, it may be that intervention evaluations may be better served by an active

inclusion of natural setting features in testing basic effects "in which the development and testing processes are moved at an early stage into clinical practice contexts, where protocol development and refinement, outcome assessment, and efforts to answer the 'how, why, and with whom' questions are all based" (Weisz, 2000, p. 838) and the typical conditions of mounting intervention programs such as school-level implementation of prevention efforts can be considered (Tolan, 2004). Although the evaluation of prevention programs typically occurs in such settings, treatment evaluation is just beginning to contemplate moving in this direction.

In addition to undertaking more intervention evaluation that combines careful and strong research designs with real-world service organization, there is increasing recognition that strong and careful methods of studying how intervention findings can be translated for practice are needed (Greenberg et al., 2003; Tolan, 2004). For example, tests of how practice and use of intervention methods typically occur may provide important clues as to how intervention tests might be undertaken so that results are more directly transferable to practice (Lonigan et al., 1998).

Challenges in Translating to Practice

Two of the most difficult challenges in transporting efficacious interventions into the community include (1) developing strategies for rigorously evaluating the effectiveness of such programs under real-world conditions that are often less controllable than typical, university-based, research conditions; and (2) maintaining the core "ingredients"—principles, strategies, and structure—of interventions while adapting them to meet the needs of the communities, while still achieving good intervention outcomes. Consensus on guidelines for evaluating intervention programs has highlighted the following criteria: (1) group design studies in which subjects are randomly assigned; (2) well-documented intervention procedures that facilitate replication (e.g., manualized, clear, and structured management approaches intervention); (3) emphasis on uniform intervention provider training; (4) evidence of provider adherence to intervention procedures; (5) tests utilizing appropriate samples; (6) multimethod outcome assessment; (7) tests of clinical significance of outcomes; (8) tests of intervention effects on real-world functional outcomes in addition to symptoms; and (9) follow-up assessment of long-term outcomes (Elliott & Tolan, 1999; Greenberg et al., 2003).

Adopting such guidelines while attempting to transport and test efficacious interventions in community settings requires collaboration efforts between researchers and communities. Pursuing such collaboration requires compromises that may be daunting to each party. Community partners may need to be willing to undertake programmatic approaches when individual provider autonomy has been their guiding principle as well as impose supervision structures and service organization procedures that may require additional resources. Intervention scientists may have to live with ambiguities or less control than they are used to regarding how interventions are done, when and how measurement of effects occurs, and what aspects of intervention are considered most critical in evaluating outcomes. Research staff must be open to hearing suggestions from community members regarding which components of the intervention merit modification and community collaborators need to respect the value of consistency even if it may conflict with a belief of matching each intervention to each client's needs. While such compromises can be challenging and may even be seen as muddying the research enterprise, we believe they provide an opportunity to wed the strength of scientific study to the public health interest of utility for addressing youth mental health problems (Tolan, 2004).

While working to integrate intervention science and general clinical practice conditions is one valuable strategy, a complementary approach is to work systematically to improve transportability of tested interventions. Connor-Smith and Weisz (2003) recently identified suggestions for adapting or transporting empirically supported therapies for clinic use, which seems applicable to both prevention and treatment. First, when using manualized interventions, it is important to maintain flexibility in their application. Because of the individual characteristics and experiences of each client, therapists must be able to adapt intervention sessions to maximize the applicability to the client.

At the same time, therapists must balance such flexibility by adhering to the core structure, skills, and concepts of the intervention. For example, with the C.A.T. Project for anxious adolescents, it may not be essential that therapists use the exact wording and/or exercises that appear in the intervention manual. However, it is crucial that therapists cover the key concepts and skills from the intervention such as the FEAR model discussed earlier. Similarly, prevention efforts may need to rearrange the order of intervention sessions to improve fit to perceived issues of participants (e.g., focusing on parenting first rather than communication or communication before parenting skills depending on community comfort with a given topic; Tolan, 2002).

Second, therapists must also be willing to adapt session structure as needed to address the multiple problems adolescents may be experiencing in addition to the target problem identified for intervention. For instance, delivering a manualized treatment for depression may not include a meeting with the youth's school. However, if the youth is struggling academically in part because of his or her depressive symptoms, it may be worthwhile to meet with the adolescent's teachers and other school faculty to develop additional strategies to help the adolescent manage his or her depression at school and increase his or her academic performance. Additional suggestions include maintaining a therapeutic alliance, addressing severe disorders and comorbidity, devoting adequate attention to case conceptualization, taking into account clients' individual characteristics and circumstances, and finally providing thorough training for therapists to ensure they feel competent and well equipped to deliver the intervention (Connor-Smith & Weisz, 2003).

Integrating Training and Community Settings

Given the limited state of knowledge about the effectiveness of empirically supported programs under more diverse implementation conditions, transporting such programs needs to be accompanied by empirical study of transportability to gain a more substantial understanding of under what variety of conditions empirically supported programs will be effective. Based on emerging data regarding the effectiveness of efficacious treatment programs in community settings when fidelity is maintained, we propose that training programs emphasize empirically based approaches. Moreover, it appears that this training is enhanced when approached within a framework that relates prevention and treatment as part of an overall developmental–ecological understanding of risk and intervention application (Kellam & Rebok, 1992; Mrazek & Haggerty, 1994: Tolan et al., 1995). This approach centers on training for use of efficacious approaches, with an emphasis on promoting the use of research to inform practice in an ongoing fashion and to press for research and evaluation that can inform what works for whom under what circumstances. This type of training approach may lead to increased use of empirically supported programs within general clinical practice. It may also promote an interdependence and collaboration between academic centers and service systems so that innovations can be incorporated, adherence to protocols well emphasized, and evaluation within actual practice settings undertaken with strong methods. In addition, within this collaborative process, it is crucial that researchers begin to explore the characteristics of the agencies and communities in which the interventions are implemented, as well as the characteristics of adolescents and families participating in these treatment programs. Exploring how these variables vary from one setting to another will increase our understanding of mediating and moderating characteristics in the process of implementing efficacious programs within community settings.

For example, we have recently undertaken a partnership with community mental health agencies and schools within Chicago to introduce evidence-based interventions for younger adolescents with CD and other disruptive behavior disorders. The academic center is responsible for the development, initial testing, and manual and training program for the intervention. In partnership with the community mental health agencies, training materials and protocol features are developed to be considerate of eventual translation/transporting to practice. The intent is to undertake strong evaluation efforts (e.g., random assignment comparison) utilizing community agency staff and organization of services but with integration of principles of fidelity and intervention structuring and previously tested efficacious interventions. By training in principles of evidence-based practice as well as integrating community partner perspectives and service delivery organization, the hope is that the evaluation results will be more directly translatable to practice than is the usual case. A second strategy may be to undertake larger multisite trials that bring the controls and strict scientific designs of efficacy trials but apply the intervention across diverse settings (Conduct Problems Prevention Research Group, 1999; Tolan, 2004).

CONCLUSION

It seems that although there have been great and very important gains in understanding of intervention, whether prevention or treatment, for most of the most prevalent disorders and associated problems affecting adolescents, these important advances comprise only a base for effective practice. It is likely that this progress will continue as the needs for moving from strong efficacy findings to effective practice are better recognized, incorporated into evaluation research, and extended into training. As the complexity and depth of knowledge expand, then effective practice will be realizable.

REFERENCES

American Psychiatric Association. (1994). *Diagnostic and statistical manual of mental disorders* (4th edition). Washington, DC: Author.

Austin, A. M., Macgowan, M. J., & Wagner, E. F. (2005). Effective family-based interventions for adolescents with substance use problems: A systematic review. *Research on Social Work Practice, 15*(2), 67–83.

Baron, R. M., & Kenny, D. A. (1986). Moderator–mediator variable distinction in social psychological research: Conceptual, strategic, and statistical considerations. *Journal of Personality and Social Psychology, 51,* 1173–1182.

Barrett, P. M., Lowry-Webster, H., & Turner, C. (2000a). *FRIENDS program for children: Group leaders manual.* Brisbane, Australia: Australian Academic Press.

Barrett, P. M., Lowry-Webster, H., & Turner, C. (2000b). *FRIENDS program for youth: Group leaders manual.* Brisbane, Australia: Australian Academic Press.

Barrett, P. M., Sonderegger, R., & Sonderegger, N. L. (2001). Evaluation of an anxiety-prevention and positive-coping program (FRIENDS) for children and adolescents of nonEnglish speaking background. *Behaviour Change, 18*(1), 78–91.

Barrett, P. M., Sonderegger, R., & Xenos, S. (2003). Using FRIENDS to combat anxiety and adjustment problems among young migrants to Australia: A national trial. *Clinical Child Psychology and Psychiatry, 8*(2), 241–260.

Beardslee, W. R, Keller, M. B, Seifer, R., Lavori, P. W., Staley, J., Podorefsky, D., & Shera, D. (1996). Prediction of adolescent affective disorder: Effects of prior parental affective disorders and child psychopathology. *Journal of the American Academy of Child and Adolescent Psychiatry, 35,* 279–288.

Beardslee, W. R, Versage, E. M., & Gladstone, T. R. (1998). Children of affectively ill parents: A review of the past 10 years. *Journal of the American Academy of Child and Adolescent Psychiatry, 37,* 1134–1141.

Beardslee, W. R, Versage, E. M., Wright, E. J., & Salt, P. (1997). Examination of preventive interventions for families with depression: Evidence of change. *Development and Psychopathology, 9,* 109–130.

Borduin, C. M., Henggeler, S. W., Blaske, D. M., & Stein, R. (1990). Multisystemic treatment of adolescent sexual offenders. *International Journal of Offender Therapy and Comparative Criminology, 35,* 105–114.

Borduin, C. M., Mann, B. J., Cone, L. T., Henggeler, S. W., Fucci, B. R., Blaske, D. M., & Williams, R. A. (1995). Multisystemic treatment of serious juvenile offenders: Long-term prevention of criminality and violence. *Journal of Consulting and Clinical Psychology, 63,* 569–578.

Brestan, E. V., & Eyberg, S. M. (1998). Effective psychosocial treatments of conduct-disordered children and adolescents: 29 years, 82 studies, and 5,272 kids. *Journal of Clinical Child Psychology, 27,* 180–189.

Brown, T. L., Swenson, C. C., Cunningham, P. B., Henggeler, S. W., Schoenwald, S. K., & Rowland, M. D. (1997). Multisystemic treatment of violent and chronic juvenile offenders: Bridging the gap between research and practice. *Administration and Policy in Mental Health, 25,* 221–238.

Brunk, M., Henggeler, S. W., & Whelan, J. P. (1987). A comparison of multisystemic therapy and parent training in the brief treatment of child abuse and neglect. *Journal of Consulting and Clinical Psychology, 55,* 311–318.

Catalano, R. F., Hawkins, J. D., Krenz, C., & Gillmore, M. (1993). Using research to guide culturally appropriate drug abuse prevention. *Journal of Consulting and Clinical Psychology, 61,* 804–811.

Chorpita, B. F. (2003). The frontier of evidence-based practice. In A. E. Kazdin & J. R. Weisz (Eds.), *Evidence-based psychotherapies for children and adolescents* (pp. 42–59). New York: Guilford Press.

Chu, B. C, & Kendall, P. C. (2004). Positive association of child involvement and treatment outcome within a manual-based cognitive-behavioral treatment for children with anxiety. *Journal of Consulting and Clinical Psychology, 72*(5), 821–829.

Clarke, G. N., Hawkins, W., Murphy, M., Sheeber, L. B., Lewinsohn, P. M., & Seeley, J. R. (1995). Targeted prevention of unipolar depressive disorder in an at-risk sample of high school adolescents: A randomized trial of group cognitive intervention. *Journal of the American Academy of Child and Adolescent Psychiatry, 34,* 312–321.

Clarke, G., Hops, H., Lewinsohn, P. M., Andrews, J., Seeley, J. R., & Williams, J. (1992). Cognitive-behavioral group treatment of adolescent depression: Prediction of outcome. *Behavior Therapy, 23,* 341–354.

Clarke, G. N., Hornbrook, M., Lynch, F., Polen, M., Gale, J., O'Connor, E., et al. (2002). Group cognitive-behavioral treatment for depressed adolescent offspring of depressed parents in a health maintenance organization. *Journal of the American Academy of Child and Adolescent Psychiatry, 41*(3), 305–313.

Clarke, G., Lewinsohn, P., & Hops, H. (1990). *Adolescent Coping with depression course: Leader's manual for adolescent groups.* Eugene, OR: Castalia.

Clarke, G. N., Rohde, P., Lewinsohn, P. M., Hops, H., & Seeley, J. R. (1999). Cognitive-behavioral treatment of adolescent depression: Efficacy of acute group treatment and booster sessions. *Journal of the American Academy of Child and Adolescent Psychiatry, 38,* 272–279.

Commission on Chronic Illness. (1957). *Chronic Illness in the United States. Volume 1. Published for the Commonwealth Fund.* Cambridge, MA: Harvard University Press.

Conduct Problems Prevention Research Group. (1999). Initial impact of the fast track prevention trial for conduct problems: I. The high risk sample. *Journal of Consulting and Clinical Psychology, 67,* 631–647.

Conduct Problems Prevention Research Group. (2002). Predictor variables associated with positive fast track outcomes at the end of third grade. *Journal of Abnormal Child Psychology, 30,* 37–52.

Connor-Smith, J. K., & Weisz, J. R. (2003). Applying treatment outcome research in clinical practice: Techniques for adapting interventions to the real world. *Child and Adolescent Mental Health, 8,* 3–10.

Cowen, E. L. (1997). On the semantics and operations of primary prevention and wellness enhancement (or will the real primary prevention please stand up?). *American Journal of Community Psychology. 25,* 245–255.

Dadds, M. R., Holland, D. E., Laurens, K. R., Mullins, M., Barrett, P. M., & Spence, S. H. (1999). Early intervention and prevention of anxiety disorders in children: Results at 2-year follow-up. *Journal of Consulting and Clinical Psychology, 67,* 145–150.

Dadds, M. R., Spence, S. H., Holland, D. E., Barrett, P. M., & Laurens, K. R. (1997). Prevention and early intervention for anxiety disorders: A controlled trial. *Journal of Consulting and Clinical Psychology, 65,* 627–635.

Durlak, J. A., Fuhrman, T., & Lampman, C. (1991). Effectiveness of cognitive-behavior therapy for maladapting children: A meta-analysis. *Psychological Bulletin, 110,* 204–214.

Durlak, J. A., & Wells, A. M. (1997). Primary prevention mental health programs for children and adolescents: A meta-analytic review. *American Journal of Community Psychology, 25,* 115–144.

Durlak, J. A., & Wells, A. M. (1998). Evaluation of indicated preventive intervention. *American Journal of Community Psychology, 26,* 775–796.

Elliott, D. S., & Mihalic, S. (2004). Issues in disseminating and replicating effective prevention programs. *Prevention Science, 5,* 47–53.

Elliott, D. S., & Tolan, P. H. (1999). Youth violence prevention, intervention, and social policy. In D. J. Flannery & C. R. Huff (Eds.), *Youth violence: Prevention, intervention and social policy.* Washington, DC: American Psychiatric Press.

Furstenberg, F. (1993). How families manage risk and opportunity in dangerous neighborhoods. In W. J. Wilson (Ed.), *Sociology and the public agenda* (pp. 231–258). Newbury Park, CA: Sage.

Gordon, R. (1983). An operational classification of disease prevention. *Public Health Reports, 98,* 107–109.

Gorman-Smith, D. (2003). Effects of teacher training and consultation on teacher behavior toward students at high risk for aggression. *Behavior Therapy, 34,* 437–452.

Gorman-Smith, D., Tolan, P. H., & Henry, D. (2000). A developmental–ecological model of the relations of family functioning to patterns of delinquency. *Journal of Family Psychology, 10,* 115–129.

Gottfredson, D. C. (2001). *Schools and delinquency.* New York: Cambridge University Press.

Greenberg, M. T., & Kusche, C. A. (1998). Preventive interventions for school-age deaf children: The PATHS curriculum. *Journal of Deaf Studies and Deaf Education, 3,* 49–63.

Greenberg, M. T., Weissberg, R. P., O'Brien, M. U., Zins, J. E., Fredericks, L., Resnik, H., & Elias, M. J. (2003). Enhancing school-based prevention and youth development through coordinated social, emotional, and academic learning. *American Psychologist, 58,* 466–474.

Guerra, N. G., Eron, L. D., Huesmann, L. R., Tolan, P. H., & Van Acker, (1997). A cognitive–ecological approach to the prevention and mitigation of violence and aggression in inner-city youth. In D. P. Fry & K. Bjorkqvist (Eds.), *Cultural variation in conflict resolution: Alternatives to violence* (pp. 199–213). Mahwah, NJ: Erlbaum.

Hanish, L. D., & Tolan, P. H. (2001). Antisocial behaviors in children and adolescents: Expanding the cognitive model. In W. J. Lyddon & J. V. Jones Jr. (Eds.), *Empirically supported cognitive therapies: Current and future applications* (pp. 182–199). New York: Springer.

Hawkins, J. D., Catalano, R. F., Kosterman, R., Abbott, R. D., & Hill, K. G. (1999). Preventing adolescent health-risk behaviors by strengthening protection during childhood. *Archives of Pediatrics and Adolescent Medicine, 153,* 226–234.

Henggeler, S. W. (2003). Commentary on Ellis et al.: Adapting multisystemic therapy for challenging clinical problems of children and adolescents. *Journal of Pediatric Psychology, 28,* 295–297.

Henggeler, S. W., Cunningham, P. B., Pickrel, S. G.,

Schoenwald, S. K., & Brondino, M. J. (1996). Multisystemic therapy: An effective violence prevention approach for serious juvenile offenders. *Journal of Adolescence, 19,* 47–61.

Henggeler, S. W., Melton, G. B., Brondino, M. J., Scherer, D. G., & Hanley, J. H. (1997). Multisystemic therapy with violent and chronic juvenile offenders and their families: The role of treatment fidelity in successful dissemination. *Journal of Consulting and Clinical Psychology, 65,* 821–833.

Henggeler, S. W., Melton, G. B., & Smith, L. A. (1992). Family preservation using multisystemic therapy: An effective alternative to incarcerating serious juvenile offenders. *Journal of Consulting and Clinical Psychology, 60,* 953–961.

Henggeler, S. W., Melton, G. B., Smith, L. A., Schoenwald, S. K., & Hanley, J. H. (1993). Family preservation using multisystemic treatment: Long-term follow-up to a clinical trial with serious juvenile offenders. *Journal of Child and Family Studies, 2,* 283–293.

Henggeler, S. W., Rodick, J. D., Borduin, C. M., Hanson, C. L., Watson, S. M., & Urey, J. R. (1986). Multisystemic treatment of juvenile offenders: Effects on adolescent behavior and family interactions. *Developmental Psychology, 22,* 132–141.

Henggeler, S. W., Schoenwald, S. K., Borduin, C. M., Rowland, M. D., & Cunningham, P. B. (1998). *Multisystemic treatment for antisocial behavior in children and adolescents.* New York: Guilford Press.

Henggeler, S. W., Schoenwald, S. K., Liao, J. G., Letourneau, E. J., & Edwards, D. L. (2002). Transporting efficacious treatments to field settings: The link between supervisory practices and therapist fidelity in MST programs. *Journal of Clinical Child and Adolescent Psychology, 31,* 155–167.

Henggeler, S. W., Schoenwald, S. K., & Pickrel, S. G. (1995). Multisystemic therapy: Bridging the gap between university- and community-based treatment. *Journal of Consulting and Clinical Psychology, 63,* 709–717.

Holmbeck, G. N. (1997). Toward terminological, conceptual, and statistical clarity in the study of mediators and moderators: Examples from the child-clinical and pediatric psychology literatures. *Journal of Consulting and Clinical Psychology, 65,* 599–610.

Holmbeck, G. N., Colder, C., Shapera, W., Westhoven, V., Kenealy, L., & Updegrove, A. (2000). Working with adolescents: Guides from developmental psychology. In P. C. Kendall (Ed.), *Child and adolescent therapy: Cognitive-behavioral procedures* (2nd ed., pp. 334–385). New York: Guilford Press.

Huey, S. J., Henggeler, S. W., Brondino, M. J., & Pickrel, S. G. (2000). Mechanisms of change in multisystemic therapy: Reducing delinquent behavior through therapist adherence and improved family and peer functioning. *Journal of Consulting and Clinical Psychology, 68,* 451–467.

Kaslow, N. J., & Thompson, M. P. (1998). Applying the criteria for empirically supported treatments to studies of psychosocial interventions for child and adolescent depression. *Journal of Clinical Child Psychology, 27,* 146–155.

Kaufman, N. K., Rohde, P., Seeley, J. R., Clarke, G. N., & Stice, E. (2005). Potential mediators of cognitive-behavioral therapy for adolescents with comorbid major depression and conduct disorder. *Journal of Consulting and Clinical Psychology, 73*(1), 38–46.

Kazdin, A. E., Bass, D., Ayers, W. A., & Rodgers, A. (1990). Empirical and clinical focus of child and adolescent psychotherapy research. *Journal of Consulting and Clinical Psychology, 57,* 522–535.

Kazdin, A. E., Siegel, T. C., & Bass, D. (1992). Cognitive problem solving skills therapy and parent management training in the treatment of antisocial behavior in children. *Journal of Consulting and Clinical Psychology, 60,* 733–747.

Kazdin, A. E., & Weisz, J. R. (2003). *Evidence-based psychotherapies for children and adolescents.* New York: Guilford Press.

Kellam, S. G., & Rebok, G. W. (1992). Building developmental and etiological theory through epidemiologically based preventive intervention trials. In J. McCord & R. E. Tremblay (Eds.), *Preventing antisocial behavior: Interventions from birth through adolescence* (pp. 162–195). New York: Guilford Press.

Kendall, P. C. (1994). Treating anxiety disorders in children: Results of a randomized clinical trial. *Journal of Consulting and Clinical Psychology, 62,* 100–110.

Kendall, P. C., Brady, E. U., & Verduin, T. L. (2001). Comorbidity in childhood anxiety disorders and treatment outcome. *Journal of the American Academy of Child and Adolescent Psychiatry, 40,* 787–794.

Kendall, P. C., Choudhury, M., Hudson, J., & Webb, A. (2002). The C.A.T. Project Manual for the cognitive behavioral treatment of anxious adolescents. Ardmore, PA: Workbook.

Kendall, P. C., Flannery-Schroeder, E., Panichelli-Mindel, S. M., Southam-Gerow, M., Henin, A., & Warman, M. (1997). Therapy for youths with anxiety disorders: A second randomized clinical trial. *Journal of Consulting and Clinical Psychology, 65,* 366–380.

Kendall, P. C., Safford, S., Flannery-Schroeder, E., & Webb, A. (2004). Child anxiety treatment: Outcomes in adolescence and impact on substance use and depression at 7.4 year follow-up. *Journal of Consulting and Clinical Psychology, 72*(2), 276–287.

Kendall, P. C., & Southam-Gerow, M. (1996). Long-term follow-up of a cognitive-behavioral therapy for anxiety-disordered youth. *Journal of Consulting and Clinical Psychology, 64,* 724–730.

Kusche, C. A., & Greenberg, M. T. (1994). *The PATHS curriculum.* Seattle, WA: Developmental Research and Programs.

Lerner, R. M., Villarruel, F. A., & Castellino, D. R. (1999). Adolescence. In W. K. Silverman & T. H. Ollendick (Eds.), *Developmental issues in the clinical treatment of children* (pp. 125–136). Needham Heights, MA: Pearson/Allyn & Bacon.

Letendre, J., Henry, D., & Tolan, P. H. (2003). Leader and therapeutic influences on prosocial skill building in school-based groups to prevent aggression. *Research on Social Work Practice, 13,* 569–587.

Lewinsohn, P. M., Clarke, G. N., Hops, H., & Andrews, J. (1990). Cognitive-behavioral treatment for depressed adolescents. *Behavior Therapy, 21,* 385–401.

Lewinsohn, P. M., Clarke, G. N., Rhode, P., Hops, H., & Seeley, J. (1996). A course in coping: A cognitive-behavioral approach to the treatment of adolescent depression. In E. D. Hibbs & P. S. Jensen (Eds.), *Psychosocial treatments for child and adolescent disorders: Empirically based strategies for clinical practice* (pp. 109–135). Washington, DC: American Psychological Association.

Lipsey, M. W., & Wilson, D. B. (1993). The efficacy of psychological, educational, and behavioral treatment: Confirmation from meta-analysis. *American Psychologist, 48,* 1181–1209.

Lonigan, C. J., Elbert, J. C., & Bennett-Johnson, S. (1998). Empirically supported psychosocial interventions for children: An overview. *Journal of Clinical Child Psychology, 27,* 138–145.

Lowry-Webster, H., Barrett, P. M., & Dadds, M. (2001). A universal prevention trial of anxiety and depressive symptomatology in childhood: Preliminary data from an Australian study. *Behaviour Change, 18*(1), 36–50.

Lowry-Webster, H., Barrett, P. M., & Lock, S. (2003). A universal prevention trial of anxiety symptomatology during childhood: Results at one-year follow-up. *Behaviour Change, 21*(1), 25–43.

MacKinnon, D. P., & Dwyer, J. H. (1993). Estimating medicated effects in prevention studies. *Evaluation Review, 17,* 144–158.

Metropolitan Area Child Study Research Group. (2002a). A cognitive–ecological approach to preventing aggression in urban settings: Initial outcomes for high-risk children. *Journal of Consulting and Clinical Psychology, 70,* 179–194.

Metropolitan Area Child Study Research Group. (2002b). *Social cognitive effects of a prevention program for elementary school urban youth.* Manuscript submitted for review.

Mrazek, P. J., & Haggerty, R. J. (1994). *Reducing risks for mental disorders: Frontiers for preventive intervention research.* Washington, DC: National Academy Press.

Nation, M., Crusto, C., Wandersman, A., Kumpfer, K. L., Seybolt, D., Morrissey-Kane, E., & Davino, K. (2003). What works in prevention: Principles of effective prevention programs. *American Psychologist, 58,* 449–456.

Olds, D. L. (2002). Prenatal and infancy home visiting by nurses: From randomized trials to community replication. *Prevention Science, 3,* 153–172.

Olds, D. L., Robinson, J., O'Brien, R., Luckey, D. W., Pettitt, L. M., Henderson, C. R. et al., (2002). Home visiting by nurses and by paraprofessionals: A randomized controlled trial. *Pediatrics, 110,* 486–496.

Ollendick, T. H., & King, N. J. (1998). Empirically supported treatments for children with phobic and anxiety disorders: Current status. *Journal of Clinical Child Psychology, 27,* 156–167.

Padilla, A. M., & Lindholm, K. J. (1995). Quantitative educational research with ethnic minorities. In J. A. Banks & C. A. McGee-Banks (Eds.), *Handbook of research on multicultural education* (pp. 97–113). New York: Macmillan.

Paul, G. (1967). Outcome research in psychotherapy. *Journal of Consulting Psychology, 31,* 109–118.

Price, R. H., & Lorion, R. P. (1989). Prevention programming on organizational reinvention: From research to implementation. In D. Schaffer, I. Philips, N. B. Enzer, & M. M. Silverman (Eds.), *Prevention of mental disorders, alcohol, and other drug use in children and adolescents* (OSAP Prevention Monograph, pp. 97–123). Rockville, MD: Office of Substance Abuse Prevention.

Reed, V., & Wittchen, H. (1998). DSM-IV panic attacks and panic disorder in a community sample of adolescents and young adults: How specific are panic attacks? *Journal of Psychiatric Research, 32,* 335–345.

Rohde, P., Clarke, G. N., Lewinsohn, P. M., Seeley, J. R., & Kaufman, N. K. (2001). Impact of comorbidity on a cognitive-behavioral group treatment for adolescent depression. *Journal of the American Academy of Child and Adolescent Psychiatry, 40,* 795–802.

Rohde, P., Clarke, G. N., Mace, D. E., Jorgensen, J. S., & Seeley, J. R. (2004). An efficacy/effectiveness study of cognitive-behavioral treatment for adolescents with comorbid major depression and conduct disorder. *Journal of the American Academy of Child and Adolescent Psychiatry, 43*(6), 660–668.

Schoenwald, S. K., Henggeler, S. W., Brondino, M. J., & Rowland, M. D. (2000). Multisystemic therapy: Monitoring treatment fidelity. *Family Process, 39,* 83–103.

Shure, M. B., & Spivack, G. (1982). Interpersonal problem-solving in young children: A cognitive approach to prevention. *American Journal of Community Psychology, 10,* 341–356.

Stoolmiller, M., Eddy, J. M., & Reid, J. B. (2000). Detecting and describing preventive intervention effects in a universal school-based randomized trial targeting delinquent and violent behavior. *Journal of Consulting and Clinical Psychology, 68,* 296–306.

Sue, S., Kuraski, K. S., & Srinivasan, S. (1999). Ethnicity, gender, and cross-cultural issues in clinical research. In P. C. Kendall, J. N. Butcher, & G. N. Holmbeck (Eds.), *Handbook of research methods in clinical psychology* (2nd ed., pp. 54–71). New York: Wiley.

Tolan, P. H. (1996). Characteristics shared by exemplary child clinical interventions for indicated populations. In M. C. Roberts (Ed.), *Model programs in child and family mental health.* Mahwah, NJ: Erlbaum.

Tolan, P. H. (2001). Emerging themes and challenges in understanding youth violence involvement. *Journal of Clinical Child Psychology. 30,* 233–239.

Tolan, P. H. (2002). Family focused prevention research: Tough but tender with family intervention research. In H. Liddle, J. Bray, D. Santesban, & R. Levant (Eds.), *Family psychology intervention science* (pp. 197–214). Washington, DC: American Psychological Association.

Tolan, P. H. (2004). Lessons learned in the Multisite Violence Prevention Project: Collaboration: Big questions require large efforts. *American Journal of Preventive Medicine, 26*(Suppl. 1), 62–71.

Tolan, P. H., & Gorman-Smith, D. (1997). Treatment of juvenile delinquency: Between punishment and therapy. In D. M. Stoff & J. Breiling (Eds.), *Handbook of antisocial behavior* (pp. 405–415). New York: Wiley.

Tolan, P. H., & Gorman-Smith, D. (2003). What violence prevention can tell us about developmental psychopathology. *Developmental and Psychopathology, 14,* 713–729.

Tolan, P. H., Gorman-Smith, D., & Henry, D. B. (2003). The developmental ecology of urban males' youth violence. *Developmental Psychology, 39,* 274–291.

Tolan, P. H., & Guerra, N. G. (1994). Prevention of delinquency: Current status and issues. *Applied and Preventive Psychology, 3,* 251–273.

Tolan, P. H., Guerra, N. G., & Kendall, P. C. (1995). A developmental ecological perspective on antisocial behavior in children and adolescents: Toward a unified risk and intervention framework. *Journal of Consulting and Clinical Psychology, 63,* 579–584.

Tolan, P. H., Hanish, L. D., McKay, M. M., & Dickey, M. H. (2002). Evaluating process in child and family interventions: Aggression prevention as an example. *Journal of Family Psychology, 16,* 220–236.

Tolan, P. H., & McKay, M. M. (1996). Preventing serious antisocial behavior in inner-city children: An empirically based family intervention program. *Family Relations: Journal of Applied Family and Child Studies, 45,* 148–155.

Treadwell, K. R. H., Flannery-Schroeder, E. C., & Kendall, P. C. (1995). Ethnicity and gender in relation to adaptive functioning, diagnostic status, and treatment outcome in children from an anxiety clinic. *Journal of Anxiety Disorders, 9,* 373–384.

Treadwell, K. R. H., & Kendall, P. C. (1996). Self-talk in youth with anxiety disorders: Content specificity and treatment outcome. *Journal of Consulting and Clinical Psychology, 64,* 941–950.

U.S. Department of Health and Human Services. (2001). *Youth violence: A report of the Surgeon General.* Washington, DC: U.S. Government Printing Office.

Weersing, V. W., & Weisz, J. R. (2002). Mechanisms of action in youth psychotherapy. *Journal of Child Psychology and Psychiatry, 43,* 3–29.

Weiss, B., & Weisz, J. R. (1990). The impact of methodological factors on child psychotherapy outcome research: A meta-analysis for researchers. *Journal of Abnormal Child Psychology, 18,* 638–670.

Weisz, J. R. (2000). Agenda for child and adolescent psychotherapy research: On the need to put science into practice. *Archives of General Psychiatry, 57,* 837–838.

Weisz, J. R., Donenberg, G. R., Han, S. S., & Kauneckis, D. (1995). Child and adolescent psychotherapy outcomes in experiments versus clinics: Why the disparity? *Journal of Abnormal Child Psychology, 23,* 83–106.

Weisz, J. R., Donenberg, G. R., Han, S. S., & Weiss, B. (1995). Bridging the gap between laboratory and clinic in child and adolescent psychotherapy. *Journal of Consulting and Clinical Psychology, 63,* 688–701.

Weisz, J. R., & Hawley, K. M. (1998). Finding, evaluating, refining, and applying empirically supported treatments for children and adolescents. *Journal of Clinical Child Psychology, 27,* 206–216.

Weisz, J. R., & Hawley, K. M. (2002). Developmental factors in the treatment of adolescents. *Journal of Consulting and Clinical Psychology, 70,* 21–43.

Weisz, J. R., & Jensen, A. L. (2001). Child and adolescent psychotherapy in research and practice contexts: Review of the evidence and suggestions for improving the field. *European Child and Adolescent Psychiatry, 10,* I/12–I/18.

Weisz, J. R., Weiss, B., Alicke, M. D., & Klotz, M. L. (1987). Effectiveness of psychotherapy with children and adolescents: A meta-analysis for clinicians. *Journal of Consulting and Clinical Psychology, 55,* 542–549.

Weisz, J. R., Weiss, B., & Donenberg, G. R. (1992). The lab versus the clinic: Effects of child and adolescent psychotherapy. *American Psychologist, 47,* 1578–1585.

Weisz, J. R., Weiss, B., Han, S. S., Granger, D. A., & Morton, T. (1995). Effects of psychotherapy with children and adolescents revisited: A meta-analysis of treatment outcome studies. *Psychological Bulletin, 117,* 450–468.

Wilson, W. J. (1987). *The truly disadvantaged: The inner city, the underclass, and public policy.* Chicago: University of Chicago Press.

Yeaton, W. H., & Sechrest, L. (1981). Critical dimensions in the choice and maintenance of successful treatments: Strength, integrity, and effectiveness. *Journal of Consulting and Clinical Psychology, 49,* 156–167.

II

EXTERNALIZING DISORDERS

4

Attention-Deficit/ Hyperactivity Disorder

Russell A. Barkley

As children enter their adolescent years, they strive for greater individuation from their families, particularly their parents, and a greater identity and social status within the peer group and the larger community. This process of progressive separation comes with greater capacities for and greater societal expectations of responsibility, self-sufficiency, and self-determination that accompany the greater freedoms and privileges teenagers seek to have from others. During these years of transition to young adulthood, more will be increasingly demanded of the individual in the already familiar domains of major life activities that include self-care and family and educational, peer, and community functioning (clubs, sports, organized entertainment, etc.). New venues of major life activities also will be opened to them for exploration and eventual mastery, including sexual–reproductive, economic–occupational, health care and maintenance, self-transportation and motor vehicle operation, and, for some teens, even marital functioning and possibly childrearing. Such varied domains of adaptive functioning pose numerous and daily challenges to the conscientiousness and self-

regulation of even average or normal teenagers, though most navigate the rocky shoals of these adaptive domains relatively unscathed. But for teenagers with a developmental disability of self-control, these numerous domains hold not only the promise of greater autonomy and self-reliance but also the threat of more varied forms of impairment and of more serious personal and societal consequences than was the case in childhood. Though diagnostic criteria for attention-deficit/hyperactivity disorder (ADHD; American Psychiatric Association, 2000), continue to emphasize symptoms of inattention, overactivity, and impulsiveness as hallmarks of the disorder in adolescence, as in childhood, research and theory on the disorder now view it as more likely involving deficiencies in self-regulation and its associated executive functioning that give rise to the more obvious yet superficial diagnostic symptoms (Barkley, 1994, 1997a, 1997b; Denckla, 1994; Douglas, 1983, 1988). This chapter discusses the nature and diagnosis of ADHD particularly as it may be manifested in adolescence, along with its probable etiologies and the various comorbid disorders and domains of adaptive impairment likely to exist alongside it. Brief attention is also given to the assessment and management of the disorder within this developmental period, though the reader is directed to far more comprehensive texts dealing with these topics for greater clinical detail than space here permits (Anastopoulos & Shelton, 2001; Barkley, 2006; Brown, 2000; DuPaul & Stoner, 2003; Goldstein, 1997; Robin, 2000). The author's theoretical model of ADHD is also briefly presented, ideally providing a more parsimonious accounting of the many cognitive and social deficits in the disorder and intimating promising directions for future research while rendering a deeper appreciation for the developmental seriousness of ADHD.

Teens who are inattentive, impulsive, and restless and who possess these attributes to a degree that is markedly deviant for their age and sufficient to create impairments in major life activities are currently diagnosed as having ADHD (American Psychiatric Association, 2000). Their problematic behavior arises early in childhood in most cases and is typically persistent over development. Some cases may arise secondary to brain injury at later stages of development but this is uncommon. The disorder is among the most well studied of our time, yet the public struggles to accept the notion that it may be a largely biologically based developmental disability. Such disbelief in ADHD as a valid disorder probably stems from popular and deeply held assumptions that child behavioral problems typically arise from bad home environments, poor parenting, faulty social learning, and other agents of socialization (Harris, 1998; Pinker, 2002; Rowe, 1995). This conflict between scientific and lay perspectives on the disorder may have served to make ADHD among the most controversial child and adolescent psychiatric disorders of the past 20 years, to judge by the all-too-common frequency with which it is covered in the media. The fact that medication constitutes the most effective treatment for the management of its symptoms only further fuels the controversial nature of ADHD in the public mind. To them, the apparent enigma is how professionals can justify prescribing drugs for an obviously socially created behavior problem. But as this chapter shows, some adolescent behavioral problems are not of a social origin, at least not this one, and thus a consideration of neurobiological interventions as part of a total treatment package is not reprehensible—at least no

more so than is insulin for diabetes or anticonvulsants for epilepsy.

A note of clarification is in order here. In virtually every topic to be covered here, much of what is known of ADHD is drawn from studies of children. Vastly fewer studies of ADHD as it occurs in adolescents have been conducted. This is particularly true concerning treatments. Research on teens with ADHD does suggest, however, that the adolescent stage of the disorder may be sufficiently continuous with the childhood stage that much of what is known about the latter can be extended upward to adolescence. Also, many treatments for childhood ADHD can likewise be extended with some modification to teens with the disorder. There is no compelling evidence at this time that ADHD in teens is qualitatively different from that seen in children or in adults for that matter. This is surely not to argue that the disorder is identical across these major stages of development.

For one thing, quantitative declines in symptom severity certainly occur (Barkley, Fischer, Edelbrock, & Smallish, 1990; Barkley, Fischer, Smallish, & Fletcher, 2002), particularly in the domain of hyperactive behavior, such that it is highly unlikely that teens with ADHD would be characterized as frequently climbing on things or unable to play quietly. Other symptoms may become more prominent such as those reflecting poor persistence of effort as well as impaired self-control and organization and deficient time management. Changes in neurological and hormonal development also likely have an impact on the neuropsychology of the disorder and the expression of its symptoms at adolescence. Cognitive domains such as verbal working memory, internalized speech, emotional self-control, and the cross-temporal organization of behavior are becoming progressively more elaborate and better developed by this age and may well be more affected by the disorder than they were in childhood. Changes in the risks for certain comorbid disorders may also occur with the progression into adolescence (conduct disorder, substance use disorders, depression, etc.). And certainly new domains of potential impairments become evident that were not available to children (dating, sexual risks, driving risks, etc.). The constructs comprising the disorder (inattention, poor inhibition) do not appear to change qualitatively, but their surface manifestations may do so owing to both biological–developmental changes and those of social expectations and responsibilities occurring at this stage. Certainly the clinical presentation of the disorder does seem to become more complex in its potential for impairments. Undoubtedly it also becomes more complicated and more difficult in its management owing to the progressive independence of teens from family influences and the increasing potential for peer influence, among other changes in the potential vectors through which treatment might occur. Moreover, few studies on the etiologies of ADHD have sought to replicate their results in teens with the disorder. Yet there is little evidence from the fields of neuroanatomy, neuroimaging, and behavioral and molecular genetics to suggest that large qualitative shifts are occurring at this age. Quantitative changes are likely to be occurring into this older age group, but these would not preclude extrapolation of childhood evidence to adolescent ADHD. In short, a wholly new disorder does not spring forth at puberty. But a widening of social ecological effects, a shifting in emphasis on some symptom constructs more than others, and a likely greater emergence of executive function deficits, coupled with a progressive capacity for self-determination, add new layers of complexity to impairments and treatments not so evident in the childhood stage of the disorder.

A BRIEF HISTORY OF ADHD

Diagnostic labels for children who are hyperactive, inattentive, and impulsive may have changed numerous times over the last century, yet the actual nature of the disorder has changed little, if at all, from descriptions nearly a century ago (Still, 1902). Teens with ADHD, however, went either largely unrecognized or were simply folded in with groups of children with ADHD in research that may have occurred on the topic. It was not until the 1970s that some attention to adolescence as a separate stage of ADHD came to be widely recognized. This may have been due in part to the historically recent recognition of adolescence as a unique stage of human development and to the long-held belief that most children outgrew the disorder. While George Still (1902) provided the first serious clinical paper on the disorder, reporting on a group of 20 children in his clinical practice whom he defined as having a deficit in "volitional inhibition" (p. 1008), he

made no specific comment on an adolescent form of the disorder. Described as aggressive, passionate, lawless, inattentive, impulsive, and overactive, many of these children today would be diagnosed not only as ADHD but also as having oppositional defiant disorder (ODD) (McMahon, Chapter 5, this volume).

Interest in children with ADHD arose in North America around the time of the great encephalitis epidemics of 1917–1918. Children, including teens surviving these brain infections, had many behavioral problems similar to those comprising contemporary ADHD (Ebaugh, 1923; Hohman, 1922; Stryker, 1925). These cases and others known to have arisen from birth trauma, head injury, toxin exposure, and infections (see Barkley, 2006) gave rise to the concept of a brain-injured child syndrome (Strauss & Lehtinen, 1947). This concept evolved into that of minimal brain damage, and eventually minimal brain dysfunction (MBD), as challenges were raised to the label in view of the dearth of evidence of obvious brain injury in most cases (see Barkley, 2006, for a more detailed history). By the 1950–1970s, focus shifted away from etiology and toward the more specific behavior of hyperactivity and poor impulse control characterizing these children, reflected in labels such as "hyperkinetic impulse disorder" or "hyperactive child syndrome" (Burks, 1960; Chess, 1960). The recognition that ADHD was not caused by brain damage seemed to follow a similar argument made somewhat earlier by the prominent child psychiatrist Stella Chess (1960). It set off a major departure between professionals in North America and those in Europe that continues, though to a far lesser extent, to the present. Europe continued to view hyperkinesis for most of the latter half of this century as a relatively rare condition of extreme overactivity often associated with mental retardation or evidence of organic brain damage. This discrepancy in perspectives has been converging over the last decade as evident in the similarity of the DSM-IV criteria (see below) with those of ICD-10 (World Health Organization, 1994). Nevertheless, the manner in which clinicians and educators view the disorder, regardless of age group, remains quite disparate; in North America, Australia, and more recently Scandinavia and the Netherlands, such children have ADHD—a developmental disorder. Elsewhere in Great Britain, Europe, and most of Asia they are viewed as having a conduct problem or disorder, if they are recognized at all, with this behavioral disturbance believed to arise largely out of poor parenting, family dysfunction, or social disadvantage. The situation in these regions is changing as of this writing to be more in accord with North American views. This is surely due in part to the Internet and the easy access to scientific information it provides, with much of that information on child and adolescent mental disorders being generated by North American scientists. There has also been the increasing adoption worldwide of DSM as the standard for diagnosis. Add to this the influence of pharmaceutical companies in foreign markets to broaden their worldwide markets for medications used in the management of the disorder. And then there is the development of parent support organizations in these regions that bring political pressure to bear on educational and governmental agencies to recognize and assist with the management of the disorder.

By the 1970s, research emphasized the problems with sustained attention and impulse control in addition to hyperactivity (Douglas, 1972, 1980, 1983). This perspective eventually led to renaming the disorder "attention-deficit disorder" (ADD) in 1980 (DSM-III; American Psychiatric Association, 1980). Eventually, concern arose that the important features of hyperactivity and impulse control were being deemphasized in this ADD label and perspective when in fact they were critically important to differentiating the disorder from other conditions and to predicting later developmental risks (Barkley, 2006). In 1987, the disorder was renamed "attention-deficit/hyperactivity disorder" in DSM-III-R (American Psychiatric Association, 1987), and a single list of items incorporating all three symptoms was specified. Also important here was the placement of the condition of ADD without hyperactivity, renamed undifferentiated attention-deficit disorder, in a separate section of the manual from ADHD with the specification that insufficient research existed to guide in the construction of diagnostic criteria for it at that time.

In the 1990s, the problems with hyperactivity and impulsivity were found to form a single dimension of behavior (Lahey et al., 1988), which others described as "disinhibition" (Barkley, 1990), that was separable from the problems with inattention. All this led to the creation of two separate lists of items and thresholds for ADHD when the DSM-IV was published later in the decade (American Psychiatric Association, 1994); one for inattention and another for hyperactive–impulsive behavior. Unlike its predecessor, DSM-III-R, the establishment of these two lists led to the creation of three subtypes of ADHD (predominantly inattentive type, predominantly hyperactive–impulsive type, and combined type). The specific criteria from DSM-IV are discussed in more detail later (see "Diagnostic Criteria and Related Issues"). Healthy debate continues to the present over the core deficit(s) in ADHD—with increasing weight being given to problems with behavioral inhibition, self-regulation, and the related domain of executive functioning (Barkley, 1997a, 2000; Douglas, 1999; Nigg, 2001; Quay, 1997).

Controversy continues to swirl around the place of a subtype composed primarily of inattention within the larger condition of ADHD, with some arguing for it being a new, unique disorder from ADHD (Barkley, 2001c; Milich, Ballentine, & Lynam, 2001) and others arguing that this distinction may be premature (Hinshaw, 2001; Lahey, 2001) or not especially important to treatment planning (Pelham, 2001). Relatively consistent across viewpoints, however, is the opinion that a subset of children having only high levels of inattention associated with cognitive sluggishness and behavioral passivity probably represents a qualitatively different attention problem than ADHD (poor persistence, inhibition, and resistance to distraction).

As noted earlier, the history of ADHD has largely focused on it being a disorder of childhood. Indeed, it was common in the 1950s–1970s for clinicians to believe that most children outgrew the disorder by puberty. Longitudinal studies of hyperactive children published over the next two decades did much to overturn this benign, transient perspective (Barkley, Fischer, et al., 1990; Mannuzza & Klein, 1992; Rasmussen & Gilberg, 2001; Weiss & Hechtman, 1993), giving rise to the realization that ADHD persisted in most children into their adolescence. The growing recognition during this time that adolescence was a separate stage of human psychological development undoubtedly contributed further to this recognition of and acceptance of an adolescent stage to ADHD as well. Even so, the scientific study of ADHD in teens (and even adults) still lags far behind what is known about children with the disorder. Fortunately, studies of clinically referred teens diagnosed with the disorder (Barkley, Anastopoulos, Guevremont, & Fletcher, 1991; Barkley, Edwards, Fletcher, Laneri, & Metevia, 2001b) as well as clinically diagnosed children followed into adolescence (Barkley, Fischer, et al., 1990; Barkley, Fischer, Smallish, & Fletcher, 2002; Biederman et al., 1996) all suggest that the disorder exists in teens and is similar to that disorder seen in childhood though the pattern of comorbid disorders and the domains of impairment may change by this developmental stage.

DESCRIPTION AND DIAGNOSIS

The Core Symptoms

Two distinct behavioral dimensions underlie the behavioral problems (symptoms) in ADHD as it occurs in both children and adolescents (Burns, Boe, Walsh, Sommers-Flanagan, & Teegarden, 2001; DuPaul et al., 1999; Lahey et al., 1994).

Inattention

Attention represents a multidimensional construct (Bate, Mathias, & Crawford, 2001; Mirsky, 1996; Strauss, Thompson, Adams, Redline, & Burant, 2000). The dimension impaired in ADHD reflects an inability to sustain attention or persist at tasks, remember and follow through on rules and instructions, and resist distractions while doing so. By adolescence, this dimension more likely reflects problems with working memory than poor attention, per se (Barkley, 1997a; Seguin, Boulerice, Harden, Tremblay, & Pihl, 1999; Wiers, Gunning, & Sergeant, 1998). Working memory is the capacity to hold information in mind and use it to guide behavior, particularly across time and toward future goals. More than in childhood, it is this ability to construct and execute complex, well-organized, goal-directed, and future-oriented behavior (stick-to-it-tiveness) along with its essential capacity for self-motivation that is disabled in the adolescent with ADHD. This inattentive and distractible behavior distinguishes ADHD from learning disabilities (Barkley, DuPaul, & McMurray, 1990) or other psychiatric disorders (Chang et al., 1999; Swaab-Barneveld et al., 2000) and does not appear to be a function of the other disorders often comorbid with ADHD (anxiety, depression, or oppositional and conduct problems) (Barkley, Edwards, et al., 2001a; Klorman et

al., 1999; Murphy, Barkley, & Bush, 2001; Newcorn et al., 2001; Nigg, 1999).

Hyperactive–Impulsive Behavior (Disinhibition)

As with attention, inhibition is a multidimensional construct (Nigg, 2000; Olson, Schilling, & Bates, 1999). The problems with inhibition seen in ADHD seem to involve voluntary or executive inhibition of prepotent responses (Nigg, 2001). More specifically, teens with ADHD manifest difficulties with restlessness (sometimes subjective or internal in form), less ability to stay seated when required, talking excessively, acting impulsively, and interrupting others' activities (American Psychiatric Association, 2000). In particular, delaying gratification and valuing future over immediate rewards is difficult for the ADHD adolescent (Barkley, Edwards, et al., 2001b; Olson et al., 1999; Solanto et al., 2001). These inhibitory deficits extend to emotional reactions to provocative social situations and to less tolerance for and inhibition of frustration. These inhibitory problems are not a function of other psychiatric disorders that may overlap with ADHD (Barkley, Edwards, et al., 2001b; Murphy et al., 2001; Nigg, 1999).

Interestingly, recent research shows that the problems with inhibition arise first (at age 3–4 years) as evident in the grossly hyperactive behavior of the preschool child. These symptoms are then compounded by an increase in those related to inattention over the next few years (by age 5–7 years). The symptoms related to sluggish cognitive tempo that may characterize the predominantly inattentive subtype arise even later (ages 8–10) (Hart, Lahey, Loeber, Applegate, & Frick, 1995; Loeber, Green, Lahey, Christ, & Frick, 1992; Milich et al., 2001). Whereas the symptoms of hyperactivity decline by adolescence, inhibitory problems remain as evidenced by difficulties with self-control, disregard for the consequences of one's impulsive actions, and a diminished valuing of future goals over immediate gratification. Those of inattention remain relatively stable during the elementary grades (Hart et al., 1995) but may grow increasingly elaborate in their cognitive nature, as noted previously (encompassing working memory, self-organization, time management, etc.). By adolescence, the problem is not so much one of excessive movement or disruptive play but poor self-regulation, impaired self-motivation, and deficient future-oriented conduct.

Situational and Contextual Factors

The symptoms comprising ADHD are greatly affected in their level of severity by a variety of situational and task-related factors: (1) Time of day (Dane, Schachar, & Tannock, 2000; Zagar & Bowers, 1983); (2) task complexity; (3) degree of restraint; (4) boredom (Antrop, Roeyers, Van Oost, & Buysse, 2000); (5) delayed consequences (Carlson & Mann, 2002; Slusarek, Velling, Bunk, & Eggers, 2001); and (6) the absence of adult supervision, among others, seem to determine how symptomatic the individual is likely to be in any given context (Adams, McCarthy, & Kelly, 1995). ADHD in teens may be most problematic when persistence in work-related tasks is required (chores, homework, school projects, etc.) or where behavioral restraint is necessary (i.e., provocation or daring from peers, risk-taking behavior, and substance experimentation).

DIAGNOSTIC CRITERIA AND RELATED ISSUES

DSM-IV Criteria

The most recent diagnostic criteria for ADHD as defined in DSM-IV (American Psychiatric Association, 2000) are set forth in Table 4.1. They were derived from a committee of some of the leading experts in the field, a literature review of ADHD, an informal survey of empirically derived rating scales assessing the behavioral dimensions related to ADHD by the committee, and from statistical analyses of the results of a field trial of the items using 380 children (ages 4–16) from 10 different sites in North America (Lahey et al., 1994). Despite its empirical basis, the DSM criteria have some problems. A critical issue for the diagnosis of teens is how well the diagnostic thresholds set for the two symptom lists apply to age groups outside those used in the field trial (ages 4–16 years, chiefly). The behavioral items comprising these lists, particularly those for hyperactivity, decline significantly with age (DuPaul et al., 1997; Hart et al., 1995). Applying the same threshold across such a declining developmental slope could produce a situation in which a smaller than expected percentage of teens and adults would meet the criteria (false negatives). One study (Murphy & Barkley, 1996b) collecting norms for DSM-IV item lists on a large sample of adults, ages 17–84 years, suggested

that the threshold needed to place an individual at the 93rd percentile for that person's age group declined to four of nine inattention items and five of nine hyperactive–impulsive items for ages 17–29 years, then declined still further every 20 years thereafter. In view of these results, it seems prudent to utilize the recommended symptom list thresholds only for children ages 4–16 years and to be more cautious in doing so with older teens and young adults until better normative data for these age groups become available.

As noted earlier, evidence is mounting that the ADHD, predominantly inattentive (ADHD-PI) type may contain a subset that have a qualitatively different disorder of attention and cognitive processing (Milich et al., 2001). This subset is probably not a subtype of ADHD but may represent a separate disorder (Barkley, 2001c, 2006; Milich et al., 2001), manifesting a sluggish cognitive style and selective attention deficit, having less comorbidity with ODD and conduct disorder (CD), demonstrating a more passive style of social relationship, having memory retrieval problems, and, owing to their lower level of impulsiveness, probably having a different, more benign, developmental course. Noteworthy is that no research appears to have been done on the nature of this cognitively sluggish subtype in adolescents. It is also unclear whether ADHD, predominantly hyperactive–impulsive (ADHD-PHI) type is really separate from the combined (ADHD-C) type or simply an earlier developmental stage of it. The field trial found that ADHD-PHI was primarily comprised of preschool-age children, whereas ADHD-C was primarily school-age children and teens.

Studies find that childhood symptoms of hyperactivity are related to adverse adolescent outcomes, such as antisocial behavior, substance abuse, and school disciplinary actions, such as suspensions/expulsions (Babinski, Hartsough, & Lambert, 1999; Molina, Smith, & Pelham, 1999). Symptoms of inattention seem to be primarily predictive of impairment in academic achievement, particularly reading, and school performance (DuPaul, Power, Anastopoulos, & Reid, 1999; Rabiner, Coie, & Conduct Problems Prevention Research Group, 2000). A recent study suggests that adolescent inattention, however, may contribute further to the risk for tobacco use beyond that risk contributed by severity of conduct disorder alone (Burke, Loeber, & Lahey, 2001), perhaps

TABLE 4.1. DSM-IV-TR Criteria for ADHD

A. Either (1) or (2):

 (1) six (or more) of the following symptoms of **inattention** have persisted for at least 6 months to a degree that is maladaptive and inconsistent with developmental level:

 Inattention
 (a) often fails to give close attention to details or makes careless mistakes in schoolwork, work, or other activities
 (b) often has difficulty sustaining attention in tasks or play activities
 (c) often does not seem to listen when spoken to directly
 (d) often does not follow through on instructions and fails to finish schoolwork, chores, or duties in the workplace (not due to oppositional behavior or failure to understand instructions)
 (e) often has difficulty organizing tasks and activities
 (f) often avoids, dislikes, or is reluctant to engage in tasks that require sustained mental effort such as schoolwork or homework)
 (g) often loses things necessary for tasks or activities (e.g., toys, school assignments, pencils, books, or tools)
 (h) is often easily distracted by extraneous stimuli
 (i) is often forgetful in daily activities
 (2) six (or more) of the following symptoms of **hyperactivity–impulsivity** have persisted for at least 6 months to a degree that is maladaptive and inconsistent with developmental level:

 Hyperactivity
 (a) often fidgets with hands or feet or squirms in seat
 (b) often leaves seat in classroom or in other situations in which remaining seated is expected
 (c) often runs about or climbs excessively in situations in which it is inappropriate (in adolescents or adults, may be limited to subjective feelings of restlessness)
 (d) often has difficulty playing or engaging in leisure activities quietly
 (e) is often "on the go" or often acts as if "driven by a motor"
 (f) often talks excessively

 Impulsivity
 (g) often blurts out answers before the questions have been completed
 (h) often has difficulty awaiting turn
 (i) often interrupts or intrudes on others (e.g., butts into conversations or games)

B. Some hyperactive–impulsive or inattentive symptoms that caused impairment were present before age 7 years.

C. Some impairment from the symptoms is present in two or more settings (e.g., at school [or work] and at home).

D. There must be clear evidence of clinically significant impairment in social, academic, or occupational functioning.

E. The symptoms do not occur exclusively during the course of a Pervasive Developmental Disorder, Schizophrenia, or other Psychotic Disorder and are not better accounted for by another mental disorder (e.g., Mood Disorder, Anxiety Disorder, Dissociative Disorder, or a Personality Disorder).

Code based on type:
314.01 Attention-Deficit/Hyperactivity Disorder, Combined Type: if both Criteria A1 and A2 are met for the past 6 months
314.00 Attention-Deficit/Hyperactivity Disorder, Predominantly Inattentive Type: if Criterion A1 is met but Criterion A2 is not met for the past 6 months
314.01 Attention-Deficit/Hyperactivity Disorder, PredominantlyHyperactive–Impulsive Type: if Criterion A2 is met but Criterion A1 is not met for the past 6 months

Coding note: For individuals (especially adolescents and adults) who currently have symptoms that no longer meet full criteria, "In Partial Remission" should be specified).

Note. From American Psychiatric Association (2000). Copyright 2000 by the American Psychiatric Association. Reprinted by permission.

as a result of attempts at self-medication. Nico-tine may be beneficial to attention span and thus teens with ADHD may find smoking to actually have some therapeutic effect on their inattention.

Another critical issue for developing diag-nostic criteria for ADHD is the appropriateness of the content of the item set for different de-velopmental periods. Inspection of the item lists suggests that the items for inattention may have a wider developmental applicability across elementary-school-age ranges and per-haps even into adolescence and young adult-hood. Those for hyperactive–impulsive behav-ior, in contrast, seem much more applicable to young children and less appropriate or not at all to teens and adults. Studies of teens with ADHD should concentrate on what other symptoms may be more sensitive to the disor-der than are those on the current DSM list to ensure that the disorder is captured well across development. As it now stands, ADHD is being defined mainly by one of its earliest develop-mental manifestations (hyperactivity) and one of its later (school-age) sequelae (inattention) and only minimally by its central features (inhi-bition, self-control, and executive functioning). For instance, problems with working memory, organization, time management, and social impulsivity might be more discerning of the ad-olescent stage of ADHD than would be the DSM symptoms such as "often climbs on things" or "cannot play quietly."

Also of concern is the absence of any re-quirement in DSM for the symptoms to be cor-roborated by someone who has known the pa-tient well, such as a parent, sibling, long-time friend, or partner. Most likely, this absence arises from the focus on children throughout much of the history of the ADHD diagnostic category. In the case of teens and particularly adults who are self-referred to professionals, this oversight could prove potentially problem-atic. For instance, available evidence suggests that children and teens with ADHD (Henry, Moffitt, Caspi, Langley, & Silva, 1994) signifi-cantly underreport the severity of their symp-toms relative to the reports of parents (Ed-wards, Barkley, Laneri, & Metevia, 2001; Fischer, Barkley, Fletcher, & Smallish, 1993b; Romano, Tremblay, Vitaro, Zoccolillo, & Pagani, 2001). This means that self-referred patients or those being evaluated in juvenile custody or detention might underestimate the severity of their disorder, resulting in a sizable number of false-negative decisions being made by clinicians.

DSM may lose some of its sensitivity to the disorder by late adolescence or young adult-hood. Recently, we found that if children who formerly had ADHD, who are now young adults (20–26), are interviewed using the DSM criteria, just 5% of them report sufficient symptoms to receive the diagnosis (Barkley et al., 2002), a figure nearly identical to that for the New York longitudinal studies (Mannuzza, Klein, Bessler, Malloy, & LaPadula, 1993, 1998). If instead the parents are interviewed, this figure rises to 46%—a ninefold difference in persistence of disorder as a function of re-porting source. If instead of the recommended DSM symptom threshold, a developmentally referenced criterion (the 98th percentile) based on same-age control adults is substituted, then 66% still have the disorder based on parental reports (Barkley et al., 2002). Though unstud-ied, this same problem of source is likely to af-fect the diagnosis of teens as well.

The requirement of an age of onset for ADHD symptoms (7 years) in the diagnostic criteria has also come under attack from its own field trial (Applegate et al., 1997), a longi-tudinal study (McGee, Williams, & Feehan, 1992), and a review of this criterion from his-torical, empirical, and pragmatic perspectives (Barkley & Biederman, 1997). It is possible that earlier onset suggests a more severe degree of disorder, but no sharp demarcation has been found in the few studies of age of onset that in-dicate the need for this precise an onset crite-rion. In the author's view, cases of ADHD in adolescence may well arise secondary to frontal lobe or cerebellar injury (see "Etiologies" sec-tion, later).

The DSM requirement that the symptoms be demonstrated in at least two of three environ-ments to establish pervasiveness of symptoms is new to this edition and problematic. DSM implies that two of three sources of informa-tion (parent, teacher, employer) must agree on the presence of the symptoms. This confounds settings with sources of information. The de-gree of agreement between parents and teacher for any dimension of child behavior is modest, often ranging between .30 and .50 (Achenbach, McConaughy, & Howell, 1987). Recent evi-dence suggests that the best discrimination of children with ADHD from other groups might be achieved by blending the reports of parents and teachers such that one counts the number of different symptoms endorsed across *both* sources of information (Crystal, Ostrander, Chen, & August, 2001; Mitsis, McKay, Schulz, Newcorn, & Halperin, 2000). The problem is likely to be further compounded in adolescence given the limited time teens spend with parents and with any single teacher and the greater time they spend with peers.

EPIDEMIOLOGY OF ADHD

Prevalence

Szatmari (1992) reviewed six large epidemiological studies and reported a prevalence ranging from a low of 2% to a high of 6.3% with most falling within the range of 4.2–6.3%. A more recent population-based study in Rochester, Minnesota, pegged the prevalence rate for definite ADHD at 7.4% using DSM-IV criteria (Barbaresi et al., 2002). Prevalence rates may be 4% in girls and 8% in boys in the preschool age group (Gadow, Sprafkin, & Nolan, 2001) yet fall to 0.9–2% in girls and 1–5.6% in boys by adolescence (Breton et al., 1999; Lewinsohn, Hops, Roberts, Seeley, & Andrews, 1993; Romano et al., 2001). Prevalence of ADHD varies as a function of age, male gender, chronic health problems, family dysfunction, low socioeconomic status, presence of a developmental impairment, and urban living (Lavigne et al., 1996; Velez, Johnson, & Cohen, 1989). The disorder is found in all countries yet surveyed with rates similar to if not higher than those found in North America (see Barkley, 2006). Differences across ethnic groups within the United States are sometimes found but seem to be more a function social class than ethnicity (Szatmari, 1992).

Sex Differences

On average, males are between 2.5 and 5.6 times more likely than females to be diagnosed with ADHD within epidemiological samples, with the average being roughly 3:1 (Breton et al., 1999; DuPaul, Barkley, & Connor, 1998; McGee et al., 1990; Szatmari, 1992). Studies of clinic-referred girls often find that they are as impaired as clinic-referred boys with ADHD, have as much comorbidity, and may even have greater deficits in intelligence, according to meta-analytic reviews of sex differences in ADHD (Carlson, Tamm, & Gaub, 1997; Gaub & Carlson, 1997; Gershon, 2002). Some stud-

ies suggest these clinic-referred girls, at least as adolescents, may have more internalizing symptoms, such as depression, anxiety, and stress, greater problems with teacher relationships, and poorer verbal abilities (vocabulary) in comparison to ADHD boys (Rucklidge & Tannock, 2001). Like the boys, girls with ADHD also manifest more conduct, mood, and anxiety disorders; have lower intelligence; and have greater academic achievement deficits than do control samples (Biederman, Faraone, et al., 1999; Hinshaw, 2002; Hinshaw, Carte, Sami, Treuting, & Zupan, 2002; Rucklidge & Tannock, 2001). No sex differences have been identified in executive functioning, with both sexes being more impaired than control samples on such measures (Castellanos et al., 2000; Murphy et al., 2001). Studies drawing their ADHD samples from the community find that girls are significantly less likely to have comorbid ODD and CD than boys with ADHD, do not have greater intellectual deficits than ADHD boys, yet may be as socially and academically impaired as boys with the disorder (Gaub & Carlson, 1997; Gershon, 2002).

DEVELOPMENTAL COURSE AND ADULT OUTCOMES

Major follow-up studies of clinically referred and community-sampled hyperactive children have been ongoing during the last 25 years. These studies cannot be viewed as representing the inattentive subtype, for which no follow-up information is currently available.

By the time children with ADHD move into adolescence, the problems with hyperactivity are declining but those with impulsive behavior are likely to continue and to be joined now by difficulties with attention, self-regulation, and executive functioning. Difficulties with work completion and productivity, distraction, forgetfulness related to what needs doing, lack of planning, poor organization of work activities, trouble meeting time deadlines associated with home chores, school assignments, and social promises or commitments to peers are now combined with the impulsive, heedless, and disinhibited behavior typifying these teens since preschool age. Problems with oppositional and socially aggressive behavior may emerge by this age in at least 40–70% of ADHD children (Barkley, 1998; Loeber et al., 1992; Taylor, Sandberg, Thorley, & Giles, 1991).

The likelihood is that 50–80% of clinically diagnosed cases of ADHD in childhood will continue to have their disorder into adolescence, with most studies supporting the higher figure (August, Stewart, & Holmes, 1983; Claude & Firestone, 1995; Barkley, Fischer, et al., 1990; Gittelman, Mannuzza, Shenker, & Bonagura, 1985; Mannuzza et al., 1993). Using the same parent rating scales at both the childhood and adolescent evaluation points, Fischer and colleagues (1993b) were able to show that inattention, hyperactive–impulsive behavior, and home conflicts declined by adolescence. The hyperactive group showed far more marked declines than the control group, mainly because the former were so far from the mean of the normative group to begin with in childhood. Nevertheless, even at adolescence, the groups remained significantly different in each domain with the mean for the hyperactives remaining two standard deviations or more above the mean for the controls. The persistence of ADHD symptoms across childhood as well as into early adolescence appears, again, to be associated with initial degree of hyperactive–impulsive behavior in childhood, the coexistence of conduct problems or oppositional hostile behavior, poor family relations, and specifically conflict in parent–child interactions, as well as maternal depression and duration of mental health interventions (Fischer et al., 1993a; Taylor et al., 1991).

COMORBID PSYCHIATRIC DISORDERS

Teens diagnosed with ADHD are often found to have a number of other disorders besides their ADHD. What is known about comorbidity is largely confined to the combined type of ADHD. In community derived samples, up to 44% of children and teens with ADHD have at least one other disorder and 43% have at least two or more additional disorders (Szatmari, Offord, & Boyle, 1989). The figure is higher, of course, for cases drawn from clinics. As many as 87% of children clinically diagnosed with ADHD may have at least one other disorder and 67% have at least two other disorders (Kadesjo & Gillberg, 2001).

Oppositional, Conduct, and Antisocial Disorders

The most common comorbid disorders with ADHD-C type in adolescents are ODD and, to a lesser extent, CD. Indeed, the presence of ADHD increases the odds of ODD/CD by 10.7-fold (95% confidence interval [CI] = 7.7–14.8) in general population studies (Angold, Costello, & Erkanli, 1999). Studies of clinic-referred children and teens with ADHD find that between 54% and 67% will meet criteria for a diagnosis of ODD by 7 years of age or later. ODD is a frequent precursor to CD, a more severe and often (though not always) later occurring stage of ODD (Loeber, Burke, Lahey, Winters, & Zera, 2000). The co-occurrence of CD with ADHD may be 20–50% in children and 44–50% in teens with ADHD (Barkley, 1998; Barkley, Fischer, et al., 1990; Biederman, Faraone, & Lapey, 1992; Lahey, McBurnett, & Loeber, 2000). By adulthood, up to 26% may continue to have CD while 12–21% will qualify for antisocial personality disorder (APD) (Biederman et al., 1992; Barkley, Fischer, Smallish, & Fletcher, 2002; Mannuzza & Klein, 1992; Rasmussen & Gillberg, 2001; Weiss & Hechtman, 1993).

One of the strongest predictors of risk for substance use and abuse disorders (SUDs) among children with ADHD upon reaching adolescence and adulthood is prior or coexisting CD or APD (Burke et al., 2001; Chilcoat & Breslau, 1999; Molina & Pelham, 1999; White, Xie, Thompson, Loeber, & Stouthamer-Loeber, 2002). Given the heightened risk for ODD/CD/APD in teens with ADHD as they mature, one would naturally expect a greater risk for SUDs as well. While an elevated risk for alcohol abuse has not been consistently documented in follow-up studies into adulthood, the risk for other SUDs among hyperactive children followed to adulthood ranges from 12 to 24% (Fischer, Barkley, Smallish, & Fletcher, 2002; Gittelman et al., 1985; Mannuzza et al., 1993, 1998; Rasmussen & Gillberg, 2001). These results are from studies following children to adulthood that gave scant attention to teen substance use and abuse at adolescence. The issue of SUDs in teens with ADHD is only now receiving concentrated research attention.

Anxiety and Mood Disorders

The overlap of anxiety disorders with ADHD has been found to be 10–40% in clinic-referred children, averaging to about 25% (see Biederman, Newcorn, & Sprich, 1991; Tannock, 2000, for reviews). In longitudinal studies of children with ADHD, however, the risk of anxiety disorders is no greater than in control groups at either adolescence or young adulthood (Fischer et al., 2002; Mannuzza et al., 1993, 1998; Russo & Biedel, 1994; Weiss & Hechtman, 1993). The disparity in findings is puzzling. Perhaps some of the overlap of ADHD with anxiety disorders in children is due to referral bias (Biederman et al., 1992; Tannock, 2000). General population studies of children, however, do suggest an elevated odds ratio of having an anxiety disorder in the presence of ADHD of 3.0 (95% CI = 2.1–4.3), with this relationship being significant even after controlling for comorbid ODD/CD (Angold et al., 1999). For the inattentive type of ADHD, higher rates of anxiety disorders have been noted in some studies (see Milich et al., 2001 for a review; Russo & Biedel, 1994), though not always (Barkley, DuPaul, & McMurray, 1990), and in their first- and second-degree relatives (Barkley, DuPaul, & McMurray, 1990; Biederman et al., 1992) again though not always (Lahey & Carlson, 1992; Milich et al., 2001).

The evidence for the co-occurrence of mood disorders, such as major depression or dysthymia (a milder form of depression), with ADHD is now fairly substantial (see Faraone & Biederman, 1997; Jensen, Martin, & Cantwell, 1997; Spencer, Wilens, Biederman, Wozniak, & Harding-Crawford, 2000, for reviews). Between 15 and 75% of those with ADHD may have a mood disorder, though most studies place the association between 20 and 30% (Biederman et al., 1992; Cuffe et al, 2001; Fischer et al., 2002). A meta-analysis of general population studies indicated that the link between ADHD and depression was entirely mediated by the linkage of both disorders to CD (Angold et al., 1999). In the absence of CD, ADHD was not more likely to be associated with depression. Given the sharp rise in risk for CD by adolescence among youth with ADHD, it would not be surprising to find an equally sharp increase in risk for comorbid depression by this developmental stage. Gender differences in risk for mood disorders are likely to exist by this age as well given the greater predisposition of females to developing depression, at least in overt form, but females have been so strikingly underrepresented in longitudinal studies to date that no solid information is available on the issue at this time.

The comorbidity of ADHD with bipolar (manic–depressive) disorder is controversial (Carlson, 1990; Geller & Luby, 1997). Some studies of children and teens with ADHD indicate that 10–20% may have bipolar disorder (Milberger, Biederman, Faraone, Murphy, & Tsuang, 1995; Spencer et al., 2000; Wozniak et al., 1995)—a figure substantially higher than the 1% risk for the general population (Lewinsohn, Klein, & Seeley, 1995). Follow-up studies of hyperactive children, however, have not documented any significant increase in risk of bipolar disorder by adulthood (Fischer et al., 2002; Mannuzza et al., 1993, 1998; Weiss & Hechtman, 1993). A 4-year follow-up of children with ADHD reported that 12% met criteria for bipolar disorder in adolescence (Biederman, Faraone, Mick, et al., 1996), but this remains to be replicated in other longitudinal research into adolescence. Children with ADHD without bipolar disorder do not have an increased prevalence of bipolar disorder among their biological relatives (Biederman et al., 1992; Faraone, Biederman, & Monuteaux, 2001; Lahey et al., 1988) while children with ADHD with bipolar disorder do (Faraone et al., 1997, 2001), suggesting that where the overlap occurs it may represent a familially distinct subset of ADHD. In any case, the overlap of ADHD with bipolar disorder appears, for now at least, to be unidirectional—a diagnosis of ADHD seems not to increase the risk for bipolar disorder much, whereas a diagnosis of childhood bipolar disorder seems to dramatically elevate the risk of a prior or concurrent diagnosis of ADHD (Geller & Luby, 1997; Spencer et al., 2000).

ASSOCIATED DEVELOPMENTAL PROBLEMS

Apart from an increased risk for various psychiatric disorders, teens with ADHD (combined type) may also more likely to experience a substantial array of developmental and health risks, discussed below. The developmental risks for the inattentive type remain unknown.

Cognitive Impairments

ADHD is often associated with deficiencies in many other cognitive abilities besides attention. Among these, are difficulties with (1) speed of color naming (Tannock, Martinussen, & Frijters, 2000); (2) verbal and nonverbal working memory and mental computation (Barkley, 1997a; McInnis, Humphries, Hogg-Johnson, & Tannock, 2003; Murphy et al., 2001); (3) story comprehension (Lorch et al.,

2000; Sanchez, Lorch, Milich, & Welsh, 1999); (4) planning and anticipation (Grodzinsky & Diamond, 1992; Klorman et al., 1999); (5) verbal fluency and confrontational communication (Grodzinsky & Diamond, 1992; Zentall, 1988); (6) developing, applying, and self-monitoring organizational strategies (Clark, Prior, & Kinsella, 2000; Purvis & Tannock, 1997); (7) the internalization of self-directed speech (Berk & Potts, 1991; Winsler, Diaz, Atencio, McCarthy, & Chabay, 2000); and (8) self-regulation of emotion (Braaten & Rosen, 2000; Maedgen & Carlson, 2000). The latter difficulties with emotional control may be especially salient in teens having ADHD with ODD (Melnick & Hinshaw, 2000). These cognitive difficulties appear to be specific to ADHD and are not a function of its commonly comorbid disorders, such as learning disabilities, depression, anxiety, or ODD/CD (Barkley, Edwards, et al., 2001b; Clark et al., 2000; Klorman et al., 1999; Murphy et al., 2001). Here, again, these findings have received less attention in teens with ADHD, but the few domains that have been studied suggest similar domains of cognitive impairment in teens as in children or adults with ADHD (Barkley, Edwards, et al., 2001b; Rucklidge & Tannock, 2001; Schmitz et al., 2002).

Impaired Academic and Intellectual Functioning

The vast majority of clinic-referred teens with ADHD have difficulties with school performance, most often underproductivity of their work. Teens with ADHD frequently fall below normal or control groups of children on standardized achievement tests (Fischer, Barkley, Edelbrock, & Smallish, 1990; Hinshaw, 1992a, 1994). Studies suggest that the risk for reading disorders in ADHD groups is 16–39%, while that for spelling disorders is 24–27%, and for math disorders, the risk is 13–33% (Barkley, 1990; Casey, Rourke, & Del Dotto, 1996; Frick et al., 1991; Semrud-Clikeman et al., 1992). Writing disorders have not received as much attention in research on ADHD, though handwriting deficits are often found with ADHD, particularly the combined type (Marcotte & Stern, 1997). A higher prevalence of speech and language disorders has also been documented in many studies of ADHD, typically ranging from 30% to 64% of the samples (see Tannock & Brown, 2000).

Social Problems

Research finds that ADHD affects social interactions with parents and, hence, the manner in which parents may respond to the affected teen (Johnston & Mash, 2001). Teens with ADHD are likely to be more talkative, negative and defiant, less compliant and cooperative, more demanding of assistance from others, and less able to work independently (Johnston, 1996; Johnston & Mash, 2001). Their mothers are less responsive to the questions of their children, more negative and directive, and less rewarding of their children's behavior (Danforth, Barkley, & Stokes, 1991; Johnston & Mash, 2001). Teens with ADHD seem to be nearly as problematic for their fathers as their mothers (Edwards et al., 2001; Johnston, 1996). Edwards (1995) analyzed data from the study by Barkley, Anastopoulos, and colleagues (1991) looking at the various issues on which parents and teens with ADHD expressed conflict relative to parents and teens in a control group using the Issues Checklist (see below). The teens with ADHD were further subdivided into those with comorbid ODD/CD. Of the 44 issues on this list, mothers reported significantly more conflict with their teens with ADHD only around 7 issues: doing homework, making too much noise at home, playing the stereo too loudly, taking care of personal possessions, getting low grades in school, and messing up the house. Fathers of teens with ADHD only reported only 4 areas of conflict: doing homework, poor or low grades in school, lying, and messing up the house. For mothers of teens with ADHD/ODD, the number of conflicts nearly doubled to 13, with the additional issues being cursing, who their friends are, getting into trouble at school, talking back to parents, bothering parents when they wish to be left alone, and smoking. The opposite pattern was seen in fathers of teens with ADHD/ODD who reported far fewer problems; indeed just one issue of conflict occurred with their teens: talking back to parents. Why this should be so is unclear but may have to do with the possibility that oppositional teens with ADHD may have less involved or more antisocial fathers who are thereby less likely to encounter conflicts with their teens. Teens in both groups having ADHD reported fewer issues of conflict with their parents than did their parents but still endorsed more conflicts than did teens in the control group. Mothers of teens with ADHD reported more arguments around these issues and hotter arguments than did fathers of these teens. The disparity was even greater if the mothers had teens with both ADHD and ODD.

Contrary to what may be seen in normal mother–teen interactions, the mother–teen conflicts in ADHD groups may actually increase when fathers join the interaction (Buhrmester, Camparo, Christensen, Gonzalez, & Hinshaw, 1992; Edwards et al., 2001). Such increased maternal negativity and acrimony toward sons in these interactions has been shown to predict greater noncompliance in school and greater covert stealing away from home (Anderson, Hinshaw, & Simmel, 1994). With increasing age, the degree of conflict in these interactions lessens but remains deviant from normal in adolescence (Barkley, Anastopoulos, Guevremont, & Fletcher, 1992; Barkley, Fischer, Edelbrock, & Smallish, 1991; Edwards et al., 2001). Negative parent–child interactions in childhood have been observed to be significantly predictive of continuing parent–teen conflicts 8–10 years later in adolescence in families with children with ADHD (Barkley, Fischer, et al., 1991). It is the presence of comorbid ODD that is associated with the highest levels of interaction conflicts between parents and their adolescents with ADHD (Barkley, Anastopoulos, et al., 1992; Barkley, Fischer, et al., 1991; Edwards et al., 2001; Fletcher, Fischer, Barkley, & Smallish, 1996).

The patterns of disruptive, intrusive, excessive, negative, and emotional social interactions of children with ADHD noted earlier have been found to occur in the interactions of children with ADHD with their teachers (Whalen, Henker, & Dotemoto, 1980) and peers (Clark, Cheyne, Cunningham, & Siegel, 1988; Cunningham & Siegel, 1987; DuPaul, McGoey, Eckert, & VanBrakle, 2001). This is likely to be so with teens with ADHD, but no studies have focused specifically on that age group. It should come as no surprise, then, that those with ADHD receive more correction, punishment, censure, and criticism than do other children from their teachers, as well as more school suspensions and expulsions, particularly if they have ODD/CD (Barkley, Fischer, et al., 1990; Whalen et al., 1980). In their social relationships, children with ADHD are less liked by peers, have fewer friends, and are overwhelmingly rejected as a consequence (Erhardt & Hinshaw, 1994), particularly if they have comorbid conduct problems (Gres-

ham, MacMillan, Bocian, Ward, & Forness, 1998; Hinshaw & Melnick, 1995). Up to 70% may be rejected by peers and have no reciprocated friendships by fourth grade (Gresham et al., 1998). Two important areas needing future research are the study of teacher–student as well as peer relations in teenagers with ADHD to see how well these findings on children can be extrapolated to the adolescent age group.

Motor Incoordination

As a group, as many as 60% of children with ADHD, compared to up to 35% of normal children, may have poor motor coordination or developmental coordination disorder (Kadesjo & Gillberg, 2001). Although gross motor incoordination may decrease across childhood, fine motor problems remain evident in adolescents with the disorder.

Accident Proneness and Injury

Most studies find children with ADHD experience more injuries of various sorts than control children (Barkley, 2001a), but no studies appear to have addressed this issue specifically with teens. The exception appears to be studies of driving. Barkley, Guevremont, Anastopoulos, DuPaul, and Shelton (1993) found that teens with ADHD had more crashes as the driver (1.5 vs. 0.4) than did control teens over their first few years of driving. Forty percent of the ADHD group had experienced at least two or more such crashes relative to just 6% of the control group. Four times more teens with ADHD were deemed to have been at fault in their crashes as the driver than control teens (48.6% vs. 11.1%) and were at fault more frequently than the controls (0.8 vs. 0.4). Teens with ADHD were more likely to get speeding tickets (65.7% vs. 33.3%) and got them more often (means = 2.4 vs. 0.6). Adults diagnosed with ADHD also manifest more unsafe motor vehicle operation and crashes (Barkley, Murphy, & Kwasnik, 1996a; Barkley, Murphy, DuPaul, & Bush, 2002). The ADHD groups had been involved in more vehicular crashes than the control teens and adults and had been held to be at fault in more crashes. The dollar damage caused in their first accidents was estimated to be more than twice as high in the ADHD than control group (means = $4,221 vs. $1,665). These studies leave little doubt that ADHD, or its symptoms of inattention and hyperactive–impulsive behavior, are associated with a higher risk for unsafe driving and motor vehicle accidents in teens and adults than in the normal population. In view of the substantial costs that must be associated with such a higher rate of adverse driving outcomes, prevention and intervention efforts are certainly called for to attempt to reduce the driving risks among teens and adults having ADHD.

THEORETICAL FRAMEWORK

Many different theories of ADHD have been proposed over the past century to account for the diversity of findings so evident in children with this disorder (Barkley, 1999). Yet only the author's model of ADHD set forth below considers changes that take place in cognitive development (specifically executive functioning) to be important in understanding the way symptoms of and impairment from the disorder is likely to change with age, particularly by adolescence. This theory argues that behavioral inhibition can be placed at a foundational starting point in its relation to four other executive functions dependent on it for their own effective execution. These four executive functions develop in a stepwise sequence across childhood into adolescence, each requiring the one before it for its own effective development and execution. This provides for the increasing development and greater complexity of self-regulation by young adulthood, bringing behavior progressively more under the control of time and the influence of future over immediate consequences. The stagewise emergence and interaction of these executive functions by adolescence permits far more effective adaptive functioning toward the social future (social self-sufficiency) than is capable in childhood. Indeed, this is the only model to argue for a qualitative change in the nature of self-control with age and to stipulate that there exist four forms of self-control evident by adolescence, not one unitary form as is commonly believed.

"Behavioral inhibition" is viewed as consisting of two related processes: (1) the capacity to inhibit prepotent responses, either prior to or once initiated, creating a delay in the response to an event (response inhibition); and (2) the protection of this delay, the self-directed actions occurring within it, and the goal-directed behaviors they create from interference by competing events and their prepotent responses (interference control). "Prepotent responses" are defined as those for which immediate reinforcement is available for their performance or for which there is a strong history of reinforcement in this context. Through the postponement of the prepotent response and the creation of this protected period of delay, the occasion is set for four other executive functions to act effectively in modifying the individual's eventual response(s) to the event allowing them to achieve a net maximization of distant consequences rather than immediate ones.

Four executive functions are believed to develop via a common process though in a stepwise sequence. All are said to represent private, covert forms of behavior by adolescence that in earlier child development (and in human evolution) were entirely publicly observable and were directed toward others and the external world at large. With maturation, this outer-directed behavior becomes turned on the self as a means to control one's own behavior. Such self-directed behaving then becomes increasingly less observable to others as the suppression of the public, peripheral musculoskeletal aspects of the behavior progresses into adolescence. The child and especially the teen are increasingly able to act toward them selves without publicly displaying the actual behavior being activated. This progressively greater capacity to suppress the publicly observable aspects of behavior is what is meant here by the terms "covert, privatized, or internalized." Teens come to be capable of behaving internally (in their brain) without showing that response through their peripheral muscles, at least not to the extent that it is visible to others. All the executive functions are theorized to follow the same general sequence as the internalization of speech (Diaz & Berk, 1992; Vygotsky, 1978, 1987), which in this model forms the second executive function. Each is hypothesized to contribute to the following developmental shifts in the sources of control over behavior from childhood to adolescence:

- From external events to mental representations related to those events
- From control by others to control by the self
- From immediate reinforcement to delayed gratification
- And from control by the temporal now to control by the conjectured social future

Nonverbal Working Memory (Sensory–Motor Action to the Self)

Humans activate and retain a mental representation of events in mind (Bronowski, 1977), typically using visual imagery and private audition. The capacity for imagery increases developmentally, forming the basis for nonverbal working memory. This activation of past images and other sensory representations for the sake of preparing a current response constitutes "hindsight" (Bronowski, 1977; Fuster, 1997) contributing to the "subjective estimation of time" (Michon, 1985). From such temporal sequences one can conjecture hypothetical future events. Anticipating these hypothetical futures gives rise to a preparation to act, or "anticipatory set" (Fuster, 1997). This extension of hindsight forward into time also underlies "forethought" (Bronowski, 1977; Fuster, 1997). And from this sense of future likely emerges the progressively greater valuation of future consequences over immediate ones that takes place throughout teen development and early adult life (Green, Fry, & Meyerson, 1994). For teens with ADHD, the model predicts that deficits in behavioral inhibition lead to deficiencies in nonverbal working memory and thus (1) particular forms of forgetfulness (forgetting to do things at certain critical points in time); (2) impaired ability to organize and execute their actions relative to time (e.g., time management); (3) reduced hindsight and forethought; and thus (4) a reduction in the anticipation of future events. Consequently, the capacity for the cross-temporal organization of behavior is diminished, disrupting the ability to string together complex chains of actions directed, over time, to a future goal.

Verbal Working Memory (Internalization of Speech)

One of the more fascinating developmental processes witnessed across childhood into early adolescence is the progressive internalization or privatization of speech (Diaz & Berk, 1992). During the early preschool years, speech, once developed, is initially employed for communication with others. By 3–5 years of age, language comes to be turned on the self. Such overt self-speech is readily observable in preschool and early school-age children. By 5–7 years of age, this speech becomes somewhat quieter and more telegraphic and shifts from being more descriptive to being more instructive. Language is now a means of reflection (self-directed description) as well as a means for controlling one's own behavior. Self-directed speech progresses from being public, to being subvocal, to finally being private by 9–12 years of age giving rise to verbal thought (Diaz & Berk, 1992; Kopp, 1982; Vygotsky, 1987). For those with ADHD, the privatization of speech should be delayed, resulting in greater public speech (excessive talking), less verbal reflection before acting, less organized and rule-oriented self-speech, a diminished influence of self-directed speech in controlling one's own behavior, and difficulties following the rules and instructions given by others (Barkley, 1997b). Substantial evidence has accumulated to support this prediction of delayed internalization of speech (Winsler et al., 2000).

Internalization and Self-Regulation of Affect

Inhibition extends to the initial emotional reaction that may have been elicited by an event. It is not that the teen does not experience emotion but that the behavioral reaction to or expression of that emotion is delayed along with any motor behavior associated with it. The delay in responding with this emotion allows time to engage in self-directed behavior that will modify both the eventual response to the event as well as the emotional reaction that may accompany it. This permits a moderating effect both on the emotion being experienced subjectively as well as on the eventual public expression of emotional behavior (Keenan, 2000). But it is not just affect that is being managed by the development of self-regulation but the underlying components of emotion as well, these being motivation (drive states) and arousal (Fuster, 1997; Lang, 1995). This internalization and self-regulation of motivation permits one to induce drive states that may be required for the initiation and maintenance of goal-directed, future-oriented behavior thereby permitting greater persistence toward tasks and activities that may offer little immediate reinforcement but for which their may be substantial delayed reinforcement. This capacity for creating intrinsic motivation becomes even more crucial by adolescence when teens are expected to engage in sustained behavior toward future goals with little or no reinforcement provided in the interim. Teens with ADHD will display (1) greater emotional expression in their reactions to events; (2) less objectivity in the selection of a response to an event; (3) diminished social perspective taking as the teens do not delay their initial emotional reaction long enough to take the view of others and their own needs into account; and (4) diminished ability to induce drive and motivational states in themselves in the service of goal-directed behavior. Those teens with ADHD remain more dependent upon the environmental contingencies within a situation or task to determine their motivation than do others (Barkley, 1997b). Those with ADHD do have significant problems with emotion regulation (Braaten & Rosen, 2000; Maedgen & Carlson, 2000), and this may be particularly so in that subset having comorbid oppositional defiant disorder (Melnick & Hinshaw, 2000).

Reconstitution (Internalization of Play)

The use of private visual imagery as well as private language to mentally represent objects, actions, and their properties provides a means by which the world can be taken apart and recombined cognitively rather than physically. Just as the parts of speech can be recombined to form new sentences, the parts of the world represented in speech and imagery are, likewise, recombined to create entirely new ideas about the world and entirely new responses to that world (Bronowski, 1977). I believe this process results from the internalization of play. This process of mental play, or reconstitution, is evident in everyday speech in its fluency and generativity (diversity), yet it is also evident in nonverbal expression as well, such as in motor and design fluency. The need for reconstitution becomes obvious when obstacles must be surmounted to accomplish a goal. In a sense, reconstitution provides for planning and problem solving to overcome obstacles and attain goals. This mental module produces rapid, efficient, and often novel combinations of speech or action into entirely new messages or behavioral sequences and so gives rise to behavioral innovation.

As applied to teens with ADHD, the model predicts a diminished use of analysis and synthesis in the formation of both verbal and nonverbal responses to events. The capacity to mentally visualize, manipulate, and then generate multiple plans of action (options) in the service of goal-directed behavior and to select from among them those with the greatest likelihood of succeeding should, therefore, be reduced. This impairment in reconstitution will be evident in everyday verbal fluency when the teen with ADHD is required by a task or situation to assemble rapidly, accurately, and efficiently the parts of speech into messages (sentences) to accomplish the goal or requirements of the task. It will also be evident in tasks where visual information must be held in mind and manipulated to generate diverse scenarios to help solve problems (Barkley, 1997b).

As children develop into adolescence and each new domain of executive functioning grows progressively more elaborate yet efficient, those with ADHD now experience an additional domain of cognitive impairment. For instance, preschool children with ADHD may merely be hyperactive and impulsive. But teens with ADHD are not only impulsive but have five distinct deficits now in executive functioning. The inability to listen and follow through on instructions, to verbally reflect on their own behavior and social situations, to develop and use a sense of time for self-management, to organize across time for future goals, to problem-solve and invent verbally mediated strategies, and to use verbal mediation for self-control would all now be problematic for the teen with ADHD. By adolescence ADHD has created a more complex and more serious suite of psychological deficits not characteristic of preschoolers with the disorder. This issue has received virtually no attention in research studies on the development of ADHD into adolescence, but such a hierarchical theory of executive functioning and, by extension, of ADHD predicts that such will be the case—a testable hypothesis worthy of future investigation.

ETIOLOGIES

Virtually all the research on the etiologies of ADHD pertains to the combined type of ADHD or what was previously considered hyperactivity in children. Readers should not extend these findings to the inattentive type of ADHD, especially that subset noted previously to have sluggish cognitive tempo that is likely a qualitatively different disorder. But for the combined type, there is even less doubt now among career investigators in this field that, while multiple etiologies may lead to ADHD, neurological and genetic factors likely play the greatest role in causing this disorder. These two areas, along with the associated field of the neuropsychology of ADHD, have witnessed enormous growth in the past decade, further refining our understanding of the neurogenetic basis of the disorder. Our knowledge of the final common neurological pathway through which these causes produce their effects on behavior has become clearer from converging lines of evidence employing a wide array of assessment tools, including neuropsychological tests sensitive to frontal lobe functioning, electrophysiological measures, measures of cerebral blood flow, and neuroimaging studies using positron emission tomography (PET), magnetic resonance imaging (MRI), and functional MRI (fMRI). Several recent studies have even identified specific protein abnormalities in specific brain regions that may be linked to possible neurochemical dysregulation in the disorder. Precise neurochemical abnormalities that may underlie this disorder have proven extremely difficult to document, but advancing psychopharmacological, neurological, and genetic evidence suggests involvement in at least two systems, these being dopaminergic and noradrenergic. Neurological evidence is converging on a highly probable neurological network for ADHD, as discussed below. Nevertheless, most findings on etiologies are correlational in nature, not permitting direct, precise, immediate molecular evidence of primary causality. But then that is the case for all psychiatric disorders and, indeed, many medical ones as well; thus ADHD is in good company. In fact, our understanding of causal factors here may be far more advanced than is the case in most other psychopathologies of adolescence. Though most of this research has been done with children having ADHD, studies of adults with ADHD find similar results, leaving little doubt that they would apply to the interim teenage years as well. Certainly, developmental changes in the brain through adolescence, including those induced by hormonal influences, likely affect not only the neurological expression of ADHD but also its phenotypical behavioral symptoms as well, though specific research on the issue is sorely wanting.

Neurological Factors

A variety of neurological etiologies have been proposed for ADHD. Several studies show that brain damage, particularly hypoxic/anoxic types of insults, is associated with greater attention deficits and hyperactivity (Cruikshank, Eliason, & Merrifield, 1988; O'Dougherty, Nuechterlein, & Drew, 1984). ADHD symptoms also occur more in children and teens with seizure disorders (Holdsworth & Whitmore, 1974) that are clearly related to underlying neurological malfunction. However, most children with ADHD have no history of significant brain injuries or seizure disorders, and thus that sort of brain damage is unlikely to account for the majority of children with ADHD (Rutter, 1977).

A large number of studies have used neuropsychological tests of frontal lobe functions and have detected deficits in children, teens, and adults, albeit inconsistently (Barkley, Edwards, et al., 2001b; Fischer et al., 1990; Mariani & Barkley, 1997; Murphy et al., 2001; Seidman, Biederman, Faraone, Weber, & Ouellette, 1997). Where consistent, the results suggest that it is poor inhibition of behavioral responses, or what Nigg (2001) has called executive inhibition, that is solidly established as impaired in this disorder, at least in the combined and hyperactive–impulsive types. As noted earlier, evidence has mounted for difficulties as well with nonverbal and verbal working memory, planning, verbal fluency, response perseveration, motor sequencing, sense of time, and other frontal lobe functions. Adults with ADHD have also been shown to display similar deficits on neuropsychological tests of executive functions (Barkley, Murphy, & Bush, 2001; Murphy et al., 2001; Seidman et al., 1997). Moreover, research shows that not only do siblings of children with ADHD who have ADHD show similar executive function deficits, but even those siblings of children with ADHD who do not actually manifest ADHD appear to have milder yet significant impairments in these same executive functions (Seidman et al., 1997). Such findings imply a possible genetically linked risk for executive function deficits in families having children with ADHD, even if symptoms of ADHD are not fully manifest in those family members. Supporting this implication is evidence that the executive deficits in ADHD arise from the same substantial shared genetic liability as do the ADHD symptoms themselves and as does the overlap of ADHD with ODD/CD (Coolidge, Thede, & Young, 2000). These inhibitory and executive deficits are not the result of comorbid disorders, such as ODD, CD, anxiety, or depression, thus giving greater confidence to their affiliation with ADHD itself (Barkley, Edwards, et al., 2001b; Barkley, Murphy, & Bush,

2001; Bayliss & Roodenrys, 2000; Chang et al., 1999; Clark et al., 2000; Klorman et al., 1999; Murphy et al., 2001; Nigg, Hinshaw, Carte, & Treuting, 1998).

Neurological Studies

Research using psychophysiological measures of nervous system (central and autonomic) electrical activity (electroencephalograms, galvanic skin responses, heart rate deceleration, etc.) have proven inconsistent in demonstrating group differences between ADHD and control children in resting arousal. Where differences from normal are found, they are consistently in the direction of diminished reactivity to stimulation in those with ADHD (Beaucheine, Katkin, Strassberg, & Snarr, 2001; Borger & van der Meere, 2000; Herpertz et al., 2001).

Far more consistent have been the results of *quantitative electroencephalograph (QEEG)* and *evoked response potential (ERP)* measures, sometimes taken in conjunction with vigilance tests (Frank, Lazar, & Seiden, 1992; Klorman, 1992; see Tannock, 1998, for a review). The most consistent pattern for EEG research is increased slow wave, or theta, activity, particularly in the frontal lobe, and excess beta activity, all indicative of a pattern of underarousal and underreactivity in ADHD (Baving, Laucht, & Schmidt, 1999; Monastra, Lubar, & Linden, 2001). ADHD is associated with smaller amplitudes in the late positive and negative components of the evoked response patterns. These late components are believed to be a function of the prefrontal regions of the brain, are related to poorer performances on inhibition and vigilance tests, and are corrected by stimulant medication (Johnstone, Barry, & Anderson, 2001; Pliszka, Liotti, & Woldorff, 2000).

Several studies have also examined *cerebral blood flow* using single-photon emission computed tomography (SPECT) in ADHD and normal groups (see Tannock, 1998; Hendren, DeBacker, & Pandina, 2000, for reviews). They have consistently shown decreased blood flow to the prefrontal regions (most recently in the right frontal area) and pathways connecting these regions to the limbic system via the striatum and specifically its anterior region known as the caudate, and with the cerebellum (Gustafson, Thernlund, Ryding, Rosen, & Cederblad, 2000; Sieg, Gaffney, Preston, & Hellings, 1995). Degree of blood flow in the right frontal region has been correlated with behavioral severity of the disorder, while that in more posterior regions and the cerebellum seems related to degree of motor impairment (Gustafson et al., 2000).

Studies using PET to assess cerebral glucose metabolism have found diminished metabolism in adults, particularly in the frontal region (Schweitzer et al., 2000; Zametkin et al., 1990), and adolescent females with ADHD (Ernst et al., 1994) but have proven negative in adolescent males with ADHD (Zametkin et al., 1993). An attempt to replicate the finding with adolescent females having ADHD in younger female children with ADHD failed to find such diminished metabolism (Ernst, Cohen, Liebenauer, Jons, & Zametkin, 1997). Such studies are plagued by their exceptionally small sample sizes that result in very low power to detect group differences and considerable unreliability in replicating previous findings. However, significant correlations have been noted between diminished metabolic activity in the anterior frontal region and severity of ADHD symptoms in adolescents with ADHD (Zametkin et al., 1993). Also, using a radioactive tracer that indicates dopamine activity, Ernst and colleagues (1999) were able to show abnormal dopamine activity in the right midbrain region and that severity of symptoms was correlated with the degree of this abnormality. These demonstrations of an association between the metabolic activity of certain brain regions and symptoms of ADHD and associated executive deficits is critical to proving a connection between the findings pertaining to brain activation and the behavior comprising ADHD.

More recent neuroimaging technologies offer a more fine-grained analysis of brain structures using the higher-resolution MRI devices. Studies employing this technology find differences in selected brain regions in those with ADHD relative to control groups (see Tannock, 1998, for a review). Children with ADHD may have a significantly smaller left caudate nucleus creating a reversal of the normal pattern of left > right asymmetry of the caudate (Hynd et al., 1993). Several more recent studies have used larger samples of ADHD and control groups using quantitative MRI technology. These studies have indicated significantly smaller anterior right frontal regions, smaller size of the caudate nucleus, reversed asymmetry of the head of the caudate, and smaller globus pallidus regions in those with ADHD compared to controls (Aylward et al., 1996; Castellanos et al., 1994, 1996; Filipek, et al., 1997). The size of the basal ganglia and right frontal lobe has been shown to correlate with the degree of impairment in inhibition and attention in ADHD (Casey et al., 1997; Semrud-Clikeman et al., 2000). Castellanos and colleagues (1996) also found smaller cerebellar volume in those with ADHD and by adolescence, teens with ADHD had 3–4% less volume overall than controls with particular underdevelopment of the frontal lobes and cerebellum. This would be consistent with recent views that the cerebellum plays a major role in executive functioning and the motor presetting aspects of sensory perception that derive from planning and other executive actions (Diamond, 2000).

Studies using fMRI find children, teens, and young adults with ADHD to have abnormal patterns of activation during attention and inhibition tasks relative to controls, particularly in the right prefrontal region, basal ganglia (striatum and putamen), and cerebellum (Rubia et al., 1999; Teicher et al., 2000; Vaidya et al., 1998). Again, the demonstrated linkage of brain structure and function with psychological measures of ADHD symptoms and executive deficits is exceptionally important in such research to permit causal inferences to be made about the role of these brain abnormalities in the cognitive and behavioral deficits comprising ADHD.

Neurotransmitter Deficiencies

Possible neurotransmitter dysfunction or imbalances have been proposed in ADHD for quite some time (see Pliszka, McCracken, & Maas, 1996, for a review). Initially, these rested chiefly on the responses of ADHD cases to differing drugs. ADHD responds remarkably well to stimulants, most of which act by increasing the availability of dopamine via various mechanisms, and producing some effects on the noradrenergic pathways as well (DuPaul et al., 1998). The disorder also responds well to tricyclic antidepressants giving further support to a possible noradrenergic basis to ADHD (Connor, 1998). Consequently, it seems sensible to hypothesize that these two neurotransmitters might be involved in the disorder. Other studies used blood and urinary metabolites of brain neurotransmitters to infer deficiencies in ADHD, largely related to dopamine regulation

(Halperin et al., 1997). What limited evidence there is from this literature seems to point to a selective deficiency in the availability of both dopamine and norepinephrine, but this evidence cannot be considered conclusive.

Pregnancy and Birth Complications

Prematurity or lower than normal birthweight results in higher risk for later hyperactivity or ADHD (Breslau et al., 1996; Schothorst & van Engeland, 1996; Sykes et al., 1997). The extent of white matter abnormalities due to birth injuries, such as parenchymal lesions and/or ventricular enlargement, seems especially contributory to later ADHD (Whittaker et al., 1997). One study found that the season of a child's birth was significantly associated with risk for ADHD, at least among those subgroups that also either had learning disability or did not have any psychiatric comorbidity (Mick, Biederman, & Faraone, 1996). Birth in September was overrepresented in this subgroup of ADHD. The authors conjecture that the season of birth may serve as a proxy for the timing of seasonally mediated viral infections to which these mothers and their fetuses may have been exposed and that this may account for approximately 10% of cases of ADHD.

Genetic Factors

Evidence for a genetic basis to ADHD is now overwhelming and comes from three sources: family studies, twin studies, and, most recently, molecular genetic studies identifying individual candidate genes. Again, nearly all this research applies to the combined type of ADHD, and most of it has occurred with children rather than adolescents.

Family Aggregation Studies

Between 10 and 35% of the immediate family members of children and teens with ADHD are also likely to have the disorder with the risk to siblings being approximately 32% (Biederman et al., 1992; Biederman, Faraone, Keenan, et al., 1990; Pauls, 1991). If a parent has ADHD, the risk to the offspring is 57% (Biederman, Faraone, Mick, et al., 1995). These elevated rates of disorders also have been noted in African American ADHD samples (Samuel et al., 1999) as well as in females with ADHD compared to males (Faraone et al., 2000). ADHD with CD may be a distinct familial subtype of ADHD. The conduct problems, substance abuse, and depression found in the parents and other relatives are related more to the presence of CD in the ADHD cases than to ADHD itself (Biederman, Faraone, Keenan, & Tsuang, 1992; Faraone et al., 1992; Faraone, Biederman, Mennin, Russell, & Tsuang, 1998). Rates of hyperactivity or ADHD remain high even in relatives of the group of children and teens with ADHD without CD (Biederman, Faraone, Keenan, et al., 1991), but depression and antisocial spectrum disorders are most likely to appear in the comorbid group. Using sib-pairs in which both siblings had ADHD, Smalley and colleagues have also recently supported this view through findings that CD significantly clusters among the families of only those sib-pairs having CD (Smalley et al., 2000). Some research has also suggested that females who manifest ADHD may need to have a greater genetic loading (higher family member prevalence) than do males with ADHD (Faraone et al., 1992; Smalley et al., 2000). Faraone and Biederman (1997) found that depression among family members of cases with ADHD might be a nonspecific expression of the same genetic contribution that is related to ADHD. This is based on their findings that family members of cases with ADHD are at increased risk for major depression while individuals having major depression have first-degree relatives at increased risk for ADHD. Even so, as noted previously, the risk for depression among family members is largely among those cases having ADHD with CD. Thus, ADHD clusters significantly among the biological relatives of children, teens, and adults with the disorder, strongly implying a hereditary basis to this condition.

Adoption Research

Cantwell (1975) and Morrison and Stewart (1973) both reported higher rates of hyperactivity in the biological parents of hyperactive children than in adoptive parents having such children. A later study (van den Oord, Boomsma, & Verhulst, 1994) using biologically related and unrelated pairs of international adoptees identified a strong genetic component (47% of the variance) for the Attention Problems dimension of the Child Behavior Checklist, a rating scale commonly used in research on ADHD. More recently, a comparison

of the families of adopted children with ADHD to those living with their biological parents and to a control group also showed the same pattern of an elevated prevalence of ADHD among just the biological parents of the children with ADHD (6% vs. 18% vs. 3%, respectively) (Sprich, Biederman, Crawford, Mundy, & Faraone, 2000). Thus, like the family association studies discussed earlier, results of adoption studies point to a strong possibility of a significant hereditary contribution to hyperactivity.

Twin Studies

Twin studies of ADHD and its underlying behavioral dimensions have proven strikingly consistent. Gilger, Pennington, and DeFries (1992) found that if one twin was diagnosed as ADHD, the concordance for the disorder was 81% in monozygotic (MZ) twins and 29% in dizygotic (DZ) twins. Sherman, McGue, and Iacono (1997) found that the concordance for MZ twins having ADHD (mother identified) was 67% versus 0% for DZ twins. Large twin studies have found a very high degree of heritability for ADHD, ranging from .75 to .97 (see Levy & Hay, 2001; Thapar, 1999, for reviews; see also Coolidge et al., 2000). The average heritability of ADHD is at least 0.80, being nearly that for human height (.80–.91) and higher than that found for intelligence (.55–.70). These studies consistently find little, if any, effect for shared (rearing) environment on the traits of ADHD while sometimes finding a small significant contribution for unique environmental events.

The twin studies cited previously have also been able to indicate the extent to which individual differences in ADHD symptoms are the result of nonshared environmental factors. Such factors not only include those typically thought of as involving the social environment but also all biological factors that are nongenetic in origin. Factors in the nonshared environment are those events or conditions that will have uniquely affected only one twin and not the other. Besides biological hazards or neurologically injurious events that may have befallen only one member of a twin pair, the nonshared environment also includes those differences in the manner in which parents may have treated each child. Twin studies to date have suggested that approximately 9–20% of the variance in hyperactive–impulsive–inattentive behavior or ADHD symptoms can be attributed to such nonshared environmental (nongenetic) factors (Levy & Hay, 2001). A portion of this variance, however, must be attributed to the error of the measure used to assess the symptoms.

Molecular Genetic Research

Most investigators suspect that multiple genes influence the disorder given the complexity of the traits underlying ADHD and their dimensional nature. The dopamine transporter gene (DAT1) has been implicated in three studies of ADHD (Cook et al., 1995; Cook, Stein, & Leventhal, 1997; Gill, Daly, Heron, Hawi, & Fitzgerald, 1997). However, other laboratories have not been able to replicate this association (Swanson et al., 1997). Another gene related to dopamine, the DRD4 (repeater gene), has been the most reliably found in samples of ADHD (Faraone et al., 1999). It is the 7-repeat form of this gene that has been found to be overrepresented in children with ADHD (Lahoste et al., 1996). Such a finding is quite interesting because this gene has previously been associated with the personality trait of high novelty-seeking behavior, this variant of the gene affects pharmacological responsiveness, and the gene's impact on postsynaptic sensitivity is primarily found in frontal and prefrontal cortical regions believed to be associated with executive functions and attention (Swanson et al., 1997). The finding of an overrepresentation of the 7-repeat DRD4 gene has now been replicated in a number of other studies using not only children with ADHD but also adolescents and adults with the disorder (Faraone et al., 1999). Working with Karen Mueller and Bradford Navia, we have recently identified the Taq1 allele of the DBH (dopamine beta hydroxylase) gene to be overrepresented in older teens and young adults with ADHD followed from childhood to young adulthood (Smith et al., 2003). This gene may function to regulate dopamine beta hydroxylase known to be involved in the conversion of dopamine to norepinephrine with this particular allele possibly increasing such turnover.

Environmental Toxins

As the twin and quantitative genetic studies have suggested, unique environmental events may play some role in individual differences in symptoms of ADHD. This should not be taken to mean only those influences within the realm of psychosocial or family influences. As noted earlier, variance in the expression of ADHD that may be due to environmental sources means all nongenetic sources more generally. These include pre-, peri-, and postnatal complications and malnutrition, diseases, trauma, toxin exposure, and other neurologically compromising events that may occur during the development of the nervous system before and after birth. Among these various biologically compromising events, several have been repeatedly linked to risks for inattention and hyperactive behavior.

One such factor is exposure to environmental toxins, specifically lead. Elevated body lead burden has been shown to have a small but consistent and statistically significant relationship to the symptoms comprising ADHD (Needleman, Schell, Bellinger, Leviton, & Alfred, 1990). However, even at relatively high levels of lead, less than 38% of children are rated as having the behavior of hyperactivity on a teacher rating scale (Needleman et al., 1979), implying that most lead-poisoned children do not develop symptoms of ADHD. Prenatal exposure to alcohol and tobacco smoke have a much stronger involvement in elevating risk for ADHD (Milberger, Biederman, Faraone, Chen, & Jones, 1996b; Streissguth, Bookstein, Sampson, & Barr, 1995). The relationship between maternal smoking during pregnancy and ADHD remains significant even after controlling for symptoms of ADHD in the parent (Milberger et al., 1996b).

Psychosocial Factors

In view of the foregoing findings and the absence of compelling theory or evidence to the contrary, purely social causes of ADHD are no longer given serious consideration. The twin studies discussed previously, for instance, show nonsignificant contributions of the common or rearing environment to the expression of symptoms of ADHD. This is not to say that the family and larger social environment do not matter. Despite the large role heredity seems to play in ADHD symptoms, they remain malleable to unique environmental influences and nonshared social learning. The actual severity of the symptoms within a particular context, the continuity of those symptoms over development, the types of comorbid disorders that will develop, the peer relationship problems that may arise, and various outcome domains of the disorder are likely to be related in varying degrees to parent, family, and larger environmental factors (Johnson, Cohen, Kasen, Smailes, & Brook, 2001; Johnston & Mash, 2001; Milberger, 1997; Pfiffner, McBurnett, & Rathouz, 2001; van den Oord & Rowe, 1997). Yet even here care must be taken in interpreting these findings as evidence of a purely social contribution to ADHD. This is because many measures of family functioning and adversity also show a strong heritable contribution to them, largely owing to the presence of similar symptoms and disorders (and genes!) in the parents as may be evident in the child (Pike & Plomin, 1996; Plomin, 1995). Thus, there is a genetic contribution to the family environment; a fact that often goes overlooked in studies of family and social factors involved in ADHD. Undoubtedly, this affects the child in both direct and indirect ways. Genetics may create a vulnerability to the disorder if not its outright manifestation, but this also means that parents likely have some variant of or even a frank case of ADHD. Parental disorder can easily contribute to a less-than-ideal household environment and disrupted parenting of the child with ADHD. That may affect severity of the disorder, though more likely it affects the risk for comorbid ODD and possibly CD.

ASSESSMENT

My intent here is not to provide a detailed review of the manner in which a thorough clinical evaluation should be conducted with adolescents having ADHD and their families. Instead, I highlight the major topics that should be covered and several methods that I recommend be employed in evaluating teens and their parents and the parent–teen conflicts they experience. More information on assessment can be found in the texts by Robin (1998), Barkley (2006), and Barkley, Edwards, and Robin (2000).

Issues

The evaluation of teens with ADHD incorporates multiple assessment methods relying on several informants concerning the nature of the adolescent's difficulties (and strengths!) across multiple situations. To do so, parent and teen interviews are conducted. Parent and teacher rating scales of the adolescent's behavioral adjustment are also obtained as are the adolescent's self-reports on these same rating scales. Parent self-report measures of relevant psychiatric conditions and of parent and family functioning should also be collected. Some clinicians may wish to collect laboratory measures of ADHD symptoms as well as direct observations of parent–teen interactions, but insurance reimbursement policies now place limits on time for evaluations for which they will provide compensation, thereby reducing the likelihood that such observations will be collected. Teens in whom intellectual or developmental delays or learning disabilities are suspected should receive brief psychological screening of intelligence and academic achievement skills, if such has not already been performed by the school system or other professionals, with more thorough follow-up testing should significant deficits be evident on any screen.

A major goal of such an assessment is not only the determination of the presence or absence of psychiatric disorders, such as ADHD, ODD, and CD, but also the differential diagnosis of ADHD from other psychiatric disorders. This requires extensive clinical knowledge of these other psychiatric disorders; the reader is referred to other chapters in this text and to the text by Mash and Barkley (2003) on child psychopathology for reviews of the major childhood disorders. In evaluating teens, it may be necessary to draw not only on measures that are normed for this age range but possibly for the individual's ethnic background, if such instruments are available, to preclude the overdiagnosis of minority adolescents when diagnostic criteria developed from Caucasian adolescents is extrapolated to them. At the very least, in interviewing the parent of a teen from a minority group, time should be taken to be sure that any symptoms of disorders that are endorsed by the parent are also viewed by the parent as (1) being significantly problematic relative to other same-age adolescents of that ethnic group and (2) resulting in significant impairment in one or more major life activities of the teenager.

A second purpose of the evaluation is to begin delineating the types of interventions that will be needed to address the psychiatric disorders and psychological, academic, and social impairments identified in the course of assessment. As noted later, these may include individual counseling, parent or family training in behavior management, problem solving, communication skills, classroom behavior modification and curriculum adjustments, psychiatric medications, and formal special educational services, to name just a few. For a more thorough discussion of treatments for childhood disorders, the reader is referred to the text on this subject by Mash and Barkley (1998).

Another important purpose of the evaluation is the determination of comorbid conditions and whether or not these may affect prognosis or treatment decision making. For instance, the presence of high levels of physically assaultive behavior by the adolescent may signal that a parent–teen training program such as those suggested below may be contraindicated, at least for the time being, because of its likelihood of temporarily increasing teen violence toward parents when limits on noncompliance with parental rules and commands are established. Or, consider the presence of high levels of anxiety specifically and internalizing symptoms more generally that may exist in some clinic-referred teens with ADHD. Research has shown that such internalizing symptoms may be a predictor of poorer responses or greater side effects to stimulant medication that otherwise is often useful for the management of ADHD (DuPaul et al., 1998). Similarly, the presence of high levels of irritable mood, severely hostile and defiant behavior, and periodic episodes of explosive physical aggression and destructive behavior may be early markers for bipolar disorder (manic–depression) in adolescents. Oppositional behavior as well as ADHD symptoms is almost universal in juvenile-onset bipolar disorder (Wozniak & Biederman, 1995). Such a disorder will likely require the use of psychiatric medications, psychotherapy, a family training program, and even occasional inpatient hospitalization, to assist with its management. Finally, more than occasional experimentation with alcohol or drugs by the adolescent would be the cause to refer the adolescent to a substance abuse treatment program, after which the family treatment might be resumed.

A further objective of the evaluation is to identify the pattern of the teen's psychological strengths and weaknesses and consider how these may affect treatment planning. This may also include some impression being gained as to the parents' own abilities to carry out the treatment program as well as the family's social and economic circumstances. The treatment resources that may (or may not) be available within the family's community and cultural group should also be ascertained. Some determination will need to be made as to the teen's eligibility for special educational services within their school district if eligible disorders, such as developmental delay, learning disabilities, or ADHD are present.

Preevaluation

At the parents' initial contact with the professional, a form is completed by the receptionist that gathers important demographic information about the adolescent and parents, the reason for the referral, and insurance information that will be cross-checked with the insurance company, where necessary, before the appointment. This form is then reviewed by the billing agent for the clinic and the clinician who will receive this case. Depending on the clinician's area of specialization, some types of referrals are inappropriate for the clinician's practice and can be screened out at this time for referral to more appropriate services. At this same time, the practice can send out a packet of questionnaires to parents and teachers to be completed and returned in advance of the scheduled appointment. I suggest the clinician consider not providing parents with an appointment date until these packets of information are completed and returned to the clinic. This ensures that the packets will be completed reasonably promptly, that the information is available for review by the clinician prior to meeting with the family and that it is current, and that the evaluation time in the clinic is used in a far more efficient way, particularly given the premium that managed health care plans often place on limiting the time used for the evaluation. Efficiency of the evaluation process is paramount. The packet of information sent to the parent will include a form cover letter from the professional asking the parent(s) to complete the packet of information and informing them that the appointment date will be set when this packet is returned. This packet contains an adolescent and family information form, and a medical and developmental history form, which can be found in the manual by Barkley and colleagues (1999). This packet also includes a reasonably comprehensive adolescent behavior rating scale that covers the major dimensions of adolescent psychopathology, such as the Child Behavior Checklist (CBCL; Achenbach, 2001) or the Behavioral Assessment System for Children (BASC-2; Reynolds & Kamphaus, 2001). Also sent in this packet is a copy of the Disruptive Behavior Disorders Rating Scale (DBDRS), provided in Barkley and colleagues. This scale permits the clinician to obtain information ahead of the appointment concerning the presence of symptoms of ODD, CD, and ADHD in the teen's behavior and their severity; these disorders are quite common among teenagers referred for defiant behavior and so deserve specific evaluation. Parents can be sent a version of the Home Situations Questionnaire (HSQ) developed by Barkley (1990) and modified for use with teens by Adams and colleagues (1995). The scale can be included in this packet to gain a quick appreciation for the pervasiveness and severity of the teen's disruptive behavior across a variety of home and public situations. Such information will be of clinical interest not only for indications of pervasiveness and severity of behavior problems but also for focusing discussions around these situations during the evaluation and subsequent family training program. This packet also should include both a teen self-report version of the broadband rating scale noted previously (BASC or CBCL) and three copies of the Issues Checklist. The latter scale focuses on a variety of topics over which parents and the teen may have disagreements, assessing their frequency and severity of disagreement. One of the three copies is for the mother to complete, the second for the father, and the third copy for the teen to complete. These rating scales are discussed below.

It is also my custom to send to the teen's math and language arts (English) teachers a packet of forms to complete, with parental written permission obtained beforehand, of course. The medical and developmental history form is not included. Instead, the teacher packet contains the teacher version of the CBCL or BASC, the School Situations Questionnaire (SSQ) developed by Barkley (1990) and modified for teens by Adams and colleagues (1995), and the DBDRS—Teacher Form. Whenever possible, clinicians can find it quite useful to contact these teachers by telephone for a brief interview prior to meeting with the family. Otherwise, this can be done following the family's appointment. It may be best to contact just one of the many teachers a teen may have and prevail on that teacher to

gather information on the teen's school functioning from the other relevant teachers to share with the clinician.

On the day of the appointment, the following still needs to be done: (1) parental and adolescent interview; (2) completion of self-report rating scales by the parents about themselves; and (3) any psychological testing that may be indicated by the nature of the referral (intelligence and achievement testing, etc.).

Parental Interview

The parental (often maternal) interview is an absolutely indispensable part of the clinical assessment of adolescents. The interview covers the major referral concerns of the parents, and of the professional referring the adolescent whenever appropriate. A sample interview form can be found in the manual by Barkley and colleagues (1999). This form contains not only major sections for the important information discussed here but also the diagnostic criteria used for ADHD as well as the other childhood disorders most likely to be seen in conjunction with it (i.e., ODD, CD, anxiety and mood disorders, and bipolar disorder). General descriptions of concerns by parents must be followed with specific questions by the examiner to elucidate the details of the problems and any apparent precipitants that can be identified. Such an interview probes for not only the specific nature, frequency, age of onset, and chronicity of the problematic behaviors but also for the situational and temporal variation in the behaviors and their consequences. If the problems are chronic, which they often are, determining what prompted the referral at this time reveals much about parental perceptions of the teen's problems, current family circumstances related to the problems' severity, and parental motivation for treatment. Following this, one should review with the parents any potential problems that might exist in the developmental domains of motor, language, intellectual, thinking, academic, emotional, and social functioning of the teen. Such information greatly aids in the differential diagnosis of the teen's problems. To accomplish this requires that the examiner have an adequate knowledge of the diagnostic features of other childhood disorders, some of which may present as ADHD. For instance many adolescents with atypical pervasive developmental disorders (childhood onset), Asperger syndrome, or early bipolar disorder may be viewed by their parents as having ADHD given that the parents are more likely to have heard about the latter disorders than the former ones and will recognize some of the qualities of the latter disorders in their teens. Questioning about inappropriate thinking, affect, social relations, and motor peculiarities may reveal a more seriously and pervasively disturbed teen. If such symptoms seem to be present, the clinician may want to employ the Children's Atypical Development Scale (see Barkley, 1990) at this point to obtain a more thorough review of these symptoms. Inquiry also must be made as to the presence or history of tics or Tourette syndrome in the adolescent or the immediate biological family members. Where noted, these would result in a recommendation for a more cautious use of stimulant drugs in the treatment of the ADHD adolescent and likely lower initial doses to preclude the exacerbation of the teen's tic disorder (DuPaul et al., 1998).

Information on the school and family histories should also be obtained. The latter includes a discussion of potential psychiatric difficulties in the parents and siblings, marital difficulties, and any family problems centered around chronic medical conditions, employment problems, or other potential stress events within the family. Of course, the examiner will want to obtain some information about prior treatments received by the adolescents and their families for these presenting problems. Where the history suggests potentially treatable medical or neurological conditions (allergies, seizures, Tourette syndrome, etc.), a referral to a physician is essential. Without evidence of such problems, however, referral to a physician for examination usually fails to reveal any further information of use in the treatment of the conduct problem adolescents. An exception to this occurs when use of psychiatric medications is contemplated, in which case a referral to a physician is clearly indicated.

As part of the general interview of the parent, the examiner needs to cover the symptoms of the major adolescent psychiatric disorders likely to be seen in defiant teens (American Psychiatric Association, 1994) in some semistructured or structured way. In using any such interview, care must be exercised in the evaluation of minority adolescents not to overdiagnose psychiatric disorders in such adolescents by virtue simply of differing cultural standards for adolescent behavior. The interviewer must ensure not only that the behaviors of adolescents are statistically deviant but that they also are associated with evidence of impairment in adaptive functioning or some other "harmful dysfunction" (Wakefield, 1992, 1997). As noted earlier, one means of partially precluding overidentification of psychopathology in minority children is to make the following adjustment in the parental interview. When reviewing the psychiatric symptoms for the childhood disorders with parents, should the parent indicate that a symptom is present, the interviewer should follow up with the question, "Do you consider this to be a problem for your adolescent compared to other adolescents of the same ethnic or minority group?" Only if the parent answers "yes" to this second question is the symptom to be considered present for purposes of psychiatric diagnosis. Of course, impairment from these symptoms must also be established before a diagnosis can be made. When applying the diagnostic criteria for ADHD to defiant adolescents, the problems noted earlier with the DSM criteria should be borne in mind and adjustments made for them as needed.

The parental interview may also reveal that one parent, usually the mother, has more difficulty managing the adolescent with ADHD than does the other. Care should be taken to discuss differences in the parents' approaches to management and any marital problems this may have spawned. Such difficulties in adolescent management can often lead to reduced leisure and recreational time for the parents and increased conflict within the marriage, and often within the extended family should relatives live nearby. It is often helpful to inquire as to what the parents attribute the causes or origins of their teen's behavioral difficulties, as this may unveil areas of ignorance or misinformation that will require attention later during the initial counseling of the family about the teen's disorder(s) and their likely causes. The examiner also should briefly inquire about the nature of parental and family social activities to determine how isolated, or insular, the parents are from the usual social support networks in which many parents are involved. Research by Wahler (1980) has shown that the degree of maternal insularity is significantly associated with failure in subsequent parent training programs. Where present to a significant degree, such a finding might suggest addressing the isolation as an initial goal of treatment rather than progressing directly to adolescent behavior management training with that family.

The parental interview can then conclude with a discussion of the teen's positive characteristics and attributes as well as potential rewards desired by the adolescent that will prove useful in later family training. Some parents of ADHD adolescents have had such chronic and pervasive management problems that upon initial questioning they may find it hard to report anything positive about their teen. Getting parents to begin thinking of such attributes is actually an initial step toward treatment as the early phases of family training will teach parents to focus on and attend to desirable adolescent behaviors.

Adolescent Interview

Some time should always be spent directly interacting with the referred teen. This time can be fruitfully spent inquiring about the teen's views of the reasons for the referral and evaluation, how the teen sees the family functioning, any additional problems the teen feels he or she may have, how well the teen is performing at school, the degree of acceptance by peers and classmates, and what changes in the family the teen believes might make life happier at home. A screening for suicidal ideation and substance use should also be conducted with the adolescent. As with the parents, the adolescent can be queried as to potential rewards he or she finds desirable that will prove useful later in this program.

Teens with ADHD are not especially reliable in their reports of their own disruptive behavior. The problem is compounded by the frequently diminished self-awareness and impulse control typical of their disorder. Such adolescents with ADHD often show little reflection about the examiner's questions and, particularly in cases of CD, may lie or distort information in a more socially pleasing direction. Some will report they have many friends, have no interaction problems at home with their parents, and are doing well at school, in direct contrast with the extensive parental and teacher complaints of inappropriate behavior by these children. Because of this tendency of adolescents with ADHD to underreport the seriousness of their behavior, particularly in the realm of disruptive or externalizing behaviors (Barkley, Fischer, et al., 1991; Fischer et al., 1993a), the diagnosis of ODD or ADHD is never based on the reports of the teen alone. Nevertheless, teens' reports of their internalizing symptoms, such as anxiety and depression, may be more reliable and so should play some role in the diagnosis of comorbid anxiety or mood disorders in adolescents with ADHD (Hinshaw, 1994). The clinician should inquire about depression, anxiety, and whether the adolescent has any present or past suicidal ideation. It is helpful to adapt the relevant sections of the parental interview for the systematic assessment of mood and anxiety disorders in the adolescent interview. The clinician should also inquire about experimentation and use of alcohol and drugs. Parents may not be aware of patterns of substance use.

While notation of the teen's behavior, compliance, attention span, activity level, and impulse control within the clinic is useful, clinicians must guard against drawing any diagnostic conclusions from the cases in which the adolescent is not problematic in the clinic or office. Many adolescents with ADHD do not misbehave in the clinicians' office and so heavy reliance on such observations would clearly lead to false negatives in the diagnosis. In some instances, the behavior of the adolescents with their parents in the waiting area prior to the appointment may be a better indication of the teen's management problems at home than is the teen's behavior toward the clinician, particularly when this involves a one-to-one interaction between adolescent and examiner. This is not to say that office behavior of an adolescent is entirely useless. When it is grossly inappropriate or extreme, it may well signal the likelihood of problems in the teen's natural settings, particularly in school. It is the presence of relatively normal conduct by the adolescent that may be an unreliable indicator of the teen's normalcy elsewhere.

Teacher Interview

At some point before or soon after the initial evaluation session with the family, contact with the teen's teachers may be helpful in further clarifying the nature of the teen's problems, especially those in the school setting. This will most likely be done by telephone unless the clinician works within the teen's school system. Interviews with teachers have all the same merits as do interviews with parents, providing a second ecologically valid source of indispensable information about the teen's psychological adjustment; in this case, in the school setting. Like parent reports, teacher reports are also subject to bias and the integrity of the reporter of information, be it parent or teacher, must always be weighed in judging the validity of the information itself. Many teens with ADHD have problems with academic performance and classroom behavior and the details of these difficulties need to be obtained from the teachers. Teachers should also be sent the rating scales mentioned earlier. These can be sent as a packet prior to the actual evaluation so that the results are available for discussion with the parents during the interview, as well as with the teacher during the subsequent telephone contact or school visit.

The teacher interview should focus on the specific nature of the teen's problems in the school environment, again following a behavioral format. The settings, nature, frequency, consequating events, and eliciting events for the major behavioral problems also can be explored. Teachers should be questioned about potential learning disabilities in the adolescent given the greater likelihood of occurrence of such disorders in this population. When evidence suggests their existence, the evaluation of the adolescent should be expanded to explore the nature and degree of such deficits as viewed by the teacher. Even when learning disabilities do not exist, adolescents who have ADHD are more likely to have problems with sloppy handwriting, careless approaches to tasks, poor organization of their work materials, and academic underachievement relative to their tested abilities. Time should be taken with the teachers to explore the possibility of these problems.

Adolescent Behavior Rating Scales for Parent and Teacher Reports

Adolescent behavior checklists and rating scales have become an essential element in the evaluation and diagnosis of adolescents with behavior problems. The availability of several scales with excellent normative data across a wide age range of children and adolescents and having acceptable reliability and validity makes their incorporation into the assessment protocol quite convenient and extremely useful. Such information is invaluable in determining the statistical deviance of the adolescent's problem behaviors and the degree to which other problems may be present. As a result, it is useful to

mail a packet of these scales to parents prior to the initial appointment asking that they be returned before the day of the evaluation, as described previously. This permits the examiner to review and score them before interviewing the parents, allows for vague or significant answers to be elucidated in the interview, and serves to focus the subsequent interview on those areas of abnormality that may be highlighted in the responses to items on these scales.

Numerous child behavior rating scales exist, and the reader is referred to other reviews (Barkley, 1990) for greater details on the more commonly used scales and for a discussion of the requirements and underlying assumptions of behavior rating scales; assumptions that are all too easily overlooked in the clinical use of these instruments. Despite their limitations, behavior rating scales offer a means of gathering information from informants who may have spent months or years with the adolescent. Apart from interviews, there is no other means of obtaining such a wealth of information for so little investment of time. The fact that such scales provide a means of quantifying the opinions of others, often along qualitative dimensions, and to compare these scores to norms collected on large groups of adolescents are further merits of these instruments. Nevertheless, behavior rating scales are opinions and are subject to the oversights, prejudices, and limitations on reliability and validity such opinions may have.

Initially, I advise using a "broadband" rating scale that provides coverage of the major dimensions of adolescent psychopathology known to exist, such as depression, anxiety, withdrawal, aggression, delinquent conduct, inattention, and hyperactive–impulsive behavior. These scales should be completed by parents and teachers. Such scales would be the BASC-2 (Reynolds & Kamphaus, 2001) and the CBCL (Achenbach, 2001), both of which have versions for parents and teachers and satisfactory normative information. (The CBCL can be obtained from Thomas Achenbach, Ph.D., Child and Adolescent Psychiatry, Department of Psychiatry, University of Vermont, 5 South Prospect St., Burlington, VT 05401. The BASC can be obtained from American Guidance Service, 4201 Woodland Rd., Circle Pines, MN 55014.) The recently revised Conners Parent and Teacher Rating Scales (Conners, 1998) can also be used for this initial screening for psychopathology, but they do not provide quite the breadth of coverage across all these dimensions of psychopathology as do the aforementioned scales.

More narrow-band scales should also be employed in the initial screening of adolescents that focus more specifically on the assessment of symptoms of ADHD. Clinicians can use the ADHD-IV Rating Scale (parent and teacher versions) and norms (DuPaul et al., 1998) or the DBDRS (Barkley & Murphy, 2006), which obtains ratings of the DSM-IV symptoms of ADHD, ODD, and CD. Norms, however, are not available for the ODD and CD sections while those for the ADHD portion are the same norms provided with the ADHD-IV Rating Scale.

The pervasiveness of the teen's behavior problems across a variety of situations within the home and school settings can also be examined. Measures of situational pervasiveness appear to have as much or more stability over time than do the aforementioned scales (Fischer et al., 1993b). The HSQ and SSQ (Barkley & Murphy, 2006) provide a means for doing so. Normative information for these scales is available for children ages 4–11 years of age (Altepeter & Breen, 1992; Barkley & Murphy, 2006). A somewhat modified form of these scales has been created for use with adolescents, ages 11–17 years, and norms are available (see Adams et al., 1995). The HSQ requires parents to rate their teen's behavior problems across 16 different home and public situations (15 in the case of teens). The SSQ similarly obtains teacher reports of problems in 12 different school situations (14 in the case of teens).

The more specialized or narrow band scales focusing on symptoms of ADHD as well as the HSQ and SSQ can be used to monitor treatment response when given prior to and at the end of parent training. They can also be used to monitor the behavioral effects of stimulant medication on adolescents with ADHD. In that case, use of the Side Effects Rating Scale is also to be encouraged (see Barkley & Murphy, 2006).

Self-Report Behavior Rating Scales for Children

Achenbach (2001) has a rating scale based on the CBCL, which is completed by adolescents ages 11–18 years (Youth Self-Report Form). Most items are similar to those on the parent and teacher forms of the CBCL, except that they are worded in the first person. Research suggests that while such self-reports of adolescents and teens with ADHD are more deviant than the self-reports of youth without ADHD, the self-reports of problems by the youth with ADHD, whether by interview or the CBCL Self-Report Form, are often less severe than the reports provided by parents and teachers (Fischer et al., 1993a; Loeber, Green, Lahey, & Stouthamer-Loeber, 1991). An adolescent self-report form is also available for the BASC, described earlier. The DBDRS can be given to adolescents to complete about themselves (or used as a basis for an interview) as a means of simply gathering the teen's own view of their disruptive behavior disorders. However, norms are not available and so the clinical utility of such self-ratings for the purpose of clinical diagnosis remains uncertain.

The reports of adolescents about internalizing symptoms, such as anxiety and depression, are more reliable and likely to be more valid than the reports of parents and teachers about these symptoms in the adolescents (Achenbach et al., 1987). For this reason, the self-reports of youth with ADHD should still be collected as such reports may have more pertinence to the diagnosis of comorbid disorders in adolescents than to their ADHD symptoms.

Peer Relationship Measures

As noted earlier, adolescents with ADHD often demonstrate significant difficulties in their interactions with peers and such difficulties are associated with an increased likelihood of persistence of their disorder (Biederman et al., 1996). A number of different methods for assessing peer relations have been employed in research with behavior problem children, such as direct observation and recording of social interactions, peer- and subject-completed sociometric ratings, and parent and teacher rating scales of children's social behavior. Most of these assessment methods have no norms and thus would not be appropriate for use in the clinical evaluation of adolescents with ADHD. Reviews of the methods for obtaining peer sociometric ratings can be found elsewhere (Newcomb, Bukowski, & Pattee, 1993). For clinical purposes, rating scales may offer the most convenient and cost-effective means for evaluating this important domain of childhood functioning. The CBCL and BASC rating forms described earlier contain scales that evaluate children's social behavior in a rather global way. As discussed previously, norms for adolescents are available for these scales, permitting their use in clinical settings.

Ratings of Family Conflict

It is important to evaluate the extent to which these conflicts exist, what particular issues or topics seem to trigger such conflicts, and how often and with what degree of negativity or hostility they occur. To do so, Prinz has developed the Issues Checklist, further normed as a rating scale by Robin and Foster (1989). This form is found in the manual by Barkley and colleagues (1999) along with its scoring instructions and norms. Parents and the teenager each complete a version of this scale. Using this scale, the therapist is able to create a hierarchy of parent–teen conflicts that will be used to focus problem-solving exercises that occur in parent–teen problem-solving and communication training (see below).

Parent Self-Report Measures

It has become increasingly apparent that child and adolescent behavioral disorders, their level of severity, and their response to interventions are, in part, a function of factors affecting parents and the family at large. Several types of psychiatric disorders are likely to occur more often among family members of an adolescent with ADHD than in matched groups of control teenagers. These problems might further influence the frequency and severity of behavioral problems in adolescents. The extent of social isolation in mothers of behaviorally disturbed children also may influence the severity of the children's behavioral disorders as well as the outcomes of parent training. Others have also shown separate and interactive contributions of parental psychopathology and marital discord on the decision to refer adolescents for clinical assistance, the degree of conflict in parent–teen interactions, and adolescent antisocial behavior (Patterson, Dishion, & Reid, 1992). The degree of resistance of parents to parent training is also dependent on such factors. Assessing the psychological integrity of parents, therefore, is an essential part of the clinical evaluation of defiant teens, the differential diagnosis of their prevailing disorders, and the planning of treatments stemming from such assessments. Thus, the evaluation of adolescents for ADHD is often a family assessment rather than one of the adolescent alone. While space does not permit a thorough discussion of the clinical assessment of adults and their disorders, brief mention will be made of some assessment methods that we have found useful in at least providing a preliminary screening for certain parent variables of import to treatment.

Parental ADHD

Family studies of the aggregation of psychiatric disorders among the biological relatives of adolescents with ADHD has clearly demonstrated an increased prevalence of ADHD among the parents of these adolescents (Biederman, Faraone, et al., 1991; Faraone et al., 1993). In general, there seems to be at least a 25–50% chance that one of the two parents of the defiant adolescent with ADHD will also have adult ADHD (approximately 15–20% of mothers and 25–30% of fathers). The manner in which ADHD in a parent might influence the behavior of an adolescent with ADHD specifically and the family environment more generally has not been studied. My clinical experience, however, suggests that it can be quite disruptive of family life and parent–teen interactions in some families. Adults with ADHD have been shown to be more likely to have problems with anxiety, depression, personality disorders, alcohol use and abuse, and marital difficulties, to change their employment and residence more often and to have less education and socioeconomic status than adults without ADHD (Barkley, Murphy, & Kwasnik, 1996a; Biederman, Milberger, Faraone, Guite, & Warburton, 1994; Murphy & Barkley, 1996b). Greater diversity and severity of psychopathology among parents is particularly apparent among the subgroup of adolescents with ADHD with comorbid ODD or CD (Barkley, Anastopoulos, et al., 1992; Lahey, Piacentini, et al., 1988). More severe ADHD seems to also be associated with younger age of parents (Murphy & Barkley, 1996a) suggesting that pregnancy during their own teenage or young adult years is more characteristic of parents of children with ADHD than children without ADHD. It is not difficult to see that these factors, as well as the primary symptoms of ADHD, could influence both the manner in which adolescent behavior is managed within the family and the quality of home life for such adolescents more generally. When the parent has ADHD, the probability that the adolescent with ADHD will also have ODD may increase markedly. Several papers have reported that ADHD in a parent may interfere with the ability of that parent to benefit from a typical behavioral parent training program (Evans, Vallano, & Pelham, 1994; Sonuga-Barke, Daley, & Thompson, 2002). Treatment of the parent's ADHD (with medication) may result in greater success in subsequent retraining of the parent (Evans et al., 1994). These preliminary findings are suggestive of the importance of determining the presence of ADHD in the parents of adolescents undergoing evaluation.

The DSM-IV symptom list for ADHD and ODD has been cast in the form of a behavior rating scale and some limited regional norms on 720 adults ages 17–84 years have been collected (Murphy & Barkley, 1996b). This rating scale for adults, entitled the Adult Behavior Rating Scale, is provided in the manual by Barkley and Murphy (2006). Adults complete the rating scale twice; once for their current behavioral adjustment and a second time for their recall of their childhood behavior between ages 5 and 12 years. Also available is the Conners Adult ADHD Rating Scale (CAARS; Conners, 1998). This scale also provides norms for the 18 DSM items for ADHD along with larger scales evaluating cognitive (inattentive–executive) symptoms, impulse control, and emotion regulation. Clinically significant scores on these scales do not, by themselves, grant the diagnosis of ADHD or ODD to a parent but should raise suspicion in the clinician's mind about such a possibility. If so, consideration should be given to referral of the parent for further evaluation and, possibly, treatment of adult ADHD or interpersonal hostility or even antisocial personality disorder, if necessary.

Marital Discord

Many instruments exist for evaluating marital discord in parents. The one most often used in research on childhood disorders has been the Locke–Wallace Marital Adjustment Scale (Locke & Wallace, 1959). Marital discord, parental separation, and parental divorce are more common in parents of adolescents with ADHD. Parents with such marital difficulties may have adolescents with more severe defiant and aggressive behavior, and such parents may also be less successful in parent training pro-

grams. Screening parents for marital problems, therefore, provides important clinical information to therapists contemplating a training program for such parents. Clinicians are encouraged to incorporate a screening instrument for marital discord into their assessment battery for parents of adolescents with defiant behavior.

Parental Depression and General Psychological Distress

Parents of adolescents with ADHD are frequently more depressed than those of normal adolescents, and this may affect their responsiveness to behavioral parent training programs. A scale often used to provide a quick assessment of parental depression is the Beck Depression Inventory (Beck Steer, & Garbin, 1988). Greater levels of psychopathology generally and psychiatric disorders specifically have been found in parents of adolescents with ADHD (Barkley, Anastopoulos, et al., 1992; Lahey, Piacentini, et al., 1988). One means of assessing this area of parental difficulties is through the use of the Symptom Checklist 90—Revised (SCL-90-R; Derogatis, 1986). This instrument not only has a scale assessing depression in adults but also scales measuring other dimensions of adult psychopathology and psychological distress. Whether clinicians use this or some other scale, the assessment of parental psychological distress generally and psychiatric disorders particularly makes sense in view of their likely impact on the teen's prognosis and the implementation of the teen's treatments typically delivered via the parents.

It should be clear from the foregoing that the assessment of adolescents is a complex and serious endeavor requiring adequate time (approximately 3 hours) and knowledge of the relevant research and clinical literature, as well as differential diagnosis, skillful clinical judgment in sorting out the pertinent issues, and sufficient resources to obtain multiple types of information from multiple sources (parents, child, teacher) using a variety of assessment methods.

TREATMENT

As with other sections of this chapter, here as well the vast majority of research has been conducted on children with ADHD with strikingly less attention to the efficacy of treatments for teens with the disorder (Smith, Waschbusch, Willoughby, & Evans, 2000). For instance, less than 5% of the studies done on medication management of children with ADHD have been done with teens having the disorder; and only a handful of family training studies have focused on this age group. There also have been just a few studies on educational management strategies with teens with ADHD (Smith et al., 2000). None of this means that there are no recommendations to make in these areas for teens with ADHD. It does mean that many will be based largely if not entirely on extrapolating (with caution!) from the child research and what little research on teens exists. That is fine up to a point, but one must always recognize that the adolescent's psychological and physical stages of maturity, his or her developing sense of autonomy, and his or her emergence into the larger community require that adjustments be made even to the most effective of the treatments for childhood ADHD. Worth noting as well is that teens are far less likely to receive mental health services of all forms than are children (Jensen et al., 1999; Kazdin, 1991), perhaps owing to their increased autonomy and capacity to counteract efforts by parents to get them treatment. But it may also arise from the greater costs likely to be associated with the more extensive treatment that teens with ADHD and their families are likely to require (Robin, 2000; Smith et al., 2000).

Here I briefly note the major interventions likely to be of benefit to teens with the disorder and raise issues that are necessary to address in treatment with this age group. It must be said at the outset, however, that no intervention has been found to cure this disorder. Treatment is therefore focused on symptom management and the reduction of secondary harms that may ensue if the disorder is left unmanaged. In this sense, treating ADHD is comparable to treating diabetes. A combination of medication and psychosocial accommodations may work very well to contain the disorder and preclude the occurrence of both secondary harms and even some comorbid disorders, but treatment only works when used and often does not produce any enduring benefits if removed.

Advances in the treatment of ADHD over the past 20 years have been relatively circumscribed and have mainly occurred in the area of psychopharmacology rather than psychosocial treatments. This is not to say that more information on the prevailing treatments has not been gained. Just that no significant breakthroughs in the psychosocial treatment of the disorder have been forthcoming. Most research has clarified the efficacy (or lack of it) of already extant treatment approaches, or their combinations. Findings concerning multimodality treatments have been especially sobering (Abikoff, Hechtman, Klein, Gallacher, et al., 2004; Abikoff, Hechtman, Klein, Weiss, et al., 2004; MTA Cooperative Group, 1999; Shelton et al., 2002) but have all been conducted with children, not teens. Before discussing the efficacy of specific treatments for ADHD, it will be helpful to reexamine some traditional assumptions about the treatment of this disorder. They are being called into question not only by newer theoretical models (Barkley, 1997a) but by the results of research on the etiologies of the disorder (behavioral genetics and neuroimaging) and on the efficacy of particular treatments (Barkley, 2006).

Reexamining Treatment Assumptions

Advances in research on the etiologies of ADHD and in theoretical models about the disorder seem to suggest why few treatment breakthroughs, especially in the psychosocial arena, have occurred. The information yielded from these sources increasingly points to ADHD as being a development disorder of probable neurogenetic origins in which some unique environmental factors play a role in expression of the disorder (including biological hazards affecting brain development), though far less than do genetic ones. Common family environment factors, once thought to have a major effect on the disorder, now appear to have a minor and often insignificant role in determining individual variation in the traits making up ADHD. Thus, new family-focused treatments are unlikely to be discovered at this time that would result in an amelioration of the disorder or even its practical containment as they are unlikely to correct the underlying neurological substrates or genetic mechanisms that are contributing so strongly to it. Contrary to the social learning models on which family interventions for ADHD were originally founded, children with ADHD are not tabula rasas on which socialization makes the major contribution to psychological development, the disorder is not learned through imitation of poor role models, and it surely does not arise from exposure to faulty contingencies such as through parenting. As with the learning disabilities and mental retardation that appear to have relatively analogous etiologies, treatment is actually symptomatic management or containment. It is management of a chronic developmental condition and involves finding means to cope with, compensate for, and accommodate to the developmental deficiencies. These means also include the provision of symptomatic relief such as that obtained by various medications. And given the greater relative contribution of genotype to environment in explaining individual differences in the symptoms of the disorder, it is highly likely that treatments for ADHD, while providing improvements in the symptoms, do little to change the rank-ordering of such individuals relative to each other in their posttreatment levels of ADHD (see Rutter, 1997, and Scarr, 1992, for a general discussion of this issue in developmental psychology and clinical interventions). It is also likely that such treatments, particularly in the psychosocial realm, will prove to be specific to the treatment setting, showing minimal generalization without actively arranging for its occurrence.

The theoretical model of ADHD proposed previously suggests other reasons why treatment effects may be so limited. This is largely because, according to this model, ADHD does not result from a lack of skill, knowledge, or information. It is, therefore, not going to respond well to interventions emphasizing the transfer of knowledge or of skills, as might occur in psychotherapy, social skills training, cognitive therapies, or academic tutoring. All these contain a tacit assumption that the client with ADHD is naïve about or ignorant of these skills. Yet no research has actually examined that issue in detail. Instead, in this model, ADHD is viewed as being a disorder of performance—of doing what one knows rather than knowing what to do. It is more a disorder of "when" behavior should be performed rather than "how" to perform it. Like patients with injuries to the frontal lobes, those with ADHD find that it has partially cleaved or dissociated intellect from action, or knowledge from performance. Thus, the individual with ADHD may know how to act but may not act that way when placed in social settings where such action would be beneficial to him or her. The timing and timeliness of behavior is being disrupted more in ADHD than is the basic knowledge or skill about that behavior.

From this vantage point, treatments for ADHD will be most helpful when they assist with the performance of a particular behavior at the *point (place and time) of performance* in the natural environments where and when such behavior should be performed. A corollary of this is that the further away in space and time a treatment is from this point of performance, the less effective it is likely to be in assisting with the management of ADHD (Goldstein & Ingersoll, 1993). This includes assistance at the "point of performance" with the time, timing, and timeliness of behavior in those with ADHD, not just in the training of the behavior itself (Barkley, 1997a). Nor will there necessarily be any lasting value or maintenance of treatment effects from such assistance if it is summarily removed within a short period once the individual is performing the desired behavior. The value of such treatments lies not only in providing assistance with eliciting behavior that is likely to already be in the individual's repertoire at the point of performance where its display is critical but in maintaining the performance of that behavior over time in that natural setting. Disorders of performance like ADHD pose great consternation for the mental health and educational arenas of service. This is because at the core of such problems is the vexing issue of just how to get people to behave in ways that they know are good for them yet which they seem unlikely, unable, or unwilling to perform. Conveying more knowledge does not prove as helpful as altering the motivational parameters associated with the performance of that behavior at its appropriate point of performance. Coupled with this is the realization that such changes in behavior are maintained only as long as those environmental adjustments or accommodations are as well. To expect otherwise would seem to approach the treatment of ADHD with outdated or misguided assumptions about its essential nature.

The conceptual model of ADHD I have developed has other implications for the management of ADHD too numerous to discuss in detail here (see Barkley, 1997a). Some of them are:

1. If the process of regulating behavior by internally represented forms of information (the internalization of behavior) is delayed in those with ADHD, then they will be best assisted by "externalizing" those forms of information; the provision of more external, physical representations of that information will be needed in the setting at the point of perfor-

mance. Because covert or private information is weak as a source of stimulus control, making that information overt and public may assist with strengthening control of behavior by that information.

2. The organization of the individual's behavior across time is one of the ultimate disabilities rendered by the disorder. ADHD is to time what nearsightedness is to spatial vision; it has created a temporal myopia in which the individual's behavior is governed even more than normal by events close to or within the temporal now and immediate context rather than by internal information that pertains to longer-term, future events. Those with ADHD could be expected to be assisted then by making time itself more externally represented, by reducing or eliminating gaps in time among the components of a behavioral contingency (event, response, outcome), and by serving to bridge such temporal gaps related to future events with the assistance of caregivers and others.

3. Given that the model hypothesizes a deficit in internally generated and represented forms of motivation that are needed to support goal-directed behavior, those with ADHD will require the provision of externalized sources of motivation. For instance, the provision of artificial rewards, such as tokens, may be needed throughout the performance of a task or goal-directed behavior when there is otherwise little or no such immediate consequences associated with that performance. Such artificial reward programs become for the teen with ADHD like prosthetic devices or mechanical limbs to the physically disabled, allowing them to perform more effectively in some tasks and settings with which they otherwise would have considerable difficulty. The motivational disability created by ADHD makes such motivational prostheses nearly essential for most of those with ADHD. Yet the greater autonomy of teens from their parents and teachers, the more numerous adults with whom teens are likely to be interacting and the increasing time spent with peers and in unsupervised community settings all make for difficulties in the provision of such prosthetic motivational devices. For instance, when a teen is driving home late on a weekend night from a dance at the high school, no one else is in the car to provide externalized information and prosthetic motivation, such as tokens, for the use of safe driving behavior. Many other such scenarios exist in the lives of ADHD teens where the delivery of psychosocial inter-

ventions is difficult if not impossible. Often, medication may be needed for such activities to insure control of the symptoms of the disorder and their impact on functioning in that setting and activity.

Ineffective or Unproved Therapies

A variety of treatments have been attempted with children with ADHD over the past century—far too numerous to review here (see Ingersoll & Goldstein, 1993). Vestibular stimulation (Arnold, Clark, Sachs, Jakim, & Smithies, 1985), running (Hales & Hales, 1985), EMG biofeedback and relaxation training (Richter, 1984), sensory integration training (Vargas & Camilli, 1999), and EEG biofeedback or neurofeedback (Loo & Barkley, 2006), among others, have been described as potentially effective in uncontrolled case reports, small series of case studies, or some treatment versus no-treatment comparisons, yet they are lacking in well-controlled experimental replications of their efficacy. Many dietary treatments, such as removal of additives, colorings, or sugar from the diet or addition of high doses of vitamins, minerals, or other "health food" supplements to the diet, have proven very popular despite minimal or no scientific support (Ingersoll & Goldstein, 1993; Milich, Wolraich, & Lindgren, 1986; Wolraich, Wilson, & White, 1995). Certainly traditional psychotherapy and play therapy have not proven especially effective for ADHD or other externalizing disorders (Weisz, Weiss, Han, Granger, & Morton, 1995).

The provision of cognitive-behavioral treatment, or cognitive therapy, was previously felt to hold some promise for children with ADHD (Kendall & Braswell, 1985; Meichenbaum & Goodman, 1971). Indeed, a few small-scale studies suggested some benefits to this form of treatment when used with children with ADHD (Fehlings, Roberts, Humphries, & Dawe, 1991). But this form of treatment has been challenged as being seriously flawed from a conceptual (Vygotskian) point of view on which the treatment was initially founded (Diaz & Berk, 1995). And its efficacy for impulsive children or those with ADHD has been repeatedly questioned by the rather poor or limited results of empirical research (Abikoff, 1985, 1987; Abikoff & Gittelman, 1985). In the most ambitious cognitive-behavioral program ever undertaken and involving the training of parents, teachers, and children, researchers found no significant treatment-specific effects on any of a variety of dependent measures with the exception of class observations of off-task/disruptive behavior (Bloomquist, August, & Ostrander, 1991). Even this treatment effect was not maintained at 6-week follow-up. Reviews of this literature using meta-analyses have typically found the effect sizes to be only about a third of a standard deviation and, in many studies, even less than this (Baer & Nietzel, 1991; Dush, Hirt, & Schroeder, 1989). Although such treatment effects may at times rise to the level of statistical significance, they are nonetheless of only modest clinical importance and usually are to be found mainly on relatively circumscribed lab measures rather than more clinically important measures of functioning in natural settings.

The theoretical model of ADHD discussed earlier may offer some explanation for such limited treatment effects. For one thing, it implies that the acquisition of skills is not likely to prove particularly useful in the treatment of ADHD given that the teen's primary problem lies more in the realm of performance than of knowledge. Cognitive-behavioral treatment is predominantly a skill-training program and does little to address the performance problems of those with the disorder. But the theoretical model also suggests that there is a developmental delay in self-speech and its internalization that makes teaching verbal self-instruction procedures questionable as a means of treatment. Such self-speech may have less stimulus control over motor behavior in these teens than in normal ones. Moreover, the problem with self-speech lies downstream from the problem with response inhibition and thus self-instruction training is focusing on a secondary consequence of ADHD rather than on its primary deficit. Such a theoretical position would tend to strongly question the utility of cognitive-behavioral therapies for children with ADHD, at least as the major modality of intervention.

All this research took place with children with ADHD, raising the possibility that teens with the disorder might have a somewhat greater likelihood of success with this treatment. That is because teens, even those with ADHD, may be more developed in their executive functions and especially the internalization of speech on which this form of treatment is predicated. Their greater cognitive maturity might make them more likely to adopt and subsequently utilize cognitive self-statements

taught in training environments later in nontreatment settings. But this is purely conjectural. And given the poor success rate of cognitive therapy for childhood ADHD, few investigators or funding agencies are likely to invest substantial time and resources in pursuing large-scale studies of this therapy with teens with ADHD. For all these reasons, then, this form of treatment will not receive any further attention here.

Similarly, social skills training (SST) receives little coverage here. Again, this is largely due to the fact that reviews of this treatment as applied specifically to children with ADHD have been quite discouraging (Hinshaw, 1992; Hinshaw & Erhardt, 1991; Shelton et al., 2002; Whalen & Henker, 1991). A recent study of SST in subtypes of children with ADHD (Antshel & Remer, 2003) found some benefit on parent- and child-rated assertion skills but no benefits on other domains of social competence. Those with comorbid ODD appeared to benefit little from the program whereas those with the inattentive type of ADHD improved more than the combined type in assertion skills (but not in other domains of social competence). By follow-up, these few gains especially in the inattentive type were not sustained. Of some concern was the small subset of inattentive-type children whose parents rated them as significantly worse following SST, perhaps owing to a social contagion effect of being in training with more aggressive peers, as Dishion and colleagues have found for antisocial youth (Dishion, McCord, & Poulin, 1999). The authors concluded that SST had little efficacy for addressing the social problems of children with ADHD, consistent with other studies (DuPaul & Eckert, 1997).

Children with ADHD certainly have serious difficulties in their social interactions with peers (Cunningham, Siegel, & Offord, 1985; Erhardt & Hinshaw, 1994). This seems to be especially so for that subgroup having significant levels of comorbid aggression (Erhardt & Hinshaw, 1994), in which more than 50% of the variance in peer ratings of children whom they disliked was predicted by this behavior alone. More recent research shows that these peer relationship problems continue into the adolescent years for many youth with ADHD, being the most pronounced in those children with ADHD whose ADHD persisted into adolescence and in those with comorbid CD (Bagwell, Molina, Pelham, & Hoza, 2001).

But as Hinshaw (1992b) has summarized, the social interaction problems of children with ADHD are quite heterogeneous and are not likely to respond to a treatment package that focuses only on social approach strategies and that treats all children with ADHD as if they shared common problems in their peer relationship difficulties. Nor is it especially clear at this time what the actual source of these peer difficulties happens to be or the mechanism by which it operates, with the exception of aggressive behavior as noted earlier. Teaching them additional skills is not so much the issue as is assisting them with the performance of the skills they have *when* it would be useful to do so *at the point of performance* where such skills are most likely to prove useful to the long-term social acceptance of the individual. Those children with ADHD with comorbid aggression may well have additional problems with peer perceptions, particularly around the motives they attribute to others for their behavior, as well as in information processing about social interactions (Dodge, 1989). This combination of both perceptual/information-processing deficits along with problems with the performance of social skills in social interactions with others may make children with ADHD with aggression particularly resistant to SST (Hinshaw, 1992b). And thus until more evidence for the efficacy of SST for children with ADHD is forthcoming, this form of treatment will receive no further coverage here.

Those treatments with some proven efficacy for assisting teens with ADHD and their families are (1) medications; (2) parent training in contingency management methods (Barkley, 1997c); (3) parent–teen training in problem-solving and communication skills (Barkley et al., 1999; Robin, 2000); (4) classroom applications of contingency management techniques (DuPaul & Eckert, 1997; Pfiffner, Barkley, & DuPaul, 2006); and (5) assorted combinations of these approaches with psychopharmacology. Besides these interventions, therapists should also be cognizant of the availability of special educational programs for children with ADHD now mandated under the Individuals with Disabilities in Education Act and Section 504 of the Civil Rights Act (DuPaul & Stoner, 2003). The determination of eligibility for such programs is often a major referral concern of parents or teachers dictating that clinicians be familiar with federal, state, and local regulations regarding placement in such programs.

Medications for Managing ADHD

Three classes of psychotropic drugs have proven useful in the management of ADHD symptoms: the stimulants, noradrenergic drugs, tricyclic antidepressants, and the anti-hypertensives. Until recently, it was not clear precisely how these medications affected brain function and particularly their sites and neuro-chemical modes of action. It now appears as if the major therapeutic effects of the stimulants, anyway, are achieved through alterations in frontal–striatal activity (Volkow et al., 1997). The rationale, then, for employing the stimulant medications with children with ADHD may be that they directly, if only temporarily, improve the deficiencies in these neural systems related to behavioral inhibition and self-regulation.

Stimulant Medication (Dopamine Agonists)

Since Bradley (1937) first (accidentally) discovered their successful use with behavior problem children, the stimulants have received an enormous amount of research—far more than any known treatment for any childhood psychiatric disorder. The results overwhelmingly indicate that these medications are quite effective for the management of ADHD symptoms in most children older than 5 years (Connor, 2005a, 2005b; Swanson, McBurnett, Christian, & Wigal, 1995). Between 4 and 5 years of age, the response rate is probably much less, and under 3 years of age, the drugs are not recommended for use. The effectiveness of these medications has led to their widespread use with children with ADHD, with approximately 2.8% of the school-age population possibly being treated with stimulants for ADHD symptoms (Zito et al., 2003). These medications may be nearly as useful with adolescents with ADHD (Smith et al., 2000), although fewer than 10 studies exist with this age group. And they are equally as useful with adults who have ADHD (Spencer et al., 1995; Wender, Reimherr, Wood, & Ward, 1985).

The most commonly prescribed stimulants are methylphenidate (Ritalin, Concerta, Medadate CD, Focalin), *d*-amphetamine (Dexedrine or Dextrostat), *d*- and *l*-amphetamine combination (Adderall, Adderall XR), and pemoline (Cylert). Methylphenidate (MPH) appears to work by slowing down dopamine reuptake from the extracellular space.

The amphetamines appear to work by primarily increasing dopamine release but may also have some effect on reuptake. It is not known how pemoline achieves its therapeutic effect. Because of the potential for liver complications (Safer, Zito, & Gardner, 2001), pemoline is no longer recommended for use with patients unless frequent monitoring of liver functioning is undertaken. It receives no further attention here given its near disuse in treating children. Adderall is a recently approved stimulant compound for use in the management of ADHD. It is a combination of different forms of amphetamine salts that is effective in the treatment of symptoms of ADHD in children (Biederman, Lopez, Boellner, & Chandler, 2002) and adults (Spencer et al., 2001).

MPH (in various forms) and amphetamine (AMP) are the most commonly prescribed medications for ADHD. In their original forms, they are rapidly acting stimulants, producing effects on behavior within 30 to 45 minutes after oral ingestion of their standard preparations and peaking in their behavioral effects within 2 to 4 hours (Connor, 2005b). Their utility in managing behavior quickly dissipates within 3–7 hours, although minuscule amounts of the medication may remain in the blood for up to 24 hours (Greenhill & Osmon, 2000; Solanto, Arnsten, & Castellanos, 2001). Because of their short halflife, they were often prescribed two to three times per day, posing great inconvenience and the requirement for school administration of at least one (noon) dose. Although once used predominantly for schooldays, there is an increasing clinical trend toward usage throughout the week as well as school vacations. This is the result of more recent discoveries that the growth of children with ADHD on stimulants is not as seriously affected as was once believed (Rapport & Moffitt, 2002; Spencer et al., 1996), and thus the rationale for universal drug holidays is no longer justifiable. Focalin, or dex-methlyphenidate, was recently approved for use in ADHD. It is simply the right-turning MPH molecule. Some research suggests this may be the effective form of this medication as opposed to the left-turning molecule (levo-methylphenidate). It is otherwise identical in effects and side effects to MPH but requires only half the typical dose of MPH.

Both MPH and AMP later came in slow release preparations (Ritalin SR; Dexedrine spansules) that reduced the number of daily doses children require for management of their ADHD. But their control of behavior was less than ideal owing to suboptimal blood levels during the sustained release of the medication. New and more effective delivery systems have been invented over the past 5 years that make these earlier slow-release formulations nearly outdated. These include Concerta, Medadate CD, and Ritalin LA for methylphenidate delivery and Adderall XR for mixed amphetamine delivery. Concerta is a miniature osmotic pump resembling a capsule that oozes liquid methyphenidate while transversing the gut for an interval of 10–12 hours (Swanson et al., 2003). Medadate CD, Focalin XR, and Ritalin LA are tiny MPH pellets having various time-release coatings applied to them such that they dissolve at increasingly longer time intervals as they course through the gut and last for roughly 8–12 hours. Medadate CD has the advantage of being able to be opened and sprinkled on soft food for easier oral ingestion in patients having difficulties swallowing tablets or capsules without affecting its pharmacokinetic properties (Pentikas, Simmons, Benedict, & Hatch, 2002). Ritalin LA likely has this same advantage.

The behavioral improvements produced by MPH and AMP occur in sustained attention, impulse control, and reduction of task-irrelevant activity, especially in settings demanding restraint of behavior (Connor, 2005b; Greenhill & Osmon, 2000). Generally noisy and disruptive behavior also diminishes with medication. Children with ADHD may become more compliant with parental and teacher commands, are better able to sustain such compliance, and often increase their cooperative behavior toward others with whom they may have to accomplish a task as a consequence of stimulant treatment (see Danforth et al., 1991, for a review). Children with ADHD are able to perceive the medication as beneficial to the reduction of ADHD symptoms and even describe improvements in their self-esteem (DuPaul, Anastopoulos, Kwasnik, Barkley, & McMurray, 1996), though they may report somewhat more side effects than do their parents and teachers.

Drug-related improvements in other domains of behavior include aggression (Barkley, McMurray, Edelbrock, & Robbins, 1990; Murphy, Pelham, & Lang, 1992); handwriting (Lerer, Lerer, & Artner, 1987); academic productivity and accuracy (Rapport, DuPaul,

Stoner, & Jones, 1986); and persistence of effort, working memory, peer relations, emotional control, and participation in sports, among others (Greenhill & Osmon, 2000; Solanto et al., 2001). The effects of medication are idiosyncratic (see Rapport et al., 1986), with some children showing maximal improvement at lower doses while others are most improved at higher doses of medication. Stimulants appear to remain useful in the management of ADHD over extended periods of time (MTA Cooperative Group, 1999; Schachar & Tannock, 1993; Zeiner, 1995) and can be used successfully into adulthood.

Side effects include mild insomnia and appetite reduction, particular at the noon meal (Barkley, McMurray, Edelbrock, & Robbins, 1990). Temporary suppression of weight gain may accompany stimulant treatment initially but is not generally severe or especially common (Spencer et al., 1996), may rebound in the second year of treatment, and can be managed by ensuring that adequate caloric and nutritional intake is maintained by shifting the distribution of food intake to other times of the day when the child is more amenable to eating. A small percentage of children with ADHD may complain of stomachaches and headaches when treated with stimulants, but these tend to dissipate within a few weeks of beginning medication or can be managed by reducing the dose. In approximately 1–2% of children with ADHD treated with stimulants, motor or vocal tics may occur (Connor, 2005b). In others where tics already exist, they can be mildly exacerbated by stimulant treatment in some cases but may even be improved in others (Gadow, Sverd, Sprafkin, Nolan, & Ezor, 1995). It now appears to be relatively safe to use stimulant medications with children with ADHD and comorbid tic disorders but to be prepared to reduce the dose or discontinue medication should the child experience a drug-related exacerbation of their tic symptoms.

There are few reliable predictors of response to stimulant medication in children with ADHD. Those characteristics having the most consistent relationship to response have been pretreatment levels of poor sustained attention and hyperactivity (Barkley, 1976; Buitelaar, van der Gaag, Swaab-Barneveld, & Kuiper, 1995). Predictors of adverse responding have not been as well studied but level of anxiety seems to be associated with poorer responding to stimulants (Buitelaar et al., 1995; DuPaul,

Barkley, & McMurray, 1994), but the finding is not reliable.

There is little doubt now that the stimulant medications are the most studied and most effective treatment for the symptomatic management of ADHD and its secondary consequences. Their side effects are relatively benign, particularly in comparison to other psychiatric drugs. For many children with moderate to severe levels of ADHD, this may be the first treatment employed in their clinical management. Other treatments may then be added adjuncts for domains of impairment unaffected by medication or when medication-free periods are required.

Norepinephrine Reuptake Inhibitors

Several medications are now available that have some therapeutic benefit for the management of ADHD and that function by slowing reuptake of norepinephrine. The noradrenergic reuptake inhibitors are Wellbutrin (bupropion) and, most recently (January 2003), atomoxetine (Strattera). Bupropion appears to affect both noradrenergic and dopaminegergic systems. Several studies with children with ADHD and one more recently with adults show that it results in significant improvement in ADHD symptoms relative to placebo (Spencer, Biederman, & Wilens, 1998). The beneficial effects are not as substantial or dramatic as those achieved by the stimulants. Potential side effects include edema, rashes, irritability, loss of appetite, seizures (rare), and insomnia. No studies have examined this medication with teens with ADHD, but there is no doubt it would prove of some effectiveness for them in view of its demonstrated efficacy with children and adults having the disorder.

Atomoxetine (Strattera) is the first new molecule for the treatment of ADHD approved by the Food and Drug Administration (FDA) since 1975. Indications have been approved for children, teens, and adults with ADHD. Over the past 7 years, Eli Lilly has conducted various placebo control studies of atomoxetine relative to placebo and to MPH using more than 6,000 patients. Further research continues to be done examining the effect of the drug on specific domains of functioning in children (family functioning) and adults (occupational functioning, driving, etc.) with ADHD. Unlike bupropion, atomoxetine works selectively on noradrenergic reuptake, thereby making more norepinephrine available outside nerve cells. Atomoxetine has been studied in six acute, large, randomized, double-blind, placebo-controlled studies (two in children, two in children and adolescents, and two in adults) (Michelson et al., 2002). One trial in children was conducted with once-daily dosing (6 weeks), while the others employed twice-daily dosing, all on weight-adjusted basis (8–9 weeks). Adults were dosed twice daily over 10 weeks in dose escalation within a fixed range. In all studies, atomoxetine was superior to placebo in reduction of mean symptom ratings for the primary outcome measure. The effect size for once-daily treatment was similar to that of twice-daily treatment. No serious safety concerns have been observed and tolerability has been good, evidenced by discontinuation rates for adverse events under 5% in the pediatric studies. The long-term safety of atomoxetine was assessed using data from clinical trials in children and adolescents treated for at least 1 year. Tolerability and safety were assessed by evaluating discontinuations, adverse events, weight, and height. Over 6,000 patients have been exposed to atomoxetine in these and other clinical trials, with over 400 treated for at least 2 years. Discontinuations due to adverse events were uncommon (< 5%). Reports of decreased appetite and weight loss, which were reported statistically significantly more often than with placebo in acute trials, continued to decline during long-term treatment, as did other adverse events. After at least 1 year of treatment, atomoxetine increased mean heart rate by 6.4 beats per minute and increased mean diastolic blood pressure by 2.8 mm Hg. For patients who lost weight, it tended to occur early in treatment (mean 0.5 kg in acute studies). Over longer treatment periods, weight increased (mean 4.0 kg after 1 year). Because 1 year is a relatively short period in the growth of many children, analyses of height increases are inconclusive and require data over longer treatment periods. Atomoxetine appears to be safe and efficacious for the treatment of ADHD in children, adolescents, and adults (Michelson et al., 2002) and of equal efficacy for the reduction of ADHD symptoms in comparison to MPH.

Antidepressant Medication

Clinicians have used the tricyclic antidepressants, such as imipramine and desipramine, for the management of ADHD symptoms (Spencer et al., 1998). In part this has been due to the occasional negative (and often undeserving) publicity in the popular media focusing on the stimulants, and especially Ritalin. But the rise in antidepressant use may also have resulted from cases in which stimulants have been contraindicated or have not been especially effective or in which significant comorbid mood disturbance may exist. Less is known about the pharmacokinetics and behavioral effects of the antidepressants in children with ADHD as compared to the stimulants. However, research on these compounds, particularly desipramine, increased in the early 1990s and generally supports their efficacy in the management of ADHD (Wilens et al., 1996). Often given twice daily (morning and evening), these medications are longer acting than the stimulants. As a result, it takes longer to evaluate the therapeutic value of any given dose (Viesselman, Yaylayan, Weller, & Weller, 1993). Some research suggests that low doses of the tricyclics may mimic stimulants in producing increased vigilance and sustained attention and decreased impulsivity. As a result, disruptive and aggressive behavior may also be reduced. Elevation in mood may also occur, particularly in those children in whom significant pretreatment levels of depression and anxiety exist (Pliszka, 1987). Ryan (1990) reported that treatment effects may diminish over time, however, such that the tricyclics cannot be used as longterm therapy for ADHD, unlike the stimulants.

The most common side effects of the tricyclics are drowsiness during the first few days of treatment, dry mouth and constipation, and flushing. Less likely yet more important are the cardiotoxic effects, such as possible tachycardia or arrhythmia, and in cases of overdose, coma or death (Viesselman et al., 1993). Some children may develop sluggish reactions in focusing of the optic lens that may mimic nearsightedness. The reaction is not permanent, dissipating when treatment is withdrawn. Skin rash is occasionally reported and usually warrants ceasing drug treatment.

In general, clinicians would find it preferable to use atomoxetine first as an alternative to the tricylcic antidepressants owing largely to the greater safety and information available on the former medication. The tricyclic antidepressants may be useful in the short-term treatment of children with ADHD when the stimulants or atomoxetine are not effective. However, care must be taken to properly evaluate the cardiac functioning of children before initiating treatment and then periodically monitor such functioning throughout the course of treatment given the apparent risks of the tricyclic antidepressants for impairing cardiac functioning (see Wilens et al., 1996, for a review and guidelines for monitoring children on tricyclic antidepressants).

Antihypertensive Medication

In the late 1980s, a small number of research papers appeared suggesting that the antihypertensive drug clonidine (Catapres), may be beneficial in the management of ADHD symptoms, particularly in the reduction of hyperactivity and overarousal (Connor, 2005a). Another antihypertensive drug, guanfacine (Tenex), may also have some utility in managing ADHD (Connor, 1998). These drugs are believed to act as alpha-2 adrenergic agonist that ultimately leads to the inhibition of the release of norepinephrine, increasing dopamine turnover, and reducing blood serotonin levels (Connor, 2005a; Werry & Aman, 1993). Some changes in behavior may be the result of the general sedation produced by the medication, but others appear to be specific to improvements in activity regulation and attention. A large-scale study in The Netherlands also reported significant improvements in behavior in hyperkinetic children placed on this medication (Gunning, 1992). The limited research to date suggests that the drug is much less effective than the stimulants at improving inattention and school productivity but may be equally as efficacious in the reduction of hyperactivity and moodiness. The drug may also be useful in managing the sleep disturbances that some children with ADHD may experience (Prince, Wilens, Diederman, Spencer, & Wozniak, 1996). Side effects include drowsiness, dizziness, weakness, and occasional sleep disturbance. Rarer side effects include nausea, vomiting, cardiac arrhythmia, irritability, and orthostatic hypotension (Connor, 1998). Werry and Aman (1993) have recommended that clonidine be employed in the treatment of ADHD only as a last line of medical management where stimulants have proven ineffective or are contraindicated. Given the recent availability and greater safety of atomoxetine, it would certainly be used ahead of the antihypertensives in the management of ADHD.

Direct Applications of Contingency Management

A number of early studies evaluated the effects of reinforcement and punishment, usually response cost, on the behavior and cognitive performance of children with ADHD. These studies usually indicated that the performance of children with ADHD on tasks measuring vigilance or impulse control or on academic-like tasks can be immediately and significantly improved by the use of stimulus control techniques (Barkley, 2006) or by the contingent application of consequences (Firestone & Douglas, 1977; Worland, 1976). In some cases, the behavior of children with ADHD approximates that of normal control children. However, none of these studies examined the degree to which such changes endured after treatment withdrawal or, more important, generalized to the natural environments of the children, calling into question the clinical efficacy of such an approach. Given the findings of highly limited generalization and maintenance of treatment effects for the classroom interventions described later, it is unlikely that behavioral techniques implemented only in the clinic or laboratory would carry over into the home or school settings of these children without formal programming for such generalization and maintenance. Consequently, they receive no further attention here.

Important to note here is that virtually no research has focused on the effectiveness of the aforementioned behavioral treatments using teens with ADHD. Given the limited success and particularly limited generalization and maintenance of such approaches they are unlikely to receive such attention in the future. The overall treatment-limiting features of these approaches, and the psychosocial ones discussed below, are telling of why they would be of limited utility with teens: (1) their reliance on the compassion and willingness of others to employ them with teenagers with ADHD when those others may have little time or inclination to do so; (2) the progressively greater time teens spend away from caregivers, often with peers, who are frequently not part of the treatment team; (3) the greater number of educators with whom teens are likely to take classes than are children and the greater likelihood they will not comply with recommendations or will do so only halfheartedly; (4) the increasing opportunity for teens to spend time with others and in places largely out of reach of psychosocial treatments (employment settings, driving, shopping at the mall, playing sports, etc.); and (5) the increasing capacity and desire for self-determination and freedom from coercion by others. Moreover, in view of the latter, teens can exert effective countercontrol against attempts by others to alter their behavior. In this case, intervening with teens becomes more akin to treating adults with mental disorders, placing far greater reliance on the willingness of the teen to cooperate with treatment recommendations. As in all other areas of adolescent medicine and clinical psychology, compliance with treatment becomes a, if not *the*, paramount issue in the management of ADHD in teens. And it is fair to say that most of these teens do not necessarily want the help or fully invest themselves in the treatments their parents may seek for them.

Training Parents in Behavior Management Methods

Despite the plethora of research on parent training in child behavior modification (Barkley, 1997c; Kazdin, 1991), only a small number of studies have examined the efficacy of this approach with children specifically selected for hyperactive or ADHD symptoms and only two have studied its efficacy specifically with teens with ADHD (Barkley et al., 1993; Barkley, Edwards, et al., 2001a). What limited research exists can be interpreted with cautious optimism as supporting the use of behavioral parent training with children with ADHD (Anastopoulos, Smith, & Wien, 1998; Strayhorn & Weidman, 1989, 1991). One of the few studies to conduct a follow-up reevaluation 1 year after treatment, however, found that the families receiving parent training were no longer different from the control group, although the child's school behavior was rated by teachers as significantly better (Strayhorn & Weidman, 1991). Far fewer studies have been done with teens with ADHD. The results for teens are less impressive but still suggest some benefits to a minority of families.

Those treatment techniques used to date with children with ADHD have primarily consisted of training parents in general contingency management tactics, such as contingent application of reinforcement or punishment following appropriate/inappropriate behaviors. Reinforcement procedures have typically relied on praise or tokens while punishment methods have usually been loss of tokens or time out from reinforcement. Why these particular methods were chosen or what specific target behaviors they were used with have often gone unreported. At least one study (Bidder et al., 1978) employed a shaping procedure to directly modify hyperactivity. Children with ADHD were required to sit for progressively longer periods while working on assigned tasks with their mother for which they were presumably reinforced.

I have developed a parent training program for children with ADHD, the methods of which have been borrowed from research indicating their efficacy in managing defiant and oppositional children (Barkley, 1997c). The program has been modified somewhat for families of teens with ADHD (Barkley et al., 1999) and even tested in combination with training of both parents and teens in problem-solving and communication skills (Barkley et al., 1993; Barkley, Edwards, et al., 2001b). Such treatments are viewed as being more relevant to the oppositional/defiant behaviors associated with ADHD in such cases rather than being likely to change the symptoms of ADHD or their underlying causes. The contingency management portion of the program consists of eight steps, with 1- to 2-hour weekly training sessions provided either in groups or to individual families. Each step is described in detail elsewhere (Barkley, 1997c; Barkley et al., 1999) but is briefly presented below:

1. *Review of information on ADHD.* This session provides a succinct overview of the nature, developmental course, prognosis, and etiologies of ADHD. Providing the parents with additional reading materials, such as a book for parents (Barkley, 2001b), can be a useful addition to this session. Professional videotapes are also available (Barkley, 1993a, 1993b, 1999) that present such an overview and can be loaned to parents for review at home and sharing with relatives or teachers, as needed. A recent study suggests that just this provision of information can result not only in improved knowledge of parents about ADHD but also in improved parental perceptions of the degree of deviance of their child's behavioral difficulties (Andrews, Swank, Foorman, & Fletcher, 1995).

2. *The causes of oppositional/defiant behavior.* This session provides parents with an

indepth discussion of those factors identified in past research as contributing to the development of defiant behavior in children (see Barkley, 1997c; Patterson, Dishion, & Reid, 1992, for reviews). Essentially, four major contributors are discussed: (1) child characteristics, such as health, developmental disabilities, and temperament; (2) parent characteristics similar to those described for the child; (3) situational consequences for oppositional and coercive behavior; and (4) stressful family events. Parents are taught that where problems exist in (1), (2), and (4), they increase the probability of children displaying bouts of coercive, defiant behavior. However, the consequences for such defiance, (3) above, seem to determine whether that behavior will be maintained or even increased in subsequent situations in which commands and rules are given. Such behavior appears to primarily function as escape/avoidance learning in which oppositional behavior succeeds in the child escaping from aversive parent interactions and task demands, negatively reinforcing the child's coercion. As in the first session, this content is covered to correct potential misconceptions that parents have about defiance (i.e., it is primarily attention getting in nature). This session can be augmented by the use of two professional videotapes on the nature of oppositional defiant behavior and its management (Barkley, 1997d, 1997e).

3. *Developing and enhancing parental attention.* Training occurs in more effective ways of attending to child behavior to enhance the value of their attention to their children. The technique consists of verbal narration and occasional positive statements to the child with attention being strategically deployed only when appropriate behavior is displayed. Parents are taught to ignore inappropriate behaviors but to greatly increase their attention to ongoing prosocial and compliant child behaviors.

4. *Attending to child compliance.* This session extends the techniques developed in Session 3 to instances in which parents issue direct commands to children. Parents are trained in methods of giving effective commands, such as reducing questionlike commands (e.g., Why don't you pick up your toys now?), increasing imperatives, eliminating setting activities that compete with task performance (e.g., television), reducing task complexity, and so on. Parents are also trained to provide more positive attention frequently and systematically when

their children are engaged in nondisruptive activities while parents must be occupied with some other work or activity.

5. *Establishing a home point system.* This session institutes a home token economy that is critical to addressing the motivational and time management difficulties associated with ADHD. Parents list most of the children's home responsibilities and privileges and then assign values of points or chips to each. The parents are encouraged to have at least 12–15 reinforcers on the menu to maintain the motivating properties of the program. Generally, points are used that are recorded in a notebook. Points are given only for obeying first requests. If a command must be repeated, it must still be obeyed but the opportunity to earn points has been forfeited. Parents are also encouraged to give bonus points for good attitude or emotional regulation in their children. For instance, if a command is obeyed quickly, without complaint, and with a positive attitude, parents may give the child additional points beyond those typically given for that job. Families are encouraged to establish and maintain such programs for at least 6–8 weeks to allow for the newly developed interaction patterns spawned by such programs to become habit patterns.

6. *Implementing time out for noncompliance.* Parents are now trained to use response cost (removal of points) contingent upon noncompliance. In addition, they are trained in a time-out-from-reinforcement technique for use with one or two serious forms of defiance that may continue to be problematic despite the use of the home token economy. For teens, parents are taught to simply have the teen go to a relatively dull room in the family home for a specified period, or, more likely, the teen is grounded for several hours of his or her leisure time during which the teen cannot leave home, communicate with peers, or enjoy electronic privileges.

7. *Extending time out to additional noncompliant behaviors.* In this session, no new material is taught to parents. Instead, any problems with previously implementing time out are reviewed and corrected. Parents may then extend their use of time out to one or two additional noncompliant behaviors with which the child may still have trouble.

8. *Managing noncompliance in public places.* Parents of children with ADHD are now taught to extrapolate their home management methods to troublesome public places, such as stores, church, restaurants, and so on.

Using a "think aloud–think ahead" transition plan, parents are taught to stop just before entering a public place, review two or three rules with the child that the child may previously have defied, explain to the child what reinforcers are available for obedience in the place, then explain what punishment may occur for disobedience, and finally assign the child an activity to perform during the outing. Parents then enter the public place and immediately begin attending to and reinforcing ongoing child compliance with the previously stated rules. Time out or response cost are used immediately for disobedience. Parents of teens are taught to review their expectations for teen conduct in a public place and then create a behavior contract with the teen concerning consequences that will ensue for compliance/noncompliance.

9. *Improving school behavior from home: The daily school behavior report card.* This session is a recent addition (Barkley, 1997c) to the original parent training program and was designed to help parents assist their child's or teen's teachers with the management of classroom behavior problems. The session focuses on training parents in the use of a home-based reward program in which children are evaluated on a daily school behavior report card by their teachers. This card serves as the means by which consequences later in the day will be dispensed at home for classroom conduct. The card can be designed to address class behavior, recess or free-time behavior, or more specific behavioral targets for any given child. The consequence provided at home typically consists of the rewarding or removal of tokens within the home token system as a function of the ratings the child has received from teachers on daily behavioral report card.

10. *One-month review/booster session.* In what is typically the final session, the concepts taught in earlier sessions are briefly reviewed, problems that have arisen in the last month are discussed, and plans are made for their correction. Other sessions may be needed to deal with additional issues that persist.

Research suggests that up to 64% of families experience clinically significant change or recovery (normalization) of their child's disruptive behavior as a consequence of this program (Anastopoulos et al., 1993). However, improvements in behavior may be more concentrated in the realm of aggressive and defiant child behavior than in inattentive–hyperactive

symptoms (Johnston, 1992). All these studies have relied on clinic-referred families most of whom sought out the assistance of mental health professionals for their children. In contrast to the results of research with such motivated families, my colleagues and I have found that if such a clinic-based parent training program is offered to parents of preschool children whose children were identified at kindergarten enrollment as having significant levels of aggressive–hyperactive–impulsive behavior, most do not attend training or attend unreliably (Barkley et al., 2000; Shelton et al., 2000). Moreover, no significant improvements in child behavior were found even among those who did attend at least some of the training sessions. Cunningham, Bremner, and Boyle (1995) have shown that parent training programs may be more cost-effective, reach more severely disruptive children and more minority families, and be more effective if they are provided as group classes offered through neighborhood schools in the evenings using paraprofessionals as trainers.

Both studies my colleagues and I conducted with this program slightly modified for teens found significant improvement at the group level of analysis. That is, all treatment groups improved from pre- to posttreatment. But at the individual level of analysis, a mixed picture emerged. While 31–70% of families were brought to within the normal range (75th percentile or lower), only 23–30% of treated families actually showed what could be considered reliable changes (unlikely to be due to unreliability of measurement alone) on measures of parent–teen conflict—results that did not differ from the problem-solving approach discussed next (Barkley et al., 1993; Barkley, Edwards, et al., 2001a).

We have also examined a family training program that includes problem-solving communication training (PSCT) program procedures developed by Robin and Foster (1989; see also Barkley et al., 1999; Forgatch & Patterson, 1989). This treatment program contains three major components for changing parent–adolescent conflict: (1) *problem solving:* training parents and teens in a five-step problem-solving approach (problem definition, brainstorming of possible solutions, negotiation, decision making about a solution, implementation of the solution); (2) *communication training:* helping parents and teens to develop more effective communication skills while discussing family conflicts, such as speaking in an even tone of voice, paraphrasing others' concerns before speaking ones' own, providing approval to others for positive communication, and avoiding insults, putdowns, ultimatums, and other poor communication skills; and (3) *cognitive restructuring*: helping families detect, confront, and restructure irrational, extreme, or rigid belief systems held by parents or teens about their own or the other's conduct. These skills are practiced with the therapist during each session using direct instruction, modeling, behavior rehearsal, roleplaying, and feedback. Homework assignments are also given that involved the family using PSCT skills during a conflict discussion at home and audiotaping these for later review by the therapist.

This procedure has been studied both separately and in combination with the aforementioned behavioral parent training procedure. The combination of the two approaches was superior to PSCT alone in just one respect, though it is an important one. Significantly more families in the combined group (receiving behavior management training [BMT] first) stayed in treatment than did those receiving just PSCT (Barkley, Edwards, et al., 2001a). Otherwise, the groups did not differ, either in their group-level improvements or in rates of normalization and reliable change. At most, 23% showed reliable change while 31–70% showed normalization. We believe the former is a better indicator of true change occurring as a function of treatment over and above the expected unreliability of the measures used to assess treatment effects. Of some concern was that up to 17% of families showed significant worsening of family conflicts as a function of treatment, especially with PSCT, perhaps because treatment forces them to confront issues of conflict that at home they may otherwise have avoided directly discussing.

In sum, family treatments do not appear to be useful for the management of symptoms of ADHD. Their utility may be in addressing the parent–child conflicts that often arise in such families, especially where ODD may be a comorbid disorder. Family training may be maximally effective for elementary-age children with ADHD. Its utility may decline for adolescents, where only a minority appear to derive clinically reliable change due to treatment. The combination of BMT with PSCT seems to be the most useful, if only in reducing rates of dropouts from treatment. Yet some families may actually show a worsening of conflicts as a function of treatment, apparently more so with PSCT.

Training Teachers in Classroom Management

More research has occurred on the application of behavior management methods in the classroom with ADHD children than with parent training. Moreover, there is a voluminous literature on the application of classroom management methods to disruptive child behaviors, many of which include the typical symptoms of ADHD. This research clearly indicates the effectiveness of behavioral techniques in the shortterm treatment of academic performance problems in children with ADHD. I am aware of no studies that have tested these procedures directly with teens with ADHD in school settings.

A meta-analysis of the research literature on school interventions for children with ADHD was conducted that comprised 70 separate experiments of various within- and between-subjects designs as well as single-case designs (DuPaul & Eckert, 1997). This review found an overall mean effect size for contingency management procedures of 0.60 for between-subject designs, nearly 1.00 for within-subject designs, and approximately 1.40 for single-case experimental designs. Interventions aimed at improving academic performance through the manipulation of the curriculum, antecedent conditions, or peer-tutoring produced approximately equal or greater effects sizes. In contrast, cognitive-behavioral treatments when used in the school setting were significantly less effective than these other two forms of interventions. Thus, despite some initial findings of rather limited impact of classroom behavior management on children with ADHD (Abikoff & Gittelman, 1984), the totality of the extant literature reviewed by DuPaul and Eckert (1997) suggest that behavioral and academic interventions in the classroom can be effective in improving behavioral problems and academic performance in children with ADHD. The behavior of these children, however, may not be fully normalized by these interventions. Though very encouraging, such results need to be directly tested with teens having ADHD in their school environments. Given the large number of teachers with whom teenagers must typically deal each week (up to six to eight), the more limited time they spend with each, the greater periods of unsupervised time at school, and the larger school buildings teens are likely to be housed within, it is not clear that similar levels of success would be achieved by these approaches when used with teens with ADHD as would be the case for children with ADHD. Only two studies have directly tested behavioral treatments with teens, mainly note-taking training in combination with an intensive summer treatment program (Evans et al., 1994), with some success.

A serious limitation to these results has been the lack of followup on the maintenance of these treatment gains over time. In addition, none of these studies examined whether generalization of behavioral control occurred in other school settings where no treatment procedures were in effect. Other studies employing a mixture of cognitive-behavioral and contingency management techniques have failed to find such generalization with children with ADHD (Barkley, Copeland, & Sivage, 1980), suggesting that improvements derived from classroom management methods are quite situation specific and may not generalize or be maintained once treatment has been terminated.

What can be drawn from this literature to date? First, contingency management methods can produce immediate, significant, short-term improvement in the behavior, productivity, and accuracy of children with ADHD in the classroom. Second, secondary or tangible reinforcers are more effective in reducing disruptive behavior and increasing performance than are attention or other social reinforcers. The use of positive reinforcement programs alone does not seem to result in as much improvement or to maintain that improvement over time as well as does the combination of token reinforcement systems with punishment, such as response cost (i.e. removal of tokens or privileges). Such findings would be expected from the model of ADHD discussed earlier that suggests a decreased power to self-regulate motivation and a delay in the development of internalized speech and the rule-governed behavior it affords in children with this disorder. Third, what little evidence there is, however, suggests that treatment gains are unlikely to be maintained in these children once treatment has been withdrawn, and that improvements in behavior probably do not generalize to other settings in which no treatment is in effect. And

fourth, none of these procedures has been scientifically evaluated with teenagers having ADHD in natural classroom settings.

One promising method deserving of further evaluation for teens is the use of home-based contingencies for inclass behavior and performance. Atkeson and Forehand (1978) have reviewed the early literature on this technique and found that the method offered some usefulness for managing disruptive classroom behavior but that much more rigorous research was required to evaluate its promise. As discussed earlier under the author's parent training program (see also Barkley, 1997c), the method involves having a teacher rate a child's daily school performance, either one or more times throughout a schoolday. These ratings are then sent home with the child for review by the parents. The parents then dispense rewards and punishments (usually response cost) at home contingent upon the content of these daily ratings. O'Leary, Pelham, Rosenbaum, and Price (1976) employed this procedure for 10 weeks with nine hyperkinetic children and documented significant improvements on teacher ratings of classroom conduct and hyperkinesis as compared to a no-treatment control group. Others have similarly found such home–school behavioral report cards to be useful, either alone or in combination with parent and teacher training in behavior management, in the treatment of children with ADHD (Pelham et al., 1988).

The range of accommodations that can be suggested for assisting individuals with ADHD in the classroom can be rather substantial. To illustrate the point, consider the list provided in Table 4.2 of various treatment recommendations that might be conveyed to school staff dealing with children or adolescents who have ADHD. Such recommendations range from altering the productivity requirements, classroom seating arrangements, and even teaching style to instituting classroom token systems and daily school report cards linked to home-based token reward programs to suggestions concerning classroom punishment methods. Some of the recommendations are based mainly on common sense and clinical wisdom while others are derived from the scientific literature on treatments used in classrooms with children with ADHD. Not all will prove appropriate or effective in all cases as any school intervention plan must be tailored to the issues involved in any particular case of ADHD.

TABLE 4.2. A Typical Range of Treatment Suggestions for Classroom Behavior Management of Children and Adolescents with ADHD

Educational management principles

1. Decrease work load to fit child's attentional capacity.
   • Smaller quotas for productivity
   • More frequent but shorter work periods
   • Lower accuracy quotas that increase over time with child's success
   • Don't send unfinished classwork home
   • Eliminate high appeal distractors

2. Alter teaching style and curriculum.
   • Allow some restlessness at work area
   • Be animated, theatrical, and responsive
   • Use participatory teaching with activities
   • Computer based drills and instructions
   • Stay flexible, open to unusual teaching approaches to lessons
   • Don't reinforce speed of responding
   • Reward thoughtful "think aloud" approach
   • Sit child close to teacher's work area
   • Intersperse low with high interest tasks
   • Use occasional brief exercise breaks
   • Schedule more difficult subjects in AM
   • Use direct instruction type curriculum materials

3. Make rules external.
   • Signs that signal rule periods
   • Posters listing rules for work periods
   • Cards on desks with rules for desk work
   • Child verbally restates rules before entering the next activity
   • Child uses self-instruction during work
   • Child recites rules to others before work
   • Use tape-recorded cues to facilitate on-task behavior that child listens to privately on a portable tapeplayer while working
   • Have child prestate goals for work periods

4. Increase frequency of rewards and fines.
   • Token economies
   • Use Attention Trainer (Gordon Systems, DeWitt, NY)
   • Use tape recorded tones for self-reward (see Barkley, Copeland, & Sivage, 1980)
   • Have access to rewards several times/day

5. Increase immediacy of consequences—act don't yack!
   • Stop repeating your commands
   • Avoid lengthy reasoning over misbehavior

6. Increase magnitude/power of rewards.
   • Token systems are great for this
   • Have parents send in preferred toys or games
   • Get a videogame donated to classroom
   • Use home-based reward program (daily school behavior report card) (see Barkley, 1997b)
   • Try group rewards if child meets quotas

(continued)

TABLE 4.2. *(continued)*

7. Set time limits for work completion.
   • Use timers if possible for external time references
   • Use tape recorded time prompts with decreasing time counts

8. Develop hierarchy of classroom punishments.
   • Head down at desk
   • Response cost (fines in token system)
   • Time out in corner
   • Time out at school office
   • Suspension to office (in school)
   • If all fail, schedule meeting with parents and consider special educational referral.

9. Coordinate home and school consequences
   • Daily school report card/rating form
   • Daily home–school journal
   • Gradually move to weekly monitoring

Tips to improve teen school performance

1. Daily school assignment notebook with verification and cross-checking.
2. In-class cueing system for off-task behavior and disruption.
3. Assign a daily "case manager" or organizational "coach."
4. Daily/weekly school conduct card with home–school point system.
5. Extra set of books maintained at home.
6. Additional school–home tutoring as needed.

Combined Interventions

Optimal treatment is likely to consist of a combination of psychosocial and medication approaches for maximal effectiveness (Carlson, Pelham, Milich, & Dixon, 1992; Horn et al., 1991; MTA Cooperative Group, 1999). Some research studies have examined the utility of such treatment packages with interesting results. None were done with teens having ADHD, however. It appears that in many studies, the combination of contingency management training of parents or teachers with stimulant drug therapies are generally little better than either treatment alone for the management of ADHD symptoms (Firestone, Kelly, Goodman, & Davey, 1981; Gadow, 1985; MTA Cooperative Group, 1999). One study (Abikoff & Gittelman, 1984) found that classroom behavioral interventions may have mildly improved the deviant behavior of children with ADHD but did not bring such levels of behavior within the normal range. Medication, in contrast, rendered most children normal in classroom behavior. Others have found more impressive results for classroom behavior management methods (DuPaul & Eckert, 1997) but also found that the addition of medication provides added improvements beyond that achieved by behavior management alone (Pelham et al., 2000). Moreover, the combination may result in the need for less intense behavioral interventions or lower doses of medication than might be the case if either intervention were used alone. Where there is an advantage to behavioral interventions, it appears to be in reliably increasing rates of academic productivity and accuracy. Yet, here too stimulant medication has shown positive effects (Pelham et al., 1988). Despite some failures to obtain additive effects for these two treatments, their combination may still be advantageous given that the stimulants are not usually used in the late afternoons or evenings when parents may need effective behavior management tactics to deal with the ADHD symptoms. Moreover, between 8 and 25% of children with ADHD do not respond positively to the stimulant medications (Barkley, 2006; Barkley, McMurray, et al., 1990), making behavioral interventions one of the few scientifically proven alternatives for these cases.

Satterfield, Satterfield, and Cantwell (1980) have attempted to evaluate the effects of individualized multimodality intervention provided over extensive periods (up to several years) on the outcome of boys with ADHD. Interventions included medication, behavioral parent training, individual counseling, special education, family therapy, and other programs as needed by the individual. Results suggest that such an individualized program of combined treatments continued over longer time intervals can produce improvements in social adjustment at home and school, rates of antisocial behavior, substance abuse, and academic achievement. These results seem to be sustained across at least a 3-year follow-up period (Satterfield, Satterfield, & Cantwell, 1981). Although such treatment suggests great promise for the possible efficacy of multimodality treatment extended over years for children with ADHD, the lack of random assignment and more adequate control procedures in this series of studies limits the ability to attribute those improvements obtained in this study directly to the treatments employed. And these limitations certainly preclude establishing which of the treatment components was most effective. Still, studies such as these and others (Carlson et al., 1992; Pelham et al., 1988) have raised hopes that multimodality treatment can be effective for ADHD if extended over long intervals of time.

To test this idea, an historic collaboration across five sites spearheaded by the National Institute of Mental Health systematically evaluated the effects of intensive, multimethod behavioral intervention alone (for 1 year), rigorous psychopharmacological testing, titration, and monitoring (1–3 years), and their combination against a community treatment group (treatment as available in the children's normal community setting (MTA Cooperative Group, 1999). The study involved 579 elementary-age children with ADHD (ages 7–9) having combined type ADHD. Results indicated that, for the management of ADHD, the medication only and combination therapy were equally effective and superior to the intensive behavioral and community control groups, which did not differ between them. Combined management may have been slightly superior to medication only for certain subgroups of children or for other outcome domains. Over the 2 years the children have been followed since intensive treatment ended, only the medication management group has continued to benefit from ongoing treatment. The results of this study continue to reinforce the notion that medication continues to provide benefit for the management of ADHD symptoms as long as it is sustained. Gains from behavioral interventions do occur but can only be sustained if the interventions are continued.

The Summer Day Treatment Program

This program was largely developed by Pelham and colleagues and is conducted in a day-treatment environment with a summer school/camp-like format. Daily activities include several hours of classroom instruction that also incorporates behavior modification methods, such as token economies, response cost, and time out from reinforcement. In addition, sports and recreational activities are arranged each day during which behavioral management programs are operative. The program also includes parent training, peer relationship training, and a follow-up protocol to enhance the likelihood that treatment gains will be maintained after leaving the program. During their stay at the camp, some children may be tested on stimulant medication using a double-blind, placebo-controlled procedure in which the child is tested on several different doses of medication while teacher ratings and behavioral observations are collected across the different camp activities. Pelham and colleagues have used this setting and larger programmatic context to conduct more focused research investigations into the effectiveness of classroom behavior management procedures alone, stimulant medication alone, and their combination in managing ADHD symptoms and improving academic performance and social behavior. Some of the components of this day-treatment program have been evaluated previously, such as classroom contingency management, and have been found to produce significant short-term improvements in children with ADHD. And so they clearly seem to do so here (Carlson et al., 1992; Pelham et al., 1988). But other components of the program have not been so well evaluated previously for their efficacy with children having ADHD, such as SST. And while results from parent ratings before and after their children's participation indicate that 86% believe their children with ADHD improved from their participation in the program, no data have been published as yet on whether the gains made during the treatment program are maintained in the normal school and home settings after the children terminate their participation in this program.

The UCI/OCDE Program

This program provides school day treatment for children with ADHD in kindergarten through fifth grades in a school-like atmosphere using classes of 12–15 children. The clinical interventions rely chiefly on a token economy program for the management of behavior in the classrooms and a parent training program conducted through both group and individual treatment sessions. Some training of self-monitoring, evaluation, and reinforcement also occurs as part of the class program. Children also receive daily group instruction in social skills as part of the classroom curriculum and some of these behaviors may be targeted for modification outside the group instruction time by using consequences within the classroom token economy. Before returning to their regular public school, some children may participate in a transition school program that focuses on more advanced social skills as well as behavior modification programs to facilitate the transfer of learning to their regular school setting. Some children within this program also may be receiving stimulant medication as needed for management of their ADHD symptoms. While this program has served as an exemplar for many others, published research on its efficacy has not been available. Granted, the parent training program and classroom behavior modification methods are highly similar to those used in published studies that have found them to be effective, at least in the short term, as long as they are in use (Barkley, 1997c; DuPaul & Eckert, 1997; Pelham & Sams, 1992). But the actual extent to which this particular program achieves its stated goals and, specifically, the generalization of treatment gains to nontreatment settings as well as the maintenance of those gains after children return to their public schools have not been systematically evaluated or published. No such program has been studied for teens with ADHD.

CONCLUSION

The treatment of ADHD requires expertise in many different treatment modalities, no single one of which can address all the difficulties likely to be experienced by such individuals. Among the available treatments, education of parents, family members, and teachers about the disorder, psychopharmacology (chiefly stimulant medications), parent training in effective behavior management methods, classroom behavior modification methods and academic interventions, and special educational placement appear to have the greatest efficacy or promise of such for dealing with children who have ADHD. To these must often be added family therapy around problem-solving and communication skills; the coordination of multiple teachers and school staff across the high school day; assisting teens with ADHD with their expanded responsibilities, opportunities, and privileges; and the preparation of the teen for eventual independent living and self-support. To be effective in altering eventual prognosis, treatments must be maintained over extended periods (months to years) with periodic reintervention as needed across the life course of the child as well as the need to increasingly enlist the individual with ADHD to cooperate with and invest in the long-term intervention program.

REFERENCES

Abikoff, H. (1985). Efficacy of cognitive training interventions in hyperactive children: A critical review. *Clinical Psychology Review, 5*, 479–512.

Abikoff, E. (1987). An evaluation of cognitive behavior therapy for hyperactive children. In B. Lahey & A. Kazdin (Eds.), *Advances in clinical child psychology* (Vol. 10, pp. 1.71–216). New York: Plenum Press.

Abikoff, H., & Gittelman, R. (1984). Does behavior therapy normalize the classroom behavior of hyperactive children? *Archives of General Psychiatry, 41*, 449–454.

Abikoff, H., & Gittelman, R. (1985). Hyperactive children treated with stimulants: Is cognitive training a useful adjunct? *Archives of General Psychiatry, 42*, 953–961.

Abikoff, H., Hechtman, L., Klein, R. G., Gallacher, R., Fleiss, K., Etcovitch, J., et al. (2004). Social functioning in children with ADHD treated with long-term methylphenidate and multimodal psychosocial treatment. *Journal of the American Academy of Child and Adolescent Psychiatry, 43*, 820–829.

Abikoff, H., Hechtman, L., Klein, R. G., Weiss, G., Fleiss, K., Etcovitch, J., et al. (2004). Symptomatic improvement in children with ADHD treated with long-term methylphenidate and multimodal psychosocial treatment. *Journal of the American Academy of Child and Adolescent Psychiatry, 43*, 802–811.

Achenbach, T. M. (2001). *Manual for the Revised Child Behavior Profile and Child Behavior Checklist.* Burlington, VT: Author.

Achenbach, T. M., McConaughy, S. H., & Howell, C. T. (1987). Child/adolescent behavioral and emotional problems: Implications of cross-informant correlations for situational specificity. *Psychological Bulletin, 101*, 213–232.

Adams, C. D., McCarthy, M., & Kelly, M. L. (1995). Adolescent versions of the Home and School Situations Questionnaires: Initial psychometric properties. *Journal of Child Clinical Psychology, 24*, 377–385.

Altepeter, T. S., & Breen, M. J. (1992). Situational variation in problem behavior at home and school in attention deficit disorder with hyperactivity: A factor analytic study. *Journal of Child Psychology and Psychiatry, 33*, 741–748.

American Psychiatric Association. (1980). *Diagnostic and statistical manual of mental disorders* (3rd ed.). Washington, DC: Author.

American Psychiatric Association. (1987). *Diagnostic and statistical manual of mental disorders* (3rd ed., rev.). Washington, DC: Author.

American Psychiatric Association. (1994). *Diagnostic and statistical manual of mental disorders* (4th ed.). Washington, DC: Author.

American Psychiatric Association. (2000). *Diagnostic and statistical manual of mental disorders* (4th ed., text rev.). Washington, DC: Author.

Anastopoulos, A., & Shelton, T. L. (2001). *Assessment of attention deficit hyperactivity disorder in children.* New York: Kluwer/Plenum Press.

Anastopoulos, A. D., Smith, J. M., & Wien, E. E. (1998). Counseling and training parents. In R. A. Barkley (Ed.), *Attention deficit hyperactivity disorder: A handbook for diagnosis and treatment* (2nd ed., pp. 373–393). New York: Guilford Press.

Anderson, C. A., Hinshaw, S. P., & Simmel, C. (1994). Mother–child interactions in ADHD and comparison boys: Relationships with overt and covert externalizing behavior. *Journal of Abnormal Child Psychology, 22*, 247–265.

Andrews, J. N., Swank, P. R., Foorman, B., & Fletcher, J. M. (1995). Effects of educating parents about ADHD. *The ADHD Report, 3*(4), 12–13.

Angold, A., Costello, E. J., & Erkanli, A. (1999). Comorbidity. *Journal of Child Psychology and Psychiatry, 40*, 57–88.

Antrop, I., Roeyers, H., Van Oost, P., & Buysse, A. (2000). Stimulant seeking and hyperactivity in children with ADHD. *Journal of Child Psychology and Psychiatry, 41*, 225–231.

Antshel, K. M., & Remer, R. (2003). Social skills training in children with attention deficit hyperactivity disorder: A randomized-controlled clinical trial. *Journal of Clinical Child and Adolescent Psychology, 32*, 153–165.

Applegate, B., Lahey, B. B., Hart, E. L., Waldman, I., Biederman, J., Hynd, G. W., et al. (1997). Validity of the age-of-onset criterion for ADHD: A report of the DSM-IV field trials. *Journal of American Academy of Child and Adolescent Psychiatry, 36*, 1211–1221.

Arnold, L. E., Clark, D. L., Sachs, L. A., Jakim, S., & Smithies, C. (1985). Vestibular and visual rotational stimulation as treatment for attention deficit and hyperactivity. *American Journal of Occupational Therapy, 39*, 84–91.

Atkeson, B. M., & Forehand, R. (1978). Parent behavioral training for problem children: An examination of studies using multiple outcome measures. *Journal of Abnormal Child Psychology, 6*, 449–460.

August, G. J., Stewart, M. A., & Holmes, C. S. (1983). A four-year follow-up of hyperactive boys with and without conduct disorder. *British Journal of Psychiatry, 143*, 192–198.

Aylward, E. H., Reiss, A. L., Reader, M. J., Singer, H. S., Brown, J. E., & Denckla, M. B. (1996). Basal ganglia volumes in children with attention-deficit hyperactivity disorder. *Journal of Child Neurology, 11*, 112–115.

Babinski, L. M., Hartsough, C. S., & Lambert, N. M. (1999). Childhood conduct problems, hyperactivity–impulsivity, and inattention as predictors of adult criminal activity. *Journal of Child Psychology and Psychiatry, 40*, 347–355.

Baer, R. A., & Nietzel, M. T. (1991). Cognitive and behavioral treatment of impulsivity in children: A meta-analytic review of the outcome literature. *Journal of Clinical Child Psychology, 20*, 400–412.

Bagwell, C. L., Molina, B. S. G., Pelham, W. E. Jr., &

Hoza, B. (2001). Attention-deficit hyperactivity disorder and problems in peer relations: Predictions from childhood to adolescence. *Journal of the American Academy of Child and Adolescent Psychiatry, 40,* 1285–1292.

Barbaresi, W., J., Katusic, S. K., Colligan, R. C., Pankratz, S., Weaver, A. L., Weber, K. J., et al. (2002). How common is attention-deficit/hyperactivity disorder? Incidence in a population-based birth cohort in Rochester, Minn. *Archives of Pediatric and Adolescent Medicine, 156,* 217–224.

Barkley, R. A. (1976). Predicting the response of hyperkinetic children to stimulant drugs: A review. *Journal of Abnormal Child Psychology, 4,* 327–348.

Barkley, R. A. (1990). *Attention-deficit hyperactivity disorder: A handbook for diagnosis and treatment.* New York: Guilford Press.

Barkley, R. A. (1993a). *ADHD: What can we do?* [Videotape]. New York: Guilford Press.

Barkley, R. A. (1993b). *ADHD: What do we know?* [Videotape]. New York: Guilford Press.

Barkley, R. A. (1994). Impaired delayed responding: A unified theory of attention deficit hyperactivity disorder. In D. K. Routh (Ed.), *Disruptive behavior disorders: Essays in honor of Herbert Quay* (pp. 11–57). New York: Plenum Press.

Barkley, R. A. (1997a). *ADHD and the nature of self-control.* New York: Guilford

Barkley, R. A. (1997b). Behavioral inhibition sustained, attention, and executive functions: Constructing a unifying theory of ADHD. *Psychological Bulletin, 121,* 65–94.

Barkley, R. A. (1997c). *Defiant children: A clinician's manual for assessment and parent training* (2nd ed.). New York: Guilford Press.

Barkley, R. A. (1997d). *Managing the defiant child: A guide to parent training* [Videotape]. New York: Guilford Press.

Barkley, R. A. (1997e). *Understanding the defiant child.* [Videotape]. New York: Guilford Press.

Barkley, R. A. (2006). *Attention-deficit hyperactivity disorder: A handbook for diagnosis and treatment* (3rd ed.). New York: Guilford Press.

Barkley, R. A. (1999). Theories of attention-deficit/hyperactivity disorder. In H. Quay & A. Hogan (Eds.), *Handbook of disruptive behavior disorders* (pp. 295–316). New York: Plenum Press.

Barkley, R. A. (2000). *Taking charge of ADHD: The complete, authoritative guide for parents* (rev. ed.). New York: Guilford Press.

Barkley, R. A. (2001a). Accidents and ADHD. *The Economics of Neuroscience, 3,* 64–68.

Barkley, R. A. (2001b). The executive functions and self-regulation: An evolutionary neuropsychological perspective. *Neuropsychology Review, 11,* 1–29.

Barkley, R. A. (2001c). The inattentive type of ADHD as a distinct disorder: What remains to be done. *Clinical Psychology: Science and Practice, 8,* 489–493.

Barkley, R. A., Anastopoulos, A. D., Guevremont, D. G., & Fletcher, K. F. (1991). Adolescents with atten-

tion deficit hyperactivity disorder: Patterns of behavioral adjustment, academic functioning, and treatment utilization. *Journal of the American Academy of Child and Adolescent Psychiatry, 30,* 752–761.

Barkley, R. A., Anastopoulos, A. D., Guevremont, D. G., & Fletcher, K. F. (1992). Adolescents with attention deficit hyperactivity disorder: Mother–adolescent interactions, family beliefs and conflicts, and maternal psychopathology. *Journal of Abnormal Child Psychology, 20,* 263–288.

Barkley, R. A., & Biederman, J. (1997). Towards a broader definition of the age of onset criterion for attention deficit hyperactivity disorder. *Journal of the American Academy of Child and Adolescent Psychiatry, 36,* 1204–1210.

Barkley, R. A., Copeland, A. P., & Sivage, C. (1980). A self-control classroom for hyperactive children. *Journal of Autism and Developmental Disorders, 10,* 75–89.

Barkley, R. A., DuPaul, G. J., & McMurray, M. B. (1990). A comprehensive evaluation of attention deficit disorder with and without hyperactivity. *Journal of Consulting and Clinical Psychology, 58,* 775–789.

Barkley, R. A., Edwards, G., Laneri, M., Fletcher, K., & Metevia, L. (2001a). The efficacy of problem-solving communication training alone, behavior management training alone, and their combination for parent–adolescent conflict in teenagers with ADHD and ODD. *Journal of Consulting and Clinical Psychology, 69,* 926–941.

Barkley, R. A., Edwards, G., Laneri, M., Fletcher, K., & Metevia, L. (2001b). Executive functioning, temporal discounting, and sense of time in adolescents with attention deficit hyperactivity disorder and oppositional defiant disorder. *Journal of Abnormal Child Psychology, 29,* 541–556.

Barkley, R. A., Edwards, G. H., & Robin, A. R. (1999). *Defiant teens: A clinicians' manual for family assessment and intervention.* New York: Guilford Press.

Barkley, R. A., Fischer, M., Edelbrock, C. S., & Smallish, L. (1990). The adolescent outcome of hyperactive children diagnosed by research criteria: I. An 8 year prospective follow-up study. *Journal of the American Academy of Child and Adolescent Psychiatry, 29,* 546–557.

Barkley, R. A., Fischer, M., Edelbrock, C. S., & Smallish, L. (1991). The adolescent outcome of hyperactive children diagnosed by research criteria: III. Mother–child interactions, family conflicts, and maternal psychopathology. *Journal of Child Psychology and Psychiatry, 32,* 233–256.

Barkley, R. A., Fischer, M., Smallish, L., & Fletcher, K. (2002). Persistence of attention deficit hyperactivity disorder into adulthood as a function of reporting source and definition of disorder. *Journal of Abnormal Psychology, 111,* 279–289.

Barkley, R. A., Guevremont, D. G., Anastopoulos, A. D., DuPaul, G. J., & Shelton, T. L. (1993). Driving-related risks and outcomes of attention deficit hyperactivity disorder in adolescents and young adults: A 3–5 year follow-up survey. *Pediatrics, 92,* 212–218.

Barkley, R. A., Guevremont, D. C., Anastopoulos, A. D., & Fletcher, K. E. (1992). A comparison of three family therapy programs for treating family conflicts in adolescents with attention-deficit hyperactivity disorder. *Journal of Consulting and Clinical Psychology, 60,* 450–462.

Barkley, R. A., McMurray, M. B., Edelbrock, C. S., & Robbins, K. (1990). The side effects of methtlphenidate in ADHD children: A systematic, placebo controlled evaluation. *Pediatrics, 86,* 184–192.

Barkley, R. A., & Murphy, K. R. (1998). *Attention deficit hyperactivity disorder: A clinical workbook* (2nd ed.). New York: Guilford Press.

Barkley, R. A., Murphy, K. R., & Bush, T. (2001). Time perception and reproduction in young adults with attention deficit hyperactivity disorder (ADHD). *Neuropsychology, 15,* 351–360.

Barkley, R. A., Murphy, K. R., DuPaul, G. R., & Bush, T. (2002). Driving in young adults with attention deficit hyperactivity disorder: Knowledge, performance, adverse outcomes and the role of executive functions. *Journal of the International Neuropsychological Society, 8,* 655–672.

Barkley, R. A., Murphy, K. R., & Kwasnik, D. (1996a). Motor vehicle driving competencies and risks in teens and young adults with attention deficit hyperactivity disorder. *Pediatrics, 98,* 1089–1095.

Barkley, R. A., Murphy, K. R., & Kwasnik, D. (1996b). Psychological functioning and adaptive impairments in young adults with ADHD. *Journal of Attention Disorders, 1,* 41–54.

Barkley, R. A., Shelton, T. L., Crosswait, C., Moorehouse, M., Fletcher, K., Barrett, S., et al. (2000). Early psycho-educational intervention for children with disruptive behavior: Preliminary post-treatment outcome. *Journal of Child Psychology and Psychiatry, 41,* 319–332.

Bate, A. J., Mathias, J. L., & Crawford, J. R. (2001). Performance of the Test of Everyday Attention and standard tests of attention following severe traumatic brain injury. *The Clinical Neuropsychologist, 15,* 405–422.

Baving, L., Laucht, M., & Schmidt, M. H. (1999). Atypical frontal brain activation in ADHD: Preschool and elementary school boys and girls. *Journal of the American Academy of Child and Adolescent Psychiatry, 38,* 1363–1371.

Bayliss, D. M., & Roodenrys, S. (2000). Executive processing and attention deficit hyperactivity disorder: An application of the supervisory attentional system. *Developmental Neuropsychology, 17,* 161–180.

Beck, A. T., Steer, R. A., & Garbin, M. G. (1988). Psychometric properties of the Beck Depression Inventory: Twenty-five years of evaluation. *Clinical Psychology Review, 8,* 77–100.

Beauchaine, T. P., Katkin, E. S., Strassberg, Z., & Snarr, J. (2001). Disinhibitory psychopathology in male adolescents: Discriminating conduct disorder from attention-deficit/hyperactivity disorder through concurrent assessment of multiple autonomic states. *Journal of Abnormal Psychology, 110,* 610–624.

Berk, L. E., & Potts, M. K. (1991). Development and functional significance of private speech among attention-deficit hyperactivity disorder and normal boys. *Journal of Abnormal Child Psychology, 19,* 357–377.

Bidder, R. T., Gray, O. P., & Newcombe, R. (1978). Behavioural treatment of hyperactive children. *Archives of Disease in Childhood, 53,* 574–579.

Biederman, J., Faraone, S. V., Keenan, K., & Tsuang, M. T. (1991). Evidence of a familial association between attention deficit disorder and major affective disorders. *Archives of General Psychiatry, 48,* 633–642.

Biederman, J., Faraone, S. V., & Lapey, K. (1992). Comorbidity of diagnosis in attention-deficit hyperactivity disorder. In G. Weiss (Ed.), *Child and adolescent psychiatric clinics of North America: Attention-deficit hyperactivity disorder* (pp. 335–360). Philadelphia: Saunders.

Biederman, J., Faraone, S. V., Mick, E., Williamson, S., Wilens, T. E., Spencer, T. J., et al. (1999). Clinical correlates of ADHD in females: Findings from a large group of girls ascertained from pediatric and psychiatric referral sources. *Journal of the American Academy of Child and Adolescent Psychiatry, 38,* 966–975

Biederman, J., Faraone, S., Mick, E., Wozniak, J., Chen, L., Ouellette, C., et al. (1996). Attention-deficit hyperactivity disorder and juvenile mania: An overlooked comorbidity? *Journal of the American Academy of Child and Adolescent Psychiatry, 35,* 997–1008.

Biederman, J., Faraone, S., Milberger, S., Curtis, S., Chen, L., Marrs, A., et al. (1996). Predictors of persistence and remission of ADHD into adolescence: Results from a four-year prospective follow-up study. *Journal of the American Academy of Child and Adolescent Psychiatry, 35,* 343–351.

Biederman, J., Lopez, F., Boellner, S., & Chandler, M. (2002). A randomized, double-blind, placebo-controlled, parellel-group study of SLI381 (Adderall XR) in children with attention-deficit/hyperactivity disorder. *Pediatrics, 110,* 258–266.

Biederman, J., Milberger, S., Faraone, S. V., Guite, J., & Warburton, R. (1994). Associations between childhood asthma and ADHD: Issues of psychiatric comorbidity and familiality. *Journal of the American Academy of Child and Adolescent Psychiatry, 33,* 842–848.

Biederman, J., Newcorn, J., & Sprich, S. (1991). Comorbidity of attention deficit hyperactivity disorder with conduct, depressive, anxiety, and other disorders. *American Journal of Psychiatry, 148,* 564–577.

Bloomquist, M. L., August, G. J., & Ostrander, R. (1991). Effects of a school-based cognitive-behavioral intervention for ADHD children. *Journal of Abnormal Child Psychology, 19,* 591–605.

Borger, N., & van der Meere, J. (2000). Visual behaviour of ADHD children during an attention test: An almost forgotten variable. *Journal of Child Psychology and Psychiatry, 41,* 525–532.

Braaten, E. B., & Rosen, L. A. (2000). Self-regulation of affect in attention deficit–hyperactivity disorder (ADHD) and non-ADHD boys: Differences in empathic responding. *Journal of Consulting and Clinical Psychology, 68,* 313–321.

Bradley, W. (1937). The behavior of children receiving benzedrine. *American Journal of Psychiatry, 94,* 577–585.

Breslau, N., Brown, G. G., DelDotto, J. E., Kumar, S., Exhuthachan, S., Andreski, P., & Hufnagle, K. G. (1996). Psychiatric sequelae of low birth weight at 6 years of age. *Journal of Abnormal Child Psychology, 24,* 385–400.

Breton, J., Bergeron, L., Valla, J. P., Berthiaume, C., Gaudet, N., Lambert, J., et al. (1999). Quebec children mental health survey: Prevalence of DSM-III-R mental health disorders. *Journal of Child Psychology and Psychiatry, 40,* 375–384.

Bronowski, J. (1977). Human and animal languages. In *A sense of the future* (pp. 104–131). Cambridge, MA: MIT Press.

Brown, T. E. (2000). *Attention deficit disorders in children, adolescents, and adults: Patterns of comorbidity.* New York: American Psychiatric Press.

Buhrmester, D., Camparo, L., Christensen, A., Gonzalez, L. S., & Hinshaw, S. P. (1992). Mothers and fathers interacting in dyads and triads with normal and hyperactive sons. *Developmental Psychology, 28,* 500–509.

Buitelaar, J. K., Van der Gaag, R. J., Swaab-Barneveld, H., & Kuiper, M. (1995). Prediction of clinical response to methylphenidate in children with attention-deficit hyperactivity disorder. *Journal of the American Academy of Child and Adolescent Psychiatry, 34,* 1025–1032.

Burke, J. D., Loeber, R., & Lahey, B. B. (2001). Which aspects of ADHD are associated with tobacco use in early adolescence? *Journal of Child Psychology and Psychiatry,* 493–502.

Burks, H. (1960). The hyperkinetic child. *Exceptional Children, 27,* 18.

Burns, G. L., Boe, B., Walsh, J. A., Sommers-Flannagan, R., & Teegarden, L. A. (2001). A confirmatory factor analysis on the DSM-IV ADHD and ODD symptoms: What is the best model for the organization of these symptoms? *Journal of Abnormal Child Psychology, 29,* 339–349.

Cantwell, D. (1975). *The hyperactive child.* New York: Spectrum.

Carlson, C. L., Pelham, W. E., Jr., Milich, R., & Dixon, J. (1992). Single and combined effects of methylphenidate and behavior therapy on the classroom performance of children with attention-deficit hyperactivity disorder. *Journal of Abnormal Child Psychology, 20,* 213–232.

Carlson, C. L., Tamm, L., & Gaub, M. (1997). Gender differences in children with ADHD, ODD, and co-occurring ADHD/ODD identified in a school population. *Journal of the American Academy of Child and Adolescent Psychiatry, 36,* 1706–1714.

Carlson, C. L., & Mann, M. (2002). Sluggish cognitive tempo predicts a different pattern of impairment in the attention deficit hyperactivity disorder, predominantly inattentive type. *Journal of Clinical Child and Adolescent Psychology, 31,* 123–129.

Carlson, G. A. (1990). Child and adolescent mania—Diagnostic considerations. *Journal of Child Psychology and Psychiatry, 31,* 331–342.

Casey, B. J., Castellanos, F. X., Giedd, J. N., Marsh, W. L., Hamburger, S. D., Schubert, A. B., et al. (1997). Implication of right frontstriatal circuitry in response inhibition and attention-deficit/hyperactivity disorder. *Journal of the American Academy of Child and Adolescent Psychiatry, 36,* 374–383.

Casey, J. E., Rourke, B. P., & Del Dotto, J. E. (1996). Learning disabilities in children with attention deficit disorder with and without hyperactivity. *Child Neuropsychology, 2,* 83–98.

Castellanos, F. X., Giedd, J. N., Eckburg, P., Marsh, W. L., Vaituzis, C., Kaysen, D., et al. (1994). Quantitative morphology of the caudate nucleus in attention deficit hyperactivity disorder. *American Journal of Psychiatry, 151,* 1791–1796.

Castellanos, F. X., Giedd, J. N., Marsh, W. L., Hamburger, S. D., Vaituzis, A. C., Dickstein, D. P., et al. (1996). Quantitative brain magnetic resonance imaging in attention-deficit hyperactivity disorder. *Archives of General Psychiatry, 53,* 607–616.

Castellanos, F. X., Marvasti, F. F., Ducharme, J. L., Walter, J. M., Israel, M. E., Krain, A., et al. (2000). Executive function oculomotor tasks in girls with ADHD. *Journal of the American Academy of Child and Adolescent Psychiatry, 39,* 644–650.

Chang, H. T., Klorman, R., Shaywitz, S. E., Fletcher, J. M., Marchione, K. E., Holahan, J. M., et al. (1999). Paired-associate learning in attention-deficit/hyperactivity disorder as a function of hyperactivity–impulsivity and oppositional defiant disorder. *Journal of Abnormal Child Psychology, 27,* 237–245.

Chess, S. (1960). Diagnosis and treatment of the hyperactive child. *New York State Journal of Medicine, 60,* 2379–2385.

Chilcoat, H. D., & Breslau, N. (1999). Pathways from ADHD to early drug use. *Journal of the American Academy of Child and Adolescent Psychiatry, 38,* 1347–1354.

Clark, C., Prior, M., & Kinsella, G. J. (2000). Do executive function deficits differentiate between adolescents with ADHD and oppositional defiant/conduct disorder? A neuropsychological study using the Six Elements Test and Hayling Sentence Completion Test. *Journal of Abnormal Child Psychology, 28,* 405–414.

Clark, M. L., Cheyne, J. A., Cunningham, C. E., & Siegel, L. S. (1988). Dyadic peer interaction and task orientation in attention-deficit-disordered children. *Journal of Abnormal Child Psychology, 16,* 1–15.

Claude, D., & Firestone, P. (1995). The development of ADHD boys: A 12-year follow-up. *Canadian Journal of Behavioural Science, 27,* 226–249.

Conners, C. K. (1998). *The Conners ADHD Rating Scales.* North Tonawanda, NY: Multi-Health Systems.

Connor, D. F. (2005a). Other medications in the treatment of child and adolescent ADHD. In R. A. Barkley (Ed.), *Attention-deficit hyperactivity disorder: A handbook for diagnosis and treatment* (3rd ed.). New York: Guilford Press.

Connor, D. F. (2005b). Stimulants. In R. A. Barkley (Ed.), *Attention-deficit hyperactivity disorder: A handbook for diagnosis and treatment* (3rd ed.). New York: Guilford Press.

Cook, E. H., Stein, M. A., Krasowski, M. D., Cox, N. J., Olkon, D. M., Kieffer, J. E., & Leventhal, B. L. (1995). Association of attention deficit disorder and the dopamine transporter gene. *American Journal of Human Genetics, 56,* 993–998.

Cook, E. H., Stein, M. A., & Leventhal, D. L. (1997). Family-based association of attention-deficit/hyperactivity disorder and the dopamine transporter. In K. Blum (Ed.), *Handbook of psychiatric genetics* (pp. 297–310). New York: CRC Press.

Coolidge, F. L., Thede, L. L., & Young, S. E. (2000). Heritability and the comorbidity of attention deficit hyperactivity disorder with behavioral disorders and executive function deficits: A preliminary investigation. *Developmental Neuropsychology, 17,* 273–287.

Cruickshank, B. M., Eliason, M., & Merrifield, B. (1988). Long-term sequelae of water near-drowning. *Journal of Pediatric Psychology, 13,* 379–388.

Crystal, D. S., Ostrander, R., Chen, R. S., & August, G. J. (2001). Multimethod assessment of psychopathology among DSM-IV subtypes of children with attention-deficit/hyperactivity disorder: self-, parent, and teacher reports. *Journal of Abnormal Child Psychology, 29,* 189–205.

Cuffe, S. P., McKeown, R. E., Jackson, K. L., Addy, C. L., Abramson, R., & Garrison, C. Z. (2001). Prevalence of attention-deficit/hyperactivity disorder in a community sample of older adolescents. *Journal of the American Academy of Child and Adolescent Psychiatry, 40,* 1037–1044.

Cunningham, C. E., Bremmer, R., & Boyle, M. (1995). Large group community-based parenting programs for families of preschoolers at risk for disruptive behaviour disorders: Utilization, cost effectiveness, and outcome. *Journal of Child Psychology and Psychiatry, 36,* 1141–1159.

Cunningham, C. E., Siegel, L. S., & Offord, D. R. (1985). A developmental dose response analysis of the effects of methylphenidate on the peer interactions of attention deficit disordered boys. *Journal of Child Psychology and Psychiatry, 26,* 955–971.

Dane, A. V., Schachar, R. J., & Tannock, R. (2000). Does actigraphy differentiate ADHD subtypes in a clinical research setting? *Journal of the American Academy of Child and Adolescent Psychiatry, 39,* 752–760.

Danforth, J. S., Barkley, R. A., & Stokes, T. F. (1991). Observations of parent–child interactions with hyperactive children: Research and clinical implications. *Clinical Psychology Review, 11,* 703–727.

Denckla, M. B. (1994). Measurement of executive function. In G. R. Lyon (Ed.), *Frames of reference for the assessment of learning disabilities: New views on measurement issues* (pp. 117–142). Baltimore: Brookes.

Derogatis, L. (1986). *Manual for the Symptom Checklist 90—Revised (SCL90–R).* Baltimore: Author.

Diamond, A. (2000). Close interrelation of motor development and cognitive development and of the cerebellum and prefrontal cortex. *Developmental Psychology, 71,* 44–56.

Diaz, R. M., & Berk, L. E. (1992). *Private speech: From social interaction to self-regulation.* Mahwah, NJ: Erlbaum.

Diaz, R. M., & Berk, L. E. (1995). A Vygotskian critique of self-instructional training. *Development and Psychopathology, 7,* 369–392.

Dishion, T. J., McCord, J., & Poulin, F. (1999). When interventions harm: Peer groups and problem behavior. *American Psychologist, 54,* 755–764.

Dodge, K. A. (1989). Problems in social relationships. In E. J. Mash & R. A. Barkley (Eds.), *Treatment of childhood disorders* (pp. 222–246). New York: Guilford Press.

Douglas, V. I. (1972). Stop, look, and listen: The problem of sustained attention and impulse control in hyperactive and normal children. *Canadian Journal of Behavioural Science, 4,* 259–282.

Douglas, V. I. (1980). Higher mental processes in hyperactive children: Implications for training. In R. Knights & D. Bakker (Eds.), *Treatment of hyperactive and learning disordered children* (pp. 65–92). Baltimore: University Park Press.

Douglas, V. I. (1983). Attention and cognitive problems. In M. Rutter (Ed.), *Developmental neuropsychiatry* (pp. 280–329). New York: Guilford Press.

Douglas, V. I. (1988). Cognitive deficits in children with attention deficit disorder with hyperactivity. In L. Blommingdale & J. Sergeant (Eds.), *Attention deficit disorder: Criteria, cognition, and intervention* (pp. 6582). New York: Pergamon Press.

Douglas, V. I. (1999). Cognitive control processes in attention-deficit/hyperactivity disorder. In H. C. Quay & A. Horgan (Eds.), *Handbook of disruptive behavior disorders* (pp. 105–138). New York: Plenum Press.

DuPaul, G. J., Anastopoulos, A. D., Kwasnik, D., Barkley, R. A., & McMurray, M. B. (1996). Methylphenidate effects on children with attention deficit hyperactivity disorder: Self-report of symptoms, side effects, and self-esteem. *Journal of Attention Disorders, 1,* 3–15.

DuPaul, G. J., Barkley, R. A., & Connor, D. F. (1998). Stimulants. In R. A. Barkley (Ed.), *Attention-deficit hyperactivity disorder: A handbook for diagnosis and treatment* (pp. 510–551). New York: Guilford Press.

DuPaul, G. J., Barkley, R. A., & McMurray, M. B. (1994). Response of children with ADHD to methylphenidate: Interaction with internalizing symptoms. *Journal of the American Academy of Child and Adolescent Psychiatry, 33,* 894–903.

DuPaul, G. J., & Eckert, T. L. (1997). The effects of school-based interventions for attention deficit hyperactivity disorder: A meta-analysis. *School Psychology Digest, 26,* 5–27.

DuPaul, G. J., McGoey, K. E., Eckert, T. L., & VanBrakle, J. (2001). Preschool children with attention-deficit/hyperactivity disorder: impairments in behavioral, social, and school functioning. *Journal of the American Academy of Child and Adolescent Psychiatry, 40,* 508–515.

DuPaul, G. J., Power, T. J., Anastopoulos, A. D., & Reid, R. (1999). *The ADHD Rating Scale-IV: Checklists, norms, and clinical interpretation.* New York: Guilford Press.

DuPaul, G. J., & Stoner, G. (2003). *ADHD in the schools: Assessment and intervention strategies* (2nd ed.). New York: Guilford Press.

Dush, D. M., Hirt, M. L., & Schroeder, H. E. (1989). Self-statement modification in the treatment of child behavior disorders: A meta-analysis. *Psychological Bulletin, 106,* 97–106.

Ebaugh, F. G. (1923). Neuropsychiatric sequelae of acute epidemic encephalitis in children. *American Journal of Diseases of Children, 25,* 89–97.

Edwards, G. (1995). Patterns of paternal and maternal conflict with adolescents with ADHD. *The ADHD Report, 3*(5), 10–12.

Edwards, G., Barkley, R., Laneri, M., Fletcher, K., & Metevia, L. (2001). Parent-adolescent conflict in teenagers with ADHD and ODD. *Journal of Abnormal Child Psychology, 29,* 557–572.

Erhardt, D., & Hinshaw, S. P. (1994). Initial sociometric impressions of attention-deficit hyperactivity disorder and comparison boys: predictions from social behaviors and from nonbehavioral variables. *Journal of Consulting and Clinical Psychology, 62,* 833–842.

Ernst, M., Cohen, R. M., Liebenauer, L. L., Jons, P. H., & Zametkin, A. J. (1997). Cerebral glucose metabolism in adolescent girls with attention-deficit/hyperactivity disorder. *Journal of the American Academy of Child and Adolescent Psychiatry, 36,* 1399–1406.

Ernst, M., Liebenauer, L. L., King, A. C., Fitzgerald, G. A., Cohen, R. M., & Zametkin, A. J. (1994). Reduced brain metabolism in hyperactive girls. *Journal of the American Academy of Child and Adolescent Psychiatry, 33,* 858–868.

Ernst, M., Zametkin, A. J., Matochik, J. A., Pascualvaca, D., Jons, P. H., & Cohen, R. M. (1999). High midbrain [^{18}F]DOPA accumulation in children with attention deficit hyperactivity disorder. *American Journal of Psychiatry, 156,* 1209–1215.

Evans, S. W., Vallano, M.D., & Pelham, W. (1994).

Treatment of parenting behavior with a psychostimulant: A case study of an adult with attention-deficit hyperactivity disorder. *Journal of Child and Adolescent Psychopharmacology, 4,* 63–69.

Faraone, S. V., & Biederman, J. (1997). Do attention deficit hyperactivity disorder and major depression share familial risk factors? *Journal of Nervous and Mental Disease, 185,* 533–541.

Faraone, S. V., Biederman, J., Chen, W. J., Krifcher, B., Keenan, K., Moore, C., et al. (1992). Segregation analysis of attention deficit hyperactivity disorder. *Psychiatric Genetics, 2,* 257–275.

Faraone, S. V., Biederman, J., Lehman, B., Keenan, K., Norman, D., Seidman, L. J., et al. (1993). Evidence for the independent familial transmission of attention deficit hyperactivity disorder and learning disabilities: Results from a family genetic study. *American Journal of Psychiatry, 150,* 891–895.

Faraone, S. V., Biederman, J., Mennin, D., Russell R., & Tsuang, M. T. (1998). Familial subtypes of attention deficit hyperactivity disorder: A 4-year follow-up study of children from antisocial–ADHD families. *Journal of Child Psychology and Psychiatry, 39,* 1045–1053.

Faraone, S. V., Biederman, J., & Monuteaux, M. C. (2001). Attention deficit hyperactivity disorder with bipolar disorder in girls: Further evidence for a familial subtype? *Journal of Affective Disorders, 64,* 19–26.

Faraone, S. V., Biederman, J., Weiffenbach, B., Keith, T., Chu, M. P., Weaver, A., et al. (1999). Dopamine D4 gene 7–repeat allele and attention deficit hyperactivity disorder. *American Journal of Psychiatry, 156,* 768–770.

Faraone, S. V., Biederman, J., Wozniak, J., Mundy, E., Mennin, D., & O'Donnell, D. (1997). Is comorbidity with ADHD a marker for juvenile-onset mania? *Journal of the American Academy of Child and Adolescent Psychiatry, 36,* 1046–1055.

Fehlings, D. L., Roberts, W., Humphries, T., & Dawe, G. (1991). Attention deficit hyperactivity disorder: Does cognitive behavioral therapy improve home behavior? *Journal of Developmental and Behavioral Pediatrics, 12,* 223–228.

Filipek, P. A., Semrud-Clikeman, M., Steingard, R. J., Renshaw, P. F., Kennedy, D. N., & Biederman, J. (1997). Volumetric MRI analysis comparing subjects having attention-deficit hyperactivity disorder with normal controls. *Neurology, 48,* 589–601.

Firestone, P., & Douglas, V. 1. (1977). The effects of verbal and material reward and punishers on the performance of impulsive and reflective children. *Child Study Journal, 7,* 71–78 .

Firestone, P., Kelly, M. J., Goodman, J. T., & Davey, J. (1981). Differential effects of parent training and stimulant medication with hyperactives. *Journal of the American Academy of Child Psychiatry, 20,* 135–147.

Fischer, M., Barkley, R. A., Edelbrock, C. S., & Smallish, L. (1990). The adolescent outcome of hyperactive children diagnosed by research criteria. II: Academic, attentional, and neuropsychological status. *Journal of Consulting and Clinical Psychology, 58,* 580–588.

Fischer, M., Barkley, R. A., Fletcher, K., & Smallish, L. (1993a). The adolescent outcome of hyperactive children diagnosed by research criteria. V: Predictors of outcome. *Journal of the American Academy of Child and Adolescent Psychiatry, 32,* 324–332.

Fischer, M., Barkley, R. A., Fletcher, K., & Smallish, L. (1993b). The stability of dimensions of behavior in ADHD and normal children over an 8 year period. *Journal of Abnormal Child Psychology, 21,* 315–337.

Fischer, M., Barkley, R. A., Smallish, L., & Fletcher, K. (2002). Young adult follow-up of hyperactive children: Self-reported psychiatric disorders, comorbidity, and the role of childhood conduct problems. *Journal of Abnormal Child Psychology, 30,* 463–475.

Fletcher, K., Fischer, M., Barkley, R. A., & Smallish, L. (1996). A sequential analysis of the mother–adolescent interactions of ADHD, ADHD/ODD, and normal teenagers during neutral and conflict discussions. *Journal of Abnormal Child Psychology, 24,* 271–298.

Forgatch, M., & Patterson, G. R. (1989). *Parents and adolescents living together.* Eugene, OR: Castalia.

Frank, Y., Lazar, J. W., & Seiden, J. A. (1992). Cognitive event-related potentials in learning-disabled children with or without attention-deficit hyperactivity disorder [Abstract]. *Annals of Neurology, 32,* 478.

Frick, P. J., Kamphaus, R. W., Lahey, B. B., Loeber, R., Christ, M. A. G., Hart, E. L., & Tannenbaum, L. E. (1991). Academic underachievement and the disruptive behavior disorders. *Journal of Consulting and Clinical Psychology, 59,* 289–294.

Fuster, J. M. (1997). *The prefrontal cortex* (3rd ed.). New York: Raven Press.

Gadow, K. D. (1985). Relative efficacy of pharmacological, behavioral, and combination treatments for enhancing academic performance. *Clinical Psychology Review, 5,* 513–533.

Gadow, K. D., Sprafkin, J., & Nolan, E. E. (2001). DSM-IV symptoms in community and clinic preschool children. *Journal of the American Academy of Child and Adolescent Psychiatry, 40,* 1383–1392.

Gadow, K. D., Sverd, J., Sprafkin, J., Nolan, E. E., & Ezor, S. N. (1995). Efficacy of methylphenidate for attention-deficit hyperactivity disorder in children with tic disorder. *Archives of General Psychiatry, 52,* 444–455.

Gaub, M., & Carlson, C. L. (1997). Gender differences in ADHD: A meta-analysis and critical review. *Journal of the American Academy of Child and Adolescent Psychiatry, 36,* 1036–1045.

Geller, B., & Luby, J. (1997). Child and adolescent bipolar disorder: A review of the past 10 years. *Journal of the American Academy of Child and Adolescent Psychiatry, 36,* 1168–1176.

Gershon, J. (2002). A meta-analytic review of gender differences in ADHD. *Journal of Attention Disorders, 5*(3), 143–154.

Gilger, J. W., Pennington, B. F., & DeFries, J. C. (1992). A twin study of the etiology of comorbidity: Attention-deficit hyperactivity disorder and dyslexia. *Journal of the American Academy of Child and Adolescent Psychiatry, 31,* 343–348.

Gill, M., Daly, G., Heron, S., Hawi, Z., & Fitzgerald, M. (1997). Confirmation of association between attention deficit hyperactivity disorder and a dopamine transporter polymorphism. *Molecular Psychiatry, 2,* 311–313.

Gittelman, R., Mannuzza, S., Shenker, R., & Bonagura, N. (1985). Hyperactive boys almost grown up: I. Psychiatric status. *Archives of General Psychiatry, 42,* 937–947.

Goldstein, S. (1997). *Management of attention deficit hyperactivity disorder in children and adolescents.* New York: Wiley.

Goldstein, S., & Ingersoll, B. (1993). Controversial treatments for ADHD: Essential information for clinicians. *The ADHD Report, 1*(3), 4–5.

Green, L., Fry, A. F., & Meyerson, J. (1994). Discounting of delayed rewards: A life-span comparison. *Psychological Science, 5,* 33–36.

Greenhill, L. L., & Osmon, B. B. (2000). *Ritalin: Theory and patient management.* New York: Mary Ann Liebert.

Gresham, F. M., MacMillan, D. L., Bocian, K. M., Ward, S. L., & Forness, S. R. (1998). Comorbidity of hyperactivity-impulsivity-inattention and conduct problems: Risk factors in social, affective, and academic domains. *Journal of Abnormal Child Psychology, 26,* 393–406.

Grodzinsky, G. M., & Diamond, R. (1992). Frontal lobe functioning in boys with attention-deficit hyperactivity disorder. *Developmental Neuropsychology, 8,* 427–445.

Gunning, B. (1992). *A controlled trial of clonidine in hyperkinetic children.* Amsterdam: University of Amsterdam.

Gustafsson, P., Thernlund, G., Ryding, E., Rosen, I., & Cederblad, M. (2000). Associations between cerebral blood-flow measured by single photon emission computed tomography (SPECT), electro-encephalogram (EEG), behavior symptoms, cognition and neurological soft signs in children with attention-deficit hyperactivity disorder (ADHD). *Acta Paediatrica, 89,* 830–835.

Hales, D., & Hales, R. (1985). Using the body to mend the mind. *American Health,* 27–31.

Halperin, J. M., Newcorn, J. H., Koda, V. H., Pick, L., McKay, K. E., & Knott, P. (1997). Noradrenergic mechanisms in ADHD children with and without reading disabilities: A replication and extension. *Journal of the American Academy of Child and Adolescent Psychiatry, 36,* 1688–1697.

Harris, J. (1998). *The nurture assumption.* New York: HarperCollins.

Hart, E. L., Lahey, B. B., Loeber, R., Applegate, B., &

Frick, P. J. (1995). Developmental changes in attention-deficit hyperactivity disorder in boys: A four-year longitudinal study. *Journal of Abnormal Child Psychology, 23,* 729–750.

Hendren, R. L., De Backer, I., & Pandina, G. J. (2000). Review of neuroimaging studies of child and adolescent psychiatric disorders from the past 10 years. *Journal of the American Academy of Child and Adolescent Psychiatry, 39,* 815–828.

Henry, B., Moffitt, T. E., Caspi A., Langley, J., & Silva, P. A. (1994). On the "remembrance of things past": A longitudinal evaluation of the retrospective method. *Psychological Assessment, 6,* 92–101.

Herpertz, S. C., Wenning, B., Mueller, B., Qunaibi, M., Sass, H., & Herpetz-Dahlmann, B. (2001). Psychological responses in ADHD boys with and without conduct disorder: Implications for adult antisocial behavior. *Journal of the American Academy of Child and Adolescent Psychiatry, 40,* 1222–1230.

Hinshaw, S. P. (1992a). Externalizing behavior problems and academic underachievement in childhood and adolescence: Causal relationships and underlying mechanisms. *Psychological Bulletin, 111,* 127–155.

Hinshaw, S. P. (1992b, October). Interventions for social competence and social skill. *Child and Adolescent Psychiatric Clinics of North America, 1*(2), 539–552.

Hinshaw, S. P. (1994). *Attention deficits and hyperactivity in children.* Thousand Oaks, CA: Sage.

Hinshaw, S. P. (2001). Is the inattentive type of ADHD a separate disorder? *Clinical Psychology: Science and Practice, 8,* 498–501.

Hinshaw, S. P. (2002). Preadolescent girls with attention-deficit/hyperactivity disorder: I. Background characteristics, comorbidity, cognitive and social functioning, and parenting practices. *Journal of Consulting and Clinical Psychology, 70,* 1086–1098.

Hinshaw, S. P., Carte, E. T., Sami, N., Treuting, J. J., & Zupan, B. A. (2002). Preadolescent girls with attention-deficit hyperactivity disorder: II. Neuropsychological performance in relation to subtypes and individual classification. *Journal of Consulting and Clinical Psychology, 70,* 1099–1111.

Hinshaw, S. P., & Erhardt, D. (1991). Attention-deficit hyperactivity disorder. In P. C. Kendall (Ed.), *Child and adolescent therapy: Cognitive-behavioral procedures* (p. 98). New York: Guilford Press.

Hinshaw, S. P., & Melnick, S. M. (1995). Peer relationships in boys with attention-deficit hyperactivity disorder with and without comorbid aggression. *Development and Psychopathology, 7,* 627–647.

Hohman, L. B. (1922). Post-encephalitic behavior disorders in children. *Johns Hopkins Hospital Bulletin, 33,* 372–375.

Holdsworth, L., & Whitmore, K. (1974). A study of children with epilepsy attending ordinary schools: I. Their seizure patterns, progress, and behaviour in school. *Developmental Medicine and Child Neurology, 16,* 746–758.

Horn, W. F., Ialongo, N., Pascoe, J. M., Greenberg, G.,

Packard, T., Lopez, M., et al. (1991). Additive effects of psychostimulants, parent training, and self-control therapy with ADHD children. *Journal of the American Academy of Child and Adolescent Psychiatry, 30,* 233–240.

Hynd, G. W., Hern, K. L., Novey, E. S., Eliopulos, D., Marshall, R., Gonzalez, J. J., & Voeller, K. K. (1993). Attention-deficit hyperactivity disorder and asymmetry of the caudate nucleus. *Journal of Child Neurology, 8,* 339– 347.

Ingersoll, B. D., & Goldstein, S. (1993). *Attention deficit disorder and learning disabilities: Realities, myths, and controversial treatments.* New York: Doubleday.

Jensen, P. S., Kettle, L., Roper, M. T., Sloan, M. T., Dulcan, M. K., Hoven, C., et al. (1999). Are stimulants overprescribed? Treatment of ADHD in four U.S. communities. *Journal of the American Academy of Child and Adolescent Psychiatry, 38,* 797–804.

Jensen, P. S., Martin, D., & Cantwell, D. P. (1997). Comorbidity in ADHD: Implications for research, practice, and DSM-V. *Journal of the American Academy of Child and Adolescent Psychiatry, 36,* 1065–1079.

Jensen, P. S., Shervette, R. E., Xenakis, S. N., & Bain, M. W. (1988). Psychosocial and medical histories of stimulant-treated children. *Journal of the American Academy of Child and Adolescent Psychiatry, 27,* 798–801.

Johnson, J. G., Cohen, P., Kasen, S., Smailes, E., & Brook, J. S. (2001). Association of maladaptive parental behavior with psychiatric disorder among parents and their offspring. *Archives of General Psychiatry, 58,* 453–460.

Johnston, C. (1992, February). *The influence of behavioral parent training on inattentive–overactive and aggressive–defiant behaviors in ADHD children.* Poster presented at the annual meeting of the International Society for Research in Child and Adolescent Psychopathology, Sarasota, FL.

Johnston, C. (1996). Parent characteristics and parent–child interactions in families of nonproblem children and ADHD children with higher and lower levels of oppositional–defiant disorder. *Journal of Abnormal Child Psychology, 24,* 85–104.

Johnston, C., & Mash, E. J. (2001). Families of children with attention-deficit/hyperactivity disorder: Review and recommendations for future research. *Clinical Child and Family Psychology Review, 4,* 183–207.

Johnstone, S. J., Barry, R. J., & Anderson, J. W. (2001). Topographic distribution and developmental timecourse of auditory event-related potentials in two subtypes of attention-deficit hyperactivity disorder. *International Journal of Psychophysiology, 42,* 73–94.

Kadesjo, B., & Gillberg, C. (2001). The comorbidity of ADHD in the general population of Swedish school-age children. *Journal of Child Psychology and Psychiatry, 42,* 487–492.

Kazdin, A. E. (1991). Effectiveness of psychotherapy

with children and adolescents. *Journal of Consulting and Clinical Psychology, 58,* 729–740.

Keenan, K. (2000). Emotion dysregulation as a risk factor for child psychopathology. *Clinical Psychology: Science and Practice, 7,* 418–434.

Kendall, P. C., & Braswell, L. (1985). *Cognitive-behavioral therapy for impulsive children.* New York: Guilford Press.

Klorman, R. (1992). Cognitive event-related potentials in attention deficit disorder. In S. E. Shaywitz & B. A. Shaywitz (Eds.), *Attention deficit disorder comes of age: Toward the twenty-first century* (pp. 221–244). Austin, TX: Pro-Ed.

Klorman, R., Hazel-Fernandez, H., Shaywitz, S. E., Fletcher, J. M., Marchione, K. E., Holahan, J. M., et al. (1999). Executive functioning deficits in attention-deficit/hyperactivity disorder are independent of oppositional defiant or reading disorder. *Journal of the American Academy of Child and Adolescent Psychiatry, 38,* 1148–1155.

Kopp, C. B. (1982). Antecedents of self-regulation: A developmental perspective. *Developmental Psychology, 18,* 199–214.

Lahey, B. B. (2001). Should the combined and predominantly inattentive types of ADHD be considered distinct and unrelated disorders? Not now, at least. *Clinical Psychology: Science and Practice, 8,* 494–497.

Lahey, B. B., Applegate, B., McBurnett, K., Biederman, J., Greenhill, L., Hynd, G. W., et al. (1994). DSM-IV field trials for attention deficit/hyperactivity disorder in children and adolescents. *American Journal of Psychiatry, 151,* 1673–1685.

Lahey, B. B., & Carlson, C. L. (1992). Validity of the diagnostic category of attention deficit disorder without hyperactivity: A review of the literature. In S. E. Shaywitz & B. A. Shaywitz (Eds.), *Attention deficit disorder comes of age: Toward the twenty-first century* (pp. 119–144). Austin, TX: Pro-Ed.

Lahey, B. B., McBurnett, K., & Loeber, R. (2000). Are attention-deficit/hyperactivity disorder and oppositional defiant disorder developmental precursors to conduct disorder? In A. J. Sameroff, M. Lewis, & S. M. Miller (Eds.), *Handbook of developmental psychopathology* (2nd ed., pp. 431–446). New York: Plenum Press.

Lahey, B. B., Pelham, W. E., Schaughency, E. A., Atkins, M. S., Murphy, H. A., Hynd, G. W., et al. (1988). Dimensions and types of attention deficit disorder with hyperactivity in children: A factor and cluster-analytic approach. *Journal of the American Academy of Child and Adolescent Psychiatry, 27,* 330–335.

Lahey, B. B., Piacentini, J. C., McBurnett, K., Stone, P., Hartdagen, S., & Hynd, G. (1988). Psychpathology in the parents of children with conduct disorder and hyperactivity. *Journal of the American Academy of Child and Adolescent Psychiatry, 27,* 163–170.

Lahoste, G. J., Swanson, J. M., Wigal, S. B., Glabe, C., Wigal, T., King, N., & Kennedy, J. L. (1996). Dopamine D4 receptor gene polymorphism is associated with attention deficit hyperactivity disorder. *Molecular Psychiatry, 1,* 121–124.

Lang, P. (1995). The emotion probe. *American Psychologist, 501,* 372–385.

Lavigne, J. V., Gibbons, R. D., Christoffel, K., Arend, R., Rosenbaum, D., Binns, H., et al. (1996). Prevalence rates and correlates of psychiatric disorders among preschool children. *Journal of the American Academy of Child and Adolescent Psychiatry, 35,* 204–214.

Levy, F., & Hay, D. (2001). *Attention, genes, and ADHD.* Philadelphia: Brunner-Routledge.

Lewinsohn, P. M., Hops, H., Roberts, R. E., Seeley, J. R., & Andrews, J. A. (1993). Adolescent psychopathology: I. Prevalence and incidence of depression and other DSM-III-R disorders in high school students. *Journal of Abnormal Psychology, 102,* 133–144.

Lewinsohn, P. M., Klein, D. N, & Seeley, J. R. (1995). Bipolar disorders in a community sample of older adolescents: Prevalence, phenomenology, comorbidity, and course. *Journal of the American Academy of Child and Adolescent Psychiatry, 34,* 454–463.

Locke, H. J., & Wallace, K. M. (1959). Short marital adjustment and prediction tests: Their reliability and validity. *Journal of Marriage and Family Living, 21,* 251255.

Loeber, R., Burke, J. D., Lahey, B. B., Winters, A., & Zera, M. (2000). Oppositional defiant and conduct disorder: A review of the past 10 years, Part I. *Journal of the American Academy of Child and Adolescent Psychiatry, 39,* 1468–1484.

Loeber, R., Green, S. M., Lahey, B. B., Christ, M. A. G., & Frick, P. J. (1992). Developmental sequences in the age of onset of disruptive child behaviors. *Journal of Child and Family Studies, 1,* 21–41.

Loeber, R., Green, S., Lahey, B. B., & Stouthamer-Loeber, M. (1991). Differences and similarities between children, mothers, and teachers as informants on disruptive behavior disorders. *Journal of Abnormal Child Psychology, 19,* 75–95.

Loo, S., & Barkley, R. A. (2005). Clinical utility of EEG in attenion deficit hyperactivity disorder. *Applied Neuropsychology, 12,* 64–76.

Lorch, E. P., Milich, M., Sanchez, R. P., van den Broek, P., Baer, S., Hooks, K., et al. (2000). Comprehension of televised stories in boys with attention deficit/hyperactivity disorder and nonreferred boys. *Journal of Abnormal Psychology, 109,* 321–330.

Maedgen, J. W., & Carlson, C. L. (2000). Social functioning and emotional regulation in the attention deficit hyperactivity disorder subtypes. *Journal of Clinical Child Psychology, 29,* 30–42.

Mannuzza, S., & Klein, R. (1992). Predictors of outcome of children with attention-deficit hyperactivity disorder. *Child and Adolescent Psychiatric Clinics of North America, 1,* 567–578.

Mannuzza, S., Klein, R., Bessler, A., Malloy, P., & LaPadula, M. (1993). Adult outcome of hyperactive boys: Educational achievement, occupational rank, and psychiatric status. *Archives of General Psychiatry, 50,* 565–576.

Mannuzza, S., Klein, R., Bessler, A., Malloy, P., & LaPadula, M. (1998). Adult psychiatric status of hyperactive boys grown up. *American Journal of Psychiatry, 155*, 493–498.

Marcotte, A. C., & Stern, C. (1997). Qualitative analysis of graphomotor output in children with attentional disorders. *Child Neuropsychology, 3*, 147–153.

Mariani, M., & Barkley, R. A. (1997). Neuropsychological and academic functioning in preschool children with attention deficit hyperactivity disorder. *Developmental Neuropsychology, 13*, 111–129.

Mash, E. J., & Barkley, R. A. (1998). *Treatment of childhood disorders* (2nd ed.). New York: Guilford Press.

Mash, E. J., & Barkley, R. A. (2003). *Child psychopathology* (2nd ed.). New York: Guilford Press.

McGee, R., Feehan, M., Williams, S., Partridge, F., Silva, P. A., & Kelly, J. (1990). DSM-III disorders in a large sample of adolescents. *Journal of the American Academy of Child and Adolescent Psychiatry, 29*, 611–619.

McGee, R., Williams, S., & Feehan, M. (1992). Attention deficit disorder and age of onset of problem behaviors. *Journal of Abnormal Child Psychology, 20*, 487–502.

McInnes, A., Humphries, T., Hogg-Johnson, S., & Tannock, R. (2003). Listening comprehension and working memory are impaired in attention-deficit/hyperactivity disorder irrespective of language impairment. *Journal of Abnormal Child Psychology, 31*, 427–444.

Meichenbaum, D., & Goodman, J. (1971). Training impulsive children to talk to themselves: A means of developing self-control. *Journal of Abnormal Psychology, 77*, 115–126.

Melnick, S. M., & Hinshaw, S. P. (2000). Emotion regulation and parenting in AD/HD and comparison boys: Linkages with social behaviors and peer preference. *Journal of Abnormal Child Psychology, 28*, 73–86.

Michelson, D., Allen, A. J., Busner, J., Casat, C., Dunn, D., Kratochwill, C., et al. (2002). One-dail atomoxetine treatment for children and adolescents with attention deficit hyperactivity disorder: A randomized, placebo-controlled study. *American Journal of Psychiatry, 159*, 1896–1901.

Michon, J. (1985). Introduction. In J. Michon & T. Jackson (Eds.), *Time, mind, and behavior*. Berlin: Springer-Verlag.

Mick, E., Biederman, J., & Faraone, S. V. (1996). Is season of birth a risk factor for attention-deficit hyperactivity disorder? *Journal of the American Academy of Child and Adolescent Psychiatry, 35*, 1470–1476.

Milberger, S. (1997, October). *Impact of adversity on functioning and comorbidity in girls with ADHD*. Paper presented at the annual meeting of the American Academy of Child and Adolescent Psychiatry, Toronto.

Milberger, S., Biederman, J., Faraone, S. V., Chen, L., & Jones, J. (1996). Is maternal smoking during pregnancy a risk factor for attention deficit hyperactivity disorder in children? *American Journal of Psychiatry, 153*, 1138–1142.

Milberger, S., Biederman, J., Faraone, S. V., Murphy, J., & Tsuang, M. T. (1995). Attention deficit hyperactivity disorder and comorbid disorders: Issues of overlapping symptoms. *American Journal of Psychiatry, 152*, 1783–1800.

Milich, R., Ballentine, A. C., & Lynam, D. (2001). ADHD combined type and ADHD predominantly inattentive type are distinct and unrelated disorders. *Clinical Psychology: Science and Practice, 8*, 463–488.

Milich, R., Wolraich, M., & Lindgren, S. (1986). Sugar and hyperactivity: A critical review of empirical findings. *Clinical Psychology Review, 6*, 493–513.

Mirsky, A. F. (1996). Disorders of attention: A neuropsychological perspective. In R. G. Lyon & N. A. Krasnegor (Eds.), *Attention, memory, and executive function* (pp. 71–96). Baltimore: Brookes.

Mitsis, E. M., McKay, K. E., Schulz, K. P., Newcorn, J. H., & Halperin, J. M. (2000). Parent–teacher concordance in DSM-IV attention-deficit/hyperactivity disorder in a clinic-referred sample. *Journal of the American Academy of Child and Adolescent Psychiatry, 39*, 308–313.

Molina, B. S. G., Smith, B. H., & Pelham, W. E. (1999). Interactive effects of attention deficit hyperactivity disorder and conduct disorder on early adolescent substance use. *Psychology of Addictive Behavior, 13*, 348–358

Monastra, V. J., Lubar, J. F., & Linden, M. (2001). The development of quantitative a electroencephalographic scanning process for attention deficit-hyperactivity disorder: Reliability and validity studies. *Neuropsychology, 15*, 136–144.

Morrison, J., & Stewart, M. (1973). The psychiatric status of the legal families of adopted hyperactive children. *Archives of General Psychiatry, 28*, 888–891.

MTA Cooperative Group. (1999). A 14-month randomized clinical trial of treatment strategies for attention-deficit/hyperactivity disorder. *Archives of General Psychiatry, 56*, 1073–1086.

Murphy, D. A., Pelham, W. E., & Lang, A. R. (1992). Aggression in boys with attention deficit-hyperactivity disorder: Methylphenidate effects on naturalistically observed aggression, response to provocation, and social information processing. *Journal of Abnormal Child Psychology, 20*, 451–465.

Murphy, K. R., & Barkley, R. A. (1996a). Attention deficit hyperactivity disorder in adults: Comorbidities and adaptive impairments. *Comprehensive Psychiatry, 37*, 393–401.

Murphy, K. R., & Barkley, R. A. (1996b). Prevalence of DSM-IV symptoms of ADHD in adult licensed drivers: Implications for clinical diagnosis. *Journal of Attention Disorders, 1*, 147–161.

Murphy, K. R., Barkley, R. A., Bush, T. (2001). Executive functioning and olfactory identification in young adults with attention deficit hyperactivity disorder. *Neuropsychology, 15,* 211–220.

Needleman, H. L., Gunnoe, C., Leviton, A., Reed, R., Peresie, H., Maher, C., & Barrett, P. (1979). Deficits in psychologic and classroom performance of children with elevated dentine lead levels. *New England Journal of Medicine, 300,* 689–695.

Needleman, H. L., Schell, A. Bellinger, D. C., Leviton, L., & Alfred, E. D. (1990). The long-term effects of exposure to low doses of lead in childhood: An 11-year follow-up report. *New England Journal of Medicine, 322,* 83–88.

Newcomb, A. F., Bukowski, W. M., & Pattee, L. (1993). Children's peer relations: A meta-analytic review of popular, rejected, neglected, controversial, and average sociometric status. *Psychological Bulletin, 113,* 99–128.

Newcorn, J. H., Halperin, J. M., Jensen, P. S., Abikoff, H. B., Arnold, L. E., Cantwell, D. P., et al. (2001). Symptom profiles in children with ADHD: Comorbidity and gender. *Journal of the American Academy of Child and Adolescent Psychiatry, 40,* 137–146.

Nigg, J. T. (1999). The ADHD response-inhibition deficit as measured by the stop task: Replication with DSM-IV Combined Type, extension, and qualification. *Journal of Abnormal Child Psychology, 27,* 393–402.

Nigg, J. T. (2000). On inhibition/disinhibition in developmental psychopathology: Views from cognitive and personality psychology and a working inhibition taxonomy. *Psychological Bulletin, 126,* 220–246.

Nigg, J. T. (2001). Is ADHD an inhibitory disorder? *Psychological Bulletin, 125,* 571–596.

Nigg, J. T., Hinshaw, S. P., Carte, E. T., & Treuting, J. J. (1998). Neuropsychological correlates of childhood attention-deficit/hyperactivity disorder: Explainable by comorbid disruptive behavior or reading problems? *Journal of Abnormal Psychology, 107,* 468–480.

O'Dougherty, M., Nuechterlein, K. H., & Drew, B. (1984). Hyperactive and hypoxic children: Signal detection, sustained attention, and behavior. *Journal of Abnormal Psychology, 93,* 178–191.

O'Leary, R. D., Pelham, W. E., Rosenbaum., A., &, Price, G. H. (1976). Behavioral treatment of hyperkinetic children: An experimental evaluation of its usefulness. *Clinical Pediatrics, 15,* 510–515.

Olson, S. L., Schilling, E. M., & Bates, J. E. (1999). Measurement of impulsivity: Construct coherence, longitudinal stability, and relationship with externalizing problems in middle childhood and adolescence. *Journal of Abnormal Child Psychology, 27,* 151–165.

Patterson, G. R., Degarmo, D. S., & Knutson, N. (2000). Hyperactive and antisocial behaviors: Comorbid or two points in the same process. *Development and Psychopathology, 12,* 91–106.

Patterson, G. R., Dishion, T., & Reid, J. (1992). *Antisocial boys.* Eugene, OR: Castalia.

Pelham, W. E., Jr. (2001). Are ADHD/I and ADHD/C the same or different? Does it matter? *Clinical Psychology: Science and Practice, 8,* 502–506.

Pelham, W. E., & Sams, S. E. (1992, October). Behavior modification. *Child and Adolescent Psychiatry Clinics of North America, 1,* 505–518.

Pelham, W. E., Schnedler, R. W., Bender, M. E., Nilsson, D. E., Miller, J., Budrow, M. S., et al. (1988). The combination of behavior therapy and methylphenidate in the treatment of attention deficit disorders: A therapy outcome study. In L. Bloomingdale (Ed.), *Attention deficit disorders* (Vol. 3, pp. 29–48) New York: Pergamon Press.

Pentikis, H. S., Simmons, R. D., Benedict, M. F., & Hatch, S. J. (2002). Methylphenidate bioavailability in adults when an extended-release multiparticulate formulation is administered sprinkled on food or as an intact capsule. *Journal of the American Academy of Child and Adolescent Psychiatry, 41,* 443–449.

Pfiffner, L., Barkley, R. A., & DuPaul, G. J. (2006). Treatment of ADHD in school settings. In R. A. Barkley (Ed.), *Attention-deficit hyperactivity disorder: A handbook for diagnosis and treatment* (3rd ed., pp. 547–590). New York: Guilford Press.

Pfiffner, L. J., McBurnett, K., & Rathouz, P. J. (2001). Father absence and familial antisocial characteristics. *Journal of Abnormal Child Psychology, 29,* 357–367.

Pike, A., & Plomin, R. (1996). Importance of nonshared environmental factors for childhood and adolescent psychopathology. *Journal of the American Academy of Child and Adolescent Psychiatry, 35,* 560–570.

Pinker, S. (2002). *The blank slate: The modern denial of human nature.* New York: Norton.

Pliszka, S. R. (1987). Tricyclic antidepressants in the treatment of children with attention deficit disorder. *Journal of the American Academy of Child and Adolescent Psychiatry, 26,* 127–132.

Pliszka, S. R., Liotti, M., & Woldorff, M. G. (2000). Inhibitory control in children with attention-deficit/hyperactivity disorder: Event-related potentials identify the processing component and timing of an impaired right-frontal response-inhibition mechanism. *Biological Psychiatry, 48,* 238–246.

Pliszka, S. R., McCracken, J. T., & Maas, J. W. (1996). Catecholamines in attention deficit hyperactivity disorder: current perspectives. *Journal of the American Academy of Child and Adolescent Psychiatry, 35,* 264–272.

Plomin, R. (1995). Genetics and children's experiences in the family. *Journal of Child Psychology and Psychiatry, 36,* 33–68.

Prince, J. B., Wilens, T. E., Biederman, J., Spencer, T. J., & Wozniak, J. (1996). Clonidine for sleep disturbances associated with attention-deficit hyperactivity disorder: A systematic chart review. *Journal of the American Academy of Child and Adolescent Psychiatry, 35,* 599–605.

Purvis, K. L., & Tannock, R. (1997). Language abilities in children with attention deficit hyperactivity disorder, reading disabilities, and normal controls. *Journal of Abnormal Child Psychology, 25,* 133–144.

Quay, H. C. (1997). Inhibition and attention deficit hyperactivity disorder. *Journal of Abnormal Child Psychology, 25,* 7–13.

Rabiner, D., Coie, J. D., & the Conduct Problems Prevention Research Group. (2000). Early attention problems and children's reading achievement: A longitudinal investigation. *Journal of the American Academy of Child and Adolescent Psychiatry, 39,* 859–867.

Rapport, M. D., DuPaul, G. J., Stoner, G., & Jones, J. T. (1986). Comparing classroom and clinic measures of attention deficit disorder: Differential, idiosyncratic, and dose–response effects of methylphenidate. *Journal of Consulting and Clinical Psychology, 54,* 334–341.

Rapport, M. D., & Moffitt, C. (2002). Attention-deficit/hyperactivity disorder and methylphenidate: A review of height/weight, cardiovascular, and somatic complaint side effects. *Clinical Psychology Review, 22,* 1107–1131.

Rasmussen, P., & Gillberg, C. (2001). Natural outcome of ADHD with developmental coordination disorder at age 22 years: A controlled, longitudinal, community-based study. *Journal of the American Academy of Child and Adolescent Psychiatry, 39,* 1424–1431.

Reynolds, C. R., & Kamphaus, R. W. (2001). *Behavioral Assessment System for Children–2.* Circle Pines, MN: American Guidance Systems.

Richter, N. C. (1984). The efficacy of relaxation training with children. *Journal of Abnormal Child Psychology, 12,* 319–344.

Robin, A. L. (2000). *ADHD in adolescents: Diagnosis and treatment.* New York: Guilford Press.

Robin, A. L., & Foster, S. L. (1989). *Negotiating parent–adolescent conflict: A behavioral–family systems approach.* New York: Guilford Press.

Romano, E., Tremblay, R. E., Vitaro, F., Zoccolillo, M., & Pagani, L. (2001). Prevalence of psychiatric diagnoses and the role of perceived impairment: findings from an adolescent community sample. *Journal of Child Psychology and Psychiatry, 42,* 451–462.

Rowe, D. C. (1995). *The limits of family influence: Genes, experience, and behavior.* New York: Guilford Press.

Rubia, K., Overmeyer, S., Taylor, E., Brammer, M., Williams, S. C. R., Simmons, A., & Bullmore, E. T. (1999). Hypofrontality in attention deficit hyperactivity disorder during higher-order motor control: A study with functional MRI. *American Journal of Psychiatry, 156,* 891–896.

Rucklidge, J. J., & Tannock, R. (2001). Psychiatric, psychosocial, and cognitive functioning of female adolescents with ADHD. *Journal of the American Academy of Child and Adolescent Psychiatry, 40,* 530–540.

Russo, M. F., & Beidel, D. C. (1994). Comorbidity of childhood anxiety and externalizing disorders: Prevalence, associated characteristics, and validation issues. *Clinical Psychology Review, 14,* 199–221.

Rutter, M. (1977). Brain damage syndromes in childhood: Concepts and findings. *Journal of Child Psychology and Psychiatry, 18,* 1–21.

Rutter, M. (1997). Nature–nurture integration: The example of antisocial behavior. *American Psychologist, 52,* 390–398.

Ryan, N. D. (1990). Heterocyclic antidepressants in children and adolescents. *Journal of Child and Adolescent Psychopharmacology, 1,* 21–32.

Safer, D. J., Zito, J. M., & Gardner, J. F. (2001). Pemoline hepatoxicity and postmarketing surveillance. *Journal of the American Academy of Child and Adolescent Psychiatry, 40,* 622–629.

Sanchez, R. P., Lorch, E. P., Milich, R., & Welsh, R. (1999). Comprehension of televised stories in preschool children with ADHD. *Journal of Clinical Child Psychology, 28,* 376–385.

Satterfield, J. H., Satterfield, B. T., & Cantwell, D. P. (1980). Multimodality treatment: A two-year evaluation of 61 hyperactive boys. *Archives of General Psychiatry, 37,* 915–919.

Satterfield, J. H., Satterfield, B. T., & Cantwell, D. P. (1981). Three-year multimodality treatment study of 100 hyperactive boys. *Journal of Pediatrics, 98,* 650–655.

Scarr, S. (1992). Developmental theories for the 1990s: Development and individual differences. *Child Development, 63,* 1–19.

Schachar, R., & Tannock, R. (1993). Childhood hyperactivity and psychostimulants: A review of extended treatment studies. *Journal of Child Adolescent Psychopharmacology, 3,* 81–97.

Schmitz, M., Cadore, L., Paczko, M., Kipper, L., Chaves, M., Rohde, L. A., et al. (2002). Neuropsychological performance in DSM-IV ADHD subtypes: An exploratory study with untreated adolescents. *Canadian Journal of Psychiatry, 47,* 863–869.

Schothorst, P. F., & van Engeland, H. (1996). Long-term behavioral sequelae of prematurity. *Journal of the American Academy of Child and Adolescent Psychiatry, 35,* 175–183.

Schweitzer, J. B., Faber, T. L., Grafton, S. T., Tune, L. E., Hoffman, J. M., & Kilts, C. D. (2000). Alterations in the functional anatomy of working memory in adult attention deficit hyperactivity disorder. *American Journal of Psychiatry, 157,* 278–280

Seidman, L. J., Biederman, J., Faraone, S. V., Weber, W., & Ouellette, C. (1997). Toward defining a neuropsychology of attention deficit-hyperactivity disorder: Performance of children and adolescence from a large clinically referred sample. *Journal of Consulting and Clinical Psychology, 65,* 150–160.

Seguin, J. R., Boulerice, B., Harden, P. W., Tremblay, R. E., & Pihl, R. O. (1999). Executive functions and physical aggression after controlling for attention deficit hyperactivity disorder, general memory, and IQ. *Journal of Child Psychology and Psychiatry, 40,* 1197–1208.

Semrud-Clikeman, M., Biederman, J., Sprich-Buckminster, S., Lehman, B. K., Faraone, S. V., & Norman, D. (1992). Comorbidity between ADDH and learning disability: A review and report in a clinically referred sample. *Journal of the American Academy of Child and Adolescent Psychiatry, 31,* 439–448.

Semrud-Clikeman, M., Steingard, R. J., Filipek, P., Biederman, J., Bekken, K., & Renshaw, P. F. (2000). Using MRI to examine brain-behavior relationships in males with attention deficit disorder with hyperactivity. *Journal of the American Academy of Child and Adolescent Psychiatry, 39,* 477–484.

Shelton, T. L., Barkley, R. A., Crosswait, C., Moorehouse, M., Fletcher, K., Barrett, S., et al. (2000). Early intervention with preschool children with aggressive and hyperactive–impulsive behavior: Two-year post-treatment follow-up. *Journal of Abnormal Child Psychology, 28,* 253–266.

Sherman, D. K., McGue, M. K., & Iacono, W. G. (1997). Twin concordance for attention deficit hyperactivity disorder: A comparison of teachers' and mothers' reports. *American Journal of Psychiatry, 154,* 532–535.

Sieg, K. G., Gaffney, G. R., Preston, D. F., & Hellings, J. A. (1995). SPECT brain imaging abnormalities in attention deficit hyperactivity disorder. *Clinical Nuclear Medicine, 20,* 55–60.

Slusarek, M., Velling, S., Bunk, D., & Eggers, C. (2001). Motivational effects on inhibitory control in children with ADHD. *Journal of the American Academy of Child and Adolescent Psychiatry, 40,* 355–363.

Smalley, S. L., McGough, J. J., Del'Homme, M., NewDelman, J., Gordon, E., Kim, T., et al. (2000). Familial clustering of symptoms and disruptive behaviors in multiplex families with attention-deficit/hyperactivity disorder. *Journal of the American Academy of Child and Adolescent Psychiatry, 39,* 1135–1143.

Smith, B. H., Waschbusch, D. A., Willoughby, M. T., & Evans, S. (2000). The efficacy, safety, and practicality of treatments for adolescents with attention-deficit/hyperactivity disorder (ADHD). *Clinical Child and Family Psychology Review, 3,* 243–260.

Smith, K. M., Daly, M., Fischer, M., Yianmoutsos, V. T., Bruer, L., Barkley R., et al. (2003). Association of the dopamine beta hydroxylase gene with attention deficit hyperactivity disorder: Genetic analysis of the Milwaukee longitudinal study. *American Journal of Medical Genetics, 119*(1), 77–85.

Solanto, M. V., Abikoff, H., Sonuga-Barke, E., Schachar, R., Logan, G. D., Wigal, T., et al. (2001). The ecological validity of delay aversion and response inhibition as measures of impulsivity in AD/HD: A supplement to the NIMH Multimodal Treatment Study of ADHD. *Journal of Abnormal Child Psychology, 29,* 215–228.

Solanto, M. V., Arnsten, A. F. T., & Castellanos, F. X. (2001). *Stimulant drugs and ADHD: Basic and clinical neuroscience.* New York: Oxford University Press.

Sonuga-Barke, E. J. S., Daley, D., & Thompson, M.

(2002). Does maternal ADHD reduce the effectiveness of parent training for preschool children's ADHD? *Journal of the American Academy of Child and Adolescent Psychiatry, 41,* 696–702.

Spencer, T. J., Biederman, J., Harding, M., O'Donnell, D., Faraone, S. V., & Wilens, T. E. (1996). Growth deficits in ADHD children revisited: Evidence for disorder-associated growth delays? *Journal of the American Academy of Child and Adolescent Psychiatry, 35,* 1460–1469.

Spencer, T. J., Biederman, J., & Wilens, T. (1998). Pharmacotherapy of ADHD with antidepressants. In R. A. Barkley (Ed.), *Attention-deficit hyperactivity disorder: A handbook for diagnosis and treatment* (2nd ed., pp. 552–563). New York: Guilford Press.

Spencer, T., Biederman, J., Wilens, T., Faraone, S., Prince, J., Gerard, K., et al. (2001). Efficacy of mixed amphetamine salts compound in adults with attention-deficit/hyperactivity disorder. *Archives of General Psychiatry, 58,* 775–782.

Spencer, T. J., Wilens, T., Biederman, J., Faraone, S. V., Ablon, J. S., & Lapey, K. (1995). A double-blind, crossover comparison of methylphenidate and placebo in adults with childhood-onset attention-deficit hyperactivity disorder. *Archives of General Psychiatry, 52,* 434–443.

Spencer, T., Wilens, T., Biederman, J., Wozniak, J., & Harding-Crawford, M. (2000). Attention-deficit/hyperactivity disorder with mood disorders. In T. E. Brown (Ed.), *Attention deficit disorders and comorbidities in children, adolescents, and adults* (pp. 79–124). Washington, DC: American Psychiatric Press.

Sprich, S., Biederman, J., Crawford, M. H., Mundy, E., & Faraone, S. V. (2000). Adoptive and biological families of children and adolescents with ADHD. *Journal of the American Academy of Child and Adolescent Psychiatry, 39,* 1432–1437.

Still, G. F. (1902). Some abnormal psychical conditions in children. *Lancet, 1,* 1008–1012, 1077–1082, 1163–1168.

Strauss, A. A., & Lehtinen, L. E. (1947). *Psychopathology and education of the brain-injured child.* New York: Grune & Stratton.

Strauss, M. E., Thompson, P., Adams, N. L., Redline, S., & Burant, C. (2000). Evaluation of a model of attention with confirmatory factor analysis. *Neuropsychology, 14,* 201–208.

Strayhorn, J. M., & Weidman, C. S. (1989). Reduction of attention deficit and internalizing symptoms in preschoolers through parent–child interaction training. *Journal of the American Academy of Child and Adolescent Psychiatry, 28,* 888–896.

Strayhorn, J. M., & Weidman, C. S. (1991). Follow-up one year after parent-child interaction training: Effects on behavior of preschool children. *Journal of the American Academy of Child and Adolescent Psychiatry, 30,* 138–143.

Streissguth, A. P., Bookstein, F. L., Sampson, P. D., & Barr, H. M. (1995). Attention: Prenatal alcohol and continuities of vigilance and attentional problems from 4 through 14 years. *Development and Psychopathology, 7,* 419–446.

Stryker, S. (1925). Encephalitis lethargica—The behavior residuals. *Training School Bulletin, 22,* 152–157.

Swaab-Barneveld, H., DeSonneville, L., Cohen-Kettenis, P., Gielen, A., Buitelaar, J., & van Engeland, H. (2000). Visual sustained attention in a child psychiatric population. *Journal of the American Academy of Child and Adolescent Psychiatry, 39,* 651–659.

Swanson, J., Gupta, S., Lam, A., Shoulson, I., Lerer, M., Modi, N., et al. (2003). Development of a new once-a-day formulation of methylphenidate for the treatment of attention-deficit/hyperactivity disorder. *Archives of General Psychiatry, 60,* 204–211.

Swanson, J. M., McBurnett, K., Christian, D. L., & Wigal, T. (1995). Stimulant medications and the treatment of children with ADHD. In T. H. Ollendick & R. J. Prinz (Eds.), *Advances in clinical child psychology* (Vol. 17, pp. 265–322). New York: Plenum Press.

Swanson, J. M., Sunohara, G. A., Kennedy, J. L., Regino, R., Fineberg, E., Wigal, E., et al. (1997). *Association of the dopamine receptor D4 (DRD4) gene with a refined phenotype of attention deficit hyperactivity disorder (ADHD): A family-based approach.* Manuscript submitted for publication, University of California at Irvine.

Sykes, D. H., Hoy, E. A., Bill, J. M., McClure, B. G., Halliday, H. L., & Reid, M. M. (1997). Behavioural adjustment in school of very low birthweight children. *Journal of Child Psychology and Psychiatry, 38,* 315–325.

Szatmari, P. (1992). The epidemiology of attention-deficit hyperactivity disorders. *Child and adolescent psychiatric clinics of North America, 1,* 361–372.

Szatmari, P., Offord, D. R., & Boyle, M. H. (1989). Correlates, associated impairments, and patterns of service utilization of children with attention deficit disorders: Findings from the Ontario Child Health Study. *Journal of Child Psychology and Psychiatry, 30,* 205–217.

Tannock, R. (1998). Attention deficit hyperactivity disorder: advances in cognitive, neurobiological, and genetic research. *Journal of Child Psychology and Psychiatry, 39,* 65–100.

Tannock, R. (2000). Attention-deficit/hyperactivity disorder with anxiety disorders. In T. E. Brown (Ed.), *Attention deficit disorders and comorbidities in children, adolescents, and adults* (pp. 125–170). Washington, DC: American Psychiatric Press.

Tannock, R., & Brown, T. E. (2000). Attention-deficit disorders with learning disorders in children and adolescents. In T. E. Brown (Ed.), *Attention deficit disorders and comorbidities in children, adolescents, and adults* (pp. 231–296). Washington, DC: American Psychiatric Press.

Tannock, R., Martinussen, R., & Frijters, J. (2000). Naming speed performance and stimulant effects indicate effortful, semantic processing deficits in attention-deficit/hyperactivity disorder. *Journal of Abnormal Child Psychology, 28,* 237–252.

Taylor, E., Sandberg, S., Thorley, G., & Giles, S. (1991). *The epidemiology of childhood hyperactivity.* Oxford, UK: Oxford University Press.

Teicher, M. H., Anderson, C. M., Polcari, A., Glod, C. A., Maas, L. C., & Renshaw, P. F. (2000). Functional deficits in basal ganglia of children with attention-deficit/hyperactivity disorder shown with functional magnetic resonance imaging relaxometry. *Nature Medicine, 6,* 470–473.

Thapar, A. J. (1999). Genetic basis of attention deficit and hyperactivity. *British Journal of Psychiatry, 174,* 105–111

Vaidya, C. J., Austin, G., Kirkorian, G., Ridlehuber, H. W., Desmond, J. E., Glover, G. H., & Gabrieli, J. D. E. (1998). Selective effects of methylphenidate in attention deficit hyperactivity disorder: A functional magnetic resonance study. *Proceedings of the National Academy of Sciences, 95,* 14494–14499.

van den Oord, E. J. C. G., Boomsma, D. I., & Verhulst, F. C. (1994). A study of problem behaviors in 10- to 15-year-old biologically related and unrelated international adoptees. *Behavior Genetics, 24,* 193–205.

van den Oord, E. J. C., & Rowe, D. C. (1997). Continuity and change in children's social maladjustment: A developmental behavior genetic study. *Developmental Psychology, 33,* 319–332.

Vargas, S., & Camilli, G. (1999). A meta-analysis of research on sensory integration treatment. *American Journal of Occupational Therapy, 53,* 189–198.

Velez, C. N., Johnson, J., & Cohen, P. (1989). A longitudinal analysis of selected risk factors for childhood psychopathology. *Journal of the American Academy of Child and Adolescent Psychiatry, 28,* 861–864.

Viesselman, J. O., Yaylayan, S., Weller, E. B., & Weller, R. A. (1993). Antidysthymic drugs (antidepressants and antimanics). In J. S. Werry & M. G. Aman (Eds.), *A practitioner's guide to psychoactive drugs for children and adolescents* (pp. 239–268). New York: Plenum Press.

Volkow, N. D., Wang, G., Fowler, J. S., Logan, J., Angrist, B., Hitzemann, R., et al. (1997). Effects of methylphenidate on regional brain glucose metabolism in humans: Relationship to dopamine D_2 receptors. *American Journal of Psychiatry, 154,* 50–55.

Vygotsky, L. S. (1978). *Mind in society.* Cambridge, MA: Harvard University Press.

Vygotsky, L. S. (1987). Thinking and speech. In *The collected works of L. S. Vygotsky: Vol. 1. Problems in general psychology* (N. Minick, Trans.). New York: Plenum Press.

Wahler, R. G. (1980). The insular mother: Her problems in parentchild treatment. *Journal of Applied Behavior Analysis, 13,* 207–219.

Wakefield, J. C. (1992). The concept of mental disorder: On the boundary between biological facts and social values. *American Psychologist, 47,* 373–388.

Wakefield, J. C. (1997). Normal inability versus pathological disability: Why Ossorio's definition of mental disorder is not sufficient. *Clinical Psychology: Science and Practice, 4,* 249–258.

Weiss, G., & Hechtman, L. (1993). *Hyperactive children grown up* (2nd ed.). New York: Guilford Press.

Weisz, J. R., Weiss, B., Han, S. S., Granger, D. A., & Morton, T. (1995). Effects of psychotherapy with children and adolescents revisited: A meta-analysis of treatment outcome studies. *Psychological Bulletin, 117,* 450–468.

Wender, P. H., Reimherr, F. W., Wood, D., & Ward, M. (1985). A controlled study of methylphenidate in the treatment of attention deficit disorder, residual type, in adults. *American Journal of Psychiatry, 142,* 547–552.

Werry, J. S., & Aman, M. G. (1993). *Practitioner's guide to psychoactive drugs for children and adolescents.* New York: Plenum Press.

Whalen, C. K., & Henker, B. (1991). Therapies for hyperactive children: Comparisons, combinations, and compromises. *Journal of Consulting and Clinical Psychology, 59,* 126–137.

Whalen, C. K., Henker, B., & Dotemoto, S. (1980). Methylphenidate and hyperactivity: Effects on teacher behaviors. *Science, 208,* 1280–1282.

White, H. R., Xie, M., Thompson, W., Loeber, R., & Southamer-Loeber, M. (2005). Psychopathology as a predictor of adolescent drug use trajectories. *Psychology of Addictive Behavior, 15,* 210–218.

Whittaker, A. H., Van Rossem, R., Feldman, J. F., Schonfeld, I. S., Pinto-Martin, J. A., Torre, C., et al. (1997). Psychiatric outcomes in low-birth-weight children at age 6 years: Relation to neonatal cranial ultrasound abnormalities. *Archives of General Psychiatry, 54,* 847–856.

Wiers, R. W., Gunning, W. B., & Sergeant, J. A. (1998). Is a mild deficit in executive functions in boys related to childhood ADHD or to parental multigenerational alcoholism. *Journal of Abnormal Child Psychology, 26,* 415–430.

Wilens, T. E., Biederman, J., Baldessarini, R. J., Geller, B., Schleifer, D., Spencer, T. J., et al. (1996). Cardiovascular effects of therapeutic doses of tricyclic antidepressants in children and adolescents. *Journal of the American Academy of Child and Adolescent Psychiatry, 35,* 1491–1501.

Winsler, A., Diaz, R. M., Atencio, D. J., McCarthy, E. M., & Chabay, L. A. (2000). Verbal self-regulation over time in preschool children at risk for attention and behavior problems. *Journal of Child Psychology and Psychiatry, 41,* 875–886.

Wolraich, M. L., Wilson, D. B., & White, J. W. (1995). The effect of sugar on behavior or cognition in children; A meta-analysis. *Journal of the American Medical Association, 274,* 1617–1621.

Worland, J. (1976). Effects of positive and negative feedback on behavior control in hyperactive and normal boys. *Journal of Abnormal Child Psychology, 4,* 315–325.

World Health Organization. (1994). *The ICD-10 classification of mental and behavioral disorders: Diagnostic criteria for research.* Geneva, Switzerland: Author.

Wozniak, J., & Biederman, J. (1995). Prepubertal mania exists (and co-exists with ADHD). *The ADHD Report, 2*(3), 5–6.

Wozniak, J., Biederman, J., Kiely, K., Ablon, S., Faraone, S. V., Mundy, E., & Mennin, D. (1995). Mania-like symptoms suggestive of childhood-onset bipolar disorder in clinically referred children. *Journal of the American Academy of Child and Adolescent Psychiatry, 34,* 867–876.

Zagar, R., & Bowers, N. D. (1983). The effect of time of day on problem-solving and classroom behavior. *Psychology in the Schools, 20,* 337–345.

Zametkin, A. J., Liebenauer, L. L., Fitzgerald, G. A., King, A. C., Minkunas, D. V., Herscovitch, P., et al. (1993). Brain metabolism in teenagers with attention-deficit hyperactivity disorder. *Archives of General Psychiatry, 50,* 333–340.

Zametkin, A. J., Nordahl, T. E., Gross, M., King, A. C., Semple, W. E., Rumsey, J., et al. (1990). Cerebral glucose metabolism in adults with hyperactivity of childhood onset. *New England Journal of Medicine, 323,* 1361–1366.

Zeiner, P. (1995). Body growth and cardiovascular function after extended treatment (1.75 years) with methylphenidate in boys with attention-deficit hyperactivity disorder. *Journal of Child and Adolescent Psychopharmacology, 5,* 129–138.

Zentall, S. S. (1988). Production deficiencies in elicited language but not in the spontaneous verbalizations of hyperactive children. *Journal of Abnormal Child Psychology, 16,* 657–673.

Zito, J., Safer, D., dosReis, S., Gardner, J., Magder, L., Soeken, K., et al. (2003). Psychotropic practice patterns for youth: A 10-year perspective. *Archives of Pediatric and Adolescent Medicine, 157,* 17–25.

5

Conduct Problems

Robert J. McMahon
Julie S. Kotler

Conduct problems in children and adolescents constitute a broad range of "acting-out" behaviors, ranging from annoying but relatively minor oppositional behaviors such as yelling and temper tantrums to more serious forms of antisocial behavior including aggression, physical destructiveness, and stealing. Typically, these behaviors do not occur in isolation but as a complex or syndrome, and there is strong evidence to suggest that oppositional behaviors (e. g., noncompliance in younger children) are developmental precursors to antisocial behaviors in adolescence. However, it is also the case that, for some youth, these behaviors first appear during adolescence. When displayed as a cluster, these behaviors have been referred to as oppositional, antisocial, conduct disordered, and, from a legal perspective, delinquent (see Hinshaw & Lee, 2003, and Tremblay, 2003, for discussions of terminology). In this chapter, we use the term conduct problems (CP) to refer to this constellation of behaviors. Terminology from the *Diagnostic and Statistical Manual of Mental Disorders* (DSM; American Psychiatric Association [APA], 1994, 2000) is used only in those instances in which a formal DSM diagnosis is being discussed or referred to (e.g., conduct disorder and oppositional defiant disorder).

The primary purposes of this chapter are to present (1) a description of CP, including diagnostic issues, associated comorbidities and child characteristics, epidemiology, contextual influences (including the family, peer group, and neighborhood), and developmental pathways; (2) a discussion of assessment procedures that are currently employed with adolescents with CP; and (3) a description of empirically based interventions currently in use for addressing CP in adolescents.

BRIEF HISTORICAL CONTEXT OF ADOLESCENT CONDUCT PROBLEMS

How to define and deal with CP in children and adolescents has a long and checkered history. Costello and Angold (2001) present an intriguing historical account from religious, legal, and medical perspectives of how society has attempted to deal with "bad" children over the centuries. They note that many of the same issues first described by Plato 2,500 years ago pertaining to how best to ascribe responsibility and culpability for such behavior and the relative roles of the family and state are still sources of debate.

The formal recognition of CP as a diagnostic entity (or entities) is fairly recent. Conduct disorder (CD) first appeared in the second edition of the *Diagnostic and Statistical Manual* (DSM-II; APA, 1968), and what was then called oppositional disorder appeared 12 years later in DSM-III (APA, 1980). It was relabeled "oppositional defiant disorder" (ODD) in DSM-III-R (APA, 1987). The specific symptoms and the number required to make these diagnoses has fluctuated across the various versions of the DSM. For example, only a single symptom was required for a CD diagnosis in DSM-III, whereas 3 of 13 symptoms were required in DSM-III-R and 3 of 15 symptoms are required in the current version of the DSM (DSM-IV—APA, 1994; DSM-IV-TR—APA 2000). The subtypes of CD presented in the DSM have also differed in various editions. For example, the DSM-III had four subtypes based on crossing aggressive/nonaggressive and socialized/undersocialized dimensions, whereas the basis for subtyping in DSM-IV has to do with age of onset (i.e., childhood vs. adolescent onset).

An issue of current concern is whether rates and severity of CP have been increasing over the past 50 years or so. One perspective on this question involves official statistics concerning juvenile crime. Rutter and colleagues (Rutter, Giller, & Hagell, 1998; Rutter & Smith, 1995) conducted an extensive analysis of crime records in both Europe and North America from 1950 through the mid-1990s. They concluded that juvenile crime did increase in these countries from the 1950s through the 1980s, with a plateau occurring in the 1990s. Findings in the 1990s are less clear-cut because of various policy changes regarding the handling of juvenile offenders. In addition, there is evidence that the proportion of violent to nonviolent crime has increased, that proportionally more juvenile crime is being committed by females, and that the peak age of offending has moved from middle to late adolescence. In the United States, both the total number and the rates of juvenile arrests for violent crime (including homicides) dropped annually from 1994 to 2000 (Howell, 2003).

Another perspective on whether there have been changes in the occurrence of CP behaviors involves data presented by Achenbach and colleagues with respect to the renorming of the Child Behavior Checklist from 1976 to 1999 (Achenbach, Dumenci, & Rescorla, 2003a). In brief, there were slight but significant increases in the various indicators of CP behavior (externalizing broadband scale, rule-breaking behavior and aggressive behavior narrow-band syndrome scales, and the oppositional defiant problems and conduct problems DSM-oriented scales) from 1976 to 1989 and decreases from 1989 to 1999. However, effect sizes (ES) ranged from 1% to 2%. Results were similar when analyses were conducted with national samples in 1989 and 1999 that included referred children. The aggressive behavior and externalizing scales had more positive scores in 1999 than in 1989; however, the DSM-oriented scale of oppositional defiant problems increased from 1989 to 1999 (ES = 1%). In contrast, the scale of conduct problems was the only DSM-oriented scale to show a significant reduction from 1989 to 1999 when percentage of scores in the deviant range was the variable of interest (from 9.2 to 6.8%). Achenbach and colleagues (2003a) concluded that there is no evidence to suggest that the overall functioning of children in the United States is steadily worsening. When their findings and those related to juvenile crime rates are considered together, a similar conclusion appears to apply with respect to CP: CP does seem to have increased from 1950 through the 1980s, but during the 1990s, it seems to have plateaued or, in some cases, decreased.

DESCRIPTION OF ADOLESCENT CONDUCT PROBLEMS

There are a number of current approaches to the description and classification of CP. We begin by first describing the diagnostic criteria delineated in DSM-IV-TR (APA, 2000) for various disorders related to CP. We then describe a number of ways in which CP (or certain aspects of CP, such as aggression) have been subtyped. This is followed by a section on the various disorders and conditions that are most commonly associated with CP.

Diagnostic Criteria

In the DSM-IV-TR (APA, 2000), CP is classified in the category of disruptive behavior disorders (see Angold & Costello, 2001, for a consideration of nosological issues related to CD and ODD). The two diagnostic categories that are most relevant to CP are ODD and CD. The essential feature of ODD is a "recurrent pattern of negativistic, defiant, disobedient, and hostile behavior toward authority figures" (p. 91). The pattern of behavior must have a duration of at least 6 months, and at least four of the following eight behaviors must be present: losing temper, arguing with grownups, defying or not complying with grownups' rules or requests, deliberately doing things that annoy other people, blaming others for own mistakes, being touchy or easily becoming annoyed by others, exhibiting anger and resentment, and showing spite or vindictiveness. The behaviors must have a higher frequency than is generally seen in other children of similar developmental level and age. Furthermore, the behaviors must lead to meaningful impairment in academic and social functioning.

Although the prototypical presentation of ODD is in a preschool-age child (e.g., McMahon & Forehand, 2003), it is possible for ODD to begin in early adolescence (APA, 2000). Because the aforementioned behaviors can be typical of many adolescents, DSM-IV-TR emphasizes the frequency and impairment criteria noted previously. This may be especially relevant when the oppositional behaviors have their initial onset during adolescence.

The essential feature of CD is a "repetitive and persistent pattern of behavior in which the basic rights of others or major age-appropriate societal norms or rules are violated" (APA, 2000, p. 98). At least 3 of the 15 behaviors listed below must have been present in the past 12 months, with at least one of the behaviors present in the past 6 months. The behaviors are categorized into four groups: aggressiveness to people and animals (bullying, fighting, using a weapon, physical cruelty to people, physical cruelty to animals, stealing with confrontation of victim, forced sexual activity); property destruction (firesetting, other destruction of property); deceptiveness or theft (breaking and entering, lying for personal gain, stealing without confronting victim); and serious rule violations (staying out at night [before age 13], running away from home, being truant [before age 13]). It is important to note that ODD includes behaviors (e.g., noncompliance) that are also included in CD. However, ODD does not involve the more serious behaviors that represent violations of either the basic rights of others or

age-appropriate societal norms or rules. Thus, if a youth meets the diagnostic criteria for both disorders, only the diagnosis of CD is made.

Two subtypes of CD are described in DSM-IV-TR (APA, 2000); these are differentiated on the basis of the child's age at the appearance of the first symptom of CD. The childhood-onset type is defined by the onset of at least 1 of the 15 behaviors prior to 10 years of age, whereas CD behavior does not appear until age 10 or older in the adolescent-onset type. It is important to note that clinicians working with adolescents with CP will encounter both subtypes. Indeed, distinguishing adolescents with CP on the basis of age of onset is one of the most clinically important tasks for the clinician, given differences in likely causal and maintaining factors and prognosis (see below).

Field trials for assessing the psychometric properties of the DSM-IV diagnoses of ODD and CD have demonstrated that the internal consistency and test–retest reliabilities of the DSM-IV versions are higher than those of their DSM-III-R counterparts (Lahey et al., 1994). The validity of the childhood-onset and adolescent-onset types of CD has also been supported in that children with the childhood-onset type were more likely to display more aggressive symptoms, to be boys, to have a family history of antisocial behavior, to experience neurocognitive and temperamental difficulties, and to have additional psychiatric diagnoses, whereas adolescent-onset type CD is more highly related to ethnic minority status and exposure to deviant peers (e.g., Lahey et al., 1998; McCabe, Hough, Wood, & Yeh, 2001; Moffitt & Caspi, 2001; Waldman & Lahey, 1994).

Subtypes of Conduct Problems

In addition to the distinction between ODD and CD and subtypes based on age of onset, several other subtypes of CP are salient when considering the diagnosis and treatment of CP. Loeber and Schmaling (1985a) proposed a bipolar unidimensional typology of "overt" and "covert" CP behaviors. Overt CP behaviors include those that involve direct confrontation with or disruption of the environment (e.g., aggression, temper tantrums, and argumentativeness), whereas covert CP behaviors include those that usually occur without the awareness of adult caretakers (e.g., lying, stealing, and firesetting).

In an extension of this investigation, Frick and colleagues (1993) conducted a meta-analysis of 60 factor analyses with more than 28,000 children. They identified a similar "overt–covert" dimension but also extracted a second bipolar dimension of "destructive–nondestructive." When individual CP behaviors were plotted, four subtypes were obtained: "property violations," "aggression," "status violations," and "oppositional" (see Figure 5.1). Symptoms of CD fall into the first three quadrants, whereas symptoms of ODD fall into the fourth quadrant. Cluster analyses of an independent sample of clinic-referred boys ages 7–12 indicated one group of boys who displayed high elevations on the oppositional quadrant score and moderate elevations on the aggression quadrant score, and another group of boys who showed high elevations on the property violations, oppositional, and aggression quadrant scores. These clusters approxi-mated those groups of boys who received diagnoses of ODD and CD, respectively.

More recent studies (e.g., Tiet, Wasserman, Loeber, Larken, & Miller, 2001; Tolan, Gorman-Smith, & Loeber, 2000; Willoughby, Kupersmidt, & Bryant, 2001) have provided additional validation for this typology. For example, the earlier phase of the developmental trajectory of childhood-onset type CD consists primarily of overt CP, followed by a rapid increase in covert CP (Patterson & Yoerger, 2002).

Noncompliance (i.e., excessive disobedience to adults) appears to be a keystone behavior in the development of both overt and covert CP. Loeber and Schmaling (1985a) found that noncompliance was positioned near the zero point of their unidimensional overt–covert scale of CP behaviors. Patterson and colleagues (e.g., Chamberlain & Patterson, 1995; Patterson, Reid, & Dishion, 1992) have developed a com-

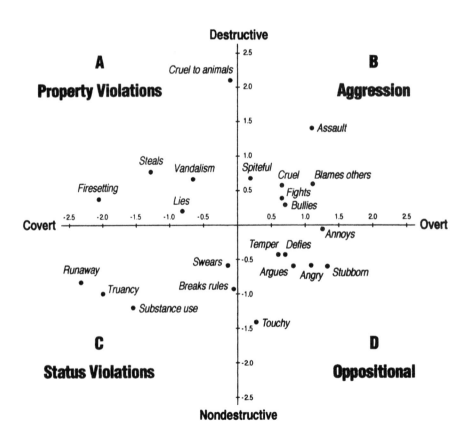

FIGURE 5.1. Meta-analysis of parent and teacher ratings of child conduct problems using multidimensional scaling. From Frick et al. (1993). Copyright 1993 by Elsevier. Reprinted by permission.

prehensive theoretical model for the development and maintenance of CP; in their model, early child noncompliance not only is the precursor of severe manifestations of CP behaviors later in childhood and adolescence but plays a role in these children's subsequent academic and peer relationship problems as well. Walker and Walker (1991) have stressed the role of compliance and noncompliance in the classroom. There is also empirical support for the premise that noncompliance appears early in the progression of CP, and continues to be manifested in subsequent developmental periods (e.g., Chamberlain & Patterson, 1995; Loeber et al., 1993; McMahon & Forehand, 2003). Low levels of compliance are also associated with referral for services in children with CP (Dumas, 1996). Furthermore, intervention research has shown that when child noncompliance is targeted, there is often concomitant improvement in other CP behaviors as well (Parrish, Cataldo, Kolko, Neef, & Egel, 1986; Russo, Cataldo, & Cushing, 1981; Wells, Forehand, & Griest, 1980).

There appear to be several different forms of aggressive behavior. One of the most robust distinctions is between "reactive" and "proactive" forms of aggression (e.g., Crick & Dodge, 1996; Dodge & Coie, 1987; Poulin & Boivin, 2000). The former is a response to perceived provocation, whereas the latter occurs as a means of obtaining some self-serving outcome or to influence and coerce others (e.g., bullying). This reactive/proactive subtype has been found to have good criterion validity, to differ in terms of antecedent characteristics (e.g., a temperament characterized by angry reactivity and emotional dysregulation and inattention is more related to reactive aggression), and to differentially predict maladaptive outcomes (e.g., proactive aggression tends to predict more delinquency and disruptive behavior) (e.g., Hubbard et al., 2002; Vitaro, Brendgen, & Tremblay, 2002; Vitaro, Gendreau, Tremblay, & Oligny, 1998; Waschbusch, Willoughby, & Pelham, 1998). Youth who display reactive aggression are more likely to display social information-processing deficits (e.g., hostile attributional bias and poor social problem-solving skills) (Crick & Dodge, 1996; Dodge, Lochman, Harnish, Bates, & Pettit, 1997). There is also a subgroup of children who are both proactively and reactively aggressive and who have more difficulties than their nonaggressive and proactively aggressive peers but

fewer difficulties than reactively aggressive children in terms of social information-processing deficits (Dodge & Coie, 1987) and on dimensions of reactivity, attention, and depression (Vitaro et al., 2002).

Bullying is a form of proactive aggression, occurring primarily in school settings, that has received increasing attention. It is notable that some authors (e.g., Pikas, 1989) have suggested that bullies may also be provoked; thus, some bullying behavior might also be appropriately categorized as reactive rather than proactive. Several authoritative reviews have appeared on the topic of bullying (e.g., Farrington, 1993; Olweus, 1993; Smith et al., 1999). The general definition of bullying has included physical, verbal, or psychological attack or intimidation that is intended to cause fear, distress, or harm to the victim. Direct bullying, which is more characteristic of boys, involves physical and direct verbal attacks. Indirect bullying, which is more characteristic of girls, includes efforts by the bully to isolate and exclude the victim from the social group and involves behaviors such as slandering, spreading rumors, and manipulating friendships (similar to the construct of "relational aggression," discussed later). In addition, whether direct or indirect, these bullying behaviors are generally carried out repeatedly over time and are characterized by an imbalance of power between the bully and the victim (Olweus, 1999). A cross-national comparison of bullying definitions demonstrated that adolescents (age 14) discriminate between direct and indirect, verbal and nonverbal bullying more effectively than do younger children (age 8), who mostly distinguish aggressive from nonaggressive acts (Smith, Cowie, Olafsson, & Liefooghe, 2002). Furthermore, according to Smith and colleagues (2002), gender differences in youths' conceptualization of bullying are much less appreciable than these developmental differences.

The prevalence of bullying is alarmingly high. A cross-national study including data from 35 countries participating in a World Health Organization survey indicated that, for adolescents ages 11–16, the prevalence rates of two or three bullying occurrences in the last month range from 2% to 37% for bullying and 2% to 36% for being victimized (Craig & Yossi, 2003). Additional data suggest that, in a given year, 75% of youth report at least one bullying incident (Glover, Gough, Johnson, & Cartwright, 2000). Further, in a recent U.S.

study that included a survey of 15,686 students in grades 6–10, Nansel and colleagues (2001) found that 29.9% of the sample reported frequent involvement in bullying, with 13% as a bully, 10.6% as a victim, and 6% as a bully–victim. Nansel et al. also found that the typical developmental trajectory of bullying included an increase and peak during early adolescence and a decrease during high school. While bullying is often studied independently from other CP behaviors, some findings suggest that it may also be a part of a more general pattern of violent and aggressive behavior (Andershed, Kerr, & Stattin, 2001; Baldry & Farrington, 2000). Researchers in this area emphasize that adults (teachers and parents) are relatively unaware of the extent of, and harm created by, the problem and that teachers intervene to help victims very infrequently. Peers intervene approximately three times more often than teachers to stop bullying (Craig & Pepler, 1995), but even they are more likely to observe or even collaborate than to help the victim. Involvement in bullying (as a bully, a victim, or a bully–victim) is associated with a range of negative psychological outcomes (e.g., anger, depression, low self-esteem, unhappiness at school, and suicidal ideation) (Bosworth, Espelage, & Simon, 1999; Duncan, 1999; Kaltiala-Heino, Rimpela, Marttunen, Rimpela, & Rantanen, 1999; Nansel et al., 2001) and youth involved in bullying are four times as likely to have criminal convictions by early adulthood (Olweus, 1993).

In contrast to proactive and reactive forms of aggression, both of which are primarily overt in nature, Crick and colleagues have identified a form of aggression, called relational aggression, that involves manipulation of relationships and may be overt or covert (e.g., Crick & Grotpeter, 1995; Crick & Werner, 1998; Geiger, Zimmer-Gembeck, & Crick, 2004). It includes strategies such as social isolation and exclusion and behaviors such as slandering, rumor spreading, and friendship manipulation. Relational aggression occurs more frequently in girls, although the evidence for this gender difference is less clear during adolescence (Underwood, 2003). Recent evidence suggests that it may be possible to divide relational aggression into proactive and reactive forms as well (Little, Jones, Henrich, & Hawley, 2003).

Some authors have proposed that unique subtypes of CP can even be identified within the childhood-onset pathway. Frick and colleagues suggest that youth described as early starters are quite a heterogeneous group and can be distinguished based on their affective and interpersonal style (Frick & Ellis, 1999). Specifically, these authors propose that two groups of youth can be identified that differ based on the presence or absence of callous and unemotional (CU) traits (e.g., lack of guilt and empathy, callous use of others) (e.g., Caputo, Frick, & Brodsky, 1999; Christian, Frick, Hill, Tyler, & Frazer, 1997; Frick, Bodin, & Barry, 2000). Within groups of youth diagnosed with CD, Frick and colleagues have identified youth who also have high scores on the dimension of CU traits and have found that these youth (1) engage in more diverse and serious CP; (2) have a more stable constellation of CP; (3) are more likely to have had police contact; (4) engage in patterns of violence that are more severe, premeditated, and instrumental; and (5) have an increased likelihood of parental antisocial personality disorder (APD) (Christian et al., 1997; Frick, Cornell, Barry, Bodin, & Dane, 2003; Kruh, Frick, & Clements, 2005). In contrast, youth with CP who are low on CU traits are less likely to be aggressive, and their aggression is more likely to be reactive in nature (Frick et al., 2003). Also, youth with CP who are low on CU traits are more likely to have experienced dysfunctional parenting practices (Oxford, Cavell, & Hughes, 2003; Wootton, Frick, Shelton, & Silverthorn, 1997) and to have deficits in verbal intelligence (Loney, Frick, Ellis, & McCoy, 1998).

There is also evidence that the subgroup of youth with CU traits may exhibit some unique temperamental attributes. In general, these youth have higher levels of behavioral dysregulation and lower levels of behavioral inhibition compared to children with CP who are low on CU traits (Frick et al., 2003). Specifically, they seem to prefer novel, exciting, and dangerous activities (Frick, Lilienfeld, Ellis, Loney, & Silverthorn, 1999; Frick et al., 2003) and are less reactive to emotionally distressing stimuli than other youth with CP (Blair, 1999; Frick et al., 2003). Further, children with CU traits have been shown to be less sensitive to punishment cues (Barry et al., 2000; Fisher & Blair, 1998), to have poor perspective-taking skills, and to expect more positive rewards from aggression (Pardini, Lochman, & Frick, 2003).

Relatively less research has been conducted on covert types of CP and has focused on youth who steal and who set fires. Lying is significantly underresearched compared to other forms of covert CP.

There is a paucity of longitudinal research on youth who steal, although retrospective reports suggest developmental sequences for stealing such that minor forms of theft (e.g., shoplifting) seem to occur prior to more serious forms of theft (e.g., car theft) (LeBlanc & Frechette, 1989; Loeber, 1988). Much of the work on stealing has been conducted by Patterson and his colleagues. Youth who steal exhibit levels of aversive behavior that are comparable to those of nonreferred youth, although youth who engage in both stealing and social aggression are even more aversive than youth who are socially aggressive but who do not steal (Loeber & Schmaling, 1985b; Patterson, 1982). It also appears that youth who steal are older at time of referral than youth referred for overt types of CP (Moore, Chamberlain, & Mukai, 1979; Reid & Hendricks, 1973) and are at greater risk for committing delinquent offenses as adolescents (Loeber & Schmaling, 1985b; Moore et al., 1979). In one study of incarcerated juvenile offenders, stealing was the most common first offense, accounting for 42% of the cases (Taylor et al., 2001).

Patterson (1982) has reported that the parents of youth who steal are more distant and less involved in interactions with their youth than parents of nonreferred youth or parents of youth who are aggressive. The mothers and siblings of youth who are aggressive are more coercive than their counterparts in nonreferred families or families in which the youth steal. Loeber and Schmaling (1985b) found that families with youth who are aggressive and those with youth who both fought and stole were more likely to demonstrate poorer monitoring skills and to have rejecting mothers. Fathers of youth who steal also appear to be less involved in the discipline process than fathers of aggressive or normal youth (Loeber, Weissman, & Reid, 1983).

Lying, defined as a "verbal statement intended to deceive" (Stouthamer-Loeber, 1986, p. 268), may be one of the first covert CP behaviors to appear (Edelbrock, 1985) and is highly correlated with stealing (especially in adolescents). For example, the correlations between lying and stealing in 4th-, 7th-, and 10th-grade boys were .39, .59, and .74, respectively (Stouthamer-Loeber & Loeber, 1986).

Based on the finding of the meta-analytic study conducted by Loeber and Schmaling (1985a), Stouthamer-Loeber (1986) concluded that although lying loads most heavily on the covert dimension of CP, it is also related (albeit less strongly) to overt CP. Lying did correlate significantly with fighting in a community sample of 4th-, 7th-, and 10th-grade boys (r's = .50–.65) (Stouthamer-Loeber & Loeber, 1986), particularly when it occurred in conjunction with stealing. Furthermore, early lying has been shown to be predictive of later recidivism (Loeber & Dishion, 1983).

Childhood firesetting is quite common and potentially very serious in its effects. Prevalence estimates have ranged from 3% to 35% across epidemiological, outpatient, and inpatient samples (Achenbach & Edelbrock, 1981; Heath, Hardesty, Goldfine, & Walker, 1983; Kolko & Kazdin, 1988). Juveniles are arrested for a greater share of arsons than any other type of crime, accounting for 50% of the firesetting arrests according to the Federal Bureau of Investigation's Uniform Crime Report (Snyder, 1999). Approximately two-thirds of those arrested are adolescents (i.e., ages 13–18).

In the last 20 years, three general domains of risk factors associated with firesetting have emerged: child characteristics, parenting, and the broader family climate (e.g., Kolko & Kazdin, 1992; McCarty, McMahon, & Conduct Problems Prevention Research Group, 2005). Child factors that have been identified as risk factors for firesetting behavior include being male (but see Saunders & Awad, 1991, for a retrospective chart study of a small sample of adolescent female firesetters), having higher impulsivity or traits of attention-deficit/hyperactivity disorder (ADHD), having social skill deficits and poor peer relations, displaying other CP behaviors, demonstrating poorer academic performance, and having been abused.

Firesetting has been consistently associated with other CP behaviors. Although only a relatively small proportion of youth with CP engage in firesetting behavior (e.g., 5% in Jacobson's, 1985, outpatient sample in London), most, but not all, firesetters demonstrate other CP behaviors (i.e., can be considered to display the "syndrome" of CP). For example, 74% of the youth who set fires in both outpatient (Jacobson, 1985) and inpatient (Kazdin & Kolko, 1986) samples received a diagnosis of CD. In addition, juvenile offenders who also set fires seem to have more severe levels of CP behavior, to have a history of previous firesetting, and to be arrested at younger ages (Becker, Stuewig, Herrera, & McCloskey, 2004; Forehand, Wierson, Frame, Kemptom, & Armistead, 1991; Hanson, Mackay-Soroka, Staley, & Poulton, 1994; Stickle & Blechman, 2002).

Parenting factors that have been empirically linked to firesetting behavior include harsh or lax discipline, lack of parental involvement, less parental acceptance of the child, and limited monitoring and supervision. Family factors associated with firesetting behavior include low socioeconomic status (SES), marital discord, parental psychopathology/depression, and stressful life events.

The number and nature of risk factors associated with firesetting may vary according to age of onset and persistence of firesetting. McCarty and colleagues (2005) classified youth from a community-based sample into four groups (nonfiresetters, desisters, late-onset firesetters, and persisters) based on their reported firesetting behavior during two developmental periods: prior to fourth grade and between fourth and sixth grade. Firesetters differed from nonfiresetters on 13 of 19 risk factors. Within firesetting groups, most of the differences were between persisters and desisters. Persisters were more likely to exhibit impulsivity/hyperactivity, and their parents demonstrated lower levels of appropriate discipline, higher levels of harsh discipline, and higher levels of maternal depression and spousal hostility. Persisters and desisters had significantly more risk factors than nonfiresetters. The cumulative number of risk factors had a linear relationship with an increased likelihood of firesetting. The percentage of youth who engaged in firesetting was 1.5%, 13.2%, 19.6%, and 40.3% for 0, 1, 2, and 3 or more risk factors.

In the clinical literature, a number of typologies of juvenile firesetting exist. For example, Humphreys, Kopet, and Lajoy (1993) described typologies that include curiosity firesetters (typically younger children), crisis firesetters (firesetting associated with stress or high negative affect), delinquent firesetters (deliberate violations of others' rights), and severely disturbed firesetters (firesetters with major affective instability or disturbed thinking). Although these typologies of firesetting have a certain appeal in terms of face validity, there has been relatively little empirical validation.

Comorbidity and Associated Characteristics

Youth with CP are at increased risk for manifesting a variety of other behavior disorders and adjustment problems as well. These include ADHD; various internalizing disorders, such as anxiety and depressive disorders; somatization disorder (e.g., Loeber & Keenan, 1994); substance use disorders; and academic underachievement (Hinshaw, 1992). In their review of the relationship of CP to various comorbid conditions, Loeber and Keenan (1994) stressed the importance of considering the temporal ordering of comorbid conditions, as well as the different patterns and influences of these comorbid disorders for boys versus girls. For example, although girls are less likely to display CP than are boys, when girls do display CP, they may be more likely than boys to develop one or more of these comorbid disorders.

ADHD is the comorbid condition most commonly associated with CP, and is thought to precede the development of CP in the majority of cases. In fact, some investigators consider ADHD (or, more specifically, the impulsivity or hyperactivity components of ADHD) to be the "motor" that drives the development of early-onset CP, especially for boys (e.g., Burns & Walsh, 2002; Coie & Dodge, 1998; Loeber, Farrington, Stouthamer-Loeber, & Van Kammen, 1998; White et al., 1994). Coexisting ADHD also predicts a more negative life outcome than does CP alone (see Waschbush, 2002). For example, children with both ADHD and CD seem to show a greater variety of delinquent acts in adolescence (Loeber, Brinthaupt, & Green, 1990), a greater number of aggressive acts in adolescence (Moffitt, 1993), and increased APD and more violent offending in adulthood (Fischer, Barkley, Smallish, & Fletcher, 2002; Klinteberg, Andersson, Magnusson, & Stattin, 1993). Some have suggested that comorbid ADHD and CP warrants separate diagnostic status (e.g., Angold & Costello, 2001).

Internalizing disorders, such as the depressive and anxiety disorders and somatization disorder, also co-occur with CP at rates higher than expected by chance (Zoccolillo, 1992). In most cases, CP precedes the onset of depressive symptoms (Loeber & Keenan, 1994), although in some cases depression may precede CP behavior (e.g., Kovacs, Paulauskas, Gatsonis,

& Richards, 1988). However, this relationship between CP and depression may be due to common risk factors as opposed to a causal relationship (Fergusson, Lynskey, & Horwood, 1996). Also, the relationship appears to differ for boys and girls, at least during middle to late adolescence. Wiesner (2003) found a reciprocal relationship between delinquent behaviors and depressive symptoms for girls, whereas for boys, there was a unidirectional effect of delinquent behavior on depressive symptoms. Risk for suicidality has been shown to increase as a function of preexisting CP (e.g., Capaldi, 1991, 1992), and this risk appears to be higher for girls than for boys (Loeber & Keenan, 1994). In addition, Loeber and Keenan (1994) indicate that the co-occurrence of anxiety disorders with CP is also especially likely for girls. In some studies, children with CP and a comorbid anxiety disorder are less seriously impaired than are children with CP alone (e.g., Walker et al., 1991); in other studies, the presence of a comorbid anxiety disorder has not been shown to have a differential effect (e.g., Campbell & Ewing, 1990); and yet in others, comorbid anxiety is associated with increased risk (e.g., Serbin, Moskowitz, Schwartzman, & Ledingham, 1991). Current investigators (e.g., Hinshaw & Lee, 2003; Lahey & Waldman, 2003) have noted the importance of distinguishing between anxiety based on inhibition and fear (which appears to be protective) and anxiety based on social withdrawal due to emotional negativity (which seems to increase risk) as a means of interpreting these apparently contradictory findings. It is notable that although the base rate of somatization disorder alone is much higher in girls than in boys, its comorbid occurrence with CP may actually be higher in boys (Lilienfeld, 1992; Offord, Alder, & Boyle, 1986).

In a review of 20 population-based studies examining the comorbidity of CD/ODD with other disorders, Angold and Costello (2001) noted that the joint odds ratios (OR) of CD/ODD with either ADHD (OR = 10.7) or depression (OR = 6.6) were significantly higher than the OR with anxiety (OR = 3.1). They concluded that the apparent comorbidity of CD/ODD with anxiety may be due to the co-occurrence of anxiety with depression and ADHD rather than representing an independent comorbid relationship with CD/ODD (Angold, Costello, & Erkanli, 1999).

Both longitudinal and cross-sectional studies have documented that preexisting CP constitutes a significant risk factor for substance use (e.g., Angold et al., 1999; Hawkins, Catalano, & Miller, 1992). This may be particularly true for girls (Loeber & Keenan, 1994). The comorbidity between CP and substance abuse is important because, when youth with CP also abuse substances, they tend to show an early onset of substance use and they are more likely to abuse multiple substances (Lynskey & Fergusson, 1995). They may be at increased risk of more serious delinquent behavior (Angold et al., 1999). Although most of the research on the association between CP and substance abuse prior to adulthood has been conducted with adolescents, the association between CP and substance use may begin much earlier in development (Van Kammen, Loeber, & Stouthamer-Loeber, 1991).

An association between CP and academic underachievement has long been noted. In a comprehensive review, Hinshaw (1992) concluded that during preadolescence, this relationship is actually a function of comorbid ADHD rather than of CP per se. In adolescence, the relationship is more complex, with preexisting ADHD (and perhaps other neuropsychological deficits), a history of academic difficulty and failure, and long-standing socialization difficulties with family and peers all playing interacting roles. It is also important to note that the relationship between CP and academic achievement is a transactional one that plays out across the developmental period (Hinshaw & Lee, 2003).

An issue of ongoing debate concerns the extent to which CP in adolescence is most appropriately conceptualized as part of a unitary behavior problem syndrome (problem behavior theory; Jessor, 1998; Jessor & Jessor, 1977) or as one of several different but related types of behavior problems (e.g., Fergusson, Horwood, & Lynskey, 1994). The range of behavior problems considered in problem behavior theory has typically included CP, various forms of substance use, and risky sexual behavior (Biglan, Brennan, Foster, & Holder, 2004), although Jessor (1998) and others (e.g., Loeber et al., 1998) have more recently broadened the theory to include ADHD and internalizing disorders, school failure, and health behavior. Space considerations preclude a thorough examination of this issue. Although it is quite clear that CP is associated with a variety of other behavior problems and disorders during childhood *and* adolescence, the evidence that this spectrum of behaviors reflects a single underlying dimension is mixed. For example, Fergusson and colleagues (1994) found four latent classes of problem behavior in their sample of 15-year-olds from New Zealand: (1) low problem behaviors of any type (85.4% of the sample); (2) high risk of precocious sexual behavior, alcohol use, and marijuana use (5.2%); (3) high risk of CP, police contact, and marijuana use (6.7%); and (4) elevated risks for all problem behaviors (2.7%). The model applied equally well for boys and girls, but among girls, the predominant pattern was that of precocious sexual activity and alcohol and marijuana use (9.4% vs. 3.6% for boys). For boys, the CP pattern was predominant (6.1% vs. 3.6% for girls). The multiproblem class included 3.3% of boys and 2.0% of girls. Fergusson and colleagues concluded that their findings were not generally supportive of problem behavior theory. Although there was a group of multiproblem youth, they accounted for less than 15% of the youth engaging in problem behaviors.

EPIDEMIOLOGY

Prevalence

CP is among the most frequently occurring child behavior disorders. However, determining accurate estimates of prevalence has proven to be quite difficult as a function of the various changes in diagnostic criteria for both ODD and CD over the various DSM revisions, whether an impairment criterion is included, the informant (i.e., youth, parent, teacher, and clinician), and the method of combining information from various informants (Essau, 2003). Averaging across 20 population-based studies conducted in the United States, Puerto Rico, Holland, and New Zealand, Angold and Costello (2001) reported that on average 5–10% of youth ages 8–16 years demonstrated CD or ODD (the diagnoses were combined in their analyses). Prevalence rates generally range from 1% to 9% for CD and 2% to 10% for ODD in various nonclinic samples (e.g., Essau, 2003; Lahey, Miller, Gordon, & Riley, 1999). Adolescents tend to report more frequent engagement in CD behaviors than do their parents. For example, in a sample of 13- to 18-

year-old Dutch adolescents, the 6-month prevalence of CD was 5.6% and 1.2% based on adolescent and parent reports, respectively (Verhulst, van der Ende, Ferdinand, & Kasius, 1997). This is likely due at least in part to parental unawareness of their offspring's engagement in covert forms of CP behavior. The prevalence figures for ODD were the same for adolescent and parent informants (0.7% and 0.6%, respectively).

Age of Onset and Sex Differences

Prevalence rates have been shown to vary as a function of age and sex of the child, as well as the type of CP behavior. For example, younger children are more likely to engage in oppositional, overt behaviors, whereas older children and adolescents are more likely to engage in more covert CP behavior (e.g., stealing) (Patterson & Yoerger, 2002). Because the specific CP behaviors required for a DSM diagnosis of CD generally occur much more frequently in older children and adolescents, it is much more difficult for younger children to receive a CD diagnosis. In fact, there is a paucity of data concerning the diagnostic criteria for ODD and CD as they might be applied to children younger than age 7 (Angold & Costello, 2001; Keenan & Wakschlag, 2002), although the ability to identify an externalizing broadband syndrome of CP is well established in these younger children (e.g., Campbell, 2002).

In general, boys are more likely to begin engaging in overt CP behaviors earlier and at higher rates than girls throughout the developmental period. In fact, gender is the most consistently documented risk factor for CP (Robins, 1991). Perhaps due to the lower rates of antisocial behavior in girls, much of the research on CP has focused exclusively on boys or, when girls have been included, has failed to consider possible gender effects. Many questions about the onset and development of CP behavior in girls remain unanswered. However, some evidence does suggest that compared to boys, girls' CP behavior tends to be less chronic, more experimental, and more likely to desist. Most of the sex differences in CD are probably due to the increased prevalence of physical aggression among boys (Angold & Costello, 2001). As noted earlier, even this sex difference may be attenuated or disappear when more socially oriented forms of aggression (e.g., relational aggression), which occur more frequently among girls, are incorporated into the definition of aggression. During adolescence, gender differences in prevalence decrease dramatically; this seems to be largely accounted for by an increase in the number of girls engaging in covert CP behaviors. However, gender differences in ODD, in which more boys than girls are diagnosed prior to adolescence, also disappear for the most part during adolescence (APA, 2000). There is an increase in oppositional behavior during adolescence for both boys and girls (e.g., McDermott, 1996). For a comprehensive discussion of CP in girls, the reader is referred to recent volumes by Putallaz and Bierman (2004); Moretti, Odgers, and Jackson (2004); Pepler, Madsen, Webster, and Levene (2005); and Underwood (2003).

Continuity and Adult Outcomes

There is a high degree of continuity in CP behaviors from infancy to early childhood (e.g., Keenan, Shaw, Delliquadri, Giovannelli, & Walsh, 1998), from early childhood to later childhood (e.g., Campbell, 1995), from childhood to adolescence (e.g., Lahey, Loeber, Burke, & Rathouz, 2002; Offord et al., 1992), and from adolescence to adulthood (e.g., Farrington, 2003; Rutter, Harrington, Quinton, & Pickles, 1994). There is also evidence for cross-generational consistency (e.g., Huesmann, Eron, Lefkowitz, & Walder, 1984; Loeber et al., 2003). Furthermore, stability appears comparable for boys and girls (e.g., Coie & Dodge, 1998; Stanger, Achenbach, & Verhulst, 1997). In general, youth with CP are at increased risk for a broad spectrum of negative outcomes that extend beyond APD and criminal activity to family instability and poor educational and health outcomes (see Maughan & Rutter, 2001, for a review). Both boys and girls with CP are at increased risk as adults for engaging in criminal activity (e.g., Keenan, Loeber, & Green, 1999; Kratzer & Hodgins, 1997; Pajer, 1998); girls also seem to be more at risk for a broad array of other adverse outcomes, including various internalizing disorders (e.g., Bardone, Moffitt, Caspi, Dickson, & Silva, 1996; Pajer, 1998). One outcome of adolescent CP in girls is increased risk for early pregnancy, which, in conjunction with other risk factors associated with adolescent pregnancy (and the mother's own CP), increases the risk for the eventual development of CP in the offspring (e.g., Stack, Serbin, Schwartzman, & Leding-

ham, 2005; Zoccolillo, Paquette, & Tremblay, 2005).

DEVELOPMENTAL COURSE, OUTCOMES, AND POTENTIAL ETIOLOGICAL FACTORS

The preceding description of CP and various comorbid conditions fails to convey three different but related considerations that must guide assessment and intervention procedures for adolescents with CP: the developmental, contextual, and transactional aspects of CP (McMahon & Estes, 1997). With respect to developmental considerations, it is clear that the behavioral manifestations of CP (as well as the base rates of various comorbid disorders) change over time. With respect to context, the development and maintenance of CP are influenced by genetic/constitutional characteristics of the child, family, peers, and broader ecologies. Ethnicity and cultural considerations may also apply to these contexts (e.g., Prinz & Miller, 1991). By "transactional," we mean that these developmental and contextual processes unfold over time and continuously influence one another.

Space considerations preclude an extensive description of the roles these various developmental, contextual, and transactional influences play in the development and maintenance of CP. Instead, we present summary descriptions of two developmental progressions of CP as a means of illustrating many of these influences. The reader is referred to several recent excellent sources for more extensive treatment of these issues (Dodge & Pettit, 2003; Lahey, Moffitt, & Caspi, 2003; Moffitt, 2003; Patterson & Yoerger, 2002; Thornberry & Krohn, 2003).

Early-Starter Pathway

The most thoroughly delineated pathway, and the one that seems to have the most negative longterm prognosis, has been referred to as the early-starter (Patterson, Capaldi, & Bank, 1991) or life-course-persistent (Moffitt, 1993, 2003) pathway. The childhood-onset type of CD in DSM-IV-TR (APA, 2000) would seem to be a likely diagnostic outcome of this pathway. The early-starter pathway is characterized by the onset of CP in the preschool and early school-age years, and by a high degree of continuity throughout childhood and into adolescence and adulthood. It is thought that these youth progress from relatively less serious to more serious CP behaviors over time; that overt behaviors appear earlier than covert behaviors; and that later CP behaviors expand the youth's behavioral repertoire rather than replacing earlier behaviors (Edelbrock, 1985; Loeber & Farrington, 2000; Patterson, Forgatch, Yoerger, & Stoolmiller, 1998; Patterson & Yoerger, 2002). Furthermore, there is an expansion of the settings in which the CP behaviors occur over time, from the home to other settings such as the school and the broader community. The risk for continuing on this developmental pathway through the elementary school years and into adolescence may be as high as 50% for children who display CP behaviors at ages 3 and 4 (Campbell, 1995). In the Dunedin study, this pathway was much more common in boys than girls (5–10% vs. 1%) (Moffitt, Caspi, Rutter, & Silva, 2001).

As we present in detail later, characteristics of the child (e.g., temperament and social cognitive skills) and the family (e.g., insecure attachment and coercive patterns of interaction) can lead to the development of high levels of child noncompliance and other CP behaviors in the preschool years. Upon school entry, the child's coercive style of interaction with parents and siblings is likely to extend to interactions with teachers and peers, resulting in frequent disciplinary confrontations with school personnel, rejection by peers, and continued coercive interchanges with parents (some of which now center around school-related problems) (e.g., Patterson et al., 1992). Difficulties in the acquisition of basic academic skills are most likely consequences of preexisting neuropsychological deficits (which now may be manifested as verbal deficits, self-control difficulties, social-cognitive deficits and biases, and/or ADHD), as well as the child's coercive interactional style. The CP behaviors may become more serious, more frequent, and more covert (e.g., stealing) during the elementary school years.

By age 10 or 11, this recurrent constellation of negative events places the child at increased risk for association with deviant peer groups in middle school and high school (with a likely escalation in the CP behaviors) and/or for depression. The role of the peer group in the maintenance and escalation of CP behaviors during middle and late childhood and early adolescence has been documented in several longitudinal investigations, in terms of both peer

rejection (e.g., Coie, Lochman, Terry, & Hyman, 1992) and subsequent involvement with antisocial peers (e.g., Dishion, Patterson, Stoolmiller, & Skinner, 1991). Peer rejection in childhood may operate to increase subsequent CP behavior by excluding the child from opportunities for peer socialization, by modeling of CP behavior by other rejected children, or by demoralization due to peer rejection (Hinshaw & Lee, 2003). Association with a deviant peer group provides multiple and repeated opportunities for the modeling of, practice in, and reinforcement of a wide variety of CP behaviors (e.g., Dishion, Patterson, & Griesler, 1994; Lacourse, Nagin, Tremblay, Vitaro, & Claes, 2003).

Children with CP are also at increased risk for depression by the time they reach adolescence. Capaldi (1991, 1992) found co-occurrence of CP and depressive symptoms in an at-risk community sample of early adolescent boys in sixth grade. Over the next 2 years, the boys with CP and depressive symptoms displayed higher levels of suicidal ideation than boys with only CP or only depressive symptoms. They also displayed poor academic achievement and a high arrest rate (65%) by eighth grade. The boys with CP who were depressed also appeared to initiate substance use at an earlier age than boys with only CP. Adolescent girls' risk for both CP and depressive behavior at age 16 was associated with family and sibling coercive processes in childhood and adolescence (Compton, Snyder, Schrepferman, Bank, & Shortt, 2003). (The coercive processes predicted CP but not depressive behavior for boys.)

Early menarche appears to be a significant risk factor for CP in adolescent girls, particularly if they already have a history of CP (Moffitt, Caspi, Belsky, & Silva, 1992). An increased likelihood of exposure to older males with CP is a potential consequence (Caspi, Lynam, Moffitt, & Silva, 1993).

It is not surprising that adolescents who have progressed along the early-starter pathway are at significant risk for continuing to engage in more serious CP behaviors throughout adolescence and into adulthood (e.g., Farrington, 2003; Moffitt, Caspi, Harrington, & Milne, 2002; Rutter et al., 1994). As adults, such individuals are not only at high risk for subsequent diagnosis of APD but also at increased risk for other psychiatric diagnoses and a variety of negative life outcomes (e.g., lower occupational adjustment and educational attainment, poorer physical health) (e.g., Farrington, 2003; Kratzer & Hodgins, 1997; Moffitt et al., 2002). For example, in the Dunedin Multidisciplinary Health Study, at age 26, males who exhibited this early-starting pattern of CP had two to three times as many convictions as adults than did the late-starting youth; were more likely to exhibit substance use problems and APD symptoms; engaged in more domestic violence; and were more likely to lack minimal education credentials; to have a poor work history in low-status, unskilled jobs; and to have married antisocial women (Moffitt et al., 2002).

Risk Factors

There is a growing body of evidence concerning the many individual, familial, and broader contextual factors that may increase the likelihood of a child's entering and progressing along the early-starter pathway (see Dodge & Pettit, 2003; Leve & Chamberlain, 2005; Loeber & Farrington, 2000; Patterson et al., 1998; Shaw, Bell, & Gilliom, 2000; for reviews). Child factors that may increase risk for entering the early-starter pathway include hyperactivity (e.g., Loeber & Keenan, 1994; Moffitt, 1993) and a difficult temperament (Frick & Morris, 2004; Moffitt, 1993). Moffitt posits that subtle neuropsychological variations in the infant's central nervous system, which could be due to a variety of prenatal, perinatal, and/or postnatal difficulties (e.g., exposure to toxic agents, birth complications, and heredity), increase the likelihood that the infant will be "temperamentally difficult," displaying characteristics such as irritability, hyperactivity, impulsivity, and the like.

The role of child temperament (usually viewed as involving relatively stable innate personality characteristics) has received increased attention from clinicians as a possible contributing factor to conduct problems (e.g., Frick & Morris, 2004). Of particular interest is the "temperamentally difficult" child who, from very early in life, is intense, irregular, negative, and nonadaptable (Thomas, Chess, & Birch, 1968). Such a child is thought to be predisposed to the development of subsequent behavior problems, due to the increased likelihood of maladaptive interactions with family members. However, temperament has often been found to have a low to moderate relation to subse-

quent CP in early and middle childhood at best (e.g., Bates, Bayles, Bennett, Ridge, & Brown, 1991), and in some cases, to have no relation (Aguilar, Sroufe, Egeland, & Carlson, 2000). Other investigators have shown that it is the combination of difficult temperament in infancy with other concurrently measured risk factors, such as maternal perception of difficulty, male gender, prematurity, and low SES (Sanson, Oberklaid, Pedlow, & Prior, 1991), or inappropriate parenting (Bates et al., 1991), that best predicts subsequent CP.

The development of the child's social-cognitive skills may also be affected by these neuropsychological deficits (e.g., Coie & Dodge, 1998; Crick & Dodge, 1994).[1] Children with CP have deficits in encoding (e.g., lack of attention to relevant social cues and hypervigilant biases), to make more hostile attributional biases and errors in the interpretation of social cues, to have deficient quantity and quality of generated solutions to social situations, to evaluate aggressive solutions more positively, and to be more likely to decide to engage in aggressive behavior. These deficiencies and biases in social-cognitive skills predict the subsequent development of CP in kindergarten and are associated with parental report of earlier harsh disciplinary practices (Weiss, Dodge, Bates, & Pettit, 1992).

These child characteristics (i.e., difficult temperamental style and deficits in social information processing) may increase risk for both the development of an insecure attachment to the parent (DeKlyen & Speltz, 2001; Greenberg, 1999) and a coercive style of interaction with family members (Patterson et al., 1992; Snyder & Stoolmiller, 2002). Both of these interaction patterns have been implicated in the development of CP. However, the relationship between security of attachment in infancy and later CP has been inconsistent. Attachment researchers (e.g., Greenberg, 1999) have noted the necessity of adopting a transactional perspective in that attachment security is likely mediated by other risk or protective factors (e.g., parenting practices, maternal depression, and family adversity) over time.

The critical role of parenting practices in the development and maintenance of CP has been well established. Types of parenting practices that have been closely associated with the development of child CP include inconsistent discipline, irritable explosive discipline, low supervision and involvement, and inflexible rigid discipline (Chamberlain, Reid, Ray, Capaldi, & Fisher, 1997). Indeed, physical abuse is a clear risk factor for the development of CP (Dodge, Bates, & Pettit, 1990; Jaffee, Caspi, Moffitt, & Taylor, 2004).

The most comprehensive family-based formulation for the early-starter pathway has been the coercion model developed by Patterson and his colleagues (e.g., Patterson, 1982, 2002; Patterson et al., 1992; Snyder, Reid, & Patterson, 2003). The model describes a process of "basic training" in CP behaviors that occurs in the context of an escalating cycle of coercive parent–child interactions in the home that begins prior to school entry. The proximal cause for entry into the coercive cycle is thought to be ineffective parental management strategies, particularly in regard to child compliance with parental directives during the preschool period. As this process continues over long periods, significant increases in the rate and intensity of these coercive behaviors occur as family members are reinforced by engaging in aggressive behaviors. Furthermore, the child also observes his or her parents engaging in coercive responses, and this provides the opportunity for modeling of aggression to occur (Patterson, 1982). Coercive interactions with siblings also play an important role in the development of CP (Garcia, Shaw, Winslow, & Yaggi, 2000; Snyder & Stoolmiller, 2002). Siblings of children with CP often engage in comparable levels of coercive behavior, and coercive parent–child interactions interact with sibling coercion and conflict to predict subsequent child CP. Although the coercion process begins early in the developmental period, it continues into adolescence (Snyder et al., 2003).

Various other risk factors that may have an impact on the family and serve to precipitate or maintain child CP have been identified. These include familial factors such as parental social cognitions, parental personal and marital adjustment, other familial stressors, and certain extrafamilial factors (e.g., Capaldi, DeGarmo, Patterson, & Forgatch, 2002; Coie & Jacobs, 1993; Ingoldsby & Shaw, 2002; Leve & Chamberlain, 2005; Wakschlag & Keenan, 2001), such as low SES, neighborhood risk, and parental insularity/low social support. Less clear are the mechanisms by which these factors exert their effects on CP and on one another, the extent to which child CP may reciprocally influence them, and the role of timing and dura-

tion (Kazdin, 1995b). For example, these risk factors may have a direct effect on child CP, or they may exert their effects by disrupting parenting practices (Patterson et al., 1992). In some cases, the "risk" factor may be a *result* of CP, rather than a potential cause. With these caveats in mind, we note some of the relationships of these factors to CP.

Parents of children with CP display more maladaptive social cognitions, and they experience more personal (e.g., depression and antisocial behavior), interparental (marital problems), and extrafamilial (e.g., isolation) distress than do parents of nonreferred children. It has been suggested that these stressors may interact to impede parental tracking of child behavior and lead to perceptual biases (Wahler & Dumas, 1989). With respect to social cognitions, Johnston (1996) has proposed a model that places parental cognitions (expectancies, perceptions, and attributions concerning child behavior and sense of parenting efficacy) in a mediational role vis-à-vis parenting behavior. Parents of clinic-referred children with CP are more likely to misperceive child behaviors (Holleran, Littman, Freund, & Schmaling, 1982; Middlebrook & Forehand, 1985; Wahler & Sansbury, 1990), to have fewer positive and more negative family-referent cognitions (Sanders & Dadds, 1992), and to perceive CP behaviors as intentional and to attribute them to stable and global causes (Baden & Howe, 1992; MacBrayer, Milich, & Hundley, 2003). Furthermore, these negative perceptions of the child are associated with higher levels of maternal anger and overreactivity in child discipline (Slep & O'Leary, 1998). Sense of parenting efficacy has been shown to relate negatively to child CP in both clinic-referred and nonreferred samples (e.g., Johnston & Mash, 1989; Roberts, Joe, & Rowe-Hallbert, 1992).

Maternal depression is related to a broad spectrum of child behavior disorders, including CP (e.g., Cummings & Davies, 1994b; Goodman & Gottlib, 1999). Some evidence suggests that not only may maternal depression have an adverse effect on the mothers' parenting behavior, but it may also negatively bias maternal perceptions of children with CP (e.g., Dumas & Serketich, 1994; Fergusson, Lynskey, & Horwood, 1993; Forehand, Lautenschlager, Faust, & Graziano, 1986). However, others have presented evidence suggesting that depressed mothers do not possess a negative perceptual bias in their reports of their children's CP behaviors and that they may be accurate reporters (Richters, 1992). There is evidence of a reciprocal relationship between maternal depression and child adjustment problems, including CP (Elgar, McGrath, Waschbusch, Stewart, & Curtis, 2004). Chronicity of maternal depression may be particularly related to child CP (Alpern & Lyons-Ruth, 1993; Fergusson & Lynskey, 1993).

Parental antisocial behavior has received increasing attention as both a direct and an indirect influence on the development and maintenance of CP. Links between parental criminality, aggressive behavior, and a diagnosis of APD and childhood delinquency, aggression, and CD/ODD diagnoses have been reported by a number of investigators (see Frick & Loney, 2002, for a review; see Leve & Chamberlain, 2005, for a consideration of this risk factor in girls). This association appears specific to CP, occurs more frequently in parents whose children are diagnosed with CD rather than ODD (but see Frick et al., 1993), and is not associated with increased occurrence of ADHD or other child disorders (Frick et al., 1992). There is some evidence to suggest that parental antisocial behavior may play a more central role than other risk factors in its effect on parenting practices and child CP (e.g., Capaldi et al., 2002; Frick et al., 1992; Leve & Chamberlain, 2005; Patterson et al., 1992). For example, in a sample of boys at high risk for CP, Patterson and colleagues (1992) reported that both paternal and maternal antisocial behavior was negatively correlated with parenting practices; furthermore, parental antisocial behavior mediated the effect of social disadvantage and divorce/remarriage transitions in predicting parental practices. Thus, parental antisocial behaviors may have a direct impact on child behavior, may have an indirect impact on child behavior through parenting, and may play a role in the relationship between other family and extrafamilial variables and parenting.

Similarly, parental substance abuse has been associated with youth CP and substance use, at least partly because of its association with disrupted parenting practices (Dishion, Reid, & Patterson, 1988; Wills, Schreibman, Benson, & Vaccaro, 1994). Observations of parent–child interactions in families with parental alcohol problems suggest that the parents are less able to engage their children and are less congenial (Jacob, Krahn, & Leonard, 1991; Whipple, Fitzgerald, & Zucker, 1995). Furthermore, alcohol consumption by parents can influence parental perceptions of children's behavior and has a negative impact on parenting behaviors displayed toward children (e.g., inadequate monitoring, inconsistent and harsh discipline, indulgence, and less problem solving) (El-Sheikh & Flanagan, 2001; Lang, Pelham, Atkeson, & Murphy, 1999; Pelham & Lang, 1993; Whipple et al., 1995). In a review of laboratory studies examining the effects of alcohol consumption on parent–child interaction, Pelham and Lang (1993) concluded not only that alcohol consumption had a deleterious effect on parenting practices but that the children's inappropriate behavior increased parental alcohol consumption (for parents with a positive family history of alcohol problems) and distress (for all parents), thus perpetuating the cycle.

Marital distress and conflict have been shown to be associated with child CP, negative parenting behavior, and parental perceptions of child maladjustment (Amato & Keith, 1991; Cummings & Davies, 1994a). The most commonly offered hypothesis for the relationship has been that marital distress or conflict interferes with the parents' ability to engage in appropriate parenting practices, which then leads to child CP (e.g., Emery, 1999); however, other explanations are possible (see Rutter, 1994). These include direct modeling of aggressive and coercive behavior and the cumulative stressful effects of such conflict, including maternal depression. It has been suggested that both child CP and parental marital distress/conflict may be the result of parental antisocial behavior (Frick, 1994). Child characteristics such as age and gender appear to moderate the relationship between specific aspects of marital adjustment and CP (Dadds & Powell, 1991; Katz & Gottman, 1993). Some investigators (e.g., Abidin & Brunner, 1995; Jouriles et al., 1991; Porter & O'Leary, 1980) have focused more narrowly on specific aspects of marital conflict that relate directly to parenting, such as disagreement over childrearing practices, marital conflict in a child's presence, or the strength of the parenting alliance. There is some indication that these more narrowly focused constructs may demonstrate stronger relationships to CP than may broader constructs such as marital distress.

Parents of children with CP also appear to experience higher frequencies of stressful events, both minor ones (e.g., daily hassles) and those of a more significant nature (e.g., unemployment and major transitions) (Capaldi et al., 2002; Leve & Chamberlain, 2005; Webster-Stratton, 1990). The effects of stress on child CP may be mediated through maladaptive parental social cognitions (e.g., Johnston, 1996; Wahler & Dumas, 1989) and parenting practices such as disrupted parental discipline (e.g., Forgatch, Patterson, & Skinner, 1988; Snyder, 1991), although the role of parenting behavior in mediating the association between parenting stress and child adjustment has not yet been rigorously tested (Deater-Deckard, 1998).

CP has been associated with a number of extrafamilial factors (Capaldi et al., 2002; Coie & Jacobs, 1993), such as low SES (Dodge, Pettit, & Bates, 1994), neighborhood risk (Ingoldsby & Shaw, 2002), and parental insularity/low social support (Jennings, Stagg, & Connors, 1991; Wahler, Leske, & Rogers, 1979). However, it is important to note that the relationship of SES with CP appears to be largely mediated by parenting practices (e.g., Capaldi & Patterson, 1994). On the other hand, neighborhood risk has been shown to operate as an independent risk factor (e.g., Gorman-Smith, Tolan, & Henry, 2000). Some parents of children with CP may be quite isolated from friends, neighbors, and the community. Wahler and his colleagues have developed a construct called "insularity," which is defined as a "specific pattern of social contacts within the community that is characterized by a high level of negatively perceived coercive interchanges with relatives and/or helping agency representatives and by a low level of positively perceived supportive interchanges with friends" (Wahler & Dumas, 1984, p. 387). Insularity is positively related to negative parent behavior directed toward children and oppositional child behavior directed toward parents (Dumas & Wahler, 1985; Wahler, 1980). It has also been associated with poor maintenance of treatment effects (e.g., Dumas & Wahler, 1983). Thus, when a mother has a large proportion of aversive interactions outside the home, the interactions between the mother and her child in the home are likely to be negative as well.

Not surprisingly, youth who follow the early-starter pathway are at greatly increased risk for negative outcomes as adults. In their follow-up of these individuals at age 26, Moffitt et al. (2002) found criminal conviction rates to be two to three times greater for the early starters than for the late starters. This was especially the case for more serious offenses, including violence. Family violence is also more common in the early starter group (Moffitt et al., 2002; Woodward, Fergusson, & Horwood, 2002). As adults, early starters were also more likely to work in low-status, unskilled jobs; to lack minimal education credentials; and to have increased levels of substance use problems.

Late-Starter Pathway

A second major pathway for the development of CP has been proposed, but there has been less consistency in how it has been described. In general, this second pathway begins in adolescence rather than early childhood; it is also thought to result in less serious forms of CP (e.g., property offenses rather than violent offenses) and to have a higher rate of desistance. However, more children are involved in this pathway than in the early-starter pathway (e.g., 24% vs. 7%, respectively, in the Dunedin study; Moffitt, Caspi, Dickson, Silva, & Stanton, 1996), and it is roughly comparable between boys and girls (Moffitt et al., 2001). It has been referred to as the late-starter (Patterson et al., 1991) or adolescence-limited (Moffitt, 1993) pathway. The adolescent-onset type of CD in DSM-IV-TR (APA, 2000) would seem to be a likely diagnostic outcome of this pathway.

Empirical support for the late-starter pathway has been provided in both epidemiological (e.g., McGee, Feehan, Williams, & Anderson, 1992; Moffitt, 1990; Moffitt et al., 1996; Piquero & Brezina, 2000) and high-risk (e.g., Loeber et al., 1993) samples. In the Dunedin sample, a large increase in nonaggressive (but not aggressive) CP behaviors was noted between ages 11 and 15 for both boys and girls (McGee et al., 1992). Moffitt (1990) found that the late starters made up 73% of her delinquent sample of boys at age 13, and had levels of CP behaviors at age 13 comparable to those displayed by the early-starter boys. However, in contrast to the early-starter boys, the late-starter boys had engaged in very low levels of CP in childhood, and there was no evidence of verbal IQ deficits, reading difficulties, preexisting family adversity, temperamental difficulty (Moffitt et al., 1996), or perinatal or motor skills difficulties. Furthermore, they were less likely to have been convicted of violent criminal offenses than were the early-starter boys (Moffitt et al., 1996). Moffitt and colleagues (2001) found that the risk factors associated with the late-starter pathway were comparable for boys and girls. Capaldi and Patterson (1994) presented data on a high-risk sample indicating that late-starter boys were less likely than early-starter boys to live in families characterized by inappropriate parental discipline practices, unemployment, divorce, parental antisocial behavior, and low SES. Association with a deviant peer group was especially salient for the late-starter boys.

Moffitt (1993, 2003) posits that participation in CP behaviors by late starters is a form of social mimicry of early starters that is one way of asserting independence from the family. Initial empirical support for this proposition was provided by Piquero and Brezina (2000), who found that late starters were more likely to commit "rebellious" rather than aggressive offenses, and that both maturational timing and aspects of personal autonomy related to peers were associated with this form of CP behavior. The basis for desistance among the late starters is thought to be the gradual increase in opportunities to engage in more legitimate adult roles and activities as these adolescents grow older. However, the likelihood of desistance is decreased to the extent that adolescents are caught in "snares" (e.g., incarceration and dropout). Patterson and colleagues (e.g., Patterson & Yoerger, 2002) have hypothesized that the process leading to the late-starter pathway begins in families that have marginally effective family management skills. Inadequate parental supervision in middle and high school increase the likelihood of significant involvement in a deviant peer group. However, because these adolescents have a higher level of social skills and a longer learning history of employing such skills successfully than do early starters, they are far less likely to continue to engage in CP behaviors than are early starters.

Nonetheless, there is evidence suggesting that adolescents who develop CP through the late-starter pathway may still be at substantial risk for future maladjustment. Moffitt and colleagues (2002) reported that at age 26, the original adolescent-limited boys had elevated convictions for property and drug offenses. They postulated that these individuals were still in a "maturity gap" that prevented them from assuming adult roles. Hämäläinen and Pulkkinen (1996) found that late starters constituted nearly one-third of their group of young adult (age 27) criminal offenders. At age 32, males classified as late starters reported that they continued to fight, commit various offenses, and abuse substances, although this was not reflected in official records (Nagin, Farrington, & Moffitt, 1995).

Other Developmental Pathways

Identification of the early-starter and late-starter pathways nearly 15 years ago has stimulated a tremendous amount of research concerning developmental pathways of CP. In addition to validating and clarifying the nature of these two pathways, this research has also identified other pathways. For example, Loeber and colleagues (1993, 2003) have identified three pathways: authority conflict (i.e., noncompliance and defiance), overt (i.e., fighting and severe violence), and covert (i.e., property damage and serious delinquency). Movement across pathways for individual youth is fluid, and some will be on more than one pathway at a given point in development. These pathways have been replicated in European American, African American, and Hispanic samples (Loeber et al., 2003; Tolan et al., 2000).

Hinshaw and Lee (2003) suggest that there are at least three developmental pathways that have childhood onset of CP as a common starting point: (1) early starters (who persist in their CP behavior), (2) desisters, and (3) "low-level chronics," who engage in relatively low but persistent levels of CP throughout the developmental period and into adulthood (e.g., Fergusson, Horwood, & Nagin, 2000). With respect to the desisters, as noted previously, it is estimated that 50% of children who demonstrate high levels of CP behavior during the preschool period will not follow the early-starter progression of increasingly severe CP as they get older (Campbell, 1995). With respect to the low-level chronic offenders, in Moffitt's earlier work (e.g., Moffitt et al., 1996) she identified a third group of youth in the Dunedin sample that were originally labeled the "recovery" group. This group was characterized by high levels of CP during childhood but only moderate levels during adolescence.

However, at the age 26 follow-up, these individuals were engaging in low but consistent levels of offending (Moffitt et al., 2002). In addition, they displayed high levels of internalizing problems such as depression and anxiety disorders and were impaired on a variety of life outcome indicators such as education, occupational status, and degree of optimism.

Other hypothesized pathways include a delayed-onset pathway for CP in girls (Silverthorn & Frick, 1999), and as noted previously, Frick and colleagues (2000) have suggested that youth with CP who display CU traits represent a specific subtype of the early-starter pathway. Other investigators have identified multiple trajectories for individual forms of CP behavior, such as physical aggression, vandalism, and stealing (e.g., Broidy et al., 2003; Lacourse et al., 2002).

Although ongoing research will most certainly lead to further development and delineation of the aforementioned pathways, current versions illustrate the value of adopting a developmental perspective for constructing an accurate and useful conceptual framework for the assessment and treatment of children and adolescents with CP. We now turn to a discussion of the assessment process itself.

ASSESSMENT

The delineation of different developmental pathways of CP has a number of important implications for the assessment of youth with CP (McMahon & Estes, 1997; McMahon & Frick, 2005). First, the assessment must be developmentally sensitive, not only with respect to the adolescent's age and sex but also in terms of the adolescent's status and progression on a particular developmental pathway of CP. The heterogeneity of CP in youth requires that the assessment of these behaviors be focused broadly. In adolescence, this also includes the assessment of delinquent behaviors. The possibility of comorbid conditions such as ADHD, internalizing disorders, and substance use should also be investigated. The assessment must also be contextually sensitive and look at CP behavior and other behavior problems as well as other youth characteristics and familial and peer influences. Furthermore, this assessment must examine the broader ecologies of home, school, neighborhood, and community to the extent that each is warranted. Cultural sensitivity in the development, administration,

and interpretation of assessment instruments also requires increased attention (Prinz & Miller, 1991). Finally, the clinician needs to recognize the transactional nature of these developmental and contextual processes and conduct the assessment accordingly. In addition to focusing on each of these issues, a proper assessment of the adolescent with CP must make use of multiple methods completed by multiple informants concerning the adolescent's behavior in multiple settings and the familial and extrafamilial context in which the adolescent functions must also be assessed (McMahon & Estes, 1997; McMahon & Frick, 2005).

CP Behavior Per Se and in an Interactional Context

To obtain an accurate representation of the referred youth's CP behavior, the therapist must rely on multiple assessment methods, including interviews with the parents, youth, and other relevant parties (e.g., teachers), and behavior rating scales completed by the same individuals. Although direct behavioral observations of adolescents in the clinic, home, and/or school settings are desirable, clinicians have somewhat fewer observational tools at their disposal than when assessing younger children (see McMahon & Estes, 1997).

Interviews

Interviews conducted with youth with CP and their families and other important adults (e.g., teachers) can be divided into two general categories: clinical interviews and structured diagnostic interviews. Clinical interviews with the parent and youth provide a method for assessing (1) the type, severity, and impairment associated with CP; (2) typical parent–child interactions that may be contributing to the CP; and (3) relevant antecedent and consequent events. An individual interview with the adolescent may or may not provide useful content-oriented information, depending on the nature of the specific behaviors. When assessing overt types of CP, Loeber and Schmaling (1985b) have suggested that maternal and teacher reports may be preferable to youth reports, as youth often underestimate or minimize their own aggressive behavior. However, when assessing covert types of CP, more valid reports are likely to be obtained from the youth.[2] When the presenting problems include classroom behavior or academic underachievement, an interview with the youth's teacher or teachers is also appropriate.

Structured interviews have been used in efforts to improve the reliability and validity of diagnostic (using DSM criteria) interviewing. They can be employed with multiple informants. Two structured diagnostic interviews that are frequently employed in the diagnosis of youth with CP are the Diagnostic Interview Schedule for Children (DISC; e.g., Shaffer, Fisher, Lucas, Dulcan, & Schwab-Stone, 2000) and the Diagnostic Interview for Children and Adolescents (DICA; e.g., Reich, 2000). For recent reviews of these and other structured diagnostic interviews, see Kamphaus and Frick (2002) and McClellan and Werry (2000).

An alternative approach to interviewing youth has been developed by McConaughy and Achenbach (2001). The Semistructured Clinical Interview for Children and Adolescents (SCICA) is a broad interview administered to children (ages 6–18) that employs a protocol of open-ended questions to assess a variety of areas of child functioning. Dimensional scores similar to those obtained from various instruments in the Achenbach System of Empirically Based Assessment (ASEBA; Achenbach & Rescorla, 2001; see below) can also be derived from these items. Kolko and colleagues have developed several semistructured interviews for parents and children that have been used to assess various aspects of firesetting and matchplay in inpatient, outpatient, and community samples of children. Examples include the Firesetting History Screen, the Firesetting Risk Interview, and the Children's Firesetting Interview (Kolko, Nishi-Strattner, Wilcox, & Kopet, 2002; Wilcox & Kolko, 2002). Evidence for the reliability and validity of these interviews is encouraging.

The interview as an assessment tool does not end with the first contact but continues throughout treatment formulation and implementation. The interview is used to obtain information necessary for the development of interventions, to assess the effectiveness of the intervention and its implementation, and to alter the intervention if necessary (Breen & Altepeter, 1990).

Behavior Rating Scales

Behavior rating scales, completed by adults or youth are very useful as screening devices, both for covering a broad range of CP behaviors and for assessing the presence of other child behavior disorders. In addition, they provide the best norm-referenced assessment concerning the youth's CP behavior. Although there are many behavior rating scales, several have been recommended as most appropriate for clinical and research use with youth with CP (McMahon & Estes, 1997; McMahon & Frick, 2005). There are a number of instruments in the ASEBA that are applicable for use with adolescents (Achenbach & Rescorla, 2001). There are parallel forms of the Child Behavior Checklist (CBCL) for parents (CBCL/6-18), teachers (Teacher's Report Form; TRF/6-18), youth (Youth Self-Report; YSR/11-18), and observers (Direct Observation Form; DOF/5-14). They are designed to be self-administered, and each can usually be completed in 15–20 minutes. The instruments include sections concerning Competence and Problem items (the DOF includes only Problem items). The ASEBA now also includes DSM-oriented scales (Achenbach, Dumenci, & Rescorla, 2003b). Other broadband rating scales include the Behavioral Assessment System for Children (BASC-2; Reynolds & Kamphaus, 2004); the Conners' Rating Scales, (Conners, 1997), the Revised Behavior Problem Checklist (RBPC; Quay & Peterson, 1996), and the Children's Symptom Inventory-4 (CSI-4; Gadow & Sprafkin, 1995).

Various other behavior rating scales, completed by parents, teachers, or adolescents, focus on specific aspects of CP. An example of an adolescent self-report measure that focuses specifically on CP is the Self-Report Delinquency Scale (SRD; Elliott, Huizinga, & Ageton, 1985). The SRD is probably the most widely used self-report measure of CP behavior. It consists of 47 items that are derived from offenses listed in the Uniform Crime Reports and covers index offenses (e.g., stole motor vehicle and aggravated assault), other delinquent behaviors (e.g., hit parent and panhandled), and drug use. The SRD is intended for use by 11- to 19-year-olds, who report on the frequency of engagement in each behavior over the past year. It has been employed primarily in epidemiological and community samples to assess prevalence of CP (e.g., Elliott et al., 1985; Loeber, Stouthamer-Loeber, Van Kammen, & Farrington, 1989), but it has also been employed as a measure of intervention outcome in clinic-referred samples (e.g., Henggeler, Melton, Brondino, Scherer, & Hanley, 1997; Kazdin, Mazurick, & Siegel, 1994; Kazdin, Siegel, & Bass, 1992). Pretreatment levels of CP behavior as assessed by the SRD were predictive of teacher ratings of child behavior problems following a cognitive-behavioral therapy intervention (Kazdin, 1995a).

Behavioral Observation

Direct behavioral observation has long been a critical component of the assessment of youth with CP and their families, both for delineating specific patterns of maladaptive parent–child or teacher–child interaction and for assessing change in those interactions as a function of treatment. More recently, observational data have been compared with data gathered via other methods to assist the clinician in determining whether the focus of treatment should be on the adult–youth interaction or on adult perceptual and/or personal adjustment issues. However, as noted previously, the majority of these observation systems have been designed for use with preadolescents (see McMahon & Estes, 1997).

For adolescents, structured clinical observational paradigms have been developed for the direct assessment of parent–youth communication and problem solving (see Foster & Robin, 1997, for a review). When behavioral observations in the school setting are indicated, the DOF/5-14 (Achenbach & Rescorla, 2001) may be used as part of a multimodal assessment with the other versions of the ASEBA described earlier. In addition, Dishion has developed a structured observational paradigm for assessing adolescent peer interactions (e.g., Dishion, Andrews, & Crosby, 1995).

An alternative to observations by independent observers in the natural setting is to train significant adults in the youth's environment to observe and record certain types of behavior. The most widely used procedure of this type is the Parent Daily Report (PDR; Chamberlain & Reid, 1987), a parent observation measure that is typically administered during brief telephone interviews. Parents are asked which of a number of overt and covert behaviors have occurred in the past 24 hours. The PDR has been employed on a pretreatment basis to assess the magnitude of CP behaviors, to monitor the progress of the family during therapy, and to assess treatment outcome (e.g., Bank, Marlowe, Reid, Patterson, & Weinrott, 1991; Chamberlain & Reid, 1991). An added advantage is its brevity and the possibility of providing more objective data than interviews or behavior rating scales.

Few assessment instruments have focused primarily on covert, as opposed to overt, forms of CP behavior (Miller & Klungness, 1989). A brief daily interview similar to the PDR for collecting parent-report data on stealing has been developed by Jones (1974). The Telephone Interview Report on Stealing and Social Aggression (TIROSSA) has adequate test–retest reliability and is sensitive to the effects of treatment procedures designed to reduce stealing (Reid, Hinojosa Rivera, & Lorber, 1980). Hinshaw and colleagues have developed and evaluated an analogue observational procedure to assess stealing and property destruction in children ages 6–12 years (Hinshaw, Heller, & McHale, 1992; Hinshaw, Simmel, & Heller, 1995; Hinshaw, Zupan, Simmel, Nigg, & Melnick, 1997). Kolko, Watson, and Faust (1991) employed a very brief (1-minute) observation to assess children's preference for fire-related stimuli. Both of these temptation provocation tasks demonstrated high interobserver agreement and sensitivity to treatment. However, their applicability to adolescents has yet to be demonstrated.

Associated Youth Characteristics

A brief developmental and medical history of the adolescent should be obtained to determine whether any medical factors might be associated with the development or maintenance of the adolescent's CP behaviors and whether the adolescent's early temperament may have contributed to the development of a coercive style of parent–child interaction. Because youth with CP may also present with a variety of other behavior disorders, behavior rating scales that provide information about a wide range of narrow-band behavior disorders (e.g., the ASEBA family of instruments; Achenbach & Rescorla, 2001) can serve as useful screening devices in addition to more open-ended interview techniques. As noted previously, ADHD, internalizing disorders, and substance use are of particular interest. The Antisocial Process Screening Device (Frick & Hare, 2002), which is a behavior rating scale completed by parents and/or teachers, can be used to identify youth with CP who also exhibit CU traits (e.g., Christian et al., 1997; Frick et al., 2000).

In addition to having comorbid behavior disorders, youth with CP frequently have problems with peer interactions and classroom behavior. Demaray and colleagues (1995) review several behavior rating scales for the assessment of social competence. Other measures, such as peer sociometric ratings, are difficult to employ outside elementary school settings. Research-based measures to assess youth's social-cognitive processes (e.g., Dodge & Coie, 1987) may have clinical utility for treatment planning, given that the processes are targeted in many cognitively oriented interventions (McMahon & Frick, 2005). Clinically useful measures to assess associations with a deviant peer group are limited currently to youth or parent report, although, as noted earlier, Dishion and colleagues (e.g., Dishion et al., 1995) have developed a structured observational paradigm for research purposes that may be adaptable to the clinical setting (McMahon & Frick, 2005).

If the presenting problem concerns classroom behavior, a functional analysis of the problem behaviors should also include an assessment of the youth's academic behavior. Although interviews, observations, and behavior rating scales can provide information concerning the youth's academic behavior, additional evaluation in the form of standardized intelligence test and academic achievement test screeners is necessary to determine whether the youth may have learning difficulties in addition to CP. Walker (1995) discusses the use of a standardized method for retrieving and using school records (School Archival Records System; Walker, Block-Pedego, Todis, & Severson, 1991) with youth with CP. Kaufman and Kaufman (2001) provide a comprehensive review of assessment strategies with which to evaluate learning problems.

Familial and Extrafamilial Factors

McMahon and Estes (1997) delineated six areas that are relevant to the assessment of youth with CP: parenting practices, parents' (and teachers') social cognitions, parents' perceptions of their own personal and marital adjustment, parental stress, parental functioning in extrafamilial social contexts, and parental satisfaction with treatment. *Parenting practices* are typically assessed via direct observation of parent–child interaction. However, questionnaire measures (e.g., Alabama Parenting Questionnaire; Frick, 1991) may often be more appropriate with parents of adolescents and in instances in which parental behaviors occur infrequently are or otherwise difficult to observe.

Although most of these measures of parenting practices have been developed for parents of children ages 2–13, some have also been employed with adolescent samples (e.g., Frick, Christian, & Wootton, 1999; Loeber Youth Questionnaire—Jacob, Moser, Windle, Loeber, & Stouthamer-Loeber, 2000).

Parents' (and teachers') perceptions of the child and social cognitions are a second important area to be assessed. Perceptions of the youth may be best assessed through the behavior rating scales described previously. Measures of parental self-esteem (e.g., Parenting Sense of Competence Scale, adapted by Johnston & Mash, 1989) may also be appropriate.

The third area involves the assessment of the role that *parents' personal and marital adjustment problems* may be playing in the adolescent's presenting behavior problems. Measures of maternal depression (e.g., Beck Depression Inventory-II; Beck, Steer, & Brown, 1996), parental antisocial behavior (e.g., Antisocial Behavior Checklist; Zucker & Fitzgerald, 1992), parental substance use (e.g., Drug Abuse Screening Test [DAST]; Skinner, 1982), marital satisfaction (e.g., Dyadic Adjustment Scale; Spanier, 1976), marital conflict (e.g., Conflict Tactics Scale—Partner [CTS-Partner]; Strauss, 1979, 1990), and parenting-related conflict (e.g., Parenting Alliance Inventory; Abidin, 1988) are some of the most widely used instruments with parents of youth with CP. Parental screening for ADHD (e.g., DSM-IV ADHD Rating Scale; Murphy & Gordon, 1998) is recommended when the adolescent presents with comorbid CP and ADHD (McMahon & Frick, 2005).

The fourth area is *parenting stress*, which includes general measures of stress (e.g., Family Events List; Patterson, 1982) and specific measures of parenting-related stress (e.g., Stress Index for Parents of Adolescents; Sheras, Abidin, & Konold, 1998). With respect to *extrafamilial functioning*, the Community Interaction Checklist (CIC; Wahler et al., 1979), which is a brief interview designed to assess maternal insularity, has been extensively employed in research with children with CP and their families. The Neighborhood Questionnaire (Greenberg, Lengua, Coie, Pinderhughes, & Conduct Problems Prevention Research Group, 1999) is a brief parent-report measure to assess the parent's perception of the family's neighborhood in terms of safety, violence, drug traffic, satisfaction, and stability. Finally, it is important to assess *parental satisfaction with treatment*, which may be assessed in terms of satisfaction with the outcome of treatment, therapists, treatment procedures, and teaching format (McMahon & Forehand, 1983). At present, no single consumer satisfaction measure is appropriate for use with all types of interventions for youth with CP and their families.

An Assessment Model

As described earlier, the assessment of youth with CP should be guided by what is currently known about the heterogeneous nature of CP, its comorbid conditions, the relevant risk and protective factors, and the different developmental pathways (McMahon & Estes, 1997; McMahon & Frick, 2005). It is readily apparent that the assessment of youth with CP must make use of multiple methods (e.g., behavior rating scales, direct observation, and interviews) completed by multiple informants (parents, teachers, the youth him- or herself) concerning the youth's behavior in multiple settings (e.g., home and school). However, in cost-effectiveness terms, to conduct such a broad-based assessment with every adolescent who is referred would be prohibitively expensive, and the incremental utility of each additional assessment measure or content area with respect to improving our treatment selecting capabilities would be suspect as well (Johnston & Murray, 2003).

"Multiple-gating" approaches to screening are an example of one strategy for employing multiple assessment measures that may prove to be cost-effective (e.g., Reid, Baldwin, Patterson, & Dishion, 1988; Walker, Ramsey, & Gresham, 2004). In this approach, less costly assessment procedures (e.g., brief interviews and broadband behavior rating scales) can be employed as screening instruments with all adolescents who are clinic-referred for the treatment of CP. More expensive methods, such as structured diagnostic interviews and observational methods, can be used to assess only that subgroup of youth for whom the less expensive methods have indicated the desirability of further assessment. An analogous strategy could be followed in the assessment of other youth characteristics and familial and extrafamilial factors, in that low-cost methods such as interview questions (e.g., concerning the child's temperament) and/or brief questionnaires (e.g., concerning the presence of substance use) would be employed as screening measures. Should additional assessment in these areas be warranted, a more thorough (and expensive) assessment could be conducted.

The ultimate goal of the assessment process is, of course, to facilitate selection of the most appropriate treatment strategy or strategies. Algorithms for matching clinic-referred families with specific interventions exist (e.g., Blechman, 1981; Embry, 1984), but they have been quite limited in scope, have not been closely tied to underlying assessment strategies, and have yet to be empirically tested. A comprehensive, empirically based treatment selection model for youth with CP is sorely needed. More clinically oriented strategies for integrating and interpreting information from comprehensive assessments, such as those presented in Kamphaus and Frick (2002), are a step in the right direction. Others have suggested that incorporation of a functional analytic approach into more traditional assessment practices will facilitate integration of information from multiple sources and the selection of appropriate treatments (e.g., Reitman & Hupp, 2003; Scotti, Morris, McNeil, & Hawkins, 1996).

Another goal of assessment is intervention monitoring and evaluating treatment outcome (McMahon & Frick, 2005). It is essential that clinicians ascertain whether interventions have brought about meaningful change in the youth's adjustment, either for better or worse (i.e., an iatrogenic effect). The very real possibility of iatrogenic effects resulting from interventions to treat CP in adolescents is discussed below. As noted previously, a variety of assessment measures have demonstrated sensitivity to intervention effects; however, there is minimal evidence of the successful use of assessment measures to monitor the effects of *ongoing* interventions for adolescents with CP.

TREATMENT AND PREVENTION

As demonstrated in the preceding material, CP is multifaceted in the diversity of specific behaviors that are manifested, the ages of the youth who engage in those behaviors, and the settings in which the behaviors occur. Not surprisingly, a plethora of interventions have been developed to deal with the various manifestations of CP during adolescence (e.g., Frick, 1998; Hill & Maughan, 2001; McMahon &

Wells, 1998). To impose some structure in our discussion of this array of interventions, we first describe three broad categories of psychosocial interventions: (1) family-based interventions, (2) skills training approaches, and (3) community-based programs. We then summarize findings from a series of meta-analytic studies on the effects of psychosocial interventions with delinquent populations. This is followed by a description of interventions that have been developed for specific subtypes of CP. In addition, we provide a brief summary of the relatively limited evidence for pharmacological interventions specific to CP behaviors. Finally, we briefly summarize evidence for the effects of preventive interventions that take place in infancy, childhood, and early adolescence on CP behavior displayed during adolescence.

Because available interventions vary widely in the extent to which they have been empirically validated, we have selected interventions that are generally considered to meet currently accepted criteria for determining whether an intervention is considered efficacious. (See Brestan and Eyberg, 1998, for a discussion of this issue specifically related to CP.) We have focused our review on interventions that are applicable to adolescents. Most of these interventions are intended for adolescents with more serious CP (e.g., a CD diagnosis), although we briefly describe an intervention (problem-solving communication training [PSCT]; Robin & Foster, 1989) that is intended primarily for dealing with parent–adolescent conflict. Finally, most of the interventions address overt, rather than covert, CP. Although covert CP behaviors (e.g., lying, stealing, and firesetting) are key components of later developmental manifestations of CD, most interventions primarily targeting covert CP do not qualify as empirically supported treatments, and many have targeted preadolescents. However, for the sake of completeness, we provide brief descriptions of interventions for these specific manifestations of CP.

Family-Based Interventions

Because of the primary role of the family in the development and maintenance of CP (e.g., Loeber & Stouthamer-Loeber, 1986; Patterson et al., 1992), we focus first on interventions directed at the youth with CP in the context of the family. We describe five intervention mod-

els: the Oregon Social Learning Center's (OSLC) parent management training model as adapted for adolescents (Bank et al., 1991), functional family therapy (Alexander & Sexton, 2002), brief strategic family therapy (Szapocznik & Williams, 2000), PSCT (Robin & Foster, 1989), and multisystemic therapy (Henggeler, Schoenwald, Borduin, Rowland, & Cunningham, 1998).

OSLC Parent Management Training

As noted previously, the work of Patterson and his associates at OSLC with children with CP and their families has been seminal in the development of the theoretical and empirical knowledge base concerning CP. Patterson's efforts over the past 30 years have also been extremely influential with respect to the development and evaluation of family-based intervention strategies for children with CP. Although nearly all that work has focused on parent training interventions for preadolescent children (3–12 years of age) who engage in overt CP, Patterson and his colleagues also modified their parent training intervention for use with adolescents with CP (Bank et al., 1991; Forgatch & Patterson, 1989; Patterson & Forgatch, 1987). Modifications for delinquent adolescents include (1) targeting any behaviors that put the adolescent at risk for further delinquency; (2) emphasizing parental monitoring/supervision; (3) revising punishment procedures to include work details, point loss, restriction of free time, and restitution of stolen/damaged property; (4) encouraging parents to report legal offenses to juvenile authorities and then to act as advocates for the adolescent in court; and (5) promoting greater involvement of the adolescent in treatment sessions (Bank et al., 1991). A study of the efficacy of this modification (Bank et al., 1991) revealed that although adolescents in the parent-training condition did have fewer offenses during the treatment year compared to the control condition (i.e., community treatment as usual), by the first year after treatment, offense rates for the two conditions were comparable, and remained so throughout the 3-year follow-up. Despite these somewhat positive findings, Bank and colleagues (1991) were pessimistic as to the feasibility of this approach on a larger scale, given the extreme distress of the families and the high likelihood of therapist burnout. Instead, they argued for intervention with these families at an earlier stage, before the problems have increased to such severity and duration.

Functional Family Therapy

A family-based intervention for adolescents engaging in CP behaviors has been developed and evaluated by Alexander and his colleagues. Functional family therapy (FFT; Alexander & Parsons, 1982; Barton & Alexander, 1981) represents a unique integration and extension of family systems and behavioral perspectives. The model has also incorporated cognitive and affective perspectives (Alexander, Jameson, Newell, & Gunderson, 1996).

FFT consists of three main components (e.g., Alexander & Sexton, 2002; Sexton & Alexander, 2002). The *engagement/motivation* phase is concerned with family members' expectations prior to therapy and in the initial sessions. Factors that enhance the perception that positive change is possible are maximized, while factors that might lessen this perception are minimized. During this phase, the clinician identifies the behavioral, cognitive, and emotional expectations of each family member and the family processes in need of change (e.g., interpersonal functions such as closeness and distance). In addition, the clinician takes steps to modify the inappropriate attributions and expectations of family members. Various cognitive therapy techniques, especially relabeling of "negative" behavior as more positive or benign, are employed. This reattribution process among family members is seen as necessary, but not sufficient, for successful treatment. Actual behavior change must follow. In the *behavior change phase*, a variety of behavioral techniques are employed, including communication skills training, behavioral contracting, and contingency management. In the *generalization phase*, the therapist's job is to facilitate maintenance of therapeutic gains while also fostering the family's independence from the therapy context through gradual disengagement. It is also during this phase that relevant extrafamilial factors (e.g., school and the legal system) are dealt with as necessary.

Much of the empirical research on the efficacy of FFT was conducted in the 1970s, prior to the inclusion of the cognitive and affective components described earlier. A series of three studies was conducted using a single sample of 86 status delinquents and their families (Alexander & Parsons, 1973; Klein, Alexander, & Parsons, 1977; Parsons & Alexander, 1973). At the conclusion of treatment, families in the FFT condition performed better than families in the comparison conditions on a number of communication variables assessed in a 20-minute family discussion. An examination of juvenile court records 6–18 months after treatment indicated that adolescents in the FFT condition had a significantly lower recidivism rate (26%), compared to adolescents in comparison conditions (50% for no-treatment controls, 47% for client-centered family groups, and 73% for eclectic psychodynamic family therapy) (Alexander & Parsons, 1973). Within the FFT condition, a poorer outcome on the behavioral family interaction measures was associated with an increased likelihood of recidivism, thus lending direct support to the relationship between the two measures.

These early investigations focused on the families of adolescent delinquents with relatively minor status offenses. The current version of FFT, in conjunction with supportive adjuncts such as remedial education and job training, has been shown to be effective with multiply offending, previously incarcerated delinquents (Barton, Alexander, Waldron, Turner, & Warburton, 1985). In this investigation, adolescents who participated in FFT were less likely to be charged with committing an offense in the 15-month follow-up period than were adolescents placed in group homes (60% vs. 93% respectively). FFT participants who did commit additional offenses committed significantly fewer offenses than adolescents in the group home condition.

Gordon, Arbuthnot, and their colleagues (Gordon, Arbuthnot, Gustafson, & McGreen, 1988; Gordon, Graves, & Arbuthnot, 1995) successfully employed a slightly modified version of FFT (longer treatment, treatment in the home as opposed to clinic, and longer training and supervision of therapists) with a sample of 27 disadvantaged, rural families with a delinquent adolescent, many of whom were multiple offenders. Recidivism rates for the FFT and comparison (probation-only) groups at a 2½-year follow-up were 11% and 67%, respectively. In a subsequent follow-up when the subjects were 20 to 22 years old, Gordon and colleagues (1995) reported recidivism rates of 9% versus 41% for the FFT and comparison groups, respectively.

A cross-cultural replication of FFT with juvenile delinquents was completed recently in Sweden by Hansson, Cederblad, and Alexander (2002). In this study, 49 youth received FFT while 40 comparison subjects received treatment as usual (e.g., counseling, case management, and referral to other treatment resources). At a 1-year follow-up, only 33% of the FFT group had relapsed compared to 65% of the comparison group. This pattern was maintained at the 2-year follow-up with a 41% relapse rate in the FFT group compared to an 83% relapse rate in the group of youth that received treatment as usual.

In addition to this body of outcome research, a number of process studies have been conducted to clarify the mechanisms of therapeutic change associated with FFT (see Sexton & Alexander, 2003, for a detailed review of both outcome and process research). Examples of this research include an examination of the complex impact of family–therapist alliances on dropout rates (Robbins, Turner, Alexander, & Perez, 2003) and an evaluation of several therapy techniques designed to reduce defensive communications between family members (Robbins, Alexander, & Turner, 2000).

When analyzed as part of a cost-benefit study conducted by the Washington State Institute of Public Policy (Aos, Lieb, Mayfield, Miller, & Pennucci, 2004), FFT was shown to save taxpayers between approximately $14,351 (in Washington State) and $26,216 (excluding Washington State) per participant in the program, compared to the cost of one offense (including the crime itself, associated law enforcement costs, adjudication, and punishment/rehabilitation).

Brief Strategic Family Therapy

Brief strategic family therapy (BSFT) began as a response to increasing drug use in the Hispanic adolescent population in the 1970s (Robbins, Szapocznik, et al., 2003; Szapocznik & Williams, 2000). The initial goal was to develop a culturally appropriate intervention for behavior problems in Cuban youths. Eventually, a time-limited treatment approach was developed and refined that included both structural and strategic interventions (Robbins, Szapocznik, et al., 2003; Szapocznik & Williams, 2000). According to Szapocznik and Williams (2000), "The goal of BSFT is to target repetitive interactions within or between systems in the family social ecology that are unsuccessful at achieving the goals of the family or its individual members" (p. 119).

BSFT interventions are strategic in that they are practical and problem focused. When selecting a practical intervention, the goal is to move the family toward desired objectives, and these interventions often involve positive or negative reframing (Szapocznik & Williams, 2000). Problem-focused interventions involve only targeting family interaction patterns that are directly relevant to the behavior problem of concern (Szapocznik & Williams, 2000).

The content of BSFT involves a number of key steps (Robbins, Szapocznik, et al., 2003). The first step is the establishment of a therapeutic alliance with each family member and the family as a whole. Steps 2–5 involve diagnosing the strengths and weaknesses of a family and developing a treatment plan. Step 6 is called restructuring and involves using change strategies to "transform" family relations. In addition to reframing, other interventions employed at this step might include (1) directing, redirecting, or blocking communication; (2) shifting family alliances; (3) giving parents more control; (4) building conflict resolution skills; (5) developing behavior management skills; and (6) fostering effective parenting skills.

The first clinical trial of BSFT compared this intervention to individual psychodynamic child-centered psychotherapy and a recreational control condition (Szapocznik et al., 1989). The sample included 69 preadolescent boys (ages 6–11 years) with moderate behavioral and/or emotional problems. Findings indicated that family retention was significantly better in the two treatment conditions compared to the recreation condition. Further, both treatment conditions were equivalent in terms of the reduction in emotional and behavior problems. However, BSFT was more effective than child-centered psychotherapy at protecting family integrity at the 1-year follow-up.

The efficacy of BSFT with adolescents was examined in a clinical trial study in which 126 adolescents (ages 12–18; 77% male) with CP and/or substance use problems were assigned to BSFT or a control group condition (Santisteban et al., 2003). In the control condition, adolescents were in a group and were encouraged to discuss and solve problems among themselves with the guidance of a facilitator.

Of the 126 families entered in the study, 79 families completed treatment. BSFT youth demonstrated significantly greater reductions in CP, socialized aggression, and delinquency (as assessed by parent report) compared to the control group. BSFT was also more effective at reducing marijuana use than the control group (although there was no treatment effect with respect to alcohol use), and families in the BSFT group also demonstrated significantly more improvement in observer ratings and self-reports of family functioning.

One of most troubling problems in treating families with adolescents with CP and/or substance abuse problems is that many of these families never become engaged in therapy (Robbins, Szapocznik, et al., 2003). To address this problem, a set of specialized engagement procedures to deal with treatment resistance was developed to add to the core BSFT intervention. These strategies include allying with the adolescent and asking the mother for permission to talk to the most "resistant" family member (Robbins, Szapocznik, et al., 2003). To test the value of these specialized engagement procedures, Szapocznik and colleagues (1988) assigned 109 families with adolescents with CP and/or substance use problems to either a BSFT-engagement as usual group (the control group) or a BSFT-enhanced-engagement group. While only 42% of the families in the control group were successfully engaged into treatment, 93% of the families in the enhanced condition were engaged into treatment. Of these engaged cases, only 59% of the control families completed treatment compared to 83% of the families in the enhanced-engagement group. Additional studies conducted by Szapocznik and colleagues have replicated these findings (Coatsworth, Santisteban, McBride, & Szapocznik, 2001; Santisteban et al., 1996).

Problem-Solving Communication Training

PSCT (Robin & Foster, 1989) is an intervention for adolescents with mild to moderate CP that directly addresses family members' discussions of conflict situations (Foster & Robin, 1998). This intervention is rooted in a behavioral–family systems model of parent–adolescent conflict that posits that family conflict is driven by a combination of adolescent developmental factors, family skill deficits and structural difficulties, and problematic interaction patterns (Robin & Foster, 1989). Specifically, family members receive direct training in (1) problem solving, (2) communications skills, and (3) cognitive restructuring in the context of sessions that focus on specific family problems (Foster & Robin, 1998; Robin & Foster, 1989). Less complex and anger-provoking issues are addressed before proceeding to more difficult issues.

Problem-solving skills are taught didactically, modeled, and rehearsed by family members. Basic problem-solving skills addressed include (1) problem definition, (2) generation of alternative solutions, (3) decision making, and (4) implementation of a solution. The therapist provides feedback on these skills and helps to guide feedback between family members. Generally, communication training is tailored to address communication deficits specific to the family. Communication problems are addressed when they occur in sessions, and instruction and modeling of more appropriate communication strategies are provided. The cognitive restructuring component of PSCT involves teaching cognitive restructuring techniques that can be used to change problematic perceptions, beliefs, and attributions. Reframing and relabeling techniques and experiments designed to disconfirm unreasonable beliefs are common therapy techniques for this intervention component. The complete treatment is generally conducted in 8–12 sessions. Homework is completed between sessions and involves communication and problem-solving practice (including implementing solutions generated during therapy).

The first studies evaluating PSCT used samples of families recruited with public notices advertising treatment for "families in conflict" (Foster, Prinz, & O'Leary, 1983; Robin, Kent, O'Leary, Foster, & Prinz, 1977). Robin and colleagues (1977) trained 12 mother–adolescent dyads (adolescents ages 11–14 years) with PSCT utilizing both hypothetical and real problems and compared this group to 12 control dyads. Compared to the control group, improvements in observed communication were noted in the intervention group. However, reports of home conflict did not decrease. Foster and colleagues (1983) replicated and extended this first study by including fathers in the treatment and focusing solely on actual problems rather than hypothetical problems ($N = 28$ families divided into a control group, a PSCT group, and a group receiving "enhanced"

PSCT [PSCT+ homework discussions and discussions of home use of communication skills]). In contrast to the previous study, results from the Foster and colleagues study showed no change in observed skills in the PSCT group or the enhanced PSCT group compared to the control group. However, intervention groups did demonstrate significant improvements in questionnaire measures assessing family relationships. Gains were maintained at a 6- to 8-week follow-up. Although the enhanced PSCT condition was designed to improve home generalization, there was no evidence that generalization in this group was superior to that of the PSCT-only intervention group.

Robin (1981) compared PSCT, an alternative family therapy (AFT) treatment, and a control condition in a sample of families with adolescents experiencing parent–adolescent conflict (N = 31 families, divided into the three groups). The AFT condition consisted of typical treatment that might be obtained from therapists with psychodynamic, family systems, or eclectic orientations. Both treatment groups improved compared to the control group on observational measures of problem-solving communication skills and on self-report conflict measures. PSCT resulted in significantly larger improvements on observational measures of problem-solving behavior compared to both AFT and the control condition. Gains on questionnaire measures were maintained at a 10-week follow-up.

More recently, Barkley, Edwards, Laneri, Fletcher, and Metevia (2001) compared 18 sessions of PSCT alone to a combined treatment composed of nine sessions of behavior management training followed by nine sessions of PSCT in a sample of 97 families with adolescents ages 12–18 years meeting criteria for both ADHD and ODD. In the discussion of results that follows, both therapies produced equivalent results except where noted. At the midpoint of treatment and at posttreatment, there were improvements on participant ratings of parent–adolescent conflicts (compared to pretreatment measures). Improvements in observational measures of communication and problem solving were evident at posttreatment but not at the midpoint of treatment, and these improvements were only significant for mothers. At a 2-month follow-up, improvements in observational measures were significant for fathers and adolescents but not for mothers.

Only 23% of families showed significant improvements on a measure of "reliable change." However, a contrasting measure of "normalization" (i.e., the percentage of families that were brought into the normal range on outcome measures as a consequence of treatment) suggested that 31–71% of families improved. It is notable that significantly more families dropped out of the PSCT-alone condition compared to the combined treatment condition.

Multisystemic Therapy

While the family unit has clearly been a successful focus of interventions for CD, adolescents with CP and their families commonly present with a range of problems that are demonstrated in multiple settings. This is especially the case with adolescents who display the early-starting manifestations of CP. There is increasing recognition of the value of multicomponent interventions that address adolescents' CP behavior in multiple settings. Multisystemic therapy (MST) is a multicomponent, family-based intervention that has been extensively tested with adolescents with CP and serious, multiproblem juvenile offenders. The MST approach to treating adolescents with CP emphasizes both the interactional nature of adolescent psychopathology and the role of multiple systems in which the adolescent is embedded, such as the family, school, and peer group (Henggeler & Borduin, 1990; Henggeler et al., 1998). The family is viewed as a core focus of the intervention. Assessment and treatment are concerned with the adolescent as an individual, his or her role in the various systems, and the interrelationships among those systems. Therapists intervene at one or more levels as required and employ a variety of therapy approaches, such as family therapy, school consultation, peer intervention strategies, marital therapy, or individual therapy. Treatment techniques are similarly wide ranging and may include traditional family therapy procedures (e.g., paradoxical intent) as well as behavioral and cognitive-behavioral techniques (e.g., reinforcement, contingency contracting, and self-instructions) (Schoenwald, Henggeler, Pickrel, & Cunningham, 1996). Clinicians are guided by a set of nine treatment principles (e.g., focus on systemic strengths, promote responsible behavior and decrease irresponsible behavior among family members, implement developmentally appropriate interventions) (Henggeler et al.,

1998; Schoenwald, Brown, & Henggeler, 2000).

MST has been evaluated in multiple studies across problems, therapists, and settings (Henggeler et al., 1998; Henggeler & Lee, 2003; Schoenwald et al., 2000). Most of the evaluations of MST have been conducted with samples of juvenile offenders (often chronic and/or violent offenders), although the efficacy of MST has also been investigated with adolescent sexual offenders, juvenile offenders who met criteria for substance abuse or dependence, youth presenting with psychiatric emergencies, and youth who have been physically abused. MST has been shown to be generally efficacious in treating youth populations (including minority populations; see Borduin et al., 1995; Henggeler, Melton, & Smith, 1992; and Henggeler, Pickrel, & Brondino, 1999; for results indicating that MST outcomes are not moderated by race). However, results regarding the effectiveness of MST in broader community applications (i.e., using community therapists rather than graduate student therapists supervised by program developers) are less robust.

In an initial examination of MST efficacy, Henggeler and colleagues (1986) conducted an evaluation of MST with inner-city adolescent delinquents, most of whom were repeat offenders, and their families (*n* = 57). At the conclusion of treatment, parents in the MST condition reported fewer CP behaviors, whereas parents of adolescents in an alternative mental health services condition (*n* = 23) and in the normal control condition (*n* = 44) reported no change. Families in the MST condition had also improved at posttreatment on several observational measures of family interaction, whereas the families in the alternative treatment condition either did not change or deteriorated on those measures from pretreatment to posttreatment.

Henggeler and colleagues (1992) assessed the efficacy of MST with a sample of 84 violent, chronic juvenile offenders (mean age = 15.2 years). The offenders were randomly assigned to receive either MST or "usual services" through the Department of Youth Services. One year following referral, youth whose families had participated in MST reported fewer CP behaviors and were less likely to have been arrested or incarcerated than youth in the comparison group. Families that received MST also reported greater cohesion and less peer aggression than families in the comparison group.

In a follow-up study conducted 2.4 years postreferral (Henggeler, Melton, Smith, Schoenwald, & Hanley, 1993), survival analyses indicated that MST continued to be the superior treatment—39% of the MST group had not been rearrested, compared to 20% of the comparison group.

In a second randomized trial with 200 seriously delinquent adolescents (mean age = 15) (Borduin et al., 1995), youth were assigned to MST or a treatment as usual condition that consisted of community individual therapy. At the end of treatment, the MST group demonstrated decreased CP, decreased parent psychopathology, and improved parent–youth interaction, whereas the treatment as usual group showed no improvement or grew worse on these measures. In a 4-year follow-up, adolescents in the MST group had much lower rates of rearrest (26% compared to 71% in the treatment as usual group), and those adolescents who were rearrested were arrested less often and for less serious and violent offenses than adolescents in the treatment as usual group.

In an application of MST to a sample of juvenile offenders with substance abuse or dependence, youth were randomly assigned to MST or community services as usual, consisting of outpatient substance use treatment (Henggeler et al., 1999). Compared to the youth receiving community services as usual, the youth receiving MST had higher treatment completion (Henggeler, Pickrel, Brondino, & Crouch, 1996) and increased mainstream school attendance (Brown, Henggeler, Schoenwald, Brondino, & Pickrel, 1999). Treatment with MST also resulted in cost savings compared to treatment with community services as usual (Schoenwald, Ward, Henggeler, Pickrel, & Patel, 1996). Although significant treatment effects for substance abuse were reported at posttreatment, they were not maintained at 6-month follow-up (Henggeler et al., 1999). A 4-year follow-up revealed significant reductions in aggressive criminal behavior (Henggeler, Clingempeel, Brondino, & Pickrel, 2002). Findings in terms of long-term reductions in illicit drug use were mixed. Although biological indices of drug use (i.e., urine and head hair samples) indicated the superiority of MST, self-report measures did not distinguish MST from community services as usual.

A cross-cultural evaluation of MST has also recently been completed in Norway (Ogden & Halliday-Boykins, 2004). Male and female adolescents (N = 100; mean age = 15.0 years) with serious antisocial behavior were randomly assigned to MST or treatment as usual (i.e., child welfare services). At posttreatment, MST was more effective than treatment as usual at reducing internalizing and externalizing behaviors and out-of-home placements. Compared to treatment as usual, MST also led to higher youth social competence, and MST families were more satisfied with treatment.

However, not all outcome research on MST has supported its effectiveness. Leschied and Cunningham (2002; Cunningham, 2002) conducted a carefully designed multisite effectiveness trial of MST using teams of community therapists at four sites in Ontario, Canada. Across the sites, 409 youth (largely probation and court referrals; mean age = 14.6 years) and their families participated in the study with half of the youth receiving community treatment as usual and half receiving MST. Based on the currently available follow-up data (collected at 6 months and 1, 2, and 3 years), the MST group and the treatment as usual group were not statistically distinguishable on any outcome measure of offending (e.g., convictions, prosecutions, time before a first conviction, time to first custody admission, overall incarceration rate, and length of sentence). Important caveats for these results include the fact that not all subjects were serious or chronic offenders (unlike most of the other MST studies). Further, broader outcome measures (e.g., school completion and need for residential treatment) were not explored and treatment fidelity was not specifically examined (Cunningham, 2002). Finally, collection and analysis of longer-term outcome data are still underway.

A meta-analysis of MST conducted by Curtis, Ronan, and Borduin (2004) may shed some light on discrepant findings related to the efficacy and effectiveness of MST. Examining seven MST treatment studies (but not including the ongoing Canadian study conducted by Leschied & Cunningham [2002; Cunningham, 2002]), Curtis and colleagues found that overall, youth and their families treated with MST were functioning better and offending less than 70% of their counterparts who received alternative treatments. These treatment effects were sustained for up to 4 years. MST demonstrated larger effects on measures of family relations than on peer measures or individual measures. However, Henggeler (2004) notes that the most significant finding from this meta-analysis

demonstrated that treatment ES was moderated by differences in study conditions (i.e., efficacy trials with MST developers as clinical supervisors and graduate student therapists had ES = .81 on average while community effectiveness trials had much lower ESs [ES = .26]). Henggeler also indicated that the results underlined the importance of (1) conducting research on optimizing treatment transportability, and (2) considering factors that may have an impact on effectiveness in real-world settings during efficacy trials (e.g., site characteristics, funding, and organizational structure).

As with FFT, process studies have also been included as part of the ongoing evaluation of MST. However, some of the most interesting process research on MST has related to issues of successful dissemination. This research is particularly relevant given the ES differences between efficacy and effectiveness trials just described. Specifically, Henggeler, Schoenwald, and Pickrel (1997) addressed aspects of MST that make it particularly effective in community settings (e.g., high levels of training and supervision for community therapists, a very structured and focused treatment model, and efforts to maximize the fit between the therapy components and client needs). Henggeler, Melton, and colleagues (1997) have also demonstrated that high adherence to treatment protocols is a key factor in the success of MST dissemination efforts.

The Aos and colleagues (2004) cost–benefit analysis suggested that MST saved taxpayers approximately \$9,316 per participant in the program. A cost-efficiency analysis for the study conducted by Leschied and Cunningham (2002) is also planned, but results are not available at this time (Cunningham, 2002).

Skills Training Approaches

Several systematic programs of research have evaluated skills training programs for adolescents with CP (see reviews by Bennett & Gibbons, 2000; Nangle, Erdley, Carpenter, & Newman, 2002; and Taylor, Eddy, & Biglan, 1999). While the particular foci of these programs may vary, they share an emphasis on remediating or changing skill deficiencies and dysfunctions displayed by the adolescent with CP. The historical evolution of this research has followed a path from early emphasis on the behavioral aspects of social skills to a later emphasis on the cognitive aspects of social/interpersonal behavior, to a most recent emphasis on comprehensive, multicomponent skills training programs. As the interventions have become more complex, so too have the theoretical models underpinning these interventions. The following is a brief overview of some of the current major skills training models of intervention for adolescents with CP.

Social Skills Training Programs

One of the first skills-based models of intervention for youth with CP was social skills training. As noted previously, youth with CP often evidence problematic peer relations (including involvement with deviant peer groups) and display social skills deficits. Theoretical models underpinning social skills training have emphasized that youth who display such skill deficits will engage in CP behavior in order to secure rewards from the social environment. Therefore, direct training in social skills was hypothesized to be a potentially viable treatment method for these youth. Social skills training typically involves modeling, role playing, coaching and practice, feedback, and positive reinforcement.

One of the first evaluations of a social skills training approach was the well-designed investigation reported by Spence and Marzillier (1981), in which 76 male delinquents (ages 10–16) were randomly assigned to a social skills training group, an attention-placebo group, or a no-treatment group. The social skills training program included 12, 1-hour sessions with youths in groups of four. Training procedures included instructions, discussion, live and videotaped modeling, role plays, videotaped feedback, social reinforcement, and homework tasks. Skills taught were individually tailored to each adolescent, based on a needs assessment. Results of both multiple-baseline-across-behaviors and group-comparison designs indicated specific improvements in many individual social skills on the analogue assessment tests for the social skills training group but not for the attention-placebo or no-treatment control groups. Furthermore, these improvements were maintained at a 3-month follow-up assessment. However, there was no evidence of generalized differential changes in social skills, according to staff ratings; self-report of social problems; observer ratings of friendliness, social anxiety, social skills, and employability; so-

cial workers' ratings of improvements in family work, school, and social relationships; self-report of delinquent offenses; or police convictions.

Cognitive-Behavioral Skills Training

Several of the programs of skills-based intervention research have been based on cognitive models of psychopathology in youth who began to gain prominence after the earlier models, which focused more exclusively on behavior (e.g., social skills). One cognitive model evolved quite directly from social skills training approaches. It was hypothesized that social skills deficits were at least partially driven by immaturity in moral reasoning and judgment (Chandler & Moran, 1990; Gregg, Gibbs, & Basinger, 1994; Nelson, Smith, & Dodd, 1990). Therefore, direct training in moral reasoning was suggested as a potentially viable treatment method. Higher levels of moral reasoning can be facilitated by relatively brief (8–20 sessions) discussion groups composed of behavior-disordered (Arbuthnot & Gordon, 1986) or incarcerated delinquent (Gibbs, Arnold, Ahlborn, & Cheesman, 1984) adolescents. However, only the Arbuthnot and Gordon (1986) study included measures of behavioral functioning to assess whether changes in moral reasoning were associated with behavior change. Following participation in a "moral dilemma discussion group" that met for 45 minutes per week over 16–20 weeks in the school, adolescents with CP had fewer referrals to the principal for disciplinary reasons, were less tardy, had higher grades in the humanities and social sciences, and had fewer police or court contacts than adolescents in a no-treatment control condition. At a 1-year follow-up, these between-group differences were still evident, although both groups had virtually eliminated any police or court contacts. It should also be noted that there were no differences between the groups on teacher ratings of the adolescents' behavior, either at posttreatment or at the 1-year follow-up.

Other studies using this approach show that while intervention may stimulate more mature moral judgment, the reduction of CP behavior does not necessarily follow (Gibbs et al., 1984; Power, Higgins, & Kohlberg, 1989). Interestingly, the Arbuthnot and Gordon (1986) study, which did find positive changes on indices of CP behavior, also included techniques to develop social skills. Insofar as the Arbuthnot and Gordon intervention included such techniques, it may be that the singular results in terms of changes in indices of CP may be mainly attributable to the social skills training rather than the moral reasoning component.

Somewhat more comprehensive cognitive models for skills deficits have been articulated most forcefully by Kendall (1985, 1991; Kendall & MacDonald, 1993) and by Dodge and his associates in the latter's social information-processing model of social competence in children (Crick & Dodge, 1994; Dodge, 2003). In these models, there is a fundamental assumption that when youth with CP encounter an anger- or frustration-arousing event (often an interpersonal interaction), their emotional, physiological, and behavioral reactions are determined by their cognitive perceptions and appraisals of that event rather than by the event itself. Intervening at the level of these cognitive processes then becomes the most important focus of treatment (e.g., Guerra & Slaby, 1990; Hudley & Graham, 1993). Evidence supporting these more complex cognitive models indicates that youth with CP appear to display both deficiencies (a lack or insufficient amount of cognitive activity in situations in which this would be useful) and distortions (active but maladaptive cognitive contents and processes) in their cognitive functioning (Crick & Dodge, 1994; Kendall, 1991; Kendall & MacDonald, 1993).

Guerra and Slaby (1990) developed and evaluated a 12-session program based on Dodge's (1986) social information-processing model and targeted toward male and female adolescents incarcerated for aggressive offenses. In this program, adolescents learned social problem-solving skills, addressed and modified beliefs that support a broad and extensive use of aggression as a legitimate activity, and learned cognitive self-control skills to control impulsive responding. Relative to an attention-placebo control group, the aggressive adolescents who received treatment showed greater social problem-solving skills, greater reductions in some beliefs associated with aggression, and greater reductions on staff ratings of aggressive, impulsive, and inflexible behavior. In addition, posttest aggression was related to change in cognitive factors. However, no differences were noted between groups on recidivism rates 24 months after release from the institu-

tion, although there seemed to be a trend toward lower recidivism for those who received the active treatment.

Multicomponent Skills Training

Because single-component programs may produce limited results, some investigators have combined different approaches to skills training into multicomponent treatment packages. Goldstein and his colleagues developed a 10-week curriculum called aggression replacement training (ART; Goldstein, Glick, & Gibbs, 1998; Goldstein, Glick, Reiner, Zimmerman, & Coultry, 1986), which combines interventions designed to enhance social skills (structured learning training; Goldstein & Pentz, 1984), anger control (anger control training; Feindler, Marriott, & Iwata, 1984; see below), and moral reasoning (moral education). The program was subsequently expanded to a 50-skill curriculum (Goldstein & Glick, 1994).

Preliminary evaluations in two juvenile correctional facilities suggested differential improvements on analogue measures of social skills (and sometimes on the moral development measure) for adolescent males who participated in ART as opposed to those in either a brief instruction or a no-treatment control group (Glick & Goldstein, 1987). Subsequent evaluations in community settings employing ART with adolescents with CP showed evidence of significantly improved skills across a variety of domains targeted in treatment (Goldstein, Glick, Irwin, McCartney, & Rubama, 1989). Evidence for generalization to the community after release was limited to global ratings completed by probation officers in initial studies. In subsequent reports, 3-month rearrest data showed significantly fewer arrests for youth receiving ART (Goldstein & Glick, 1994). At a 1-year follow-up, social workers rated youth who had received ART more highly on a variety of indices of adjustment.

Independent investigators have also conducted evaluations of ART (as reported by Goldstein et al., 1998). Coleman, Pfeiffer, and Oakland (1991) evaluated the effectiveness of a 10-week ART program for behaviorally disordered adolescents in a residential treatment center. Improvements in skills knowledge were evident but there were no significant changes in overt skill behaviors. However, Jones (1990) compared ART to moral education and a no-treatment control in a sample of aggressive male high school students in Brisbane, Australia, and found that students in the ART program showed significant decreases in aggressive behavior and significant improvements in coping behaviors and social skills.

Taken together, this body of research suggests that ART does have the potential for facilitating improvement across a broad array of skills deficits and may also be useful for reducing recidivism rates in offending adolescents with CP. When analyzed as part of the Aos and colleagues (2004) cost–benefit study, ART was shown to be cost-effective as well. It saved taxpayers between approximately $8,805 (in Washington state) and $14,846 (excluding Washington state) per participant in the program.

Another multicomponent skills training approach that integrates methods from ART with the positive peer culture approach has been described by Gibbs, Potter, Barriga, and Liau (1996). This treatment model, called EQUIP, combines social skills training, moral reasoning, and problem solving in group meetings that emphasize positive peer culture. Behavioral methods such as self-monitoring in daily homework assignments are also included. The effectiveness of EQUIP has been evaluated in a controlled outcome study with 15- to 18-year old incarcerated juvenile male offenders (Leeman, Gibbs, & Fuller, 1993). The experimental condition was compared to both no-treatment and attention-placebo (a brief motivational induction) control conditions. Outcome measures assessed institution and postrelease conduct, as well as mediating processes of social skills and moral judgment. Improvements in institutional conduct were highly significant for the EQUIP group relative to the control groups in terms of self-reported misconduct, staff-filed incident reports, and unexcused absences from schools. Twelve months after subjects' release from the institution, the recidivism rate for EQUIP participants remained low and stable (15%), whereas the likelihood of recidivism for untreated subjects (41%) climbed. Social skills also improved significantly for EQUIP participants and were significantly correlated with self-reported improvements in institutional conduct. Both the ART and the EQUIP studies of intervention efficacy suggest that multicomponent skills training programs are more effective than single-component programs and may result in more significant long-term effects as well.

While skills training approaches are quite commonly used to treat CP in youth, reviews of the literature in this area indicate that there is generally weak empirical support for the use of skills training as an isolated intervention for the treatment of serious CP (Taylor et al., 1999). Specifically, Taylor and colleagues (1999) reviewed several of the interventions discussed previously and concluded that although they appeared to result in short-term improvements for minor CP, there was little empirical evidence for longer-term improvements in more serious CP (e.g., violence, property damage, and parole violations). In addition, Bennett and Gibbons (2000) conducted a meta-analysis of 30 skills training studies for children and adolescents and generally found that skills training interventions resulted in a fairly small treatment effect (mean weighted ES = .23). However, it is notable that Bennett and Gibbons also identified a trend in the studies they evaluated, suggesting that skills training may be more effective with older children and adolescents as compared to younger children. Finally, results from a cost-efficacy study provide some evidence that skills training may be useful even in adolescents with more serious CP as compared to other possible community treatments. Blechman, Maurice, Bueker, and Helberg (2000) found that a skills training program with a juvenile offender population was more cost-effective than a mentoring approach or a standard juvenile-diversion program. Specifically, the skills training program reduced the recidivism rate of juveniles in the study to 37% (vs. 51% and 46% for the other two programs, respectively), resulting in a cost savings of approximately $33,600 per 100 youths.

Clinicians who employ skills training interventions with adolescents with CP must be aware of, and take steps to minimize, the possibility of iatrogenic effects for group-based approaches to training. Dishion and colleagues (Dishion, McCord, & Poulin, 1999) have reviewed evidence suggesting that the placement of high-risk adolescents in at least some peer-group interventions may result in increases in both CP behavior and negative life outcomes compared to control youth. For example, Poulin, Dishion, and Burraston (2001) demonstrated that increases in both teacher-reported delinquency and self-report of smoking were associated with participation in prevention-oriented groups of high-risk youth 3 years earlier. The putative mechanism of influence is so-called deviancy training, in which youth receive group attention for engaging in various problem behaviors. These findings have led to the development and promotion of interventions that minimize the influence of groups of high-risk adolescent peers and involve the youngsters in conventional peer activities (e.g., sports teams and school clubs) with low-risk peers. At this point, it is not known whether such iatrogenic effects occur with groups of younger children at risk for CP, or the extent to which this phenomenon is occurring in other interventions with at-risk adolescents. Nevertheless, these findings indicate the need to minimize the risk of unintended negative effects and, in some cases, consider alternatives to group-based interventions for at-risk adolescents.

Community-Based Programs

The systematic development and evaluation of community-based residential programs for aggressive and delinquent adolescents began over 35 years ago, arising from several national directives (e.g., The Presidential Commission on Law Enforcement and the Administration of Justice, 1967) that highlighted the inhumane, expensive, and ineffective nature of traditional institutional programs. Since that time, numerous programs have been developed to address the challenges presented by juvenile offenders who also often display other emotional or behavioral conditions.

Achievement Place/Teaching Family Model

The Achievement Place model (currently known as the teaching family model; TFM) was originally developed in 1967 and has become the prototypical community-based residential program for aggressive and delinquent adolescents (Fixsen, Blase, Timbers, & Wolf, 2001). Each TFM group home is run by a young married couple, referred to as "teaching parents," who undergo a rigorous 1-year training program. While living in the group home, the adolescents, most of whom are adjudicated delinquents, attend local schools and are involved in community activities. The primary treatment components of the TFM include a multilevel point system, self-government procedures, social skills training, academic tutoring, and a home-based reinforcement system for monitor-

ing school behavior. The average stay for a participant in the program is about 1 year (Kirigin, 1996).

In terms of effectiveness, the TFM approach appears to be more effective than comparison programs while the adolescents are active participants. Specifically, the developers of the TFM compared the TFM to other community-based programs (nearly all of which were group homes) and found that, during treatment, a lower percentage of the TFM participants engaged in offenses and fewer offenses were recorded (Kirigin, Braukmann, Atwater, & Wolf, 1982). Independent evaluators (Weinrott, Jones, & Howard, 1982) found that participants in the TFM showed slightly more academic improvement compared to participants in community-based comparison programs. However, once the adolescents complete treatment and leave the group home setting, these differences have generally been found to disappear (Kirigin, 1996). It is notable that results from a recent evaluation of the TFM at Girls and Boys Town (Larzelere et al., 2001) suggest that some improvements in youth functioning are maintained at a 10-month follow-up. However, as this study did not include a control group, it is difficult to compare these results to those of youth in other types of treatment settings. With respect to cost-effectiveness, the TFM is cheaper than alternative group homes. However, both approaches are very expensive; only 45% of the adolescents complete treatment; and by 2 to 3 years later, there are few meaningful differences between treatment completers and dropouts (Weinrott et al., 1982).

A cross-cultural replication of the TFM was conducted in The Netherlands (Slot, Jagers, & Dangel, 1992). Comparisons of pre- and posttreatment scores indicated that the 58 adolescents (ages 14–19 years) in the program showed improvements in social competence and decreases in delinquent behavior. An analysis of program costs indicated that the TFM program was about one-quarter as costly as placements in a Dutch correctional institute.

Multidimensional Treatment Foster Care

Treatment foster care models are seeing a proliferation in use and evaluation. In a meta-analytic review, Reddy and Pfeiffer (1997) analyzed 40 published studies encompassing 12,282 subjects that employed some kind of treatment foster care model for a variety of child and adolescent populations. There were large positive effects on increasing placement permanency of difficult-to-place and difficult-to-maintain youth and on social skills and medium positive effects on reducing behavior problems, improving psychological adjustment, and reducing restrictiveness of postdischarge placement.

Over the past decade, Chamberlain and her colleagues at OSLC have developed and systematically evaluated a multicomponent intervention for youth with CP that is called the multidimensional treatment foster care (MTFC) model (e.g., Chamberlain, 1994, 2003; Chamberlain & Moore, 1998; Chamberlain & Reid, 1994, 1998; Eddy & Chamberlain, 2000). This model is based on previous intervention work at OSLC and was also influenced by the work of Hawkins and colleagues (Hawkins, 1989; Hawkins, Meadowcroft, Trout, & Luster, 1985), who were the first to use treatment foster care in community-based settings. The key components of MTFC include (1) recruitment and up to 20 hours of preservice training for foster parents in a social learning-based parent training model; (2) ongoing case management consisting of individualized consultation to foster parents, weekly group foster parent meetings, and 24-hour on-call services for crisis management and support to foster parents; (3) daily structure and telephone contact support; (4) school consultation consisting of teaching foster parents school advocacy skills and setting up a home–school daily report card for the adolescent; (5) family therapy with biological parents (or relatives) to coordinate gradual transfer of care from the MTFC parents to the home, if possible; and (6) individual therapy for skills training in problem solving, anger management, educational issues, and other individual issues. A hallmark of the program is the provision of some adjunctive services that are individualized to meet the needs of youth and their families, similar to MST.

The MTFC program has been evaluated in a number of experimental trials. In an early pilot study of the program, Chamberlain and Reid (1991) randomly assigned 19 adolescents with CP discharged from the state hospital to postdischarge MTFC or control treatment consisting of traditional community placements (e.g., group homes and training school). There were significantly greater reductions in PDR ratings of behavior problems at 3 months for MTFC compared to control subjects and a trend for differences at 7 months. There was a significantly shorter time from referral to placement for MTFC subjects with associated cost savings. However, social competency and problem-solving skills did not improve for either group.

Another study was conducted with a sample of regular foster parents and the children placed in their care (Chamberlain, Moreland, & Reid, 1992). This study compared one group of foster parents who received the MTFC model of training and support plus a small increase in their monthly stipend to a control group of foster parents who received only the increased stipend. The enhanced MTFC group had increased foster parent retention rates, increased ability to manage child CP, decreased reports of child CP, and decreased number of disrupted placements over the 2-year study period.

In more recent work, Chamberlain and Reid (1998) randomly assigned 79 boys referred for out-of-home care due to chronic delinquency to either MTFC or one of 11 group care (GC) placements. During the 1-year follow-up, significant differences were found in length of time in placement, runaway rates, arrest rates, days incarcerated, and self-reported delinquency, all in favor of MTFC. Four-year follow-up data showed that boys in MTFC continued to have significantly fewer arrests (Chamberlain, Fisher, & Moore, 2002). Family management skills and peer associations mediated the effect of MFTC on antisocial behavior and delinquency, accounting for approximately one-third of the variance in boys' subsequent antisocial behavior (Eddy & Chamberlain, 2000).

Chamberlain and colleagues (Chamberlain & Smith, 2003; Leve & Chamberlain, 2005) have also just completed a 5-year randomized trial of MTFC with 12- to 17-year-old females who had, on average, 11 offenses prior to referral. Girls were randomly assigned to MTFC or treatment as usual settings (e.g., group home, hospital, and inpatient drug and alcohol treatment). Preliminary 12-month follow-up data for 61 girls showed a greater decrease in arrests and fewer days in the hospital for mental health-related problems for girls treated with MTFC compared to girls receiving treatment as usual. Notably, however, girls in MTFC still reported participating in high-risk sexual activities and using alcohol and drugs at high rates. Chamberlain and colleagues (Chamberlain & Smith, 2003; Leve & Chamberlain, 2005) are currently conducting a study in which they have added components to MTFC to address these concerns.

With respect to the financial benefits of MTFC, the Aos and colleagues (2004) cost–benefit analysis estimated that the MTFC model saved taxpayers approximately $24,290 per participant in the program. In sum, these studies indicate that MTFC is an efficacious and cost-effective intervention for seriously delinquent and aggressive youth requiring out-of-home placement. Although the program is staff- and time-intensive, it still results in greater cost savings than traditional group home and residential placements.

A Broader Perspective on Psychosocial Intervention Efficacy: Meta-Analytic Research

In the previous sections on psychosocial interventions, we have presented a range of psychosocial interventions for adolescents with CP and, in each case, have attempted to summarize the available research on program efficacy (and where available, on effectiveness), noting both program strengths and limitations. However, given the substantial body of research on interventions for CP that currently exists, it also seems reasonable to wonder about the comparable efficacy of different types of interventions for CP. What magnitude of effect sizes is typically associated with different types of interventions? On the whole, do some categories of intervention seem to be more efficacious than others? Are particular interventions clearly more useful with mild to moderate CP as opposed to severe CP? How do individual characteristics (e.g., age and ethnicity) and particular intervention characteristics (e.g., type of service provider and duration of intervention) affect efficacy? Meta-analytic research is one approach to comparing a variety of interventions. (Meta-analysis can also be used to summarize data from multiple studies focused on a given intervention, as highlighted elsewhere in this chapter.) While meta-analysis has demonstrated utility in that it can certainly afford a broader perspective on a large body of research, it can also gloss over the details of individual studies including important strengths and limitations of a given intervention protocol or research design. Thus, the meta-analytic studies that follow complement the individual analyses of intervention results presented in the preceding sections. With this caveat in mind, we consider a number of meta-analytic studies reviewing psychosocial interventions for delinquent adolescent populations.

Lipsey has conducted some of the most extensive and in-depth meta-analytic research on interventions for CP. Several studies have been conducted examining the efficacy (and where available, effectiveness) of a range of interventions for delinquency in juveniles between the ages of 12 and 21 (Lipsey, 1992, 1995; Lipsey & Wilson, 1998). Over 500 intervention studies with data relevant to juvenile delinquency were incorporated into these meta-analyses, and 200 of these studies included results for serious juvenile offenders (Lipsey, 1999).

In a report on 400 of these intervention studies for juvenile delinquency (Lipsey, 1995), recidivism rates in treated groups (at about 6 months posttreatment) were 45% (compared to 50% in control groups). This decrease represents a 10% reduction compared to control groups. Compared to controls, treatment also leads to (1) a 28% relative improvement in psychological outcomes (e.g., attitudes, self-esteem, and clinical scales); (2) a 12% relative improvement in interpersonal adjustment (e.g., peer or family relationships and interpersonal skills); (3) a 12% relative improvement in school participation (e.g., attendance and dropout); (4) a 14% relative improvement in academic performance (e.g., grades and achievement tests); and (5) a 10% relative improvement in vocational accomplishment (e.g., job status and wages). Moving beyond these overall results, Lipsey (1995) found that older juveniles with more severe histories showed somewhat larger reductions in delinquency as a result of treatment compared to younger juveniles with less severe histories. However, these findings may be due to the fact that more serious offenders have more room for improvement (Lipsey, 1995). More significant differences in treatment efficacy were attributable to the type of treatment. Interventions that were skill oriented (e.g., some cognitively oriented skills training approaches as well as vocational training), multimodal (e.g., broad groups of services that usually combined a number of interventions), and behavioral (e.g., some more behaviorally oriented, skills training approaches as well as some family and community interventions) resulted in a 20–30% improvement compared to control groups. Several forms of individual counseling were at the other end of the spectrum, resulting in no significant improvement compared to controls. Other factors related to more positive outcomes included high researcher involvement in treatment design and implementation as well as high dosages of treatment (i.e., more than 100 hours of contact).

Examining the subset of intervention studies with at least a partial focus on serious juvenile offenders (n = 200 studies, as noted earlier), Lipsey (1999) found that treated serious juvenile offenders had a 44% recidivism rate compared to a 50% recidivism rate for untreated serious juvenile offenders. This result, although modest, is actually quite encouraging because it is almost identical to the recidivism rates for the broader group of juveniles discussed above, suggesting that serious delinquents are as "treatable" as other delinquents. In addition, as expected from the previous results, the meta-analytic findings from this study indicated that there was large heterogeneity in the ESs in the 200 studies. Thus, Lipsey and colleagues conducted further analyses to better understand the factors influencing intervention efficacy. Studies with institutionalized offenders (n = 83) were separated from studies with noninstitutionalized juveniles (n = 117).

Lipsey (1999) found that for both noninstitutionalized juveniles and institutionalized juveniles, interpersonal skills training (e.g., many of the social and cognitive-behavioral skills training intervention strategies discussed previously were included in this category) resulted in consistently positive effects. For the noninstitutionalized juveniles, "individual counseling" approaches (e.g., MST) and behavioral programs (e.g., FFT) also produced consistently positive effects. In contrast, for the institutionalized juveniles, behavioral programs produced less consistent positive effects (community residential programs and programs providing a variety of community services also produced only moderately consistent positive effects) while teaching family homes (e.g., TFM) produced consistently positive effects.

For both groups of juveniles, several overall factors were also important in terms of positive effects. Notably lower recidivism rates were associated with (1) juveniles receiving the full number of intervention sessions prescribed by treatment authors and (2) with program lengths of more than 6 months. Recidivism was not affected by the gender, ethnicity, or age composition of the juveniles in the samples. For institutionalized juveniles only, recidivism rates were also improved when juveniles participated in programs that (1) had been in use for 2 or more years (i.e., programs that had been in place longer were more successful at improving recidivism) and (2) had service providers who were not juvenile justice personnel. In the institutionalized sample, it is also notable that recidivism rates were not affected by the extent or type of prior offenses or the extent of aggressive history (although variation in prior offenses and aggressive history was somewhat limited because all of the studies focused on severe delinquency).

Wilson, Lipsey, and Soydan (2003) also conducted a meta-analysis examining whether interventions for juvenile delinquency were less effective with minority youth. Examining results from 305 intervention studies, these authors found that interventions generally had positive effects for minority youth and these effects did not differ significantly from the effects of intervention on nonminority youth.

Psychosocial Interventions for Specific Subtypes of Conduct Problems

Anger

A number of interventions have been designed to specifically address issues with anger control. Sukhodolsky, Kassinove, and Gorman (2004) conducted a meta-analysis to examine intervention results for anger-related problems. This analysis involved 50 studies (21 published and 19 unpublished) that used cognitive-behavioral therapy to treat anger in children and adolescents. Youth age ranged from 7 to 17.2 years (mean age = 12.5). In all, there were 51 treatment versus control comparisons, and approximately 25 of these involved adolescents. Overall, the mean ES for the cognitive-behavioral interventions was in the medium range (ES = 0.67). Age of subjects in the studies and the magnitude of ES were not correlated. However, the authors conducted a qualitative examination of ES means for the first age quartile and the fourth age quartile and found that there was a $0.2d$ increase in ES for the older age group. Skills training, problem-solving, and multimodal interventions were more effective than affective education. Skills training and multimodal interventions were particularly effective in reducing aggressive behavior and improving social skills. Problem-solving interventions were more effective in reducing youths' self-reports of anger. Specific treatment techniques involving modeling, feedback, and homework were related to larger ESs.

Feindler has developed and refined an anger-control training program for adolescents, the "Chill Out" program (Feindler, 1990, 1991, 1995; Feindler & Guttman, 1994), that includes many of the efficacious characteristics (skills training, problem solving, multiple intervention targets) described in the Sukholdolsky and colleagues (2004) meta-analysis. The Chill Out program is anchored in a model that assumes that anger motivates much of aggressive behavior, and, thus, interventions for anger problems will reduce aggressive behavior. Furthermore, the program is based on Novaco's (1978) model of anger arousal, in which anger is thought to consist of physiological, cognitive, and behavioral components; the program has more recently incorporated findings from research on the social information-processing model (Crick & Dodge, 1994). Following from the tripartite model of anger, the Chill Out program focuses on three major intervention target categories: arousal management training (relaxation training procedures), cognitive restructuring (addressing hostile and dysfunctional attributions), and behavioral skills training (assertion, communication, and problem-solving skills).

Although there have been increasing theoretical and technical refinements to the Chill Out program over recent years, the empirical foundation of the program rests on two studies conducted in the 1980s. In the first study (Feindler et al., 1984), 36 junior high school students with a history of high rates of classroom and/or community disruption were randomly assigned to the treatment program (10, 50-minute Chill Out sessions) or a no-treatment control condition. Data collected at a 5-week follow-up provided minimal support for the efficacy of the treatment program. Students who received anger-control training did perform better than the students in the no-treatment control condition on self-report measures of problem solving, and teachers rated the former more highly on a self-control measure. However, there were no between-group differences on fines for aggressive behavior in an ongoing contingency management system (the most direct measure of behavior in this study), or on self-report measures of locus of control and impulsivity.

This program was also adapted for use with male adolescent psychiatric inpatients, most of whom had been diagnosed with CD (Feindler, Ecton, Kingsley, & Dubey, 1986). Although there were significant posttreatment differences between the Chill Out and no-treatment control groups on the Matching Familiar Figures Test and child care staff ratings of self-control, the groups differed on only 3 of 11 behavioral measures in role-play tests at posttreatment. Daily records of discipline interactions on the ward indicated a significant decrease in general rule violations for the Chill Out group and an increase in those violations for the control group. There were no group differences at posttreatment with respect to violations for physical aggression. Thus, this study produced mixed results on behavioral outcomes; the broad-based efficacy of this anger-control training program for adolescents has yet to be clearly demonstrated.

Bullying

Bullying interventions have, for the most part, been implemented in the school setting. Large-scale efforts to introduce and evaluate schoolwide antibullying programs have occurred in Scandinavia (Olweus, 1993), England (Smith & Sharp, 1994a), Canada (Pepler, Craig, Ziegler, & Charach, 1993, 1994), and Belgium (Stevens, De Bourdeaudhuij, & Van Oost, 2000). These programs are both systems and person oriented (Olweus, 1992); that is, they are directed at both the school as a system and at the level of individual bullies, victims, and their parents. Although component analyses have not been conducted, Olweus believes that both major components are necessary, and that the typical clinical approach of intervening at the individual level will not be sufficient to achieve a meaningful outcome.

Key elements of the whole-school approach are the school taking responsibility for bullying and giving it a high priority; increasing awareness of bullying by teachers, peers, and parents; publicizing explicit school policies and classroom rules that devalue and communicate low tolerance and negative consequences for bullying; discussing bullying in the curriculum; encouraging peer disapproval of bullying; and encouraging bystanders to help victims and report bullying to teachers (Farrington, 1993; Olweus, 1992). Examples of interventions at the individual level include serious talks with bullies; letters home to parents and parent meetings; implementation of negative consequences for bullying (e.g., privilege removal); social skills training for victims; encouraging victims to report bullying incidents to adults; and assigning older children to "shadow" victims to observe the bullying and report it to teachers (Farrington, 1993; Pepler et al., 1993).

The first large-scale evaluation of the whole-school approach to bullying was conducted by Olweus (1990, 1991, 1996) in Norway. Olweus's intervention, the *Core Program Against Bullying and Antisocial Behavior*, was a nationwide campaign to intervene in grades 4–7 with an antibullying, whole-school approach to intervention following the suicides of several victims of bullies. This program aimed to "restructure the social environment" by targeting the school, classroom, and individuals, in order to provide fewer opportunities and rewards for aggression and bullying. The intervention emphasized positive teacher and parent involvement; enhanced communication, awareness, and supervision; set firm limits to unacceptable behavior; and devised consistent, nonphysical sanctions for rule breaking. At the school level, components included dissemination of an anonymous student questionnaire that assessed the extent of bullying in each school, formalized discussion of the problem, formation of a committee to plan and deliver the program, and a system of supervision of students between classes and during recess. At the classroom level, teachers provided clear, "no tolerance" rules for bullying and held regular classroom meetings for students and parents. Finally, individual interventions were provided for bullies, victims, and parents to ensure that the bullying stopped and that victims were supported and protected.

Evaluation of the effects of the intervention was based on data from approximately 2,500 students in Bergen schools using a quasi-experimental design. Outcome data were derived from a student self-report questionnaire. Results after 8 months and 20 months of intervention showed marked reductions in the level of bully/victim problems for both boys and girls. Similar effects were found on an aggregated peer-rating variable. There was also a reduction in covert CP behaviors such as vandalism, theft, and truancy. This is an interesting,

unintended effect that may have arisen from the general increase in adult monitoring and supervision. Finally, there was an increase in student satisfaction with school life. Marked reductions in aggressive behavior have been demonstrated in a subsequent intervention trial, with effects maintained 2 years later (see Olweus, 2001, for an overview).

A similar program, based closely on the model implemented in Norway, was introduced in 23 schools in the United Kingdom by Smith and his colleagues (Smith & Sharp, 1994a, 1994b). In addition to the basic Olweus program elements, this variation also included bully courts and the "Heartstone Odyssey" (a story that introduces experiences of racial harassment). The U.K. program has produced results similar to those presented by Olweus (Smith & Sharp, 1994a) although, in contrast with the results from Olweus and colleagues, there were larger program outcomes in primary schools compared to secondary schools. In addition, Eslea and Smith (1998) followed up four of the original primary schools and found that the program had been effective in reducing boys' bullying but not girls' bullying.

Pepler, Craig, and their colleagues (Pepler et al., 1993, 1994) conducted an evaluation of the Toronto Anti-Bullying Intervention, a whole-school approach modeled after Olweus's program and developed and implemented with the cooperation of the Toronto Board of Education. As with the Olweus program, the Toronto program involved intervention components at the school, parent, classroom/peer, and individual levels, similar to those described earlier. Results of this study confirmed that bullying is a stable and pervasive problem in schools. Over an 18-month whole-school intervention program implemented in four Toronto schools, there were some improvements in students' reports of bullying as assessed at individual, peer, and school levels and increases in teachers' interventions to stop bullying. However, there were no differences in students' discussions of bully/victim problems with their parents, and, unfortunately, victim reports of racial bullying increased.

While the programs described have tested school bullying interventions on a substantial number of youth, Stevens and colleagues (2000) also included a nonintervention control group in their study of a whole-school bullying program in primary and secondary schools. They found significant improvements in the experimental group but only in the primary school setting. These authors suggested that the lack of results in the secondary school setting may be due in part to adolescents' tendency to conform less with antibullying rules (a key component of these programs). They also commented that administering and maintaining these interventions in secondary schools was much more complicated, because of the less-structured secondary school setting. Taken together, this group of studies suggests that whole-school bullying interventions may have promise, but their efficacy in adolescent populations has not been clearly demonstrated.

In a somewhat more individualistic approach to a bullying intervention, Baldry (2001) developed a program that was directed toward students and their peer groups and was designed to enhance awareness about violence and its negative effects. Using videos and a three-part booklet combined with role playing, group discussions and focus groups, participants were taught about the negative effects of bullying, and intervention components focused on enhancing empathy, building perspective-taking skills, and encouraging peers to support victims rather than ignoring or downplaying bullying. Baldry and Farrington (2004) evaluated this intervention with 237 students (control *n* = 106, intervention *n* = 131) ages 11–15. Victimization (e.g., direct victimization, having belongings stolen, and being called nasty names) decreased for older students but not for younger students.

Gender-Specific Interventions for Girls

Recognizing that much of what is currently known about the development of, and intervention with, CP has been based on research with boys, there has been a recent explosion of interest in, and research on, CP in girls (see Moretti et al., 2004; Pepler et al., 2005; Putallaz & Bierman, 2004; Underwood, 2003; for comprehensive reviews). Appropriately, most of that research has focused on the phenomenology of CP in girls, rather than on intervention. However, as the knowledge base expands, implications for intervention are beginning to emerge. First, it is still unclear as to the extent that gender-specific interventions for girls are indicated and the nature of their content (Antonishak, Reppucci, & Mulford, 2004; Craig, 2005; Underwood & Coie, 2004). On the other hand, it is clear that there is a dearth

of interventions that are specifically targeted to relational and other "social" forms of CP. Because at least during some developmental periods girls are more likely to engage in these forms of CP rather than in physical aggression, they are more likely to be adversely affected by the absence of these types of interventions.

General suggestions for intervention include (1) increased awareness of parents and teachers of the seriousness of relational aggression; (2) adaptation and expansion of existing interventions for bullying and other forms of CP to directly target relational aggression; and (3) increased focus on gender-specific interventions targeted to girls as they approach adolescence (Geiger et al., 2004; Underwood, 2003; Underwood & Coie, 2004). With respect to the latter, interventions might target relational aggression (and, more generally, the development of positive same-sex friendships), the tendency of adolescent girls with CP to associate with adolescent males, romantic relationships, and sexual risk taking (Craig, 2005; Leve & Chamberlain, 2005; Underwood & Coie, 2004). Thus, interventions might focus on relationship enhancement strategies and the prevention of relationship violence (e.g., anger management skills and conflict resolution strategies). The common thread underlying all these suggestions is the emphasis placed on relationship-based issues and interventions. Underwood (2003) provides a thoughtful discussion about a number of content areas for gender-specific interventions with girls. Preliminary or interim reports from several gender-specific interventions for girls have recently presented promising results: the Earlscourt Girls Connection for preadolescents (Levene, Walsh, Augimeri, & Pepler, 2004; Pepler, Walsh, & Levene, 2004); the Friend to Friend Program for relationally and physically aggressive elementary-school-age girls (Leff, Angelucci, Grabowski, & Weil, 2004); and the adaptation of MTFC for adolescent girls (Leve & Chamberlain, 2005).

Covert Conduct Problems

Whereas psychosocial interventions for overt CP behaviors have been evaluated extensively in home, school, and community settings, there are relatively few data concerning interventions of any type for covert types of CP behavior, especially with respect to adolescents. However, the attention being given to some of these covert behaviors, especially firesetting, and their treatment is increasing due to the rising recognition that when both overt and covert behaviors are present, the youth's CP is more serious and may have a poorer long-term outcome. In addition, covert CP often represents serious violations of the rights of others, provoking concern from the community. In this section of the chapter, we describe interventions that have been designed to treat stealing, lying, and firesetting.

Stealing

There is a consensus that the identification/labeling of stealing is the key to developing a successful intervention for this behavior (Barth, 1987; Miller & Klungness, 1989; Patterson, Reid, Jones, & Conger, 1975). Because of its low base rate and covert nature, firsthand, immediate detection of all stealing events by parents, teachers, or others is not a feasible goal. Therefore, stealing is operationally defined as "the child's taking, or being in possession of, anything that does not clearly belong to him [or her]" (Barth, 1987, p. 151). Table 5.1 contains an elaboration of this definition, as well as instructions for caregivers on how to respond to stealing behavior. Although adoption of this definition of stealing may result in instances in which the youth is incorrectly labeled as having stolen, the alternative of not being able to treat the stealing behavior effectively is regarded as the greater of the two evils.

The most systematic work on the treatment of covert CP had been conducted by Patterson, Reid, and their colleagues at OSLC with respect to family-based interventions for treating stealing. The OSLC group developed a specialized approach to parent management training with youth who display stealing and other covert CP behaviors (Patterson et al., 1975; Reid et al., 1980) that takes into account the definitional and detection problems inherent in treating covert CP behaviors and also attempts to impact directly on the parenting variables strongly associated with delinquency (i.e., parental involvement, monitoring, and parental discipline practices). The failure of parents of youth who steal to monitor their youth's whereabouts or to be involved with the youth to any great extent compounds the difficulty of designing effective family-based interventions.

In the OSLC approach to the treatment of stealing, the standard parent training program for treating overt CP behaviors is implemented

TABLE 5.1. Instructions to Caregivers for Defining and Providing Consequences for Stealing

1. The most important part of working to decrease stealing is *defining stealing as stealing. Stealing is defined as the child's taking, or being in possession of, anything that does not clearly belong to him.* Parents, teachers, or other adults are the only judges. They may label an act as stealing by observing it, by having it reported to them, or by noticing that something is missing. There is no arguing about guilt or innocence. It is the child's job to be sure that he is not accused. The value of the object is irrelevant. Trading and borrowing are not permissible. Any "purchases" that the child brings home must be accompanied by a receipt. Otherwise they are to be returned and consequences instituted.

2. Once the behavior of stealing has been labeled, then the consequences are to be applied. Avoid discussions, shaming, or counseling.

3. *Every* stealing event must be so labeled and consequences given.

4. Avoid using excessive detective tactics (such as searches); just keep your eyes open, and investigate the origins of new property.

5. Consequences for stealing should be work restrictions and loss of privileges for the day of the stealing, and basic privileges only on the following weekend. There should be no other consequences such as humiliations or beatings. Special privileges can be earned again on the following day.

6. *Remember*: Stealing goes hand in hand with wandering and with your not knowing the whereabouts of your child. Check-in times are recommended if stealing is a problem.

7. Do not tempt your child. Keep items like those that your child has stolen in the past away from him or her. For example, avoid leaving your wallet or cigarette packs in view or unwatched.

8. Stealing may occur no matter how many possessions your child has, so giving him or her everything is not a successful approach to ending stealing. Your child should, however, have some way of earning his or her own money so that he or she may have a choice of things to buy.

Note. From Barth (1987). Copyright 1987 by Plenum Publishing Corporation. Reprinted with permission from the author and Springer Science and Business Media.

first, because these behaviors covary with the lower-rate covert CP behaviors in many youth. In addition, the standard OSLC program addresses two important parenting practices (i.e., poor discipline practices and parental involvement with the child). Next, parents are taught to identify stealing using an operational definition similar to the one presented earlier, and to monitor its occurrence on a daily basis. Much discussion and role playing of these procedures occur in therapy sessions.

Once the operational definition of stealing is accepted by the parents, parents are taught to administer a mild consequence immediately contingent upon each and every suspected stealing event. The consequence (e.g., 1–2 hours of hard work around the home) is kept at a mild level because the youth will be inaccurately accused from time to time. The implementation of this approach involves much support, telephone contact, and discussion. Check-in systems are instituted for families in which infrequent monitoring occurs. In addition, it would seem important to incorporate therapeutic strategies for involving fathers in the therapy process, given the relationship between uninvolved fathers and stealing (Frick, 1994; Loeber et al., 1983).

In a study that remains the most systematic evaluation of treatment focused specifically on stealing behavior, Reid and colleagues (1980) evaluated the effectiveness of this modified approach to parent management training for 5- to 14-year-old youth with CP who were referred for stealing. In this study, 28 families of children with CP who stole received treatment. The mean amount of therapist contact was 32 hours. Outcome measures consisted of parent reports of stealing on the TIROSSA, parent reports of other referral problems on the PDR, and a deviant behavior summary score in home observations conducted by trained independent observers. There were significant decreases in parent-reported stealing events and other referral problems from pre- to posttreatment and at a 6-month follow-up. Observed deviant behavior scores decreased nonsignificantly. However, as might be expected, aversive social behaviors in the families were not high to begin with in this sample of youth who stole. A waiting-list control group, in which parent-report data on stealing were collected at baseline, at the end of the parent training program for dealing with overt CP, and following the treatment package for stealing, indicated that significant reductions in parent-reported stealing did not occur until after the treatment for stealing was implemented. However, large differences in baseline levels of stealing limit the utility of this comparison.

In another study with chronic delinquents from the OSLC group, described earlier in this chapter, Bank and colleagues (1991) found some empirical support for the efficacy of this family-based approach with the subset of adolescents who engaged in both overt and covert CP behaviors. Parent-reported stealing (as noted on the PDR) was reduced to zero at treatment termination. In addition, the preventive intervention implemented by Tremblay and colleagues (see below), which employed an adaptation of the OSLC model of parent management training and children's social skills training, successfully reduced stealing through age 17 (e.g., Lacourse et al., 2002).

Stealing has also been approached from a more traditional family therapy model. Seymour and Epston (1989) treated 45 consecutive cases (20% of whom were adolescents ages 13–15) of childhood stealing with an approach that "regraded" the child from "stealer" to "honest person." Therapists focused questions in such a way as to "externalize the symptom," a framework promulgated by White (1986), and assisted the child and the parents to engage together in working against the stealing. Thereafter, techniques were very similar to those employed by Reid and colleagues (1980). Emphasis was placed on suspicion of stealing, on responding to stealing with work chore consequences, and on "honesty tests" in which items of interest were left around the house, and the child was reinforced by parents for not stealing. Although no control group was employed, Seymour and Epston reported significant pre- to posttreatment changes in stealing. Fifty-four percent of the cases reported no stealing at a 2-month follow-up, and an additional 40% reported only one to three instances. At a 1-year follow-up, levels of stealing remained low. Sixty-two percent of parents reported no instances of stealing and 19% of parents reported that stealing was "substantially reduced." A similar family-based intervention is described by Pawsey (1996). An initial period of parental monitoring of stealing was followed by the sequential presentation of up to four additional interventions: contracting, restitution, punishment, and honesty tests. The intervention was successful for 12 of 14 youth (ages 7–15 years) referred to an outpatient child psychiatry clinic; effects were maintained for 10 of the 12 youth at a 3-month follow-up. Effects were comparable for preadolescents and adolescents. More recently, Venning, Blampied, and France (2003) presented a case study describing the positive effects of the Triple P parenting program (Sanders, Turner, &

Markie-Dadds, 2002) on stealing with two preadolescent boys. Using similar procedures to those described previously, they reported rapid cessation of stealing that was maintained at a 10-week follow-up.

Although the results of family-based intervention studies are suggestive, the effects of treatment on stealing were assessed primarily from parent-report measures. Given the problems these parents have with respect to effective monitoring of their children's behavior, future investigators should attempt to include some treatment component directed specifically to parental monitoring (see Dishion & McMahon, 1998). Not only is this a worthwhile target of intervention in its own right, but effective monitoring of the youth's behavior and whereabouts would seem to be a prerequisite for accurate recording on measures such as the TIROSSA and PDR. Another critical issue that must be addressed pertains to the generalizability of family-based interventions for stealing in other settings, such as the school or the community at large. Although there are effective treatment procedures for dealing with stealing in the elementary school setting (see below), identifying and stopping stealing in public places such as stores is very difficult.

Henderson (1981, 1983) developed an "individualized combined treatment" (ICT) program for children and adolescents who report that they want to stop stealing. This approach has three broad components: (1) self-control of the internal environment, (2) adult or responsible-other control of the external environment, and (3) personalization of the program by the therapist. In the first component, Henderson teaches relaxation skills in an effort to countercondition internal arousal stimuli, which he maintains are often associated with stealing. In therapy sessions, the youth is asked to imagine him- or herself in theft situations and then to relax and imagine walking away. In this way, relaxation and imagery are also conceptualized as self-control techniques, which are later extended to the external environment. Heart-rate biofeedback is used to facilitate relaxation. Parents are asked to provide stealing opportunities or "traps" for the youth in the home so that the youth has an opportunity to practice self-control strategies. Bonuses in a reward system are provided for not stealing. The "traps" are gradually made less obvious and easier to take without being caught.

To provide external controls for not stealing, some system for monitoring "not stealing" must be implemented. Henderson (1981) advocates the use of a "not-stealing diary." Two types of entries are made in the diary: (1) any length of time that the stealer has been observed by a responsible adult not to have stolen; and (2) times of departure and arrival noted by responsible adults at both ends of a journey (e.g., from home to school). If the times logged in conform to appropriate travel time, an assumption is made that no stealing has occurred. Daily time "not stealing" is computed, and nonstealing time is rewarded with backup privileges and activities. These reinforcers are selected so that they are related in some way to the youth's motive for stealing (see Barth, 1987). For example, if the youth seems to steal for "kicks," an appropriate backup reinforcer might be a roller-coaster ride at an amusement park.

Henderson (1981, 1983) presented descriptive data on 10 youth (8–15 years of age) who were treated using the ICT program. Compared to 17 other youth who were treated for stealing at the same clinic using a variety of other treatment procedures, only 20% of the youth who received the ICT program were reported to have stolen in the 2-year period following treatment, whereas 60–75% of the other youth were reported to have stolen. Although the descriptive data on this approach to treatment are certainly encouraging, systematic evaluation of the program with appropriate controls needs to be undertaken.

A few studies have focused on the reduction of stealing in elementary school classrooms. To our knowledge, similar work has not been conducted with adolescent samples in school settings. Because of its relatively controlled and geographically confined nature, the classroom may be amenable to more systematic monitoring of stealing behavior and to the implementation of differential reinforcement procedures for not stealing than is the case when treatment is implemented in the home (cf. Reid, 1984). Classroom interventions have included some form of response cost for stealing and positive reinforcement for periods of nonstealing (Brooks & Snow, 1972; Rosen & Rosen, 1983; Switzer, Deal, & Bailey, 1977). In all cases, the frequency of stealing was significantly reduced when either group or individual contingencies were applied. Group contingencies that are applied to an entire classroom may be considered as adjuncts to individualized sets of contingencies when designing an intervention for stealing by an individual youth. Behavioral generalization of the effects of other school-based interventions to stealing has been demonstrated in at least one instance. As noted previously, reductions in stealing at school (as well as other covert behaviors such as vandalism and truancy) were found as a result of implementing the antibullying program designed by Olweus (1990, 1991, 1996).

Miller and Klungness (1989) make several recommendations about interventions to reduce the occurrence of stealing. First, they recommend that therapists emphasize the accurate labeling and consistent detection of stealing. Second, therapists should emphasize the promotion of effective child management skills with parents. Third, with motivated youth, Miller and Klungness recommend the use of self-control procedures by the youth in addition to external controls employed by parents. Fourth, the intervention should designate alternative behaviors to reinforce in order to counteract the withdrawal of reinforcement that has been attendant to stealing. Fifth, it is important to implement systemic-level changes in the school setting such as increased supervision of youth at recess and in school hallways. Although the recommendations of Miller and Klungness have not been evaluated, they are consistent with the treatment package designed and evaluated by Reid and colleagues (1980), and seem applicable to adolescents as well as younger children.

Lying

Stouthamer-Loeber (1986) has suggested that younger children, whose lies are more transparent and easily detectable, should be easier to treat. She advocates an educational approach in which the parent instructs the child in the difference between what is true and not true and provides training in empathy and/or perspective taking. For older children and adolescents, she suggests an approach similar to that described previously by Reid and colleagues (1980) for stealing. If the parent suspects that the child is lying, the child must prove that he or she is being truthful to avoid a negative consequence. Stouthamer-Loeber also stresses the necessity of focusing on increasing parental monitoring of the child in interventions designed to decrease lying. To our knowledge,

there has only been a single report of a formalized intervention to deal with lying. Venning and colleagues (2003) presented data in which the Triple P parenting intervention (Sanders et al., 2002) was used to successfully decrease lying (and stealing, as described earlier) in a 10-year-old male. Intervention procedures paralleled those employed to decrease stealing and included good-behavior charts, immediate parental response when lying was suspected, and consequences such as time out, restitution, and loss of privileges. At a 10-week follow-up, parental concerns about lying had been eliminated over the 3-week data-collection period.

Firesetting

Although firesetting is often (but not always) associated with a diagnosis of CD and indicates a more advanced, extreme, or complex form of CP (Forehand et al., 1991; Hanson et al., 1994; Stickle & Blechman, 2002), it has been recognized as requiring a specific treatment focus in addition to standard psychosocial treatments for CP.

There are a number of case studies and a few experimental studies involving both behavioral and nonbehavioral treatments (see Kolko, 2002b, and Stadolnik, 2000, for reviews). Treatments have included contingency management procedures, negative practice in firesetting as a satiation and extinction procedure, prosocial skills training in the expression of anger and other emotional arousal, and family therapy. A brief cognitive-behavioral skills training curriculum implemented with psychiatrically hospitalized children (ages 4–8) was associated with significantly greater reductions in contact with fire-related toys and matches in an analogue task and an increase in firesetting knowledge compared to a firesetting discussion group control (Kolko et al., 1991). At a 6-month follow-up, parents reported less involvement with fire for children in the cognitive-behavioral condition.

In addition to the psychological treatments just reviewed, another approach to intervention has been developed by the Fire Service and is implemented by trained firefighters in the community. These programs emphasize detection and assessment of the firesetter and rely heavily on fire-safety education and mentoring (Kolko, 1988). In addition, several states (e.g., Oregon and Massachusetts) have developed statewide interagency intervention programs (Okulitch & Pinsonneault, 2002), and increasing attention is being paid to residential (Pelletier-Parker, Slate, Moriarity, & Personneault, 1999; Richardson, 2002) and juvenile justice diversion and intervention (Elliott, 2002) programs for adolescents.

Unfortunately, systematic, controlled evaluations of these programs are scarce. An evaluation of educational materials (a brief brochure) alone or in conjunction with an adaptation of the Federal Emergency Management Agency (FEMA) program or referral to a mental health specialist showed statistically and clinically significant reductions in frequency and seriousness of firesetting in a sample of 5- to 16-year-olds at a 1-year follow-up assessment, regardless of intervention condition (Adler, Nunn, Northam, Lebnan, & Ross, 1994). Thus, the multicomponent FEMA intervention was no more effective than the provision of educational materials.

Because fire-safety education alone provides for significant reductions in firesetting, Kolko (2001) conducted an experiment to test the comparative effects of fire-safety education as implemented in community settings (such as the FEMA program) and psychosocial treatment as implemented in mental health settings. In this study, psychosocial treatment consisted of cognitive-behavioral procedures designed to modify the characteristics and correlates of firesetting. Specifically, children learned graphing techniques to relate firesetting motives to specific events or affective states, problem-solving skills, and assertion skills. Parents received parent management training with special emphasis on child monitoring and consequences. (See Kolko, 2002a, for an extended description of these procedures.) Five- to 13-year old boys who set fires were randomly assigned to the two treatments, each of which consisted of eight sessions. In addition, a third condition, consisting of nonrandomly assigned participants received two fire-safety education home visits from a firefighter. All three interventions were associated with significant decreases in a number of indices of firesetting behavior at both posttreatment and 1-year follow-up. The cognitive-behavioral and fire-safety education interventions demonstrated greater effects than the firefighter-visit intervention on several additional indices of firesetting behavior. This study suggests that brief interventions conducted by a trained firefighter are effective in reducing firesetting behavior in preadolescent males, but that more intensive cognitive-behavioral and fire-safety education interventions are even more effective.

Psychopharmacological Treatment

Use of psychopharmacological treatment for adolescents with primary CP has been steadily increasing over the last two decades. Here, we briefly review several pharmacological treatments for adolescents with CP for which some empirical support is available. We also recommend two useful reviews, which detail the available literature in this area (Connor, 2002; Waslick, Werry, & Greenhill, 1998). Before considering specific classes of drugs often used to treat aspects of CP, an important caveat should be noted: In general, studies on this topic have included only small numbers of children from a wide age range (i.e., preschoolers or young school-age children through adolescents). Furthermore, in the majority of studies, preadolescents (i.e., 11- and 12-year-olds) are the oldest children included. Thus, in reviewing specific studies, age and sample size have been noted where appropriate so that this information can be considered in weighing the applicability of the current research to adolescents with CP.

Psychostimulants

Psychostimulants (e.g., methylphenidate, dextroamphetamine, and pemoline) have been shown to reduce aggressive behavior as well as some covert problem behaviors in children and adolescents with ADHD. For example, Hinshaw, Henker, Whalen, Erhardt, and Dunnington (1989) examined 25 children with ADHD (ages 6–12 years) and found significant improvements in aggression and related behaviors. Extending these findings into adolescence, Kaplan, Busner, Kupietz, Wasserman, and Segal (1990) examined six 13- to 16-year-olds and also found improvements in aggression. Hinshaw and colleagues (1992) assessed the effects of methylphenidate on covert CP in boys with ADHD in a laboratory paradigm designed to provide an occasion for stealing, cheating, and property destruction. In a drug-placebo crossover design, drug treatment resulted in significant decreases in stealing and property destruction, observed surreptitiously in the laboratory. However, cheating *increased* when the children were taking methylphenidate. Although ADHD is the only behavioral disorder for which psychostimulants have been clearly shown to be efficacious, this class of drugs may also be useful in the treatment of CP (with or without comorbid ADHD) (Barkley, McMurray, Edelbrock, & Robbins, 1989; Connor, Glatt, Lopez, Jackson, & Melloni, 2002; Hinshaw, Buhrmester, & Heller, 1989; Hinshaw, Henker, et al., 1989). Furthermore, because comorbidity of ADHD and CP is probably the rule rather than the exception in clinical samples (Abikoff & Klein, 1992), findings suggesting that psychostimulants may be helpful in cases in which CP and ADHD are co-occurring (e.g., Abikoff, Klein, Kass, & Ganeles, 1987; Connor, Barkley, & Davis, 2000; MTA Cooperative Group, 1999) have significance when considering treatment options for youth with CP. Klein, Abikoff, and colleagues have conducted two of the only studies focusing on the use of psychostimulants in youth with CD. Klein, Abikoff, Klass, Shah, and Seese (1994) compared methylphenidate, lithium, and placebo, and found that methylphenidate produced improvement over placebo in measures of CP in 80 children and adolescents diagnosed with CD. In addition, Klein and colleagues (1997), examining 84, 6- to 15-year-olds, found that treatment with methylphenidate resulted in reduced aggression and improved symptoms of antisocial behavior in youth diagnosed with CD regardless of their level of ADHD symptoms (i.e., 69% of the youth in the study met criteria for ADHD, but when ADHD was controlled for in the analyses, all findings remained significant, and there was no significant interaction between ADHD and treatment outcome, indicating that initial ADHD ratings did not have a significant impact on youths' response to methylphenidate). Taken together, these studies provide increasing support for the conclusion that stimulant medications produce reductions in CP in children and adolescents selected on the basis of primary diagnoses of ADHD or CD.

Lithium

Lithium carbonate has been used in children and adolescents for control of severe aggression with an affective component. However, limited and mixed findings regarding efficacy (see qualitative review by Connor, 2002, for a complete survey of studies involving the use of lithium in reducing aggression in children and adolescents) and concerns about serious toxicity and side effects have led psychopharmacologists to recommend that lithium be used to treat CP only in a very specific circumstance— with explosively aggressive youth who have failed to improve with other treatments (e.g., Waslick et al., 1998). Recommendations for its use come primarily from the work of Campbell and colleagues, who have conducted two separate, large-scale, double-blind, placebo-controlled studies in preadolescents diagnosed with CD that was characterized by aggressive and explosive behaviors, and who were hospitalized following outpatient treatment failure (Campbell et al., 1984: 21 children ages 5–12; Campbell et al., 1995: 20 children ages 5–12). In both studies, lithium was superior to placebo in reducing aggressive behavior and produced fewer side effects than haloperidol (a commonly prescribed neuroleptic). More recently, Campbell and colleagues (Malone, Delaney, Luebbert, Cater, & Campbell, 2000) have extended these findings into adolescence, again showing lithium to be superior to placebo in reducing aggression and related behaviors in a sample of 20 youth ages 10–17. In contrast to the positive results reported in studies conducted by Campbell and colleagues, Klein and colleagues (1994) completed a study in which 80 outpatient children and adolescents with diagnoses of CD were randomly assigned to lithium, methylphenidate, or placebo. Lithium did not produce improvement compared to placebo. However, it is notable that in this study children were outpatients and "only a few" displayed "explosively dangerous outbursts" (Klein, 1991, p. 120) as opposed to the inpatient population in the Campbell and colleagues (1984, 1995) studies, for whom "explosiveness" was one of the selection criteria.

Antipsychotics (Neuroleptics)

Antipsychotic medications (e.g., chlorpromazine, risperidone, and haloperidol) have been used historically to treat CP in children and adolescents, especially those who are hospitalized chronically or who display mental retardation. Several controlled trials have demonstrated the efficacy of antipsychotics in reducing aggression, fighting, explosiveness, and hostility, mostly with hospitalized inpatient youth populations (e.g., Campbell et al., 1984; Findling, Aman, & Derivan, 2000; Greenhill, Solomon, Pleak, & Ambrosini, 1985). However, it should be noted that of these controlled trials, only Findling and colleagues (2000) included adolescents in their study (20 youth ages 5–15 were examined). Thus, the applicability of these findings to adolescent populations remains unclear. In addition, concern about serious adverse side effects (e.g., tardive and withdrawal dyskinesias and neuroleptic malignant syndrome) has limited both the use of neuroleptics in treating CP and research in this area.

Any consideration of use of drugs with youth must include careful review of their putative effects against their side effects. Physicians considering pharmacological treatments are referred to other authoritative reviews of drug side effects (Kruesi & Lelio, 1996; Werry & Aman, 1993). Likewise, all clinicians prescribing drugs to children must familiarize themselves with Food and Drug Administration (FDA) regulations and *Physicians' Desk Reference* guidelines. In addition, Bloomquist and Schnell (2002) and Bukstein (2003) both provide excellent summaries of practical issues worthy of consideration and related "best practices" in the administration and management of psychopharmacological treatments in childhood and adolescence.

Prevention

Although the focus of this chapter is on the *treatment* of adolescents with CP, we feel that it is important to briefly describe more preventively oriented interventions that are either intended, or have been shown, to *prevent* subsequent CP. The prevention of CP has received increasing interest and attention over the past 15 years. This has been partly due to advances made in the delineation of developmental pathways of CP (especially the early-starter pathway) and the risk and protective factors associated with progression on this pathway. Increased interest in prevention has also evolved from the successes and limitations of the treatment-focused interventions described in earlier sections of this chapter.

To a certain extent, the distinction between treatment and prevention of CP is often difficult to make, because preventive interventions have usually (although not always) targeted younger children who are already engaging in some type of CP behavior (Coie & Dodge, 1998). One distinction is that treatment involves referral for assistance, whereas partici-

pation in prevention is usually done by screening. This is a somewhat tenuous distinction. For example, a number of family-based interventions that were developed as treatments for CP have been identified as model family programs for delinquency prevention (Alvarado, Kendall, Beesley, & Lee-Cavaness, 2000). Such programs include the parent training programs for younger (age 3–8 years) children developed by Forehand and McMahon (1981; McMahon & Forehand, 2003) and Webster-Stratton (1996), and treatments for adolescents described in this chapter such as FFT (Alexander & Sexton, 2002), BSFT (Szapocznik & Williams, 2000), MST (Henggeler et al., 1998), and MTFC (Chamberlain, 1994).

There are two broad classes of interventions that are applicable to the prevention of CP: early intervention programs with infants and preschool-age children that are not focused on CP per se and interventions that specifically target the prevention of CP. The latter type of preventive interventions has focused on youth ranging from preschool age to early adolescence. Space considerations preclude a detailed description of the many programs that have been developed or that are in progress for the prevention of CP. Reviews of such efforts may be found in Lemarquand, Tremblay, and Vitaro (2001); McMahon and Rhule (2005); Webster-Stratton and Taylor (2001); and Yoshikawa (1994).

Broad-Based Early Interventions

There is growing evidence that early intervention programs (i.e., those that are implemented during the infancy and/or preschool periods) can have long-term effects on the reduction of CP in adolescence and into adulthood (for reviews, see Yoshikawa, 1994; Zigler, Taussig, & Black, 1992). These long-term effects have been noted in later childhood and adolescence, and in at least one case, into adulthood (Schweinhart, Barnes, & Weikart, 1993). This is of particular interest, because prevention of CP has not typically been an explicit goal of these interventions. Yoshikawa noted four common elements of these interventions: (1) inclusion of both family support and child education components; (2) implementation during the child's first 5 years; (3) at least 2 years duration (range = 2–5 years); and (4) short- to medium-term effects on risk factors shown to be associated with CP.

One of the best-known of these early intervention programs is the Infancy and Early Childhood Visitation Program developed by Olds and colleagues (Olds, Kitzman, Cole, & Robinson, 1997), which offered extensive home visits from nurses to low-income, first-time mothers and their babies. To reduce risk factors for infant prematurity, low birthweight, and neurodevelopmental impairment, visits during pregnancy addressed women's health behaviors such as smoking, drug and alcohol use, and nutrition. Visitation continued until the children were 2 years old and focused on improving caregiving and reducing child maltreatment, preventing future unplanned pregnancies, and promoting the mothers' completion of school and participation in the work force.

Several controlled studies have demonstrated the program's effectiveness in meeting these objectives. In comparison to mothers in the control groups, mothers who received visitation had heavier and fewer preterm babies and showed a greater reduction in smoking. Fifteen years later, visited mothers had fewer subsequent births, fewer reports of child maltreatment and child injuries, a greater increase in labor force participation and decrease in welfare dependence, and fewer arrests. Of particular interest (although not specifically targeting child CP), the visitation program successfully reduced the children's early antisocial behavior, juvenile delinquency, and other problem behaviors, including arrests, running away, number of sexual partners, smoking and alcohol use, and substance-related behavioral problems (e.g., Olds et al., 1998). The program had its greatest impact on the most at-risk families (low-income, unmarried women) and offered relatively little benefit for the broader population.

Preventive Interventions Focused on Conduct Problems

There have been at least two generations of preventive interventions that have been designed specifically to prevent CP. First-generation interventions implemented in the 1980s have now reported on long-term outcomes, whereas second-generation interventions implemented in the 1990s have reported short- to medium-term outcomes to date. The Montreal and Seattle prevention trials were conducted in the 1980s and are representative examples of the first generation of preventive interventions.

Montreal Longitudinal–Experimental Study. The Montreal Longitudinal–Experimental Study (see Tremblay, Vitaro, Nagin, Pagani, & Seguin, 2003, for a summary) evaluated the effects of a two-component intervention in preventing CP in boys identified as aggressive and disruptive during kindergarten in a randomized trial. The program offered parent training, based on the OSLC model developed by Patterson and colleagues (Patterson et al., 1975), and classroom-based child social skills training, focusing on prosocial skills and self-control. Services were provided for 2 years, beginning when boys were in second grade.

By early adolescence (to age 15), boys who received the intervention were less disruptive, showed better elementary school adjustment, and reported fewer delinquent behaviors of their own (including stealing, gang membership, and substance use) and friends' arrests than did boys in the control condition (Tremblay et al., 1992; Tremblay, Masse, Pagani, & Vitaro, 1996; Tremblay, Pagani-Kurtz, Masse, Vitaro, & Pihl, 1995). The combined effects of decreases in postintervention disruptiveness (based on teacher reports) and association with deviant peers over the next 3 years mediated intervention effects in obtaining a diagnosis of CD at age 13 (Vitaro, Brendgen, Pagani, Tremblay, & McDuff, 1999). In a growth curve analysis, Vitaro, Brengden, and Tremblay (2002) demonstrated that the level of self-reported delinquency at age 13 was lower for the intervention than control boys, and this difference was maintained over the next 3 years. Decreases in disruptiveness and increased parental monitoring at age 11 and association with deviant peers at age 12 mediated the intervention effects at age 13. However, the intervention did not significantly affect delinquency as measured by juvenile court records or early sexual intercourse. Although the earlier positive effects in elementary school on school adjustment were not maintained, intervention boys were much less likely than control boys to have dropped out of school by age 17 (10.5% vs. 21.6%) (Vitaro, Brendgen, & Tremblay, 1999). The intervention also altered trajectories of physical aggression, vandalism, and stealing from ages 11 to 17 (Lacourse et al., 2002).

Seattle Social Development Project (SSDP). The SSDP (Hawkins et al., 1992, 2002) was a universal intervention implemented in regular classrooms in the Seattle public school system. The intervention offered a combination of teacher training, parent training, and social-cognitive skills training for children in grades 1–6. Teachers were instructed in the use of proactive classroom management, interactive teaching, and cooperative learning and in the implementation of a social-cognitive skills training program, based on the interpersonal cognitive problem solving curriculum (Shure & Spivack, 1980). Tailored to the children's developmental level, the parent component provided skills training in effective monitoring, reinforcement, and consequences; having clear expectations; and the encouragement of greater parental involvement and support of the children's academic success.

At the end of grade 6, girls in the intervention program reported significantly more classroom participation, bonding, and commitment to school and showed a trend to less initiation of alcohol and marijuana use. Boys showed better social and academic skills, reported more commitment and bonding to school and less initiation of delinquency, and were rated as having fewer antisocial friends (O'Donnell, Hawkins, Catalano, Abbott, & Day, 1995). Six years after the program ended, intervention students reported less school misbehavior, violent delinquent behavior, alcohol use, and sexual activity, as well as greater academic achievement and commitment to school (Hawkins, Catalano, Kosterman, Abbott, & Hill, 1999). In addition, the intervention demonstrated a dose-dependent effect in that the group that received the comprehensive, 6-year intervention showed better outcomes than those that received the intervention in grades 5 and 6 only.

Fast Track Project. There is a second generation of prevention trials specifically focused on CP that are currently underway. These trials tend to provide more comprehensive intervention components and to implement the intervention for a longer period than the earlier prevention trials. One example is the Fast Track Project (Conduct Problems Prevention Research Group, 1992, 2000). This multisite collaborative study is following a high-risk sample of almost 900 children who have been identified by both teachers and parents as displaying high rates of CP behavior during kindergarten, as well as 387 children who comprise a representative sample from the same schools as the

high-risk children. The neighborhoods in which these children live are in urban, suburban, and rural communities. There is adequate representation of girls (approximately 30%) and minorities (approximately 50%, most of whom are African American), so that it will be possible to examine both the developmental course and the effects of intervention with various subgroups of children.

Half the children in the high-risk sample participated in an intensive and long-term intervention that was designed to address the developmental issues involved in the early-starter pathway of CP. The Fast Track project is unique in the size, scope, and duration of the intervention. The intervention began in first grade and continued through grade 10. However, there were two periods of more intensive intervention: school entry (first and second grade) and the transition into middle school (fifth and sixth grade). The intervention at school entry targeted proximal changes in six domains: (1) disruptive behaviors in the home; (2) disruptive and off-task behaviors in the school; (3) social-cognitive skills facilitating affect regulation and social problem-solving skills; (4) peer relations; (5) academic skills; and (6) the family–school relationship. Integrated intervention components included parent training, home visiting, social skills training, academic tutoring, and a teacher-based classroom intervention. (See Bierman, Greenberg, & Conduct Problems Prevention Research Group, 1996; and McMahon, Slough, & Conduct Problems Prevention Research Group, 1996; for detailed descriptions of the first phase of the intervention.) The intervention at the entry into middle school (and through grade 10) included interventions with increasing emphasis on parent/adult monitoring and positive involvement, peer affiliation and peer influence, academic achievement and orientation to school, and social cognition and identity development.

Evaluations of the effects of the intervention through elementary school have been encouraging, with hypothesized changes in the domains described previously being obtained, and with other analyses suggesting that changes in child CP behavior and related outcomes are accounted for by changes in the hypothesized parent and child mediating variables (Conduct Problems Prevention Research Group, 1999, 2002a, 2002b, 2004). To date, the intervention appears to have been equally effective across child gender, ethnicity, and site location.

Adolescent Transitions Program. Another example of a second-generation prevention trial is the adolescent transitions program (ATP; Dishion & Kavanagh, 2002). ATP is a family-based intervention (integrated into a school setting) that is designed specifically to reduce problem behavior in adolescents. It originated out of more than a decade of efforts to combine family treatment experience with research on problem behavior. This "tiered" intervention includes three levels of service for families: a universal intervention, a selected intervention, and an indicated intervention (Dishion & Kavanagh, 2002, 2003). The universal intervention, which is provided to all parents in a school setting, consists of a Family Resource Center. The Family Resource Center is intended to (1) provide an infrastructure for school–parent collaboration; (2) disseminate information and norms about protective parenting practices and family management practices that promote school success; and (3) educate school and community professionals about accurate assessment of problem behavior and empirically supported treatments and reach parents with information about available services. Specific Family Resource Center services include school orientation meetings for parents with a self-checkup, books, and videotapes; media on effective parenting and parenting norms; classroom-based parent–child exercises that support and enhance family management practices; child-specific communication with parents about attendance, behavior, and work completion; and screening and assessment.

For families identified as having at-risk youth, a selected intervention (i.e., the Family Check-Up) is available. This three-session intervention is based on motivational interviewing techniques (Miller & Rollnick, 1991) and offers families (1) an initial interview, (2) a comprehensive assessment, and (3) a feedback session utilizing motivational skills to encourage maintenance of current positive parenting skills and change of problematic parenting practices.

For families with youth having ongoing problem behavior, an indicated level of intervention is available. A menu of family interventions allows for the provision of direct professional support to parents in dealing with youth adjustment and CP. The available interventions include a brief family intervention, a school monitoring system, parent groups, behavioral family therapy, and case management services. These core intervention components are offered to families as part of the family management curriculum (FMC), which provides a framework for working with families in groups or individually. This curriculum could include a family management group, a home–school card, sessions on special topics, monthly monitoring, individual family management therapy, and referrals to more intensive services.

In an early component analysis of ATP involving 120 families with high-risk adolescents (Dishion & Andrews, 1995), two cognitive-behavioral curricula were examined. The first curriculum was a group intervention for adolescents aimed at improving self-regulation. The second curriculum evaluated was the FMC for parents (described as the main component in the ATP indicated level of intervention). Early outcome analyses showed that contrary to expectations, problem behaviors in the adolescent group intervention were escalated compared to the control group (i.e., the adolescent group intervention resulted in iatrogenic effects, as discussed earlier). Thus, this adolescent group intervention was dropped from the ATP intervention model. However, the FMC intervention was associated with reductions in parent–child coercion as measured from videotaped parent–child interactions and reductions in teacher-reported antisocial behavior. Reductions in substance use for the FMC group were also noted at immediate follow-up but faded by the 1-year follow-up and were not evident in later follow-ups. Irvine, Biglan, Metzler, Smolkowski, and Ary (1999) replicated these FMC intervention effects in a sample of high-risk rural families. At the conclusion of the intervention, they found that families in the FMC group showed improved childrearing practices and reduced adolescent problem behavior.

Project Alliance, a prevention trial initiated in 1996, is currently underway to test the full ATP model (Dishion & Kavanagh, 2003). Two cohorts of sixth-grade youth (N = 999 families) in three middle schools were randomly assigned to intervention or control conditions. Initial findings with the first cohort (n = 672) indicated that ATP produced a reliable reduction in substance use for both typically developing and high-risk students (Dishion, Kavanagh, Schneiger, Nelson, & Kaufman, 2002). Effects did not differ significantly by ethnicity or gender. Outcomes related to CP have not yet been reported.

In a recent study, the impact of the Family Check-Up (the selected intervention in the ATP model) on parental monitoring was examined in a subset of the Project Alliance sample ($N = 71$ families) (Dishion, Nelson, & Kavanagh, 2003). Families receiving the Family Check-Up intervention increased their monitoring from seventh to eighth grade whereas control families decreased their monitoring during this period. Further, this increase in monitoring mediated an association between membership in the Family Check-Up intervention group and reduced substance use.

ATP has also been identified as a cost-effective intervention. The Aos and colleagues (2004) cost–benefit analysis showed that ATP saved taxpayers approximately $1,938 per participant in the program.

CURRENT NEEDS AND FUTURE DIRECTIONS

Needs in Conceptualizing and Understanding Conduct Problems in Adolescents

The heterogeneity of CP is perhaps the greatest stumbling block to advancement of knowledge in this area (Bloomquist & Schnell, 2002; Hinshaw & Lee, 2003; McMahon & Frick, 2005). It relates to issues of diagnosis, subtyping, and developmental pathways. It even relates to the question whether current approaches to describing and classifying CP behavior adequately cover CP behaviors that occur more frequently, or perhaps even primarily, in girls. In adolescence, issues about the definition of delinquency, and its partial overlap with the construct of CP, also become salient.

The heterogeneity of CP behaviors included in the DSM-IV categories of ODD and CD is especially problematic. There are several ways in which this issue could be addressed. First, increased attention to subtyping approaches for CP will help. One of the most promising is the childhood- versus adolescent-onset subtyping. However, as currently employed in DSM-IV, it is extremely underdeveloped, simply stating that childhood onset is characterized by the presence of a single CD symptom prior to age 10. The extensive literature on the early-starter and late-starter developmental pathways should guide refinement of this subtyping approach in the next revision of DSM (see below). In addition, examining the extent to which different subtyping approaches overlap or intersect would be beneficial. The Frick and

colleagues (1993) meta-analytic study is one example of such an approach.

Heterogeneity is also an issue in at least two other domains with respect to CP: comorbidity and risk/protective factors. Youth with CP often present with additional difficulties, including ADHD, internalizing disorders, and substance use. In addition, youth with CP (especially adolescents) are functioning in multiple social settings and groups, some or all of which may be playing a role in the development or maintenance of the CP behavior.

An overarching difficulty is that research concerning diagnosis, subtypes, comorbidity, and risk and protective factors has too often occurred in a vacuum. We have stressed here and elsewhere (e.g., McMahon & Frick, 2005) the need to employ a developmental pathways perspective as an organizational schema for integrating knowledge about these various aspects of CP in children and adolescents. Although great progress has been made in the past 15 years in the identification and subsequent delineation of some key developmental pathways (most notably the early- and late-starter pathways), it is clear that there is much more to be learned about these pathways, and that identification of additional pathways is needed to provide a more complete picture about the phenomenology of CP.

Specific areas that warrant further investigation include the need for additional information concerning covert forms of CP, especially with respect to lying and cheating, which have been significantly underresearched compared to stealing and firesetting. As noted previously, ways in which girls develop and manifest CP has also been quite underresearched. We are optimistic that the many research groups that have made this topic a focus of their work will make significant advances in knowledge about this very important issue in the years to come. Similarly, testing of the applicability of various developmental pathways to various cultural groups is essential (Dodge & Pettit, 2003).

Needs Related to Assessment and Intervention

Assessment

General issues and needs with respect to the assessment of CP in youth have recently been delineated by McMahon and Frick (2005). They stress the importance of a developmentally sensitive assessment, not only with respect to age and sex but also with respect to progression along a particular developmental pathway. They also stress the importance of assessing broadly as a means of addressing the heterogeneity of CP, comorbid conditions, and contextual factors discussed previously. The clinician needs to recognize the transactional nature of these developmental and contextual processes and conduct the assessment accordingly. Finally, use of multiple methods completed by multiple informants in relevant settings is crucial to the success of the assessment process.

With respect to assessment issues specific to adolescents with CP, we identify the following as in need of further attention. With few exceptions (e.g., the SRD), most measures of CP are typically intended for youth from ages 2 to 18. Well-validated measures that focus more specifically and thoroughly on CP behaviors known to occur frequently during adolescence (especially covert CP) are needed. Similarly, there is a paucity of measures concerning parenting practices during the adolescent period. Most current measures have focused on parenting of preschool or elementary-school-age children. A third area of needed development concerns clinician-friendly observation paradigms that can be employed to assess parent–adolescent interaction. Again, most paradigms have been designed for assessing parent–child interactions prior to adolescence. Finally, increased attention must be paid to ongoing intervention monitoring and evaluation of intervention effects. Given the documented possibility of iatrogenic effects from at least some forms of intervention for adolescents with CP, this becomes paramount.

Intervention

Numerous psychosocial interventions have been shown to be efficacious with adolescents with CP, and a smaller number have demonstrated effectiveness as well. At present, there is some limited support for the use of psychopharmacological treatment specifically for CP. However, it is also the case that the question of efficacy of such medications for treating CP in adolescents has not been addressed satisfactorily, given that most of the research has been focused on preadolescents.

Psychosocial treatments for CP that work (or that seem to have the best chance of working) share a number of attributes. First, they

are based on empirically supported developmental approaches to CP, including coercion theory and social–ecological perspectives of risk and protection. Second, they consider developmental pathways of CP, target both risk and protective factors, and address multiple socialization and support systems (e.g., Bloomquist & Schnell, 2002; Conduct Problems Prevention Research Group, 1992, 2000). In general, multicomponent interventions seem to be particularly indicated for adolescents, primarily because of the multiple social contexts in which they function. These multicomponent interventions should always include family-based interventions as a core component, and it is important for the various intervention components to be well integrated with each other (Conduct Problems Prevention Research Group, 1992, 2000; Rutter et al., 1998).

Finally, it is clear that *prevention* of CP can play an important role in adolescent CP. Data from both early interventions (i.e., infancy and preschool) and interventions implemented during preadolescence (and even early adolescence) indicate that they can have important effects on decreasing the frequency and severity of CP during adolescence. Furthermore, as the boundaries between prevention and treatment become increasingly blurred, a related issue is the need for an increased focus on developing coherent continua of service and transitioning from prevention efforts to treatment efforts when appropriate (see Prinz & Dumas, 2004).

There are several areas concerning intervention with adolescents with CP that we feel are in need of greater attention. The long-term effects of efficacious treatments for adolescents with CP are relatively unknown, so increased attention to conducting these follow-ups is needed. Although there is growing documentation of the cost-effectiveness of some of these interventions (e.g., MST, FFT, and MTFC), little evidence is available to determine what treatment may be most cost-effective for a given population of adolescents with serious CP (see Aos et al., 2004).

Whereas most of the treatments presented in this chapter have shown documented improvements under controlled and ideal conditions (i.e., efficacy), it is essential to know whether effects can be maintained when the interventions are transitioned to real-world settings (i.e., effectiveness). Some of the treatments presented in this chapter (e.g., MST, FFT, and MTFC) have studies to support effectiveness, and process research has been conducted to examine factors that may impact treatment success once it is implemented outside the relatively controlled environment of efficacy trials. However, in most cases, adequate effectiveness trials have yet to be conducted.

Another set of issues deserving increased attention relates to the question whether interventions that are specifically targeted to subgroups of adolescents or to subtypes of CP are warranted. With respect to targeting interventions to subgroups of adolescents, whether gender-specific interventions for girls with CP are indicated is currently a topic of great interest and discussion (e.g., Craig, 2005; Underwood & Coie, 2004). Preliminary reports from several gender-specific interventions for girls have recently presented promising results, although most of them are with preadolescents (Leve & Chamberlain, 2005, is an exception).

It is well established that most interventions for adolescents with CP have been based primarily on research with European American, middle-class families (Kerns & Prinz, 2002; Kumpfer, Alvarado, Smith, & Bellamy, 2002). Important questions that need to be addressed are the extent to which these interventions work with other cultural groups, whether there is a need to adapt these interventions, or whether culturally specific interventions need to be developed. Unfortunately, there is a paucity of data that address these questions, and the field is divided on this issue (Kumpfer et al., 2002). It is the case that many of the interventions described in this chapter have included other ethnic groups in their program evaluations, and some have noted the generalization of effects across groups (i.e., a lack of moderation), including MST, Fast Track, and ATP. The Wilson and colleagues (2003) meta-analysis found that interventions for juvenile delinquency generally had positive effects for minority youth, and that these effects were comparable to those found for nonminority youth. However, that is not to say that culturally adapted versions of these interventions would not be even more effective.

With respect to subtypes of CP, treatments for stealing, reactive/proactive aggression, and CU traits require additional attention. There is some empirical support for interventions that specifically target stealing, but they have not tended to be of the same methodological quality or sophistication that characterizes many of the general outcome studies for CP. Further-

more, these treatments for stealing have been targeted primarily at preadolescents rather than adolescents.

Smithmyer, Hubbard, and Simons (2000) have proposed using the cognitive deficits that are differentially associated with reactive and proactive aggression to select intervention strategies. Based on their findings with a sample of incarcerated delinquent adolescent males, they suggested that contingency management systems may be more effective for proactive aggression, whereas interventions designed to decrease attributes of hostile intent (e.g., Hudley & Graham, 1993) may be more effective for reactive aggression.

To our knowledge, no specific treatments have been developed for CP in the population of youth identified as having CU traits (Stickle & Frick, 2002). However, Stickle and Frick (2002), building on treatment recommendations for adults with psychopathic traits proposed by Wong and Hare (2005), suggest a number of treatment strategies that might be more effective with youth with CU traits. These strategies include (1) early intervention to promote the development of empathy; (2) motivational intervention strategies that will engage youth with a reward-oriented response style; and (3) interventions that focus on relationship development and supervision rather than on discipline and structure.

Conclusions

Substantial progress has been made in the development and evaluation of efficacious interventions for adolescents with CP. In home and community settings, a variety of evidence-based approaches are currently available. However, a number of factors, including the cost and the availability of these treatments and preventive interventions, preclude many youth from receiving the help they need. In addition, even the well-validated treatments presented in this chapter may not result in the elimination of CP behaviors. Thus, the continued development, evaluation, and dissemination of effective interventions that are sensitive to our growing knowledge about the various developmental pathways of CP and that are designed to address the wide array of CP behaviors should be primary goals for researchers and clinicians.

In closing, we wish to present the following guidelines for clinicians who work with adolescents with CP. First, know the problem! By that, we mean that the clinician should stay up-to-date with respect to current knowledge about developmental phenomenology, assessment, and intervention for youth with CP. Second, it is essential to screen and assess broadly with adolescent clients with CP, including the CP behaviors, comorbid conditions, risk and protective factors, and, most important, developmental pathways. Third, multicomponent interventions are most likely going to be needed. While the family-based intervention is core, it is also likely that intervention will also need to be introduced in other settings as well.

NOTES

1. It should be noted that some recent research has brought the neuropsychological risk hypothesis into question, finding that neuropsychological deficits may not develop until late childhood or adolescence, sometime after entry onto the early-starter pathway (Aguilar et al., 2000).
2. However, given the strong positive correlations between stealing and lying noted previously, children who steal may not be veridical in their self-reports.

REFERENCES

Abidin, R. R. (1988). *Parenting Alliance Inventory*. Unpublished scale, University of Virginia, Charlottesville.

Abidin, R. R., & Brunner, J. F. (1995). Development of a parenting alliance inventory. *Journal of Clinical Child Psychology, 24*, 31–40.

Abikoff, H., & Klein, R. G. (1992). Attention-deficit hyperactivity and conduct disorder: Comorbidity and implications for treatment. *Journal of Consulting and Clinical Psychology, 60*, 881–892.

Abikoff, H., Klein, R., Klass, E., & Ganeles, D. (1987, October). Methylphenidate in the treatment of conduct disordered children. In H. Abikoff (Chair), *Diagnosis and treatment issues in children with disruptive behavior disorders*. Symposium conducted at the meeting of the American Academy of Child and Adolescent Psychiatry, Washington, DC.

Achenbach, T. M., Dumenci, L., & Rescorla, L. A. (2003a). Are American children's problems still getting worse? A 23-year comparison. *Journal of Abnormal Child Psychology, 31*, 1–11.

Achenbach, T. M., Dumenci, L., & Rescorla, L. A. (2003b). DSM-oriented and empirically based approaches to constructing scales from the same item pools. *Journal of Clinical Child and Adolescent Psychology, 32*, 328–340.

Achenbach, T. M., & Edelbrock, C. S. (1981). Behavioral problems and competencies reported by parents of normal and disturbed children aged four through sixteen. *Monographs of the Society for Research in Child Development* (No. 188). Chicago: Society for Research in Child Development.

Achenbach, T. M., & Rescorla, L. A. (2001). *Manual for the ASEBA school-age forms and profiles*. Burlington: University of Vermont, Research Center for Children, Youth, & Families.

Adler, R., Nunn, R., Northam, E., Lebnan, V., & Ross, R. (1994). Secondary prevention of childhood firesetting. *Journal of the American Academy of Child and Adolescent Psychiatry, 33*, 1194–1202.

Aguilar, B., Sroufe, A., Egeland, B., & Carlson, E. (2000). Distinguishing the early-onset/persistent and adolescence-onset antisocial behavior types: From birth to 16 years. *Development and Psychopathology, 12*, 109–132.

Alexander, J. F., Jameson, P. B., Newell, R. M., & Gunderson, D. (1996). Changing cognitive schemas: A necessary antecedent to changing behaviors in dysfunctional families? In K. S. Dobson & K. D. Craig (Eds.), *Advances in cognitive-behavioral therapy* (pp. 174–191). Thousand Oaks, CA: Sage.

Alexander, J. F., & Parsons, B. V. (1973). Short-term behavioral intervention with delinquent families: Impact on family process and recidivism. *Journal of Abnormal Psychology, 81*, 219–225.

Alexander, J. F., & Parsons, B. (1982). *Functional family therapy*. Monterey, CA: Brooks/Cole.

Alexander, J. F., & Sexton, T. L. (2002). Functional Family Therapy (FFT): A model for treating high-risk, acting-out youth. In F. W. Kaslow (Ed.), *Comprehensive handbook of psychotherapy: Vol. 4. Integrative/eclectic* (pp. 111–132). New York: Wiley.

Alpern, L., & Lyons-Ruth, K. (1993). Preschool children at social risk: Chronicity and timing of maternal depressive symptoms and child behavior problems at school and at home. *Development and Psychopathology, 5*, 371–387.

Alvarado, R., Kendall, K., Beesley, S., & Lee-Cavaness, C. (2000). *Strengthening America's Families: Model family programs for substance abuse and delinquency prevention*. Salt Lake City: University of Utah.

Amato, P. R., & Keith, B. (1991). Parental divorce and the well-being of children: A meta analysis. *Psychological Bulletin, 110*, 26–46.

American Psychiatric Association. (1968). *Diagnostic and statistical manual of mental disorders* (2nd ed.). Washington, DC: Author

American Psychiatric Association. (1980). *Diagnostic and statistical manual of mental disorders* (3rd ed.). Washington, DC: Author.

American Psychiatric Association. (1987). *Diagnostic and statistical manual of mental disorders* (3rd ed., rev.). Washington, DC: Author.

American Psychiatric Association. (1994). *Diagnostic and statistical manual of mental disorders* (4th ed.). Washington, DC: Author.

American Psychiatric Association. (2000). *Diagnostic and statistical manual of mental disorders* (4th ed., text rev.). Washington, DC: Author.

Andershed, H. Kerr, M., & Stattin, H. (2001). Bullying in school and violence on the streets: Are the same people involved? *Journal of Scandinavian Studies of Criminology and Crime Prevention, 2,* 31–49.

Angold, A., & Costello, E. J. (2001). The epidemiology of disorders of conduct: Nosological issues and comorbidity. In J. Hill & B. Maughan (Eds.), *Conduct disorders in childhood and adolescence* (pp. 126–168). Cambridge, UK: Cambridge University Press.

Angold, A., Costello, E. J., & Erkanli, A. (1999). Comorbidity. *Journal of Child Psychology and Psychiatry, 40,* 57–87.

Antonishak, J., Reppucci, N. D., & Mulford, C. F. (2004). Girls in the justice system: Treatment and intervention. In M. M. Moretti, C. L. Odgers, & M. A. Jackson (Eds.), *Girls and aggression: Contributing factors and intervention principles* (pp. 165–180). New York: Kluwer/Plenum Press.

Aos, S., Lieb, R., Mayfield, J., Miller, M., & Pennucci, A. (2004). *Benefits and costs of prevention and early intervention programs for youth* [On-line]. Available: http://www.wsipp.wa.gov/rptfiles/04-07-3901. pdf

Arbuthnot, J., & Gordon, D. A. (1986). Behavioral and cognitive effects of a moral reasoning development intervention for high-risk behavior-disordered adolescents. *Journal of Consulting and Clinical Psychology, 54,* 208–216.

Baden, A. D., & Howe, G. W. (1992). Mothers' attributions and expectancies regarding their conduct-disordered children. *Journal of Abnormal Child Psychology, 20,* 467–485.

Baldry, A. C. (2001). Italy. In R. Summers & A. Hoffman (Eds.), *Teen violence: Global perspective* (pp. 144–196). Westport, CT: Greenwood.

Baldry, A. C., & Farrington, D. P. (2000). Bullies and delinquents: Personal characteristics and parental styles. *Journal of Community and Applied Social Psychology, 10,* 17–31.

Baldry, A. C., & Farrington, D. P. (2004). Evaluation of an intervention program for the reduction of bullying and victimization in schools. *Aggressive Behavior, 30,* 1–15.

Bank, L., Marlowe, J. H., Reid, J. B., Patterson, G. R., & Weinrott, M. R. (1991). A comparative evaluation of parent training interventions for families of chronic delinquents. *Journal of Abnormal Child Psychology, 19,* 15–33.

Bardone, A. M., Moffit, T. E., Caspi, A., Dickson, N., & Silva, P. A. (1996). Adult mental health and social outcomes of adolescent girls with depression and conduct disorder. *Development and Psychopathology, 8,* 811–829.

Barkley, R. A., Edwards, G., Laneri, M., Fletcher, K., & Metevia, L. (2001). The efficacy of Problem-Solving Communication Training alone, behavior manage-ment training alone, and their combination for parent–adolescent conflict in teenagers with ADHD and ODD. *Journal of Consulting and Clinical Psychology, 69,* 926–941.

Barkley, R. A., McMurray, M. B., Edelbrock, C. S., & Robbins, K. (1989). The response of aggressive and nonaggressive ADHD children to two doses of methylphenidate. *Journal of the American Academy of Child and Adolescent Psychiatry, 28,* 873–881.

Barry, C. T., Frick, P. J., DeShazo, T. M., McCoy, M. G., Ellis, M. L., & Loney, B. R. (2000). The importance of callous–unemotional traits for extending the concept of psychopathy to children. *Journal of Abnormal Psychology, 109,* 335–340.

Barth, R. P. (1987). Assessment and treatment of stealing. In B. B. Lahey & A. E. Kazdin (Eds.), *Advances in clinical child psychology* (Vol. 10, pp. 137–170). New York: Plenum Press.

Barton, C., & Alexander, J. F. (1981). Functional Family Therapy. In A. S. Gurman & D. P. Kniskern (Eds.), *Handbook of family therapy* (pp. 403–443). New York: Brunner/Mazel.

Barton, C., Alexander, J. F., Waldron, H., Turner, C. W., & Warburton, J. (1985). Generalizing treatment effects of Functional Family Therapy: Three replications. *American Journal of Family Therapy, 13,* 16–26.

Bates, J. E., Bayles, K., Bennett, D. S., Ridge, B., & Brown, M. M. (1991). Origins of externalizing behavior problems at eight years of age. In D. J. Pepler & K. H. Rubin (Eds.), *The development and treatment of childhood aggression* (pp. 93–120). Hillsdale, NJ: Erlbaum.

Beck, A. T, Steer, R. A., & Brown, G. K. (1996). *Beck Depression Inventory manual* (2nd ed.). San Antonio, TX: Psychological Corporation.

Becker, K. D., Stuewig, J., Herrera, V. M., & McCloskey, L. A. (2004). A study of firesetting and animal cruelty in children: Family influences and adult outcomes. *Journal of the American Academy of Child and Adolescent Psychiatry, 43,* 905–912.

Bennett, D. S., & Gibbons, T. A. (2000). Efficacy of child cognitive-behavioral interventions for antisocial behavior: A meta-analysis. *Child & Family Behavior Therapy, 22,* 1–15.

Bierman, K. L., Greenberg, M. T., & Conduct Problems Prevention Research Group. (1996). Social skills training in the Fast Track program. In R. DeV. Peters & R. J. McMahon (Eds.), *Preventing childhood disorders, substance abuse, and delinquency* (pp. 65–89). Thousand Oaks, CA: Sage.

Biglan, A., Brennan, P. A., Foster, S. L., & Holder, H. D. (2004). *Helping adolescents at risk: Prevention of multiple problem behaviors.* New York: Guilford Press.

Blair, R. J. R. (1999). Responsiveness to distress cues in the child with psychopathic tendencies. *Personality and Individual Differences, 27,* 135–145.

Blechman, E. A. (1981). Toward comprehensive behavioral family intervention: An algorithm for matching families and interventions. *Behavior Modification, 5,* 221–236.

Blechman, E. A., Maurice, A., Buecker, B., & Helberg, C. (2000). Can mentoring or skill training reduce recidivism? Observational study with propensity analysis. *Prevention Science, 1,* 139–155.

Bloomquist, M. L., & Schnell, S. V. (2002). *Helping children with aggression and conduct problems: Best practices for intervention.* New York: Guilford Press.

Borduin, C. M., Mann, B. J., Cone, L. T., Henggeler, S. W., Fucci, B. R., Blaske, D. M., & Williams, R. A. (1995). Multisystemic treatment of serious juvenile offenders: Long-term prevention of criminality and violence. *Journal of Consulting and Clinical Psychology, 63,* 569–578.

Bosworth, K., Espelage, D. L., & Simon, T. (1999). Factors associated with bullying behavior in middle school students. *Journal of Early Adolescence, 19,* 341–362.

Breen, M. J., & Altepeter, T. S. (1990). *Disruptive behavior disorders in children: Treatment-focused assessment.* New York: Guilford Press.

Brestan, E. V., & Eyberg, S. M. (1998). Effective psychosocial treatments of conduct-disordered children and adolescents: 29 years, 82 studies, and 5,272 kids. *Journal of Clinical Child Psychology, 27,* 180–189.

Broidy, L. M., Nagin, D. S., Tremblay, R. E., Bates, J. E., Brame, B., Dodge, K. A., et al. (2003). Developmental trajectories of childhood disruptive behaviors and adolescent delinquency: A six-site, cross-national study. *Developmental Psychology, 39,* 222–245.

Brooks, R. B., & Snow, D. L. (1972). Two case illustrations of the use of behavior modification techniques in the school setting. *Behavior Therapy, 3,* 100–103.

Brown, T. L., Henggeler, S. W., Schoenwald, S. K., Brondino, M. J., & Pickrel, S. G. (1999). Multisystemic treatment of substance abusing and dependent juvenile delinquents: Effects on school attendance at posttreatment and 6–month follow-up. *Children's Services Social Policy Research and Practice, 2,* 81–93.

Bukstein, O. G. (2003). Psychopharmacology of disruptive behavior disorders. In C. A. Essau (Ed.), *Conduct and oppositional defiant disorders: Epidemiology, risk factors, and treatment* (pp. 319–355). Mahwah, NJ: Erlbaum.

Burns, L. G., & Walsh, J. A. (2002). The influence of ADHD–hyperactivity/impulsivity symptoms on the development of oppositional defiant disorder symptoms in a 2-year longitudinal study. *Journal of Abnormal Child Psychology, 30,* 245–256.

Campbell, M., Adams, P. B., Small, A. M., Kafantaris, V., Silva, R. R., Shell, J., et al. (1995). Lithium in hospitalized aggressive children with conduct disorder: A double-blind and placebo-controlled study. *Journal of the American Academy of Child and Adolescent Psychiatry, 34,* 445–453.

Campbell, M., Small, A. M., Green, W. H., Jennings, S. J., Perry, R., Bennett, W. G., & Amderson, L. (1984).

Behavioral efficacy of haloperidol and lithium carbonate: A comparison in hospitalized aggressive children with conduct disorder. *Archives of General Psychiatry, 41,* 650–656.

Campbell, S. B. (1995). Behavior problems in preschool children: A review of recent research. *Journal of Child Psychology and Psychiatry and Allied Disciplines, 36,* 113–149.

Campbell, S. B. (2002). *Behavior problems in preschool children: Clinical and developmental issues* (2nd ed.). New York: Guilford Press.

Campbell, S. B., & Ewing, L. J. (1990). Follow up of hard to manage preschoolers: Adjustment at age 9 and predictors of continuing symptoms. *Journal of Child Psychology and Psychiatry and Allied Disciplines, 31,* 871–889.

Capaldi, D. M. (1991). Co-occurrence of conduct problems and depressive symptoms in early adolescent boys: I. Familial factors and general adjustment at age 6. *Development and Psychopathology, 3,* 277–300.

Capaldi, D. M. (1992). Co-occurrence of conduct problems and depressive symptoms in early adolescent boys: II. A 2-year follow-up at grade 8. *Development and Psychopathology, 4,* 125–144.

Capaldi, D., DeGarmo, D., Patterson, G. R., & Forgatch, M. (2002). Contextual risk across the early life span and association with antisocial behavior. In J. B. Reid, G. R. Patterson, & J. Snyder (Eds.), *Antisocial behavior in children and adolescents: A developmental analysis and model for intervention* (pp. 123–146). Washington, DC: American Psychological Association.

Capaldi, D. M., & Patterson, G. R. (1994). Interrelated influences of contextual factors on antisocial behavior in childhood and adolescence for males. In D. C. Fowles, P. Sutker, & S. H. Goodman (Eds.), *Progress in experimental personality and psychopathology research* (pp. 165–198). New York: Springer.

Caputo, A. A., Frick, P. J., & Brodsky, S. L. (1999). Family violence and juvenile sex offending: Potential mediating roles of psychopathic traits and negative attitudes toward women. *Criminal Justice and Behavior, 26,* 338–356.

Caspi, A., Lynam, D., Moffitt, T. E., & Silva, P. (1993). Unraveling girls' delinquency: Biological, dispositional, and contextual contributions to adolescent misbehavior. *Developmental Psychology, 29,* 19–30.

Chamberlain, P. (1994). *Family connections.* Eugene, OR: Castalia.

Chamberlain, P. (2003). *Treating chronic juvenile offenders: Advances made through the Oregon Multidimensional Treatment Foster Care model.* Washington, DC: American Psychological Association.

Chamberlain, P., Fisher, P. A., & Moore, K. (2002). Multidimensional Treatment Foster Care: Application of the OSLC intervention model to high-risk youth and their families. In J. B. Reid, G. R. Patterson, & J. Snyder (Eds.), *Antisocial behavior in children and adolescents: A developmental analysis and model for intervention* (pp. 203–218). Washington, DC: American Psychological Association.

Chamberlain, P., & Moore, K. J. (1998). Models of community treatment for serious juvenile offenders. In J. Crane (Ed.), *Social programs that really work* (pp. 258–276). New York: Russell Sage.

Chamberlain, P., Moreland, S., & Reid, K. (1992). Enhanced services and stipends for foster parents: Effects on retention rates and outcomes of children. *Child Welfare, 71,* 387–401.

Chamberlain, P., & Patterson, G. R. (1995). Discipline and child compliance in parenting. In M. H. Bornstein (Ed.), *Handbook of parenting: Vol. 4. Applied and practical parenting* (pp. 205–225). Hillsdale, NJ: Erlbaum.

Chamberlain, P., & Reid, J. B. (1987). Parent observation and report of child symptoms. *Behavioral Assessment, 9,* 97–109.

Chamberlain, P., & Reid, J. B. (1991). Using a specialized foster care community treatment model for children and adolescents leaving the state mental health hospital. *Journal of Community Psychology, 19,* 266–276.

Chamberlain, P., & Reid, J. B. (1994). Differences in risk factors and adjustment for male and female delinquents in treatment foster care. *Journal of Child and Family Studies, 3,* 23–39.

Chamberlain, P., & Reid, J. B. (1998). Comparison of two community alternatives to incarceration for chronic juvenile offenders. *Journal of Consulting and Clinical Psychology, 66,* 624–633.

Chamberlain, P., Reid, J. B., Ray, J., Capaldi, D. M., & Fisher, P. (1997). Parent inadequate discipline (PID). In T. A. Widiger, A. J. Frances, H. A. Pincus, R. Ross, M. B. First, & W. Davis (Eds.), *DSM-IV sourcebook* (Vol. 3, pp. 569–629). Washington, DC: American Psychiatric Association.

Chamberlain, P., & Smith, D. K. (2003). Antisocial behavior in children and adolescents: The Oregon Multidimensional Treatment Foster Care model. In A. E. Kazdin & J. R. Weisz (Eds.), *Evidence-based psychotherapies for children and adolescents* (pp. 282–300). New York: Guilford Press.

Chandler, M., & Moran, T. (1990). Psychopathy and moral development: A comparative study of delinquent and nondelinquent youth. *Development and Psychopathology, 2,* 227–246.

Christian, R. E., Frick, P. J., Hill, N. L., Tyler, L., & Frazer, D. R. (1997). Psychopathy and conduct problems in children: II. Implications for subtyping children with conduct problems. *Journal of the American Academy of Child and Adolescent Psychiatry, 36,* 233–241.

Coatsworth, J. D., Santisteban, D. A., McBride, C. K., & Szapocznik, J. (2001). Brief Strategic Family Therapy versus community control: Engagement, retention, and an exploration of the moderating role of adolescent symptom severity. *Family Process, 40,* 313–332.

Coie, J. D., & Dodge, K. A. (1998). Aggression and antisocial behavior. In W. Damon (Series Ed.) & N. Eisenberg (Vol. Ed.), *Handbook of child psychology: Vol. 3. Social, emotional, and personality development* (5th ed., pp. 779–862). New York: Wiley.

Coie, J. D., & Jacobs, M. R. (1993). The role of social context in the prevention of conduct disorder. *Development and Psychopathology, 5,* 263–275.

Coie, J. D., Lochman, J. E., Terry, R., & Hyman, C. (1992). Predicting early adolescent disorder from childhood aggression and peer rejection. *Journal of Consulting and Clinical Psychology, 60,* 783–792.

Coleman, M., Pfeiffer, S., & Oakland, T. (1991). *Aggression replacement training with behavior disordered adolescents.* Unpublished manuscript, University of Texas.

Compton, K., Snyder, J., Schrepferman, L., Bank, L., & Shortt, J. (2003). The contribution of parents and siblings to antisocial and depressive behavior in adolescents: A double jeopardy coercion model. *Development and Psychopathology, 15,* 163–182.

Conduct Problems Prevention Research Group. (1992). A developmental and clinical model for the prevention of conduct disorder: The FAST Track program. *Development and Psychopathology, 4,* 509–527.

Conduct Problems Prevention Research Group. (1999). Initial impact of the Fast Track prevention trial of conduct problems: I. The high-risk sample. *Journal of Consulting and Clinical Psychology, 67,* 631–647.

Conduct Problems Prevention Research Group. (2000). Merging universal and indicated prevention programs: The Fast Track model. *Addictive Behaviors, 25,* 913–927.

Conduct Problems Prevention Research Group. (2002a). Evaluation of the first three years of the Fast Track prevention trial with children at high risk for adolescent conduct problems. *Journal of Abnormal Child Psychology, 30,* 19–35.

Conduct Problems Prevention Research Group. (2002b). Using the Fast Track randomized prevention trial to test the early-starter model of the development of serious conduct problems. *Development and Psychopathology, 14,* 925–943.

Conduct Problems Prevention Research Group. (2004). The effects of the Fast Track program on serious problem outcomes at the end of elementary school. *Journal of Clinical Child and Adolescent Psychology, 33,* 650–661.

Conners, C. K. (1997). *Conners Rating Scales—Revised manual.* New York: Multi-Health Systems.

Connor, D. F. (2002). *Aggression and antisocial behavior in children and adolescents: Research and treatment.* New York: Guilford Press.

Connor, D. F., Barkley, R. A., & Davis, H. T. (2000). A pilot study of methylphenidate, clonidine, or the combination in ADHD comorbid with aggressive oppositional defiant or conduct disorder. *Clinical Pediatrics, 39,* 15–25.

Connor, D. F., Glatt, S. J., Lopez, I. D., Jackson, D., & Melloni, R. H. (2002). Psychopharmacology and aggression. I: A meta-analysis of stimulant effects on over/covert aggression-related behaviors in ADHD. *Journal of the American Academy of Child and Adolescent Psychiatry, 31,* 253–261.

Costello, E., & Angold, A. (2001). Bad behaviour: An historical perspective on disorders of conduct. In J. Hill & B. Maughan (Eds.), *Conduct disorders in childhood and adolescence* (pp. 1–31). Cambridge, UK: Cambridge University Press.

Craig, W. M. (2005). The treatment of aggressive girls: Same but different? In D. J. Pepler, K. C. Madsen, C. Webster, & K. S. Levene (Eds.), *The development and treatment of girlhood aggression* (pp. 217–221). Mahwah, NJ: Erlbaum.

Craig, W. M., & Pepler, D. J. (1995). Peer processes in bullying and victimization: An observational study. *Exceptionality Education Canada, 5,* 81–95.

Craig, W. M., & Yossi, H. (2003). Bullying and fighting: Results from the World Health Organization Health and Behavior Survey of school aged children. *International Report for World Health Organization.*

Crick, N. R., & Dodge, K. A. (1994). A review and reformulation of social information-processing mechanisms in children's social adjustment. *Psychological Bulletin, 115,* 74–101.

Crick, N. R., & Dodge, K. A. (1996). Social information-processing mechanisms in reactive and proactive aggression. *Child Development, 67,* 993–1002.

Crick, N. R., & Grotpeter, J. K. (1995). Relational aggression, gender, and social-psychological adjustment. *Child Development, 66,* 710–722.

Crick, N. R., & Werner, N. E. (1998). Response decision processes in relational and overt aggression. *Child Development, 69,* 1630–1639.

Cummings, E. M., & Davies, P. (1994a). *Children and marital conflict: The impact of family dispute resolution.* New York: Guilford Press.

Cummings, E. M., & Davies, P. T. (1994b). Maternal depression and child development. *Journal of Child Psychology and Psychiatry, 35,* 73–112.

Cunningham, A. (2002). *Lessons learned from a randomized study of multisystemic therapy in Canada* [Online]. Available: http://www.lfcc.on.ca/One_Step_Forward.pdf

Curtis, N. M., Ronan, K. R., & Borduin, C. M. (2004). Multisystemic treatment: A meta-analysis of outcome studies. *Journal of Family Psychology, 18,* 411–419.

Dadds, M. R., & Powell, M. B. (1991). The relationship of interparental conflict and global marital adjustment to aggression, anxiety, and immaturity in aggressive and nonclinic children. *Journal of Abnormal Child Psychology, 19,* 553–567.

Deater-Deckard, K. (1998). Parenting stress and child adjustment: Some old hypotheses and new questions. *Clinical Psychology: Science and Practice, 5,* 314–332.

DeKlyen, M., & Speltz, M. L. (2001). Attachment and conduct disorder. In J. Hill & B. Maughan (Eds.), *Conduct disorders in childhood and adolescence* (pp. 320–345). Cambridge, UK: Cambridge University Press.

Demaray, M. K., Ruffalo, S. L., Carlson, J., Busse, R. T., Olson, A. E., McManus, S. M., et al. (1995). Social skills assessment: A comparative evaluation of six published rating scales. *School Psychology Review, 24,* 648–671.

Dishion, T. J., & Andrews, D. W. (1995). Preventing escalation in problem behaviors with high-risk young adolescents: Immediate and 1-year outcomes. *Journal of Consulting and Clinical Psychology, 63,* 538–548.

Dishion, T. J., Andrews, D. W., & Crosby, L. (1995). Antisocial boys and their friends in early adolescence: Relationship characteristics, quality, and interactional process. *Child Development, 66,* 139–151.

Dishion, T. J., & Kavanagh, K. (2002). The Adolescent Transitions Program: A family-centered prevention strategy for schools. In J. B. Reid, G. R. Patterson, & J. Snyder (Eds.) *Antisocial behavior in children and adolescents: A developmental analysis and model for intervention* (pp. 257–272). Washington, DC: American Psychological Association.

Dishion, T. J., & Kavanagh, K. (2003). *Intervening in adolescent problem behavior: A family-centered approach.* New York: Guilford Press.

Dishion, T. J., Kavanagh, K., Schneiger, A., Nelson, S., & Kaufman, N. (2002). Preventing early adolescent substance use: A family-centered strategy for the public middle-school ecology. *Prevention Science, 3,* 191–201.

Dishion, T. J., McCord, J., & Poulin, F. (1999). When interventions harm: Peer groups and problem behavior. *American Psychologist, 54,* 755–764.

Dishion, T. J., & McMahon, R. J. (1998). Parental monitoring and the prevention of child and adolescent problem behavior: A conceptual and empirical formulation. *Clinical Child and Family Psychology Review, 1,* 61–75.

Dishion, T. J., Nelson, S. E., & Kavanagh, K. (2003). The Family Check-Up with high-risk young adolescents: Preventing early-onset substance use by parental monitoring. *Behavior Therapy, 34,* 553–571.

Dishion, T. J., Patterson, G. R., & Griesler, P. C. (1994). Peer adaptation in the development of antisocial behavior: A confluence model. In L. R. Huesmann (Ed.), *Current perspectives on aggressive behavior* (pp. 61–95). New York: Plenum Press.

Dishion, T. J., Patterson, G. R., Stoolmiller, M., & Skinner, M. L. (1991). Family, school, and behavioral antecedents to early adolescent involvement with antisocial peers. *Developmental Psychology, 27,* 172–180.

Dishion, T. J., Reid, J. B., & Patterson, G. R. (1988). Empirical guidelines for a family intervention for adolescent drug use. *Journal of Chemical Dependency Treatment, 1,* 189–224.

Dodge, K. A. (1986). A social information processing model of social competence in children. In M. Perlmutter (Ed.), *Minnesota Symposium on Child*

Psychology (Vol. 18, pp. 77–125). Hillsdale, NJ: Erlbaum.

Dodge, K. A. (2003). Do social information-processing patterns mediate aggressive behavior? In B. B. Lahey, T. E. Moffitt, & A. Caspi (Eds.), *Causes of conduct disorder and delinquency* (pp. 254–274). New York: Guilford Press.

Dodge, K A., Bates, J. E., & Pettit, G. S. (1990). Mechanisms in the cycle of violence. *Science, 250,* 1678–1683.

Dodge, K. A., & Coie, J. D. (1987). Social-information processing factors in reactive and proactive aggression in children's peer groups. *Journal of Personality and Social Psychology, 53,* 1146–1158.

Dodge, K. A., Lochman, J. E., Harnish, J. D., Bates, J. E., & Pettit, G. S. (1997). Reactive and proactive aggression in school children and psychiatrically impaired chronically assaultive youth. *Journal of Abnormal Psychology, 106,* 37–51.

Dodge, K. A., & Pettit, G. S. (2003). A biopsychosocial model of the development of chronic conduct problems in adolescence. *Developmental Psychology, 39,* 349–371.

Dodge, K. A., Pettit, G. S., & Bates, J. E. (1994). Socialization mediators of the relation between socioeconomic status and child conduct problems. *Child Development, 65,* 649–665.

Dumas, J. E. (1996). Why was this child referred? Interactional correlates of referral status in families of children with disruptive behavior problems. *Journal of Clinical Child Psychology, 25,* 106–115.

Dumas, J. E., & Serketich, W. J. (1994). Maternal depressive symptomatology and child maladjustment: A comparison of three process models. *Behavior Therapy, 25,* 161–181.

Dumas, J. E., & Wahler, R. G. (1983). Predictors of treatment outcome in parent training: Mother insularity and socioeconomic disadvantage. *Behavioral Assessment, 5,* 301–313.

Dumas, J. E., & Wahler, R. G. (1985). Indiscriminate mothering as a contextual factor in aggressive-oppositional child behavior: "Damned if you do and damned if you don't." *Journal of Abnormal Child Psychology, 13,* 1–17.

Duncan, R. D. (1999). Maltreatment by parents and peers: The relationship between child abuse, bully victimization, and psychological distress. *Child Maltreatment, 4,* 45–55.

Eddy, J. M., & Chamberlain, P. (2000). Family management and deviant peer association as mediators of the impact of treatment condition on youth antisocial behavior. *Journal of Consulting and Clinical Psychology, 68,* 857–863.

Edelbrock, C. (1985). *Conduct problems in childhood and adolescence: Developmental patterns and progressions.* Unpublished manuscript.

Elgar, F. J., McGrath, P. J., Waschbusch, D. A., Stewart, S. H., & Curtis, L. J. (2004). Mutual influences on maternal depression and child adjustment problems. *Clinical Psychology Review, 24,* 441–459.

Elliott, D. S., Huizinga, D., & Ageton, S. S. (1985). *Explaining delinquency and drug use.* Beverly Hills, CA: Sage.

Elliott, E. J. (2002). Juvenile justice diversion and intervention. In D. Kolko (Ed.), *Handbook on firesetting in children and youth* (pp. 383–394). San Diego, CA: Academic Press.

El-Sheikh, M., & Flanagan, E. (2001). Parental problem drinking and children's adjustment: Family conflict and parental depression as mediators and moderators of risk. *Journal of Abnormal Child Psychology, 29,* 417–432.

Embry, L. H. (1984). What to do? Matching client characteristics and intervention techniques through a prescriptive taxonomic key. In R. F. Dangel & R. A. Polster (Eds.), *Parent training: Foundations of research and practice* (pp. 443–473). New York: Guilford Press.

Emery, R. E. (1999). *Marriage, divorce, and children's adjustment* (2nd ed.). Thousand Oaks, CA: Sage.

Eslea, M., & Smith, P. K. (1998). The long term effectiveness of anti-bullying work in primary schools. *Educational Research, 40,* 203–218.

Essau, C. A. (2003). Epidemiology and comorbidity. In C. A. Essau (Ed.), *Conduct and oppositional defiant disorders: Epidemiology, risk factors, and treatment* (pp. 33–59). Mahwah, NJ: Erlbaum.

Farrington, D. P. (1993). Understanding and preventing bullying. In M. Tonry (Ed.), *Crime and justice: A review of research* (Vol. 17, pp. 381–458). Chicago: University of Chicago Press.

Farrington, D. P. (2003). Key results from the first forty years of the Cambridge Study in Delinquent Development. In T. P. Thornberry & M. D. Krohn (Eds.), *Taking stock of delinquency: An overview of findings from contemporary longitudinal studies* (pp. 137–183). New York: Kluwer/Plenum Press.

Feindler, E. L. (1990). Adolescent anger control: Review and critique. In M. Hersen, R. M. Eisler, & P. M. Miller (Eds.), *Progress in behavior modification* (Vol. 26, pp. 11–59). Newbury Park, CA: Sage.

Feindler, E. L. (1991). Cognitive strategies in anger control interventions for children and adolescents. In P. C. Kendall (Ed.), *Child and adolescent therapy: Cognitive-behavioral procedures* (pp. 66–97). New York: Guilford Press.

Feindler, E. L. (1995). An ideal treatment package for children and adolescents with anger disorders. In H. Kassinove (Ed.), *Anger disorders: Definition, diagnosis, and treatment* (pp. 173–195). Washington, DC: Taylor & Francis.

Feindler, E. L., Ecton, R. B., Kingsley, D., & Dubey, D. R. (1986). Group anger-control training for institutionalized psychiatric male adolescents. *Behavior Therapy, 17,* 109–123.

Feindler, E. L., & Guttman, J. (1994). Cognitive-behavioral anger control training for groups of adolescents: A treatment manual. In C. W. LeCroy (Ed.), *Handbook of child and adolescent treatment manuals* (pp. 170–199). New York: Free Press.

Feindler, E. L., Marriott, S. A., & Iwata, M. (1984). Group anger control training for junior high school delinquents. *Cognitive Therapy and Research, 8,* 299–311.

Fergusson, D. M., Horwood, L. J., & Lynskey, M. T. (1994). The comorbidities of adolescent problem behaviors: A latent class model. *Journal of Abnormal Child Psychology, 22,* 339–354.

Fergusson, D. M., Horwood, L. J., & Nagin, D. S. (2000). Offending trajectories in a New Zealand birth cohort. *Criminology, 38,* 401–427.

Fergusson, D. M., & Lynskey, M. T. (1993). The effects of maternal depression on child conduct disorder and attention deficit behaviours. *Social Psychiatry and Psychiatric Epidemiology, 28,* 116–123.

Fergusson, D. M., Lynskey, M. T., & Horwood, L. J. (1993). The effect of maternal depression on maternal ratings of child behavior. *Journal of Abnormal Child Psychology, 21,* 245–269.

Fergusson, D. M., Lynskey, M. T., & Horwood, L. J. (1996). Origins of comorbidity between conduct and affective disorders. *Journal of the American Academy of Child and Adolescent Psychiatry, 35,* 451–460.

Findling, R. L., Aman, M., & Derivan, A. (2000). Long-term safety and efficacy of risperidone in children with significant conduct problems and borderline IQ or mental retardation. *Scientific Proceedings of the 39th Annual Meeting of the American College of Neuropsychopharmacology,* 224.

Fischer, M., Barkley, R. A., Smallish, L., & Fletcher, K. (2002). Young adult follow-up of hyperactive children: Self-reported psychiatric disorders, comorbidity, and the role of childhood conduct problems and teen CD. *Journal of Abnormal Child Psychology, 30,* 463–475.

Fisher, L., & Blair, R. J. R. (1998). Cognitive impairment and its relationship to psychopathic tendencies in children with emotional and behavioral difficulties. *Journal of Abnormal Child Psychology, 26,* 511–519.

Fixsen, D. L., Blase, K. A., Timbers, G. D., & Wolf, M. M. (2001). In search of program implementation: 792 replications of the Teaching Family Model. In G. A. Bernfield, D. P. Farrington, & A. W. Leschied (Eds.), *Offender rehabilitation in practice: Implementing and evaluating effective programs* (pp. 149–166). London, UK: Wiley.

Forehand, R., Lautenschlager, G. J., Faust, J., & Graziano, W. G. (1986). Parent perceptions and parent–child interactions in clinic-referred children: A preliminary investigation of the effects of maternal depressive moods. *Behaviour Research and Therapy, 24,* 73–75.

Forehand, R. L., & McMahon, R. J. (1981). *Helping the noncompliant child: A clinician's guide to parent training.* New York: Guilford Press.

Forehand, R., Wierson, M., Frame, C. L., Kemptom, T., & Armistead, L. (1991). Juvenile firesetting: A unique syndome or an advanced level of antisocial behavior? *Behaviour Research and Therapy, 29,* 125–128.

Forgatch, M., & Patterson, G. R. (1989). *Parents and adolescents living together. Part 2: Family problem solving.* Eugene, OR: Castalia.

Forgatch, M. S., Patterson, G. R., & Skinner, M. L. (1988). A mediational model for the effect of divorce on antisocial behavior in boys. In E. M. Hetherington & J. D. Arasteh (Eds.), *Impact of divorce, single parenting, and stepparenting on children* (pp. 135–154). Hillsdale, NJ: Erlbaum.

Foster, S. L., Prinz, R. J., & O'Leary, K. D., (1983). Impact of Problem-Solving Communication Training and generalization procedures on family conflict. *Child & Family Behavior Therapy, 5,* 1–23.

Foster, S. L., & Robin, A. L. (1997). Family conflict and communication in adolescence. In E. J. Mash & L. G. Terdal (Eds.), *Assessment of childhood disorders* (3rd ed., pp. 627–682). New York: Guilford Press.

Foster, S. L., & Robin, A. L. (1998). Parent–adolescent conflict and relationship discord. In E. J. Mash & R. A. Barkley (Eds.), *Treatment of childhood disorders* (2nd ed., pp. 601–686). New York: Guilford Press.

Frick, P. J. (1991). *The Alabama Parenting Questionnaire.* Unpublished rating scale. Department of Psychology, University of New Orleans.

Frick, P. J. (1994). Family dysfunction and the disruptive behavior disorders: A review of recent empirical findings. In T. H. Ollendick & R. J. Prinz (Eds.), *Advances in clinical child psychology* (Vol. 16, pp. 203–226). New York: Plenum Press.

Frick, P. J. (1998). *Conduct disorders and severe antisocial behavior.* New York: Plenum Press.

Frick, P. J., Bodin, S. D., & Barry, C. T. (2000). Psychopathic traits and conduct problems in community and clinic-referred samples of children: Further development of the Psychopathy Screening Device. *Psychological Assessment, 12,* 382–393.

Frick, P. J., Christian, R. E., & Wootton, J. M. (1999). Age trends in the association between parenting practices and conduct problems. *Behavior Modification, 23,* 106–128.

Frick, P. J., Cornell, A. H., Barry, C. T., Bodin, S. D., & Dane, H. A. (2003). Callous–unemotional traits and conduct problems in the prediction of conduct problem severity, aggression, and self-report of delinquency. *Journal of Abnormal Child Psychology, 31,* 457–470.

Frick, P. J., & Ellis, M. (1999). Callous–unemotional traits and subtypes of conduct disorder. *Clinical Child and Family Psychology Review, 2,* 149–168.

Frick, P. J., & Hare, R. D. (2002). *Antisocial Process Screening Device.* Toronto, ON, Canada: Multi-Health Systems.

Frick, P. J., Lahey, B. B., Loeber, R., Stouthamer-Loeber, M., Christ, M. A. G., & Hanson, K. (1992). Familial risk factors to conduct disorder and oppositional defiant disorder: Parental psychopathology and maternal parenting. *Journal of Consulting and Clinical Psychology, 60,* 49–55.

Frick, P. J., Lahey, B. B., Loeber, R., Tannenbaum, L. E., Van Horn, Y., Christ, M. A. G., et al. (1993). Oppositional defiant disorder and conduct disorder: A meta-analytic review of factor analyses and cross-validation in a clinic sample. *Clinical Psychology Review, 13,* 319–340.

Frick, P. J., Lilienfeld, S. O., Ellis, M. L, Loney, B. R., & Silverthorn, P. (1999). The association between anxiety and psychopathy dimensions in children. *Journal of Abnormal Child Psychology, 27,* 381–390.

Frick, P. J., & Loney, B. R. (2002). Understanding the association between parent and child antisocial behavior. In R. J. McMahon & R. DeV. Peters (Eds.), *The effects of parental dysfunction on children* (pp. 105–126). New York: Kluwer/Plenum Press.

Frick, P. J., & Morris, A. S. (2004). Temperament and developmental pathways to conduct problems. *Journal of Clinical Child and Adolescent Psychology, 33,* 54–68.

Gadow, K. D., & Sprafkin, J. (1995). *Manual for the Child Symptom Inventory—4th ed.* Stony Brook, NY: Checkmate Plus.

Garcia, M. M., Shaw, D. S., Winslow, E. B., & Yaggi, K. E. (2000). Destructive sibling conflict and the development of conduct problems in young boys. *Developmental Psychology, 36,* 44–53.

Geiger, T. C., Zimmer-Gembeck, M. J., & Crick, N. R. (2004). The science of relational aggression: Can we guide intervention? In M. M. Moretti, C. L. Odgers, & M. A. Jackson (Eds.), *Girls and aggression: Contributing factors and intervention principles* (pp. 27–40). New York: Kluwer/Plenum Press.

Gibbs, J. C., Arnold, K. D., Ahlborn, H. H., & Cheesman, F. L. (1984). Facilitation of sociomoral reasoning in delinquents. *Journal of Consulting and Clinical Psychology, 52,* 37–45.

Gibbs, J. C., Potter, G. B., Barriga, A. Q., & Liau, A. K. (1996). Developing the helping skills and prosocial motivation of aggressive adolescents in peer group programs. *Aggression and Violent Behavior, 1,* 283–305.

Glick, B., & Goldstein, A. P. (1987). Aggression replacement training. *Journal of Counseling and Development, 65,* 356–362.

Glover, D., Gough, G., Johnson, M., & Cartwright, N. (2000). Bullying in 25 secondary schools: Incidence, impact, and intervention. *Educational Research, 42,* 141–156.

Goldstein, A. P., & Glick, B. (1994). Aggression replacement training: Curriculum and evaluation. *Simulation and Gaming. 25,* 9–26.

Goldstein, A. P., Glick, B., & Gibbs, J. C. (1998). *Aggression Replacement Training: A comprehensive intervention for aggressive youth.* Champaign, IL: Research Press.

Goldstein, A. P., Glick, B., Irwin, M. J., McCartney, C., & Rubama, I. (1989). *Reducing delinquency: Intervention in the community.* New York: Pergamon Press.

Goldstein, A. P., Glick, B., Reiner, S., Zimmerman, D., & Coultry, T. (1986). *Aggression replacement training.* Champaign, IL: Research Press.

Goldstein, A. P., & Pentz, M. A. (1984). Psychological skill training and the aggressive adolescent. *School Psychology Review, 13,* 311–323.

Goodman, S., & Gotlib, I. (1999). Risk for psychopathology in the children of depressed mothers: A developmental model for understanding mechanisms of transmission. *Psychological Review, 106,* 485–490.

Gordon, D. A., Arbuthnot, J., Gustafson, K. E., & McGreen, P. (1988). Home-based behavioral-systems family therapy with disadvantaged juvenile delinquents. *American Journal of Family Therapy, 16,* 243–255.

Gordon, D. A., Graves, K., & Arbuthnot, J. (1995). The effect of Functional Family Therapy for delinquents on adult criminal behavior. *Criminal Justice and Behavior, 22,* 60–73.

Gorman-Smith, D., Tolan, P. H., & Henry, D. B. (2000). A developmental–ecological model of the relations of family functioning to patterns of delinquency. *Journal of Quantitative Criminology, 16,* 169–198.

Greenburg, M. T. (1999). Attachment and psychopathology in childhood. In J. Cassidy & P. R. Shaver (Eds.), *Handbook of attachment: Theory, research, and clinical applications* (pp. 469–496). New York: Guilford Press.

Greenberg, M. T., Lengua, L. J., Coie, J., Pinderhughes, E., & Conduct Problems Prevention Research Group. (1999). Predicting developmental outcomes at school entry using a multiple-risk model: Four American communities. *Developmental Psychology, 35,* 403–417.

Greenhill, L. L., Solomon, M., Pleak, R., & Ambrosini, P. (1985). Molindine hydrochloride treatment of hospitalized children with conduct disorder. *Journal of Clinical Psychiatry, 46,* 20–25.

Gregg, V., Gibbs, J. C., & Basinger, K. S. (1994). Patterns of delay in male and female delinquents' moral judgment. *Merrill-Palmer Quarterly, 40,* 538–553.

Guerra, N. G., & Slaby, R. G. (1990). Cognitive mediators of aggression in adolescent offenders: 2. Intervention. *Developmental Psychology, 26,* 269–277.

Hämäläinen, M., & Pulkkinen, L. (1996). Problem behavior as a precursor of male criminality. *Development and Psychopathology, 8,* 443–455.

Hanson, M., Mackay-Soroka, S., Staley, S., & Poulton, L. (1994). Delinquent firesetters: A comparative study of delinquency and firesetting histories. *Canadian Journal of Psychiatry, 39,* 230–232.

Hansson, K., Cederblad, M., & Alexander, J. F. (2002). *A method for treating juvenile delinquents—A cross-cultural comparison.* Manuscript submitted for publication.

Hawkins, J. D., Catalano, R. F., Kosterman, R., Abbott, R., & Hill, K. G. (1999). Preventing health-risk behaviors by strengthening protection during childhood. *Archives of Pediatrics and Adolescent Medicine, 153,* 226–234.

Hawkins, J. D., Catalano, R. F., & Miller, J. Y. (1992).

Risk and protective factors for alcohol and other drug problems in adolescence and early adulthood: Implications for substance abuse prevention. *Psychological Bulletin, 112,* 64–105.

Hawkins, J. D., Smith, B. H., Hill, K. G., Kosterman, R., Catalano, R. F., & Abbott, R. D. (2002). Understanding and preventing crime and violence. In T. P. Thornberry & M. D. Krohn (Eds.), *Taking stock of delinquency: An overview of findings from contemporary longitudinal studies* (pp. 255–312). New York: Kluwer/Plenum Press.

Hawkins, R. P. (1989). The nature and potential of therapeutic foster family care programs. In R. P. Hawkins & J. Breiling (Eds.), *Therapeutic foster care: Critical issues* (pp. 17–36). Washington, DC: Child Welfare League of America.

Hawkins, R. P., Meadowcroft, P., Trout, B. A., & Luster, W. C. (1985). Foster family-based treatment. *Journal of Clinical Child Psychology, 14,* 220–228.

Heath, G. A., Hardesty, V. A., Goldfine, P. E., & Walker, A. M. (1983). Childhood firesetting: An empirical study. *Journal of the American Academy of Child Psychiatry, 22,* 370–374.

Henderson, J. Q. (1981). A behavioral approach to stealing: A proposal for treatment based on ten cases. *Journal of Behavior Therapy and Experimental Psychiatry, 12,* 231–236.

Henderson, J. Q. (1983). Follow-up of stealing behavior in 27 youths after a variety of treatment programs. *Journal of Behavior Therapy and Experimental Psychiatry, 14,* 331–337.

Henggeler, S. W. (2004). Decreasing effect sizes for effectiveness studies—Implications for the transport of evidence-based treatments: Comments on Curtis, Ronan, and Borduin (2004). *Journal of Family Psychology, 18,* 420–423.

Henggeler, S. W., & Borduin, C. M. (1990). *Family therapy and beyond: A multisystemic approach to treating the behavior problems of children and adolescents.* Pacific Grove, CA: Brooks/Cole.

Henggeler, S. W., Clingempeel, G. W., Brondino, M. J., & Pickrel, S. G. (2002). Four-year follow-up of multisystemic therapy with substance-abusing and substance-dependent juvenile offenders. *Journal of the American Academy of Child and Adolescent Psychiatry, 41,* 868–874.

Henggeler, S. W., & Lee, T. (2003). Multisystemic treatment of serious clinical problems. In A. E. Kazdin & J. R. Weisz (Eds.), *Evidence-based psychotherapies for children and adolescents* (pp. 301–322). New York: Guilford Press.

Henggeler, S. W., Melton, G. B., Brondino, M. J., Scherer, D. G., & Hanley, J. H. (1997). Multisystemic Therapy with violent and chronic juvenile offenders and their families: The role of treatment fidelity in successful dissemination. *Journal of Consulting and Clinical Psychology, 65,* 821–833.

Henggeler, S. W., Melton, G. B., & Smith, L. A. (1992). Family preservation using multisystemic therapy: An effective alternative to incarcerating serious juvenile offenders. *Journal of Consulting and Clinical Psychology, 60,* 953–961.

Henggeler, S. W., Melton, G. B., Smith, L. A., Schoenwald, S. K., & Hanley, J. H. (1993). Family preservation using multisystemic treatment: Long-term follow-up to a clinical trial with serious juvenile offenders. *Journal of Child and Family Studies, 4,* 283–293.

Henggeler, S. W., Pickrel, S. G., & Brondino, M. J. (1999). Multisystemic treatment of substance abusing and dependent delinquents: Outcomes, treatment fidelity, and transportability. *Mental Health Services Research, 1,* 171–184.

Henggeler, S. W., Pickrel, S. G., Brondino, M. J., & Crouch, J. L. (1996). Eliminating (almost) treatment dropout of substance abusing or dependent delinquents through home-based multisystemic therapy. *American Journal of Psychiatry, 153,* 427–428.

Henggeler, S. W., Rodick, J. D., Borduin, C. M., Hanson, C. L., Watson, S. M., & Urey, J. R. (1986). Multisystemic treatment of juvenile offenders: Effects on adolescent behavior and family interaction. *Developmental Psychology, 22,* 132–141.

Henggeler, S. W., Schoenwald, S. K., Borduin, C. M., Rowland, M. D., & Cunningham, P. B. (1998). *Multisystemic treatment of antisocial behavior in children and adolescents.* New York: Guilford Press.

Henggeler, S. W., Schoenwald, S. K., & Pickrel, S. G. (1997). Multisystemic therapy: Bridging the gap between university- and community-based treatment. *Journal of Consulting and Clinical Psychology, 63,* 709–717.

Hill, J., & Maughan, B. (2001). *Conduct disorders in childhood and adolescence.* Cambridge, UK: Cambridge University Press.

Hinshaw, S. P. (1992). Externalizing behavior problems and academic underachievement in childhood and adolescence: Causal relationships and underlying mechanisms. *Psychological Bulletin, 111,* 127–155.

Hinshaw, S. P., Buhrmester, D., & Heller, T. (1989). Anger control in response to verbal provocation: Effects of stimulant medication for boys with ADHD. *Journal of Abnormal Child Psychology, 17,* 393–407.

Hinshaw, S. P., Heller, T., & McHale, J. P. (1992). Covert antisocial behavior in boys with attention-deficit hyperactivity disorder: External validation and effects of methylphenidate. *Journal of Consulting and Clinical Psychology, 60,* 274–281.

Hinshaw, S. P., Henker, B., Whalen, C. K., Erhardt, D., & Dunnington, R. E. (1989). Aggressive, prosocial, and nonsocial behavior in hyperactive boys: Dose effects of methylphenidate in naturalistic settings. *Journal of Consulting and Clinical Psychology, 57,* 636–643.

Hinshaw, S. P., & Lee, S. S. (2003). Conduct and oppositional defiant disorders. In E. J. Mash & R. A. Barkley (Eds.), *Child psychopathology* (2nd ed., pp. 144–198). New York: Guilford Press.

Hinshaw, S. P., Simmel, C., & Heller, T. L. (1995). Multimethod assessment of covert antisocial behavior in children: Laboratory observation, adult ratings, and child self-report. *Psychological Assessment,* 7, 209–219.

Hinshaw, S. P., Zupan, B. A., Simmel, C., Nigg, J. T., & Melnick, S. (1997). Peer status in boys with and without attention-deficit hyperactivity disorder: Predictions from overt and covert antisocial behavior, social isolation, and authoritative parenting beliefs. *Child Development,* 68, 880–896.

Holleran, P. A., Littman, D. C., Freund, R. D., & Schmaling, K. B. (1982). A signal detection approach to social perception: Identification of negative and positive behaviors by parents of normal and problem children. *Journal of Abnormal Child Psychology,* 10, 547–557.

Howell, J. C. (2003). *Preventing and reducing juvenile delinquency: A comprehensive framework.* Thousand Oaks, CA: Sage.

Hubbard, J. A., Smithmyer, C. M., Ramsden, S. R., Parker, E. H., Flanagan, K. D., Dearing, K. F., & Relyea, N. (2002). Observational, physiological, and self-report measures of children's anger: Relations to reactive versus proactive aggression. *Child Development,* 73, 1101–1118.

Hudley, C., & Graham, S. (1993). An attributional intervention to reduce peer-directed aggression among African-American boys. *Child Development,* 64, 124–138.

Huesmann, L. R., Eron, L. D., Lefkowitz, M. M., & Walder, L. O. (1984). Stability of aggression over time and generations. *Developmental Psychology,* 20, 1120–1134.

Humphreys, J., Kopet, T., & Lajoy, R. (1993). Clinical considerations in the treatment of juvenile firesetters. *Clinical Child Psychology Newsletter, 9,* 2–3.

Ingoldsby, E. M., & Shaw, D. S. (2002). The role of neighborhood contextual factors on early-starting antisocial behavior. *Clinical Child and Family Psychology Review, 6,* 21–65.

Irvine, A. B., Biglan, A., Metzler, C. W., Smolkowski, K., & Ary, D. V. (1999). The effectiveness of a parenting skills program for parents of middle school students in small communities. *Journal of Consulting and Clinical Psychology, 67,* 811–825.

Jacob, T., Krahn, G. L., & Leonard, K. (1991). Parent–child interactions in families with alcoholic fathers. *Journal of Consulting and Clinical Psychology, 59,* 176–181.

Jacob, T., Moser, R. P., Windle, M., Loeber, R., & Stouthamer-Loeber, M. (2000). New measure of parenting practices involving preadolescent- and adolescent-aged children. *Behavior Modification, 24,* 611–634.

Jacobson, R. R. (1985). Child firesetters: A clinical investigation. *Journal of Child Psychology and Psychiatry, 26,* 759–768.

Jaffee, S. R., Caspi, A., Moffitt, T. E., & Taylor, A. (2004). Physical maltreatment victim to antisocial child: Evidence of an environmentally mediated process. *Journal of Abnormal Psychology, 113,* 44–55.

Jennings, K. D., Stagg, V., & Connors, R. E. (1991). Social networks and mothers' interactions with their preschool children. *Child Development, 62,* 966–978.

Jessor, R. (Ed.). (1998). *New perspectives on adolescent risk behavior.* New York: Cambridge University Press.

Jessor, R., & Jessor, S. L. (1977). *Problem behavior and psychosocial development: A longitudinal study of youth.* New York: Academic Press.

Johnston, C. (1996). Addressing parent cognitions in interventions with families of disruptive children. In K. S. Dobson & K. D. Craig (Eds.), *Advances in cognitive-behavioral therapy* (pp. 193–209). Thousand Oaks, CA: Sage.

Johnston, C., & Mash, E. J. (1989). A measure of parenting satisfaction and efficacy. *Journal of Clinical Child Psychology, 18,* 167–175.

Johnston, C., & Murray, C. (2003). Incremental validity in the psychological assessment of children and adolescents. *Psychological Assessment, 15,* 496–507.

Jones, R. R. (1974). *"Observation" by telephone: An economical behavior sampling technique* (Oregon Research Institute Technical Report No. 1411). Eugene: Oregon Research Institute.

Jones, Y. (1990). *Aggression replacement training in a high school setting.* Unpublished manuscript, Center for Learning and Adjustment Difficulties, Brisbane, Australia.

Jouriles, E. N., Murphy, C. M., Farris, A. M., Smith, D. A., Richters, J. E., & Waters, E. (1991). Marital adjustment, parental disagreements about child rearing, and behavior problems in boys: Increasing the specificity of the marital assessment. *Child Development, 62,* 1424–1433.

Kaltiala-Heino, R., Rimpela, M., Marttunen, M., Rimpela, A., & Rantanen, P. (1999). Bullying, depression, and suicidal ideation in Finnish adolescents: School survey. *British Medical Journal, 319,* 348–351.

Kamphaus, R. W., & Frick, P. J. (2002). *Clinical assessment of child and adolescent personality and behavior* (2nd ed.). Boston: Allyn & Bacon.

Kaplan, S. L., Busner, J., Kupietz, S., Wassermann, E., & Segal, B. (1990). Effects of methylphenidate on adolescents with aggressive conduct disorder and ADHD: A preliminary report. *Journal of the American Academy of Child and Adolescent Psychiatry, 29,* 719–723.

Katz, L. F., & Gottman, J. M. (1993). Patterns of marital conflict predict children's internalizing and externalizing behavior. *Developmental Psychology, 29,* 940–950.

Kaufman, A. S., & Kaufman, N. L. (Eds.). (2001). *Specific learning disabilities and difficulties in children and adolescents: Psychological assessment and evaluation.* New York: Cambridge University Press.

Kazdin, A. E. (1995a). Child, parent and family dysfunction as predictors of outcome in cognitive-behavioral treatment of antisocial children. *Behaviour Research and Therapy, 33,* 271–281.

Kazdin, A. E. (1995b). *Conduct disorders in childhood and adolescence* (2nd ed.). Thousand Oaks, CA: Sage.

Kazdin, A. E., & Kolko, D. J. (1986). Parent psychopathology and family functioning among childhood firesetters. *Journal of Abnormal Child Psychology, 14,* 315–329.

Kazdin, A. E., Mazurick, J. L., & Siegel, T. C. (1994). Treatment outcome among children with externalizing disorder who terminate prematurely versus those who complete psychotherapy. *Journal of the American Academy of Child and Adolescent Psychiatry, 33,* 549–557.

Kazdin, A. E., Siegel, T. C., & Bass, D. (1992). Cognitive problem-solving skills training and parent management training in the treatment of antisocial behavior in children. *Journal of Consulting and Clinical Psychology, 60,* 733–747.

Keenan, K., Loeber, R., & Green, S. (1999). Conduct disorder in girls: A review of the literature. *Clinical Child and Family Psychology Review, 2,* 3–19.

Keenan, K., Shaw, D., Delliquadri, E., Giovannelli, J., & Walsh, B. (1998). Evidence for the continuity of early problem behaviors: Application of a developmental model. *Journal of Abnormal Child Psychology, 26,* 441–454.

Keenan, K., & Wakschlag, L. S. (2002). Can a valid diagnosis of disruptive behavior disorder be made in preschool children? *American Journal of Psychiatry, 159,* 351–358.

Kendall, P. C. (1985). Toward a cognitive-behavioral model of child psychopathology and a critique of related interventions. *Journal of Abnormal Psychology, 13,* 357–372.

Kendall, P. C. (1991). Guiding theory for therapy with children and adolescents. In P. C. Kendall (Ed.), *Child and adolescent therapy: Cognitive-behavioral procedures* (pp. 3–22). New York: Guilford Press.

Kendall, P. C., & MacDonald, J. P. (1993). Cognition in the psychopathology of youth and implications for treatment. In K. S. Dobson & P. C. Kendall (Eds.), *Psychopathology and cognition* (pp. 387–426). San Diego, CA: Academic Press.

Kerns, S. E., & Prinz, R. J. (2002). Critical issues in the prevention of violence-related behavior in youth. *Clinical Child and Family Psychology Review, 5,* 133–160.

Kirigin, K. A. (1996). Teaching-family model of group home treatment of children with severe behavior problems. In M. C. Roberts (Ed.), *Model programs in child and family mental health* (pp. 231–247). Mahwah, NJ: Erlbaum.

Kirigin, K. A., Braukmann, C. J., Atwater, J. D., & Wolf, M. M. (1982). An evaluation of Teaching-Family (Achievement Place) group homes for juvenile offenders. *Journal of Applied Behavior Analysis, 15,* 1–16.

Klein, N. C., Alexander, J. F., & Parsons, B. V. (1977). Impact of family systems intervention on recidivism and sibling delinquency: A model of primary prevention and program evaluation. *Journal of Consulting and Clinical Psychology, 45,* 469–474.

Klein, R. G. (1991). Preliminary results: Lithium effects in conduct disorders. *CME Syllabus and Proceedings Summary, 144th Annual Meeting of the American Psychiatric Association,* pp. 119–120.

Klein, R., Abikoff, H., Klass, E., Ganales, D., Seese, L., & Pollack, S. (1997). Clinical efficacy of methylphenidate in conduct disorder with and without attention deficit hyperactivity disorder. *Archives of General Psychiatry, 54,* 1073–1080.

Klein, R. G, Abikoff, H., Klass, E., Shah, M., & Seese, L. (1994). *Controlled trial of methylphenidate, lithium, and placebo in children and adolescents with conduct disorders.* Paper presented at the meeting of the Society for Research in Child and Adolescent Psychopathology, London.

Klinteberg, B. A., Andersson, T., Magnusson, D., & Stattin, H. (1993). Hyperactive behavior in childhood as related to subsequent alcohol problems and violent offending: A longitudinal study of male subjects. *Personality and Individual Differences, 15,* 381–388.

Kolko, D. J. (1988). Community interventions for childhood firesetters: A comparison of two national programs. *Hospital and Community Psychiatry, 39,* 973–979.

Kolko, D. J. (2001). Efficacy of cognitive-behavioral treatment and fire safety education for children who set fires: Initial and follow-up outcomes. *Journal of Child Psychology and Psychiatry and Allied Disciplines, 42,* 359–369.

Kolko, D. J. (2002a). Child, parent, and family treatment: Cognitive-behavioral interventions. In D. Kolko (Ed.), *Handbook on firesetting in children and youth* (pp. 305–336). San Diego, CA: Academic Press.

Kolko, D. J. (2002b). Research studies on the problem. In D. Kolko (Ed.), *Handbook on firesetting in children and youth* (pp. 33–56). San Diego, CA: Academic Press.

Kolko, D. J., & Kazdin, A. E. (1988). Prevalence of firesetting and related behaviors among child psychiatric inpatients. *Journal of Consulting and Clinical Psychology, 56,* 628–630.

Kolko, D. J., & Kazdin, A. E. (1992). The emergence and recurrence of child firesetting: A one-year prospective study. *Journal of Abnormal Child Psychology, 20,* 17–37.

Kolko, D. J., Nishi-Strattner, L., Wilcox, D. K., & Kopet, T. (2002). Clinical assessment of juvenile firesetters and their families: Tools and tips. In D. J. Kolko (Ed.), *Handbook on firesetting in children and youth* (pp. 177–212). San Diego, CA: Academic Press.

Kolko, D. J., Watson, S., & Faust, J. (1991). Fire safety/prevention skills training to reduce involvement with fire in young psychiatric inpatients: Preliminary findings. *Behavior Therapy, 22,* 269–284.

Kovacs, M., Paulauskas, S., Gatsonis, C., & Richards, C. (1988). Depressive disorders in childhood. *Journal of Affective Disorders, 15,* 205–217.

Kratzer, L., & Hodgins, S. (1997). Adult outcomes of child conduct problems: A cohort study. *Journal of Abnormal Child Psychology, 25,* 65–81.

Kruesi, M. J. P., & Lelio, D. F. (1996). Disorders of conduct and behavior. In J. M. Wiener (Ed.), *Diagnosis and psychopharmacology of childhood and adolescent disorders* (2nd ed., pp. 401–447). New York: Wiley.

Kruh, I. P., Frick, P. J., & Clements, C. B. (2005). Historical and personality correlates to the violence patterns of juveniles tried as adults. *Criminal Justice and Behavior, 32,* 69–96.

Kumpfer, K. K., Alvarado, R., Smith, P., & Bellamy, N. (2002). Cultural sensitivity and adaptation in family-based prevention interventions. *Prevention Science, 3,* 241–246.

Lacourse, E., Cote, S., Nagin, D. S., Vitaro, F., Brendgen, M., & Tremblay, R. E. (2002). A longitudinal–experimental approach to testing theories of antisocial behavior development. *Development and Psychopathology, 14,* 909–924.

Lacourse, E., Nagin, D., Tremblay, R. E., Vitaro, F., & Claes, M. (2003). Developmental trajectories of boys' delinquent group membership and facilitation of violent behaviors during adolescence. *Development and Psychopathology, 15,* 183–197.

Lahey, B. B., Applegate, B., Barkley, R. A., Garfinkel, B., McBurnett, K., Kerdyck, L., et al. (1994). DSM-IV field trials for oppositional defiant disorder and conduct disorder in children and adolescents. *American Journal of Psychiatry, 151,* 1163–1171.

Lahey, B. B., Loeber, R., Burke, J., & Rathouz, P. J. (2002). Adolescent outcomes of childhood conduct disorder among clinic-referred boys: Predictors of improvement. *Journal of Abnormal Child Psychology, 30,* 333–348.

Lahey, B. B, Loeber, R., Quay, H. C., Applegate, B., Shaffer, D., Waldman, I., et al. (1998). Validity of the DSM-IV subtypes of conduct disorder based on age of onset. *Journal of the American Academy of Child and Adolescent Psychiatry, 37,* 435–442.

Lahey, B. B., Miller, T. L., Gordon, R. A., & Riley, A. W. (1999). Developmental epidemiology of the disruptive behavior disorders. In H. C. Quay & A. E. Hogan (Eds.), *Handbook of disruptive behavior disorders* (pp. 23–48). New York: Kluwer/Plenum Press.

Lahey, B. B., Moffitt, T. E., & Caspi, A. (Eds.). (2003). *Causes of conduct disorder and juvenile delinquency.* New York: Guilford Press.

Lahey, B. B., & Waldman, I. D. (2003). A developmental propensity model of the origins of conduct problems during childhood and adolescence. In B. B. Lahey, T. E. Moffitt, & A. Caspi (Eds.), *Causes of conduct disorder and juvenile delinquency* (pp. 76–117). New York: Guilford Press.

Lang, A. R., Pelham, W. E., Atkeson, B. M., & Murphy, D. A. (1999). Effects of alcohol intoxication on parenting behavior and interactions with child confederates exhibiting normal or deviant behavior. *Journal of Abnormal Child Psychology, 27,* 177–189.

Larzelere, R. E., Dinges, K., Schmidt, M. D., Spellman, D. F., Criste, T. R., & Connell, P. (2001). Outcomes of residential treatment: A study of the adolescent clients of Girls and Boys Town. *Child and Youth Care Forum, 30,* 175–185.

Le Blanc, M., & Frechette, M. (1989). *Male criminal activity from childhood to adulthood: Multilevel and developmental perspectives.* New York: Springer-Verlag.

Leeman, L. W., Gibbs, J. C., & Fuller, D. (1993). Evaluation of a multicomponent group treatment program for juvenile delinquents. *Aggressive Behavior, 19,* 281–292.

Leff, S. S., Angelucci, J., Grabowski, L., & Weil, J. (2004, July). Using school and community partners to design, implement, and evaluate a group intervention for relationally aggressive girls. In S. S. Leff (Chair), *Using partnerships to design, implement, and evaluate aggression prevention programs.* Symposium conducted at the meeting of the American Psychological Association, Honolulu.

LeMarquand, D., Tremblay, R. E., & Vitaro, F. (2001). The prevention of conduct disorder: A review of successful and unsuccessful experiments. In J. Hill & B. Maughan (Eds.), *Conduct disorders in childhood and adolescence* (pp. 449–477). Cambridge, UK: Cambridge University Press.

Leschied, A. W., & Cunningham, A. (2002). *Seeking effective interventions for young offenders: Interim results for a four-year randomized study of multisystemic therapy in Ontario, Canada.* London, ON, Canada: Centre for Children and Families in the Justice System.

Leve, L. D., & Chamberlain, P. (2005). Girls in the juvenile justice system: Risk factors and clinical implications. In D. Pepler, K. Madsen, C. Webster, & K. Levine (Eds.), *Development and treatment of girlhood aggression.* Mahwah, NJ: Erlbaum.

Levene, K. S., Walsh, M. M., Augimeri, L. K., & Pepler, D. J. (2004). Linking identification and treatment of early risk factors for female delinquency. In M. M. Moretti, C. L. Odgers, & M. A. Jackson (Eds.), *Girls and aggression: Contributing factors and intervention principles* (pp. 147–163). New York: Kluwer/Plenum Press.

Lilienfeld, S. O. (1992). The association between antisocial personality and somatization disorders: A review and integration of theoretical models. *Clinical Psychology Review, 12,* 641–662.

Lipsey, M. W. (1992). Juvenile delinquency treatment: A meta-analytic inquiry into the variability of effects. In T. D. Cook, H. Cooper, D. S. Cordray, H. Hartmann, L. V. Hedges, R. J. Light, et al. (Eds.), *Meta-analysis for explanation: A casebook* (pp. 83–127). New York: Russell Sage.

Lipsey, M. W. (1995). What do we learn from 400 research studies on the effectiveness of treatment with juvenile delinquents? In J. McGuire (Ed.), *What works? Reducing reoffending* (pp. 63–78). New York: Wiley.

Lipsey, M. W. (1999). Can intervention rehabilitate serious delinquents? *Annals of the American Academy of Political and Social Science, 564,* 142–166.

Lipsey, M. W., & Wilson, D. B. (1998). Effective intervention for serious juvenile offenders: A synthesis of research. In R. Loeber & D. P. Farrington (Eds.), *Serious and violent juvenile offenders: Risk factors and successful interventions* (pp. 313–345). Thousand Oaks, CA: Sage.

Little, T. D., Jones, S. M., Henrich, C. C., & Hawley, P. H. (2003). Disentangling the "whys" from the "whats" of aggressive behavior. *International Journal of Behavioural Development, 27,* 122–133.

Loeber, R. (1988). Natural histories of conduct problems, delinquency, and associated substance use: Evidence for developmental progressions. In B. B. Lahey & A. E. Kazdin (Eds.), *Advances in clinical child psychology* (Vol. 11, pp. 73–124). New York: Plenum Press.

Loeber, R., Brinthaupt, V. P., & Green, S. M. (1990). Attention deficits, impulsivity, and hyperactivity with or without conduct problems: Relationships to delinquency and unique contextual factors. In R. J. McMahon & R. DeV. Peters (Eds.), *Behavior disorders of adolescence: Research, intervention, and policy in clinical and school setting* (pp. 39–61). New York: Plenum Press.

Loeber, R., & Dishion, T. S. (1983). Early predictors of male delinquency: A review. *Psychological Bulletin, 94,* 68–99.

Loeber, R., & Farrington, D. P. (2000). Young children who commit crime: Epidemiology, developmental origins, risk factors, early interventions, and policy implications. *Development and Psychopathology, 12,* 737–762.

Loeber, R., Farrington, D. P., Stouthamer-Loeber, M., Moffitt, T. E., Caspi, C., White, H. R., et al. (2003). The development of male offending: Key findings from fourteen years of the Pittsburgh Youth Study. In T. P. Thornberry & M. D. Krohn (Eds.), *Taking stock of delinquency: An overview of findings from contemporary longitudinal studies* (pp. 93–136). New York: Kluwer/Plenum Press.

Loeber, R., Farrington, D. P., Stouthamer-Loeber, M., & Van Kammen, W. B. (1998). Multiple risk factors for multi-problem boys: Co-occurrence of delinquency, substance use, attention deficit, conduct problems, physical aggression, covert behavior, depressed mood, and shy/withdrawn behavior. In R. Jessor (Ed.), *New perspectives on adolescent risk behavior* (pp. 90–149). New York: Cambridge University Press.

Loeber, R., & Keenan, K. (1994). Interaction between conduct disorder and its comorbid conditions: Effects of age and gender. *Clinical Psychology Review, 14,* 497–523.

Loeber, R., & Schmaling, K. B. (1985a). Empirical evidence for overt and covert patterns of antisocial conduct problems: A meta-analysis. *Journal of Abnormal Child Psychology, 13,* 337–352.

Loeber, R., & Schmaling, K. B. (1985b). The utility of differentiating between mixed and pure forms of antisocial child behavior. *Journal of Abnormal Child Psychology, 13,* 315–336.

Loeber, R., & Stouthamer-Loeber, M. (1986). Family factors as correlates and predictors of juvenile conduct problems and delinquency. In M. Tonry & N. Morris (Eds.), *Crime and justice* (Vol. 7, pp. 29–149). Chicago: University of Chicago Press.

Loeber, R., Stouthamer-Loeber, M., Van Kammen, W. B., & Farrington, D. P. (1989). Development of a new measure of self-reported antisocial behavior for young children: Prevalence and reliability. In M. W. Klein (Ed.), *Cross national research and self-reported crime and delinquency* (pp. 203–225). Dordrecht, The Netherlands: Kluwer-Nijhoff.

Loeber, R., Weissman, W., & Reid, J. B. (1983). Family interactions of assaultive adolescents, stealers, and nondelinquents. *Journal of Abnormal Child Psychology, 11,* 1–14.

Loeber, R., Wung, P., Keenan, K., Giroux, B., Stouthamer-Loeber, M., Van Kammen, W. B., et al. (1993). Developmental pathways in disruptive child behavior. *Development and Psychopathology, 5,* 101–131.

Loney, B. R., Frick, P. J., Ellis, M., & McCoy, M. G. (1998). Intelligence, psychopathy, and antisocial behavior. *Journal of Psychopathology and Behavioral Assessment, 20,* 231–247.

Lynskey, M. T., & Fergusson, D. M. (1995). Childhood conduct problems, attention deficit behaviors, and adolescent alcohol, tobacco, and illicit drug use. *Journal of Abnormal Child Psychology, 23,* 281–302.

MacBrayer, E. K., Milich, R., & Hundley, M. (2003). Attributional biases in aggressive children and their mothers. *Journal of Abnormal Psychology, 112,* 698–708.

Malone, R. P., Delaney, M. A., Luebbert, J. F, Cater, J., & Campbell, M. (2000). A double-blind placebo-controlled study of lithium in hospitalized aggressive children and adolescents with conduct disorder. *Archives of General Psychiatry, 57,* 649–654.

Maughan, B., & Rutter, M. (2001). Antisocial children grown up. In J. Hill & B. Maughan (Eds.), *Conduct disorders in childhood and adolescence* (pp. 507–552). Cambridge, UK: Cambridge University Press.

McCabe, K. M., Hough, R., Wood, P. A., & Yeh, M. (2001). Childhood and adolescent onset conduct disorder: A test of the developmental taxonomy. *Journal of Abnormal Child Psychology, 29,* 305–316.

McCarty, C. A., McMahon, R. J., & Conduct Problems Prevention Research Group. (2005). Domains of risk in the developmental continuity of firesetting. *Behavior Therapy, 36,* 185–195.

McClellan, J. M., & Werry, J. S. (2000). Introduction to special section: Research psychiatric diagnostic interviews for children and adolescents. *Journal of the American Academy of Child and Adolescent Psychiatry, 39,* 19–27.

McConaughy, S. H., & Achenbach, T. M. (2001). *Manual for the Semistructured Clinical Interview for Children and Adolescents* (2nd ed.). Burlington: University of Vermont, Center for Children, Youth, & Families.

McDermott, P. A. (1996). A nationwide study of development and gender prevalence for psychopathology in childhood and adolescence. *Journal of Abnormal Child Psychology, 24,* 53–66.

McGee, R., Feehan, M., Williams, S., & Anderson, J. (1992). DSM-III disorders from age 11 to age 15 years. *Journal of the American Academy of Child and Adolescent Psychiatry, 31,* 50–59.

McMahon, R. J., & Estes, A. M. (1997). Conduct problems. In E. J. Mash & L. G. Terdal (Eds.), *Assessment of childhood disorders* (3rd ed., pp. 130–193). New York: Guilford Press.

McMahon, R. J., & Forehand, R. (1983). Consumer satisfaction in behavioral treatment of children: Types, issues, and recommendations. *Behavior Therapy, 14,* 209–225.

McMahon, R. J., & Forehand, R. L. (2003). *Helping the noncompliant child: Family-based treatment for oppositional behavior* (2nd ed.). New York: Guilford Press.

McMahon, R. J., & Frick, P. J. (2005). Evidence-based assessment of conduct problems in children and adolescents. *Journal of Clinical Child and Adolescent Psychology, 34,* 477–505.

McMahon, R. J., & Rhule, D. M. (2005). The prevention of conduct problems. In P. Graham (Ed.), *Cognitive behaviour therapy for children and families* (2nd ed., pp. 481–503). Cambridge, UK: Cambridge University Press.

McMahon, R. J., Slough, N. M., & Conduct Problems Prevention Research Group. (1996). Family-based intervention in the Fast Track program. In R. DeV. Peters & R. J. McMahon (Eds.), *Preventing childhood disorders, substance abuse, and delinquency* (pp. 90–110). Thousand Oaks, CA: Sage.

McMahon, R. J., & Wells, K. C. (1998). Conduct problems. In E. J. Mash & R. A. Barkley (Eds.), *Treatment of childhood disorders* (2nd ed., pp. 111–207). New York: Guilford Press.

Middlebrook, J. L., & Forehand, R. (1985). Maternal perceptions of deviance in child behavior as a function of stress and clinic versus non-clinic status of the child: An analogue study. *Behavior Therapy, 16,* 494–502.

Miller, G. E., & Klungness, L. (1989). Childhood theft: A comprehensive review of assessment and treatment. *School Psychology Review, 18,* 82–97.

Miller, W. R., & Rollnick, S. (1991). *Motivational interviewing: Preparing people to change addictive behavior.* New York: Guilford Press.

Moffitt, T. E. (1990). Juvenile delinquency and attention deficit disorder: Boys' developmental trajectories from age 3 to age 15. *Child Development, 61,* 893–910.

Moffitt, T. E. (1993). "Adolescence-limited" and "life-course-persistent" antisocial behavior: A developmental taxonomy. *Psychological Review, 100,* 674–701.

Moffitt, T. E. (2003). Life-course persistent and adolescence-limited antisocial behavior: A 10-year research review and research agenda. In B. B. Lahey, T. E. Moffitt, & A. Caspi (Eds.), *Causes of conduct disorder and juvenile delinquency* (pp. 49–75). New York: Guilford Press.

Moffitt, T. E., & Caspi, A. (2001). Childhood predictors differentiate life-course persistent and adolescence-limited antisocial pathways in males and females. *Development and Psychopathology, 13,* 355–376.

Moffitt, T. E., Caspi, A., Belsky, J., & Silva, P. A. (1992). Childhood experience and the onset of menarche: A test of a sociobiological model. *Child Development, 63,* 47–58.

Moffitt, T. E., Caspi, A., Dickson, N., Silva, P., & Stanton, W. (1996). Childhood-onset versus adolescent-onset antisocial conduct problems in males: Natural history from ages 3 to 18 years. *Development and Psychopathology, 8,* 399–424.

Moffitt, T. E., Caspi, A., Harrington, H., & Milne, B. (2002). Males on the life-course persistent and adolescence-limited antisocial pathways: Follow-up at age 26. *Development and Psychopathology, 14,* 179–206.

Moffitt, T. E., Caspi, A., Rutter, M., & Silva, P. A. (2001). *Sex differences in antisocial behaviour.* Cambridge, UK: Cambridge University Press.

Moore, D., Chamberlain, P., & Mukai, L. (1979). Children at risk for delinquency: A follow-up comparison of aggressive children and children who steal. *Journal of Abnormal Child Psychology, 7,* 345–355.

Moretti, M. M., Odgers, C. L., & Jackson, M. A. (Eds.). (2004). *Girls and aggression: Contributing factors and intervention principles.* New York: Kluwer/Plenum Press.

MTA Cooperative Group. (1999). Moderators and mediators of treatment response for children with attention-deficit/hyperactivity disorder. *Archives of General Psychiatry, 56,* 1088–1096.

Murphy, K. R., & Gordon, M. (1998). Assessment of adults with ADHD. In R. A. Barkley (Ed.), *Attention-deficit hyperactivity disorder: A handbook for diagnosis and treatment* (2nd ed., pp. 345–369). New York: Guilford Press.

Nagin, D. S., Farrington, D. M., & Moffitt, T. E. (1995). Life-course trajectories of different types of offenders. *Criminology, 33,* 111–139.

Nangle, D. W., Erdley, C. A., Carpenter, E. M., & Newman, J. E. (2002). Social skills training as a treatment for aggressive children and adolescents: A developmental–clinical integration. *Aggression and Violent Behavior, 7,* 169–199.

Nansel, T. R., Overpeck, M., Pilla, R. S., Ruan, W. J.,

Simmons-Morton, B., & Scheidt, P. C. (2001). Bullying behaviors among US youth: Prevalence and association with psychological adjustment. *Journal of the American Medical Association, 285,* 2094–2100.

Nelson, J. R, Smith, D. J., & Dodd, J. (1990). The moral reasoning of juvenile delinquents: A meta analysis. *Journal of Abnormal Child Psychology, 18,* 231–239.

Novaco, R. W. (1978). Anger and coping with stress: Cognitive-behavioral interventions. In J. P. Foreyet & D. P. Rathjen (Eds.), *Cognitive behavioral therapy: Research and application* (pp. 135–173). New York: Plenum Press.

O'Donnell, J., Hawkins, J. D., Catalano, R. F., Abbott, R. D., & Day, L. E. (1995). Preventing school failure, drug use, and delinquency among low-income children: Long-term intervention in elementary schools. *American Journal of Orthopsychiatry, 65,* 87–100.

Offord, D. R., Alder, R. J., & Boyle, M. H. (1986). Prevalence and sociodemographic correlates of conduct disorder. *American Journal of Social Psychiatry, 6,* 272–278.

Offord, D. R., Boyle, M. H., Racine, Y. A., Fleming, J. E., Cadman, D. T., Blum, H. M., et al. (1992). Outcome, prognosis, and risk in a longitudinal follow-up study. *Journal of the American Academy of Child and Adolescent Psychiatry, 31,* 916–923.

Ogden, T., & Halliday-Boykins, C. A. (2004). Multisystemic treatment of antisocial adolescents in Norway: Replication of clinical outcomes outside of the U. S. *Child and Adolescent Mental Health, 9,* 77–83.

Okulitch, J., & Pinsonneault, I. (2002). The interdisciplinary approach to juvenile firesetting: A dialogue. In D. Kolko (Ed.), *Handbook on firesetting in children and youth* (pp. 57–74). San Diego, CA: Academic Press.

Olds, D., Henderson, C. R., Cole, R., Eckenrode, J., Kitzman, H., Luckey, D., et al. (1998). Long-term effects of nurse home visitation on children's criminal and antisocial behavior: 15-year follow-up of a randomized trial. *Journal of the American Medical Association, 280,* 1238–1244.

Olds, D., Kitzman, H., Cole, R., & Robinson, J. (1997). Theoretical foundations of a program of home visitation for pregnant women and parents of young children. *Journal of Community Psychology, 25,* 9–25.

Olweus, D. (1990). Bullying among children. In K. Hurrelmann & F. Losel (Eds.), *Health hazards in adolescence: Prevention and intervention in childhood and adolescence* (Vol. 8, pp. 259–297). Berlin: Walter de Gruyter.

Olweus, D. (1991). Bully/victim problems among schoolchildren: Basic facts and effects of a school based intervention program. In D. J. Pepler & K. H. Rubin (Eds.), *The development and treatment of childhood aggression* (pp. 411–488). Hillsdale, NJ: Erlbaum.

Olweus, D. (1992). Bullying among schoolchildren: Intervention and prevention. In R. DeV. Peters, R. J. McMahon, & V. L. Quinsey (Eds.), *Aggression and violence throughout the lifespan* (pp. 100–125). Newbury Park, CA: Sage.

Olweus, D. (1993). *Bullying at school: What we know and what we can do.* Maiden, MA: Blackwell.

Olweus, D. (1996). Bullying at school: Knowledge base and an effective intervention program. *Annals of the New York Academy of Sciences, 794,* 265–276.

Olweus, D. (1999). Sweden. In P. K. Smith, Y. Morita, J. Junger-Tas, D. Olweus, R. Catalano, & P. Slee (Eds.), *The nature of school bullying: A cross-national perspective* (pp. 7–27). New York: Routledge.

Olweus, D. (2001). Peer harassment: A critical analysis and some important issues. In J. Juvonen & S. Graham (Eds.), *Peer harassment in school: The plight of the vulnerable and victimized* (pp. 3–20). New York: Guilford Press.

Oxford, M., Cavell, T. A., & Hughes, J. N. (2003). Callous–unemotional traits moderate the relation between ineffective parenting and child externalizing problems: A partial replication and extension. *Journal of Clinical Child and Adolescent Psychology, 32,* 577–585.

Pajer, K. A. (1998). What happens to "bad" girls? A review of the adult outcomes of antisocial adolescent girls. *America Journal of Psychiatry, 155,* 862–870.

Pardini, D. A., Lochman, J. E., & Frick, P. J. (2003). Callous/unemotional traits and social cognitive processes in adjudicated youth. *Journal of the American Academy of Child and Adolescent Psychiatry, 42,* 364–371.

Parrish, J. M., Cataldo, M. F., Kolko, D. J., Neef, N. A., & Egel, A. L. (1986). Experimental analysis of response covariation. *Journal of Applied Behavior Analysis, 19,* 241–254.

Parsons, B. V., & Alexander, J. F. (1973). Short-term family intervention: A therapy outcome study. *Journal of Consulting and Clinical Psychology, 41,* 195–201.

Patterson, G. R. (1982). *Coercive family process.* Eugene, OR: Castalia.

Patterson, G. R. (2002). The early development of coercive family process. In J. B. Reid, G. R. Patterson, & J. Snyder (Eds.), *Antisocial behavior in children and adolescents: A developmental analysis and model for intervention* (pp. 25–44). Washington, DC: American Psychological Association.

Patterson, G. R., Capaldi, D., & Bank, L. (1991). An early starter model for predicting delinquency. In D. J. Pepler & K. H. Rubin (Eds.), *The development and treatment of childhood aggression* (pp. 139–168). Hillsdale, NJ: Erlbaum.

Patterson, G. R., & Forgatch, M. (1987). *Parents and adolescents living together. Part 1: The basics.* Eugene, OR: Castalia.

Patterson, G. R., Forgatch, M. S., Yoerger, K. L., & Stoolmiller, M. (1998). Variables that initiate and maintain an early-onset trajectory for juvenile offending. *Development and Psychopathology, 10,* 531–547.

Patterson, G. R., Reid, J. B., & Dishion, T. J. (1992). *Antisocial boys.* Eugene, OR: Castalia.

Patterson, G. R., Reid, J. B., Jones, R. R., & Conger, R. R. (1975). *A social learning approach to family intervention: Families with aggressive children* (Vol. 1). Eugene, OR: Castalia.

Patterson, G. R., & Yoerger, K. (2002). A developmental model for early and late-onset delinquency. In J. B. Reid, G. R. Patterson, & J. Snyder (Eds.), *Antisocial behavior in children and adolescents: A developmental analysis and model for intervention* (pp. 147–172). Washington, DC: American Psychological Association.

Pawsey, R. (1996). A family behavioural treatment of persistent juvenile theft. *Australian Psychologist, 31,* 28–33.

Pelham, W. E., & Lang, A. R. (1993). Parental alcohol consumption and deviant child behavior: Laboratory studies of reciprocal effects. *Clinical Psychology Review, 13,* 763–784.

Pelletier-Parker, A. Slate, F. Moriarty, D., & Pinsonneault, I. (1999). *The best practice treatment guidelines for adolescent firesetters in residential treatment.* Boston: Option/Commonworks.

Pepler, D. J., Craig, W. M., Ziegler, S., & Charach, A. (1993). A school-based anti-bullying intervention: Preliminary evaluation. In D. Tattum (Ed.), *Understanding and managing bullying* (pp. 76–91). Oxford, UK: Heinemann.

Pepler, D. J., Craig, W. M., Ziegler, S., & Charach, A. (1994). An evaluation of an anti-bullying intervention in Toronto schools. *Canadian Journal of Community Mental Health, 13,* 95–110.

Pepler, D. J., Madsen, K. C., Webster, C., & Levene, K. S. (Eds.). (2005). *The development and treatment of girlhood aggression.* Mahwah, NJ: Erlbaum.

Pepler, D. J., Walsh, M. M., & Levene, K. S. (2004). Interventions for aggressive girls: Tailoring and measuring the fit. In M. M. Moretti, C. L. Odgers, & M. A. Jackson (Eds.), *Girls and aggression: Contributing factors and intervention principles* (pp. 131–145). New York: Kluwer/Plenum Press.

Pikas, A. (1989). A pure conception of mobbing gives the best results for treatment. *School Psychology International, 10,* 95–104.

Piquero, A., & Brezina, T. (2000). Testing Moffitt's account of adolescence-limited delinquency. *Criminology, 39,* 353–370.

Porter, B., & O'Leary, K. D. (1980). Marital discord and childhood behavior problems. *Journal of Abnormal Child Psychology, 8,* 287–295.

Poulin, F., & Boivin, M. (2000). Reactive and proactive aggression: Evidence of a two-factor model. *Psychological Assessment, 12,* 115–122.

Poulin, F., Dishion, T. J., & Burraston, B. (2001). 3-year iatrogenic effects associated with aggregating high-risk adolescents in cognitive-behavioral preventive interventions. *Applied Developmental Science, 5,* 214–224.

Power, C., Higgins, A., & Kohlberg, L. (1989). *Lawrence Kohlberg's approach to moral education.* New York: Columbia University Press.

Presidential Commission on Law Enforcement and the Administration of Justice. (1967). *Task force report: Juvenile delinquency and youth crime.* Washington, DC: U.S. Government Printing Office.

Prinz, R. J., & Dumas, J. E. (2004). Prevention of oppositional defiant disorder and conduct disorder in children and adolescents. In P. M. Barrett & T. H. Ollendick (Eds.), *Handbook of interventions that work with children and adolescents: Prevention and treatment* (pp. 475–488). Chichester, UK: Wiley.

Prinz, R. J., & Miller, G. E. (1991). Issues in understanding and treating childhood conduct problems in disadvantaged populations. *Journal of Clinical Child Psychology, 20,* 379–385.

Putallaz, M., & Bierman, K. L. (Eds.). (2004). *Aggression, antisocial behavior, and violence among girls: A developmental perspective.* New York: Guilford Press.

Quay, H. C., & Peterson, D. (1996). *Revised Behavior Problem Checklist, PAR Edition: Professional manual.* Odessa, FL: Psychological Assessment Resources.

Reddy, L. A., & Pfeiffer, S. I. (1997). Effectiveness of treatment foster care with children and adolescents: A review of outcome studies. *Journal of the American Academy of Child and Adolescent Psychiatry, 36,* 581–588.

Reich, W. (2000). Diagnostic Interview for Children and Adolescents (DICA). *Journal of the American Academy of Child and Adolescent Psychiatry, 39,* 59–66.

Reid, J. B. (1984, November). Stealing and other clandestine activities among antisocial children. In D. J. Kolko (Chair), *Child antisocial behavior research: Current status and implications.* Symposium conducted at the meeting of the Association for Advancement of Behavior Therapy, Philadelphia.

Reid, J. B., Baldwin, D. V., Patterson, G. R., & Dishion, T. J. (1988). Observations in the assessment of childhood disorders. In M. Rutter, A. H. Tuma, & I. S. Lann (Eds.), *Assessment and diagnosis in child psychopathology* (pp. 156–195). New York: Guilford Press.

Reid, J. B., & Hendricks, A. F. C. J. (1973). A preliminary analysis of the effectiveness of direct home intervention for treatment of pre-delinquent boys who steal. In L. A. Hamerlynck, L. C. Handy, & E. J. Mash (Eds.), *Behavior change: Methodology, concepts, and practice* (pp. 209–220). Champaign, IL: Research Press.

Reid, J. B., Hinojosa Rivera, G., & Lorber, R. (1980). *A social learning approach to the outpatient treatment of children who steal.* Unpublished manuscript, Oregon Social Learning Center, Eugene.

Reitman, D., & Hupp, S. D. A. (2003). Behavior problems in the school setting: Synthesizing structural and functional assessment. In M. L. Kelley, D. Reitman, & G. H. Noell (Eds.), *Practitioner's guide to empiri-*

cally based measures of school behavior (pp. 23–36). New York: Kluwer Academic/Plenum.

Reynolds, C. R., & Kamphaus, K. W. (2004). *Behavioral assessment system for children* (2nd ed.). Circle Pines, MN: American Guidance Service.

Richardson, J. P. (2002). Secure residential treatment for adolescent firesetters. In D. Kolko (Ed.), *Handbook on firesetting in children and youth* (pp. 353–381). San Diego, CA: Academic Press.

Richters, J. E. (1992). Depressed mothers as informants about their children: A critical review of the evidence for distortion. *Psychological Bulletin, 112,* 485–499.

Robbins, M. S., Alexander, J. F., & Turner, C. W. (2000). Disrupting defensive family interactions in family therapy with delinquent adolescents. *Journal of Family Psychology, 14,* 688–701.

Robbins, M. S., Szapocznik, J., Santisteban, D. A., Hervis, O. E., Mitrani, V. B., & Schwartz, S. J. (2003). Brief strategic family therapy for Hispanic youth. In A. E. Kazdin & J. R. Weisz (Eds.), *Evidence-based psychotherapies for children and adolescents* (pp. 407–424). New York: Guilford Press.

Robbins, M. S., Turner, C. W., Alexander, J. F., & Perez, G. A. (2003). Alliance and dropout in family therapy for adolescents with behavior problems: Individual and systemic effects. *Journal of Family Psychology, 17,* 534–544.

Roberts, M. W., Joe, V. C., & Rowe-Hallbert, A. (1992). Oppositional child behavior and parental locus of control. *Journal of Clinical Child Psychology, 21,* 170–177.

Robin, A. L. (1981). A controlled evaluation of problem-solving communication training with parent–adolescent conflict. *Behavior Therapy, 12,* 593–609.

Robin, A. L., & Foster, S. L. (1989). *Negotiating parent–adolescent conflict: A behavioral–family systems approach.* New York: Guilford Press.

Robin, A. L., Kent, R., O'Leary, K. D., Foster, S. L., & Prinz, R. J. (1977). An approach to teaching parents and adolescents problem-solving communication skills: A preliminary report. *Behavior Therapy, 8,* 639–643.

Robins, L. N. (1991). Conduct disorder. *Journal of Child Psychology and Psychiatry, 32,* 193–209.

Rosen, H. S., & Rosen, L. A. (1983). Eliminating stealing: Use of stimulus control with an elementary student. *Behavior Modification, 7,* 56–63.

Russo, D. C., Cataldo, M. F., & Cushing, P. J. (1981). Compliance training and behavioral covariation in the treatment of multiple behavior problems. *Journal of Applied Behavior Analysis, 14,* 209–222.

Rutter, M. (1994). Family discord and conduct disorder: Cause, consequence, or correlate? *Journal of Family Psychology, 8,* 170–186.

Rutter, M., Giller, H., & Hagell, A. (1998). *Antisocial behavior by young people.* Cambridge, UK: Cambridge University Press.

Rutter, R., Harrington, R., Quinton, D., & Pickles, A. (1994). Adult outcome of conduct disorder in childhood: Implications for concepts and definitions of patterns of psychopathology. In R. D. Ketterlinus & M. E. Lamb (Eds.), *Adolescent problem behaviors: Issues and research* (pp. 57–80). Hillsdale, NJ: Erlbaum.

Rutter, M., & Smith, D. J. (1995). *Psychosocial disorders in young people: Time, trends, and their causes.* Chichester, UK: Wiley.

Sanders, M. R., & Dadds, M. R. (1992). Children's and parents' cognitions about family interaction: An evaluation of video-mediated recall and thought listing procedures in the assessment of conduct-disordered children. *Journal of Clinical Child Psychology, 21,* 371–379.

Sanders, M. R., Turner, K. M. T., & Markie-Dadds, C. (2002). The development and dissemination of the Triple P-Positive Parenting Program: A multilevel, evidence-based system of parenting and family support. *Prevention Science, 3,* 173–189.

Sanson, A., Oberklaid, F., Pedlow, R., & Prior, M. (1991). Risk indicators: Assessment of infancy predictors of pre-school behavioural maladjustment. *Journal of Child Psychology and Psychiatry, 32,* 609–626.

Santisteban, D. A., Coatsworth, J. D., Perez-Vidal, A., Kurtines, W. M., Schwartz, S. J., LaPerriere, A., & Szapocznik, J. (2003). Efficacy of brief strategic family therapy in modifying Hispanic adolescent behavior problems and substance use. *Journal of Family Psychology, 17,* 121–133.

Santisteban, D. A., Szapocznik, J., Perez-Vidal, A., Kurtines, W. M., Murray, E. J., & LaPerriere, A. (1996). Efficacy of intervention for engaging youth and families into treatment and some variables that may contribute to differential effectiveness. *Journal of Family Psychology, 10,* 35–44.

Saunders, E. B., & Awad, G. A. (1991). Adolescent female firesetters. *Canadian Journal of Psychiatry, 36,* 401–404.

Schoenwald, S. K., Brown, T. L., & Henggeler, S. W. (2000). Inside multisystemic therapy: Therapist, supervisory, and program practices. *Journal of Emotional and Behavioral Disorders, 8,* 113–127.

Schoenwald, S. K., Henggeler, S. W., Pickrel, S. G., & Cunningham, P. B. (1996). Treating seriously troubled youths and families in their contexts: Multisystemic therapy. In M. C. Roberts (Ed.), *Model programs in child and family mental health* (pp. 317–332). Mahwah, NJ: Erlbaum.

Schoenwald, S. K., Ward, D. M., Henggeler, S. W., Pickrel, S. G., & Patel, H. (1996). MST treatment of substance abusing or dependent adolescent offenders: Costs of reducing incarceration, inpatient, and residential placement. *Journal of Child and Family Studies, 5,* 431–444.

Schweinhart, L. J., Barnes, H. V., & Weikart, D. P. (Eds.). (1993). *Significant benefits: The High/Scope Perry Preschool Study through age 27.* Ypsilanti, MI: High/Scope Press.

Scotti, J. R., Morris, T. L., McNeil, C. B., & Hawkins, R. P. (1996). DSM-IV and disorders of childhood and adolescence: Can structural criteria be functional? *Journal of Consulting and Clinical Psychology, 64*, 1177–1191.

Serbin, L. A., Moskowitz, K. S., Schwartzman, A. E., & Ledingham, J. E. (1991). Aggressive, withdrawn, and aggressive/withdrawn children in adolescence: Into the next generation. In D. J. Pepler & K. H. Rubin (Eds.), *The development and treatment of childhood aggression* (pp. 55–70). Hillsdale, NJ: Erlbaum.

Sexton, T. L., & Alexander, J. F. (2002). Functional Family Therapy for at-risk adolescents and their families. In T. Patterson (Ed.), *Comprehensive handbook of psychotherapy: Vol. 2. Cognitive-behavioral approaches* (pp. 117–140). New York: Wiley.

Sexton, T. L., & Alexander, J. F. (2003). Functional Family Therapy: A mature clinical model for working with at-risk adolescents and their families. In T. L. Sexton, G. R. Weeks, & M. S. Robbins (Eds.), *Handbook of family therapy: The science and practice of working with families and couples* (pp. 323–348). New York: Brunner-Routledge.

Seymour, F. W., & Epston, D. (1989). An approach to childhood stealing with evaluation of 45 cases. *Australian and New Zealand Journal of Family Therapy, 10*, 137–143.

Shaffer, D., Fisher, P., Lucas, C. P., Dulcan, M. K., & Schwab-Stone, M. E. (2000). NIMH Diagonstic Interview Schedule for Children—Version IV (NIMH DISC-IV): Description, differences from previous versions, and reliability of some common diagnoses. *Journal of the American Academy of Child and Adolescent Psychiatry, 39*, 28–38.

Shaw, D. S., Bell, R. Q., & Gilliom, M. (2000). A truly early starter model of antisocial behavior revisited. *Clinical Child and Family Psychology Review, 3*, 155–172.

Sheras, P. L., Abidin, R. R., & Konold, T. R. (1998). *Stress Index for Parents of Adolescents: Professional manual*. Odessa, FL: Psychological Assessment Resources.

Shure, M. B., & Spivack, G. (1980). Interpersonal problem solving as a mediator of behavioral adjustment in preschool and kindergarten children. *Journal of Applied Developmental Psychology, 1*, 29–44.

Silverthorn, P., & Frick, P. J. (1999). Developmental pathways to antisocial behavior: The delayed-onset pathway in girls. *Development and Psychopathology, 11*, 101–126.

Skinner, H. A. (1982). The Drug Abuse Screening Test. *Addictive Behaviors, 7*, 363–371.

Slep, A. M., & O'Leary, S. G. (1998). The effects of maternal attributions on parenting: An experimental analysis. *Journal of Family Psychology, 12*, 234–243.

Slot, N. W., Jagers, H. D., & Dangel, R. F. (1992). Cross-cultural replication and evaluation of the Teaching Family Model of community-based residential treatment. *Behavioral Residential Treatment, 7*, 341–354.

Smith, P. K., Cowie, H., Olafsson, R. F., & Liefooghe, P. D. (2002). Definitions of bullying: A comparison of terms used, and age and gender differences, in a fourteen-country international comparison. *Child Development, 73*, 1119–1133.

Smith, P. K., Morita, Y., Junger-Tas, J., Olweus, D., Catalano, R., & Slee, P. (Eds.). (1999). *The nature of school bullying: A cross-national perspective*. New York: Routledge.

Smith, P. K., & Sharp, S. (Eds.). (1994a). *School bullying: Insights and perspectives*. London: Routledge.

Smith, P. K., & Sharp, S. (Eds.). (1994b). *Tackling bullying in your school: A practical handbook for teachers*. London: Routledge.

Smithmyer, C. M., Hubbard, J. A., & Simons, R. F. (2000). Proactive and reactive aggression in delinquent adolescents: Relations to aggression outcome expectancies. *Journal of Clinical Child Psychology, 29*, 86–93.

Snyder, H. N. (1999). *Juvenile arson, 1997*. Fact Sheet #91. Washington, DC: U. S. Department of Justice, Office of Justice Programs, Office of Juvenile Justice and Delinquency Prevention.

Snyder, J. (1991). Discipline as a mediator of the impact of maternal stress and mood on child conduct problems. *Development and Psychopathology, 3*, 263–276.

Snyder, J., Reid, J., & Patterson, G. (2003). A social learning model of child and adolescent antisocial behavior. In B. B. Lahey, T. E. Moffitt, & A. Caspi (Eds.), *Causes of conduct disorder and juvenile delinquency* (pp. 27–48). New York: Guilford Press.

Snyder, J., & Stoolmiller, M. (2002). Reinforcement and coercion mechanisms in the development of antisocial behavior: The family. In J. B. Reid, G. R. Patterson, & J. Snyder (Eds.), *Antisocial behavior in children and adolescents: A developmental analysis and model for intervention* (pp. 65–100). Washington, DC: American Psychological Association.

Spanier, G. B. (1976). Measuring dyadic adjustment: New scales for assessing the quality of marriage and similar dyads. *Journal of Marriage and the Family, 38*, 15–28.

Spence, S. H., & Marzillier, J. S. (1981). Social skills training with adolescent male offenders: II. Short-term, long-term, and generalized effects. *Behaviour Research and Therapy, 19*, 349–368.

Stack, D. M., Serbin, L. A., Schwartzman, A. E., & Ledingham, J. (2005). Girls' aggression across the life course: Long-term outcomes and intergenerational risk. In D. J. Pepler, K. C. Madsen, C. Webster, & K. S. Levene (Eds.), *The development and treatment of girlhood aggression* (pp. 253–283). Mahwah, NJ: Erlbaum.

Stadolnik, R. F. (2000). *Drawn to the flame: Assessment and treatment of juvenile firesetting behavior*. Sarasota, FL: Professional Resource Press.

Stanger, C., Achenbach, T. M., & Verhulst, F. C. (1997). Accelerated longitudinal comparisons of aggressive versus delinquent syndromes. *Development and Psychopathology, 9*, 43–58.

Stevens, V., De Bourdeaudhuij, I., & Van Oost, P.

(2000). Bullying in Flemish schools: An evaluation of anti-bullying intervention in primary and secondary schools. *British Journal of Educational Psychology, 70,* 195–210.

Stickle, T. R., & Blechman, E. A. (2002). Aggression and fire: Antisocial behavior in firesetting and nonfiresetting juvenile offenders. *Journal of Psychopathology and Behavioral Assessment, 24,* 177–193.

Stickle, T. R., & Frick, P. J. (2002). Developmental pathways to severe antisocial behavior: Interventions for youth with callous–unemotional traits. *Expert Review of Neurotherapeutics, 2,* 511–522.

Stouthamer-Loeber, M. (1986). Lying as a problem behavior in children: A review. *Clinical Psychology Review, 6,* 267–289.

Stouthamer-Loeber, M., & Loeber, R. (1986). Boys who lie. *Journal of Abnormal Child Psychology, 14,* 551–564.

Straus, M. A. (1979). Measuring intrafamily conflict and violence: The Conflict Tactics (CT) Scales. *Journal of Marriage and the Family, 41,* 75–88.

Straus, M. A. (1990). The Conflict Tactics Scales and its critics: An evaluation and new data on validity and reliability. In M. A. Straus & R. J. Gelles (Eds.), *Physical violence in American families: Risk factors and adaptations to violence in 8,145 families* (pp. 49–73). New Brunswick, NJ: Transaction.

Sukhodolsky, D. G., Kassinove, H., & Gorman, B. S. (2004). Cognitive-behavioral therapy for anger in children and adolescents: A meta-analysis. *Aggression and Violent Behavior, 9,* 247–269.

Switzer, E. B., Deal, T. E., & Bailey, J. S. (1977). The reduction of stealing in second graders using a group contingency. *Journal of Applied Behavior Analysis, 10,* 267–272.

Szapocznik, J., Perez-Vidal, A., Brickman, A., Foote, F. H., Santisteban, D. A., Hervis, O. E., & Kurtines, W. M.. (1988). Engaging adolescent drug abusers and their families in treatment: A strategic structural systems approach. *Journal of Consulting and Clinical Psychology, 56,* 552–557.

Szapocznik, J., Rio, A., Murray, E., Cohen, R., Scopetta, M., Rivas-Vasquez, A., et al. (1989). Structural family versus psychodynamic child therapy for problematic Hispanic boys. *Journal of Consulting and Clinical Psychology, 57*(5), 571–578.

Szapocznik, J., & Williams, R. A. (2000). Brief Strategic Family Therapy: Twenty-five years of interplay among theory, research and practice in adolescent behavior problems and drug abuse. *Clinical Child and Family Psychology Review, 3,* 117–134.

Taylor, E. R., Kelly, J., Valescu, S., Reynolds, G. S., Sherman, J., & German, V. (2001). Is stealing a gateway crime? *Community Mental Health Journal, 37,* 347–358.

Taylor, T. K., Eddy, J. M., & Biglan, A. (1999). Interpersonal skills training to reduce aggressive and delinquent behavior: Limited evidence and the need for an evidence-based system of care. *Clinical Child and Family Psychology Review, 2,* 169–182.

Thomas, A., Chess, S., & Birch, H. G. (1968). *Temperament and behavior disorders in children.* New York: University Press.

Thornberry, T. P., & Krohn, M. D. (Eds.). (2003). *Taking stock of delinquency: An overview of findings from contemporary longitudinal studies.* New York: Kluwer/Plenum Press.

Tiet, Q. Q., Wasserman, G. A., Loeber, R., Larken, S. M., & Miller, L. S. (2001). Developmental and sex differences in types of conduct problems. *Journal of Child and Family Studies, 10,* 181–197.

Tolan, P. H., Gorman-Smith, D., & Loeber, R. (2000). Developmental timing of onsets of disruptive behaviors and later delinquency of inner-city youth. *Journal of Child and Family Studies, 9,* 203–220.

Tremblay, R. E. (2003). Why socialization fails: The case of chronic physical aggression. In B. B. Lahey, T. E. Moffitt, & A. Caspi (Eds.), *Causes of conduct disorder and delinquency* (pp. 182–224). New York: Guilford Press.

Tremblay, R. E., Masse, L. C., Pagani, L., & Vitaro, F. (1996). From childhood physical aggression to adolescent maladjustment. In R. DeV. Peters & R. J. McMahon (Eds.), *Preventing childhood disorders, substance abuse, and delinquency* (pp. 268–299). Thousand Oaks, CA: Sage.

Tremblay, R. E., Pagani-Kurtz, L., Masse, L. C., Vitaro, F., & Pihl, R. O. (1995). A bimodal preventive intervention for disruptive kindergarten boys: Its impact through mid-adolescence. *Journal of Consulting and Clinical Psychology, 63,* 560–568.

Tremblay, R. E., Vitaro, F., Bertrand, L., LeBlanc, M., Beauchesne, H., Boileau, H., et al. (1992). Parent and child training to prevent early onset of delinquency: The Montreal Longitudinal–Experimental Study. In J. McCord & R. E. Tremblay (Eds.), *Preventing antisocial behavior: Interventions from birth through adolescence* (pp. 117–138). New York: Guilford Press.

Tremblay, R. E., Vitaro, F., Nagin, D., Pagani, L., & Seguin, J. R. (2003). The Montreal Longitudinal and Experimental Study: Rediscovering the power of descriptions. In T. P. Thornberry & M. D. Krohn (Eds.), *Taking stock of delinquency: An overview of findings from contemporary longitudinal studies* (pp. 205–254). New York: Kluwer/Plenum Press.

Underwood, M. K. (2003). *Social aggression among girls.* New York: Guilford Press.

Underwood, M. K., & Coie, J. D. (2004). Future directions and priorities for prevention and intervention. In M. Putallaz & K. L. Bierman (Eds.), *Aggression, antisocial behavior, and violence among girls: A developmental perspective* (pp. 289–301). New York: Guilford Press.

Van Kammen, W. B., Loeber, R., & Stouthamer-Loeber, M. (1991). Substance use and its relationship to conduct problems and delinquency in young boys. *Journal of Youth and Adolescence, 20,* 399–413.

Venning, H. B., Blampied, N. M., & France, K. G. (2003). Effectiveness of a standard parenting-skills program in reducing stealing and lying in two boys. *Child & Family Behavior Therapy, 25*(2), 31–44.

Verhulst, F. C., van der Ende, J., Ferdinand, R. F., & Kasius, M. C. (1997). The prevalence of DSM-III-R diagnoses in a national sample of Dutch adolescents. *Archives of General Psychiatry, 54,* 329–336.

Vitaro, F., Brendgen, M., Pagani, L., Tremblay, R. E., & McDuff, P. (1999). Disruptive behavior, peer association, and conduct disorder: Testing the developmental links through early intervention. *Development and Psychopathology, 11,* 287–304.

Vitaro, P., Brendgen, M., & Tremblay, R. E. (1999). Prevention of school dropout through the reduction of disruptive behaviors and school failure in elementary school. *Journal of School Psychology, 37,* 205–226.

Vitaro, F., Brendgen, M., & Tremblay, R. E. (2002). Reactively and proactively aggressive children: Antecedent and subsequent characteristics. *Journal of Child Psychology and Psychiatry, 43,* 495–505

Vitaro, F., Gendreau, P. L., Tremblay, R. E., & Oligny, P. (1998). Reactive and proactive aggression differentially predict later conduct problems. *Journal of Child Psychology and Psychiatry and Allied Disciplines, 39,* 377–385.

Wahler, R. G. (1980). The insular mother: Her problems in parent–child treatment. *Journal of Applied Behavior Analysis, 13,* 207–219.

Wahler, R. G., & Dumas, J. E. (1984). Changing the observational coding styles of insular and noninsular mothers: A step toward maintenance of parent training effects. In R. F. Dangel & R. A. Polster (Eds.), *Parent training: Foundations of research and practice* (pp. 379–416). New York: Guilford Press.

Wahler, R. G., & Dumas, J. E. (1989). Attentional problems in dysfunctional mother–child interactions: An interbehavioral model. *Psychological Bulletin, 105,* 116–130.

Wahler, R. G., Leske, G., & Rogers, E. S. (1979). The insular family: A deviance support system for oppositional children. In L. A. Hamerlynck (Ed.), *Behavioral systems for the developmentally disabled: Vol. 1. School and family environments* (pp. 102–127). New York: Brunner/Mazel.

Wahler, R. G., & Sansbury, L. E. (1990). The monitoring skills of troubled mothers: Their problems in defining child deviance. *Journal of Abnormal Child Psychology, 18,* 577–589.

Wakschlag, L. S., & Keenan, K. (2001). Clinical significance and correlates of disruptive behavior in environmentally at-risk preschoolers. *Journal of Clinical Child Psychology, 30,* 262–275.

Waldman, I. D., & Lahey, B. B. (1994). Design of the DSM-IV disruptive behavior disorder field trials. *Child and Adolescent Psychiatric Clinics of North America, 3,* 195–208.

Walker, H. M. (1995). *The acting-out child: Coping with classroom disruption* (2nd ed.). Longmont, CO: Sopris West.

Walker, H. M., Block-Pedego, A., Todis, B., & Severson, H. (1991). *School archival records search (SARS):* *User's guide and technical manual.* Longmont, CO: Sopris West.

Walker, H. M., Ramsey, E., & Gresham, F. M. (2004). *Antisocial behavior in school: Evidence-based practices* (2nd ed.). Belmont, CA: Thomson/Wadsworth Learning.

Walker, H. M., & Walker, J. E. (1991). *Coping with noncompliance in the classroom: A positive approach for teachers.* Austin, TX: Pro-Ed.

Walker, J. L., Lahey, B. B., Russo, M. F., Frick, P. J., Christ, M. A., McBurnett, K., et al. (1991). Anxiety, inhibition, and conduct disorder in children: I. Relations to social impairment. *Journal of the American Academy of Child and Adolescent Psychiatry, 30,* 187–191.

Waschbusch, D. A. (2002). A meta-analytic examination of comorbid hyperactive–impulsive–attention problems and conduct problems. *Psychological Bulletin, 128,* 118–50.

Waschbusch, D. A., Willoughby, M. T., & Pelham, W. E. (1998). Criterion validity and the utility of reactive and proactive aggression: Comparisons to attention deficit hyperactivity disorder, oppositional defiant disorder, conduct disorder, and other measures of functioning. *Journal of Clinical Child Psychology, 27,* 396–405.

Waslick, B., Werry, J. S., & Greenhill, L. L. (1998). Pharmacology and toxicology of oppositional defiant disorder and conduct disorder. In H. C. Quay & A. E. Hogan (Eds.), *Handbook of disruptive behavior disorders* (pp. 455–474). New York: Kluwer/Plenum Press.

Webster-Stratton, C. (1990). Stress: A potential disruptor of parent perceptions and family interactions. *Journal of Clinical Child Psychology, 19,* 302–312.

Webster-Stratton, C. H. (1996). Early intervention with videotape modeling: Programs for families of children with oppositional defiant disorder or conduct disorder. In E. S. Hibbs & P. S. Jensen (Eds.), *Psychosocial treatments for child and adolescent disorders: Empirically-based strategies for clinical practice* (pp. 435–474). Washington, DC: American Psychological Association.

Webster-Stratton, C., & Taylor, T. (2001). Nipping early risk factors in the bud: Preventing substance abuse, delinquency, and violences in adolescence through interventions targeted at young children (0–8 years). *Prevention Science, 2,* 165–192.

Weinrott, M. R., Jones, R. R., & Howard, J. R. (1982). Cost-effectiveness of teaching family programs for delinquents: Results of a national evaluation. *Evaluation Review, 6,* 173–201.

Weiss, B., Dodge, K. A., Bates, J. E., & Pettit, G. S. (1992). Some consequences of early harsh discipline: Child aggression and a maladaptive social information processing style. *Child Development, 63,* 1321–1335.

Wells, K. C., Forehand, R., & Griest, D. L. (1980). Generality of treatment effects from treated to untreated behaviors resulting from a parent training program. *Journal of Clinical Child Psychology, 9,* 217–219.

Werry, J. S., & Aman, M. G. (1993). *Practitioner's guide to psychoactive drugs for children and adolescents.* New York: Plenum Press.

Whipple, E. E., Fitzgerald, H. E., & Zucker, R. A. (1995). Parent–child interactions in alcoholic and nonalcoholic families. *American Journal of Orthopsychiatry, 65,* 153–159.

White, J. L., Moffitt, T. E., Caspi, A., Bartusch, D. J., Needles, D., & Stouthamer-Loeber, M. (1994). Measuring impulsivity and examining its relationship to delinquency. *Journal of Abnormal Psychology, 103,* 1922–1205.

White, M. (1986). Negative explanation, restraint and double description: A template for family therapy. *Family Process, 25,* 169–184.

Wiesner, M. (2003). A longitudinal latent variable analysis of reciprocal relations between depressive symptoms and delinquency during adolescence. *Journal of Abnormal Psychology, 112,* 633–645.

Wilcox, D. K., & Kolko, D. J. (2002). Assessing recent firesetting behavior and taking a firesetting history. In D. J. Kolko (Ed), *Handbook on firesetting in children and youth* (pp. 161–175). San Diego, CA: Academic Press.

Willoughby, M., Kupersmidt, J., & Bryant, D. (2001). Overt and covert dimensions of antisocial behavior in early childhood. *Journal of Abnormal Child Psychology, 29,* 177–187.

Wills, T. A., Schreibman, D., Benson, G., & Vaccaro, D. (1994). Impact of parental substance use on adolescents: A test of a mediational model. *Journal of Pediatric Psychology, 19,* 537–555.

Wilson, S. J., Lipsey, M. W., & Soydan, H. (2003). Are mainstream programs for juvenile delinquency less effective with minority youth than majority youth? A meta-analysis of outcomes research. *Research on Social Work Practice, 13,* 3–26.

Wong, S., & Hare, R. D. (2005). *Guidelines for Psychopathy Treatment Program.* Toronto, ON, Canada: Multi-Health Systems.

Woodward, L. J., Fergusson, D. M., & Horwood, L. J. (2002). Romantic relationships of young people with early and late onset antisocial behavior problems. *Journal of Abnormal Child Psychology, 30,* 231–243.

Wootton, J. M., Frick, P. J., Shelton, K. K., & Silverthorn, P. (1997). Ineffective parenting and childhood conduct problems: The moderating role of callous–unemotional traits. *Journal of Consulting and Clinical Psychology, 65,* 301–308.

Yoshikawa, H. (1994). Prevention as a cumulative protection: Effects of early family support and education on chronic delinquency and its risks. *Psychological Bulletin, 115,* 28–54.

Zigler, E., Taussig, C., & Black, K. (1992). Early childhood intervention: A promising preventative for juvenile delinquency. *American Psychologist, 47,* 997–1006.

Zoccolillo, M. (1992). Co-occurrence of conduct disorder and its adult outcomes with depressive and anxiety disorders: A review. *Journal of the American Academy of Child and Adolescent Psychiatry, 31,* 547–556.

Zoccolillo, M., Paquette, D., & Tremblay, R. (2005). Maternal conduct disorder and the risk for the next generation. In D. J. Pepler, K. C. Madsen, C. Webster, & K. S. Levene (Eds.), *The development and treatment of girlhood aggression* (pp. 225–252). Mahwah, NJ: Erlbaum.

Zucker, R. A., & Fitzgerald, H. E. (1992). *The Antisocial Behavior Checklist.* East Lansing: Michigan State University Family Study, Department of Psychology.

6

Substance Use Disorders

Sandra A. Brown
Ana M. Abrantes

Substance use disorders (SUDs) among adolescents are an important public health concern. Twenty-six percent of high school seniors report having used a substance in the last month, with alcohol and tobacco being the most commonly reported substance (Johnston, O'Malley, & Bachman, 2002). Significant impairments are associated with SUDs among adolescents, such as poor academic functioning (e.g., Chatlos, 1997), family dysfunction (e.g., Dakof, 2000), health problems (Brown & Tapert, 2004), and psychiatric comorbidity (e.g., Abrantes, Brown, Tomlinson, in press). In addition, SUDs during adolescence predict adversity in adulthood such as unstable work patterns, higher divorce rates, delinquent behaviors, and physical and psychological disturbances (e.g., Aarons et al., 1999; Kandel, Davies, Karus, & Yamaguchi, 1986; Newcomb & Bentler, 1988).

Although SUDs have been less extensively studied in adolescents than adults, the last two decades of research with substance-abusing adolescents has resulted in significant advances in the field. Historically, SUDs among adolescents have been considered and treated as if similar to SUDs in adults. However, important developmental distinctions exist for SUDs in adolescence compared to SUDs in adulthood. The course of SUDs, characteristics of substance involvement, context of relapse, and temporal patterns of use differ between adults and adolescents (Deas, Riggs, Langenbucher, Goldman, & Brown, 2000). Perhaps because of the restricted availability and illegal nature of substances for adolescents, youth drink less often but in larger amounts than adults. In addition, adolescents consume substances in different social and developmental contexts (Bukstein, 1995). Adolescents' use is highly influenced by peer use, desire for autonomy and experimentation with alternative attitudes and lifestyles, level of supervision from parents, and other psychosocial factors (Bukstein, 1995). These important differences need to be taken into account when assessing the disorder among youth and developing prevention and treatment programs.

This chapter addresses the nature of SUDs among adolescents by examining etiological pathways, risk and protective factors, assessment approaches, and treatment and prevention efforts.

DESCRIPTION OF THE DISORDER AMONG ADOLESCENTS

SUDs in adolescence involve the self-administration of any substance that alters mood, perception, or brain functioning (Brown, Aarons,

& Abrantes, 2001). In general, substances are used in order to produce a change in affective state or consciousness. Whereas almost all abused substances can lead to psychological dependence, some also extend to physical dependence. Psychological dependence refers to the subjective feeling of needing the substance to adequately function. Physical dependence occurs when the body adapts to the substance's presence. For example, tolerance refers to requiring more of the substance in order to experience an effect once obtained at a lower dose. Another aspect of physical dependence involves the experience of adverse physiological symptoms, referred to as withdrawal, when consumption of an abused substance is abruptly ended and thus removed from the body.

Indicators of substance use among adolescents often involve physical, socioemotional, and health changes. Physical changes include deterioration in appearance such as rapid weight loss, unusual breath and body odors, and unexplained cuts and bruises. In addition, bloodshot eyes, very large or small pupils, and watery or blank stares are physical indicators of substance use. Examples of socioemotional changes include increased energy or lethargy, insomnia or excessive sleep, clinically significant levels of depression or anxiety, deviant behaviors not evident in childhood, decreases in school grades, and changes in social activities or peer groups. Health changes may include chronic coughing or sniffing, skin boils or sores, nasal bleeding, and evidence of intravenous drug use (needle tracks) or inhalation (perforated nasal septum).

Following is a brief description of the most commonly abused drugs and their effects on adolescents. Physiological and behavioral effects of substances vary according to length of use, dose, environment, and health of user. Also, adolescent substance abusers typically use multiple substances, which complicates the clinical picture.

Substances of Abuse

Alcohol

The most commonly used and abused substance by adolescents is alcohol, a central nervous system (CNS) depressant (Johnston et al., 2002). The short-term psychological effects of alcohol can include euphoria, increased sense of well-being, decreased anxiety, decreased inhibition, and increased self-confidence. However, there are also negative psychological effects, usually experienced at higher doses and during decreasing blood alcohol levels that include confusion, memory loss, irritability and dysphoria, poor judgment, and even violent behavior. With increasing doses of alcohol, physical effects include impaired coordination, slowed reaction time, slurred speech, nausea, and vomiting. Much more serious effects of alcohol use include depression, anxiety, respiratory failure, coma, and death. Furthermore, alcohol-abusing adolescents, when compared to nonabusing adolescents, self-report more symptoms of health problems (e.g., sleep, heart and lung, metabolism and bleeding, neurological, and urinary) and have increased serum liver enzyme levels as well as dental abnormalities in oral examinations (Clark, Lynch, Donovan, & Block, 2001). Common withdrawal symptoms among adolescent heavy drinkers include nausea, vomiting, depression, irritability, and muscle aches (Stewart & Brown, 1995).

Nicotine

Cigarette use is second only to alcohol use among adolescents. The rates of current smoking are very high among youth in substance abuse treatment (84%; Myers & Brown, 1994) and inpatient mental health programs (60%; Brown, Ramsey, Strong, & Sales, 2000). Nicotine is the active drug in cigarettes and common acute effects of smoking include increased mental alertness and concentration. Tolerance and withdrawal symptoms are common among adolescents dependent on nicotine. Withdrawal symptoms include protracted craving, irritability, frustration, anxiety, depression, poor concentration, restlessness, and decreased heart rate. There is some evidence that health-related consequences of smoking can begin as early as adolescence. For example, smoking has been associated with respiratory problems among substance-abusing adolescents over a 2-year period (Myers & Brown, 1994).

Marijuana

Among adolescents, marijuana is the most commonly used illicit substance. The psychoactive element in marijuana, delta-9-tetrahydrocannabinol (THC), has often been considered of low addictive potential and relatively harmless. With increasing potency of marijuana plants over the last 25 years, the addictive potential of THC has been well documented (Substance Abuse and Mental Health Services Administration [SAMHSA], 1999b). A substantial amount of research has identified potential dangers of both acute and chronic use of marijuana (Brown, Mott, & Stewart, 1992; Tapert & Brown, 1999). The desired effects of intoxication may include euphoria, relaxation, enhanced sensory perception, and sensation of slowed time. The negative effects of intoxication are anxiety, decreased concentration, short-term memory impairment, confusion, panic reactions, paranoia, and hallucinations. The physical effects of marijuana use consist of increased appetite, decreased muscle strength, bloodshot eyes, dry mouth, and autonomic dysfunction (e.g., increased heart rate and respiratory rate). There are significant health risks associated with chronic use of marijuana such as lung damage, decreased sperm production, decreased size of prostate and testes in males, blocked ovulation in females, weight gain, and amotivational syndrome (Cohen, 1981; McGlothin & West, 1968). In addition, among adolescents, protracted use of marijuana has been found to be predictive of deterioration of neurocognitive functioning, especially attention (Tapert & Brown, 1999).

Stimulants

The most commonly abused stimulants by adolescents include amphetamines (e.g., methamphetamine, Benzedrine, Dexedrine), cocaine, crack, and MDMA (i.e., Ecstasy). Although MDMA is most often classified a stimulant, it also possesses hallucinogenic properties. The route of ingestion for stimulants varies across drugs. For example, cocaine is obtained in a powder form and inhaled through the nose. Crack, a crystallized form of cocaine, is typically smoked and results in a more rapid and intense effect than cocaine. Amphetamines can be taken orally, intravenously, or through inhalation. MDMA is typically taken orally in the form of a pill. Despite the varied forms of ingestion, stimulants have similar psychological and physiological effects. The desired effect of these substances include exhilaration, euphoria, increased energy, self-confidence, and sense of well-being. Chronic use and use at higher doses can result in irritability, aggression, anxiety, depression, confusion, panic, paranoia, de-

lusions of persecution, and hallucinations. At very high doses of stimulants, cardiac arrest and seizures are possible. Withdrawal from stimulants includes depression, fatigue, prolonged sleep, irritability, and potentially violent or aggressive behavior.

Inhalants

These substances are primarily abused among children and younger adolescents and in economically disadvantaged areas, possibly due to high availability and low cost. Inhalants include substances in industrial and household compounds such as glue, typewriter correction fluid, aerosol spray cans, paint, paint thinner, nail polish remover, gasoline, and nitrous oxide ("laughing gas"). These substances are often sniffed from a soaked rag and produce effects lasting from a few minutes to an hour. Psychological effects of inhalant use include euphoria, floating sensation, disorientation, confusion, irritability and anxiety. Physical effects may include dizziness, headache, slurred speech, lethargy, nausea, and vomiting. Inhalant abuse has been found to be associated with serious physiological problems, including respiratory damage, kidney, liver, heart, gastrointestinal, and nervous system damage (Morton, 1990). In addition, significant neurological and cognitive deficits have been identified for inhalant abusers such as abnormal tandem gait, finger-to-nose movements, postural tremor, cortical atrophy, ventricular dilation, and poor performance on neuropsychological tests measuring concentration, attention, memory, and coordination (Fornazzari, 1990; Maruff, Burns, Tyler, Currie, & Currie, 1998).

Hallucinogens

These substances, usually taken orally, produce dramatic changes in perception and sensory awareness. Commonly abused hallucinogens include lysergic acid diethylamide (LSD), mescaline, psilocybin, dimethyltryptamine (DMT), 2,5-dimethodxy-4-methylamphetamine (STP), and methylene dioxyamphetamine (MDA). The effects of hallucinogen use include hallucinations, detachment, and euphoria, as well as fluctuations in emotion, anxiety, paranoia, panic, confusion, and sadness. Physical effects may include tachycardia, dilated pupils, tremors, and nausea. These substances also produce adverse neurocognitive consequences. A significant risk associated with hallucinogen abuse involves acting on hallucinations or delusional belief such as the ability to fly.

Opiates

The most commonly abused opiates, derivatives of the opium poppy, include heroin, morphine, opium, codeine, Percodan, and compounds synthesized to have opiate-like properties such as Darvon, and Demerol. Each of these substances acts as an analgesic and depresses most bodily functions (e.g., respiration and gag reflex). Opiates can be self-administered in a variety of means including orally, snorted, smoked, and injected. Opiates produce intense euphoria, relaxation, drowsiness, apathy, slurred speech, constricted pupils, and constipation. A tolerance for opiates develops very quickly and overdose can result in respiratory arrest and even death. In addition, the use of unclean needles when injecting may result in several medical complications such as HIV (human immunodeficiency virus), hepatitis B, and skin or muscle infections. Opiate withdrawal is associated with very painful muscle spasms, flu-like symptoms, tremors, weakness, nausea, vomiting, and diarrhea.

Sedatives

Because these substances are CNS depressants as well, their psychological and physical effects are very similar to alcohol. Most commonly abused sedatives include barbiturates (e.g., Amytal, Nembutal, Seconal, and Phenobarbital), benzodiazepines (e.g., Ativan, Halcion, Librium, Valium, Xanax, and Rohypnol) and methaqualone (e.g., Quaalude, Sopor, and Parest). These substances are usually taken orally but may also be injected or snorted, and they carry risks associated with these forms of administration. Sedative substances demonstrate cross-tolerance and high potential for overdose and are especially dangerous in combination with other CNS depressants such as alcohol.

DIAGNOSTIC CRITERIA AND NEEDS

The most prevalent diagnostic criteria for alcohol and other substance use disorders is based on the fourth edition, text revision of the *Diagnostic and Statistical Manual of Mental Disor-*

ders (DSM-IV-TR; American Psychiatric Association [APA], 2000; see Tables 6.1 and 6.2). The two types of SUDs (abuse and dependence) are characterized by a maladaptive pattern of use and symptoms that result in clinical impairment or distress. A diagnosis of substance abuse is not assigned if criteria for substance dependence is met. Substance dependence is also characterized as with or without physiological dependence (i.e., with or without evidence of tolerance or withdrawal).

Because DSM-IV criteria were developed with adults, concern has been raised regarding their appropriateness for diagnoses of SUDs among adolescents. While there are benefits to using DSM-IV criteria to diagnose SUDs, such as improving reliable communication between clinicians and researchers (Connors & Volk, 1995), there are also significant limitations. These criteria do not take into consideration important developmental differences between adults and adolescents (Brown, Aarons, & Abrantes, 2001). As previously mentioned,

---

TABLE 6.1. DSM-IV-TR Criteria for Substance Abuse

A. A maladaptive pattern of substance use leading to clinically significant impairment or distress, as manifested by one (or more) of the following, occurring within a 12-month period:

   (1) recurrent substance use resulting in a failure to fulfill major role obligations at work, school, or home (e.g., repeated absences or poor work performance related to substance use; substance-related absences, suspensions, or expulsions from school; neglect of children or household)

   (2) recurrent substance use in situations in which it is physically hazardous (e.g., driving an automobile or operating a machine when impaired by substance use)

   (3) recurrent substance-related legal problems (e.g., arrests for substance-related disorderly conduct)

   (4) continued substance use despite having persistent or recurrent social or interpersonal problems caused or exacerbated by the effects of the substance (e.g., arguments with spouse about consequences of intoxication, physical fights)

B. The symptoms have never met the criteria for Substance Dependence for this class of substance.

Note. From American Psychiatric Association (2000). Copyright 2000 by the American Psychiatric Association. Reprinted by permission.

TABLE 6.2. DSM-IV-TR Criteria for Substance Dependence

A. A maladaptive pattern of substance use, leading to clinically significant impairment or distress, as manifested by three (or more) of the following, occurring at any time in the same 12-month period:

(1) tolerance, as defined by either of the following:

(a) a need for markedly increased amounts of the substance to achieve intoxication or desired effect

(b) markedly diminished effect with continued use of the same amount of the substance

(2) withdrawal, as manifested by either of the following:

(a) the characteristic withdrawal syndrome for the substance . . .

(b) the same (or a closely related) substance is taken to relieve or avoid withdrawal symptoms

(3) the substance is often taken in larger amounts or over a longer period then was intended

(4) there is a persistent desire or unsuccessful efforts to cut down or control substance use

(5) a great deal of time is spent in activities necessary to obtain the substance (e.g., visiting multiple doctors or driving long distances), use the substance (e.g., chain-smoking), or recover from its effects

(6) important social, occupational, or recreational activities are given up or reduced because of substance use

(7) the substance is continued despite knowledge of having a persistent or recurrent physical or psychological problem that is likely to have been caused or exacerbated by the substance (e.g, current cocaine use despite recognition of cocaine-induced depression, or continued drinking despite recognition that an ulcer was made worse by alcohol consumption)

Note. American Psychiatric Association (2000). Copyright 2000 by the American Psychiatric Association. Reprinted by permission.

substance use patterns and progression of substance involvement and related problems differ between adults and adolescents resulting in different associated characteristics. For example, while withdrawal symptoms are common among substance-abusing adolescents (Stewart & Brown, 1995), physiological dependence is less prevalent than among adults (Chassin, 1984; Kaminer, 1994). Among adolescents, cognitive and affective features are much more prevalent during withdrawal than physiological symptoms. Therefore, clinicians should not rely on physiological symptoms to determine dependence in adolescents.

Another diagnostic issue for youth is that DSM-IV criteria for abuse and dependence can result in no disorder diagnosis (i.e., "diagnostic orphans") even when youth exhibit multiple problems. Because there is no overlap between dependence and abuse symptoms, it is possible for an adolescent to have multiple substance-related problems (e.g., two dependence symptoms and no abuse symptoms) and not meet criteria for either abuse or dependence whereas other youth may exhibit one abuse symptom and meet criteria for substance abuse. In a study of adolescent regular drinkers, Pollack and Martin (1999) found that 31% had alcohol dependence symptoms but did not meet criteria for either abuse or dependence. Furthermore, when these adolescents were followed up 1 year later, they resembled abusers, in terms of outcome measures, rather than the nonabusers. In another example, Aarons, Brown, Hough, Garland, and Wood (2001) determined rates of DSM-IV substance use disorders among adolescents in substance abuse treatment programs and found that although all exhibited multiple problems, only 82.6% met DSM-IV criteria for an SUD. Therefore, DSM-IV abuse and dependence criteria may not be optimal to identify substance use problems in adolescents.

Alternative approaches to the DSM-IV diagnostic structure have been suggested as a means of categorizing substance use problems in adolescents. In the broader study of child psychopathology, there has been evidence to support the prognostic utility of viewing psychopathology from a continuous perspective (Angold, Costello, Farmer, Burns, & Erkanli, 1999; Lewinsohn, Solomon, Seeley, & Zeiss, 2000). Similarly, in the addiction arena, some researchers have suggested combining abuse and dependence symptoms to reflect a continuous measure of the disorder (Harrison, Fulkerson, & Beebe, 1998). Further work will be necessary to determine the validity of using DSM criteria for making diagnoses of adolescent substance abuse or dependence.

EPIDEMIOLOGY

Prevalence

Substance use during adolescence is highly prevalent. Monitoring the Future, a study funded by the National Institute on Drug Abuse, conducts nationwide surveys of high school students to assess use of alcohol and other drugs. Table 6.3 depicts drug use trends among high school seniors over a 10-year period, from 1991 to 2001 (Johnston et al., 2002). Of all substances, alcohol emerges as most prevalent, with 79.7% of high school seniors reporting lifetime use in 2001 and 50% of seniors having drunk alcohol in the last 30 days. Of particular concern, one-third of adolescents report a history of binge drinking (i.e., episodic heavy drinking of five or more drinks in a row). A study of high school students in San Diego County found that 51% of current (last month) drinkers were characterized as bingers (D'Amico et al., 2001)

According to Monitoring the Future (Johnston et al., 2002), the second most commonly used substance among adolescents is cigarettes with 61% of high school seniors reporting lifetime use of nicotine and one-third smoking cigarettes in the last month. While cigarette smoking in adults has decreased over the last decade, use among adolescents increased,

although modest reductions in prevalence has been observed recently.

The rates of illicit substance use are also very high, with 53.9% of high school seniors reporting the lifetime use of a drug other than alcohol or cigarettes. The most widely used illicit substance by adolescents is marijuana. In 2001, half of high school seniors reported lifetime use of marijuana and 22.4% smoked marijuana in the prior month. While rates of marijuana use among adolescents has not fluctuated over the last few years, marijuana use increased among adolescents during the 1990s. Of note, the greatest increase of any substance use among adolescents over the last several years has been that of MDMA (i.e., Ecstasy). While 6.9% of high school seniors reported use of Ecstasy in 1997, by 2001 that number had increased to 11.7%. Over the last decade, there has been a trend for increased use of "hard" drugs (e.g., opiates, cocaine, and crack), while hallucinogens and inhalants displayed marked decreases.

Although these prevalence rates are high, they may underestimate actual prevalence among youth. It is often the case that adolescents with problematic substance involvement are truant, suspended, or expelled from school (Brown et al., 1992). For example, among adolescents involved in substance abuse treatment in San Diego County, California, 61% reported

TABLE 6.3. Trends in Lifetime Prevalence (Percentage) of Substance Use among High School Seniors from 1991 to 2001

Substance	1991	1993	1995	1997	1999	2001
Alcohol[a]	88.0	80.0	80.7	81.7	80.0	79.7
Cigarettes	63.1	61.9	64.2	65.4	64.6	61.0
Marijuana	36.7	35.3	41.7	49.6	49.7	49.0
Amphetamines	15.4	15.1	15.3	16.5	16.3	16.2
Inhalants	17.6	17.4	17.4	16.1	15.4	13.0
Hallucinogens	9.6	10.9	12.7	15.1	13.7	12.8
MDMA (Ecstasy)	—	—	—	6.9	8.0	11.7
Opiates[b]	6.6	6.4	7.2	9.7	10.2	9.9
Tranquilizers	7.2	6.4	7.1	7.8	9.3	9.2
Barbiturates	6.2	6.3	7.4	8.1	8.9	8.7
Cocaine	7.8	6.1	6.0	8.7	9.8	8.2
Crack	3.1	2.6	3.0	3.9	4.6	3.7
Steroids	2.1	2.0	2.3	2.4	2.9	3.7
Heroin	0.9	1.1	1.6	2.1	2.0	1.8

Note. Data from Johnston, O'Malley, and Bachman (2002).
[a]In 1993, lifetime prevalence alcohol questions changes to from previous years to define a drink as "more than a few sips."
[b]Does not include heroin.

not attending school prior to admission to treatment. Adolescents in substance abuse treatment programs are more likely to regularly use multiple substances and in significantly greater quantities than in community or school samples. For example, in this treatment sample, alcohol, marijuana, amphetamines, and cigarettes had been used by approximately 90% of adolescents. Approximately 75% of youth reported at least weekly use of marijuana prior to substance abuse treatment, and 20% reported abuse of prescription medication by either purposefully taking more than the prescribed dose or acquiring prescription medication for recreational use.

In addition, to the high rates of substance use among adolescents, a significant portion meet criteria for a substance abuse or dependence diagnosis. For example, among a community sample of 1,506 high school students, approximately 9% met criteria for a substance use disorder (Lewinsohn, Rohde, & Seeley, 1995). More recently, the 2001 National Household Survey on Drug Abuse (NHSDA), found that 7.8% of adolescents ages 12–17 met criteria for substance abuse or dependence with prevalence rates increasing from early to late adolescence (SAMHSA, 2002). Aarons and colleagues (2001) examined the prevalence of adolescent substance use disorders among youth ages 13–18 years in five sectors of public service care: mental health, alcohol and drug, child welfare, juvenile justice, and severely emotionally disturbed in schools. Table 6.4 displays lifetime rates of substance use diagnosis for each of these settings. Across all sectors of care, 35% of adolescents met diagnostic criteria for either substance abuse or substance dependence. Meeting diagnostic criteria for an alcohol and marijuana use disorder was more common among mental health settings, while other illicit substance use disorders were more prevalent in juvenile justice settings.

Age of Onset

Clearly, not all adolescents who experiment with a psychoactive substance develop SUDs. However, previous research has identified age of first use as a risk factor for the onset of substance use problems and later disorders. For example, data from the National Household Survey on Drug Abuse showed that while 11.8% of adolescents whose first use of marijuana was before age 15 developed dependence, only 2.1% of those whose first use of marijuana was after age 17 went on to meet criteria for dependence. Early onset of alcohol and marijuana use has also been found to be predictive of binge drinking in adolescence (D'Amico et al., 2001). In addition, in the National Longitudinal Survey of Youth (NLSY), the odds of developing alcohol dependence decreased by 9% for each year that the onset of drinking was delayed (Grant, Stinson, & Harford, 2001). Among adolescents in substance abuse treatment programs, age of alcohol initiation has been reported at 11 years with progression to weekly alcohol use by age 13 years, while other drug use was initiated by age 13.7 years and progressed to regular use within a year (Brown, Gleghorn, Schuckit, Myers, & Mott, 1996). Among substance-abusing adolescents with comorbid psychopathology, the

TABLE 6.4. Percentage of Adolescents Who Meet Diagnostic Criteria for an SUD across Five Sectors of Care

	Alcohol/ drug (*n* = 137)	Juvenile justice (*n* = 419)	Mental health (*n* = 547)	Severely emotionally disturbed (*n* = 230)	Child welfare (*n* = 190)	Total (*n* = 1,036)
Any substance	82.6	62.1	40.8	23.6	19.2	39.5
Alcohol	68.9	48.6	32.2	19.1	16.6	31.5
Cannabis	54.3	44.5	29.1	14.6	8.3	26.6
Amphetamine	37.8	22.6	13.8	4.9	3.7	12.8
Hallucinogen	19.6	9.0	5.8	2.8	.09	5.2
Cocaine	13.0	2.2	1.3	0.0	0.5	1.2
Opiate	2.2	0.5	0.2	0.0	0.0	0.3

Note. Data from Aarons, Brown, Hough, Garland, and Wood (2001).

age of onset of drug initiation is earlier with onset of drug use at 12.4 years and weekly use at 13.3 years (Abrantes et al., 2004).

Gender, Racial, and Ethnic Differences

Historically, the prevalence of substance involvement has been higher for adolescent males than for females. However, recent trends in substance involvement have demonstrated few prevalence differences between males and females. For example, in the years from 1996 to 2000, data from the Monitoring the Future study show few differences between males and females in the lifetime prevalence rates of substance use (Wallace et al., 2003). Increases in drug use among girls have resulted in converging prevalence rates for males and females (Wallace et al., 2003) and recent data from the NHSDA demonstrated that among adolescents ages 12–17, rates of substance dependence did not differ significantly between boys and girls (7.6% vs. 8.0%, respectively).

Differences in prevalence rates of substance use across racial and ethnic groups have been observed. American Indian high school seniors have the greatest lifetime and 30-day prevalence rates of any illicit substance and alcohol use (Wallace et al., 2002), and Asian American adolescents display the lowest prevalence rates of substance use. White, Mexican American, Cuban American, and Puerto Rican high school seniors display comparable rates of use, while African American use rates are somewhat lower than these groups. When gender and ethnic differences were examined concurrently, Wallace and colleagues (2003) found that Native American girls displayed the highest rates of alcohol and drug use whereas African American and Asian American girls demonstrated the lowest rates of use.

ETIOLOGY

Considerable research has been devoted to understanding the onset of substance use, abuse, and dependence among adolescents. While several theories explain youth behavior more generally, others specifically address substance involvement. The most prevalent etiological theories of substance use among adolescents include theory of planned behavior (TPB), social learning theory (SLT), prob-lem behavior theory (PBT), domain model, and maturation theory.

Theory of Planned Behavior

TPB (Ajzen, 1988), which is a derivative of theory of reasoned action (Ajzen & Fishbein, 1980), can be used to explain why individuals engage in varied addictive behaviors. In this theory, attitudes about using substances, perceived social norms of using, and self-efficacy in potential use situations influence intentions to engage in substance use, which, in turn, influence actual behavior. Substance-specific attitudes result from expectations about personal consequences (i.e., costs and benefits) associated with substance use and the value placed on these consequences (Ajzen & Fishbein, 1980; Petraitis, Flay, & Miller, 1995). Normative beliefs about substance use are determined by the perception that others want the individual to use in addition to personal motivation to please others. Self-efficacy about substance use refers to whether the adolescent feels control over the behavior. Two types of self-efficacy related to substance use intentions include use self-efficacy (i.e., belief about the ability to successfully obtain and use substances) and refusal self-efficacy (i.e., ability to resist pressures to use) (Ajzen, 1988). Petraitis and colleagues (1995) argue that although there has been strong support for TPB in explaining experimental substance use, it does not address whether substance-specific beliefs are a cause or a consequence of substance use.

Social Learning Theory

SLT was first developed by Akers (1977) and further developed into social cognitive/learning theory by Bandura (1986). Both of these theories focus on the relation of the substance-using model and the substance use of the adolescent. From this perspective, adolescents develop outcome expectations about the effects of substance use by observing (e.g., watching a parent have a drink after a long, stressful day at work) or hearing about (e.g., a peer discusses how he was able to ask someone on date after drinking at a party) the effects of substance use. SLT posits that positive social, personal, and physiological expectations resulting from attending to influential social role models are predictive of adolescent substance use.

Problem Behavior Theory

PBT considers substance involvement as one of a number of deviant behaviors that typically co-occur among adolescents (Jessor & Jessor, 1977). All adolescent deviant behavior reflects unconventionality, such that if an adolescent is prone to engage in one deviant behavior, he or she will likely engage in other deviant behaviors. Donovan and Jessor (1985) found that in a high school sample, the use of marijuana and alcohol was significantly related to being sexually active, illegal activity, truancy, and fighting but not to health-promoting behaviors or conventional behaviors such as church attendance (Donovan, Jessor, & Costa, 1991). Also, PBT posits that adolescents at risk for deviant behaviors are more detached from their parents and more influenced by their peers.

Domain Model

Huba, Wingard, and Bentler (1980) developed an interactive theory where biological, intrapersonal, interpersonal, and sociocultural domains jointly influence adolescents' substance use behavior. Biological contributors consist of genetic susceptibility, physiological reactions to substance use, and general health. The intrapersonal domain that influences use decisions includes psychological status, cognitive style, personality traits, and personal values. Interpersonal characteristics, including social support, modeling, social reinforcement, and sense of identity and belonging, all contribute to substance involvement. Finally, prevalent social sanctions of substance use, degree of availability of substances, social expectations, and environmental stressors operate at a sociocultural level to impact the development of substance involvement of youth.

Maturation Theory

Maturation theory (Tarter et al., 1999) is a recent description of the development of early onset of substance use disorders. This heuristic posits that deviations in somatic and neurological maturation, along with stressful, adverse environments, predispose children to difficulties in regulating affect and behavior, which result in "difficult temperaments." Children with "difficult temperaments" in infancy are predisposed to oppositional behaviors, leading to conduct problems, and in turn to SUDs and ul-

timately comorbid antisocial personality disorder in adulthood (Dawes, et al., 2000; Tarter et al., 1999). Maturation theory incorporates an epigenetic perspective where from the moment of conception, genetic and environmental interactions result in a developmental sequence of events leading to increased risk for the onset of substance use disorders.

RISK AND PROTECTIVE FACTORS

Biological

Through family, twin, adoption and genetic studies, a link between parental alcohol and drug abuse and risk for alcohol and drug dependence in offspring, especially males, has been demonstrated (e.g., Dinwiddie & Cloninger, 1991; Rose et al., 1997; Schuckit, 1988, Sher, 1993). Although associated risks (e.g., conduct disorder) may influence outcomes, differences in behavioral, cognitive, and neurological measures have been observed between offspring of alcoholics (family history positive, or FHP) and offspring of non-alcoholics (family history negative, or FHN). For example, when FHP adolescents are compared to FHN teens, they demonstrate greater impulsivity, rebelliousness (Knop, Teasdale, Schulsinger, & Goodwin, 1985), poorer neuropsychological performance (Tapert & Brown, 1999; Tarter & Edwards, 1988), and less physiological and subjective effects of alcohol (Newlin, 1994; Schuckit; 1988). Cadoret, Yates, Troughton, Woodworth, and Stewart (1995) found two genetic pathways that independently predicted drug abuse among male adoptees: (1) a direct pathway from the biological parent's alcoholism to drug abuse and dependency in offspring; and (2) an indirect pathway from antisocial personality disorder in the biological parent to externalizing behaviors and, eventually, drug abuse and dependence in the offspring. Similarly, developmentally focused cross-cultural research supports multiple genetically influenced pathways to addiction (e.g., Rose, Dick, Viken, & Kaprio, 2001). Recent advances in genetic mapping and genetic engineering suggest that several brain proteins and receptor sites are implicated in sensitivity to preference for alcohol and other drugs (e.g., Schuckit, 2002) and highlight the heterogeneity of genetic risks for substance abuse. However, despite these genetic influences on the development of alcohol and other substance use disorders, the majority of FHP offspring do not become substance dependent. A number of individual and environmental factors moderate the risk for initiation of substance involvement and progression of use.

Individual

Personality

Personality characteristics may directly and indirectly influence substance involvement of adolescents (Sher, 1994; ; Windle, 1990; Zucker & Gomberg, 1986). Personality characteristics most consistently associated with increased risk for adolescent substance use problems include high sensation seeking (Cloninger, Sigvardsson, & Bohman, 1988; Zuckerman, 1994); behavioral disinhibition (McGue, Slutske, Taylor, & Iacono, 1997); impulsivity (Baker & Yardley, 2002); aggression (Kuo, Yang, Soong, & Chen, 2002); behavioral undercontrol (Colder & Chassin, 1993); and antisocial patterns (Zucker et al., 2000). For example, in a study of Taiwanese adolescents, personality factors most often associated with substance use included higher extraversion, higher novelty seeking, and aggressive behavior (Kuo et al., 2002). In addition, Comeau, Stewart, and Loba (2001) have demonstrated that trait anxiety and anxiety sensitivity were also predictive of adolescents' motivations for alcohol, cigarette, and marijuana use.

Psychopathology

Although it is often difficult to determine the extent to which SUDs and concomitant mental health problems develop independently, one causes or exacerbates the other, or common underlying mechanisms are present for both (Meyer, 1986), there is substantial evidence that high rates of comorbidity are present in both community and clinical samples. For example, lifetime comorbid psychiatric disorders were examined in a community sample of 1,507 adolescents ages 14–18 years, and found that 66% of adolescents who met diagnostic criteria for SUDs also met criteria for at least one other Axis I disorder (Lewinsohn et al., 1995). The Methods for the Epidemiology of Child and Adolescent Mental Disorders (MECA) study obtained similar rates with a community sample of 1,285 children and adolescents ages 9–18 years old (Kandel et al.,

1997). They found that 66% of weekly drinkers also met diagnostic criteria for a psychiatric disorder, as did 85% of females and 56% of males who used illicit drugs three or more times in the past year. A subsequent report on the MECA study found that three times as many adolescents with current SUDs (compared to those without) met criteria for another current psychiatric disorder (Kandel et al., 1999). In a review of all community samples, Armstrong and Costello (2002) found that 60% of adolescent substance users had an additional comorbid disorder.

As expected, rates of psychiatric disorders in inpatient substance-abusing adolescents tend to be even higher than those reported in community samples and vary across types of clinical settings (Abrantes et al., 2004). Studies of adolescents in inpatient substance abuse treatment report high rates of comorbidity ranging from 68% (Novins, Beals, Shore, & Manson, 1996) and 82% of adolescents (Stowell & Estroff, 1992). Recent studies have documented the co-occurrence of SUDs in adolescents hospitalized for a psychiatric problem, reporting that from 33% to 50% of adolescents admitted to an adolescent acute-care psychiatric inpatient unit also met criteria for one or more SUD (Deas-Nesmith, Campbell, & Brady, 1998; Grilo et al., 1995). Similarly elevated rates of SUDs in psychiatrically hospitalized adolescents have been found elsewhere (Bukstein, Brent, & Kaminer, 1989; Greenbaum, Foster-Johnson, & Petrila, 1996; Piazza, 1996). While relatively few studies have examined rates of adolescent comorbidity in outpatient settings, they are likely to be lower (Wilens, Biederman, Abrantes, & Spencer, 1997).

As noted in recent reviews of SUDs and psychiatric disorders (Abrantes et al., 2004; Bukstein, 1995) the psychiatric disorders commonly co-occurring with substance use disorders among adolescents include both externalizing disorders (e.g., conduct disorder, attention-deficit/hyperactivity disorder, and oppositional defiant disorder) and internalizing disorders (e.g., depression and anxiety). In addition to high rates of internalizing and externalizing disorders, a history of physical and/or sexual abuse is also prevalent among adolescent substance abusers. For example, in a multisite study of 803 adolescents in drug treatment, 59% of girls and 39% of boys reported a history of physical and/or sexual abuse (Grella & Joshi, 2003).

Alcohol and Drug Expectancies

Alcohol and drug outcome expectancies refer to anticipated effects of using a specific substance (Brown, 1993). Expectancies develop as a result of both direct and vicarious learning experiences with substances, including peer and parental modeling and media exposure (Goldman, Brown, Christiansen, & Smith, 1991). Alcohol and drug expectancies have been found to mediate the relationship between family history of substance problems and substance involvement in offspring (Goldman & Rather, 1993; Sher, 1994). In addition, progression from initiation of use to problematic use is more likely to occur among adolescents who expect more global positive effects, increased social facilitation, and enhancement of cognitive and motor performance with alcohol (Brown, Creamer, & Stetson, 1987; Christiansen, Smith, Roehling, & Goldman, 1989; Smith, Goldman, Greenbaum, & Christiansen, 1995). Alcohol and drug expectancies have also been found to be related to poorer outcomes among substance-abusing adolescents (Vik, Brown, & Myers, 1997). In general, positive alcohol and drug expectancies are related to accelerate substance involvement and substance-related problems, whereas negative outcome expectancies may operate as a protective factor against the initiation of substance use (Brown, 1993).

Environmental

Family Functioning

Disruption in family relations and functioning have been identified as precursors, correlates, and consequences of adolescent substance abuse problems (Stewart & Brown, 1995; Zucker et al., 2000). Parental deviance (e.g., antisocial behaviors and substance abuse), lack of parental involvement, and lack of parent–child affection are associated with increased risk of adolescent substance use problems (Sadava, 1987). More recently, inconsistent parental discipline, poor monitoring of behavior, excessive punishing, hostile environment, permissiveness, and negative parent–child interactions have also been found to be risk factors for substance use problems among adolescents (Brody & Forehand, 1993; Chilcoat & Anthony, 1996; Gilvarry, 2000; Williams & Hine, 2002). In addition, Zucker and colleagues have found that family conflict is predictive of more disruptive behavior in children, which elevates

the risk for substance involvement in adolescence (Loukas, Zucker, Fitzgerald, & Krull, 2003; Zucker et al., 2000). Furthermore, the extent to which parents monitor an adolescent's activities may indirectly influence selection of peers (Brown et al., 1992; Chassin, Pillow, Curran, Molina, & Barrera, 1993). While poorer cohesion and expressiveness as well as more conflict are relationship features that elevate risk for early substance abuse, these aspects of interactions improve with the resolution of youth substance involvement (Stewart & Brown, 1995).

Peers

Peer influences have been identified as one of the most significant risk factors for adolescent substance involvement (Bates & Labouvie, 1995; Fergusson, Horwood, & Lynskey, 1995). Adolescents with earlier and greater use of alcohol and/or drugs report higher perception of peer use and more friends who engage in substance use and deviant behaviors (Barnes, Farrell, & Banerjee, 1994; Epstein & Botvin, 2002; Vik, Grizzle, & Brown, 1992). Social networks of substance-abusing peers not only create greater access to substances but also lead to the adoption of beliefs and values consistent with a drug use lifestyle (Tapert, Stewart, & Brown, 1999). For example, Bryant and Zimmerman (2002) found that African American students who perceived negative school attitudes in their peers were more likely to show increases in use of cigarettes and marijuana. Recent research also indicates that association with substance-abusing and deviant peers mediates the relationship between parental alcoholism, low socioeconomic status, and family conflict and substance abuse in adolescence (Fergusson & Horwood, 1999). Furthermore, such peer associations facilitate access to substances, exposure to stressful situations, and modeling of maladaptive coping efforts (Richter, Brown, & Mott, 1991).

Stress

Stressful life experiences increase substantially during adolescence, as does heightened reactivity to stress, especially for girls (Vik & Brown, 1998). Stressful life events (e.g., end of relationship, automobile accidents, and academic failure) have been associated with substance use. There is evidence that psychosocial stress, as well as economic adversity, is associated with risk factors for early substance use involvement and progression of use (McCubbin, Needle, & Wilson, 1985; Pandina & Schuele, 1983; Wills, Vaccaro, & McNamara, 1992). In addition, Brown (1989) found that youth from alcohol-abusing families experience more life stress and rate stressful life events as more negative than youth from families with no parental alcohol or substance abuse. The association is bidirectional, as alcohol and drug involvement also provoke substantial stress in the form of subsequent physical, academic, legal, family, peer, and emotional problems (Vik et al., 1997).

Protective Factors

Protective factors are not simply the absence of risk factors but, instead, distinctive characteristics or circumstances associated with decreased likelihood of engaging in health-damaging behaviors (Jessor et al., 1995). Protective factors associated with decreased likelihood of engaging in problematic substance use among adolescents include positive temperament, high intelligence, social support, involvement with conventional peers, and low risk taking (Brown, Schulenberg, Bachman, O'Malley, & Johnston, 2001; Fergusson & Lynskey, 1996; Gilvarry, 2000). In a recent study, Epstein, Griffin, and Botvin (2002) identified competence skills (e.g., decision making and self-efficacy) and psychological wellness as protective against alcohol involvement among 1,459 middle to junior high school students. Recently, genetic variations in enzymes for alcohol metabolism, in particular, aldehyde dehydrogenase (ALDH) and alcohol dehydrogenase (ADH), have been found to protect against the development of alcohol abuse and dependence in Asians (e.g., Wall, Shea, Chan, & Carr, 2001). Some researchers have argued the importance of the interaction between risk and protective factors has been demonstrated through predictors of future substance use and misuse (Brown, Aarons, & Abrantes, 2001; Glantz & Leshner, 2000).

In summary, research on the development of substance use problems among adolescents has identified multiple factors that set the stage for alcohol and drug abuse in the teenage years. Biological, individual, and environmental factors each contribute to the initiation of substance use and progression to substance abuse and dependence. Further, previous studies have also identified important factors that protect against the development of problematic substance involvement among youth.

DEVELOPMENTAL COURSE AND OUTCOMES

Across species, increases in exploration, risk taking, and independence increase during adolescence to experiment with different lifestyles. Thus it is not surprising that middle school and high school students explore new activities and, during this stage, youth typically seek autonomy and independence from their parents and experimentation with substance use as a possible part of this process (Schinke, Botvin, & Orlandi, 1991). For example, several studies have found that experimental alcohol and marijuana use in adolescence were not associated with poorer psychosocial adjustment in adulthood (Newcomb & Bentler, 1988, Shelder & Block, 1990). However, although some experimentation with substances may be normative in adolescence, there is a substantial evidence that early onset of use is associated with increased risk for the development of abuse and dependence (e.g., Grant et al., 2001).

Epidemiological studies indicate that the initiation of substance use typically occurs with the gateway substances of cigarettes and alcohol in early to middle adolescence (Kandel, Yamaguchi, & Chen, 1992). A predictable sequence of use emerges with marijuana initiation following alcohol and tobacco, followed by other illegal drugs in late adolescence (Kandel et al., 1992; Kandel & Yamaguchi, 1993). Despite this gateway sequence of drug initiation, not all adolescents will progress to other substances. The sequence effect from cigarettes to alcohol has been found to occur among different ethnic groups and among multiethnic adolescents (Chen et al., 2002).

Escalation to more frequent and diversified substance use may occur in late adolescence and early adulthood (Chen & Kandel, 1995). This may be due to transitions from living with parental figures to independent and less restrictive living situations where there is greater access to and approval of substance involvement (Chassin & Ritter, 2001; Kypri, McCarthy, Coe, & Brown, 2004). However, with the adoption of adult roles including work, marriage, and parenthood, there is often a significant decline in substance involvement and abuse/dependence symptoms (Chilcoat &

Breslau, 1996; Gotham, Sher, & Wood, 1997). As a result, some researchers have found that a portion of substance abusing youth will "mature out" of problematic use when anticipating or transitioning into adult responsibilities (Chassin & Ritter, 2001; Zucker, Fitzgerald, & Moses, 1995) or changing environments (Schulenberg et al. 1996).

Developmental Pathways

Although the identification of biological, individual, and environmental risk factors is important in understanding the etiology of substance abuse in adolescence, their independent contributions only partially predict substance involvement during adolescence. However, conceptual models that include these factors as mediators and moderators enhance efforts to explain initiation and progression of adolescent substance involvement. As a result, multiple developmental pathways to substance involvement in adolescence have been proposed and are summarized below.

Deviance Proness Pathway

Zucker and colleagues' (2000) research has demonstrated that parental alcoholism is a risk factor for behavioral difficulties (e.g., disruptive behavior disorders) in their children. These behavioral problems are associated with an increased risk for subsequent substance involvement and deviant behaviors in adolescence. Similarly, Sher (1994) proposed that ineffective parenting increases the risk for temperamental difficulties, cognitive deficits, and school failure in their offspring. These, in turn, result in emotional distress and affiliation with substance-using, deviant peers and eventually the offspring's own substance involvement and problematic behaviors. A key feature of this model involves the child's inability to self-regulate his or her emotional distress and externalizing behavior tendencies, which elevate risk for the development of substance use problems in adolescence. In addition, difficulties in self-regulation have been associated with higher-order executive functioning deficits that have been demonstrated in neuropsychological studies of adolescent substance abusers (e.g., Giancola & Parker, 2001). Furthermore, Rose and colleagues (1997) conducted behavioral genetic studies with adolescent twins in Finland

exploring the extent to which behavioral difficulties in childhood were associated with an increased risk of alcohol dependence during adolescence. They found that monozygotic twins display greater behavioral difficulty similarity than dizygotic twins, suggesting that genetic factors do contribute to these developing behavioral problems.

Negative Affect Pathway

In addition to the aforementioned developmental pathway, adolescents may come to use and abuse substances in order to regulate negative affect resulting from exposure to environmental stressors or temperament-based emotionality (Colder & Chassin, 1993; Cooper, Frone, Russell, & Muldar, 1995). This pathway is further mediated by peer use and may partially account for the elevated incidence of substance use by youth with mental health disorders (Abrantes et al., 2004). Although this pathway has received support with cross-sectional and cross-cultural research (e.g., Rose et al., 1997), weaker associations between negative affectivity and substance involvement have been identified in prospective high-risk studies (Chassin & Ritter, 2001). Of note, this pathway is supported for adolescents who demonstrate a predisposition toward negative affectivity while possessing poor self-regulation and coping skills (Colder & Chassin, 1997; Cooper et al., 1995).

Enhanced Reinforcement Pathway

Some youth are more sensitive to the reinforcing effects of substances and, consequently, will use substances more frequently and in greater quantities (Chassin & Ritter, 2001). This pathway appears to be genetically based on physiological differences experienced from the pharmacological effects of substances (e.g., Schuckit & Smith, 2001) and related expectancies that develop as a result of these genetically based responses (McCarthy, Brown, Carr & Wall, 2001). Animal studies support this pathway through reduced sedation during adolescence. Thus, in addition to the physiological effects of the substances, positive, reinforcing cognitions and outcome expectancies of substance use have been found to predict continued drinking and escalation to abuse (Schuckit & Smith, 2001).

Outcomes

Varied trajectories unfold for youth with heavy substance involvement. For a substantial portion of youth, substance involvement and related problems peak during late adolescence and young adulthood and resolve without emerging again (Zucker et al., 1995). However, their substance involvement may progress into a recurrent pattern of abuse, persistent problems, and dependence, which may require treatment. For these youth, substance-related negative consequences accumulate during adolescence and adulthood. For example, Newcomb and Bentler (1988) followed 654 adolescents over 8 years and found that heavy drug use during adolescence predicted health problems, family problems, dysphoric emotional functioning, and troubled romantic relationships in adulthood.

For youth whose problems are so severe as to bring them into treatment settings (e.g., alcohol and drug, mental health, and juvenile justice), the course of substance use may vary markedly (Brown, Aarons, & Abrantes, 2001). One way to classify these patterns in use over time is developmental trajectories. In a recent study of long-term outcomes of treated substance-abusing adolescents, youth were classified as abstainers (22%), infrequent users (24%), worse with time (36%), and frequent users (18%) according to alcohol use over an 8-year period (Abrantes, McCarthy, Aarons, & Brown, 2002). Alcohol trajectories were associated with level of substance involvement across time and important functional outcomes such as family, emotional, relationship, and interpersonal functioning in late adolescence and young adulthood. Similar longitudinal patterns have been replicated in multiple studies (e.g., Chung et al., 2003).

One at-risk behavior commonly correlated with substance involvement among adolescents is sexual behavior. Substance-abusing adolescents are more likely to engage in unsafe sexual behaviors and have adverse consequences when compared to similar youth with no substance abuse history. For example, Tapert, Aarons, Sedlar, and Brown (2001) found that when compared to sociodemographically similar community youth, substance use–disordered adolescents reported more sexual partners, less consistent use of condoms, more sexually transmitted diseases, and greater HIV

testing in the 6 years after inpatient treatment. Similarly, Otto, Laura, Gore-Felton, McGarvey, and Canterbury (2002) found that higher levels of alcohol use among incarcerated adolescents were associated with HIV risk behavior. More recently, adolescents presenting at an urban health clinic were assessed for substance involvement and body modification (e.g., piercings and tattoos). Adolescents who had engaged in body modification, compared to those without body modification, were three times more likely to demonstrate problematic substance use (Brooks, Woods, Knight, & Sheir, 2003). In addition, heavy alcohol and drug use among males has been found to be predictive of engaging in illegal activities and association with similarly deviant peers (White, Tice, Loeber, & Stouthamer-Loeber, 2002).

SUDs in adolescence have also been associated with substantially elevated health problems. Substance involvement contributes to the top three causes of death for youth: accidents, homicide, and suicide (Aarons et al., 1999). Clark and colleagues (2001) report that adolescents with alcohol use disorders are more likely to present with health-related problems than nonabusing adolescents (e.g., sleep, dental, metabolism and bleeding, neurological, and urinary). Aarons and colleagues (1999) found that substance-abusing youth compared to community controls experienced more health problems over a 5-year period. In addition, a history of stimulant use among boys and alcohol use among girls was associated with trauma-related injuries (e.g., broken bones, puncture wounds, and contusions). Cigarette smoking, which is a concomitant behavior for alcohol and other drug involvement, is related to respiratory problems in late adolescence and young adulthood (Myers & Brown, 1994). In addition, Johnson and Richter (2002) found that cigarette and alcohol use was predictive of poorer overall health among community adolescents.

Recent research has examined the impact of substance involvement during adolescence on neuropsychological functioning in young adulthood. Tapert, Graham, Leedy, and Brown (2002) compared youth with a history of SUDs to matched controls on neuropsychological functioning measures over the course of 8 years. After controlling for baseline functioning, they found that substance use over the 8 years predicted poorer performances on memory and attention measures at the end of this time. In addition, they found that withdrawal symptoms were most related to problems in visuospatial functioning. More research will be necessary to examine mechanisms whereby substance involvement influences neurocognitive performance as adolescents transition into young adulthood.

Psychiatric comorbidity and symptomatology has been found to be an adverse outcome of early substance involvement. Because the etiology of symptoms is often unclear, identification of independent psychiatric disorders from substance-induced disorders is difficult for both researchers and clinicians. For example, alcohol and drug intoxication and withdrawal may result in symptoms of depressive, anxiety, or psychotic disorders (Brown et al., 1995; Brown, Irwin, & Schuckit, 1991; Schuckit, Irwin, & Brown, 1990). Several weeks of abstinence are often necessary before adults can be ideally diagnosed with an independent psychiatric disorder (Brown & Schuckit, 1988). However, no research to date has examined the period of time necessary for differentiating independent psychiatric diagnoses among adolescent substance abusers.

ASSESSMENT

Treatment improvement protocols (TIPs) sponsored by SAMHSA's Center for Substance Abuse Treatment (CSAT) (1999a) provides a multiple assessment model for assessing substance abuse in adolescence including content, methods, and sources. In this model, content focuses on the assessment of important clinical characteristics such as substance use severity, risk factors, psychiatric comorbidity, and validity of self-report. Method refers to procedures whereby the content is assessed such as questionnaires, structured interviews, and biochemical testing. Finally, sources of the information may consist of the adolescent, parents, teachers, peers, and public records. Therefore, a comprehensive assessment of adolescent substance abuse involves collecting information on relevant clinical characteristic through the use of reliable and developmentally appropriate instruments that are administered to multiple sources.

Major content areas of assessment important in youth substance abuse include changes in behavioral functioning among adolescents in the following domains: school, family, social, activities, and physical and emotional health (Brown, Aarons, & Abrantes, 2001); while these domains are reviewed elsewhere (e.g., Brown, 1993), examples within domains have been well documented. For example, within the school domain, decreased grades, truancy, suspension, and conflict with teachers may occur. Changes in the family domain may include decreased contact, cohesion, expressiveness, increased conflicts, arguments, and running away from home. Social changes in peer group affiliation, fighting, sexual activity, and gang involvement may be associated with substance involvement. Within the activities domain, changes in school involvement, work absenteeism, illegal activities, and reckless behavior may reflect substance abuse. Finally, physical problems (e.g., accidents, injuries, sleep, dental, and withdrawal symptoms) and emotional problems (e.g., anxiety, agitation, depression, and suicidal ideation) may be related to alcohol or drug use problems. Therefore, decreased functioning or impairment in these domains may reflect indicators of abuse and that further assessment and treatment for SUDs is necessary.

Assessment of youth substance abuse most commonly involves the use of two types of assessment instruments: screening and comprehensive measures. Screening instruments are specifically designed to identify individuals who are currently experiencing substance-related problems or are at risk for such difficulties but have not yet received any addiction treatment (Connors & Volk, 1995). Screening instruments are not designed to diagnose or explain substance abuse or dependence in great depth but instead provide information about who needs to receive further, more in-depth assessment of the problem. Because of the high prevalence rates of experimentation in normal adolescent development, screening is most effectively implemented when targeted to at-risk adolescents (Bukstein, 1995). Screening instruments can also serve as an early detection technique that can often alleviate later economic costs of alcohol and drug use. Screening instruments are useful tools because they are generally easy and inexpensive to administer (Leccese & Waldron, 1994). In addition, they can be used in a variety of settings such as juvenile justice system, adolescent psychiatry units, and primary care facilities.

Several well-validated substance abuse screening instruments exist that are designed specifically for adolescents. The Personal Experience Screening Questionnaire (PESQ; Winters, 1992) is a short, 40-item, self-report questionnaire that screens for severity, psychosocial problems, frequency of use, and faking responses. Psychometric properties of the PESQ include high internal consistency, good criterion validity (.90), and 87% sensitivity (Winters, 1992). The Drug Use Screening Inventory—Revised (DUSI-R; Kirisci, Mezzich, & Tarter, 1995) is a longer 159-item, self-report instrument that assesses for level of substance involvement and related consequences, in addition to a variety of psychosocial functioning domains (e.g., family system, school work, peer relationships, and behavior patterns). The DUSI has demonstrated high test–retest reliability, internal consistency, and content validity (Tarter, Mezzich, Kirisci, & Kaczynksi, 1997) as well as 86% sensitivity (Kirisci et al., 1995). The Problem Oriented Screening Instrument for Teenagers (POSIT; Rahdert, 1991) is a 139-item, self-report instrument designed to identify potential problems and treatment needs in 10 different problem areas including substance use and abuse, physical health, mental health, family relations, peer relations, and educational status. The POSIT is 84% accurate in identifying substance abuse and has demonstrated good criterion validity (Rahdert, 1991). The Teen Addiction Severity Index (T-ASI; Kaminer, Wagner, Plummer, & Seifer, 1993) is a brief assessment instrument that is interviewer administered. The T-ASI was developed to collect basic information from substance-abusing adolescents admitted to inpatient facilities. The T-ASI provides a global measure of substance use and substance-related functional impairment in seven domains (e.g., school status, family relationships, peer relationships, and psychiatric status). Good psychometric properties have been demonstrated for the T-ASI (Kaminer et al., 1993).

Adolescent substance abuse screening instruments have limitations. First, screening instruments are often self-report. As a result, there are concerns about the validity of the information gathered due to comfort with self-disclosure, recall bias, and honesty in reporting. Second, brief screening instruments are often unidimensional in focus. Although, this allows for quick and easy administration, it restricts the detail and breadth of information that can be gathered. Finally, screening measures, especially in clinical settings, are used to make dichotomous choices (e.g., further assessment or intervention) even when measures often yield dimensional scores. Consequently, unfortunate decisions can be made if cutoffs are not appropriately established for the age group, sex, or ethnic/cultural group. In addition, important information may be lost when the information gathered is simply used for cutoff distinctions.

Although screening instruments are an effective means of identifying adolescents at high risk for SUDs, comprehensive instruments are used for a more detailed, extensive assessment of substance involvement and related problems. A primary purpose of these instruments is to assess DSM-IV diagnostic criteria for substance use disorders and associated life problems used for treatment planning. There are also several well-validated substance abuse diagnostic instruments that have been designed specifically for adolescents. The Adolescent Diagnostic Interview (ADI; Winters & Henly, 1993) is a structured interview that assesses DSM-IV criteria for SUDs along with functioning in several domains such as relationships with peers and family, school performance, and stressful life events. The ADI has demonstrated test–retest reliability for alcohol abuse (.64), alcohol dependence (.60), cannabis abuse (.70), and cannabis dependence (.66), in addition to criterion validity (Winters, Stinchfield, Fulkerson, & Henly, 1993). The Customary Drinking and Drug Use Record (CDDR; Brown et al., 1998) is a structured interview that provides a detailed assessment of substance use patterns, abuse and dependence symptoms, and substance-related consequences for alcohol and eight different substances. With both lifetime and current use versions, the CDDR has well demonstrated psychometric validation for use with both Caucasian and African American adolescents (Brown et al., 1998). Finally, the Personal Experiences Inventory (PEI; Winters & Henly, 1989) is an instrument that assesses substance use in addition to psychological variables such as an adolescent's perceptions of family and peer functioning. The PEI has also been used to determine the appropriateness of inpatient or outpatient substance abuse treatment (Winters, Stinchfield, & Henly, 1996).

The extent to which adolescents are accurately assessed often depends on the sources of information. Although there has been debate about the validity of adolescent self-report of the substance use, Winters (2001) outlines the following summary of why researchers can feel confident about adolescent self-report of substance use: (1) in clinically referred settings, a large portion of adolescents report use; (2) higher rates of drug use are reported in clinical samples compared to community samples; (3) low rates of endorsing "faking bad" items; and (4) general consistency of disclosures across time. However, corroborating sources of information (e.g., parents, treatment providers, and toxicology screens) can be instrumental in more accurately assessing substance involvement among youth particularly in clinical settings (Brown, Aarons, & Abrantes, 2001).

Corroborating sources of information are especially important when assessing substance-abusing adolescents with comorbid mental health problems in psychiatric, juvenile justice, and other service sectors (e.g., child welfare). For example, in the child and adolescent psychopathology literature, limited parent–offspring reliability has been demonstrated for such disorders as depression, anxiety, and alcohol dependence (Cantwell, Lewinsohn, Rohde, & Seeley, 1997). In general, adolescents are more likely to report internalizing symptoms on structured interviews whereas externalizing symptoms are more evident to parents (Bird, Gould, & Staghezza, 1992). As noted by Cantwell and colleagues (1997), adolescents may not acknowledge socially undesirable symptoms, parents may be less aware of internalizing symptoms, adolescents may behave differently based on the setting (e.g., school vs. home), and parents and adolescents may differ in their interpretation of the severity or impact of symptoms. Furthermore, studies have shown individuals with both a SUD and a psychiatric disorder tend to underreport both their substance involvement and their psychiatric symptoms (Bryant, Rounsaville, Spitzer, & Williams, 1992; Carey & Correia, 1998; Corty, Lehman, & Myers, 1993). Therefore, it has become standard in childhood psychopathology research to collect information about symptoms from multiple sources, and this may be especially important for adolescent substance abusers with concomitant psychopathology.

In addition to using collateral sources of information when assessing comorbid, substance-abusing adolescents, determining the temporal sequencing of disorders may help clarify the etiological and developmental factors influencing comorbidity and may be of prognostic value in the treatment of substance-abusing youth. For example, information about the chronology of disorders may facilitate disentangling the possible direct, indirect, and interactive influences psychopathology has on adolescent problem substance use (Stice, Myers, & Brown, 1998). Furthermore, clarification of the primary and secondary disorders may provide useful clinical information regarding potential substance-induced disorders among youth. In particular, SUDs developing during adolescence may result in psychophysiological effects that either provoke or exacerbate symptoms of mood or anxiety disorders. In such cases, no medication may be necessary for the psychiatric symptoms to abate. By contrast, medication as well as cognitive and behavioral interventions may be necessary to resolve psychiatric disorders predating substance involvement. There may exist additional distinguishing features of those comorbid adolescents with primary SUDs compared to secondary SUDs such as severity of substance involvement, which may influence course of disorders, treatment needs, and treatment outcome (e.g., Brown et al., 1995).

TREATMENT

The development of effective intervention approaches to address adolescent substance use problems must be considered a very high priority. However to date, successful treatment outcomes have eluded both researchers and clinicians in this field with approximately half of adolescents receiving treatment for SUDs relapsing within the first 3 months following treatment (Brown, Mott, & Myers, 1990; Cornelius et al., 2003). In addition, only approximately 10% of adolescents who endorse SUD symptoms in the past year actually receive any treatment (Dennis & McGreary, 1999). Until recently, youth with such problems were typically treated outside specialized alcohol/drug treatment programs or in adult substance abuse programs (Brown et al., 1990). Because adolescent substance abusers differ from adult substance abusers with respect to use patterns, prevalent problems, and developmental and social factors, it is important to take these characteristics into consideration when developing interventions for adolescent substance abuse problems (Deas et al., 2000). Therefore, a significant discrepancy exists between the need for adolescent treatment services and the existence and provision for these services (Brown et al. 2000).

Interventions for adolescent substance use vary according to treatment modality and type of setting. The most common interventions include 12-step programs, system-oriented approaches, brief interventions, cognitive-behavioral therapy, therapeutic communities, and pharmacotherapy. Interventions can be conducted in schools, outpatient, partial hospitalization, or residential settings. Several organization (e.g., SAMSHA, 1999b) and individuals (e.g., Winters, 1999) have presented guidelines for tailoring treatment to adolescents based on a continuum of intensity of involvement and problems. Primary prevention and early intervention efforts, often conducted in school settings, can be geared toward adolescents with modest experience with substances. Outpatient settings are more appropriate for adolescents experiencing low to moderate substance-related problems and with fairly stable home environments. Residential settings are typically reserved for adolescents experiencing severe problems due to substance use, concomitant psychiatric problems, unstable home environment, and requiring medical monitoring of withdrawal symptoms. Results of a comprehensive assessment of substance use and consequences should guide decisions regarding intervention.

Type of Interventions

12-Step Programs

Derived from the philosophy of Alcoholics Anonymous (AA), 12-step programs, are an integral part of most substance abuse treatment programs for adults and adolescents in the United States (Brown, 1999; Bukstein, 1994). Participation in 12-step programs involves learning and practicing the 12 steps, or sequential recommendations for abstinence, sharing experiences with others with similar problems in a group setting, and receiving guidance and help from an another member designated as a sponsor. There is a focus on anonymity and complete abstinence in 12-step programs. Despite the long history and popularity of 12-step programs as intervention for SUDs, empirical research on efficacy has only recently begun.

In one study, Brown (1993) examined the rates of adolescents who participated in 12-step programs in the year following inpatient treatment for substance use problems. Of the 57% who youth who attended at least 25 12-step meetings in the year following treatment, a majority (69%) demonstrated positive substance outcomes. By contrast, only 31% of adolescents who did not attend 12-step meetings regularly demonstrated positive outcomes in the year after treatment. In addition to positive outcomes, another study found that attending 12-step meetings was associated with increased motivation for abstinence, which predicted reductions in subsequent drug involvement among substance-abusing adolescents (Kelly, Myers, & Brown, 2000).

Whereas 12-step approaches appear to be related to positive outcomes among adolescents, there is a need for controlled studies to test the efficacy and effectiveness of this approach. Furthermore, 12-step approaches were originally designed for substance-abusing adult populations. It is unclear whether the specific developmental needs of adolescents are addressed in this approach (Brown, 1999). For example, the strong commitment to total abstinence in 12-step approaches may be less palatable to adolescents who, in their youth, view it as an unattainable and unrealistic goal. It does appear that youth are more likely to sustain AA attendance if other adolescents are in attendance and if youth perceive more similarity to other group members (Vik et al., 1997).

System-Oriented Approaches

Unlike the limited study of 12-step approaches, system-oriented interventions have been the most widely evaluated treatments for adolescent substance abuse problems. Family-oriented approaches were originally developed to treat behavioral problems (e.g., conduct disorder) in youth but showed such promising results that they were applied to substance use problems in adolescents (Liddle & Dakof, 1995). Current family-based approaches are multidimensional in nature, including all family members and, when appropriate, peers (Liddle, 1995). The fundamental assumptions in system-oriented approaches are that dysfunctional relationships between adolescents and their family may result in the initiation and maintenance of substance use problems. The focus of family therapy is to identify and change negative interactions between family members, to improve communication between members, and to learn effective problem-solving skills to address areas of conflict.

Early studies examining the efficacy of family therapy for the treatment of adolescent substance abuse found significant reductions in substance use and problem behaviors in addition to overall improved family functioning at 6- and 12- month follow-ups (Szapocznik, Kurtines, Foote, Perez-Vidal, & Hervis, 1986; Szapocznik, Kurtines, & Hervis, 1983). More recently, family therapy for adolescent substance abuse has been compared to several other available treatments. For example, family-based therapy was associated with more positive substance use outcomes than peer group therapy (Joanning, Quinn, Thomas, & Mullen, 1992) or parent education (Joanning et al., 1992; Lewis, Piercy, Sprenkle, & Trepper, 1990).

Another systems oriented approach that has demonstrated efficacy for treating adolescents with substance use disorder is multisystemic therapy (MST). Pickrel and Henggeler (1996) describe MST's capacity to address multiple determinants of clinical problems with ecological validity. MST interventions are intensive and target family, peer, school, and community systems. MST has been especially effective in the treatment of SUDs among delinquent adolescents (Henggeler, 1998; Pickrel & Henggeler, 1996). Recently, Randall, Henggeler, Cunningham, Rowland, and Swenson (2001) implemented MST with a community reinforcement approach to more effectively treat adolescent substance abuse.

Brief Interventions

Brief interventions range in duration anywhere from a single session lasting a few minutes to five sessions (Bien, Miller, & Tonigan, 1993). Brief interventions are low intensity and consist of providing feedback, encouraging acceptance of responsibility for change, and providing a menu of change options. Brief interventions are conducted by using motivational interviewing techniques such as empathic understanding, reflective listening, and optimism toward the possibility of change (Colby, Lee, Lewis-Esquerre, Esposito, & Monti, 2004; Winters, 1999). Because adolescents are often poorly motivated for substance abuse treatment, a brief, motivationally based intervention may result in less resistance (Myers, Brown, Tate, Abrantes, & Tomlinson, 2001). In addition, brief interventions are less expensive than other substance abuse treatments and can be implemented across a variety of settings including, primary care, emergency rooms, and schools.

Although a fair amount of research on the utility of brief interventions to treat alcohol and drug abuse has been conducted with adult populations, much less has been conducted with adolescents. Recent efforts to study the efficacy of brief interventions among substance-abusing adolescent have demonstrated promising results. For example, Monti and colleagues (1999) found that a motivational, brief alcohol intervention conducted in a hospital emergency room was associated with decreased alcohol-related problems. Similarly, in a primary care setting, Breslin, Sdao-Jarvie, and Pearlman (1998) demonstrated that a brief cognitive-behavioral outpatient intervention for youth was effective in motivating behavioral change in substance involvement. In addition, D'Amico and Fromme (2002) found that a 50-minute risk skills training program (RSTP) conducted in a high school setting was associated with decreased drinking and driving after drinking. Tubman, Wagner, Gil, and Pate (2002) developed a guided self-change brief motivational intervention for substance abuse among delinquent adolescents that focuses on skill building to help youth understand their use and identify supports and barriers to substance use reduction attempts.

Cognitive-Behavioral Therapy

Cognitive-behavioral therapy (CBT) for substance use problems is based on the premises that substance use is conditioned behavior that plays a functional role in an individual's life and is influenced by social and cognitive factors (Deas & Thomas, 2001). In CBT, high-risk situations (i.e., triggers for substance use) are identified and alternative responses (i.e., coping strategies) to handle these situations are developed. The alternative coping strategies skill building can be both behavioral (e.g., avoiding substance-using peers and participating in substance-free activities) and cognitive (e.g., changing maladaptive beliefs about substance use and utilizing images to moderate affect).

In a controlled study, Kaminer, Burleson, Blitz, Sussman, and Rounsaville (1998) compared the efficacy of CBT to interactional group therapy among adolescent substance abusers with concomitant psychiatric disorders. They predicted that CBT would be more efficacious for adolescents with comorbid externalizing disorders whereas those with internalizing disorder would display better substance use outcomes in the interactional group. Although this matching hypothesis was not supported, they found that CBT, regardless of comorbid disorder, was associated with less severe substance use 3 months later than the interactional group. In addition, the CBT group showed trends for improvements in family functioning, peer relationships, legal problems, and psychiatric functioning. Recent studies have combined CBT with family therapy and found improved substance use outcomes when compared to CBT alone (Waldron, Slesnick, Brody, & Peterson, 2001).

Therapeutic Communities

Therapeutic communities are residential programs with lengths of stay from 6 months to 1 year. These types of programs have historically treated the most severe adolescent substance abusers with significant behavioral difficulties, including conduct and oppositional behaviors, and have often treated youth mandated to attend by the legal system. The therapeutic community (i.e., residents and staff) serves as therapists in the treatment process and operates within a highly structured program where residents are involved in both group therapy and chores necessary to maintain the facility (Winters, 1999). There are a limited number of studies that have examined the efficacy of therapeutic communities in the treatment of adolescent substance abuse problems. Jainchill, Hawke, DeLeon, and Yagelka (2000) reported a study of 485 adolescents in therapeutic communities and found that 31% completed the program, 52% dropped out, and the rest were terminated. Those who completed the program showed significantly better substance use outcomes and reductions in criminal activity than dropouts or those terminated.

Pharmacotherapy

Efficacy trials of pharmacological agents for the treatment of substance use disorders or co-occuring mental health problems is in its infancy in adolescents (Solhkhah & Wilens, 1998). Kaminer (1995) highlights the concerns associated with treating substance-abusing ad-

olescents with pharmacotherapy, including developmental risks, uncertainty of long-term consequences, potential for abuse of medications, stigma associated with medicating children and adolescents, issues of consent, and lack of knowledge about the pharmacokinetic properties of certain medications. Despite the limited research and unknown compliance, medications are commonly prescribed for youth for reduction of craving (e.g., naltrexone), substitution therapy (e.g., nicotine gum and methadone), aversive therapy (e.g., Antabuse), and treatment for comorbid psychiatric condition such as depression or attention-deficit/hyperactivity disorder (ADHD) (Brown, 2001; Bukstein, 1995; Solhkhah & Wilens, 1998).

Recent studies of pharmacotherapy have demonstrated efficacy for treatment of substance use problems among adolescents with psychiatric comorbidity. For example, Cornelius and colleagues (2001) evaluated the efficacy of fluoxetine for treating substance-abusing adolescents with concomitant major depression. They found significant reductions in both depressive symptoms and quantity and frequency of alcohol use after 12 weeks. Also, a study examining the effects of buproprion for adolescents with comorbid ADHD and SUDs demonstrated reductions in both ADHD symptoms and substance involvement (Riggs, Leon, Mikulich, & Pottle, 1998). However, when considering the clinical utility of psychopharmacological agents in treating adolescents, issues of medication compliance are salient. One study found that 25% of alcohol-abusing adolescents were noncompliant with taking their prescribed medication (Wilens et al., 1997). Future research will be necessary to identify predictors of medication noncompliance among adolescents along with strategies to facilitate compliance within a developmental framework.

Self-Change

While substantial proportions of adults can successfully change problematic alcohol and other substance consumption use without formal treatment, the self-change process among adolescent populations has received limited investigation (Brown, 2001). In a recent study, Brown and colleagues reported that approximately half of adolescent problem drinkers were able to resolve their excessive drinking and alcohol-related problems for a 2-year period without receiving any formal treatment (Wagner, Brown, Monti, Myers, & Waldron, 1999). In addition, 25% of current drinkers reported that they had made a personal attempt to stop or cut down their drinking. In several samples, youth have been found to report efforts to change (Brown, 2001; Wagner et al., 1999) and demonstrated changes in substance involvement (Stice et al., 1998). For example, Stice and colleagues (1998) prospectively studied a group of adolescent drinkers and found that 20% of drinkers reduced their drinking over the school year. Similarly, 21% of drug users stopped drug use. In another high school sample, heavy drinking (five or more drinks per occasion) has been shown prospectively to remit for 17% of high school students each year (D'Amico & Fromme, 2002).

S. A. Brown (2001) developed a motivational enhancement-focused secondary intervention, (i.e., Project Options) designed to facilitate interest in reducing and/or stopping substance involvement among high school students. The theoretical underpinnings are derived from social-cognitive learning theory (Bandura, 1986) and information-processing principles. Project Options targets prevalent concerns of youth while providing practical information, resources, and socially acceptable behavioral strategies for adolescents motivated to make changes in their use of substances. Interested students self-select to participate in the secondary prevention through one or more adolescent-preferred formats (i.e., group discussion, individual sessions, or interactive website).

Treatment Outcome

Although the study of treatment outcome of substance abusers adolescents has lagged considerably behind that of adult substance abuse treatment outcome research (Brown, 1993; Winters, 1999) substantial advances have been made in the last decade. There exists a great deal of descriptive work on the approaches to treating adolescents but a limited number of studies that have empirically tested distinct treatment models. Many studies that have rigorously evaluated the effectiveness of specific interventions are limited by methodological problems such as small sample sizes and lack of randomized assignment (Muck et al., 2001; Williams & Chang, 2000). Therefore, although

research in this area is expanding, efficacious, well-specified, and innovative treatment approaches to address adolescent substance use and abuse are sorely needed.

In several reviews of adolescent substance abuse treatment outcome studies, youth receiving treatment show significant reductions in substance use and problems in other life areas (e.g., Chung et al., 2003; Grella, Hser, Joshi, & Rounds-Bryant, 2001; Tomlinson, Abrantes & Brown, 2004). Relapses often occur early after treatment, and between 20 and 32% of adolescents remain abstinent for 1 year. Completion of treatment programs, lower pretreatment substance use severity, peer/parent social support, lack of psychiatric comorbidity, and participation in aftercare/12-step groups are associated with positive substance use outcomes among adolescents (e.g., Brown, 1999; Grella et al., 2001). Due to limitations in methodology of many studies, it is not clear whether one treatment modality is better than any other, although family therapy above or in conjunction with other modalities appears to be superior to other therapeutic approaches in treating substance use problems among adolescents (Williams & Chang, 2000).

Several important factors influence the way treatment outcome studies are conducted among adolescents. First, although a substantial number of adolescents experience substance use problems and possess concerns about their use, very few will seek help (e.g., Brown, 1999; Johnson, Stiffman, Hadley-Ives, & Elze, 2001) and many substance-abusing youth who receive treatment do so in systems not primarily focusing on substance abuse (e.g., juvenile justice and mental health; Aarons et al., 2001). Though little is known about adolescent choices regarding substance abuse treatment services, youth may be resistant to seeking treatment for substance use–related problems because of lack of knowledge about available programs, fears of confidentiality, embarrassment, and worries about provider confidence (Brown, 2001). As a result, multiple options or choices may increase the likelihood of service utilization and be a more effective approach for engaging youth (Brown, 2001). Similarly, a significant problem among adolescents receiving services for substance use problems is treatment retention. This has been hypothesized to be related to low adolescent motivation for treatment and family barriers (Colby et al., 2004). Some youth intervention researchers purport that treatments that focus on retention (e.g., MST) have the greatest likelihood for long-term behavioral changes (e.g., Henggeler, 1998).

Second, whether adolescents are treated in a group or individually may influence outcomes. For example, Dishion, McCord, and Poulin (1999) have reported that peer-group interventions can result in iatrogenic effects such as increases in adolescent problem behavior and negative life outcomes in adulthood. However, other work has found that adolescents prefer group formats to discuss problems related to drinking and drug use (Brown, 2001; O'Leary et al., 2002). Therefore, future work is necessary to identify under which conditions adolescents should and should not be treated in group formats. Another important consideration in treating substance use disorders among adolescents is comorbid psychopathology. As mentioned previously, psychiatric comorbidity complicates the clinical presentation of adolescent substance abusers. Concomitant psychopathology among substance-abusing adolescents is associated with worse treatment outcomes such as earlier relapse and greater frequency of use in the follow-up period (Grella et al., 2001; Tomlinson et al., 2004). Tailored, integrated interventions designed to address both substance use and mental health problems among youth need to be developed and studied.

PREVENTION

Given that substance abuse among youth is considered a major public health concern, prevention efforts have received increased attention over the last several decades. Prevention programs vary according to their target population. For example, universal prevention programs are aimed at all youth, regardless of level of substance involvement. By contrast, selective prevention programs focus on youth who are at higher risk for early substance involvement or progression to substance use disorder. Indicated prevention efforts are designed for youth who have begun to express substance use problems but have not demonstrated a persistent pattern of abuse requiring treatment. However, there is recent evidence that suggests that a universal drug abuse prevention approach may also be effective for youth at high risk for early substance use initiation (Griffin, Botvin, Nichols, & Doyle, 2003).

The most common types of programs developed for preventing substance abuse among youth have been universal, school-based programs. The prevention approaches in school settings have been categorized as (1) information dissemination approaches, (2) affective education approaches, (3) social influences approaches, and (4) social influence and competence enhancement approaches (Botvin, Botvin, & Ruchlin, 1998). Information dissemination approaches consist of providing education about the consequences of substance use with intent of producing fear about using substances. The affective education approach focuses on building self-esteem, personal insight, and self-awareness in order to decrease risk for substance involvement (Botvin et al., 1998). There has been very little evidence that either of these two approaches is effective in reducing the risk for substance involvement among adolescents (Botvin et al., 1998; Cuijpers, 2002). Botvin (2000) argues that these approaches have not been effective because they have not taken into account the heterogeneity of substance users and multiple, etiological pathways to substance involvement.

Social influence approaches have received empirical support as effective for the prevention of substance use among youth (Tobler et al., 2000). Social influence approaches are based on social-cognitive learning theory (Bandura, 1986), which posits that social factors are highly influential in the initiation of substance involvement for youth. Social influence approaches consist of "psychological inoculation" (i.e., exposure to initially weak prosmoking messages with gradual increase to stronger prosmoking messages), correcting normative expectations about actual rates of peer use, and resistance skills training. In addition, social influences approaches in combination with competence enhancement consist of learning general life skills such as assertiveness, communication skills, social skills, problem-solving capabilities, and coping strategies to deal with anxiety and stress. Competence enhancement is conducted using such techniques as instruction, feedback, reinforcement, and behavioral rehearsal (Botvin et al., 1998). Although, a significant concern about school-based prevention programs is lack of evidence of their long-term efficacy, Botvin, Baker, Dusenbury, Botvin, and Diaz (1995) demonstrated reductions in alcohol, marijuana, and tobacco use 6 years after participation in this type of prevention program (e.g., life-skills training).

In a comprehensive review of the school-based prevention literature, Cuijpers (2002) outlined a set of criteria for effective drug abuse prevention programs. Programs that implemented interactive (e.g., exchange of ideas between participants and practicing drug refusal skills) versus noninteractive (e.g., instructional) delivery methods were more effective in reducing rates of substance initiation. Programs incorporating the social influences approach and with a focus on norms, personal commitment, and intention not to use were most effective. In addition, adding community-level components to interventions and life-skills training may strengthen the effects of the prevention programs. Finally, the utilization of peer leaders rather than adult leaders results in greater short-term effects. While Cuijpers (2002) concluded there was not sufficient evidence to support the use of booster sessions, future studies will be necessary to determine whether they can significantly contribute to the long-term efficacy of programs.

While considerable progress has been achieved in the development of effective school-based prevention programs (e.g., Project Alert—Ellickson, Bell, & Harrison, 1993; Project Northland—Perry et al., 1996), there have also been attempts to build on this work by extending the social environment beyond school and into the home, mass media, and the community (Flay, 2000). For example, studies that have included parent training components within classroom prevention programs have demonstrated positive effects on substance use (Battistich, Schaps, Watson, & Solomon, 1996; Hawkins, Catalano, Kosterman, Abbott, & Hill, 1999). In addition, in a study conducted by Flynn and colleagues (1994), a mass media campaign consisting of counteracting perceived smoking norms, pros and cons of smoking, and how to refuse a cigarette was related to 35% less smoking than a school prevention program alone. The Midwestern Prevention Project (MPP, also known as Project STAR; Pentz et al., 1989) is a comprehensive prevention program that included school, media, parent, community organizing, and health policy components designed to target the gateway substances of cigarette, alcohol, and marijuana use. The MPP project has demonstrated efficacious outcomes with significantly lower rates of substance involvement than comparison students

(Johnson et al., 1990). In addition, in a meta-analysis conducted by Tobler and Stratton (1997), MPP was associated with much higher effect sizes than those with only school-based programs.

CURRENT NEEDS AND FUTURE DIRECTIONS

Substance involvement among adolescents continues to be a significant public health concern. Although experimentation with tobacco, alcohol, and marijuana may not be uncommon during the second decade of life, other substance involvement among adolescents has been associated with significant psychosocial and neurocognitive impairments and predictive of poorer adult functioning. Although considerable strides have been made in the understanding of unique features of substance use problems in adolescence, a great need for research on developmentally appropriate assessment, treatment, and prevention efforts remains.

Research focusing on enhanced validity of assessment instrumentation and procedures is needed. Incorporation of both continuous and dichotomous measures of use, identification of substance-related problems across multiple adolescent-specific life domains, examination of corroborating sources of information, and consideration of the influence of concomitant psychiatric symptoms on the presentation of substance use problems of youth would aid the development of the field. Furthermore, the reliability and validity of screening and assessment instruments is needed for specific cultural and ethnic groups.

Although several empirically validated preventions and interventions for adolescent substance use exist, considerable treatment-related research is needed for adolescent substance abusers. For example, innovative techniques for improving access to treatment, engagement in treatment retention, and the development of efficacious approaches for addressing concomitant mental health problems are critical areas of future study. In addition, consideration should be given to the public health perspective on sequential treatment goals. For example, programs designed to interest youth or address substance-related problems (rather than use) may increase rates of treatment engagement and retention and serve as platforms for subsequent abstention efforts.

REFERENCES

Aarons, G. A., Brown, S. A., Coe, M. T., Myers, M. G., Garland, A. F., Ezzet-Lofstram, R., et al. (1999). Adolescent alcohol and drug abuse and health. *Journal of Adolescent Health, 24,* 412–421.

Aarons, G. A., Brown, S. A., Hough, R. L., Garland, A. F., & Wood, P. A. (2001). Prevalence of adolescent substance use disorders across five sectors of care. *Journal of the American Academy of Child and Adolescent Psychiatry, 40,* 419–426.

Abrantes, A. M., Brown, S. A., & Tomlinson, K. L. (2004). Psychiatric comorbidity among inpatient substance-abusing adolescents. *Journal of Child and Adolescent Substance Abuse, 13,*(2), 83–101.

Abrantes, A. M., McCarthy, D. M., Aarons, G. A., & Brown, S. A. (2002). *Trajectories of alcohol involvement following addiction treatment through 8–year follow-up in adolescents.* Paper presented in a symposium at the 25th annual scientific meeting of the Research Society for Alcoholism, San Francisco.

Ajzen, I. (1988). *Attitudes, personality, and behavior.* Homewood, IL: Dorsey Press.

Ajzen, I., & Fishbein, M. (1980). *Understanding attitudes and predicting social behavior.* Englewood Cliffs, NJ: Prentice-Hall.

Akers, R. L. (1977). *Deviant behavior: A social learning approach* (2nd ed.). Belmont, CA: Wadsworth.

American Psychiatric Association. (2000). *Diagnostic and statistical manual of mental disorders* (4th ed., text rev.). Washington, DC: Author.

Angold, A., Costello, E. J., Farmer, E., Burns, B. J., & Erkanli, A. (1999). Impaired but undiagnosed. *Journal of the American Academy of Child and Adolescent Psychiatry, 38,* 129–137.

Armstrong, T. D., & Costello, E. J. (2002). Community studies on adolescent substance use, abuse, or dependence and psychiatric comorbidity. *Journal of Consulting and Clinical Psychology, 70,* 1224–1239.

Baker, J. R., & Yardley, J. K. (2002). Moderating effect of gender on the relationship between sensation seeking-impulsivity and substance use in adolescents. *Journal of Child and Adolescent Substance Abuse, 12,* 27–43.

Bandura, A. (1986). *Social foundations of thought and action: A social cognitive theory.* Englewood Cliffs, NJ: Prentice Hall.

Barnes, G. M., Farrell, M. P., & Banerjee, S. (1994). Family influence on alcohol abuse and other problem behaviors among black and white adolescents in a general population sample. *Journal of Research on Adolescence, 4,* 183–201.

Bates, M. E., & Labouvie, E. W. (1995). Personality–environment constellation and alcohol use: A process-oriented study of intraindividual change during adolescence. *Psychology of Addictive Behaviors, 9,* 23–35.

Battistich, V., Schaps, E., Watson, M., & Solomon, D. (1996). Prevention effects of the Child Development Project: Early findings from an ongoing multisite demonstration trial. *Journal of Adolescent Research, 11,* 12–35.

Bien, T. H., Miller, W. R., & Tonigan, J. S. (1993). Brief interventions for alcohol problems: A review. *Addiction, 88,* 315–336.

Bird, H. R., Gould, M. S., & Staghezza, B. (1992). Aggregating data from multiple informants in child psychology epidemiological research. *Journal of the American Academy of Child and Adolescent Psychiatry, 31,* 78–85.

Botvin, G. J. (2000). Preventing drug abuse in schools: Social and competence enhancement approaches targeting individual-level etiological factors. *Addictive Behaviors, 25,* 887–897.

Botvin, G. J., Baker, E., Dusenbury, L., Botvin, E. M., & Diaz, T. (1995). Long-term follow-up results of a randomized drug abuse prevention trial in a white middle-class population. *Journal of the American Medical Association, 273,* 1106–1112.

Botvin, G. J., Botvin, E. M., & Ruchlin, H. (1998). School-based approaches to drug abuse prevention: Evidence for effectiveness and suggestions for determining cost-effectiveness. In W. J. Bukoski & R. I. Evans (Eds.), *Cost–benefit/cost-effectiveness research of drug prevention. Implication for programming and policy* (NIDA Research Monograph, 176, NIH Publication No. 98-4021, pp 59–82). Rockville, MD: National Institute on Drug Abuse.

Breslin, C., Sdao-Jarvie, K., & Pearlman, S. (1998). *Brief treatment for youth* (3rd ed.). Toronto, ON, Canada: Center for Addiction and Mental Health, Addiction Research Foundation.

Brody, G. H., & Forehand, R. (1993). Prospective associations among family form, family process, and adolescents' alcohol and drug use. *Behaviour Research, and Therapy, 31,* 587–593.

Brooks, T. L., Woods, E. R., Knight, J. R., & Shrier, L. A. (2003). Body modification and substance use in adolescents: Is there a link? *Journal of Adolescent Health, 32,* 44–49.

Brown, S. A. (1989). Life events of adolescents in relation to personal and parental substance abuse. *American Journal of Psychiatry, 146,* 484–489.

Brown, S. A. (1993). Drug effect expectancies and addictive behavior change. *Experimental and Clinical Psychopharmacology, 1,* 55–67.

Brown, S. A. (1999). Treatment of adolescent alcohol problems: Research review and appraisal. In National Institute on Alcohol Abuse and Alcoholism Extramural Scientific Advisory Board (Ed.), *Treatment* (pp. 1–26). Bethesda, MD: National Institute on Alcohol Abuse and Alcoholism.

Brown, S. A. (2001). Facilitating change for adolescent alcohol problems: A multiple options approach. In E. F. Wagner & H. B. Waldron (Eds.), *Innovations in adolescent substance abuse interventions* (pp. 169–187). Oxford, UK: Elsevier Science.

Brown, S. A., Aarons, G. A., & Abrantes, A. M. (2001). Adolescent alcohol and drug abuse. In C. E. Walker & M. C. Roberts (Eds.), *Handbook of clinical child psychology* (3rd ed., pp. 757–775). New York: Wiley.

Brown, S. A., Creamer, V. A., & Stetson, B. A. (1987). Adolescent alcohol expectancies in relation to personal and parental drinking patterns. *Journal of Abnormal Psychology, 96,* 117–121.

Brown, S. A., Gleghorn, A., Schuckit, M. A., Myers, M. G., & Mott, M. A. (1996). Conduct disorder among adolescent alcohol and drug abusers. *Journal of Studies on Alcohol, 57,* 314–324.

Brown, S. A., Inaba, R. K., Gillin, J. C., Schuckit, M. A., Stewart, M. A., & Irwin, M. R. (1995). Alcoholism and affective disorder: Clinical course of depressive symptoms. *American Journal of Psychiatry, 152,* 45–52.

Brown, S. A., Irwin, M., & Schuckit, M. A. (1991). Changes in anxiety among abstinent male alcoholics. *Journal of Studies on Alcohol, 52,* 55–61.

Brown, S. A., Mott, M. A., & Myers, M. G. (1990). Adolescent alcohol and drug treatment outcome. In R. R. Watson (Ed.), *Drug and alcohol abuse prevention* (pp. 373–403). Totowa, NJ: Humana.

Brown, S. A., Mott, M. A., & Stewart, M. A. (1992). Adolescent alcohol and drug abuse. In C. E. Walker & M. C. Roberts (Eds.), *Handbook of clinical child psychology* (2nd ed., pp 677–693). New York: Wiley.

Brown, S. A., Myers, M. G., Lippke, L., Tapert, S. F., Stewart, D., & Vik, P. (1998). Psychometric evaluation of the Customary Drinking and Drug Use Record (CDDR): A measure of adolescent alcohol and drug involvement. *Journal of Studies on Alcohol, 59,* 427–438.

Brown, S. A., & Schuckit, M. A. (1988). Changes in depression among abstinent alcoholics. *Journal of Studies on Alcohol, 49,* 412–417.

Brown, S. A., & Tapert, S. F. (2004). Health consequences of adolescent alcohol involvement. In *Reducing underage drinking: A collective responsibility* (pp. 383–401). Washington, DC: National Academy Press.

Brown, R. A., Ramsey, S. E., Strong, D. R., & Sales, S. D. (2000). *Cigarette smoking among adolescent psychiatric inpatients.* Arlington, VA: Society for Research on Nicotine and Tobacco.

Brown, T. N., Schulenberg, J., Bachman, J. G., O'Malley, P. M., & Johnston, L. D. (2001). Are risk and protective factors for substance use consistent across historical time?: National data from the high school classes of 1976 through 1997. *Prevention Science, 2,* 29–43.

Bryant, A. L., & Zimmerman, M. A. (2002). Examining the effects of academic beliefs and behaviors on changes in substance use among urban adolescents. *Journal of Educational Psychology, 94,* 621–637.

Bryant, K. J., Rounsaville, B., Spitzer, R. L., & Williams, J. B. (1992). Reliability of dual diagnosis: Substance dependent and psychiatric disorders. *Journal of Nervous and Mental Disorders, 180,* 251–257.

Bukstein, O. (1994). Treatment of adolescent alcohol abuse and dependence. *Alcohol Health and Research World, 18,* 296–301.

Bukstein, O. (1995). *Adolescent substance abuse: Assessment, prevention, and treatment.* New York: Wiley.

Bukstein, O. G., Brent, D. A., & Kaminer, Y. (1989). Comorbidity of substance abuse and other psychiatric disorders in adolescents. *American Journal of Psychiatry, 146*(9), 1131–1141.

Cadoret, R. J., Yates, W. R., Troughton, E., Woodworth, G., & Stewart, M. A. (1995). Adoption study demonstrating two genetic pathways to drug abuse. *Archives of General Psychiatry, 52,* 42–52.

Cantwell, D., Lewinsohn, P. M., Rohde, P., & Seeley, J. (1997). Correspondence between adolescent report and parent report of psychiatric diagnostic data. *Journal of the American Academy of Child and Adolescent Psychiatry, 36*(5), 610–620.

Carey, K. B., & Correia, C. J. (1998). Severe mental illness and addictions: Assessment considerations. *Addictive Behaviors, 23*(6), 735–748.

Chassin, L. (1984). Adolescent substance use and abuse. *Advances in Child Behavioral Analysis and Therapy, 3,* 99–152.

Chassin, L., Pillow, D. R., Curran, P. J., Molina, B. S., & Barrera, M. (1993). Relation of parental alcoholism to early adolescent substance use: A test of three mediating mechanisms. *Journal of Abnormal Psychology, 102,* 3–19.

Chassin, L., & Ritter, J. (2001). Vulnerability to substance use disorders in childhood and adolescence. In R. E. Ingram & J. M. Price (Eds.), *Vulnerability to psychopathology: Risk across the lifespan* (pp. 107–134). New York: Guilford Press.

Chatlos, J. C. (1997). Substance use and abuse and the impact on academic difficulties. *Journal of the American Academy of Child and Adolescent Psychiatry, 6,* 545–568.

Chen, K., & Kandel, D. B. (1995). The natural history of drug use from adolescence to the mid-thirties in a general population sample. *American Journal of Public Health, 85,* 41–47.

Chen, X., Unger, J. B., Palmer, P., Weiner, M. D., Johnson, C. A., Wong, M. A., & Austin, G. (2002). Prior cigarette smoking initiation predicting current alcohol use: Evidence for a gateway drug effect among California adolescents from eleven ethnic groups. *Addictive Behaviors, 27,* 799–817.

Chilcoat, H. D., & Anthony, J. C. (1996). Impact of parent monitoring on initiation of drug use through late childhood. *Journal of the American Academy of Child and Adolescent Psychiatry, 35,* 91–100.

Chilcoat, H., & Breslau, N. (1996). Alcohol disorders in young adulthood: Effects of transitions into adult roles. *Journal of Health and Social Behavior, 37,* 339–349.

Christiansen, B. A., Smith, G. T., Roehling, P. V., & Goldman, M. S. (1989). Using alcohol expectancies to predict adolescent drinking behavior after one year. *Journal of Consulting and Clinical Psychology, 57,* 93–99.

Chung, T., Martin, C. S., Grella, C. E., Winters, K. C.,

Abrantes, A. M., & Brown, S. A. (2003). Course of alcohol problems in treated adolescents. *Alcoholism: Clinical and Experimental Research, 27*(2), 253–261.

Clark, D. B., Lynch, K. G., Donovan, J. E., & Block, G. D. (2001). Health problems in adolescents with alcohol use disorders: Self-report, liver injury, and physical examination findings and correlates. *Alcoholism: Clinical and Experimental Research, 25,* 1350–1359.

Cloninger, C. R., Sigvardsson, S., & Bohman, M. (1988). Childhood personality predicts alcohol abuse in young adults. *Alcoholism: Clinical and Experimental Research, 12,* 494–505.

Cohen, S. (1981). Cannabis: Impact on motivation, Part I. *Drug Abuse and Alcoholism Newsletter, 10,* 1–3.

Colby, S. M., Lee, C. S., Lewis-Esquerre, J., Esposito, C., & Monti, P. M. (2004). Adolescent alcohol misuse, abuse, and dependence: Methodological issues for enhancing treatment research. *Addiction, 99*(Suppl. 2), 47–62.

Colder, C., & Chassin, L. (1993). The stress and negative affect model of adolescent alcohol use and the moderating effects of behavioral undercontrol. *Journal of Studies on Alcohol, 54,* 326–333.

Colder, C., & Chassin, L. (1997). Affectivity and impulsivity: Temperamental risk for adolescent alcohol involvement. *Psychology of Addictive Behaviors, 11,* 83–87.

Comeau, N., Stewart, S. H., & Loba, P. (2001). The relations of trait anxiety, anxiety sensitivity and sensation seeking to adolescents' motivations for alcohol, cigarette, and marijuana use. *Addictive Behaviors, 26,* 803–825.

Connors, G. J., & Volk, R. J. (2003). Self-report screening for alcohol problems among adults. In J. P. Allen & V. B. Wilson (Eds.), *Assessing alcohol problems* (pp. 21–35). Bethesda, MD: National Institutes of Health.

Cooper, M. L., Frone, M., Russell, M., & Muldar, P. (1995). Drinking to regulate positive and negative emotions: A motivational model of alcohol use. *Journal of Personality and Social Psychology, 69,* 990–1005.

Cornelius, J. R., Bukstein, O. G., Birmaher, B., Salloum, I. M., Lynch, K., Pollock, N. K., et al. (2001). Fluoxetine in adolescents with major depression and an alcohol use disorder: An open-label trial. *Addictive Behaviors, 26,* 735–739.

Cornelius, J. R., Maisto, S. A., Pollock, N. K., Martin, C. S., Salloum, I. M., Lynch, K. G., & Clark, D. B. (2003). Rapid relapse generally follows treatment for substance use disorders among adolescents. *Addictive Behaviors, 28,* 381–386.

Corty, E., Lehman, A. F., & Myers, C. F. (1993). Influence of psychoactive substance use on the reliability of psychiatric diagnosis. *Journal of Consulting and Clinical Psychology, 61,* 165–170.

Cuijpers, P. (2002). Effective ingredients of school-based drug prevention programs: A systematic review. *Addictive Behaviors, 27,* 1009–1023.

D'Amico, E. J., & Fromme, K. (2002). Brief prevention for adolescents. *Addiction, 97,* 563–574.

D'Amico, E. J., Metrik, J., McCarthy, D. M., Frissell, K. C., Appelbaum, M., & Brown, S. A. (2001). Progression into and out of binge drinking among high school students. *Psychology of Addictive Behaviors, 15,* 341–349.

Dawes, M. A., Antelman, S. M., Vanyukov, M. M., Giancola, P., Tarter, R. E., Susman, E. J., et al. (2000). Developmental sources of variation in liability to adolescent substance use disorders. *Drug and Alcohol Dependence, 61,* 3–14.

Deas, D., Riggs, P., Langenbucher, J., Goldman, M., & Brown, S. (2000). Adolescents are not adults: Developmental consideration in alcohol users. *Alcoholism: Clinical and Experimental Research, 24,* 232–237.

Deas, D., & Thomas, S. E. (2001). An overview of controlled studies of adolescent substance abuse treatment. *The American Journal on Addictions, 10,* 178–189.

Deas-Nesmith, D., Campbell, S., & Brady, K. T. (1998). Substance use disorders in adolescent inpatient psychiatric population. *Journal of the National Medical Association, 90,* 233–238.

Dennis, M. L., & McGreary, K. A. (1999). Adolescent alcohol and marijuana treatment: Kids need it now. In *TIE communiqe* (pp. 10–12). Rockville, MD: Center for Substance Abuse Treatment.

Dinwiddie, S. H., & Cloninger, C. R. (1991). Family and adoption studies in alcoholism and drug addiction. *Psychiatric Annals, 21,* 206–214.

Dishion, T. J., McCord, J., & Poulin, F. (1999). Why interventions harm: Peer groups and problem behavior. *American Psychologist,* 755–764.

Donovan, J. E., & Jessor, R. (1985). Structure of problem behavior in adolescence and young adulthood. *Journal of Consulting and Clinical Psychology, 53,* 890–904.

Donovan, J. E., Jessor, R., & Costa, F. M. (1991). Adolescent health behavior and conventionality–unconventionality: An extension of problem-behavior theory. *Health Psychology, 10,* 52–61.

Ellickson, P. L., Bell, R. M., & Harrison, E. R. (1993). Changing adolescent propensities to use drugs: Results from Project ALERT. *Health Education Quarterly, 20,* 227–242.

Epstein, J. A., & Botvin, G. J. (2002). The moderating role of risk-taking tendency and refusal assertiveness on social influences in alcohol use among inner-city adolescents. *Journal of Studies on Alcohol, 63,* 456–459.

Epstein, J. A., Griffin, K. W., & Botvin, G. J. (2002). Positive impact of competence skills and psychological wellness in protecting inner-city adolescents from alcohol use. *Prevention Science, 3,* 95–104.

Fergusson, D. M., & Horwood, L. J. (1999). Prospective childhood predictors of deviant peer affiliations in adolescence. *Journal of Child Psychology and Psychiatry, 40,* 581–592.

Fergusson, D., Horwood, J., & Lynskey, M. (1995). The

prevalence and risk factors associated with abusive or hazardous alcohol consumption in 16–year-olds. *Addiction, 90,* 935–946.

Fergusson, D. M., & Lynskey, M. T. (1996). Adolescent resiliency to family adversity. *Journal of Child Psychology and Psychiatry, 37,* 281–292.

Flay, B. R. (2000). Approaches to substance use prevention utilizing school curriculum plus environmental change. *Addictive Behaviors. Special Addictions 2000: Prevention of Substance Abuse Problems: Directions for the Next Millennium, 25*(6), 861–885.

Flynn, B. S., Worden, J. K., Secker-Walker, R. H., Pirie, P. L., Badger, G. L., Carpenter, J. H., & Geller, B. M. (1994). Mass media and school interventions for cigarette smoking prevention: Effects 2 years after completion. *American Journal of Public Health, 84,* 1148–1150.

Fornazzari, L. (1990). The neurotoxicity of inhaled toluene. *Canadian Journal of Psychiatry, 35,* 723.

Giancola, P. R., & Parker, A. (2001). A six year prospective study of pathways toward drug use in adolescent boys with and without a family history of substance use disorder. *Journal of Studies on Alcohol, 62,* 166–178.

Gilvarry, E. (2000). Substance abuse in young people. *Journal of Child Psychology and Psychiatry, 41,* 55–80.

Glantz, M. D., & Leshner, A. I. (2000). Drug abuse and developmental psychopathology. *Development and Psychopathology, 12,* 795–814.

Goldman, M. S., Brown, S. A., Christiansen, B. A., & Smith, G. T. (1991). Alcoholism and memory broadening the scope of alcohol-expectancy research. *Psychological Bulletin, 110,* 137–146.

Goldman, M. S., & Rather, B. C. (1993). Substance use disorders: Cognitive models and architecture. In P. C. Kendall & K. Dobson (Eds.), *Psychopathology and cognition* (pp. 245–292). New York: Academic Press.

Gotham, H. Sher, K., & Wood, P. (1997). Predicting stability and change in frequency of intoxication from the college years to beyond: Individual difference and role transition variables. *Journal of Abnormal Psychology, 106,* 619–629.

Grant, B. F., Stinson, F. S., & Harford, T. C. (2001). Age of onset of alcohol use and DSM-IV alcohol abuse and dependence: A 12–year follow-up. *Journal of Substance Abuse, 13,* 493–504.

Greenbaum, P. E., Foster-Johnson, L., & Petrila, A. (1996). Co-occurring addictive and mental disorders among adolescents: Prevalence research and future directions. *American Journal of Orthopsychiatry, 66,* 52–60.

Grella, C. E., Hser, Y., Joshi, V., & Rounds-Bryant, J. (2001). Drug treatment outcomes for adolescents with comorbid mental and substance use disorders. *Journal of Nervous and Mental Disease, 189,* 384–392.

Grella, C. E., & Joshi, V. (2003). Treatment processes and outcomes among adolescents with a history of abuse who are in drug treatment. *Child Maltreatment: Journal of the American Professional Society on the Abuse of Children, 8,* 7–18.

Griffin, K. W., Botvin, G. J., Nichols, T. R., & Doyle, M. M. (2003). Effectiveness of a universal drug abuse prevention approach for youth at high risk for substance use initiation. *Prevention Medicine, 36,* 1–7.

Grilo, C. M., Becker, D. F., Walker, M. L., Levy, K. N., Edell, W. S., & McGlashan, T. H. (1995). Psychiatric comorbidity in adolescent inpatients with substance use disorder. *Journal of the American Academy of Child and Adolescent Psychiatry, 34*(8), 1085–1091.

Harrison, P. A., Fulkerson, J. A., & Beebe, T. J. (1998). DSM-IV substance use disorder criteria for adolescents: A critical examination based on statewide school survey. *American Journal of Psychiatry, 155,* 486–492.

Hawkins, J. D., Catalano, R. F., Kosterman, R., Abbott, R., & Hill, K. G. (1999). Preventing adolescent health-risk behaviors by strengthening protection during childhood. *Archives of Pediatrics and Adolescent Medicine, 153,* 226–234.

Henggeler, S. W. (1998). *Multisystemic therapy.* Denver, CO: C&M Press.

Huba, G. J., Wingard, J. A., & Bentler, P. M. (1980). Framework for an interactive theory of drug use. *NIDA Research Monograph, 30,* 95–101.

Jainchill, N., Hawke, J., DeLeon, G., & Yagelka, J. (2000). Adolescents in therapeutic communities: one-year posttreatment outcomes. *Journal of Psychoactive Drugs, 32,* 81–94.

Jessor, R., & Jessor, S. L. (1977). *Problem behavior and psychosocial development.* New York: Academic Press.

Joanning, H., Quinn, W., Thomas, F., & Mullen, R. (1992). Treating adolescent drug abuse: A comparison of family systems therapy, group therapy, and family drug education. *Journal of Marital and Family Therapy, 18,* 345–356.

Johnson, C. A., Pentz, M. A., Weber, M. D., Dwyer, J. H., Baer, N., MacKinnon, D. P., et al. (1990). Relative effectiveness of comprehensive community programming for drug abuse prevention with high-risk and low-risk adolescents. *Journal of Consulting and Clinical Psychology, 58,* 447–456.

Johnson, P. B., & Richter, L. (2002). The relationship between smoking, drinking, and adolescents' self-perceived health and frequency of hospitalization: Analyses from the 1997 National Household Survey on Drug Abuse. *Journal of Adolescent Health, 30,* 175–183.

Johnson, S. D., Stiffman, A., Hadley-Ives, E., & Elze, D. (2001). An analysis of stressors and co-morbid mental health problems that contribute to youth's paths to substance-specific services. *Journal of Behavioral Health Services Research, 28,* 412–426.

Johnston, L. D., O'Malley, P. M., & Bachman, J. (2002). *Monitoring the Future national results on adolescent drug use: Overview of key findings, 2001* (NIH Publication No. 02-5105). Bethesda, MD: National Institute on Drug Abuse.

Kaminer, Y. (1994). *Adolescent substance abuse: A comprehensive guide to theory and practice.* New York: Plenum Press.

Kaminer, Y. (1995). Issues in the pharmacological treatment of adolescent substance abuse. *Journal of Child and Adolescent Psychopharmacology, 5,* 93–106.

Kaminer, Y., Burleson, J., Blitz, C., Sussman, J., & Rounsaville, B. J. (1998). Psychotherapies for adolescent substance abusers: A pilot study. *Journal of Nervous and Mental Disease, 186,* 684–690.

Kaminer, Y., Wagner, E., Plummer, B., & Seifer, R. (1993). Validation of the Teen Addiction Severity Index (T-ASI). *The American Journal on Addictions, 2,* 250–254.

Kandel, D. B., Davies, M., Karus, D., & Yamaguchi, K. (1986). The consequences in young adulthood of adolescent drug involvement. *Archives of General Psychiatry, 43,* 746754.

Kandel, D. B., Johnson, J. G., Bird, H. R., Canino, G., Goodman, S. H., Lahey, B. B., et al. (1997). Psychiatric disorders associated with substance use among children and adolescents: Findings from the Methods for the Epidemiology of Child and Adolescent Mental Disorders (MECA) study. *Journal of Abnormal Child Psychology, 25,* 121–132.

Kandel, D. B., Johnson, J. G., Bird, H. R., Weissman, M. M., Goodman, S. H., Lahey, B. B., et al. (1999). Psychiatric comorbidity among adolescents with substance use disorders: Findings from the MECA study. *Journal of the American Academy of Child and Adolescent Psychiatry, 38,* 693–699.

Kandel, D. B., & Yamaguchi, K. (1993). From beer to crack: Developmental patterns of drug involvement. *American Journal of Public Health, 83,* 851–855.

Kandel, D. B., Yamaguchi, K., & Chen, K. (1992). Stages of progression in drug involvement from adolescence to adulthood: Further evidence for the gateway theory. *Journal of Studies on Alcohol, 53,* 447–457.

Kelly, J. F., Myers, M. G., & Brown, S. A. (2000). A multivariate process model of adolescent 12–step attendance and substance use outcome following inpatient treatment. *Psychology of Addictive Behaviors, 14,* 376–389.

Kirisci, L., Mezzich, A., & Tarter, R. (1995). Norms and sensitivity of the adolescent version of the Drug Use Screening Inventory. *Addictive Behaviors, 20,* 149–157.

Knop, J., Teasdale, T. W., Schulsinger, F., & Goodwin, D. W. (1985). A prospective study of young men at high risk for alcoholism: School behavior and achievement. *Journal of Studies on Alcohol, 46,* 273–278.

Kuo, P. H., Yang, H. J., Soong, W. T., & Chen, W. J. (2002). Substance use among adolescents in Taiwan: Associated personality traits, incompetence, and behavioral/emotional problems. *Drug and Alcohol Dependence, 67,* 27–39.

Kypri, K., McCarthy, D. M., Coe, M. T., & Brown, S. A. (2004). Transition to independent living and substance involvement of treated and high-risk youth. *Journal of Child and Adolescent Substance Abuse, 13,* 85–100.

Leccese, M., & Waldron, H. B. (1994). Assessing adolescent substance use: A critique of current measurement instruments. *Journal of Substance Abuse Treatment, 11,* 553–563.

Lewinsohn, P. M., Rohde, P., & Seeley, J. R. (1995). Adolescent psychopathology: III. The clinical consequences of comorbidity. *Journal of the American Academy of Child and Adolescent Psychiatry, 34,* 510–519.

Lewinsohn, P. M., Solomon, A., Seeley, J. R., & Zeiss, A. (2000). Clinical implications of "subthreshold" depressive symptoms. *Journal of Abnormal Psychology, 109,* 345–351.

Lewis, R. A., Piercy, F. P., Sprenke, D. H., & Trepper, T. S. (1990). Family-based interventions for helping drug abusing adolescents. *Journal of Adolescent Research, 50,* 82–95.

Liddle, H. A. (1995). Conceptual and clinical dimensions of a multidimensional, multisystems engagement strategy in family-based adolescent treatment. *Psychotherapy, Research, and Practice, 32,* 39–58.

Liddle, H. A., & Dakof, G. A. (1995). Family-based treatment for adolescent drug use: State of the science. In E. R. D. Czechowicz (Ed.), *Adolescent drug abuse: Clinical assessment and therapeutic interventions* (NIH Publication No. 95-3908). Rockville, MD: National Institute on Drug Abuse.

Loukas, A., Zucker, R. A., Fitzgerald, H. E., & Krull, J. L. (2003). Developmental trajectories of disruptive behavior problems among sons of alcoholics effects of parent psychopathology, family conflict, and child undercontrol. *Journal of Abnormal Psychology, 112,* 119–131.

Maruff, P., Burns, C. B., Tyler, P., Currie, B. J., & Currie, J. (1998). Neurological and cognitive abnormalities associated with chronic petrol sniffing. *Brain, 121,* 1903–1917.

McCarthy, D. M., Brown, S. A., Carr, L. G., & Wall, T. L. (2001). ALDH2 Status, alcohol expectancies and alcohol response: Preliminary evidence for a mediation model. *Alcoholism Clinical and Experimental Research, 25,* 11, 1558–1563.

McCubbin, H. I., Needle, R. H., & Wilson, M. (1985). Adolescent health risk behaviors: Family stress and adolescent coping as critical factors. *Family Relations, 34,* 51–62.

McGlothin, W. H., & West, L. J. (1968). The marijuana problem: An overview. *American Journal of Psychiatry, 125,* 1126–1134.

McGue, M., Slutske, W., Taylor, J., & Iacono, W. (1997). Personality and substance use disorders: I. Effects of gender and alcoholism subtype. *Alcoholism: Clinical and Experimental Research, 21,* 513–520.

Meyer, R. E. (1986). *Psychopathology and addictive disorders.* New York: Guilford Press.

Monti, P. M., Colby, S. M., Barnett, N. P., Spirito, A.,

Rohsenow, D. J., Myers, M. G., et al. (1999). Brief interventions for harm reduction with alcohol-positive older adolescents in a hospital emergency department. *Journal of Consulting and Clinical Psychology, 67,* 989–994.

Morton, H. G., (1990). Occurrence and treatment of solvent abuse in children and adolescents. In D. J. K. Balfour (Ed.), *Psychotropic drugs of abuse* (pp. 431–451). New York: Pergamon Press.

Muck, R., Zempolich, K. A., Titus, J. C., Fishman, M., Godley, M. D., & Schwebel, R. (2001). An overview of the effectiveness of adolescent substance abuse treatment models. *Youth and Society, 33,* 143–168.

Myers, M. G., & Brown, S. A. (1994). Smoking and health in substance-abusing adolescents: A two-year follow-up. *Pediatrics, 93,*561–566.

Myers, M. G., Brown, S. A., Tate, S., Abrantes, A., & Tomlinson, K. (2001). Toward brief interventions for adolescents with substance abuse and comorbid psychiatric problems. In P. M. Monti, S. M. Colby, & T. A. O'Leary (Eds.), *Adolescents, alcohol, and substance abuse: Reaching teens through brief interventions* (pp. 275–296). New York: Guilford Press.

Newcomb, M., & Bentler, P. (1988). *Consequences of teenage drug use: Impact on the lives of young adults.* Newbury Park, CA: Sage.

Newlin, D. B. (1994). Alcohol challenge in high-risk individuals. In R. Zucker, G. Boyd, & J. Howard (Eds.), *The development of alcohol problems: Exploring the biopsychosocial matrix of risk* (DHHS Publication No. ADM 94-3495, pp. 47–68). Washington, DC: U.S. Government Printing Office.

Novins, D. K., Beals, J., Shore, J. H., & Manson, S. M. (1996). Substance abuse treatment of American Indian adolescents: Comorbid symptomatology, gender differences, and treatment patterns. *Journal of the American Academy of Child and Adolescent Psychiatry, 35*(12), 1593–1601.

O'Leary, T. A., Brown, S. A., Colby, S. M., Cronce, J. M., D'Amico, E. J., Fader, J. S., et al. (2002). Treating adolescents together or individually? Issues in adolescent substance abuse interventions. *Alcoholism: Clinical and Experimental Research, 26,* 890–899.

Otto, S., Laura, L., Gore-Felton, C., McGarvey, E., & Canterbury, R. J. (2002). Psychiatric functioning and substance use: Factors associated with HIV risk among incarcerated adolescents. *Child Psychiatry and Human Development, 33,* 91–106.

Pandina, R. J., & Schuele, J. A. (1983). Psychosocial correlates of alcohol and drug use of adolescent students and adolescents in treatment. *Journal of Studies on Alcohol, 44,* 950–973.

Pentz, M. A., Dwyer, J. H., MacKinnon, D. P., Flay, B. R., Hansen, W. B., Wang, E. Y., & Johnson, A. (1989). A multicommunity trial for primary prevention of adolescent drug abuse. *Journal of the American Medical Association, 261,* 3259–3266.

Perry, C., L., Williams, C. L., Veblen-Mortenson, S., Toomey, T. L., Komro, K. A., Anstine, P. S., et al. (1996). Project Northland: Outcomes of a community wide alcohol use prevention program during early adolescence. *American Journal of Public Health, 86,* 956–965.

Petraitis, J., Flay, B. R., & Miller, T. Q. (1995). Reviewing theories of adolescent substance use: Organizing pieces of the puzzle. *Psychological Bulletin, 117,* 67–86.

Piazza, N. J. (1996). Dual diagnosis and adolescent psychiatric inpatients. *Substance Use and Misuse, 31,* 215–223.

Pickrel, S. G., & Henggeler, S. W. (1996). Multisystemic therapy for adolescent substance abuse and dependence. *Child and Adolescent Psychiatric Clinics of North America, 5,* 201–211.

Rahdert, E. R. (1991). *The adolescent assessment/referral system manual* (DHHS Publication No. ADM91-1735). Rockville, MD: National Institute on Drug Abuse.

Randall, J., Henggeler, S. W., Cunningham, P. B., Rowland, M. D., & Swenson, C. C. (2001). Adapting multisystemic therapy to treat adolescent substance abuse more effectively. *Cognitive and Behavioral Practice, 8,* 359–366.

Richter, S. S., Brown, S. A., & Mott, M. A. (1991). The impact of social support and self-esteem on adolescent substance abuse treatment outcome. *Journal of Substance Abuse, 3,* 371–385.

Riggs, P. D., Leon, S. L., Mikulich, S. K., & Pottle, L. C. (1998). An open trial of buproprion for ADHD in adolescents with substance use disorders and conduct disorder. *Journal of the American Academy of Child and Adolescent Psychiatry, 37,* 1271–1278.

Rose, R. J., Dick, D. M., Viken, R. J., & Kaprio, J. (2001). Gene-environment interaction patterns of adolescent drinking: Regional residency moderates longitudinal influences on alcohol use. *Alcoholism: Clinical and Experimental Research, 25,* 637–643.

Rose, R. J., Kaprio, J., Pulkkinen, L., Koskenvuo, M., Viken, R. J., & Bates, J. E. (1997). FinnTwin 12 and FinnTwin 16: Longitudinal twin-family studies in Finland. *Behavior Genetics, 27,* 603–604.

Sadava, S. W. (1987). Interactionist theories. In H. T. Blane & K. E. Leonard (Eds.), *Psychological theories of drinking and alcoholism* (pp. 90–130). New York: Guilford Press.

Schinke, S. P., Botvin, G. J., & Orlandi, M. A. (1991). *Substance abuse in children and adolescents: Evaluation and intervention.* Newbury Park, CA: Sage.

Schuckit, M. (1988). Reactions to alcohol in sons of alcoholics and controls. *Alcoholism: Clinical and Experimental Research, 12,* 465–470.

Schuckit, M. (2002). Vulnerability factors for alcoholism. In K. L. Davis, D. Charney, J. T. Coyle, & Nemeroff, C. (Eds.) *Neuropsychopharmacology: The fifth generation of progress* (pp. 1399–1411). New York: Lippincott Williams & Wilkins

Schuckit, M. A., Irwin, M., & Brown, S. A. (1990). The history of anxiety symptoms among 171 primary alcoholics. *Journal of Studies on Alcohol, 51,* 34–41.

Schuckit, M. A., & Smith, T. L. (2001). The clinical

course of alcohol dependence associated with a low level of response to alcohol. *Addiction, 96,* 903–910.

Shelder, J., & Block, J. (1990). Adolescent drug use and psychological health. *American Psychologist, 45,* 612–630.

Sher, K. J. (1993). Children of alcoholics and the intergenerational transmission of alcoholism: A biopsychosocial perspective. In J. S. Baer, G. A. Marlatt, & R. J. McMahon (Eds.), *Addictive behaviors across the lifespan* (pp. 3–33). Newbury Park, CA: Sage.

Sher, K. J. (1994). Individual-level risk factors. In R. Zucker, G. Boyd, & J. Howard (Eds.), *The development of alcohol problems: Exploring the biopsychosocial matrix of risk* (DHHS Publication No. ADM 94-2495, pp. 77-108). Washington, DC: U.S. Government Printing Office.

Smith, G. T., Goldman, M. S., Greenbaum, P. E., & Christiansen, B. A. (1995). Expectancy for social facilitation from drinking: The divergent paths of high-expectancy and low-expectancy adolescents. *Journal of Abnormal Psychology, 104,* 32–40.

Solhkhah, R., & Wilens, T. E. (1998). Pharmacotherapy of adolescent AOD use disorders. *Alcohol Health and Research World, 22,* 12–126.

Stewart, D. G., & Brown, S. A. (1995). Withdrawal and dependency symptoms among adolescent alcohol and drug abusers. *Addiction, 90,* 627–635.

Stice, E., Myers, M. G., & Brown, S. A. (1998). Relations to delinquency to adolescent substance use and problem use: A prospective study. *Psychology of Addictive Behaviors, 12,* 136–146.

Stowell, R. J., & Estroff, T. W. (1992). Psychiatric disorders in substance-abusing adolescent inpatients: A pilot study. *Journal of the American Academy of Child and Adolescent Psychiatry, 31*(6), 1036–1040.

Substance Abuse and Mental Health Services Administration. (1999a). *Screening and assessing adolescents for substance use disorders: Treatment improvement protocol (TIP) Series 31.* Rockville, MD: Department of Health and Human Services.

Substance Abuse and Mental Health Services Administration. (1999b). *Treatment of adolescents with substance use disorders: Treatment improvement protocol (TIP) Series 32.* Rockville, MD: Department of Health and Human Services.

Substance Abuse and Mental Health Services Administration. (2002). *Results from the 2001 National Household Survey on Drug Abuse: Volume 1. Summary of national findings* (Office of Applied Studies, NHSDA Series H-17, DHHS Publication No. SMA 02-3758). Rockville, MD: Author.

Szapocznik, J., Kurtines, W. M., Foote, F., Perez-Vidal, A., & Hervis, O. (1986). Conjoint versus one-person family therapy: Further evidence for the effectiveness of conducting family therapy through one person with drug-abusing adolescents. *Journal of Consulting and Clinical Psychology, 54,* 395–397.

Szapocznik, J., Kurtines, W. M., & Hervis, O. (1983). Conjoint versus one-person family therapy: Some evidence for the effectiveness of conducting family therapy through one person. *Journal of Consulting and Clinical Psychology, 51,* 889–899.

Tapert, S. F., Aarons, G. A., Sedlar, G. R., & Brown, S. A. (2001). Adolescent substance use and sexual risk-taking behavior. *Journal of Adolescent Health, 28,* 181–189.

Tapert, S. F., & Brown, S. A. (1999). Neuropsychological correlates of adolescent substance abuse: Four year outcomes. *Journal of the International Neuropsychological Society, 5,* 475–487.

Tapert, S. F., Granholm, E., Leedy, N. G., & Brown, S. A. (2002). Substance use and withdrawal: Neuropsychological functioning over 8 years in youth. *Journal of the International Neuropsychological Society, 8*(7), 873–883.

Tapert, S. F., Stewart, D. G., & Brown, S. A. (1999). Drug abuse in adolescence. In A. J. Goreczny & M. Hersen (Eds.), *Handbook of pediatric and adolescent health psychology* (pp. 161–178). Boston: Allyn & Bacon.

Tarter, R. E., & Edwards, K. (1988). Psychological factors associated with the risk for alcoholism. *Alcoholism: Clinical and Experimental Research, 12,* 471–480.

Tarter, R. E., Mezzich, A. C., Kirisci, L., & Kaczynksi, N. (1997). Reliability of the Drug Use Screening Inventory among adolescent alcoholics. *Journal of Child and Adolescent Substance Abuse, 3,* 25–36.

Tarter, R., Vanyukov, M., Giancola, P., Dawes, M., Blackson, T., Mezzich, A., & Clark, D. (1999). Etiology of early age onset substance use disorder: A maturational perspective. *Development and Psychopathology, 11,* 657–683.

Tobler, N. S., Roona, M. R., Ochshorn, P., Marshall, D. G., Streke, A. V., & Stackpole, K. M. (2000). School-based adolescent drug prevention programs: 1998 meta-analysis. *Journal of Primary Prevention, 20,* 275–336.

Tobler, N. S., & Stratton, H. H. (1997). Effectiveness of school-based drug prevention programs: A meta-analysis of the research. *Journal of Primary Prevention, 18,* 71–128.

Tomlinson, K., Brown, S. A., & Abrantes, A. M. (2004). Psychiatric comorbidity and substance use treatment outcomes of adolescents. *Psychology of Addictive Behaviors, 13*(2), 83–101.

Tubman, J. G., Wagner, E. F., Gil, A. G., & Pate, K. N. (2002). Brief motivational intervention for substance-abusing delinquent adolescents: Guided self-change as a social work practice innovation. *Health and Social Work, 27,* 208–212.

Vik, P. W., & Brown, S. A. (1998). Life events and substance abuse during adolescence. In T. W. Miller (Ed.), *Children of trauma: Stressful life events and their effects on adolescents* (pp. 179–205). Madison, CT: International Universities Press.

Vik, P. W., Brown, S. A., & Myers, M. G. (1997). Adolescent substance abuse problems. In E. J. Mash & L. G. Terdal (Eds.), *Assessment of childhood disorders* (3rd ed., pp. 717–748). New York: Guilford Press.

Vik, P. W., Grizzle, K. L., & Brown, S. A. (1992). Social resource characteristics and adolescent substance abuse relapse. *Journal of Adolescent Chemical Dependency, 2,* 59–74.

Wagner, E. F., Brown, S. A., Monti, P. M., Myers, M. G., & Waldron, H. B. (1999). Innovations in adolescent substance abuse intervention. *Alcoholism: Clinical and Experimental Research, 23,* 236–249.

Waldron, H. B., Slesnick, N., Brody, J. L., & Peterson, T. R. (2001). Treatment outcomes for adolescent substance abuse 4- and 7-month assessments. *Journal of Consulting and Clinical Psychology, 69,* 802–813.

Wall, T. L., Shea, S. H., Chan, K. K., & Carr, L. G. (2001). A genetic association with the development of alcohol and other substance use behavior in Asian Americans. *Journal of Abnormal Psychology, 110*(1), 173–178.

Wallace, J. M., Jr., Bachman, J. G., O'Malley, P. M., Johnston, L. D., Schulenberg, J. E., & Cooper, S. M. (2002). Tobacco, alcohol, and illicit drug use: Racial and ethnic differences among U.S. high school seniors, 1976–2000. *Public Health Reports, 117*(Suppl. 1), S67–S75.

Wallace, J. M., Jr., Bachman, J. G., O'Malley, P. M., Schulenberg, J. E., Cooper, S. M., & Johnston, L. D. (2003). Gender and ethnic differences in smoking, drinking, and illicit drug use among American 8th, 10th, and 12th grade students, 1976–2000. *Addiction, 98,* 225–234.

White, H. R., Tice, P. C., Loeber, R., Stouthamer-Loeber, M. (2002). Illegal acts committed by adolescents under the influence of alcohol and drugs. *Journal of Research in Crime and Delinquency, 39,* 131–152.

Wilens, T. E., Biederman, J., Abrantes, A. M., & Spencer, T. J. (1997). Clinical characteristics of psychiatrically referred adolescent outpatients with substance use disorder. *Journal of the American Academy of Child and Adolescent Psychiatry, 36,* 941–947.

Williams, P. S., & Hine, D. W. (2002). Parental behaviour and alcohol misuse among adolescents: A path analysis of mediating influences. *Australian Journal of Psychology, 54,* 17–24.

Williams, R. J., & Chang, S. Y. (2000). A comprehensive and comparative review of adolescent substance abuse treatment outcome. *Clinical Psychology: Science and Practice, 7,* 138–166.

Wills, T. A., Vaccaro, D., & McNamara, G. (1992). The role of life events, family support, and competence in adolescent substance use: A test of vulnerability and protective factors. *American Journal of Community Psychology, 20,* 349–374.

Windle, M. (1990). Temperament and personality attributes of children of alcoholics. In M. Windle & J. S. Searles (Eds.), *Children of alcoholics: Critical perspectives* (pp. 129–167). New York: Guilford Press.

Winters, H. (1992). Development of an adolescent drug abuse screening scale: Personal Experience Screening Questionnaire. *Addictive Behaviors, 17,* 479–490.

Winters, K. C. (1999). Treating adolescents with substance use disorders: An overview of practice issues and treatment outcome. *Substance Abuse, 20,* 203–225.

Winters, K. C. (2001). Assessing adolescent substance use problems and other areas of functioning: State of the art. In P. M. Monti, S. M. Colby, & T. A. O'Leary (Eds.), *Adolescents, alcohol, and substance abuse: Reaching teens through brief interventions* (pp. 80–108). New York: Guilford Press.

Winters, K. C., & Henly, G. A. (1989). *The Personal Experience Inventory manual.* Los Angeles: Western Psychological Services.

Winters, K. C., & Henly, G. A. (1993). *The Adolescent Diagnostic Interview manual.* Los Angeles: Western Psychological Services.

Winters, K. C., Stinchfield, R. D., Fulkerson, J., & Henly, G. A. (1993). Measuring alcohol and cannabis use disorders in an adolescent clinical sample. *Psychology of Addictive Behaviors, 7,* 185–196.

Winters, K. C., Stinchfield, R. D., & Henly, G. A. (1996). Convergent and predictive validity of scales measuring adolescent substance abuse. *Journal of Child and Adolescent Substance Abuse, 5,* 37–55.

Zucker, R. A., Fitzgerald, H. E., & Moses, H. D. (1995). Emergence of alcohol problems and the several alcoholisms: A developmental perspective on etiological theory and life course trajectory. In D. Cicchetti & D. Cohen (Eds.), *Manual of developmental psychopathology* (Vol. 2, pp. 677–711). New York: Wiley.

Zucker, R. A., Fitzgerald, H. E., Refior, S. K., Puttler, L. I., Pallas, D. M., & Ellis, D. A. (2000). The clinical and social ecology of childhood for children of alcoholics: Description of a study and implications for a differentiated social policy. In H. E. Fitzgerald, B. M. Lester, & B. S. Zuckerman (Eds.), *Children of addiction: Research, health, and public policy issues* (pp. 109–141). New York: Routledge Falmer.

Zucker, R. A., & Gomberg, E. S. (1986). Etiology of alcoholism reconsidered: The case for a biopsychosocial process. *American Psychologist, 41,* 783–793.

Zuckerman, M. (1994). *Behavioral expressions and biosocial bases of sensation seeking.* New York: Cambridge University Press.

III

INTERNALIZING DISORDERS

7

Anxiety Disorders

Philip C. Kendall
Kristina A. Hedtke
Sasha G. Aschenbrand

Adolescence is a crossroads from childhood to adulthood that has only been viewed as a separate developmental phase worthy of investigation in the past century. Although historically this developmental period has been perceived as a time of great emotional upheaval and turmoil, research on the development and maintenance of psychopathology specific to adolescence is scant. The research that has been conducted concerning adolescence focuses to a large extent on the normative developmental pathways of the period. Nevertheless, we have gained some knowledge concerning the nature of psychopathology in adolescence, but the literature in this area focuses to a great degree on externalizing behaviors. Until recently, internalizing problems have been largely overlooked. The study of this broad category of psychopathology has recently received attention in the field of developmental psychology, but research in clinical psychology on the nature of specific internalizing disorders in adolescence is lacking. Specifically, we are facing a huge knowledge gap when it comes to adolescents with anxiety disorders.

The lack of research on anxiety disorders in adolescents is surprising, as large epidemiologi-cal studies of anxiety disorders in adults have consistently shown ages of onset in childhood and adolescence (e.g., Kessler et al., 1994). Anxiety not only is prevalent in adolescent populations but also has significant psychosocial implications in multiple domains, including academic work, peer relationships, and social competence (Ialongo, Edelsohn, Werthamer-Larsson, Crockett, & Kellam, 1995; Kashani & Orvaschel, 1990; Strauss, Lease, Kazdin, Dulcan, & Last, 1989). Data suggest that the majority of anxiety disorders do not simply remit with the passage of time and may even become chronic and developmentally dysfunctional (Barrett, 2000; Keller et al., 1992). Despite these findings, the systematic investigation of anxiety disorders in adolescents lags far behind that of adults.

One problem that impedes the progression of knowledge in the field of adolescent anxiety relates to what Kendall termed the "developmental uniformity myth" (Kendall, 1984). That is, researchers may implicitly believe that children and adolescents are a homogeneous group. Given this erroneous assumption, researchers may tend to lump the age groups together in studies and/or apply research findings concerning one age group to another, ignoring the fact that the groups may be qualitatively different. For instance, recent epidemiological research has found that specific subtypes of anxiety have differential peak periods of onset. Specifically, separation anxiety and specific phobias peak in middle childhood, whereas overanxious disorder/generalized anxiety disorder typically peaks in late childhood, and social phobia and panic disorder peak uniquely in adolescence (Cohen et al., 1993; Compton, Nelson, & March, 2000; Costello, 1989; Last, Perrin, Hersen, & Kazdin, 1996; Pine, Cohen, Gurley, Brook, & Ma, 1998). Moreover, little is known as to whether the experience and expression of anxiety disorders differ across developmental periods. This developmental difference seems quite likely, given that adolescents typically have greater cognitive maturity and insight into their thoughts and feelings, and that concerns about self-presentation and evaluation by others normatively increase in adolescence. Given that evidence seems to point to differences between childhood and adolescent anxiety and given that adolescent anxiety has been largely overlooked, it is imperative that we consider the social and developmental factors unique to adolescence that may play a crucial role in the nature of adolescent anxiety disorders.

DESCRIPTION OF THE DISORDER

An understanding of the nature of adolescent anxiety begins with a grasp of the core symptoms and characteristics of anxiety disorders. Separation anxiety disorder (SAD), generalized anxiety disorder (GAD), social phobia (SoP), specific phobia, obsessive–compulsive disorder (OCD), panic disorder (PD), posttraumatic stress disorder (PTSD), and acute stress disorder (ASD) collectively fall under the umbrella phrase "anxiety disorders." Anxiety disorders are often referred to as a group, despite the fact that each disorder has its own diagnostic criteria in the *Diagnostic and Statistical Manual of Mental Disorders* (DSM-IV-TR; American Psychiatric Association [APA], 2000) and can be manifested quite differently. The tendency to view the anxiety disorders as a unified group may be partially due to their shared etiological factors (e.g., specific temperamental and familial influences as well as cognitive biases), high comorbidity with each other (e.g., Brady &

Kendall, 1992), and the overlap of symptomatology. To illustrate, the core feature of the various anxiety disorders is an intense fear or worry associated with emotional distress and/or avoidance behavior. Considering the core feature, anxiety disorders are viewed as similar to each other yet are perceived as distinct from other disorders that share similar etiological factors and with which anxiety is comorbid, such as depression, its core feature being sad mood.

The diagnostic system for classifying anxiety in youth changed from the third edition (DSM-III; APA, 1980) to the fourth edition of DSM (DSM-IV; APA, 1994). Specifically, the category "anxiety disorders of childhood and adolescence," along with the diagnoses of avoidant disorder and overanxious disorder, were eliminated from DSM, with SAD the only anxiety disorder unique to childhood remaining within DSM's "disorders usually first diagnosed in infancy, childhood or adolescence." In DSM-IV, the anxiety disorders in youth are considered much the same as anxiety disorders in adults with only a few minor exceptions (e.g., classification of SAD). In this section, we review the core symptoms for each anxiety disorder, followed by a discussion of the sensitivity and developmental appropriateness of the current criteria in identifying and diagnosing adolescents.

SAD remains a disorder of childhood and, as opposed to the other anxiety disorders, requires an age of onset before age 18. The central feature of SAD is unrealistic or excessive anxiety about separating from major caregivers or attachment figures, usually, but not limited to, parents. Youth with SAD generally fear that loss or harm will befall themselves (e.g., getting lost, being kidnapped) or those to whom they are attached (e.g., car accident, abandonment), and therefore they do whatever they can to be near those for whom they care. It is not unusual for a child or teen with SAD to complain of stomachaches, headaches, or other physical symptoms in anticipation of separating from a caregiver and/or to refuse to leave home or be alone in the house without a loved one. Youth with SAD often avoid "sleepovers," visiting others at their home, and being alone in their bedroom or another room in the house. Many times, youth with SAD require that a caregiver or loved one sleep next to them at bedtime and, in school-age youth, SAD can lead to school refusal behavior. Although DSM lists nightmares about separating from caregivers as a potential criterion, we have not found this symptom to be frequently reported by youth with SAD or their parents. Children and teens may respond differently to anticipation of or upon actual separation from an attachment figure. Younger children with SAD may cry or throw temper tantrums, whereas older children and teens may tend to seek excessive reassurance from caregivers before separating and/or may require caregivers to "check in" frequently while separated.

As described in DSM-IV, GAD is characterized by excessive, uncontrollable worry about multiple events or daily activities, which lasts more days than not for at least 6 months and causes significant interference or impairment. In adults, work performance, family health, community affairs, world issues, and finance are typically areas of excessive worry. Although somewhat surprising, youth with GAD show similar areas of worry, as well as worry about school performance. Although adults with GAD seem to worry excessively about events or activities that most adults think about or worry about once in awhile, youth with GAD sometimes appear to be "little adults," being overly concerned about topics that other children do not consider or shrug off easily; topics such as weather conditions, family finances, tardiness, and/or natural or man-made disasters (Southam-Gerow, 2001). Youth with GAD typically seek reassurance from parents and friends (e.g., ask for weather updates, frequently ask the time) and ask "what-if" questions almost incessantly. For a diagnosis, the worry and anxiety characteristic of GAD must be associated with at least one physical symptom in youth (three are required for adults) such as restlessness, fatigue, difficulty concentrating, irritability, muscle tension, and/or sleep problems.

In previous diagnostic systems, youth who displayed symptoms now labeled GAD would have been classified as having overanxious disorder (OAD). The overlap in symptoms between OAD and GAD was likely the reason for eliminating OAD from DSM-IV in favor of considering both children and adults who are excessive worriers as suffering from GAD. However, as Southam-Gerow (2001) noted, although GAD and OAD share considerable overlap, they differ on important details. For instance, the presence of a physical symptom was not required for a diagnosis of OAD (see also Kendall & Pimentel, 2003). Also as part of

OAD, worried youth did not have to experience the worry as uncontrollable, as is required for a GAD diagnosis. Finally, OAD symptoms were described with more detail than GAD symptoms and the broader scope of the GAD description may not fully capture certain aspects of the child-like experience (e.g., need for reassurance, self-consciousness). Despite the differences between OAD and GAD, there is some evidence of consistency between the older and the newer diagnostic systems. Specifically, one study found that a child once diagnosed with OAD according to DSM-III-R (APA, 1987) would quite likely receive a GAD diagnosis as described in DSM-IV (Kendall & Warman, 1996).

SoP, also referred to as social anxiety disorder, was previously diagnosed in children as avoidant disorder (AvD). Similar to the reported consistency between OAD and GAD, Kendall and Warman (1996) also reported that a child diagnosed AvD would most likely receive a DSM-IV diagnosis of SoP, although the agreement between these diagnoses was not as strong as the OAD–GAD agreement.

The core feature of SoP is a strong or persistent fear of social or performance situations in which a person is exposed to unfamiliar people or is being observed or evaluated by others. In these situations, the individual is afraid that he or she will embarrass or humiliate him- or herself. SoP can be limited to one social or performance situation or be generalized to a variety of situations, but the feared situation(s) is almost always anxiety provoking and either avoided altogether or endured with extreme distress. DSM-IV qualifies some of the SoP criteria for youth, noting that there must be the capacity for developmentally appropriate social relationships in order to give a SoP diagnosis. Also, anxiety cannot only occur in interactions with adults to be considered SoP, as many youth are nervous when interacting with adults; anxiety must occur in peer settings as well. Another key difference between diagnosing adults and youth with SoP is that, unlike adults, youth with SoP may not recognize that their social or performance fears are excessive or unreasonable and may express these fears quite differently than adults (e.g., crying, defiance or "acting out" in social situations). Finally, as a criterion for a diagnosis, the excessive social and performance fears must last at least 6 months in youth under 18, as transient social and performance fears are generally considered normative during childhood and especially adolescence.

Specific phobias, formerly called simple phobias, are excessive fears of certain specific objects or events such as flying, animals, seeing blood, heights, and storms. The actual presence of the object or event, or anticipation of the event or coming into contact with the object is almost always anxiety provoking. Similar to SoP, children diagnosed with a specific phobia may express their fear by crying, screaming, and/or throwing temper tantrums and may not recognize that their fear is excessive or unreasonable. Also, youth under 18 years of age must show phobic symptoms related to the object or event for 6 months prior to receiving a diagnosis of specific phobia.

The core characteristics of OCD are essentially the same for youth and adults and include obsessions, compulsions, or, as is usually the case, both obsessions and compulsions (that are time-consuming, taking up more than 1 hour a day). Obsessions are recurrent thoughts, images, and/or impulses that do not make sense and are often intrusive, distressing, and difficult to control (e.g., thoughts of leaving appliances turned on, thoughts of contracting germs, and thoughts of causing accidental harm to others). Whereas obsessions are mental events, compulsions can be mental events or actions. Specifically, compulsions are repetitive behaviors (e.g., washing hands, checking locks) or repetitive mental activities (e.g., repeating phrases) that individuals feel driven to perform excessively, generally in response to an obsession and to prevent a negative consequence or dreaded event. Compulsions are usually thought of as "neutralizing" activities carried out to reduce distress. An important distinguishing element of OCD is that the obsessions are not simply everyday worries about real-life problems. They are thoughts, images, or impulses that "stretch the logic" beyond the realm of everyday worries. As is true for some other diagnoses, children who experience OCD symptoms need not recognize that the obsessions or compulsions are excessive or unreasonable.

PD is defined by recurrent attacks, in a short period of time (usually about 10 minutes or less), of intense fear or discomfort when there is no real danger present (panic attacks). Panic attacks are accompanied by intense cognitive and/or physical symptoms such as heart palpitations, shortness of breath, sweating, chest pain, fear of dying, and feelings of being unreal or detached from oneself, to name a few. Because panic attacks can occur as a response to a feared object or event and can be a part of any anxiety disorder, the key feature of PD is that (1) the panic attacks are seemingly unexpected and come "out of the blue" and (2) at least one of the attacks has been followed by 1 month or more of concern about having another attack, worry about the implications of an attack (e.g., heart attack, "going crazy," losing control), and/or a change in behavior associated with having an attack (e.g., avoiding places or situations in which a panic attack occurred, not engaging in activities that create panic-like symptoms such as exercise, sexual activity, watching thrilling movies).

PD is classified as either occurring in conjunction with agoraphobic symptoms or without agoraphobic symptoms. Individuals with PD who display agoraphobia feel intense anxiety in places or situations in which they anticipate/fear that a panic attack may occur and escape or attainment of help might be difficult. Such situations might include being in crowds, leaving home, waiting in lines, and traveling on public transportation. Because of the intense fear of incapacitating panic symptoms produced in these situations, individuals who have PD with agoraphobia tend to avoid such situations or are only willing to engage in or endure certain situations in the presence of a "safe" person, a trusted person who may be able to help in the event of an attack. It is important to note that agoraphobia can occur outside the context of PD, because the central feature of agoraphobia is fear of developing incapacitating panic symptoms and not actually experiencing panic symptoms or panic attacks.

It was only recently considered that PD occurs in children and adolescents. In fact, some researchers and theorists claim that PD cannot occur in young children and younger adolescents due to their lack of cognitive sophistication, which is purported as necessary to misinterpret bodily sensations and experience the cognitive symptoms of panic attacks (Chorpita, Albano, & Barlow, 1996). Although some evidence suggests that PD does occur in younger populations (Kessler et al., 1998; Last & Strauss, 1989), community prevalence rates for PD are low and PD in children and younger adolescents is still considered rare (Ollendick, Mattis, & King, 1994; Verhulst, van der Ende, Ferdinand, & Kasius, 1997).

Both PTSD and ASD are anxiety disorders that are characterized by significant functional impairment following the witnessing or experiencing of a traumatic or life-threatening event. For both disorders, the trauma produces intense fear, helplessness, or horror and is persistently reexperienced in at least one of a variety of ways. In children, reexperiencing may occur through repetitive play thematically related to the trauma, reenactment of the trauma, and/or having scary nightmares. Individuals with PTSD and ASD tend to avoid objects and/or situations associated with the trauma and show heightened autonomic nervous system arousal, which can be manifested as difficulty falling asleep, irritability, hypervigilance of surroundings, concentration difficulties, and a quick startle response. One additional feature of ASD is that either during the trauma or after the trauma, the individual may demonstrate dissociative symptoms (e.g., feeling "dazed," not being able to recall the trauma or important aspects of the trauma). Also, the duration of PTSD and ASD differ. For ASD, impairment or distress associated with the trauma must begin within 4 weeks of the traumatic event and last between 2 days and 4 weeks. PTSD is longer in duration, lasting greater than 1 month, and onset of symptoms can occur immediately following the event or with delayed onset (i.e., at least 6 months after the event).

DIAGNOSTIC CRITERIA: NEEDS AND CONSIDERATIONS

Despite some evidence challenging the assumption, the diagnostic criteria for anxiety disorders largely assumes that both the presentation and relative contribution of anxiety symptoms to achieve an anxiety diagnosis are continuous and equally weighted throughout the lifespan. A lifespan developmental approach would suggest variations in presentation. For instance, evidence shows that certain SAD symptoms are more prevalent for different ages: younger children tend to experience fewer and less distressing symptoms of SAD (e.g., fewer physical symptoms) than adolescents who demonstrate greater avoidance, distress, and more frequent physical symptoms related to separating from attachment figures (Francis, Last, & Strauss, 1987; Last, Hersen, Kazdin, Orvaschel, & Perrin 1991). With regard to GAD, Tracey, Chorpita, Douban, and Barlow (1997) re-

ported that when endorsed by youth (7- to 17-year-olds), the GAD physical symptom of feeling restless or keyed up was predictive of a GAD diagnosis. In the same study, parental endorsement of irritability in their child/teen was predictive of GAD. In a similar study, Piña, Silverman, Alfano, and Saavedra (2002) suggested that although all GAD symptoms were useful for diagnosing 6- to 17-year-olds, the symptoms varied in the degree to which they contributed to a GAD diagnosis. Also, symptoms predictive of a GAD diagnosis varied depending on youth or parental report. Further research is needed to ascertain whether or not it is appropriate to differentially weight certain anxiety symptoms for specific ages or developmental levels.

"Children" and "adolescents" are not uniform groups. Indeed, the phrase "developmental uniformity myth" was proposed (Kendall, 1984) to help prevent the unwanted lumping of developmentally diverse groups under a single label. Although DSM-IV makes some qualifications for children with regard to diagnosing anxiety, the specific qualifications are generally in a "Note" embedded within the diagnostic criteria and, in general, these qualifications are more applicable to younger children than to adolescents (e.g., anxiety expressed as throwing temper tantrums) and they are rarely based on empirical research. Also, DSM-IV does not explicitly state the definition of a child and/or whether or not the qualifications apply to children and adolescents or only to children. Both the definitions of anxiety disorders and their diagnostic criteria require adaptations to prevent falling into the uniformity myth.

We also propose that explicit attention be paid to normative development and/or developmental milestones during adolescence when considering anxiety and the diagnostic criteria for disorders. For example, it is important to understand that emotional disruptions are normative for adolescents and it is typical for adolescents to report more extreme negative and positive emotions than other age groups (Larson, Csikszentmihalyi, & Graef, 1980; Larson & Richards, 1994). Adolescents report feeling self-conscious and embarrassed up to three times more often than their parents and are more likely than their parents to feel awkward, lonely, and nervous (Larson & Richards, 1994). Adolescents also report feeling "very happy," "proud," and "in control" less frequently than younger children (Larson & Richards, 1994). Such changes in emotional expression may be viewed as alarming in a young child, because emotional fluctuations are generally not considered normative during childhood but less alarming in an adolescent. Understanding normative fluctuations in adolescent emotions provides a perspective that is needed before one assigns a diagnosis.

Because cognitive functioning varies with age, another important consideration in the diagnosis of adolescent anxiety concerns cognitive development. Level of cognitive development (e.g., ability to reason abstractly) may be important when considering the nature and severity of anxiety symptoms in youth. It is not until adolescence that fairly sophisticated thinking develops, thinking that is characterized by abstraction, consequential thinking, and hypothetical reasoning. Awareness of the development of these cognitive processes during adolescence is essential to understanding anxiety disorders during this time. Adolescents are better able to interpret or misinterpret what their peers, family members, and other individuals are thinking, possibly leaving them at increased risk for cognitive distortions characteristic of GAD, SoP, and PD. Indeed, and perhaps not surprisingly, rates of both SoP and PD increase dramatically during adolescence (e.g., Compton et al., 2000) and at least two studies examining diagnostic differences in youth showed that older youth report a greater number of overanxious symptoms and have generally higher levels of anxiety (Strauss, Lease, Last, & Francis, 1988) than younger children, and that a greater variety of worries, more complex worries, and an increased ability to elaborate on worry outcomes are more common in youth over 8 years old (Vasey, Crnic, & Carter, 1994).

Other central aspects of adolescent development, such as the increasing importance of peer relationships and the development of autonomy from parents, should also be considered when diagnosing adolescents with anxiety disorders. Although the relative contribution of these factors to the development and maintenance of anxiety are described more fully later in this chapter, assessing impairment in these domains is essential when considering diagnosing adolescents with an anxiety disorder as the development of autonomy and the nurturance of peer relationships are so crucial to this developmental period (as compared with adulthood and early childhood).

EPIDEMIOLOGY

Prevalence

Findings from community studies indicate that anxiety disorders are the most common disorder in the general population of adolescents. Considering all anxiety disorders, prevalence rates range between 9 and 19% in adolescent populations (Essau, Conradt, & Petermann, 2000; Lewinsohn, Hops, Roberts, Seeley, & Andrews, 1993), with some variations according to the specific anxiety disorder and the methodology used. A number of studies have found phobias to be the most common anxiety disorders in adolescents, though the category of phobia is generally quite broad and may include phobia not otherwise specified (NOS), specific phobia, SoP, and/or agoraphobia, depending on the study (Essau et al., 2000; Reinherz, Giaconia, Lefkowitz, Pakiz, & Frost, 1993; Verhulst et al., 1997; Wittchen, Nelson, & Lachner, 1998). Prevalence rates for phobia NOS in adolescent populations range from 5.2% (Wittchen et al., 1998) to 11.9% (Essau et al., 2000). Rates of specific/simple phobia range from 2.3% (Wittchen et al., 1998) to 12.7% (Verhulst et al., 1997). Considering SoP, Essau and colleagues (2000) found the lowest prevalence rates (1.6%) and Verhulst and colleagues (1997) found the highest prevalence rates (9.2%). SAD is the next most frequent anxiety disorder in adolescents, with rates of 2–5%, though higher in younger adolescents (Cohen et al., 1993; Costello et al., 1988; Lewinsohn et al., 1993; McGee et al., 1990). Interestingly, studies using earlier DSM criteria show higher rates of certain subtypes of anxiety. For example, Verhulst and colleagues found 6-month prevalence rates of 3.1% for OAD and 1.3% for GAD among 13- to 18-year-olds. McGee and colleagues (1990) reported a prevalence rate of 5.9% in a sample of 15-year-olds, whereas another study reported rates of OAD as high as 14.1% in adolescent girls (Velez, Johnson, & Cohen, 1989). Rates of GAD in adolescents, however, using current criteria, are generally considered at 1% (Essau et al., 2000; Wittchen et al., 1998). Higher rates of OAD as compared to GAD may be observed partially because the criteria for GAD, although seemingly more broad, may actually be more restrictive for youth (e.g., requiring at least one physical symptom and uncontrollable worry to obtain a GAD diagnosis). As mentioned previously, OAD may capture more fully certain aspects of youth experiences (e.g., need for reassurance, self-consciousness) and thus result in more youth receiving a diagnosis of OAD. PD, OCD, and PTSD are relatively rare, with studies generally reporting prevalence rates ranging from < 1% to approximately 2% (Essau et al., 2000; Reinherz et al., 1993; Verhulst et al., 1997; Wittchen et al., 1998).

Age of Onset

Individual anxiety disorders have unique ages of onset and may be expressed in different ways across development. Specific phobias have an early age of onset. Öst (1987, 1991) reported onset for phobias between the ages of 7 and 12 years and Burke, Burke, Rae, and Regier (1991) found the hazard rate for developing phobias is the highest in 10- to 14-year-olds. SAD is also usually found in younger children, though some middle children and adolescents also exhibit separation anxious symptomatology. SAD appears to have different symptom expression in younger and older children. Whereas younger children present with more symptoms and extreme distress upon separation, adolescents are more likely to present with physical complaints on schooldays (Francis et al., 1987). GAD, SoP, and PD can have onsets in middle childhood, but more often onset is in later childhood and early adolescence. For example, although GAD is sometimes reported in younger children, research suggests that risk for GAD increases with age and may be linked to cognitive gains (Vasey, 1993). A study examining diagnostic differences in OAD among children ages 5–19 years reported no differences at the diagnostic level but did find that older children reported more symptoms and higher anxiety levels (Strauss et al., 1988). Vasey and colleagues (1994) found greater variety, elaboration, and complexity of worries in children older than 8 years of age. This evidence is consistent with the notion that GAD can have an early age of onset but that symptom expression increases with age.

Considering SoP, retrospective reports from adults indicate that the average age of onset is midadolescence (Liebowitz, Gorman, Fyer, & Klein, 1985), with studies using samples of children reporting even earlier age of onsets. Strauss and Last (1993) reported a mean age of onset of 12.3 years and Beidel and Turner (1998) reported that children as young as 8

years of age met criteria for SoP. According to Sweeney and Rapee (2001), it is possible that social concerns are present at an early age, yet these concerns are only characterized as SoP when they begin to be tied to avoidance and cause interference in functioning. Finally, evidence indicates that prior to puberty, panic attacks are rare (Hayward et al., 1992). After puberty, the frequency of panic attacks increases, especially for girls, and by older adolescence approaches the frequency of panic attacks reported by adults (Essau, Conradt, & Petermann, 1999). Although prepubertal panic attacks and PD can occur, the frequency appears to be low compared to the frequency in post-pubertal adolescents (Hayward & Essau, 2001).

Gender Differences

Several studies have reported gender differences in the rates of adolescent anxiety disorders (Essau et al., 2000; Lewinsohn, Gotlib, Lewinsohn, Seeley, & Allen, 1998; Reinherz et al., 1993). Results are fairly consistent, indicating significantly higher rates of anxiety disorders in female adolescents than in males. In the Essau and colleagues (2000) study, the frequency of anxiety disorders increased with age, with the greatest increase occurring between ages 12–13 and 14–15 years. Considering the rates of anxiety disorders by age and gender, results showed significant gender differences beginning at age 14, with significantly higher rates found in females than in males, and with the suggestion that the higher prevalence was associated with female's physical maturity. Lewinsohn and colleagues (1998) also found gender differences, but an earlier age of divergence, with twice as many girls than boys having experienced an anxiety disorder by age 6. Boys and girls, however, did not differ with respect to age of onset or duration of their first anxiety episode.

Most research also shows gender differences in the rates of specific anxiety disorders. SAD has been reported as more commonly observed in girls (e.g., Last, Perrin, Hersen, & Kazdin, 1992), whereas studies of panic attack frequencies in adolescents and young adults find relatively equal rates in males and females (Essau et al., 2000; King, Gullone, Tonge, & Ollendick, 1993). However, when considering the severity of panic attacks or number of symptoms, female adolescents tend to be more represented in the severe and four-symptom groups (e.g., Hayward, Killen, & Taylor, 1989; King, Ollendick, Mattis, Yang, & Tonge, 1996). Considering specific phobias, girls report more fears than boys in community samples, but gender differences are not generally seen in clinical samples (Essau et al., 2000; Kendall et al., 1997; Strauss & Last, 1993). Similarly, in community samples of children, a greater proportion of females than males meet criteria for SoP (e.g., Anderson, Williams, McGee, & Silva, 1987), but clinical samples generally find no gender differences (e.g., Kendall et al., 1997; Last et al., 1992). Community studies of adolescents suggest that SoP may be more frequent in females than in males (Essau et al., 2000; Verhulst et al., 1997). Research suggests no discernible gender differences in rates of OAD and GAD in adolescents (Essau et al., 2000).

DEVELOPMENTAL COURSE AND OUTCOMES

Other sections of this chapter touch on topics associated with the developmental course of anxiety disorders. Nevertheless, a few topics merit more focused attention. One developmental consideration is that if left untreated, anxiety disorders do not remit with the passage of time but instead run a chronic and fluctuating course into adulthood (e.g., Achenbach, Howell, McConaughy, & Stanger, 1995; Costello & Angold, 1995; Keller et al., 1992; Pine et al., 1998). Several follow-up studies of children and adolescents have shown that anxiety disorders are highly stable, though there may be some switching between categories of anxiety disorders over time (Cantwell & Baker, 1989; Ialongo et al., 1995). One study found that anxiety disorders were more stable from adolescence to adulthood than any other major diagnostic subtype (Newman et al., 1996). An epidemiological study examining the relationships between adolescent and early adult anxiety or depressive disorders reported that adolescent anxiety or depressive disorders predicted an approximate two- to threefold increased risk for adulthood anxiety or depressive disorders (Pine et al., 1998). Moreover, there was evidence of specificity in the course of simple and SoP, but less specificity in the course of other disorders. Also, whereas most adolescent disorders were no longer present in young adulthood, most adult disorders were

preceded by adolescent disorders (Pine et al., 1998). In sum, it appears that anxiety disorders are highly stable over time. There is also some evidence that simple (specific) phobia and SoP may be consistent across time/ages, but overall the type of adolescent anxiety disorder does not necessarily predict the type of adult disorder.

Anxiety in adulthood may not be the only possible outcome of youth anxiety. Youth anxiety disorders have also been identified as potential risk factors affecting the development and course of substance use disorders (e.g., Compton et al., 2000; Kessler et al., 1996). Research suggests a temporal relationship: early onset of anxiety disorders increases the risk of developing a substance use disorder in adolescence and adulthood (e.g., Abraham & Fava, 1999; Christie et al., 1988; Deas-Nesmith, Brady, & Campbell, 1998; Greenbaum, Prange, Friedman, & Silver, 1991). For instance, Christie and colleagues (1988) reported that the risk of subsequent substance abuse in adolescents and young adults who have had earlier depressive or anxiety disorders is doubled. Similarly, Regier and colleagues (1993) have reported that having an anxiety disorder increases the risk for alcoholism by 50% and the risk for substance use disorder by 70%. This temporal relationship suggests that at least some anxious adolescents use alcohol and other drugs to "self-medicate" or reduce their anxiety symptoms (Manassis & Monga, 2001). In another study, researchers examined the relation between early anxiety symptomotology (GAD and SAD) and initiation of alcohol use 4 years later in an epidemiological sample of 936 youth assessed at ages 9, 11, and 13 while controlling for the effects of depression (Kaplow, Curran, Angold, & Costello, 2001). Youth with early symptoms of GAD were found to be at increased risk for initiation of alcohol use (Kaplow et al., 2001).

Depressed mood is another problem that has been linked to anxiety disorders in youth. Although the data do not eliminate all rival hypotheses, the data are consistent in pointing to anxiety as a precursor to depression, with high rates of comorbidity (Brady & Kendall, 1992). Pine and colleagues (1998) found broad associations among major depression, OAD, and SP. Interestingly, major depression in adolescence predicted later GAD. The reverse also seemed to be true, in that OAD predicted major depression, in addition to SP, GAD, and PD. The association between adolescent OAD and adult major depression was comparable in size with the association between adolescent depression and adult GAD. Another prospective study of adolescents and young adults found that SoP in nondepressed adolescents at baseline was associated with an increased likelihood of depressive disorder onset during the follow-up period (Stein et al., 2001). Moreover, comorbid SoP and depression at baseline was associated with a worse prognosis, compared with depressive disorder without comorbid social anxiety disorder at baseline. The fact that adolescent anxiety disorders are predictive of depression in adulthood suggests that early intervention for anxiety disorders is warranted. However, additional research is needed to better understand the developmental links between anxiety in youth and later depression.

Another developmental consideration merits mention. Klein (1964) proposed that SAD in childhood was associated with PD in adulthood. Some studies have provided evidence suggestive of support for this hypothesized relationship (e.g., Battaglia et al., 1995; Pine et al., 2000; Silove et al., 1995). Recently, a 7.4 year follow-up was conducted of youth who had received treatment for an anxiety disorder in childhood. Those who were initially identified as SAD were compared to those initially identified with other anxiety disorders (GAD, SoP) and the frequency of panic problems was examined (Aschenbrand, Kendall, Webb, Safford, & Flannery-Schroeder, 2003). SAD was predictive of more anxiety disorders 7.4 years later but not predictive specifically of panic problems. The lack of prediction held for cases whose treatment was deemed effective and for those whom treatment was less effective. Although studies of untreated SAD cases are needed, as well as studies that follow cases for even more than 7 years, it appears that the developmental trajectory for SAD youth is not automatically tied to PD.

ETIOLOGY

Genetics

Although it would be inaccurate to claim that anxiety disorders are genetic, research does suggest that there is a genetic predisposition for the development of some anxiety disorders. The genetic contribution to anxiety disorders has primarily been studied via (1) research on familial aggregation of anxiety disorders, including both top-down and bottom-up studies, (2) twin studies of adult and childhood anxiety disorders, and (3) adoption studies of anxiety disorders.

Familial Aggregation Studies

Familial aggregation studies are either top down or bottom up. Top-down studies examine the children of anxiety-disordered parents to determine whether these children have higher rates of anxiety disorders than the general population. Bottom-up studies examine the rates of psychopathology in the parents of youth with anxiety disorders. Although genetics are not the sole explanation for the observations, the results of both types of studies indicate that anxiety disorders tend to run in families.

Considering top-down studies, a large literature indicates an increased risk for anxiety disorders in youth whose parents have anxiety or mood disorders. For example, Weissman, Leckman, Merikangas, Gammon, and Prusoff (1984) found significantly higher rates of anxiety disorders in children of parents with major depression and PD than in children of normal controls. Turner, Beidel, and Costello (1987) examined the children of parents with an anxiety disorder, dysthymia, and no psychiatric disorder, and the results indicated that children of anxiety-disordered parents were seven times more likely to be diagnosed with an anxiety disorder than children of parents without a psychiatric disorder. Children of anxiety-disordered parents and dysthymic parents did not significantly differ in their risk for an anxiety disorder. In fact, the disorders in children of dysthymic parents were all anxiety disorders (Turner et al., 1987). Another study examined the children of parents with major depressive disorder (MDD), PD (with and without MDD), and no diagnosis (Warner, Mufson, & Weissman, 1995). When compared with the children of never mentally ill parents, the children of parents with early-onset MDD had significantly higher rates of MDD, dysthymia, any anxiety disorder, and panic spectrum disorders. In addition, children of parents who had PD plus MDD had higher rates of SAD and panic spectrum disorders (Warner et al., 1995). Biederman, Rosenbaum, Bolduc, Faraone, and Hirshfeld (1991) assessed the children of parents with PD and agoraphobia (PDAG), children of parents with PDAG plus MDD, and children of parents with MDD only and found that children of parents with PDAG, both with and without comorbid depression, were at increased risk for an anxiety disorder. In addition, in contrast to other top-down studies, the children of depressed parents did not exhibit an increased risk for anxiety disorders. Taken together, the majority of findings from top-down studies indicate that the children of parents with both anxiety and mood disorders are at increased risk for the development of anxiety disorders.

Bottom-up studies examining the parents of anxious children also support the notion that anxiety disorders have a familial pattern. For example, Last, Hersen, Kazdin, Francis, and Grubb (1987) compared maternal lifetime psychiatric illness for children with SAD and/or OAD and for children who were psychiatrically disturbed but did not manifest an anxiety or affective disorder. Results indicated that the majority of mothers in each of the anxiety groups had a lifetime history of at least one anxiety disorder and when compared to the control group, mothers of anxious children exhibited significantly higher rates of anxiety disorders. In a later study, Last and colleagues (1991) compared the first- and second-degree relatives of children with anxiety disorders to the relatives of children with attention-deficit/hyperactivity disorder (ADHD) and children with no diagnoses for lifetime rates of psychopathological conditions, particularly anxiety disorders. Results indicated an increased prevalence of anxiety disorders in the first-degree relatives of children with an anxiety disorder compared with relatives of both children with ADHD and normal control children. Taken together, the results support a familial aggregation of anxiety disorders in children and parents and, though not the only etiology, are consistent with a genetic contribution to anxiety disorders.

Twin Studies

Much of the knowledge about the genetic contributions to adult anxiety disorders is derived from twin studies. Kendler and colleagues conducted a series of such studies with a large group of female twins (Kendler, Heath, Martin, & Eaves, 1987; Kendler, Neale, Kessler, Heath, & Eaves, 1992a, 1992b, 1992c, 1993a, 1993b;

Kendler et al., 1995). The results of one study suggest a modest genetic contribution to GAD and specific phobias (30–35% of the explained variance) and a moderate genetic contribution to PD (41–44% of the explained variance). A later study showed a more modest heritability estimate for GAD of approximately 15–20%, with no difference by gender (Hettema, Prescott, & Kendler, 2001). Studies by Scandinavian researchers reported a genetic contribution to posttraumatic stress disorder (PTSD), in addition to a genetic contribution to PD and GAD (Skre, Onstad, Torgersen, Lygren, & Kringlen, 1993).

Adoption Studies

Studies of adoption can shed light on the genetic and environmental contributions to psychopathology. In a study of adoptees in The Netherlands, van den Oord, Boomsma, and Verhulst (1994) reported that genetics were important for the development of attention problems and for externalizing behaviors but not for internalizing behaviors (including anxiety disorders). Specifically, genetic influences explained 65% of the variance in externalizing behaviors and approximately 0% of the variance in internalizing behaviors. The results of Van den Oord and colleagues are discrepant from the results of some twin studies that had suggested a modest genetic contribution. Accordingly, it is reasonable to use caution when making statements about genetic causes, and we encourage additional adoption and twin studies to better understand the genetic and environmental contributions to anxiety disorders.

Biological Factors

Temperament

Substantial evidence points to temperamental factors that are related to risk for the development of anxiety (Lonigan & Philips, 2001). Both cross-sectional and longitudinal studies have shown a consistent relationship between the temperamental factor known as negative affect (NA), a general factor of subjective distress (e.g., fear, anxiety, hostility, scorn, and disgust), and anxiety disorders in youth (Chorpita et al., 1996; Joiner, Catanzaro, & Laurent, 1996; Lonigan, Carey, & Finch, 1994; Lonigan, Hooe, David, & Kistner, 1999).

Studies have also shown a relationship between anxiety disorders and the temperamental factor known as effortful control (EC), the ability to employ self-regulative processes (Caspi, Henry, McGee, Moffitt, & Silva, 1995; Robins, John, Caspi, Moffitt, & Stouthamer-Loeber, 1996). According to Lonigan and Phillips (2001), a variety of evidence indicates that youth and adults with anxiety show attentional biases toward threatening stimuli, consistent with the suggestion that anxiety disorders are associated with impaired or low levels of EC. Considering both temperamental factors together, individuals high in NA have a greater need for EC because more stimuli are aversive and/or they react more strongly to aversive stimulation (Lonigan & Phillips, 2001). In this conceptualization, a combination of low EC and high NA is implicated as a causal factor in the development and/or maintenance of anxiety and anxiety disorders.

A large literature surrounds another temperamental concept, behavioral inhibition (BI), and its relationship with anxiety disorders. BI is defined as a consistent tendency to display fear and withdrawal in situations that are novel, unfamiliar, and stressful (Kagan, 1997). Several studies have investigated BI and its relationship to the predisposition for anxiety disorders. Rosenbaum and colleagues (1988) investigated BI as an early temperamental characteristic of youth at risk for adult PDAG and found that the rates of behavioral inhibition in youth of probands with PDAG, with or without comorbid MDD, were significantly higher than for the comparison group without PDAG. Biederman and colleagues (1993) investigated the psychopathologic correlates of BI 3 years after the initial assessment in two samples of children: (1) the high-risk offspring of parents with PDAG and other psychiatric disorders from the Rosenbaum and colleagues study, and (2) children followed longitudinally since infancy by Kagan and colleagues. The 3-year follow-up indicated that children with BI had significantly higher rates of many anxiety disorders, including avoidant disorder, SAD, and agoraphobia compared to non-BI children. Whereas initial assessments showed that the increased risk for anxiety disorders was accounted for by higher rates of AvD, OAD, and phobic disorders (Biederman et al., 1990), the follow-up findings indicated that the increased risk was accounted for by higher rates of AvD

and SAD. These studies and others suggest that BI is a predisposition or risk for the development of anxiety disorders.

Neurobiology

Significant advances have been made in recent years in the understanding of the neurobiology of anxiety disorders. Most of these advances have involved the study of adults, but some studies have also been conducted to understand the neurobiology of childhood anxiety disorders. Research has examined the role of neurotransmitter systems, the hypothalamic–pituitary–adrenal (HPA) axis, and neuropeptides in the pathogenesis of childhood anxiety (Sallee & Greenawald, 1995). Findings from these studies are briefly reviewed here.

Considering neurotransmitter systems, the major systems associated with anxiety include the GABAergic, noradrenergic, and serotonergic diatheses. Evidence also suggests the involvement of certain neuropeptides, including cholecystokinin (CCK), neuropeptide Y (NPY), and corticotropin-releasing factor (CRF) (Sallee & Greenawald, 1995). The involvement of the noradrenergic system has been implicated in pathological anxiety due to the key role of this system in the fear response. However, examination of the peripheral markers for noradrenergic activity in children and adolescents is lacking. Pharmacological probes, such as clonidine and yohimbine, which have been used extensively to examine neurotransmitter reactions in anxious adults, have not been as widely utilized with anxious children and adolescents (Cummins & Ninan, 2002). One exception is a study by Sallee and colleagues (1998), which found no blunting of growth hormone response to clonidine in a group of children with mixed anxiety disorders. Chemoreceptor function has also been studied in children with mixed anxiety disorders, with anxious children exhibiting greater changes in somatic anxiety symptoms in response to a CO_2 challenge as compared to nonanxious children (Pine et al., 2000). The serotonergic system also appears to play a key role in the pathogenesis of anxiety disorders. The involvement of this system has been investigated with regard to panic disorder, OCD, SoP, and GAD, to name a few. Much of the knowledge of serotonin's involvement in anxiety disorders has been deduced from treatment studies showing efficacy of selective serotonin reuptake inhibitors (SSRIs) in anxiety disorders (Sallee & Greenawald, 1995). Several neuropeptides, including NPY and CCK, have also been implicated in the pathogenesis of anxiety (Sallee & Greenawald, 1995).

Researchers have also gathered neurobiological data on childhood anxiety disorders by examining the involvement of the HPA axis. Perhaps most indicative of this research are the studies by Kagan and colleagues concerning behaviorally inhibited children. In one such study, Kagan, Reznick, and Snidman (1988) found salivary cortisol (the "stress" hormone) to be elevated in behaviorally inhibited children. Research has also suggested that CRF and growth hormone play a role in childhood anxiety (Sallee & Greenawald, 1995).

Knowledge of the neurobiological pathways involved in childhood anxiety disorders differs by each disorder. The greatest number of studies on the neurobiology of pediatric anxiety has been conducted using populations of children with OCD. There are virtually no studies involving the neurobiology of SoP in pediatric populations (Cummins & Ninan, 2002). In addition, there have been very few studies exploring the neurobiology of GAD and SAD in children and adolescents. According to Greenhill, Pine, March, Birmaher, and Riddle (1998), one impediment to the study of GAD is the poor reliability of measures of this disorder in childhood.

Although the study of the neurobiology of youth anxiety disorders has advanced in recent years, progress lags behind the study of adult anxiety disorders. Further research is needed to better understand the pathogenesis and treatment of youth anxiety disorders.

Psychological Factors: Cognitive Functioning

For adults, a substantial body of work indicates that the variety of anxiety disorders involve biases in information processing (Barlow, 1988). Similarly, accumulating evidence indicates that anxious youth display patterns of selective information processing (e.g., Vasey & Macleod, 2001). Work in this area has focused mainly on selective attention processes, but research has also shown evidence of interpretation and judgment biases.

Studies of the attentional biases in anxious youth have generally used one of two paradigms: a modified Stroop task or a probe detection task. The modified Stroop task is used to compare a person's average latencies to name the color in which threat-relevant and nonthreatening words are written and provides a measure of the interference caused by threatening words. Longer color-naming latencies on threatening words, as opposed to neutral words, are interpreted as evidence that the threat words captured greater attention than did the neutral words. Studies using related tasks have yielded evidence for an attentional bias in anxious youth (e.g., Martin, Horder, & Jones, 1992; Martin & Jones, 1995; Moradi, Neshat Doost, Taghavi, Yule, & Dagleish, 1999; Moradi, Taghavi, Neshat Doost, Yule, & Dagleish, 1999), yet other reports suggest a lack of attentional differences between anxious and nonanxious youth (e.g., Kindt, Brosschot, & Everaerd, 1997).

Studies using the probe detection task with anxious youth have consistently provided evidence of an attentional bias toward threat stimuli (Vasey & Macleod, 2001). The probe detection task involves two words presented one above the other on a computer screen. On certain trials, subsequent to the appearance of a threat-relevant and an emotionally neutral word, a small dot appears in the position previously occupied by one of the two words. The latency to detect this "dot probe" is said to provide a measure of the extent to which attention was direction toward the words that have just appeared in this location. Hence, faster latencies to detect the dot probe in areas in which threatening words had just appeared would indicate an attentional bias toward threat (Vasey & Macleod, 2001). Studies have found that anxious youth (ages 9–14 years) display an attentional bias toward threatening words (Vasey, Daleiden, Williams, & Brown, 1995), and youth (ages 9–14 years) with low levels of trait anxiety exhibit an attentional bias away from threat cues (Schippell, Vasey, Cravens-Brown, & Bretveld, 2003).

Anxious youth tend to display an information-processing bias in which they disproportionately impose negative interpretations upon ambiguous stimuli or situations. For example, Taghavi, Moradi, Neshat Doost, Yule, and Dagleish (2000) used a homograph task to compare the processing of anxious and nonanxious youth, ages 9–16 years. Anxious youth were more likely to produce sentences based on the threatening interpretation of the homographs when compared to control participants. In another study, socially phobic youth, ages 7–14 years, underestimated the future likelihood of positive social events relative to control children (Spence, Donovan, & Brechman-Toussaint, 1999). Moreover, Barrett, Rapee, Dadds, and Ryan (1996) presented ambiguous situations to anxious youth, oppositional youth, and normal control youth and their families. These researchers found that anxious youth perceived the situations to be more threatening than control youth, a result that was replicated in a similar study by Chorpita and colleagues (1996). In the Barrett, Rapee, and colleagues study, anxious youth also showed an increased tendency to choose avoidant solutions to situations they perceived as threatening, when compared with both oppositional and control youth.

The aforementioned studies reviewed strongly suggest that anxious youth display many of the cognitive biases that characterize anxious adults. These biases include favoring threatening interpretations of ambiguity, a selective preference for maladaptive coping responses, overestimation of the likelihood of threatening events, and an attentional bias toward threatening stimuli (Vasey & Macleod, 2001). However, we must be cautious in the application of these findings to adolescents, as most of the studies utilized combined samples of children and adolescents. Moreover, the adolescents included in these studies were generally younger (ages 13–14), to the exclusion of older ages. Although adolescents experience dramatic changes in cognitive functioning, we remain uninformed about both the nature of cognitive biases in anxious adolescents and the developmental course of the cognitive processes that are associated with anxiety because very few studies focus on anxious adolescents.

Familial Influences

Given the substantial role that families play in the lives of youth, it is not surprising that research has focused on parenting behaviors and family influences as contributors to the development and/or maintenance of anxiety. Accumulated evidence supports the integral role of family and parenting behavior in youth anxiety. Although typically limited to maternal influences, findings in family functioning research cluster within several themes: (1) parents of anxious youth tend to be overly controlling and intrusive, overprotective, less

granting of psychological autonomy, and less accepting than parents of nonanxious youth (Dumas & LaFreniere, 1993; Hudson & Rapee, 2001; Last & Strauss, 1990; Siqueland, Kendall, & Steinberg, 1996; Whaley, Pinto, & Sigman, 1999); (2) higher levels of parental rejection and criticism are associated with higher levels of youth anxiety (Dumas, LaFreniere, & Serketich, 1995; Hibbs et al., 1991; Hibbs, Hamburger, Kruesi, & Lenane, 1993; Leib et al., 2000), but studies focusing on parental negative affect and degree of emotional warmth have been mixed (Dadds, Barrett, Rapee, & Ryan, 1996; Dumas et al., 1995; Leib et al., 2000; McClure, Brennan, Hammen, & Le Brocque, 2001; Siqueland et al., 1996); (3) parents of anxious youth model and reinforce anxious and/or avoidant behavior (Barrett, Rapee, et al., 1996; Chorpita et al., 1996; and (4) families of anxious youth are more conflictual and less cohesive and have poor problem-solving and communication skills (Ginsburg, Silverman, & Kurtines, 1995; Stark, Humphrey, Crook, & Lewis, 1990). Unfortunately, because the large majority of the aforementioned studies focus exclusively on childhood, we are uninformed about these issues with regard to families of anxious adolescents.

Developmental psychologists have noted that parent–child relationships remain important well beyond the childhood years (Steinberg & Silk, 2002), but the character of parent–child relationships changes during adolescence (Collins & Laursen, 2004). For example, there is increased emotional distance in the parent–adolescent relationship, as well as transformations in attachments to parents. In addition, the nature of parent–adolescent conflict is changed. Parent–adolescent conflict, which may be high in early adolescence, decreases through mid and late adolescence, although the anger surrounding these conflicts may linger (Collins & Laursen, 2004). Some disagreements focus on mundane topics (Hill, 1988) and conflict may actually contribute to positive aspects of development, allowing for greater individuation in the context of a warm parental relationship (Hill, 1988). Other changes that occur in family relationships during adolescence include decreases in time spent with parents (Youniss & Smollar, 1985) and yielding to parents in decision making (Hill, 1988; Montemayor & Hanson, 1985). It is important during this period that parents and adolescents work together to manage the transition from childhood dependency to adolescent autonomy. In the majority of families, adolescents gradually take on more responsibility for managing their own activities.

The transformation in parent–adolescent relationships and conflicts may be important in understanding developmental processes in adolescent anxiety disorders. For example, although an increase in conflict is normative, families of anxious early adolescents may have difficulty tolerating this level of conflict and surrounding emotionality. Such families may not allow conflict to occur at all or may make conflict so aversive that the adolescent is robbed of any resulting positive consequences. In short, problems in dealing with normative parent–adolescent disagreements may have a negative impact on the process of individuation for anxious adolescents. Parents of anxious adolescents may have trouble allowing other normative developmental processes to occur as a result of their overinvolved, overprotective, and enmeshed nature. The interaction between such parental characteristics and existing adolescent anxiety may foster a discrepancy between how much autonomy the parent is willing to grant and the amount of autonomy the adolescent is able to manage. Adolescents, in turn, may experience difficulty in making decisions for themselves and becoming more autonomous, thereby creating and/or exacerbating symptoms of anxiety.

Peer Relationships

Peer relationships play a critical role in adolescent social and emotional development—adolescents spend approximately one-third of their waking hours with their friends (Hartup & Stevens, 1997). Successful peer relations positively contribute to the development of social skills and feelings of personal competence that are essential for adult functioning (Ingersoll, 1989). During adolescence, peer relationships play are integral in identity formation and increasing independence (Ingersoll, 1989), so much so that the transition from childhood into adolescence has been described as a trading of dependency on parents for dependency on peers (Steinberg & Silverberg, 1986). Disruptions in this process can lead to peer rejection, peer neglect, and membership in low-status peer crowds and related/subsequent adjustment difficulties. The ability to maintain

close friends is important in adolescence, and one might expect that adolescents who do not have close friends may be at risk for loneliness, anxiety, and related internalizing problems (La Greca, 2001).

SoP is perhaps the most likely anxiety-related outcome of poor peer relationships in adolescence; negative, aversive, or exclusionary experiences with peers can lead to avoidance of social interactions. As a result of this avoidance, adolescents miss out on opportunities for positive social interactions that are crucial for successful social and emotional development (La Greca, 2001). This cycle of poor peer interactions and avoidance behavior may lead to further problems with peer relationships and negative mental health outcomes. In addition, new dyadic relationships can form during adolescence (e.g., romantic relationships) that can also have vast implications for social and emotional development. Research is needed to examine the bidirectional impacts of anxiety and social relationships.

Socioeconomic Status, Ethnicity, Culture, and Neighborhoods

A comprehensive study of adolescent development includes examining the broader contexts in which this development occurs, including socioeconomic status (SES); racial, ethnic, and cultural considerations; and neighborhood influences. Due to interrelationships among these aspects of the social environment, we discuss them together. Studies of adults show that rates of anxiety disorders are greater among individuals of lower SES (Horwath & Weissman, 1995). Similarly, with respect to youth, Pine and colleagues (1998) found higher rates of phobias among youth in lower SES families. Considering race, greater rates of phobic disorders have been observed in African American populations (Eaton, Dryman, & Weissman, 1991). Compton and colleagues (2000) reported that African American youth are more likely to exhibit SAD symptoms and Caucasian youth are more likely to show symptoms of SoP (see also Weems et al., 2002). This is a new area of research, and little is known about the mechanism by which SES and race may be associated with anxiety in youth.

Two neglected areas of research are the impact of culture and neighborhoods on the development and/or maintenance of anxiety symptoms. To our knowledge there are currently no published studies investigating the role of culture in the development and/or maintenance of adolescent anxiety and only a few studies investigating neighborhoods. The studies of neighborhoods have shown that living in low SES neighborhoods is predictive of youth engaging in criminal and delinquent behavior (Loeber & Wikstrom, 1993; Peeples & Loeber, 1994), although these neighborhood effects can be viewed as indirect, operating through processes such as parenting, peer, and SES variables (Leventhal & Brooks-Gunn, 2004). In sum, there is no information regarding the mechanism by which SES and anxiety may be related and no research establishing a link between neighborhood and adolescent anxiety disorders.

ASSESSMENT

The goals of assessment are to classify, evaluate, and investigate (Kendall & Flannery-Schroeder, 1998). To attain these goals, multiple methods are used for measuring anxiety problems in youth, including self-report measures, diagnostic interviews, observational methods, and, in rare instances, physiological assessments. In this section we provide an overview followed by a discussion of the special needs and considerations in assessing anxiety in adolescents. The methods and measures we review were selected to be a representative, but not exhaustive, sample of the instruments currently implemented and only measures for which psychometric data is available for both younger and older adolescents are included.

Self-Report Measures

Self-report remains a common method to measure youth anxiety, probably because it is time- and cost-efficient. Most self-report questionnaires can be completed in under 20 minutes and require minimal staff time or training. In addition, many of the self-report instruments provide useful normative data, are easily scored, are reasonably reliable, can discriminate between anxious and normal youth, and are sensitive for assessing treatment outcome (Schniering, Hudson, & Rapee, 2000). Self-report measures of youth anxiety also have limitations including a lack of adequate discriminant validity (Schniering et al., 2000) and poor parent–child agreement across a vari-

ety of self-report measures (Kenny & Faust, 1997). Another consideration when using anxiety self-report instruments is that while self-report measures are useful for obtaining information about anxiety symptoms and severity, they generally are not used to assign a DSM diagnosis. The following instruments have been used extensively and possess acceptable psychometric properties for adolescents of all ages.

Multidimensional Anxiety Scale for Children

The Multidimensional Anxiety Scale for Children (MASC; March, Parker, Sullivan, Stallings, & Conners, 1997) is a 39-item, 4-point Likert self-report rating scale that can be completed by youth ages 8–16 and their parents. MASC items are not intended to map directly onto DSM diagnoses but are made up of four factors: physical symptoms (tense/restless and somatic/autonomic), social anxiety (humiliation/ rejection and public performance), harm avoidance (anxious coping and perfectionism), and separation/panic anxiety. The MASC demonstrated high internal consistency (March et al., 1997; March, Sullivan, & Parker, 1999), and 3-week test–retest reliability for the MASC is .79 in clinical (March et al., 1997) and .88 in school-based samples (March et al., 1999). Currently the MASC is being evaluated for convergent validity and discriminant validity.

Revised Children's Manifest Anxiety Scale

The Revised Children's Manifest Anxiety Scale (RCMAS; Reynolds & Richmond, 1978) assesses anxiety symptoms with 37 items to which youth ages 6–19 respond "yes" or "no." The RCMAS contains three factors: physiological manifestations of anxiety, worry and oversensitivity, and fear/concentration (Finch, Kendall, & Montgomery, 1974; Reynolds & Richmond, 1979). To assess invalid responding, the RCMAS also includes a "lie" scale. Scoring and interpretation (see the RCMAS manual; Reynolds & Richmond, 1985) includes reference to normative data from a large national sample by sex, gender, and age. Internal consistency for the RCMAS is in the .8 range (Witt, Heffer, & Pfeiffer, 1990) and test–retest reliability ranges from .68 to .90 (Reynolds, 1982; Reynolds & Paget, 1983). The RCMAS has differentiated between clinically anxious youth and nonanxious controls

(Stark, Kaslow, & Laurent, 1993) and has shown reductions in anxiety following treatment (Barrett, Dadds, & Rapee, 1996). However, the RCMAS did not discriminate anxious youth from youth with other disorders (e.g., Hoehn-Saric, Maisami, & Wiegand, 1987), specifically depressed youth (e.g., Hodges, 1990) and youth with ADHD (Perrin & Last, 1992).

Screen for Child Anxiety Related Emotional Disorders

The Screen for Child Anxiety Related Emotional Disorders (SCARED; Birmaher et al., 1997, 1999) measures anxiety symptoms. It is a 41-item self-report instrument that assesses DSM symptoms of panic, SAD, SoP, GAD, and symptoms of school phobia. The SCARED can be completed by both parent and child, allowing for multi-informant assessment with the same scale. In a sample of 190 outpatient youth ages 9–18, the SCARED demonstrated good internal consistency (Birmaher et al., 1999) and retest reliability of .86 (5 weeks; Birmaher et al., 1997). Preliminary evidence using the SCARED shows good discriminant validity both between anxiety and nonanxiety disorders and within anxiety disorders (Birmaher et al., 1999).

Fear Survey Schedule for Children—Revised

The Fear Survey Schedule for Children—Revised (FSSC-R; Ollendick, 1983) consists of 80 items describing fears scored on a 3-point Likert scale. Factor analyses suggest five factors including fear of failure and criticism, fear of the unknown, fear of injury and small animals, fear of danger and death, and medical fears (Ollendick, 1983). Normative data exist for youth ages 7–18 (Ollendick, Matson, & Helsel, 1985). Ollendick (1983) reports internal consistency in the .9 range and retest reliability of .55 (3 months) to .82 (1 week). Evidence suggests that the FSSC-R differentiates clinically anxious youth from nonanxious controls (Ollendick, 1983) and is sensitive to reductions in anxiety following treatment (Barrett, Dadds, & Rapee, 1996). However, the FSSC-R did not discriminate between anxious youth and youth with other diagnoses (Hoehn-Saric et al., 1987) as well differentiate subtypes of anxiety disorders in youth (Last, Francis, & Strauss, 1989).

Self-Report Considerations

There are commonalities and differences among the self-report measures. The measures tap multiple anxiety domains and demonstrate adequate psychometric properties. A decision to use one self-report instrument over another might depend on the question being asked. For instance, if multi-informant assessment is important, perhaps the MASC or SCARED would be chosen because both can be completed by youth and their parents. If one is interested in measuring DSM-IV anxiety symptoms/disorders, the Spence Children's Anxiety Scale (SCAS) or SCARED may be appropriate.

Self-report measures with a more specific or broader focus can be used to assess youth anxiety. Although it is beyond the scope of this chapter to review all alternative measures, a few are mentioned. The Social Phobia and Anxiety Inventory for Children (SPAI-C; Beidel, Turner, & Morris, 1995) specifically discriminates between youth with SoP and both normal youth and youth with externalizing problems (Beidel, Fink, & Turner, 1996). In addition, the Social Anxiety Scale for Adolescents (SAS-A; LaGreca, 1998) was designed to measure social anxiety symptoms specifically in adolescents and preliminary evidence indicates adequate psychometric properties (LaGreca, 1998). For younger adolescents, the SCAS (Spence, 1997, 1998) and State–Trait Anxiety Inventory for Children (STAIC; Spielberger, Edwards, & Lushene, 1973) can be used. Broader measures of internalizing symptoms can also be implemented, such as the Child Behavior Checklist (CBCL; Achenbach, 1991) and Youth Self-Report Form (YSR; Achenbach, 1991) completed by parents and youth, respectively.

Interviews

Interviews are crucial for adequate assessment of youth anxiety. Various types of interviews are available (e.g., unstructured, semistructured, and structured). Although unstructured interviews have been used, their lack of standardization poses a problem—the need for uniform evaluation and classification (Stallings & March, 1995). Both structured and semistructured interviews consist of a standardized, predetermined set of inquires that the assessor uses to make an informed diagnostic evaluation. Semistructured interviews are generally clinician administered and provide the assessor with opportunities for elaboration, probing, and application of clinical judgment. Structured interviews can be administered by trained assistants but may limit interviewer flexibility by not allowing for deviation from the predetermined set of questions.

Interviews are more time-consuming and costly than self-report instruments; however, interviews offer distinct advantages over self-reports. First, the information gained by using an interview is often more "rich" than that from self-report questionnaires; youth can elaborate during an interview and assessors can ask for clarifications. Second, whereas self-report instruments typically measure anxiety symptoms, interviews allow for diagnoses of anxiety disorders and other disorders. Finally, the standardized administration of semistructured and structured interviews helps to increase the reliability of diagnostic assessment.

The following interviews are illustrative examples for use with adolescents. Because the Anxiety Disorders Interview Schedule for DSM-IV—Child and Parent Versions (ADIS-C/P; Silverman & Albano, 1996) has been described as the premier instrument for assessing anxiety disorders in youth (Silverman, 1991; Stallings & March, 1995) and it is most often used, more attention is directed to this interview. Other interviews are described as a group and more briefly.

Anxiety Disorders Interview Schedule for DSM-IV—Child and Parent Versions

Based on the adult ADIS (DiNardo, O'Brien, Barlow, Waddell, & Blanchard, 1983) the child and adolescent version was developed for diagnoses of anxiety disorders in youth (e.g., Costello, Edelbrock, Dulcan, Kalas, & Klaric, 1987). The current version of the ADIS-C/P relies on DSM-IV criteria and implements a semistructured, interviewer–observer format through which the user can draw on information obtained in the interview as well as information gained through direct observation (Stallings & March, 1995). The ADIS-C/P focuses on assessing anxiety symptoms in depth but also allows for diagnoses of mood and externalizing disorders and screens for other disorders.

Each of the ADIS interviews, child and parent, takes approximately 1.5–2 hours to administer. There is considerable overlap between the parent and child versions; however, the parent interview addresses externalizing disorders in more depth and screens for developmental disorders, whereas the child interview focuses in greater detail on anxiety symptoms. Both interviews assess duration of the disorder, age of onset, and avoidance behavior and ask the parent and child to provide impairment ratings. The same clinician may interview the child and the parent, but in some cases different clinicians interview the child and parent simultaneously.

When assigning diagnoses, the clinician generates an impairment rating, the Clinician Severity Rating (CSR; 0 to 8) for each ADIS diagnosis. A rating of greater than 4 is necessary to assign a DSM-IV diagnosis. Ratings of less than 4 are usually referred to as subclinical. Diagnoses are typically derived separately based on parent report and child report; then, using an algorithm outlined in the ADIS-C/P Manual (Silverman & Albano, 1996), a composite diagnosis is assigned.

Earlier versions of the ADIS-C/P possess the best psychometric data of available diagnostic measures for the diagnostic assessment of anxiety disorders in youth (Silverman & Eisen, 1992; Silverman & Nelles, 1988). Studies showed previous versions to have high interrater reliability for both the parent ($r = .98$) and child ($r = .93$) interviews (Silverman & Nelles, 1988) and high retest reliability for the parent interview (Silverman & Eisen, 1992). Psychometric data for the ADIS-IV-C/P is still accumulating but looks promising to date. In a recent study, Silverman, Saavedra, and Piña (2001) reported anxiety disorder diagnoses over an interval of 7 to 14 days for the ADIS-IV-C/P to be highly reliable. Specifically, kappa coefficients for SAD, SoP, and GAD were all in the excellent range (.80-.92).

Current and previous versions of the ADIS-C/P have been used extensively with anxious youth as young as age 6 and as old as age 17 (e.g., Piña et al., 2002). The ADIS-C/P is often implemented in treatment outcome research and has shown sensitivity to treatment effects in studies of youth with anxiety disorders (e.g., Dadds, Heard, & Rapee, 1991; Kendall et al., 1997; Leger, Ladouceur, Dugas, & Freeston, 2003). In addition, the ADIS-C/P has also been used as the gold standard of diagnostics by which self-reports are compared and evaluated (e.g., Dierker et al., 2001).

Other Interviews

In addition to the ADIS-C/P, there are many more semistructured and structured interviews available to assess anxiety in youth. Whereas the ADIS-C/P places a particular emphasis on assessing anxiety disorders, most other interviews are designed to screen for a wide range of disorders in youth and contain a subset of questions devoted to the assessment of anxiety. Interviews such as these with the most promising psychometric data include the semistructured Schedule for Affective Disorders and Schizophrenia for School-Age Children-Present and Lifetime Version (K-SADS-PL; Kaufman, Birmaher, Brent, Rao, & Ryan, 1997), the NIMH Diagnostic Interview Schedule for Children version IV (NIMH DISC-IV; Shaffer, Fisher, Lucas, Dulcan, Schwab-Stone, 2000), and the Diagnostic Interview for Children and Adolescents (DICA; Herjanic & Reich, 1982). Other less researched and/or recognized interviews used to assess youth anxiety include the Children's Anxiety Evaluation Form (CAEF; Hoehn-Saric et al., 1987), developed specifically to assess anxiety in youth through a semistructured interview, chart review, and direct observation and the Child and Adolescent Psychiatric Assessment (CAPA; Angold & Costello, 2000; Angold et al., 1995), a semistructured interview developed to assess the presence and level of severity of anxiety disorders and other psychiatric disorders in youth according to DSM-III-R, DSM-IV, and International Classification of Diseases (ICD-10; World Health Organization, 1993) criteria.

Clinician-rated scales and more narrowly focused interviews are also available to assess anxious adolescents. For instance, the Pediatric Anxiety Rating Scale (PARS; RUPP Anxiety Study Group, 2002; Walkup, Davies, & RUPP Anxiety Study Group, 1999) is a clinician-rated anxiety severity rating scale for youth, which specifically addresses the combined severity of SAD, SoP, and GAD symptoms. The PARS is both narrow in focus and only takes approximately 30 minutes to complete, making it an attractive alternative to a more time-consuming diagnostic interview. As another example, the Childhood PTSD Interview (Fletcher, 1997), a semistructured interview, can be used in populations of adolescents who may have experienced or witnessed a traumatic event, thereby reducing the time and cost associated with administration of a more comprehensive interview.

Interviews: Summary and Conclusions

Using an interview format for assessment of adolescent anxiety is necessary to evaluate diagnostic status; all the interviews presented are adequate for this purpose and are the most commonly used in anxiety research with youth. It is important to note that currently there are no interviews designed for use solely with adolescents, and most interviews currently employed were not developed specifically for use with anxious populations. Notwithstanding, overall the use of semistructured and structured interviews, as compared to self-reports, has increased the reliability of diagnosing anxious youth according to DSM criteria. To reflect changes in diagnostic classification systems, most interviews have undergone revisions in recent years, potentially improving diagnostic reliability further (e.g., ADIS-C/P and K-SADS; Schniering et al., 2000). In addition, there is some evidence suggesting that diagnostic interviews are moderately sensitive to various diagnostic groups (Fisher et al., 1993; Sylvester, Hyde, & Reichler, 1987), yet there is still a need for research addressing the discriminant validity of interviews. There is also a problem with cross-informant agreement, which presents a major obstacle in drawing diagnostic conclusions. Studies of parent–child diagnostic agreement have provided mixed results; some studies report poor agreement (Boyle et al., 1993) and other studies report moderate to high agreement (Welner, Reich, Herjanic, Jung, & Amado, 1987), depending on which instrument is used.

Behavioral and Physiological Measures

Behavioral and physiological measurements are alternatives to self-reports and interviews. Both provide a perspective measure on anxiety that cannot be obtained through self-report or interview yet, for several reasons, neither has been fully developed with adolescents. Behavioral assessment of anxiety can be done with a behavioral avoidance test (BAT). BATs involve placing an individual in an anxiety-provoking situation (under controlled conditions) for a few minutes and recording (1) approach behavior, (2) verbal responses, (3) facial expression, and (4) posture

(Schniering et al., 2000). Unfortunately, there are no standardized, psychometrically evaluated BATs. BATs can be useful when a specific situation, event, or object can be identified as anxiety provoking (e.g., fear of public speaking, fear of dogs), and observations can be made of the approach or avoidance behavior. BATs are more difficult to implement when worries are pervasive, as in GAD.

Physiological measurements have been used in the assessment of anxious youth, although their use is also infrequent (King, 1994; March & Albano, 1998). Nevertheless, some studies have found that physiological responses indicate an anxious predisposition in youth. Anxious youth have shown increased adrenergic activity (Rogeness, Cepeda, Macedo, Fischer, & Harris, 1990), increased baseline zygomatic muscle tension (Turner, Beidel, & Epstein, 1991), and increased heart rate during socially relevant challenges (Beidel, 1991). However, one study found no difference between anxious and nonanxious youth on baseline measures of heart rate (Beidel, 1991) and another study found no meaningful differences on physiological measures in response to treatments for phobias (Öst, 1998). More work is needed to establish the clinical utility of physiological measurement in the assessment of anxious youth. Furthermore, no study has assessed physiological responses in an anxiety-disordered adolescent population. Clearly additional research is needed in this area.

Assessment Needs and Considerations

For the most part, the assessment of anxiety in youth has been characterized by insufficient attention to developmental issues. Even though there are multiple methods and many instruments available, most instruments were created for use with both children and adolescents and were not designed specifically for the special needs of adolescents. To our knowledge, no research exists evaluating differences in child and adolescent assessment of anxiety, despite the differences in psychological factors, emotional expressiveness, cognitive processing, and social development between the two age groups. It is important to consider factors unique to adolescence that may impact adequate assessment of anxiety.

Assessment of anxiety in adolescents can be rather straightforward. Unlike children, adolescents are more able to read and understand the questions being asked and typically have the cognitive maturity to accurately respond to inquiries about their thoughts and feelings (Essau & Barrett, 2001). Indeed, adolescents are often considered accurate reporters of their internal state (Essau & Barrett, 2001) and sometimes considered more accurate reporters than parents or teachers. For instance, Cantwell, Lewinsohn, Rohde, and Seeley (1997) found that adolescents ages 14–18 endorsed more core symptoms and disorders than their parents on the K-SADS, particularly for anxiety and depression. Specifically, 58% of diagnoses were based on adolescent report only and only 15% of diagnoses were based solely on parent report. The self-awareness that accompanies adolescent development may contribute to an adolescent's increased reporting of anxiety symptoms. Also, because increasingly more time is spent outside the family and with peers during adolescence, parents may not be the best informants about their adolescent's behavior, emotions, and/or feelings. To date there is insufficient research and multimethod, multi-informant assessment is still considered necessary when evaluating youth (Kazdin, 1986; Ollendick, 1986).

The interpretation of instrument scores is another important consideration when assessing adolescent anxiety. Recall that emotional disruptions are normative for adolescents and it is typical of adolescents to report variability, extremes of emotions (both positive and negative), and emotional disruptions more often than preadolescents (Larson & Richards, 1994; Larson et al., 1980). Increased self-awareness and increased focus on social/peer acceptance issues are also normative. When interpreting self-report scores or assessing diagnostic symptoms in adolescents it is important to keep in mind that increased levels of anxiety symptoms may be a part of normal development and not pathological. Normative data that are based on samples including youth of a wide range ages may be misleading—what is considered normative for a 7-year-old is not normative for a 17-year-old. With adolescents, in addition to measuring anxiety symptomatology, it is especially important to assess impairment and associated disability in multiple domains (e.g., in peer groups). Future assessment studies should aim to establish normative data for adolescents.

TREATMENT AND PREVENTION

Psychosocial Interventions

Individual Interventions for Children and Adolescents

There has been progress in the treatment of anxiety in youth. In the recent past, a series of studies that were conducted by various clinical researchers and used similar intervention procedures (cognitive-behavioral) were reviewed (Kazdin & Weisz, 1998; Ollendick & King, 1998), and cognitive-behavioral treatment of youth anxiety has been deemed empirically supported. We describe here one of the cognitive-behavioral programs in detail, as well as review the variety of studies of this and related and derivative interventions.

A cognitive-behavioral program for treating anxiety in youth, "The Coping Cat program" (Kendall, 2000; Kendall & Hedtke, 2006a; Kendall, Kane, Howard, & Siqueland, 1989;) includes a therapist's treatment manual and a workbook for participant youth (Kendall & Hedtke, 2006b; see www.workbookpublishing. com). The treatment program is designed for youth ages 8–13 and can be used with early adolescents. Note that a separate version, "The C.A.T. project" (Kendall, Choudhury, Hudson, & Webb, 2002), is quite similar but is designed specifically for adolescents. In this section, we first discuss the Coping Cat program because it is the basis for the C.A.T. Project and has been empirically demonstrated to be effective for treating anxious children and young adolescents. The more recently developed C.A.T. Project is described in more detail later in the section.

The overall treatment approach in is cognitive-behavioral. That is, the program integrates the demonstrated efficiencies of a behavioral approach (e.g., rewards, exposure tasks, relaxation training, and role-play opportunities) with an emphasis on the participant's cognitive information processing of social and emotional factors that contribute to and/or maintain anxiety. The typically 16-session treatment is divided into two segments. The first eight sessions are educational and the second eight are for practice (exposure tasks).

The first concept that is introduced to youth in the educational phase is an awareness of bodily reactions to feelings and recognition of those bodily reactions that are specific to anxiety. Throughout, the workbook provides youth with exercises and assignments that facilitate their learning. Next, youth come to recognize and focus on anxious "self-talk," which includes both expectations and fears about what will happen, as well as the role the child/teen sees for him- or herself. The third concept has to do with the modification of anxious self-talk into coping self-talk and the development of plans for coping effectively in anxiety-producing situations. Fourth, youth are introduced to the concepts of evaluating the results and dispensing of self-reward for effort. These concepts are summarized in the acronym FEAR, which helps youth recall the treatment plan: "F" for Feeling frightened?, "E" for Expecting bad things to happen?, "A" for Attitudes and Actions that will help, and "R" for Results and Rewards. After several weeks, with therapist and workbook and practice assignments, youth master the FEAR plan and have improved confidence.

The second segment of the treatment is devoted to exposure tasks and the application and practice of the FEAR skills in these anxiety-provoking situations. Training strategies such as coping modeling, role-play, and "Show-That-I-Can" (STIC) assignments are employed. Youth begin with imaginal exposures to nonstressful situations and progress to *in vivo* exposure tasks in highly stressful situations. Participants experience anxiety in real situations (out-of-the-office situations) and experience the pleasure and confidence that accompanies the mastery. Although planned over several sessions, the last session provides youth with the opportunity of videotaping a "commercial," an individualized and creative "message" about learning to cope with anxiety. In a nutshell, the youth shares what he or she has learned and found useful in the treatment program.

The first randomized clinical trial of cognitive-behavioral therapy (CBT) using the manualized treatment just described (Kendall, 1994) included 47 youth with anxiety disorders, ages 9–13 years, who were referred from multiple community sources. Of these 47 youth, 27 received active treatment and 20 were wait-list controls (receiving treatment after the wait period). Youth had received a primary anxiety disorder diagnosis, as assessed by the ADIS-C and the ADIS-P, of OAD ($n = 30$), SAD ($n = 8$), or AvD ($n = 9$). Cases were randomly assigned to the 16-week treatment program or the wait-list. All treated cases were randomly assigned to therapists. Participants received an average of 17, 50–60 minutes session over a 5–6-month period. Results indicated that compared to wait-list controls, those who received CBT evidenced a significant positive change from pre- to posttreatment on self-report, parent report, and behavioral observation measures as well as their diagnostic status. Both youth and parent diagnostic interview data indicated that 64% of the treated cases no longer met diagnostic criteria at posttreatment. One-year follow-up data suggested the maintenance of the treatment-produced gains, and a 3.35-year follow-up (Kendall & Southam-Gerow, 1996) examining 36 of the original 47 youth indicated that the child and adolescent clients largely maintained their gains over anxiety-related disorders.

A second randomized clinical trial with 94 youth ages 9–13 years again supported the efficacy of CBT for anxiety in youth, with over 50% of treated cases being free of the primary anxiety disorder at posttreatment (Kendall et al., 1997). Youth who received the Coping Cat treatment were also found to have significant positive change on self-report, parent report, and some behavioral observation measures. Clinically significant gains were maintained at 1-year follow-up and at 7.4-year follow-up (Kendall, Safford, Flannery-Schroeder & Webb, 2004).

Other evaluations of CBT (e.g., Barrett, 1998; Barrett, Dadds, & Rapee, 1996; Cobham, Dadds, & Spence, 1998; Mendlowitz et al., 1999; Silverman et al., 1999), including some in other countries and cultures, in combination with the work already described, have led to the designation that the treatment is probably efficacious (according to APA guidelines; Chambless & Hollon, 1998). According to Chambless and Hollon (1998), a treatment may be considered efficacious if it has been found to be more effective than no treatment, a placebo, or an alternate treatment across multiple trials conducted by different investigative teams.

Family-Focused Interventions for Children and Adolescents

Several researchers and clinicians have noted the need for more rigorous evaluation of the role of parental involvement in the outcome of treatment for anxiety in youth. Research on the etiology and maintenance of anxiety in youth

suggests that involvement of parents in treatment could be appropriate and worthwhile.

A few evaluations involving the families of youth with anxiety disorders have been reported. Howard and Kendall (1996) used a multiple-baseline design to evaluate a family-based intervention with six youth, ages 9–13 years, who met diagnostic criteria for an anxiety disorder. A manualized 18-session family-based CBT (Howard & Kendall, 1992) was the treatment. The manualized family-based intervention made the family a part of the solution. Family members were actively involved in evaluating their own experiences with anxiety and their own attempts to cope with anxious situations. Families received an average of 18, 50-minutes sessions, each of which included at least one parent. The results were favorable, with meaningful gains from pre- to posttreatment indicated on parent report, child report, and teacher report measures, as well as on independent clinicians' diagnostic ratings for four of the six subjects. The remaining two subjects showed improvement on most but not all ratings. Treatment gains were generally maintained, except for one youth who experienced parental separation and family violence during follow-up.

CBT, CBT plus family anxiety management (CBT + FAM), and a wait-list control (WLC) condition were compared in a study by Barrett, Dadds, and Rapee (1996). Seventy-nine youth, ages 7–14 years, with primary diagnoses of OAD, SAD, or SoP participated. The FAM component ran parallel with an Australian adaptation of Coping Cat called the Coping Koala. In the CBT + FAM condition, after each youth completed an individual session, the child and parents would have a FAM session. The FAM component had three aims: (1) training parents to reward courageous behavior and extinguish excessive anxiety; (2) teaching parents how to deal with their own emotional upsets, to gain awareness of their own anxiety responses in stressful situations, and to model problem-solving and proactive responses to feared situations; and (3) brief training in communication and problem-solving skills (Barrett, Dadds, & Rapee, 1996). The outcomes indicated that both active treatments produced significant change in comparison to the wait list. At posttreatment, 57% of youth who had received CBT only no longer met diagnostic criteria. 71% of youth were free of diagnoses at 6-month follow-up, and 70% were free of diagnoses at 12 months. For youth receiving CBT + FAM, 84% were diagnosis free at posttreatment, 84% at 6-month follow-up, and 95% at 12-month follow-up. Different treatment success rates by age and gender were evident in response to the two active conditions, with younger children and females responding better in the CBT + FAM condition. The age effect might be due to the fact that enhancing parenting skills is important for younger children (and less needed for adolescents) but cognitive treatment and exposure tasks remain important for older children and adolescents.

Barrett (1998) extended this work using a randomized clinical trial to investigate whether the CBT + FAM intervention presented in a group format was as effective as individual CBT + FAM interventions (Barrett, Dadds, & Rapee, 1996). The three treatment conditions in this study were a group cognitive-behavioral therapy condition (GROUP-CBT), a group cognitive-behavioral therapy plus family management condition (GROUP-FAM), and a WLC condition. Participants were 60 youth ranging in age from 7 to 14 years, with diagnoses of OAD, SAD, or SoP. Both active treatments produced significant change on the dependent variables in contrast to the WLC condition. Improvement was evident across measures and was maintained at 12-month follow-up. Moreover, the group intervention with the FAM component showed some slight improvement over the cognitive-behavioral group intervention on some measures (e.g., parent reports supported the extra benefits of the GROUP-FAM intervention). The results are encouraging, suggesting that group treatment including the family can be effective.

Cobham and colleagues (1998) focused their family intervention on the parental anxiety management component. Participants were 67 youth ranging in age from 7 to 14 years and diagnosed with SAD, OAD/GAD, simple phobia with severe impairment, or SoP. On the basis of parents' scores on the Trait Anxiety scale of the STAI, families were assigned to either the child-anxiety-only condition or to the child + parental anxiety condition. Within the two anxiety conditions, the families were randomly assigned to either CBT for the child or CBT for the child + parental anxiety management (CBT + PAM). Thus, there were four conditions: child anxiety only/CBT, child anxiety only/CBT + PAM, child + parental anxiety/CBT, and child + parental anxiety/CBT + PAM. Treatment was

conducted in 10 groups ranging in size from five to eight families and was based on the Australian adaptation of the treatment program. The CBT program consisted of 10 sessions spread across 14 weeks. The CBT + PAM program consisted of 10 sessions of CBT for the child and four sessions of PAM. These sessions involved psychoeducation about the etiology of youth anxiety (with particular emphasis on the role of the family), cognitive restructuring, relaxation training, and contingency management. The PAM program had two aims: (1) to make parents aware of their possible role in the development and/or maintenance of their children's anxiety; and (2) to teach parents how to recognize and manage their own anxiety and to model effective coping strategies for their children.

In terms of diagnostic status, the results indicated that youth who had one or more anxious parents responded less favorably to child-focused CBT compared with youth whose parents were both nonanxious. That is, the added PAM component enhanced the efficacy of child-focused CBT for youth with one or more anxious parents but not for youth with nonanxious parents. In the child-anxiety-only condition, 82.4% of youth who received CBT only and 80% of youth who received CBT + PAM were free of their diagnosis at posttreatment. In the child + parental anxiety condition, 38.9% of youth who received CBT only and 76.5% of youth who received CBT + PAM were diagnosis free. Although these diagnostic results are encouraging, neither the clinicians' ratings of improvement nor the youth self-report measures differentiated between the four groups at follow-up.

Interventions for Children and Adolescents with OCD

Though fewer than the empirical evaluations of psychosocial treatments for anxious youth with GAD, SoP, and/or SAD, some studies have evaluated psychotherapeutic interventions for youth with OCD. The literature suggests that CBT is the psychotherapeutic treatment of choice for this disorder. CBT for OCD generally involves graded exposure and response prevention, with some cognitive techniques and family involvement.

March, Mulle, and Herbel (1994) conducted an open trial of CBT for 15 children and adolescents, ages 8–18 years, with OCD. Their treatment manual was written to facilitate patient and parental compliance, exportability, and empirical evaluation. Most of the participants were also treated with medication. Treatment length ranged from 3 to 21 months and the follow-up ranged from 1 to 21 months. Significant effects of treatment were demonstrated at posttreatment and at follow-up. Nine participants experienced at least a 50% reduction in symptoms on the Children's Yale–Brown Obsessive–Compulsive Scale (CYBOCS) at posttreatment. In addition, at this time point, scores on the National Institute of Mental Health Global Obsessive Compulsive Scale showed that six patients were symptom free. None of the participants experienced relapse at subsequent follow-up assessments. Six patients who received booster behavioral sessions at follow-up points were able to discontinue medication use. March and colleagues concluded that CBT, alone or in combination with medication, showed promise as a safe and effective treatment for youth with OCD.

Another open clinical trial, reported by Franklin and colleagues (1998), also examined the efficacy of CBT involving exposure and ritual prevention for youth with OCD. Participants were 14 youth, ages 10–17 years, who were diagnosed with OCD. Seven participants received intensive treatment (mean = 18 sessions over 1 month) and seven participants received weekly treatment (mean = 16 sessions over 4 months). Six participants received CBT alone and eight participants received CBT + an SSRI. Results showed that CBT was effective in treating the symptoms of OCD, as 12 participants were at least 50% improved on YBOCS scores at posttreatment. Improvements were maintained at follow-up. The mean reduction in YBOCS scores was 67% at posttreatment and 62% at follow-up. Franklin and colleagues concluded that exposure and ritual prevention represents an efficacious treatment for youth with OCD.

In addition to individual treatment, CBT for OCD has also been conducted in group settings. One study examined the efficacy of a 14-week group format CBT program using 18 adolescents, ages 13–17 years (Thieneman, Martin, Cregger, Thompson, & Dyer-Friedman, 2001). The group CBT program, based on March and Mulle's (1998) treatment protocol, was conducted over a 1-year period. OCD symptoms, as measured by the CYBOCS, evidenced both statistical and clinical significance.

Thieneman and colleagues (2001) reported that participants consistently shared information and helped to design exposures for themselves and other group members. Self-report measures indicated that participants were satisfied with the treatment program. Thieneman and colleagues suggested that this pilot study demonstrates that a manual-based treatment protocol may be exported for clinical use, adaptable for the end user's needs, and palatable to adolescent patients. The authors called for further investigation of group CBT for OCD in a controlled study.

Himle and colleagues (Fischer, Himle, & Hanna, 1998; Himle, Fischer, Van Etten, Janeck, & Hanna, 2003) have conducted two studies to examine the efficacy of group behavioral therapy for adolescents with OCD. In the first study, 15 adolescents (ages 12–17 years) with OCD participated in a 7-week treatment program that included group sessions with therapist-assisted exposure and response prevention exercises, information regarding OCD, and the extensive use of behavioral homework assignments (Fischer et al., 1998). An additional family session was conducted to educate families about OCD and to encourage participation in the group member's behavioral program. At posttreatment, all clients showed improvement on CYBOCS, with even further improvement at 6-month follow-up. Another study examined whether response to psychosocial treatment differs in adolescents, depending on the presence of comorbid tics (Himle et al., 2003). Nineteen adolescents, 12–17 years of age, participated in 7-week, uncontrolled trial of group CBT for OCD. Significant improvement was observed for all subjects on the CYBOCS, with similar outcomes for subjects with tic-related and non-tic-related OCD.

Exposure and response prevention has also been used in conjunction with medication in the treatment of youth with OCD. Neziroglu, Yaryura-Tobias, Walz, and McKay (2000) explored whether adding behavior therapy to medication would enhance treatment efficacy. Ten patients with OCD, ages 10–17 years, who had not previously responded to behavior therapy, were randomly assigned to two groups: fluvoxamine alone or fluvoxamine with behavior therapy. All 10 participants received fluvoxamine for 10 weeks; five of these participants continued only with the medication for a year and five received 20 additional sessions of behavior therapy. Eight of the participants improved on fluvoxamine at week 10 on the CYBOCS, but improvement was not as impressive on other OCD measures. According to the CYBOCS, those who received a combination of fluvoxamine and exposure with response prevention showed the most improvement. At 2-year follow-up, all participants continued to improve, with those in the combined approach improving more than those in the medication-alone group.

Overall, these results argue for the efficacy of CBT for the treatment of youth with OCD. Only a handful of these studies (Fischer et al., 1998; Himle et al., 2003; Thieneman et al., 2001) used a solely adolescent sample; however, the encouraging results support further study of CBT for adolescents with OCD.

Special Considerations in Treating Anxious Adolescents

Given the developmental differences between children and adolescents, and a connection between psychological development and adolescent treatment, a great deal more effort needs to be directed toward interventions for youth anxiety disorders that vary according to age/developmental levels. Empirically supported treatments for adolescents are often either downward adaptations of adult treatments or upward adaptations of child treatments (Weisz & Hawley, 2002), and more attention is needed to take into account the biological, psychological, and social dimensions of adolescent development. Each of these aspects of development is relevant when treating anxious adolescents.

For example, adolescence is a time of biological change, with spurts in growth; changes in body shape, facial features, and hormone levels; and the emergence of sexual and reproductive capacity. Adolescents have a variety of reactions to these changes, some of which may include heightened self-consciousness and even distress. It makes sense for treatments for adolescent anxiety disorders to include content about maturational change. Contexts have been cited as important factors in adolescent treatment (Holmbeck et al., 2000). For instance, peer relationships become increasingly important and peer problems and increased social anxiety can be common among referred adolescents. Conflict between adolescents and their parents increases in early adolescence

(Steinberg, 1981) and treatments that address interpersonal skills and relationships during adolescence are needed (Weisz & Hawley, 2002).

Adolescence is also a time of rapid cognitive development and Holmbeck and colleagues (2000) suggested that abstraction, consequential thinking, and hypothetical reasoning are relevant. CBT, which often requires hypothetical reasoning, problem solving, anticipation of consequences for actions, and metacognition may be especially well suited for adolescents, fitting in well with their newly developing cognitive skills. Finally, motivation for change is important when treating anxious adolescents: Some may be highly motivated, whereas others will offer motivational challenges to the therapist (Weisz & Hawley, 2002). Special attention to involvement and the therapeutic relationship may be needed for effective treatment of anxious adolescents.

Psychosocial Interventions Specifically Designed for Adolescents

Although interventions have been designed for children and young adolescents as a group, treatments designed solely for adolescents are less frequent. Albano, Marten, Holt, Heimberg, and Barlow (1995) described a cognitive-behavioral group treatment for social phobic adolescents (CBGT-A). Their CBGT-A is based on the successful adult SoP program developed by Heimberg and colleagues (Heimberg et al., 1990; Hope & Heimberg, 1985) and incorporates skill-building components for increasing social functioning and prosocial behavior. According to Albano and colleagues, the goals of CBGT-A are to teach adolescents to master their SoP by learning to (1) identify specific triggers to anxiety; (2) recognize and examine anxious responses across cognitive, physiological, and behavioral components of anxiety; (3) learn and apply appropriate anxiety management skills across the three components; and (4) accept and cope with normal, expected levels of social anxiety. CBGT-A incorporates psychoeducation about the nature of anxiety, skill building, modeling and role playing, cognitive restructuring, and both within- and between-session exposure to anxiety-provoking social situations. The program is designed for groups of adolescents between the ages of 13 and 17 years, and for delivery by trained co-therapists. CBGT-A has two phases, with sessions 1 through 8 focusing on the introduction and review of skills to reduce anxiety and facilitate social interactions and sessions 9 through 14 devoted to simulated within-session exposures, cognitive restructuring, and *in vivo* exposures unique to each group member. Session 15 involves exposures in front of parents and session 16 focuses on termination, final exposures, and celebration of success (Albano & Barlow, 1996)

Preliminary data (Albano et al., 1995) have been provided on CBGT-A with five adolescents, ages 13–16 years, with a principal DSM-III-R diagnosis of SoP, generalized type. All five adolescents also met criteria for comorbid disorders (e.g., OAD and mood disorders). At 3-month follow-up, SoP was subclinical for all but one adolescent. By 12-month follow-up, four participants no longer received any psychiatric diagnoses, and the fifth participant received a subclinical SoP diagnosis. In addition, positive changes were reported in participants' cognitive functioning (change from a negative self-focus to a nonthreatening, nonanxious focus during socially challenging tasks).

Hayward and colleagues (2000) investigated the efficacy of CBGT-A in females with SoP (and its effects on the risk for major depression). Thirty-five female adolescents with SoP were randomly assigned to treatment ($n = 12$) or no-treatment ($n = 23$) groups. Eleven of the 12 participants completed the CBGT-A program and the results indicated that 16 weeks of treatment produced a significant improvement in interference and reduction in symptoms of social anxiety. The number of participants meeting DSM-IV criteria for SoP was significantly reduced in the CBGT-A condition versus the no-treatment condition. Results also suggested that treatment reduced the risk of relapse in depression among those participants with a history of depression. However, at 1-year follow-up, there were nonsignificant differences between conditions. Hayward and colleagues concluded that their pilot study provided some evidence for a short-term effect in using CBGT-A to treat adolescents suffering from SoP and that treatment may reduce the likelihood of future depressive episodes.

Masia, Klein, Storch, and Corda (2001) extended treatment for socially phobic adolescents by integrating treatment into the school setting. According to Masia and colleagues,

school intervention for SoP may be important for several reasons, including (1) teacher education and school screening may identify adolescents not receiving services, (2) a frequent concern regarding behavioral treatment programs is that skills acquired in the clinic do not generalize to the natural environment, and (3) treatment itself can be designed to include therapeutic features such as access to peer support and teacher assistance for practice exercises. Six adolescents with SoP were treated in a group treatment conducted at school. The intervention, Skills for Academic and Social Success (SASS), was composed of 14 group sessions: one educational session, one session on realistic thinking, four social-skills-training sessions, five sessions of exposure, and one session on relapse prevention. Two additional meetings were included for practicing social skills in an unstructured environment. Assessments were conducted at pre- and posttreatment. All participants were classified as treatment responders, showing moderate to marked improvement, and three out of the six adolescents no longer met diagnostic criteria for SoP at posttreatment. The severity of SoP symptoms also significantly decreased after the intervention. Masia and colleagues concluded that their behavioral intervention, consisting mainly of exposure and social-skills training, demonstrated promising treatment effects, and they reported that conducting group treatment at school was feasible.

Although empirical data have not yet been published, Scapillato and Manassis (2002) reported their clinical experience with mixed-gender groups of young adolescents (ages 12–15 years) with a DSM-IV anxiety disorder (SAD, OAD, SoP, or simple phobia) and treated with a 20-session, manual-based, cognitive-behavioral/interpersonal group intervention. The intervention emphasizes cognitive-behavioral approaches for anxiety management and problem solving within an interpersonal group context. Scapillato and Manassis theorized that the presentation of anxiety management early in the group permitted ongoing reinforcement of cognitive skills throughout the duration of treatment and speculated that group interactions that may have contributed to anxiety reduction include cohesion-building activities, psychoeducation about anxiety, opportunities for observational learning, exposure to peer models, and general group therapeutic factors.

Recently, Leger and colleagues (2003) reported on a cognitive-behavioral treatment targeting GAD among seven adolescents. The treatment consisted of awareness training, worry interventions, and relapse prevention. The worry interventions involved targeting intolerance of uncertainty, reevaluation of beliefs about worry, problem-solving training, and cognitive exposure to threatening mental images. Based on the diagnostic criteria for GAD, three of the seven participants showed a large decrease in GAD symptoms that was maintained at 6- and 12-month follow-up. Two other participants showed a moderate decrease in GAD symptoms, one participant failed to improve, and one participant dropped out of treatment at session 5. These results, as has been the case with other small sample reports of work with adolescents, suggest further evaluation of CBT for adolescents.

The empirically supported Coping Cat program was recently modified to focus specifically on adolescents (see the "C.A.T. Project"; Kendall et al., 2002) Adolescents participating in the C.A.T. Project receive 16, 60-minute sessions over a 16-week period. The first eight sessions explore the nature of the adolescent's difficulties, increasing flexibility in thinking about problems, and learning active strategies to change the adolescent's and parents' ways of reacting when the adolescent becomes anxious. The second eight sessions are devoted to the application and practice of the newly acquired skills in increasingly anxiety-provoking situations, both within session and *in vivo*. The main principles of the C.A.T. Project are (1) recognizing anxious feelings and somatic reactions to anxiety, (2) identifying cognition in anxiety-provoking situations (i.e., unrealistic or negative expectations), (3) developing a plan to cope with the situation (i.e., modifying anxious self-talk into coping self-talk as well as determining what coping actions might be effective, (4) behavioral exposure, and (5) evaluating performance and self-reinforcement. To help reinforce and generalize the skills, specific homework tasks are assigned. In addition, parents are minimally involved in the adolescent's treatment. Parents are scheduled for meetings with the therapist at the fourth and ninth sessions and prior to the end of treatment.

The C.A.T. Project, though consistent with the Coping Cat, includes adjustments made specifically for adolescents. Adolescents can be unwilling to participate in activities that they see as immature or childish; thus the treatment manual (Kendall et al., 2002) includes strategies that are matched to the developmental level of the adolescent participant. For instance, the C.A.T. Project provides adult-like information about the nature of anxiety, and provides for a more strategic use of the FEAR plan. Also, the manual addresses several "thinking traps" and refers to them in a more cognitively mature manner. There is less emphasis on affect recognition (adolescents know more about different feelings) and the C.A.T. Project uses a point system (not stickers) for keeping track of success and select from age-appealing rewards (e.g., small gift certificates). Importantly, the C.A.T. project encourages independence. The C.A.T. Project treatment is implemented flexibly yet, within the fidelity of the manual, supporting adjustments to individualize the program to the needs of the adolescent.

In a pilot evaluation, using a multiple baseline strategy, the C.A.T. Project protocol was used to treat three adolescents, two with a principal diagnosis of GAD and one with a principal diagnosis of SoP. Adolescents participated in a 16-week treatment (50–60-minute sessions/week). Treatment began after varied baselines of 2, 4, and 6 weeks. Structured clinical interviews (blind evaluator), a clinician-rated global adjustment scale, adolescent self-report instruments, and parent reports were administered at the start of the baselines, at the start of treatment, and following treatment. In addition, several measures were taken weekly throughout treatment.

At the end of their respective baseline periods, adolescents continued to meet diagnostic criteria for their principal diagnosis, based on parent and child reports. Similarly, clinician-rated global adjustment, parent report of adolescent, and adolescent self-report showed no meaningful change during baseline. These data suggest the stability of the problems and the absence of change that may be associated with seeking treatment. Following treatment, the data suggested that the adolescents who participated in treatment showed an alleviation of their target diagnosis/symptoms. Specifically, engaging in treatment was associated with changes in principal diagnoses for all three participants. Clinician-rated global adjustment, parent report measures, and adolescent self-report also showed marked improvement following treatment using the C.A.T. Project manual.

Summary

The small sample studies that have been reported are promising, but the field of research on interventions designed specifically for adolescents with anxiety disorders is in its infancy. Preliminary results are encouraging but randomized clinical trials are needed, and treatments with a special focus on the features of adolescents are likely to optimize outcomes. Stated directly: (1) interventions for adolescents need to incorporate and address physical, social, and cognitive development and (2) there is a need for interventions addressing other anxiety disorders as most psychosocial interventions for adolescent anxiety have targeted SoP exclusively.

Pharmacological Treatment

Pharmacological treatment has also been investigated as a means of alleviating anxiety in adolescents. The classes of drugs that have been investigated include benzodiazepines, tricyclic antidepressants (TCAs), SSRIs, and buspirone. Medications that are typically considered third-line medications for youth anxiety disorders, including monoamine oxidase inhibitors (MAOIs), antihistamines, and beta-blockers will not be included in this review.

Despite approximately 40 years of controlled trials in pediatric populations, none of the aforementioned medications has definitive evidence of its efficacy for adolescent anxiety disorders, except for OCD (e.g., Apter et al., 1994; Liebowitz et al., 2002; March et al., 1998; Riddle et al., 1996; Tollefson et al., 1994). Nevertheless, medications with Food and Drug Administration (FDA) indications for adults with anxiety disorders are often utilized and said to be of some benefit for anxious children and adolescents (Labellarte, Ginsburg, Walkup, & Riddle, 1999).

Benzodiazepines

The benzodiazepines used to treat anxiety include alprazolam, clonazepam, and lorazepam. These drugs have been widely studied in adults, yet the conclusions of the few controlled studies in pediatric populations are limited by small sample sizes, short duration of medication trials, low dosages, and high placebo response rates (Riddle et al., 1999). Simeon and Ferguson (1987) reported a 4-week, placebo–drug–placebo crossover trial of alprazolam with 12 youth, ages 8–16 years, who met DSM-III criteria for OAD or AvD. The results of this study showed significant improvements on clinician, parent, and teacher ratings that continued through the posttreatment placebo phase. Another open trial of a benzodiazepine, clonazepam, was conducted with four adolescents, ages 16–19 years, who met DSM-III criteria for PD (Kutcher & Mackenzie, 1988). The results showed an improvement in anxiety symptoms and a decrease in the frequency of panic attacks. Bernstein, Garfinkel, and Borchardt (1990) reported on the use of alprazolam and imipramine in an open trial with 17 patients, ages 9–17. Fifteen of these youth met criteria for a depressive or anxiety disorder and two of the participants did not meet criteria for a DSM-III diagnosis but were experiencing symptoms of depression and anxiety. All participants were not attending school and were enrolled in a school reentry program. Participants received either alprazolam or imipramine, and the duration of the medication treatment was individualized for each youth. Results indicated that 55% of the participants in the alprazolam group returned to school, whereas 50% returned to school in the imipramine group. Overall, two-thirds of the participants who completed the trial in both drug groups showed moderate to marked global improvement in symptoms of anxiety and depression. However, caution is warranted in interpreting the results of this study, as participants received psychotherapy and were involved in a school reentry program, in addition to medication treatment.

Several studies investigating the efficacy of benzodiazepines have found less favorable results. A second investigation by Bernstein and colleagues (1990), an 8-week, double-blind, placebo-controlled study, examined the efficacy of alprazolam and imipramine with 24 youth, ages 7–17 years, with school refusal and a diagnosis of an anxiety or depressive disorder. At the end of the study, scores on a clinician rating scale of anxiety significantly differentiated between the placebo and medication groups (Bernstein et al., 1990). However, the findings of this study are difficult to interpret, as the largest improvement was seen in the group that had a greater level of severity in symptomatology at baseline and the treatment groups did not differ significantly on measures of child anxiety and depression. Another study used alprazolam in a 4-week, double-blind, placebo-controlled study with 30 participants, ages 8–16 years, with a primary diagnosis of OAD or AvD (Simeon et al., 1992). When considering study completers, 88% of youth on alprazolam improved versus 62% on placebo, but this difference was not statistically significant. Another trial of clonazepam, a 4-week, double-blind, crossover trial, with 15 youth ages 7–13 years who met criteria for an anxiety disorder, also reported nonsignificant differences between clonazepam and placebo (Graae, Milner, Rizzotto, & Klein, 1994).

The lack of definitive support for benzodiazepines in the treatment of child and adolescent anxiety disorders is inconsistent with the evidence found in adult trials (Labellarte et al., 1999). According to Velosa and Riddle (2000), due to the unproven efficacy of benzodiazepines in pediatric populations and the potential for abuse and difficulty with discontinuation, this class of drugs should be considered for the treatment of adolescent anxiety disorders only when other approaches and medications have been unsuccessful.

Tricyclic Antidepressants

TCAs have been investigated for the treatment of child and adolescent anxiety disorders with inconsistent results (Velosa & Riddle, 2000). Clinicians have raised concerns about the use of TCAs with youth, due to several reports of sudden death in youth taking these medications (Popper & Ziminitzky, 1995; Riddle, Geller, & Ryan, 1993; Riddle et al., 1991). TCAs have been investigated primarily for the treatment of OCD and SAD/school refusal.

Three controlled double-blind studies of clomipramine have been conducted for youth with OCD. Two studies demonstrated efficacy for pediatric OCD when compared with placebo (DeVeaugh-Geiss et al., 1992; Flament et al., 1985), and another study found benefit when compared with desipramine (Leonard et al., 1989). In the study by Flament and colleagues (1985), approximately 75% of youth showed a moderate to marked response to clomipramine within 5 weeks. Leonard and colleagues (1989) replicated this result and also found that 66% of youth relapsed after they were switched from clomipramine to desipramine.

Four placebo-controlled studies examined the efficacy of TCAs for SAD or school refusal.

Gittelman-Klein and Klein (1971, 1973) conducted a double-blind, placebo-controlled study of imipramine in a group of 35 school phobic youth ages 6–14 years. Imipramine was superior to placebo in terms of the number of youth returning to school and symptom improvement, as measured by self-report, parent report, and clinician ratings. Klein, Koplewicz, and Kanner (1992) were unsuccessful in replicating their earlier findings in a group of 20 youth with SAD. Another placebo-controlled trial using clomipramine with 51 school phobic youth, ages 9–14 years, also failed to find evidence of efficacy (Berney et al., 1981). Findings from this study indicated no difference between clomipramine and placebo, though this might have been due to the fact that many of the patients also had depressive symptoms or to inadequate dosing. Finally, as described earlier, Bernstein and colleagues (1990) compared alprazolam and imipramine in a double-blind study of youth with school refusal. In the open study with 17 youth, two-thirds of those completing a trial of either medication reported improvement in their anxiety symptoms. Results from a placebo-controlled study with 24 youth were less clear.

Considering the results of TCA trials, this class of medications has been found to be efficacious in treating OCD and may be helpful in treating SAD and school refusal. Given the ambiguous results, as well as the potential for unwanted side effects, the literature suggests that TCAs not be considered a first-line treatment for pediatric anxiety disorders.

Selective Serotonin Reuptake Inhibitors

The SSRIs include citalopram, fluoxetine, fluvoxamine, paroxetine, and sertraline. This class of drugs selectively inhibits the reuptake of serotonin into the presynaptic terminal, which results in an increase in serotonin in the synaptic cleft. The SSRIs' therapeutic effects are hypothesized to involve neuroadaptive changes of a specific receptor subtype, which results in a net increase in serotonergic neurotransmission (Velosa & Riddle, 2000). In studies of adults, SSRIs are said to have broad anxiolytic effects (Labellarte et al., 1999) and are increasingly being considered for the treatment of anxiety disorders in youth (Velosa & Riddle, 2000).

Pediatric SSRI trials have focused on OCD. Three medications, clomipramine (a TCA with serotonergic properties), fluvoxamine, and sertraline, have evidenced sufficient safety and efficacy to warrant FDA approval for youth with OCD (Labellarte et al., 1999). Fluvoxamine has been shown to be safe, effective, and well tolerated in several open-label and placebo-controlled trials with children and adolescents with OCD (e.g., Apter et al., 1994; Riddle et al., 1996). A multisite, placebo-controlled trial of sertraline with 187 patients, ages 6–17 years, found the drug to also be safe and effective in treating pediatric OCD (March et al., 1998). Fluoxetine has also been investigated in the treatment of OCD in children and adolescents. In a multisite trial of OCD patients ages 15–70 years, fluoxetine was found to significantly improve OCD symptoms (Tollefson et al., 1994). Liebowitz and colleagues (2002) also reported fluoxetine to be well tolerated, safe, and superior to placebo for youth with OCD. Two small controlled trials of fluoxetine in youth with OCD and Tourette syndrome reported a modest effect on OCD symptoms, as symptoms improved from baseline but there was no difference from placebo, and no exacerbation of tics (Kurlan, Como, Deeley, McDermott, & McDermott, 1993; Scahill et al., 1997). Notably, in two trials of fluoxetine, Geller, Biederman, Reed, Spencer, and Wilens (1995; Geller et al., 2001) found that treatment response in children and in adolescents was comparable. Based on the results of trials for OCD, SSRIs have been used for other anxiety disorders, including SoP, selective mutism, SAD, GAD, and PD. Open fluoxetine trials in children and adolescents suggested benefits in 21 youth with SoP, SAD, OAD, or a combination of these disorders (Birmaher et al., 1994), and in 16 youth with SAD, SoP, PD, and GAD (Fairbanks et al., 1997). A small controlled trial (Black & Uhde, 1994) and an open-pilot study of fluoxetine (Dummit, Klein, Tancer, Asche, & Martin, 1996) provided some support for the efficacy of this medication in the treatment of selective mutism, sometimes considered to be a severe form of SoP. A large, multisite placebo-controlled trial of fluvoxamine with 128 youth, ages 6–17 years, who met the criteria for SoP, SAD, or GAD, concluded that fluvoxamine was effective for children and adolescents with these disorders (RUPP Anxiety Study Group, 2001). In addition to fluoxetine and fluvoxamine, two trials of sertraline have been reported: Compton and colleagues (2001) conducted an open-label study of sertraline in youth, ages 10–17 years, with social anxiety disorder and concluded that this medication resulted in a significant improvement in anxiety symptoms, and Rynn, Siqueland, and Rickels (2001) conducted a placebo-controlled trial of sertraline in the treatment of youth, ages 5–17 years, with GAD and reported that sertraline was safe and efficacious in the treatment of GAD in children and adolescents.

There is research support for the use of SSRIs in youth suffering from anxiety. Of all the anxiety disorders, the most robust evidence is for OCD. Nevertheless, there is evidence for the use of SSRIs in the treatment of pediatric GAD, SoP, selective mutism, SAD, and PD (but no reports on the use of SSRIs to treat specific phobias or PTSD in youth). Considering safety and efficacy, the SSRIs appear to be a useful medication for anxiety disorders in youth.

Buspirone

Buspirone is a nonbenzodiazepine anxiolytic that affects the serotonin neurotransmitter system. Currently, data on the use of buspirone with anxious youth is sparse. Available information regarding the use of buspirone in children and adolescents is based on open data and age-downward extension of studies in adults. One open trial of buspirone with patients ages 6–14 years found significant improvement in anxiety and only brief, mild side effects (Simeon et al., 1994). Widespread use of buspirone for the treatment of youth anxiety disorders should await more stringent evidence of safety and efficacy through placebo-controlled trials.

SUMMARY

Riddle, Subramaniam, and Walkup (1998) proposed criteria for assessing the adequacy of pediatric psychopharmacological trials. Their criteria include clear methodological details, such as diagnostic procedures and primary outcome measures, placebo-controlled design, adequate medication dose and duration, participants younger than 18 years of age, sample size of 40 in parallel groups designs and 20 in crossover groups designs, and medication impact not due to sedation. Pharmacological trials have only recently begun to meet these criteria, so it is difficult to judge the efficacy of medications in the treatment of youth anxiety disorders. Based on current knowledge, CBT can be recommended as treatment for anxious youth, with potential use of medication, preferably with SSRIs when appropriate (Labellarte et al., 1999). An area in need of research is the investigation of combined CBT and medication treatments for the treatment of anxious youth; currently, a multisite trial (i.e., Child and Adolescent Anxiety Multimodal Study, or CAMS) is ongoing for this purpose. The results should add meaningfully to our knowledge regarding the treatment of youth anxiety disorders.

Prevention Programs

Although a good deal has been written about the need to prevent youth anxiety disorders, little research has been reported evaluating the effectiveness of prevention programs. However, the results of a few rigorous studies examining prevention programs are favorable, suggesting that early intervention for youth anxiety disorders can be effective.

LaFreniere and Capuano (1997) evaluated a program that sought to prevent childhood anxiety disorders in preschool children showing anxious–withdrawn behavior. The intervention aimed to increase the mother's understanding of her child's needs, to promote sensitive parenting skills, to reduce parental stress, and to enhance the family's social support. Forty-three children were randomly assigned to the intervention group or to a no-treatment control. The treated families received 19 home visits. Treated mothers showed lower levels of intrusive control and their children showed increased cooperative behavior, and teacher ratings evidenced improvements in social competence for the treated children. However, improvements were also seen in the no-treatment controls, including reductions in anxious–withdrawn behavior and decreased maternal stress. Therefore, the results cannot be said to support the specific intervention that was used.

Supportive preventive outcomes were reported from the Queensland Early Intervention and Prevention of Anxiety Project (Dadds, Spence, Holland, Barrett, & Laurens, 1997; Dadds et al., 1999). This intervention was geared toward children showing early symptoms of anxiety. Children were identified as being at risk for the development of anxiety disorders based on a screening process designed to detect the presence of high levels of anxiety symptoms. Of the children identified, 75% met diagnostic criteria for an anxiety disorder and 25% showed symptoms of anxiety but did not yet meet diagnostic criteria. Sixty-one children received intervention and 67 children were monitored. The treatment used the Coping Koala manual, the Australian modification of the Coping Cat (Kendall, 2000), and presented the treatment in 10 group format sessions. Both child and parental sessions were conducted in children's schools. Results indicated that the program reduced the rate of existing anxiety disorders and prevented the onset of new anxiety disorders. Results at 2-year follow-up indicated that the school-based intervention produced durable reductions in anxiety problems (Dadds et al., 1999).

Although research on prevention of youth anxiety disorders is sparse, continued efforts are worthwhile. Evidence suggests that risk factors for youth anxiety can be identified and, in some cases, successfully modified. Additional research evaluations are needed before we can draw conclusions as to preventability of anxiety disorders through early intervention.

CONCLUSIONS AND FUTURE DIRECTIONS

Interest in anxiety in adolescents has peaked and research is beginning to emerge. Although much work lies ahead, it is an exciting time for researchers and clinicians who study and treat adolescents with anxiety. Knowledge across domains of adolescent anxiety (e.g., assessment, diagnosis, and treatment) has had to rely on research that involved both children and adolescents, with little known about anxiety in adolescence as a distinct developmental period.

We suggest three main areas for research. First, there is a critical need to evaluate the current diagnostic taxonomy as applied to anxious adolescents. Research could be aimed at determining whether special considerations, separate from children and adults, apply in the diagnostic classification of adolescents (e.g., should certain symptoms be weighted more heavily than others when assessing adolescents?). Second, there is a clear need for the development, evaluation, and implementation of developmentally informed measures and diagnostic interviews. Psychometric and normative data for teenagers should remain distinct from the analogous data for both children and adults. Also related to assessment/diagnosis, increased consideration should be given to adolescents' cognitive and social advances (adolescents may be more accurate reporters than others and than previously thought to be). Third, developmentally sensitive programs and methodologically sound research on the treatment of anxious adolescents is desperately needed.

Efforts in this direction have begun (e.g., the C.A.T. Project), but there are currently no empirically supported treatments for adolescent anxiety. Studies examining psychosocial treatments for adolescent anxiety have reported positive results, but they have been limited by sample size (e.g., Albano et al., 1995; Leger et al., 2003), have focused mostly on SoP (e.g., Albano et al., 1995; Hayward et al., 2000; Masia et al., 2001), and have usually implemented a group format (e.g., Albano et al., 1995; Hayward et al., 2000; Masia et al., 2001). Randomized clinical trials are sorely needed. Future research in the field of adolescent anxiety (diagnosis, assessment, and treatment) should be active in building on not only our understanding of the nature of anxiety but also our current understanding of the nature of adolescence.

REFERENCES

Abraham, H. D., & Fava, M. (1999). Order of onset of substance abuse and depression in a sample of depressed outpatients. *Comprehensive Psychiatry, 40,* 44–50.

Achenbach, T. M. (1991). *Manual for the Child Behavior Checklist 4–18 and 1991 Profile.* Burlington: Department of Psychiatry, University of Vermont.

Achenbach, T. M., Howell, C. T., McConaughy, S. H., & Stanger, C. (1995). Six-year predictors of problems in a national sample of children and youth: I. Cross-informant syndromes. *Journal of the American Academy of Child and Adolescent Psychiatry, 34,* 336–347.

Albano, A. M., & Barlow, D. H. (1996). Breaking the vicious cycle: Cognitive-behavioral group treatment for socially anxious youth. In E. D. Hibbs & P. S. Jensen (Eds.), *Psychosocial treatments for child and adolescent disorders: Empirically based strategies for clinical practice* (pp. 43–62). Washington DC: American Psychological Association.

Albano, A. M., Marten, P. A., Holt, C. S., Heimberg, R. G., & Barlow, D. H. (1995). Cognitive-behavioral group treatment for social phobia in adolescents: A preliminary study. *Journal of Nervous and Mental Disease, 183,* 649–656.

American Psychiatric Association. (1980). *Diagnostic and statistical manual of mental disorders* (3rd ed.). Washington, DC: Author.

American Psychiatric Association. (1987). *Diagnostic and statistical manual of mental disorders* (3rd ed. rev.). Washington, DC: Author.

American Psychiatric Association. (1994). *Diagnostic and statistical manual of mental disorders* (4th ed.). Washington, DC: Author.

American Psychiatric Association. (2000). *Diagnostic and statistical manual of mental disorders* (4th ed., text rev.). American Psychiatric Association: Washington D. C.

Anderson, J. C., Williams, S., McGee, R., & Silva, P. A. (1987). DSM-III-R disorders in preadolescent children: Prevalence in a large sample from the general population. *Archives of General Psychiatry, 44,* 69–76.

Angold, A., & Costello, E. J. (2000). The Child and Adolescent Psychiatric Assessment (CAPA). *Journal of the American Academy of Child and Adolescent Psychiatry, 39,* 39–48.

Angold, A., Prendergast, M., Cox, A., Harrington, R., Simonoff, E., & Rutter, M. (1995). The Child and Adolescent Psychiatric Assessment (CAPA). *Psychological Medicine, 25,* 739–753.

Apter, A., Ratzoni, G., King, R. A., Weizman, A., Iancu, I., Binder, M., & Riddle, M. A. (1994). Fluvoxamine open-label treatment of adolescent inpatients with obsessive–compulsive disorder or depression. *Journal of the American Academy of Child and Adolescent Psychiatry, 33,* 342–348.

Aschenbrand, S. G., & Kendall, P. C., Webb, A., Safford, S. M., & Flannery-Schroeder, E. (2003). Is separation anxiety disorder a predictor of adult panic disorder and agoraphobia?: A seven-year longitudinal study. *Journal of the American Academy of Child and Adolescent Psychiatry, 42,* 1478–1485.

Barlow, D. H. (1988). *Anxiety and its disorders.* New York: Guilford Press.

Barrett, P. M. (1998). Evaluation of cognitive-behavioral group treatments for childhood anxiety disorders. *Journal of Clinical Child Psychology, 27,* 459–468.

Barrett, P. M. (2000). Treatment of childhood anxiety: Developmental aspects. *Clinical Psychology Review, 20,* 479–494.

Barrett, P. M., Dadds, M. R., & Rapee, R. M. (1996). Family treatment of childhood anxiety: A controlled trial. *Journal of Consulting and Clinical Psychology, 64,* 333–342.

Barrett, P. M., Rapee, R. M., Dadds, M. M., & Ryan, S. M. (1996). Family enhancement of cognitive style in anxious and aggressive children. *Journal of Abnormal Child Psychology, 1996, 24,* 187–203.

Battaglia, M., Bertella, S., Politi, E., Bernardeschi, L., Perna, G., Gabriele, A., & Bellodi, L. (1995). Age of onset of panic disorder: Influence of familial liability to the disease and of childhood separation anxiety disorder. *American Journal of Psychiatry, 152,* 1362–1364.

Beidel, D. C. (1991). Social phobia and overanxious disorder in school-age children. *Journal of the American Academy of Child and Adolescent Psychiatry, 30,* 545–552.

Beidel, D. C., Fink, C. M., & Turner, S. M. (1996). Stability of anxious symptomatology in children. *Journal of Abnormal Child Psychology, 24,* 257–269.

Beidel, D. C., & Turner, S. M. (1998). *Shy children, phobic adults: Nature and treatment of social phobia.* Washington, DC: American Psychiatric Association.

Beidel, D. C., Turner, S. M., & Morris, T. L. (1995). A new inventory to assess childhood social anxiety and phobia: The Social Phobia and Anxiety Inventory for Children. *Psychological Assessment, 7,* 73–79.

Berney, T., Kolvin, I., Bhate, S. R., Garside, R. F., Jeans, J., Kay, B., & Scarth, L. (1981). School phobia: A therapeutic trial with clomipramine and short-term outcome. *British Journal of Psychiatry, 138,* 110–118.

Bernstein, G. A., Garfinkel, B. D., & Borchardt, C. M. (1990). Comparative studies of pharmacotherapy for school refusal. *Journal of the American Academy of Child and Adolescent Psychiatry, 29,* 773–781.

Biederman, J., Rosenbaum, J. F., Bolduc, E. A., Faraone, S. V., & Hirshfeld, D. R. (1991). A high risk study of young children of parents with panic disorder and agoraphobia with and without comorbid major depression. *Psychiatry Research, 37,* 333–348.

Biederman, J., Rosenbaum, J. F., Bolduc-Murphy, E. A., Faraone, S. V., Chaloff, J., Hirshfeld, D. R., & Kagan, J. (1993). A 3-year follow-up of children with and without behavioral inhibition. *Journal of the American Academy of Child and Adolescent Psychiatry, 32,* 814–821.

Biederman, J., Rosenbaum, J. F., Hirshfeld, D. R., Faraone, S. V., Bolduc, E. A., Gersten, M., et al. (1990). Psychiatric correlates of behavioral inhibition in young children of parents with and without psychiatric disorders. *Archives of General Psychiatry, 47,* 21–26.

Birmaher, B., Brent, D. A., Chiappetta, L., Bridge, J., Monga, S., & Baugher, M. (1999). Psychometric properties of the Screen for Child Anxiety Related Emotional Disorders (SCARED): A replication study. *Journal of the American Academy of Child and Adolescent Psychiatry, 38,* 1230–1236.

Birmaher, B., Khetarpal, S., Brent, D., Cully, M., Balach, L., Kaufman, J., & McKenzie Neer, S. (1997). The Screen for Child Anxiety Related Emotional Disorders (SCARED): Scale construction and psychometric characteristics. *Journal of the American Academy of Child and Adolescent Psychiatry, 36,* 545–553.

Birmaher, B., Waterman, G. S., Ryan, N., Cully, M., Balach, L., Ingram, J., & Brodsky, M. (1994). Fluoxetine for childhood anxiety disorders. *Journal of the American Academy of Child and Adolescent Psychiatry, 33,* 993–999.

Black, B., & Uhde, T. W. (1994). Treatment of elective mutism with fluoxetine: Double-blind, placebo-controlled study. *Journal of the American Academy of Child and Adolescent Psychiatry, 33,* 1000–1006.

Boyle, M. H., Offord, D. R., Racine, Y., Sanford, M., Szatmari, P., Fleming, J. E., & Price-Munn, N. (1993). Evaluation of the Diagnostic Interview for Children and Adolescents for use in general population samples. *Journal of Abnormal Child Psychology, 21,* 663–681.

Brady, E. U., & Kendall, P. C. (1992). Comorbidity of anxiety and depression in children and adolescents. *Psychological Bulletin, 111,* 244–255.

Burke, K. C., Burke, J. D., Rae, D. S., & Regier, D. A. (1991). Comparing the age of onset of major depression and other psychiatric disorders by birth cohorts in five U. S. community populations. *Archives of General Psychiatry, 48,* 789–795.

Cantwell, D. P., & Baker, L. (1989). Stability and natural history of DSM-III childhood diagnoses. *Journal of the American Academy of Child and Adolescent Psychiatry, 28,* 691–700.

Cantwell, D. P., Lewinsohn, P. M., Rohde, P., & Seeley, J. R. (1997). Correspondence between adolescent report and parent report of psychiatric diagnostic data. *Journal of the American Academy of Child and Adolescent Psychiatry, 36,* 610–618.

Caspi, A., Henry, B., McGee, R. O., Moffitt, T. E., & Silva, P. A. (1995). Temperamental origins of child and adolescent behavior problems: From age three to age fifteen. *Child Development, 66,* 55–68.

Chambless, D., & Hollon, S. (1998). Defining empirically supported treatments. *Journal of Consulting and Clinical Psychology, 66,* 5–17.

Chorpita, B. F., Albano, A. M., & Barlow, D. H. (1996). Cognitive processing in children: Relationship to anxiety and family influences. *Journal of Clinical Child Psychology, 25,* 170–176.

Christie, K. A., Burke, J. D., Regier, D. A., Rae, D. S., Boyd, J. H., & Locke, B. Z. (1988). Epidemiologic evidence for early onset of mental disorders and higher risk of drug abuse in young adults. *American Journal of Psychiatry, 145,* 971–975.

Cobham, V. E., Dadds, M. R., & Spence, S. H. (1998). The role of parental anxiety in the treatment of childhood anxiety. *Journal of Consulting and Clinical Psychology, 66,* 893–905.

Cohen, P., Cohen, J., Kasen, S., Velez, C. N., Hartmark, C., Johnson, J., et al. (1993). An epidemiological study of disorders in late childhood and adolescence-I: Age and gender-specific prevalence. *Journal of Child Psychology and Psychiatry and Allied Disciplines, 34,* 851–867.

Collins, W. A., & Laursen, B. (2004). Parent–adolescent relationships and influences. In R. Lerner & L. Steinberg (Eds.), *Handbook of adolescent psychology* (pp. 331–362). New York: Wiley.

Compton, S. N., Grant, P. J., Chrisman, A. K., Gammon, P. J., Brown, V. L., & March, J. S. (2001). Sertraline in children and adolescents with social anxiety disorder: An open trial. *Journal of the American Academy of Child and Adolescent Psychiatry, 40,* 564–571.

Compton, S. N., Nelson, A. H., & March, J. S. (2000). Social phobia and separation anxiety symptoms in community and clinical samples of children and adolescents. *Journal of the American Academy of Child and Adolescent Psychiatry, 39,* 1040–1046.

Costello, E. J. (1989). Child psychiatric disorders and their correlates: A primary care pediatric sample. *Journal of the American Academy of Child and Adolescent Psychiatry, 28,* 851–855.

Costello, E. J., & Angold, A. (1995). Epidemiology. In J. S. March (Ed.), *Anxiety disorders in children and adolescents* (pp. 109–124). New York: Guilford Press.

Costello, E. J., Costello, A. J., Edelbrock, C., Burns, B. J., Dulcan, M. K., Brent, D., & Janiszewski, S. (1988). Psychiatric disorders in pediatric primary care: Prevalence and risk factors. *Archives of General Psychiatry, 45,* 1107–1116.

Costello, E. J., Edelbrock, C., Dulcan, M. K., Kalas, R., & Klaric, S. (1987). *The Diagnostic Interview Schedule for Children (DISC).* Pittsburgh, PA: University of Pittsburgh Press.

Cummins, T. K., & Ninan, P. T. (2002). The neurobiology of anxiety in children and adolescents. *International Review of Psychiatry, 14,* 114–128.

Dadds, M. R., Barrett, P. M., Rapee, R. M., & Ryan, S. (1996). Family process and child anxiety and aggression: An observational analysis. *Journal of Abnormal Child Psychology, 24,* 715–734.

Dadds, M., Heard, P., & Rapee, R. (1991). Anxiety disorders in children. *International Review of Psychiatry, 3,* 231–241.

Dadds, M. R., Spence, S. H., Holland, D. E., Barrett, P. M., & Laurens, K. (1997). Prevention and early intervention for anxiety disorders: A controlled trial. *Journal of Consulting and Clinical Psychology, 65,* 627–635.

Dadds, M. R., Spence, S. H., Holland, D., Laurens, K., Mullins, M., & Barrett, P. M. (1999). Early intervention and prevention of anxiety disorders: Results of a two-year follow-up. *Journal of Consulting and Clinical Psychology, 67,* 145–150.

Deas-Nesmith, D., Brady, K. T., & Campbell, S. (1998). Comorbid substance use and anxiety disorders in adolescents. *Journal of Psychopathology and Behavioral Assessment, 20,* 139–148.

DeVeaugh-Geiss, J., Moroz, G., Biederman, J., Cantwell, D., Fontaine, R., Greist, J. H., et al. (1992). Clomipramine hydrochloride in childhood and adolescent obsessive–compulsive disorder—A multicenter trial. *Journal of the American Academy of Child and Adolescent Psychiatry, 31,* 45–49.

Dierker, L. C., Albano, A. M., Clarke, G. N., Heimberg, R. G., Kendall, P. C., Merikangas, K. R., et al. (2001). Screening for anxiety and depression in early adolescence. *Journal of the American Academy of Child and Adolescent Psychiatry, 40,* 929–936.

DiNardo, P. A., O'Brien, G. T., Barlow, D. H., Waddell, M. T., & Blanchard, E. B. (1983). Reliability of DSM-III anxiety disorder categories using a new structured interview. *Archives of General Psychiatry, 35,* 837–844.

Dumas, J. E., & LaFreniere, P. J. (1993). Mother-child relationships as sources of support or stress: A comparison of competent, average, aggressive, and anxious dyads. *Child Development, 64,* 1732–1754.

Dumas, J., LaFreniere, P. J., & Serketich, W. (1995). "Balance of power": Transactional analysis of control in mother–child dyads involving socially competent, aggressive, and anxious children. *Journal of Abnormal Psychology, 104,* 104–113.

Dummit, E. S., Klein, R. G., Tancer, N. K., Asche, B., & Martin, J. (1996). Fluoxetine treatment of children with selective mutism, an open trial. *Journal of the American Academy of Child and Adolescent Psychiatry, 35,* 615–621.

Eaton, W. W., Dryman, A., & Weissman, M. M. (1991). Panic and phobia. In L. N. Robins & D. A. Regier (Eds.), *Psychiatric disorders in America: The Epidemiologic Catchment Area study* (pp. 151–179). New York: Free Press.

Essau, C. A., & Barrett, P. (2001). Developmental issues in the assessment of anxiety. In C. A. Essau & F. Petermann (Eds.), *Anxiety disorders in children and adolescents* (pp. 75–110). New York: Taylor & Francis.

Essau, C. A., Conradt, J., & Petermann, F. (1999). Frequency of panic attacks and panic disorder in adolescents. *Depression and Anxiety, 9,* 19–26.

Essau, C. A., Conradt, J., & Petermann, F. (2000). Frequency, comorbidity, and psychosocial impairment of anxiety disorder in German adolescents. *Journal of Anxiety Disorders, 14,* 263–279.

Fairbanks, J. M., Pine, D. S., Tancer, N. K., Dummit E. S. III, Kentgen, L. M., Martin, J., et al. (1997). Open fluoxetine treatment of mixed anxiety disorders in children and adolescents. *Journal of Child and Adolescent Psychopharmacology, 7,* 17–29.

Finch, A. J., Jr., Kendall, P. C., & Montgomery, L. E. (1974). Multidimensionality of anxiety in children: Factor structure of the Children's Manifest Anxiety Scale. *Journal of Abnormal Child Psychology, 2,* 331–336.

Fischer, D. J., Himle, J. A., & Hanna, G. L. (1998). Group behavioral therapy for adolescents with obsessive–compulsive disorder: Preliminary outcomes. *Research on Social Work Practice, 8,* 629–636.

Fisher, P. W., Shaffer, D., Piacentini, J., Lapkin, J., Kafantaris, L. H., & Herzog, D. B. (1993). Sensitivity of the Diagnostic Interview Schedule for Children, 2nd edition (DISC-2. 1) for specific diagnoses of children and adolescents. *Journal of the American Academy of Child and Adolescent Psychiatry, 32,* 666–673.

Flament, M. F., Rapoport, J. L., Berg, C. J., Sceery, W., Kilts, C., Mellstrom, B., & Linnoila, M. (1985). Clomipramine treatment of childhood obsessive–compulsive disorder: A double-blind controlled study. *Archives of General Psychiatry, 42,* 977–983.

Fletcher, K. (1997). Childhood PTSD Interview (CPTSDI)—Child Form. In E. B. Carlson (Ed.), *Trauma assessments: A clinician's guide* (pp. 248–250). New York: Guilford Press.

Francis, G., Last, C. G., & Strauss, C. C. (1987). Expression of separation anxiety disorder: The roles of gender and age. *Child Psychiatry and Human Development, 18,* 82–89.

Franklin, M. E., Kozak, M. J., Cashman, L. A., Coles, M. E., Rheingold, A. A., & Foa, E. B. (1998). Cognitive-behavioral treatment of pediatric obsessive–compulsive disorder: An open clinical trial. *Journal of the American Academy of Child and Adolescent Psychiatry, 37,* 412–419.

Geller, D. A., Biederman, J., Reed, E. D., Spencer, T., & Wilens, T. E. (1995). Similarities in response to fluoxetine in the treatment of children and adolescents with obsessive–compulsive disorder. *Journal of the American Academy of Child and Adolescent Psychiatry, 34,* 36–44.

Geller, D. A., Hoog, S. L., Heilingentein, J. H., Ricardi, R. K., Tamura, R., Kluszynski, S., & Jacobson, J. G. (2001). Fluoxetine treatment for obsessive–compulsive disorder in children and adolescents: A placebo-controlled clinical trial. *Journal of the American Academy of Child and Adolescent Psychiatry, 40,* 773–779.

Ginsburg, G. S., Silverman, W. K., & Kurtines, W. M. (1995). Family involvement in treating children with anxiety and phobic disorders: A look ahead. *Clinical Psychology Review, 15,* 457–473.

Gittelman-Klein, R., & Klein, D. F. (1971). Controlled imipramine treatment of school phobia. *Archives of General Psychiatry, 25,* 204–207.

Gittelman-Klein, R., & Klein, D. F. (1973). School phobia: Diagnostic considerations in the light of imipramine effects. *Journal of Nervous and Mental Disease, 156,* 199–215.

Graae, F., Milner, J., Rizzotto, L., & Klein, R. G. (1994). Clonazepam in childhood anxiety disorders. *Journal of the American Academy of Child and Adolescent Psychiatry, 33,* 372–376.

Greenbaum, P. E., Prange, M. E., Friedman, R. M., & Silver, S. E. (1991). Substance abuse prevalence and comorbidity with other psychiatric disorders among adolescents with severe emotional disturbances. *Journal of the American Academy of Child and Adolescent Psychiatry, 30,* 575–583.

Greenhill, L. L., Pine, D. S., March, J., Birmaher, B., & Riddle, M. (1998). Assessment issues in treatment research on pediatric anxiety disorders, what is working, what is not working, and what needs improvement. *Psychopharmacology Bulletin, 34,* 155–164.

Hartup, W. W., & Stevens, N. (1997). Friendships and adaptation in the life course. *Psychological Bulletin, 121,* 355–370.

Hayward, C., & Essau, C. A. (2001). Panic attacks and panic disorder. In C. A. Essau & F. Petermann (Eds.), *Anxiety disorders in children and adolescents: Epidemiology, risk factors, and treatment* (pp. 143–161). New York: Taylor & Francis.

Hayward, C., Killen, J. D., Hammer, L. D., Litt, I. F., Wilson, D. M., Simmonds, B., & Taylor, C. B. (1992). Pubertal stage and panic attack history in sixth- and seventh-grade girls. *American Journal of Psychiatry, 149,* 1239–1243.

Hayward, C., Killen, J. D., & Taylor, C. B. (1989). Panic attacks in young adolescents. *American Journal of Psychiatry, 146,* 1061–1062.

Hayward, C., Varady, S., Albano, M., Thienemann, M., Henderson, L., & Schatzberg, A. F. (2000). Cognitive-behavioral group therapy for social phobia in female adolescents: Results of a pilot study. *Journal of the American Academy of Child and Adolescent Psychiatry, 39,* 721–726.

Heimberg, R. G., Dodge, C. S., Hope, D. A., Kennedy, C. R., Zollo, L. J., & Becker, R. J. (1990). Cognitive behavioral group treatment for social phobia: Comparison with a credible placebo control. *Cognitive Therapy and Research, 14,* 1–23.

Herjanic, B., & Reich, W. (1982). Development of a structured psychiatric interview for children: Agreement between child and parent on individual symptoms. *Journal of Abnormal Child Psychiatry, 10,* 307–324.

Hettema, J. M., Prescott, C. A., & Kendler, K. S. (2001). A population-based twin study of generalized anxiety disorder in men and women. *Journal of Nervous and Mental Disease, 189,* 413–420.

Hibbs, E. D., Hamburger, S. D., Kruesi, M. J., & Lenane, M. (1993). Factors affecting expressed emotion in parents of ill and normal children. *American Journal of Orthopsychiatry, 63,* 103–112.

Hibbs, E. D., Hamburger, S. D., Lenane, M., Rapoport, J. L., Kruesi, M. J. P., Keysor, C. S., & Goldstein, M. J. (1991) Determinants of Expressed Emotion in Families of Disturbed and Normal Children. *Journal of Child Psychology and Psychiatry, 32,* 757–770.

Hill, J. P. (1988). Adapting to menarche: Familial control and conflict. In M. R. Gunnar & W. A. Collins (Eds.), *Development during the transition to adolescence: Minnesota Symposia on Child Psychology* (Vol. 21, pp. 43–77). Hillsdale, NJ: Erlbaum.

Himle, J. A., Fischer, D. J., Van Etten, M. L., Janeck, A. S., & Hanna, G. L. (2003). Group behavioral therapy for adolescents with tic-related and non-tic-related obsessive–compulsive disorder. *Depression and Anxiety, 17,* 73–77.

Hodges, K. (1990). Depression and anxiety in children: A comparison of self-report questionnaires to clinical interview. *Psychological Assessment, 2,* 376–381.

Hoehn-Saric, E., Maisami, M., & Weigand, D. (1987). Measurement of anxiety in children and adolescents using semistructured interviews. *Journal of the American Academy of Child and Adolescent Psychiatry, 28,* 541–545.

Holmbeck, G. N., Colder, C., Shapera, W., Westhoven, V., Kenealy, L., & Updegrove, A. (2000). Working with adolescents: Guides from developmental psychology. In P. C. Kendall (Ed.), *Child and adolescent therapy: Cognitive-behavioral procedures* (2nd ed., pp. 334–385). New York: Guilford Press.

Hope, D. A., & Heimberg, R. G. (1985). Social phobia and social anxiety. In D. H. Barlow (Ed.), *Clinical handbook of psychological disorders: A step-by-step treatment manual* (pp. 99–136). New York: Guilford Press.

Horwath, E., & Weissman, M. M. (1995). Epidemiology of depression and anxiety disorder. In M. T. Tsuang, M. Tohen, & G. E. P. Zahner (Eds.), *Textbook in psychiatric epidemiology* (pp. 317–343). New York: Wiley-Liss.

Howard, B. L., & Kendall, P. C. (1992). *Family-based cognitive-behavioral intervention for anxious children: A therapy manual.* Available from P. C. Kendall, Department of Psychology, Temple University, Philadelphia, PA 19122.

Howard, B. L., & Kendall, P. C. (1996). Cognitive-behavioral family therapy for anxiety-disordered children: A multiple-baseline evaluation. *Cognitive Therapy and Research, 20,* 423–443.

Hudson, J. L., & Rapee, R. M. (2001) Parent–child interactions and anxiety disorders: An observational study. *Behaviour Research and Therapy, 39,* 1411–1427.

Ialongo, N., Edelsohn, G., Werthamer-Larsson, L., Crockett, L., & Kellam, S. (1995). The significance of self-reported anxious symptoms in first grade children: Prediction to anxious symptoms and adaptive functioning in fifth grade. *Journal of Child Psychology and Psychiatry and Allied Disciplines, 36,* 427–437.

Ingersoll, G. M. (1989) *Adolescents* (2nd ed.). Englewood Cliffs, NJ: Prentice Hall.

Joiner, T. E., Catanzaro, S., & Laurent, J. (1996). The tripartite structure of positive and negative affect, depression, and anxiety in adolescent psychiatric inpatients. *Journal of Abnormal Psychology, 105,* 401–409.

Kagan, J. (1997). Temperament and the reactions to unfamiliarity. *Child Development, 68,* 139–143.

Kagan, J., Reznick. J. S., & Snidman, N. (1988). Biological bases of childhood shyness. *Science, 240,* 167–171.

Kaplow, J. B., Curran, P. J., Angold, A., & Costello, E. J. (2001). The prospective relation between dimensions of anxiety and the initiation of adolescent alcohol use. *Journal of Clinical Child Psychology, 30,* 316–326.

Kashani, J. H., & Orvaschel, H. (1990). A community study of anxiety in children and adolescents. *American Journal of Psychiatry, 147,* 313–318.

Kaufman, J., Birmaher, B., Brent, D., Rao, U., & Ryan, N. (1997). Schedule for Affective Disorders and Schizophrenia for School-Age Children-Present and Lifetime version (K-SADS-PL): Initial reliability and validity data. *Journal of the American Academy of Child and Adolescent Psychiatry, 36,* 980–988.

Kazdin, A. E. (1986). Research designs and methodology. In S. Garfield & A. Bergin (Eds.), *Handbook of psychotherapy and behavior change* (3rd ed., pp. 85–99). New York: Wiley.

Kazdin, A., & Weisz, J. (1998). Identifying and developing empirically supported child and adolescent treatments. *Journal of Consulting and Clinical Psychology, 66,* 100–110.

Keller, M. B., Lavori, P. W., Wunder, J., Beardsless, W. R., Schwartz, C. E., & Roth, J. (1992). Chronic course of anxiety disorders in children and adolescents. *Journal of the American Academy of Child and Adolescent Psychiatry, 31,* 595–599.

Kendall, P. C. (1984). Social cognition and problem solving: A developmental and child–clinical interface. In B. Gholson & T. L. Rosenthal (Eds.), *Applications of cognitive-developmental theory* (pp. 115–148). New York: Academic Press.

Kendall, P. C. (1994). Treating anxiety disorders in children: Results of a randomized clinical trial. *Journal of Consulting and Clinical Psychology, 62,* 100–110.

Kendall, P. C. (2000). *Cognitive-behavioral therapy for anxious children: Therapist manual* (2nd ed.). Ardmore, PA: Workbook Publishing.

Kendall, P. C., Choudhury, M. A., Hudson, J., & Webb, A. (2002). *The C.A.T. Project Manual.* Ardmore, PA: Workbook Publishing.

Kendall, P. C., & Flannery-Schroeder, E. C. (1998). Methodological issues in treatment research for anxiety disorders in youth. *Journal of Abnormal Child Psychology, 26,* 27–38.

Kendall, P. C., Flannery-Schroeder, E., Panichelli-Mindell, S. M., Southam-Gerow, M., Henin, A., & Warman, M. (1997). Therapy for youths with anxiety disorders: A second randomized clinical trial. *Journal of Consulting and Clinical Psychology, 65,* 366–380.

Kendall, P. C., & Hedtke, K. A. (2006a). *Cognitive-behavioral therapy for anxious children: Therapist manual* (3rd ed.). Ardmore, PA: Workbook Publishing.

Kendall, P. C., & Hedtke, K. A. (2006b). *The Coping Cat workbook* (2nd ed.). Ardmore, PA: Workbook Publishing.

Kendall, P. C., Kane, M., Howard, B., & Siqueland, L. (1989). *Cognitive-behavioral therapy for anxious children: Treatment manual.* Available from P. C. Kendall, Department of Psychology, Temple University, Philadelphia, PA 19122.

Kendall, P. C., & Pimentel, S. S. (2003). On the physiological symptom constellation in youth with generalized anxiety disorder (GAD). *Journal of Anxiety Disorders, 17,* 211–221.

Kendall, P. C., Safford, S., Flannery-Schroeder, E., & Webb, A. (2004). Child anxiety treatment: Outcomes in adolescence and impact on substance abuse and depression at 7.4-year follow-up. *Journal of Consulting and Clinical Psychology, 72,* 276–287.

Kendall, P. C., & Southam-Gerow, M. (1996). Long-term follow-up of a cognitive-behavioral therapy for anxiety-disordered youth. *Journal of Consulting and Clinical Psychology, 64,* 724–730.

Kendall, P. C., & Warman, M. J. (1996). Anxiety disorders in youth: Diagnostic consistency across DSM-III-R and DSM-IV. *Journal of Anxiety Disorders, 10,* 453–463.

Kendler, K. S., Heath, A. C., Martin, N. G., & Eaves, L. J. (1987). Symptoms of anxiety and symptoms of depression. *Archives of General Psychiatry, 44,* 451–457.

Kendler, K. S., Neale, M. C., Kessler, R. C., Heath, A. C., & Eaves, L. J. (1992a). Generalized anxiety disorder in women. *Archives of General Psychiatry, 49,* 267–272.

Kendler, K. S., Neale, M. C., Kessler, R. C., Heath, A. C., & Eaves, L. J. (1992b). The genetic epidemiology of phobias in women: The interrelationship of agoraphobia, social phobia, situational phobia, and simple phobia. *Archives of General Psychiatry, 49,* 273–281.

Kendler, K. S., Neale, M. C., Kessler, R. C., Heath, A. C., & Eaves, L. J. (1992c). Major depression and generalized anxiety disorder. *Archives of General Psychiatry, 49,* 716–722.

Kendler, K. S., Neale, M. C., Kessler, R. C., Heath, A. C., & Eaves, L. J. (1993a). Major depression and phobias: The genetic and environmental sources of comorbidity. *Psychological Medicine, 23,* 361–371.

Kendler, K. S., Neale, M. C., Kessler, R. C., Heath, A. C., & Eaves, L. J. (1993b). Panic disorder in women: A population based twin study. *Psychological Medicine, 23,* 397–406.

Kendler, K. S., Walters, E. E., Neale, M. C., Kessler, R. C., Heath, A. C., & Eaves, L. J. (1995). The structure of the genetic and environmental risk factors for six major psychiatric disorders in women. *Archives of General Psychiatry, 52,* 374–383.

Kenny, M., & Faust, J. (1997). Mother–child agreement on self-report of anxiety in abused children. *Journal of Anxiety Disorders, 11,* 463–472.

Kessler, R. C., McGonagle, K. A., Zhao, S., Nelson, C. B., Hughes, M., Eshleman, S., et al. (1994). Lifetime and 12-month prevalence of DSM-III-R psychiatric disorders in the United States: Results from the National Comorbidity Survey. *Archives of General Psychiatry, 51,* 8–19.

Kessler, R. C., Nelson, C. B., McGonagle, K. A., Edlund, M. J., Frank, R. G., & Leaf, P. J. (1996). The epidemiology of co-occurring addictive and mental disorders: Implications for prevention and service utilization. *American Journal of Orthopsychiatry, 66,* 17–31.

Kessler, R. C., Stang, P. E., Wittchen, H. U., Bedirhan, U. T., Roy-Burne, P. P., & Walters, E. E. (1998). Lifetime panic-depression comorbidity survey. *Archives of General Psychiatry, 55,* 801–808.

Kindt, M., Brosschot, J. S., & Everaerd, W. (1997). Cognitive processing bias in spider fear and control children: Assessment of emotional interference by a card format and a single-trial format of the Stroop. *Journal of Experimental Child Psychology, 66,* 163–179.

King, N. J. (1994). Physiological assessment. In T. H. Ollendick, N. J. King, & W. Yule (Eds.), *International handbook of phobic and anxiety disorders in children and adolescents* (pp. 365–379). New York: Plenum Press.

King, N. J., Gullone, E., Tonge, B. J., & Ollendick, T. H. (1993). Self-reports of panic attacks and manifest anxiety in adolescents. *Behaviour Research and Therapy, 31,* 111–116.

King, N. J., Ollendick, T. H., Mattis, S. G., Yang, B., & Tonge, B. (1996). Nonclinical panic attacks in adolescents: Prevalence, symptomatology, and associated features. *Behavioral Change, 13,* 171–183.

Klein, D. F. (1964). Delineation of two drug-responsive anxiety syndromes. *Psychopharmacologia, 3,* 397–408.

Klein, R. G., Koplewicz, H. S., & Kanner, A. (1992). Imipramine treatment in children with separation anxiety disorder. *Journal of the American Academy of Child and Adolescent Psychiatry, 31,* 21–28.

Kurlan, R., Como, P. G., Deeley, C., McDermott, M., & McDermott, M. P. (1993). A pilot controlled study of fluoxetine for obsessive–compulsive symptoms in children with Tourette's syndrome. *Clinical Neuropharmacology, 16,* 167–172.

Kutcher, S. P., & Mackenzie, S. (1988). Successful clonazepam treatment of adolescents with panic disorder. *Journal of Clinical Psychopharmacology, 8,* 299–301.

Kutcher, S. P., Reiter, S., Gardner, D. M., & Klein, R. G. (1992). The pharmacotherapy of anxiety disorders in children and adolescents. *Psychiatric Clinics of North America, 15,* 41–67.

Labellarte, M. J., Ginsburg, G. S., Walkup, J. T., & Riddle, M. A. (1999). The treatment of anxiety disorders in children and adolescents. *Biological Psychiatry, 46,* 1567–1578.

LaFreniere, P. J., & Capuano, F. (1997). Preventive intervention as means of clarifying direction of effects in socialization: Anxious–withdrawn preschoolers case. *Development and Psychopathology, 9,* 551–564.

LaGreca, A. (1998). *Manual for the Social Anxiety Scales for Children and Adolescents.* Miami, FL: University of Miami.

LaGreca, A. M. (2001). Friends of foes? Peer influences on anxiety among children and adolescents. In W. K. Silverman & P. D. A. Treffers (Eds.), *Anxiety disorders in children and adolescents* (pp. 159–186). Cambridge, UK: Cambridge University Press.

Larson, R. W., Csikszentmihalyi, M., & Graef, R. (1980). Mood variability and the psychosocial adjustment of adolescents. *Journal of Youth and Adolescence, 9,* 469–490.

Larson, R., & Richards, M. H. (1994). *Divergent realities: The emotional lives of mothers, fathers, and adolescents.* New York: Basic Books.

Last, C. G., Francis, G., & Strauss, C. C. (1989). Assessing fears in anxiety-disordered children with the Revised Fear Survey Schedule for Children (FSSC-R). *Journal of Clinical Child Psychology, 18,* 137–141.

Last, C. G., Hersen, M., Kazdin, A. E., Francis, G., & Grubb, H. J. (1987). Psychiatric illness in the mothers of anxious children. *American Journal of Psychiatry, 144,* 1580–1583.

Last, C. G., Hersen, M., Kazdin, A. E., Orvaschel, H., & Perrin, S. (1991). Anxiety disorders in children and their families. *Archives of General Psychiatry, 48,* 928–934.

Last, C. G., Perrin, S., Hersen, M., & Kazdin, A. E. (1992). DSM-III-R anxiety disorders in children: Sociodemographic and clinical characteristics. *Journal of the American Academy of Child and Adolescent Psychiatry, 31,* 1070–1076.

Last, C. G., Perrin, S., Hersen, M., & Kazdin, A. E. (1996). A prospective study of childhood anxiety disorders. *Journal of the American Academy of Child and Adolescent Psychiatry, 35,* 1502–1510.

Last, C. G., & Strauss, C. C. (1989). Panic disorder in children and adolescents. *Journal of Anxiety Disorders, 3,* 87–95.

Last, C. G., & Strauss, C. C. (1990). School refusal in anxiety-disordered children and adolescents. *Journal of the American Academy of Child and Adolescent Psychiatry, 29,* 31–35.

Leger, E., & Ladouceur, R., Dugas, M. J., & Freeston, M. H. (2003). Cognitive-behavioral treatment of generalized anxiety disorder among adolescents: A case series. *Journal of the American Academy of Child and Adolescent Psychiatry, 42,* 327–330.

Leib, R., Wittchen, H., Hofler, M., Fuetsch, M., Stein, M., & Merikangas, K. (2000). Parental psychopathology, parenting styles, and the risk of social phobia in offspring: A prospective, longitudinal community study. *Archives of General Psychiatry, 57,* 859–866.

Liebowitz, M. R., Gorman, J. M., Fyer, A. J., & Klein, D. F. (1985). Social phobia: Review of a neglected anxiety disorder. *Archives of General Psychiatry, 42,* 669–677.

Liebowitz, M. R., Turner, S. M., Piacentini, J., Beidel, D. C., Clarvit, S. R., Davies, S. O., et al. (2002). Fluoxetine in children and adolescents with OCD: A placebo-controlled trial. *Journal of the American Academy of Child and Adolescent Psychiatry, 41,* 1431–1438.

Leonard, H. L., Swedo, S. E., Rapoport, J. L., Koby, E. V., Lenane, M. C., Cheslow, D. L., & Hamburger, S. D. (1989). Treatment of obsessive–compulsive disorder with clomipramine and desipramine in children and adolescents. A double-blind crossover comparison. *Archives of General Psychiatry, 46,* 1088–1092.

Leventhal, T., & Brooks-Gunn, J. (2004). Diversity in developmental trajectories across adolescence: Neighborhood influences. In R. M. Lerner & L. Steinberg (Eds.), *Handbook of adolescent psychology* (451–486). New York: Wiley.

Lewinsohn, P. M., Gotlib, I. H., Lewinsohn, M., Seeley, J. R., & Allen, N. B. (1998). Gender differences in anxiety disorders and anxiety symptoms in adolescents. *Journal of Abnormal Psychology, 107,* 109–117.

Lewinsohn, P. M., Hops, H., Roberts, R. E., Seeley, J. R., & Andrews, J. A. (1993). Adolescent psychopathology: I. Prevalence and incidence of depression and other DSM-III-R disorders in high school students. *Journal of Abnormal Psychology, 102,* 133–144.

Loeber, R., & Wikstrom, P.-O. H. (1993). Individual pathways to crime in different types of neighborhoods. In D. P. Farrington, R. J. Sampson, & P. -O. H. Wikstrom (Eds.), *Integrating individual and ecological aspects of crime* (pp. 169–204). Stockholm, Sweden: National Council for Crime Prevention.

Lonigan, C. J., Carey, M. P., & Finch, A. J., Jr. (1994). Anxiety and depression in children and adolescents: Negative affectivity and the utility of self-reports. *Journal of Consulting and Clinical Psychology, 62,* 1000–1008.

Lonigan, C. J., Hooe, E. S., David, C. F., & Kistner, J. A. (1999). Positive and negative affectivity in children: Confirmatory factor analysis of a two-factor model and its relation to symptoms of anxiety and depression. *Journal of Consulting and Clinical Psychology, 67,* 374–386.

Lonigan, C. J., & Phillips, B. M. (2001). Temperamental influences on the development of anxiety disorders. In M. W. Vasey & M. R. Dadds (Eds.), *The developmental psychopathology of anxiety* (pp. 60–91). New York: Oxford University Press.

Manassis, K., & Monga, S. (2001). A therapeutic approach to children and adolescents with anxiety disorders and associated comorbid conditions. *Journal of the American Academy of Child and Adolescent Psychiatry, 40,* 115–117.

March, J. S., & Albano, A. M. (1998). Advances in the assessment of pediatric anxiety disorders. *Advances in Clinical Child Psychology, 20,* 213–241.

March, J. S., Biederman, J., Wolkow, R., Safferman, A., Mardekian, J., Cook, E. H., et al. (1998). Sertraline in children and adolescents with obsessive–compulsive disorder, a multicenter randomized controlled trial. *Journal of the American Medical Association, 280,* 1752–1756.

March, J. S., & Mulle, K. (1998). *OCD in children and adolescents: A cognitive-behavioral treatment manual.* New York: Guilford Press.

March, J. S., Mulle, K., & Herbel, B. (1994). Behavioral psychotherapy for children and adolescents with obsessive–compulsive disorder: An open trial of a new protocol driven treatment package. *Journal of the American Academy of Child and Adolescent Psychiatry, 33,* 333–341.

March, J. S., Parker, J. D. A., Sullivan, K., Stallings, P., & Conners, K. (1997). The Multidimensional Anxiety Scale for Children (MASC): Factor structure, reliability, and validity. *Journal of the American Academy of Child and Adolescent PsySchiatry, 36,* 554–565.

March, J. S., Sullivan, K., & Parker, J. (1999). Test–retest reliability of the Multidimensional Anxiety Scale for Children. *Journal of Anxiety Disorders, 13,* 349–358.

Martin, M., Horder, P., & Jones, G. V. (1992). Integral bias in naming of phobia-related words. *Cognition and Emotion, 6,* 479–486.

Martin, M., & Jones, G. V. (1995). Integral bias in the cognitive processing of emotionally linked pictures. *British Journal of Psychology, 86,* 419–435.

Masia, C. L., Klein, R. G., Storch, E. A., & Corda, B. (2001). School-based behavioral treatment for social anxiety disorder in adolescents: Results of a pilot study. *Journal of the American Academy of Child and Adolescent Psychiatry, 40,* 780–786.

McClure, E. B., Brennan, P., Hammen, C., & Le Brocque, R. M. (2001). Parental anxiety disorders, child anxiety disorders, and the perceived parent–child relationship in and Australian high-risk sample. *Journal of Abnormal Child Psychology, 29,* 1–10.

McGee, R., Feehan, M., Williams, S., Partridge, F., Silva, P. A., & Kelly, J. (1990). DSM-III disorders in a large sample of adolescents. *Journal of the American Academy of Child and Adolescent Psychiatry, 36,* 554–565.

Mendlowitz, S. L., Manassis, K., Bradley, S., Scapillato, D., Miezitis, S., & Shaw, B. F. (1999). Cognitive-behavioral group treatments in childhood anxiety disorders: The role of parental involvement. *Journal of the American Academy of Child and Adolescent Psychiatry, 38,* 1223–1229.

Montemayor, R., & Hanson, E. (1985). A naturalistic view of conflict between adolescents and their parents and siblings. *Journal of Early Adolescence, 5,* 23–30.

Moradi, A. R., Neshat Doost, H. T., Taghavi, R., Yule, W., & Dagleish, T. (1999). Performance of children of adults with PTSD on the Stroop color-naming task: A preliminary study. *Journal of Traumatic Stress, 12,* 663–672.

Moradi, A. R., Taghavi, R., Neshat Doost, H. T., Yule, W., & Dagleish, T. (1999). Performance of children and adolescents with PTSD on the Stroop colour-naming task. *Psychological Medicine, 29,* 415–419.

Newman, D. L., Moffitt, T. E., Caspi, A., Magdol, L., Silva, P. A., & Stanton, W. R. (1996). Psychiatric disorder in a birth cohort of young adults: Prevalence, comorbidity, clinical significance, and new case incidence from ages 11–21. *Journal of Consulting and Clinical Psychology, 64,* 552–562.

Neziroglu, F., Yaryura-Tobias, J. A., Walz, J., & McKay, D. (2000). The effect of fluvoxamine and behavior therapy on children and adolescents with obsessive–compulsive disorder. *Journal of Child and Adolescent Psychopharmacology, 10,* 295–306.

Ollendick, T. H. (1983). Reliability and validity of the Revised Fear Survey Schedule for Children (FSSC-R). *Behaviour Research and Therapy, 21,* 685–692.

Ollendick, T. H. (1986). Behavior therapy with children. In S. Garfield & A. Bergin (Eds.), *Handbook of psychotherapy and behavior change* (3rd ed., pp. 97–113). New York: Wiley.

Ollendick, T. H., & King, N. J. (1998). Empirically supported treatments for children with phobic and anxiety disorders: Current status. *Journal of Clinical Child Psychology, 27,* 156–167.

Ollendick, T. H., Matson, J. L., & Hesel, W. J. (1985). Fears in children and adolescents: Normative data. *Behaviour Research and Therapy, 4,* 465–467.

Ollendick, T. H., Mattis, S. G., & King, N. J. (1994).

Panic in children and adolescents: A review. *Journal of Child Psychology and Psychiatry, 35,* 113–134.

Öst, L. G. (1987). Age of onset in different phobias. *Journal of Abnormal Psychology, 96,* 223– 229.

Öst, L. G. (1991). Acquisition of blood and injection phobia and anxiety response patterns in clinical patients. *Behaviour Research and Therapy, 29,* 323–332.

Öst, L. G. (1998, November). *Evaluations of the treatment of phobias in children.* Colloquium presented at Temple University.

Peeples, F., & Loeber, R. (1994). Do individual factors and neighborhood context explain ethnic differences in juvenile delinquency? *Journal of Quantitative Criminology, 10,* 141–157.

Perrin, S., & Last, C. G. (1992). Do childhood anxiety measures measure anxiety? *Journal of Abnormal Child Psychology, 20,* 567–578.

Pina, A. A., Silverman, W. K., Alfano, C. A., & Saavedra, L. M. (2002). Diagnostic efficiency of symptoms in the diagnosis of DSM-IV: Generalized anxiety disorder in youth. *Journal of Child Psychology and Psychiatry, 43,* 959–967.

Pine, D. S., Cohen, P., Gurley, D., Brook, J., & Ma, Y. (1998). The risk for early-adulthood anxiety and depressive disorders in adolescents with anxiety and depressive disorders. *Archives of General Psychiatry, 55,* 56–64.

Pine, D. S., Klein, R. G., Coplan, J. D., Papp, L. A., Hoven, C. W., Martinez, J. M., et al. (2000), Differential carbon dioxide sensitivity in childhood anxiety disorders and no null comparison group. *Archives of General Psychiatry, 57,* 96–967.

Popper, C. W., & Ziminitzky, B. (1995). Sudden death putatively related to desipramine treatment in youth: A fifth case and a review of speculative mechanisms. *Journal of Child and Adolescent Psychopharmacology, 5,* 283–300.

Regier, D. A., Narrow, W. E., Rae, D. S., Manderscheid, R. W., Locke, B. Z., & Goodwin, F. K. (1993). The de facto US mental and addictive disorders service system: Epidemiologic Catchment Area prospective 1-year prevalence rates of disorders and services. *Archives of General Psychiatry, 50,* 85–94.

Reinherz, H. Z., Giaconia, R. M., Lefkowitz, E. S., Pakiz, B., & Frost, A. K. (1993). Prevalence of psychiatric disorders in a community population of older adolescents. *Journal of the American Academy of Child and Adolescent Psychiatry, 32,* 369–377.

Reynolds, C. R. (1982). Convergent and divergent validity of the Revised Children's Manifest Anxiety Scale. *Educational and Psychological Measurement, 42,* 1205–1212.

Reynolds, C. R., & Paget, K. D. (1983). National normative and reliability data for the Revised Children's Manifest Anxiety Scale. *School Psychology Review, 12,* 324–336.

Reynolds, C. R., & Richmond, B. O. (1978). What I Think and Feel: A revised measure of children's manifest anxiety. *Journal of Abnormal Child Psychology,* 6, 271–280.

Reynolds, C. R., & Richmond, B. O. (1979). Factor structure and construct validity of "What I Think and Feel": The Revised Children's Manifest Anxiety Scale. *Journal of Personality Assessment,* 43, 281–283.

Reynolds, C. R., & Richmond, B. O. (1985). *Revised Children's Manifest Anxiety Scale (RCMAS) manual.* Los Angeles: Western Psychological Services.

Riddle, M. A., Bernstein, G. A., Cook, E. H., Leonard, H. L., March, J. S., & Swanson, J. M. (1999). Anxiolytics, adrenergic agents, and naltrexone. *Journal of the American Academy of Child and Adolescent Psychiatry,* 38, 546–556.

Riddle, M. A., Claghorn, J., Gaffney, G., Griest, J. H., Holland, D., Landbloom, R., et al. (1996). A controlled trial of fluvoxamine for obsessive–compulsive disorder in children and adolescents. *Psychopharmacology Bulletin,* 32, 399.

Riddle, M. A., Geller, B., & Ryan, N. (1993). Case study: Another sudden death in a child treated with desipramine. *Journal of Child and Adolescent Psychiatry,* 32, 792–797.

Riddle, M. A., Nelson, J. C., Kleinman, C. S., Rasmusson, A., Leckman, J. F., King, R. A., & Cohen, D. J. (1991). Case study: Sudden death in children receiving Norpramin: A review of three reported cases and commentary. *Journal of the American Academy of Child and Adolescent Psychiatry,* 30, 104–108.

Riddle, M. A., Subramaniam, G., & Walkup, J. T. (1998). Efficacy of psychiatric medications in children and adolescents: A review of controlled studies. *Psychiatric Clinics of North America (Annual Drug Therapy),* 5, 269–285.

Robins, R. W., John, O. P., Caspi, A., Moffitt, T. E., & Stouthamer-Loeber, M. (1996). Resilient, overcontrolled, and undercontrolled boys: Three replicable personality types. *Journal of Personality and Social Psychology,* 70, 157–171

Rogeness, G. A., Cepeda, C., Macedo, C. A., Fischer, C., & Harris, W. R. (1990). Differences in heart rate and blood pressure in children with conduct disorder, major depression, and separation anxiety. *Psychiatry Research,* 33, 199–206.

Rosenbaum, J. F., Biederman, J., Gersten, M., Hirshfeld, D. R., Meminger, S. R., Herman, J. B., et al. (1988). Behavioral inhibition in children of parents with panic disorder and agoraphobia: A controlled study. *Archives of General Psychiatry,* 45, 463–470.

RUPP Anxiety Study Group. (2001). An eight-week placebo-controlled trial of fluvoxamine for anxiety disorders in children and adolescents. *New England Journal of Medicine,* 344, 1279–1285.

RUPP Anxiety Study Group. (2002). The Pediatric Anxiety Rating Scale: Development and psychometric properties. *Journal of the American Academy of Child and Adolescent Psychiatry,* 41, 1061–1069.

Rynn, M. A., Siqueland, L., & Rickels, K. (2001). Placebo-controlled trial of sertraline in the treatment of children with generalized anxiety disorder. *American Journal of Psychiatry,* 158, 2008–2014.

Sallee, F. R., & Greenawald, J. (1995). Neurobiology. In J. S. March (Ed.), *Anxiety disorders in children and adolescents* (pp. 3–34). New York: Guilford Press.

Sallee, F. R., Richman, H., Sethuraman, G., Dougherty, D., Sine, L., Altman-Hamamdzic, S. (1998). Clonidine challenge in childhood anxiety disorder. *Journal of the American Academy of Child and Adolescent Psychiatry,* 37, 655–662.

Scahill, L., Riddle, M. A., King, R. A., Hardin, M. T., Rasmusson, A., Makuch, R. W., & Leckman, J. F. (1997). Fluoxetine has no marked effect on tic symptoms in patients with Tourette's syndrome: A double-blind placebo-controlled study. *Journal of Child and Adolescent Psychopharmacology,* 7, 75–85.

Scapillato, D., & Manassis, K. (2002). Cognitive-behavioral/interpersonal group treatment for anxious adolescents. *Journal of the American Academy of Child and Adolescent Psychiatry,* 41, 739–741.

Schippell, P. L., Vasey, M. W., Cravens-Brown, L. M., & Bretveld, R. A. (2003). Suppressed attention to rejection, ridicule, and failure cues: A unique correlate of reactive but not proactive aggression in youth. *Journal of Clinical Child and Adolescent Psychology,* 32, 40–55.

Schniering, C. A., Hudson, J. L., & Rapee, R. M. (2000). Issues in the diagnosis and assessment of anxiety disorders in children and adolescents. *Clinical Psychology Review,* 20, 453–478.

Shaffer, D., Fisher, P., Lucas, C., Dulcan, M., & Schwab-Stone, M. (2000). NIMH Diagnostic Interview Schedule for Children version IV (NIMH DISC-IV): Description, differences from previous versions, and reliability of some common diagnoses. *Journal of the American Academy of Child and Adolescent Psychiatry* 39, 28–38.

Silove, D., Harris, M., Morgan, A., Boyce, P., Manicavasagar, V., Hadzi-Pavlovic, D., & Wilhelm, K. (1995). Is early separation anxiety a specific precursor of panic disorder-agoraphobia? A community study. *Psychological Medicine,* 25, 405–411.

Silverman, W. K. (1991). *Guide to use the Anxiety Disorders Interview Schedule for Children—Revised (Child and Parent versions).* Albany, NY: Graywind.

Silverman, W. K., & Albano, A. M. (1996). *Manual for the Anxiety Disorders Interview Schedule for DSM-IV: Child version.* Albany, NY: Graywind Publications.

Silverman, W. K., & Eisen, A. R. (1992). Age differences in the reliability of parent and child reports of child anxious symptomatology using a structured interview. *Journal of the American Academy of Child and Adolescent Psychiatry,* 31, 117–124.

Silverman, W. K., Kurtines, W. M., Ginsburg, G. S., Weems, C. F., Rabian, B., & Serafini, L. T. (1999). Contingency management, self-control, and education support in the treatment of childhood phobic disorders: A randomized clinical trial. *Journal of Consulting and Clinical Psychology, 67,* 675–687.

Silverman, W. K., & Nelles, W. B. (1988). The Anxiety Disorders Interview Schedule for Children. *Journal of the American Academy of Child and Adolescent Psychiatry, 27,* 772–778.

Silverman, W. K., Saavedra, L. M., & Pina, A. A. (2001). Test–retest reliability of anxiety symptoms and diagnoses using the Anxiety Disorders Interview Schedule for DSM-IV (ADIS for DSM-IV C/P): Child and parent version. *Journal of the American Academy of Child and Adolescent Psychiatry, 40,* 937–944.

Simeon, J. G., & Ferguson, H. B. (1987). Alprazolam effects in children with anxiety disorders. *Canadian Journal of Psychiatry, 32,* 570–574.

Simeon, J. G., Ferguson, H. B., Knott, V., Roberts, N., Gautheir, B., Dubois, C., & Wiggins, D. (1992). Clinical, cognitive, and neurophysiological effects of alprazolam in children and adolescents with overanxious and avoidant disorders. *Journal of the American Academy of Child and Adolescent Psychiatry, 31,* 29–33.

Simeon, J. G., Knott, V. J., Dubois, C., Wiggins, D., Geraets, I., Thatte, S., & Miller, W. (1994). Buspirone therapy of mixed anxiety disorders in childhood and adolescence: A pilot study. *Journal of Child and Adolescent Psychopharmacology, 4,* 159–170.

Siqueland, L., Kendall, P. C., & Steinberg, L. (1996) Anxiety in children: Perceived family environments and observed family interaction. *Journal of Clinical Child Psychology, 25,* 225–237.

Skre, I., Onstad, S., Torgersen, S., Lygren S., & Kringlen E. (1993). A twin study of DSM-III-R anxiety disorders. *Acta Psychiatrica Scandinavica, 88,* 85–92.

Southam-Gerow, M. A. (2001). Generalized anxiety disorder. In C. A. Essau & F. Petermann (Eds.), *Anxiety disorders in children and adolescents: Epidemiology, risk factors, and treatment* (pp. 219–260). New York: Taylor & Francis.

Spence, S. H. (1997). Structure of anxiety symptoms in children: A confirmatory factor-analytic study. *Journal of Abnormal Psychology, 106,* 280–297.

Spence, S. H. (1998). A measure of anxiety symptoms among children. *Behaviour Research and Therapy, 36,* 545–556.

Spence, S. H., Donovan, C., & Brechma-Toussaint, M. (1999). Social skills, social outcomes, and cognitive features of childhood social phobia. *Journal of Abnormal Psychology, 108,* 211–221.

Spielberger, C. D., Edwards, C. D., & Lushene, R. E. (1973). *State–Trait Anxiety Inventory for Children.* Palo Alto, CA: Consulting Psychologists Press.

Stallings, P., & March, J. S. (1995). Assessment. In J. S. March (Ed.), *Anxiety disorders in children and adolescents* (pp. 125–147). New York: Guilford Press.

Stark, K. D., Humphrey, L. L., Crook, K., & Lewis, K. (1990). Perceived family environments of depressed and anxious children: Child's and maternal figure's perspectives. *Journal of Abnormal Child Psychology, 18,* 527–547.

Stark, K. D., Kaslow, N. L., & Laurent, J. (1993). The assessment of depression in children: Are we assessing depression or the broad-band construct of negative affectivity? *Journal of Emotional and Behavioral Disorders, 1,* 149–154.

Stein, M. B., Fuetsch, M., Mueller, N., Hoefler, M., Lieb, R., & Wittchen, H. (2001). Social anxiety disorder and the risk of depression: A prospective community study of adolescents and young adults. *Archives of General Psychiatry, 58,* 251–256.

Steinberg, L. D. (1981). Transformations in family relations at puberty. *Developmental Psychology, 17,* 833–840.

Steinberg, L., & Silk, J. S. (2002). Parenting adolescents. In M. H. Bornstein (Ed.), *Handbook of parenting* (Vol. 1, pp. 103–134). Mahwah, NJ: Erlbaum.

Steinberg, L., & Silverberg, S. B. (1986). The vicissitudes of autonomy in early adolescence. *Child Development, 57,* 841–851.

Strauss, C. C., & Last, C. G. (1993). Social and simple phobias in children. *Journal of Anxiety Disorders, 1,* 141–152.

Strauss, C. C., Lease, C. A., Kazdin, A. E., Dulcan, M., & Last, C. (1989). Multi-method assessment of the social competence of anxiety disordered children. *Journal of Consulting and Clinical Psychology, 18,* 184–190.

Strauss, C. D., Lease, C. A., Last, C. G., & Francis, G. (1988). Overanxious disorder: An examination of developmental differences. *Journal of Abnormal Child Psychology, 16,* 433–443.

Sweeney, L., & Rapee, R. (2001). Social phobia. In C. A. Essau & F. Petermann (Eds.), *Anxiety disorders in children and adolescents: Epidemiology, risk factors, and treatment* (pp. 163–192). New York: Taylor & Francis.

Sylvester, C., Hyde, T. S., & Reichler, R. J. (1987). The diagnostic interview for children and personality inventory for children in studies of children at risk for anxiety disorders or depression. *Journal of the American Academy of Child and Adolescent Psychiatry, 26,* 668–675.

Taghavi, R., Moradi, A. R., Neshat Doost, H. T., Yule, W., & Dagleish, T. (2000) Interpretation of ambiguous emotional information in clinically-anxious children and adolescents. *Cognition and Emotion, 14,* 809–822.

Thieneman, M., Martin, J., Cregger, B., Thompson, H. B., & Dyer-Friedman, J. (2001). Manual-driven group cognitive-behavioral therapy for adolescents with obsessive–compulsive disorder: A pilot study. *Journal of the American Academy of Child and Adolescent Psychiatry, 40,* 1254–1260.

Tollefson, G. D., Rampey Jr., A. H., Potvin, J. H., Jenike, M. A., Rush, A. J., Dominguez, R. A., et al. (1994). A multicenter investigation of fixed-dose fluoxetine in the treatment of obsessive–compulsive disorder. *Archives of General Psychiatry, 51,* 559–567.

Tracey, S. A., Chorpita, B. F., Douban, J., & Barlow, D. H. (1997). Empirical evaluation of DSM-IV generalized anxiety disorder criteria in children and adolescents. *Journal of Clinical Child Psychology, 26,* 404–414.

Turner, S. M., Beidel, D. C., & Costello, A. (1987). Psychopathology in the offspring of anxiety disorders inpatients. *Journal of Consulting and Clinical Psychology, 55,* 229–235.

Turner, S. M., Beidel, D. C., & Epstein, L. H. (1991). Vulnerability and risk for the anxiety disorders. *Journal of Anxiety Disorders, 5,* 151–166.

van den Oord, E. J. C. G., Boomsma, D. I., & Verhulst, F. C. (1994). A study of problem behaviors in 10–15-year-old biologically related and unrelated international adoptees. *Behavior Genetics, 24,* 193–205.

Vasey, M. W. (1993). Development and cognition in childhood anxiety: The example of worry. In T. H. Ollendick & R. Prinz (Eds.), *Advances in clinical child psychology* (Vol. 15, pp. 1–39). New York: Plenum Press.

Vasey, M. W., Crnic, K. A., & Carter, W. G. (1994). Worry in childhood: A developmental perspective. *Cognitive Therapy and Research, 18,* 529–549.

Vasey, M. W., Daleiden, E. L., Williams, L. L., & Brown, L. M. (1995). Biased attention in childhood anxiety disorders: A preliminary study. *Journal of Abnormal Child Psychology, 23,* 267–279.

Vasey, M. W., & Macleod, C. (2001). Information-processing factors in childhood anxiety: A review and developmental perspective. In M. W. Vasey & M. R. Dadds (Eds.), *The developmental psychopathology of anxiety* (pp. 253–277). New York: Oxford University Press.

Velez, C. N., Johnson, J., & Cohen, P. (1989). A longitudinal analysis of selected risk factors for childhood psychopathology. *Journal of the American Academy of Child and Adolescent Psychiatry, 28,* 861–864.

Velosa, J. F., & Riddle, M. A. (2000). Pharmacologic treatment of anxiety disorders in children and adolescents. *Child and Adolescent Psychiatric Clinics of North America, 9,* 119–133.

Verhulst, F. C., van der Ende, J., Ferdinand, R. F., & Kasius, M. C. (1997). The prevalence of DSM-III-R diagnoses in a national sample of Dutch adolescents. *Archives of General Psychiatry, 54,* 329–336.

Walkup, J., Davies, M., & RUPP Anxiety Study Group.

(1999, October). *The Pediatric Anxiety Rating Scale (PARS): A reliability study.* Poster presented at the annual meeting of the American Academy of Child and Adolescent Psychiatry, Chicago.

Warner, V., Mufson, L., & Weissman, M. M. (1995). Offspring at high and low risk for depression and anxiety: Mechanisms of psychiatric disorder. *Journal of the American Academy of Child and Adolescent Psychiatry, 34,* 786–797.

Weems, C. F., Hayward, C., Killen, J., & Taylor, C. B. (2002). A longitudinal investigation of anxiety sensitivity in adolescence. *Journal of Abnormal Psychology, 111,* 471–477.

Weissman, M. M., Leckman, J. F., Merikangas, K. R., Gammon, G. D., & Prusoff, B. A. (1984). Depression and anxiety disorders in parents and children: Results from the Yale family study. *Archives of General Psychiatry, 41,* 845–852.

Weisz, J. R., & Hawley, K. M. (2002). Developmental factors in the treatment on adolescents. *Journal of Consulting and Clinical Psychology, 70,* 21–43.

Welner, Z., Reich, W., Herjanic, B., Jung, K. G., & Amado, H. (1987). Reliability, validity, and parent–child agreement studies of the Diagnostic Interview for Children and Adolescents (DICA). *Journal of the American Academy of Child and Adolescent Psychiatry, 26,* 649–653.

Whaley, S. E., Pinto, A., & Sigman, M. (1999). Characterizing interactions between anxious mothers and their children. *Journal of Consulting and Clinical Psychology, 67,* 826–836.

Witt, J. C., Heffer, R. W., & Pfeiffer, J. P. (1990). Structured rating scales: A review of self-report and informant rating processes, procedures, and issues. In C. R. Reynolds & R. W. Kamphaus (Eds.), *Handbook of psychological and educational assessment of children: Personality, behavior, and context* (pp. 364–394). New York: Guilford Press.

Wittchen, H. U., Nelson, C. B., & Lachner, G. (1998). Prevalence of mental disorders and psychosocial impairments in adolescents and young adults. *Psychological Medicine, 28,* 109–126.

World Health Organization. (1993). *The ICD-10 classification of mental and behavioural disorders.* Geneva, Switzerland: Author.

Youniss, J., & Smollar, J. (1985). *Adolescent relations with mothers, fathers, and friends.* Chicago: University of Chicago Press.

8

Mood Disorders

Karen D. Rudolph
Constance Hammen
Shannon E. Daley

Depression is one of the most common psychiatric disorders and is associated with a great deal of personal distress and disruption in people's lives. Because depression often emerges during adolescence, understanding the disorder during this developmental stage is critical for determining its etiology and course, and for developing early identification and intervention strategies. Despite this need, few comprehensive reviews of adolescent depression are available. This chapter details the phenomenology, clinical course and correlates, etiology, consequences, assessment, and treatment of adolescent depression. Importantly, unique aspects of adolescence are considered to fully understand depression within a developmental context. The chapter also summarizes the recently emerging body of knowledge concerning the expression and treatment of bipolar disorder in adolescents.

HISTORICAL CONTEXT OF ADOLESCENT DEPRESSION

Early theories of depression discounted the validity of the disorder in childhood, suggest-ing that the psychological mechanisms were not yet in place for the experience of depression, or that depression was "masked" in the form of other disturbances. Once these myths were dispelled, research on childhood depression burgeoned, resulting in the growth of both theory and an empirical database. Yet, some unique obstacles existed in the pursuit of knowledge about adolescent depression. Specifically, early "storm and stress" theories of development depicted adolescence as a period of upheaval that resulted in psychological disruption reflected in such problems as confusion about identity, family discord, social stress, emotional distress, and behavior problems (for a review, see Arnett, 1999). In line with these theories, many of the problems associated with depression, such as experiences of sadness, moodiness, self-doubt and self-critical thoughts, and social withdrawal, were viewed as normative expressions of adolescent angst. It has become clear, however, that depression can be a serious disorder during adolescence, often heralding a chronic or recurrent course of disruption and impairment into adulthood.

NEED FOR A DEVELOPMENTAL PSYCHOPATHOLOGY FRAMEWORK OF ADOLESCENT DEPRESSION

In the past two decades, the field of child depression research has advanced from applying simple extensions of descriptions and theories developed in adults to generating an increasingly sophisticated understanding of depression informed by the emerging field of developmental psychopathology (e.g., Cicchetti & Toth, 1998; Garber & Horowitz, 2002; Hammen & Rudolph, 2003; Kaslow, Adamson, & Collins, 2000). This perspective takes into account the intersection between normative developmental processes and the development of psychopathology. Accordingly, research adopting this framework has considered normative developmental influences that may create differences in the phenomenology, correlates, etiology, and outcomes of depression in childhood versus adulthood. Often, however, this new generation of research does not differentiate among particular stages of development throughout childhood. Although some continuity is likely across childhood and adolescence in the experience of depression, the processes underlying risk, and the consequences of depression, some differences also may arise. In this chapter, we consider how the special circumstances of adolescence may influence such aspects of depression as its expression and associated characteristics, course, etiology, assessment, and treatment.

A complicated question that arises when applying a developmental perspective on psychopathology concerns how to conceptualize different life stages. For example, definitions of adolescence can be based on a variety of factors, including chronological age, physical maturation, or underlying biological changes of puberty. Furthermore, there is considerable interindividual variability in the timing and overlap of different markers of adolescence. Although each marker of adolescence is important, in this chapter we use age and grade as the boundaries within which to define adolescence. This decision was based on pragmatic reasons, namely, that information about physical maturational and hormonal status of participants is available in only a limited number of studies. Specifically, we focus primarily on youth between the ages of 11 and 18, or fifth and twelfth grades. In some cases, however, studies are reviewed that include samples with a subgroup that lies outside this age range due to some unique aspect of the studies (e.g., high-risk studies that typically involve large age ranges).

DESCRIPTION OF ADOLESCENT DEPRESSION

Clinical Depression: Symptoms and Associated Characteristics

Diagnostic criteria for major depressive episode (MDE) include depressed mood and/or loss of pleasure plus at least four somatic or cognitive symptoms, including weight or appetite changes, changes in sleep, psychomotor changes (agitation or retardation), loss of energy, worthlessness or guilt, concentration problems or indecisiveness, and thoughts of death or suicide. Symptoms must persist at least 2 weeks and cause impaired functioning or clinically significant distress. Dysthymic disorder requires persisting mood symptoms plus at least two somatic or cognitive symptoms, including several of those characteristic of MDE, as well as poor self-esteem or hopelessness. Diagnoses of MDE and dysthymic disorder are based on similar diagnostic criteria for adolescents and adults with two exceptions. First, the fourth edition, text revision of *Diagnostic and Statistical Manual of Mental Disorders* (DSM-IV-TR; American Psychiatric Association, 2000) allows substitution of irritability for depressed mood in adolescents. Second, the duration criterion for dysthymic disorder in adolescents is one instead of 2 years.

It might be noted that the validity of distinguishing between major depressive disorder (MDD) and dysthymic disorder as two separate entities in youngsters has been called into question by the NIMH Methods for the Epidemiology of Child and Adolescent Mental Disorders (MECA) study (Goodman, Schwab-Stone, Lahey, Shaffer, & Jensen, 2000). This study revealed that children and adolescents with either condition alone could not be distinguished on clinical or demographic features or on correlates. However, those with both diagnoses were significantly more impaired than those with either diagnosis alone. At the present time, however, no formal changes have been suggested for the DSM criteria, and the status of the diagnosis of dysthymia in youth awaits further research.

Although symptoms of depressive syndromes in adolescents are similar to those of adults (Kovacs, 1996; Lewinsohn & Essau, 2002), several symptoms or correlates of depression may be particularly noteworthy among adolescents. Suicidal thoughts and behaviors are especially elevated in depressed youth (Lewinsohn, Rohde, & Seeley, 1996; Lewinsohn, Rohde, Seeley, & Baldwin, 2001), and rates of suicide in adolescents have increased markedly in the past few decades (Harrington & Vostanis, 1995). Social withdrawal also is reported as a common correlate of adolescent depression (e.g., Goodyer & Cooper, 1993). Moreover, depressed adolescent girls are particularly likely to report distress over negative body image (e.g., Petersen, Sarigiani, & Kennedy, 1991), weight/appetite disturbance, and worthlessness/guilt (Lewinsohn, Rohde, & Seeley, 1998).

Some subtypes of depression, including psychotic depression, seasonal affective disorder, premenstrual dysphoric disorder, and atypical depression emerge in adolescence, but there is relatively little research on these disorders in youth (Birmaher, Ryan, Williamson, Brent, Kaufman, Dahl, et al., 1996). Psychotic depression in adolescents may be especially predictive of bipolar disorder (Strober, Lampert, Schmidt, & Morrell, 1993), as discussed in a later section. In view of the accepted belief that depression is highly heterogeneous in presentation and etiology, additional research that sheds light on possible subtypes in adolescents is needed.

Subclinical Depression

It is increasingly recognized that subclinical depression in the form of persistent elevated symptoms may be associated with significant impairment of functioning and increased risk for future diagnosis of depression. For example, youth with elevated symptoms but who fail to meet diagnostic criteria for depression have been found to demonstrate significant clinical and role dysfunction (Gotlib, Lewinsohn, & Seeley, 1995). Similarly, in a longitudinal study of Swiss adolescents, subsyndromal depression was a strong predictor of the onset of major depression (Angst, Sellaro, & Merikangas, 2000; see also Pine, Cohen, Cohen, & Brook, 1999). As later sections attest, nonclinically depressed youth show an array of social, cognitive, and coping difficulties and may be at risk for depressive episodes following stressors. Thus, mild but persisting depressive symptoms may be significant and detrimental.

Comorbidity

Depressive disorders in children and adolescents are highly likely to co-occur with other disorders, either concurrently or over time. A meta-analysis of comorbidity in community studies of child and adolescent samples revealed a median odds ratio (degree of association) of 8.2 for depression and anxiety disorders, 6.6 for depression and conduct disorder (CD)/oppositional defiant disorder (ODD), and 5.5 for depression and attention-deficit/hyperactivity disorder (ADHD) (Angold, Costello, & Erkanli, 1999; see also reviews by Birmaher, Ryan, Williamson, Brent, Kaufman, Dahl, et al., 1996; Kovacs, 1996).

Among adolescent samples, lifetime anxiety disorders are the most likely disorders to co-occur with MDEs, especially for females (Angold, Costello, & Erkanli, 1999; Birmaher, Ryan, Williamson, Brent, Kaufman, Dahl, et al., 1996; Kovacs, 1996). Lewinsohn, Hops, Roberts, Seeley, and Andrews (1993) reported that 21% of those with MDD also had a lifetime anxiety disorder (and among those with anxiety disorders, 49% had MDD; see also Pine, Cohen, Gurley, Brook, & Ma, 1998). It has been proposed that anxiety and depression are etiologically related (e.g., Avenevoli, Stolar, Li, Dierker, & Merikangas, 2001; Kovacs, 1990; Pine et al., 1998). Adolescent women also show relatively high rates of comorbidity between depression and eating disorders; for example, in one study, 69% of those with eating disorders also had diagnoses of unipolar depression (e.g., Lewinsohn et al., 1993; see also Lewinsohn, Striegel-Moore, & Seeley, 2000). Comorbidity of depression with disruptive behavior and substance use disorders also is common in adolescence, especially for males. Lewinsohn and colleagues reported that about 12% of adolescents with depressive disorders also had a diagnosable disruptive behavior (attention deficit, conduct, and oppositional defiant) disorder, and 20% had a substance use disorder.

Several researchers have suggested that, because depression commonly follows other disorders, it often might be a consequence of the earlier disorder. Conceptualizations of the meaning of comorbidity in children and adolescents, and analyses of the fairly sparse research examining different hypotheses are presented more fully by Angold, Costello, and Erkanli (1999). Generally, there is agreement that the implications of depression comorbidity are significant in youth given evidence that this pattern often is associated with more severe symptoms and correlates, as well as worse clinical course and treatment outcomes (Birmaher, Ryan, Williamson, Brent, Kaufman, Dahl, et al., 1996; Lewinsohn, Rohde, & Seeley, 1995).

EPIDEMIOLOGY OF ADOLESCENT DEPRESSION

Prevalence and Incidence

Rates of diagnosed depression among adolescents are comparable to those of adults. The National Comorbidity Study (NCS) is the only U.S. nationally representative community epidemiological survey that included adolescents (age 15 and above). *Lifetime prevalence* of major depression in the 15–18-year-olds was 14%, with an additional 11% reporting minor depression (Kessler & Walters, 1998). Lewinsohn and colleagues (1993) reported a lifetime MDD rate of 18% in their large community study of adolescents. These rates are relatively comparable to those in smaller community surveys of adolescents (e.g., Cohen et al., 1993). Lewinsohn and colleagues (1998) reported a rate of 5.7% of first incidence in a 1-year period and suggested that the great majority of episodes observed during follow-up were recurrences. These investigators estimated that approximately 28% of youth would experience an episode of MDD by age 19 (35% of young women, and 19% of young men). Similar rates were reported by Rao, Hammen, and Daley (1999) for a smaller community sample of young women. Lewinsohn and Essau (2002) summarized *point prevalence* rates of MDE from epidemiological studies in North America, New Zealand, Great Britain, and the Netherlands, noting rates ranging from 0.7 to 9.8%, based mostly on DSM-III-R criteria. Importantly, these data do not necessarily indicate that first onset occurred during adolescence.

There is ample evidence that rates of depression in adolescence have increased in recent years compared to those of previous decades. Earlier reports of birth-cohort effects showing growing rates of major depression in those born in more recent decades have been replicated in the United States and internationally by the Cross-National Collaborative Group (1992). Recent results from the NCS also show clear evidence of increasing prevalence of MDE, as well as minor depression, in adolescence, especially in those born since 1965 (Kessler, Avenevoli, & Merikangas, 2001). Various analyses of the sources of such increased rates generally have ruled out methodological artifacts, such as memory or increasing willingness to admit to depressive experiences (e.g., Murphy, Laird, Monson, Sobol, & Leighton, 2000), and the rates are paralleled by behavioral correlates of depression, such as suicide. The cause of the increase is not known, but often it is suggested that at least some of it may be due to social changes that contribute to vulnerability to depression, such as family disruption and exposure to greater stressors, along with reduced access to resources and supports.

The prevalence of depression is even greater when considering subsyndromal depressive symptoms. Cooper and Goodyer (1993) reported that 20.7% of their female sample of 11- to 16-year-olds had significant symptoms but fell short of diagnostic criteria. Moreover, when *self-report symptom scores*, rather than diagnostic information, are used to indicate depressive experiences, approximately 10–40% of adolescents exceed cutoffs for high levels (e.g., Roberts, Lewinsohn, & Seeley, 1991). Rather than mere "adolescent turmoil," elevated self-report scores indicate high levels of distress and impaired functioning and may portend the later development of diagnosable disorders, as noted previously.

Age of Onset

Various research designs have yielded consistent evidence that early adolescence marks the most common time for a first episode of MDD or significant symptoms. Most studies suggest that the typical onset of diagnosable major depression is around 13–15 years (e.g., Angold & Rutter, 1992; Cohen et al., 1993; Cooper & Goodyer, 1993; Petersen et al., 1991). In the Oregon Adolescent Depression Project, mean age of onset of MDD was 14.8 for girls and 15.3 for boys, a nonsignificant difference (Lewinsohn & Essau, 2002). In the NCS, meaningful risk of onset started in the early teens and increased in a linear fashion into the early 20s (Kessler et al., 2001).

Sex Differences

The emergence of higher rates of depressive symptoms and diagnoses in girls during adolescence is well established (e.g., Hankin et al., 1998; Nolen-Hoeksema & Girgus, 1994). There are divergent findings about the exact age at which adolescent girls' rates of depressive symptoms increase and sex differences appear, but most studies concur that it is around 12–14 years (e.g., Angold & Rutter, 1992; Cohen et al., 1993; Cooper & Goodyer, 1993; Petersen et al., 1991). Hankin and colleagues (1998) noted that the greatest increases in diagnosable depression in young women occurred between 15 and 18 years in a New Zealand sample. A recent cross-national survey of depressive symptoms in youth found that the sex difference emerged by age 14 (Wade, Cairney, & Pevalin, 2002). It should be noted, however, that sex differences in developmental precursors of depression may emerge at even earlier ages. For instance, Rudolph and colleagues (2005) found that sex differences emerged as early as 10 years of age in symptoms such as fearfulness, negative self-evaluation, concerns with personal inadequacy, sensitivity to social evaluation, and depressive affect, with girls reporting significantly higher rates than boys.

The issues of why sex differences occur and why they emerge in adolescence have been explored from numerous perspectives, which variously focus on hormonal changes, stress and coping processes, social roles and affiliative concerns, and interactions among these variables (for reviews, see Cyranowski, Frank, Young, & Shear, 2000; Hankin & Abramson, 2001; Nolen-Hoeksema & Girgus, 1994; Nolen-Hoeksema, 2002; Rudolph, 2002). These perspectives are described in more detail in later sections.

Social Class Effects

Social class effects on depression have been well documented in adults, and similar patterns have been observed in children and adolescents. Specifically, studies of both symptom levels (e.g., Gore, Aseltine, & Colton, 1992) and diagnoses (e.g., Bird et al., 1988; Costello et al., 1996) have linked depression to lower income and socioeconomic status (SES). However, low SES may be a marker of specific risk factors for depression, rather than exerting a direct influence on depression. For example, low SES may be linked to chronic stress due to economic difficulties, exposure to stressful life events associated with adverse environmental conditions, and family disruption, which all are predictors of depression.

Ethnic and Cultural Differences

Few studies have included sufficient ethnically diverse samples to examine differences in depression rates. One of the largest studies to date (5,423 students in grades 6–8) reported comparable rates of major depression in nine ethnic groups, except for higher rates among adolescents of Mexican descent (Roberts, Roberts, & Chen, 1997). Most studies generally have found few differences in depression between white and African American youth (e.g., Costello et al., 1996). One study found that African American girls did not show the same puberty-related increases in depression that commonly are found in white girls (Hayward, Gotlib, Schraedley, & Litt, 1999).

Examining symptoms rather than diagnoses, a large epidemiological survey of high school students (the National Longitudinal Study of Adolescent Health) revealed that nonwhite (African American, Hispanic, and Asian) adolescents reported significantly higher levels of depressive symptoms than did white adolescents (Rushton, Forcier, & Schectman, 2002), but these differences may have been due to SES effects. However, race and socioeconomic status did not predict persistence of symptoms over time. Further studies are needed to explore other race and ethnicity effects and to separate out effects that might be caused by different cultural expressions of depressive symptoms and adverse conditions that might be associated with ethnic status.

DEVELOPMENTAL COURSE AND OUTCOMES OF ADOLESCENT DEPRESSION

Episode Duration

Considerable variation has been found in the duration of major depression in community samples of untreated depressed youth. Lewinsohn, Rohde, and Seeley (1994) reported a range of 2 to 250 weeks in their community sample, with a median of 8 weeks (mean of 26 weeks). A survival function predicted that 25% would recover by 3 weeks, 50% by 8 weeks, and 75% by 24 weeks. Longer mean durations (e.g., 7 to 9 months) for major depression generally are found in clinical than community samples, although these durations are still somewhat shorter than those observed in adults (e.g., Kovacs, 1996; Rao et al., 1995). Clinical samples have a 90% likelihood of remission within 1½–2 years (for a review, see Birmaher, Ryan, Williamson, Brent, Kaufman, Dahl, et al., 1996).

In a recent review of predictors of the duration of episodes in depressed adolescents, Kaminski and Garber (2002) observed that one relatively reliable predictor of longer episodes is parental history of depression. Other predictors of episode duration across various samples are greater severity of the depression and the presence of comorbid disorders.

Developmental Pathways: Continuity between Childhood and Adolescent Depression

Given the high rates of recurrence, depression onset during childhood is likely to be followed by depressive experiences during adolescence (see Avenevoli & Steinberg, 2001). This developmental continuity may reflect, in part, an underlying stability in vulnerability factors, such as a genetic predisposition to depression or a depressogenic cognitive style. However, continuity in depression across the lifespan also may reflect the detrimental influence of depression on development. That is, depression may leave a developmental "scar" (Rohde, Lewinsohn, & Seeley, 1990), which increases risk for future episodes. More research is needed to identify the processes underlying depression continuity.

Whereas some depressive disorders emerge in childhood and recur during adolescence, others do not emerge, at least in diagnosable form, until adolescence. Little is known about the similarities and differences between childhood-onset and adolescent-onset depression. However, early research suggests that depressive disorders with onsets in childhood versus adolescence may have somewhat different predictors, correlates, and outcomes (Kaufman, Martin, King, & Charney, 2001; Weissman, Wolk, Wickramaratne, et al., 1999), indicating the need for more careful discrimination between these types of onsets in future research.

Recurrence and Continuity into Adulthood

Adolescent-onset depression is likely to recur, further supporting its similarity to adult depression. Research has shown that about 40% of adults experience a recurrence of major depression within 2 years and over 80% within 5–7 years (e.g., Coryell et al., 1994; Solomon et al., 2000). Studies of clinical samples of depressed adolescents cite nearly identical figures (Birmaher, Ryan, Williamson, Brent, Kaufman, Dahl, et al., 1996; Kovacs, 1996). A follow-up by Emslie and colleagues (1997) suggested similar rates of recurrence in a hospitalized sample, with equal rates in those with and without medication treatment (Emslie et al., 1997). Studies of community samples of diagnosed adolescents also have indicated high rates of recurrence, with approximately 40% having a recurrence over 3–5 years (Lewinsohn, Clarke, Seeley, & Rohde, 1994; Rao et al., 1999). There is some disagreement about whether sex differences in recurrence exist. Lewinsohn and Essau (2002) reported that adolescent females in the Oregon study were more likely to have recurring major depression than were males, but studies of recurrence in adults generally fail to find sex differences (e.g., Kessler, McGonagle, Swartz, Blazer, & Nelson, 1993).

Follow-up studies of depressed adolescents also have provided information about the specificity of outcomes in adulthood. There is general agreement that adolescent-onset depression specifically predicts continuing depression into adulthood. For instance, Rao and colleagues (1995) reported that 69% of a clinically ascertained sample of depressed adolescents experienced MDEs, but not nonaffective psychopathology, over a 7-year follow-up into adulthood (mean age 22). Similarly, Weissman, Wolk, Goldstein, and colleagues (1999) found increased risk for recurrence of MDEs (63%) but not other psychopathology compared to controls in an adolescent sample followed for 10–15 years (to mean age 26). Several large-scale studies of community samples also have reported high levels of continuity of adolescent major depression into adulthood. The Dunedin (New Zealand) Multidisciplinary Health and Development Study (Bardone, Moffitt, Caspi, Dickson, & Silva, 1996), the Ontario Child Health Study (Fleming, Boyle, & Offord, 1993), the Oregon Adolescent Depression Project (Lewinsohn, Rohde, Klein, & Seeley, 1999), and the Upstate New York Study (Pine et al., 1998) all reported high rates of recurrence of major depression in young adulthood. Pine and colleagues (1999) also showed that subclinical depressive symptoms in adolescence predicted adult major depression. Moreover, adolescent depression predicts considerable psychosocial maladjustment associated with the transition to adulthood, including marital and relationship discord, unwanted pregnancies, and occupational and economic impairment (Bardone et al., 1996; Gotlib, Lewinsohn, & Seeley, 1998; Rao et al., 1999; Weissman, Wolk, Wickramaratne, et al., 1999).

In contrast to adolescent-onset depression, some evidence suggests that childhood-onset depression is not necessarily predictive of depression in adulthood; except for a subsample of "true" depressives, many depressed children go on to display varied nondepressive disorders, which also are associated with considerable functional impairment (e.g., Harrington, Fudge, Rutter, Pickles, & Hill, 1990; Hofstra, van der Ende, & Verhulst, 2000; Weissman, Wolk, Wickramaratne, et al., 1999).

THEORIES AND ETIOLOGY OF ADOLESCENT DEPRESSION

Theories of adolescent depression need to take into account several characteristics of this developmental stage. Most important, adolescence has been identified as a pivotal stage of development that is marked by a confluence of normative biological, psychological, and social challenges (Eccles & Midgley, 1989; Ge, Lorenz, Conger, Elder, & Simons, 1994). These challenges are produced by major physical maturational changes (e.g., the onset of puberty), social-cognitive advances (e.g., ability for more abstract thinking and generalization across situations and time), interpersonal transitions (e.g., changes in social roles in the family and peer group), and social-contextual changes (e.g., school transitions). These normative adolescent transitions may serve as a developmental context of risk for the onset of psychopathology, particularly depression. Indeed, comprehensive theories of depression should be able to account for two of its most notable features: (1) the significant rise in rates of depression during adolescence; and (2) the emergence or enhancement of sex differences in

depression during adolescence (Angold & Rutter, 1992; Hankin et al., 1998; Nolen-Hoeksema & Girgus, 1994; Petersen et al., 1991).

In this section of the chapter, we consider how normative developmental transitions associated with adolescence act as sensitive periods for the activation of particular processes involved in depression onset, persistence, and recurrence. Specifically, we review key theories of depression and discuss empirical support for these theories in adolescents. Following the discussion of each theory, we consider the stage-specific issues that are critical to understanding the etiology and course of depression during adolescence. In the final summary section, we present a conceptual framework that highlights the role of normative developmental transitions in creating risk for depression. Throughout, we emphasize possible mechanisms underlying the rise in depression during adolescence, especially in girls. When relevant, we point out differences in theoretical models of depression or in the available empirical support for these models in preadolescents versus adolescents.

Genetic/Biological Models

Significant advances have been made in understanding the biological correlates of adult depression, and this research increasingly has included an investigation of similar processes in adolescents. Preliminary data have indicated some consistencies across development, but the presence of some differences has highlighted the need to consider developmental influences on the nature and strength of biological vulnerability to depression, as well as the extent to which biological factors may contribute to sex differences in depression that emerge during adolescence.

Genetic and Family Studies

The risk of depression and other disorders in child and adolescent offspring of depressed parents is well established. Indeed, having a parent with major depression is one of the strongest predictors of childhood or adolescent depression (for a review, see Beardslee, Versage, & Gladstone, 1998). Longitudinal studies have established that children of depressed parents have persisting and recurring depressive disorders that are associated with considerable impairment (e.g., Hammen,

Burge, Burney, & Adrian, 1990). Recently, Klein, Lewinsohn, Seeley, and Rohde (2001) found evidence of specificity of family patterns. Youth in the Oregon Adolescent Depression Project with major depressive disorders had first-degree relatives with elevated rates of MDD and dysthymia, whereas youth with nondepressive disorders did not have family members with elevated rates of depressive disorders, compared with nondisordered youth. Moreover, depressed adolescents who had recurrent episodes of depression were especially likely to have family members with high rates of MDD (Klein, Lewinsohn, Rohde, Seeley, & Durbin, 2002).

Although genetic transmission of depression may be one explanation for such risk, these designs cannot rule out the influence of adverse psychosocial factors such as disordered parent–child relationships, stressful life events and conditions, and marital discord, which are common in families with depressed parents (Goodman & Gotlib, 1999). The most compelling designs for establishing genetic influences on unipolar depression have involved biometric modeling studies of monozygotic (MZ) and dizygotic (DZ) twins. Such studies of adults have established a moderate level of heritability (for a review, see Sullivan, Neale, & Kendler, 2000), as well as a substantial effect of nonshared environment (e.g., personal stressors). However, even identical twins may have different relationships with their parents that contribute to depression outcomes, as indicated by a recent study of MZ twins who were discordant for depressive disorders (Kendler & Gardner, 2001). Some twin studies have suggested higher levels of heritability for more severely ill depressives (for a review, see Wallace, Schneider, & McGuffin, 2002).

Several studies have explicitly addressed heritability issues in child/adolescent samples, and such studies are consistent with the hypothesis of different origins of childhood-onset and adolescent-onset depression. A study of depressive symptoms in 411 British child and adolescent twin pairs by Thapar and McGuffin (1994) revealed much stronger evidence of heritability in adolescents, whereas children's depressive symptoms were strongly associated with environmental factors. Eaves and colleagues (1997) reported on a sample of 1,412 8–16-year-old twin pairs in the Virginia Twin Study of Adolescent Behavioral Development. They found a moderate genetic effect and also

significant individual environmental effects; however, the results differed by informant and no age effects were reported. In a later analysis of the Virginia Twin data, Silberg and colleagues (1999) found increased heritability effects for pubertal girls but not prepubertal girls or boys at any age. About 30% of the variance in adolescent girls' depression was attributable to genetic effects, with the rest due to individual environmental effects.

More recent research on genetic liability to depression has turned to the question of *what* is inherited. Several possibilities are being explored, including aspects of temperament related to emotionality and emotion regulation; a tendency toward stress exposure, generation, and reactivity; and disordered neurobiological processes, but considerable progress is still needed in this area.

Neuroendocrine Regulation and Neurotransmitters

There has been considerable interest in abnormalities of the hypothalamic–pituitary–adrenal (HPA) axis in adult depression, consistent with the possibility that depression is linked to dysregulation of the processes associated with responses to stress (e.g., Plotsky, Owens, & Nemeroff, 1998; Thase, Jindal, & Howland, 2002). Adult depressives commonly demonstrate higher basal cortisol, abnormal cortisol regulation indicated by the dexamethasone suppression test (DST), and abnormalities of corticotropic-releasing hormone (CRH). As reviewed by Birmaher and colleagues (1996) and Kaufman and colleagues (2001), however, similar patterns have not been observed consistently in child and adolescent samples. In particular, few differences in basal cortisol have been observed between depressed and nondepressed adolescents; when group differences have been found, they tend to be subtle alterations in normal diurnal patterns (Kaufman et al., 2001; see Goodyer, Herbert, Tamplin, & Altham, 2000a, 2000b). The few adolescent studies of CRH infusion have failed to show the same blunted corticotropin secretion responses as those found in depressed adults (Kaufman et al., 2001).

Although data on HPA dysregulation in youngsters have been inconsistent, there is considerable interest in the influence of exposure to severe stress on the developing brains of infants and children as a possible predictor of depression. Both human and preclinical research suggests that early exposure to adverse conditions, including maternal prenatal stress, negative parenting, and abuse, promotes alterations in CRH circuits and behavioral changes consistent with depression and anxiety (for reviews, see Goodman, 2002; Heim & Nemeroff, 2001). It is speculated that early adversity may be associated with abnormalities of HPA functioning, which sensitize the organism to subsequent stress. Failure to find clear evidence of HPA axis abnormalities in youth may not be surprising. As Kaufman and colleagues (2001) point out, brain and neuroregulatory processes are incompletely developed in children and adolescents. Moreover, youth may have experienced only a single episode rather than recurrent episodes and therefore may not show the same patterns as those of depressed adults. Kaufman and colleagues urge further neuroimaging studies to help identify possible neural circuits relevant to stress and depression processes in adolescents.

An additional biological marker possibly relevant to depression is growth hormone (GH), which is secreted by the anterior pituitary and follows a circadian pattern with increased secretion during slow wave sleep. To date, the precise role of GH secretion is unknown, but it appears to be a marker of central noradrenergic and serotonergic processes (Birmaher, Dahl, et al., 2000). Adult depressives have been found to hyposecrete GH after various pharmacological challenges, and blunted GH response also has been observed during remission from depressive episodes, suggesting that it may be a stable marker or "scar" of depression (Dinan, 1998). Interestingly, studies of responses to GH challenges have indicated that depressed children, but not depressed adolescents, show similar patterns as adults (for a review, see Kaufman et al., 2001). It is possible that differences have not been detected due to the small samples of adolescents studied. Similarly, studies of serotonergic neurotransmitter processes—although strongly implicated in adult depression—have yielded mixed data in child and adolescent samples. Few studies of serotonergic probes have been conducted on adolescent depressed samples, although in contrast to past studies of traditional tricyclic antidepressant medications that showed poor results, more recent studies of medications that target serotonergic systems have suggested positive effects (e.g., Emslie et al., 1997).

Sleep–Wake Cycle

Studies of dysfunction in sleep behaviors and electroencephalographic (EEG) patterns have been well established in depressed adults. Sleep disturbances may result from dysregulation of serotonergic and other neurotransmitter systems and also are affected by glucocorticoid activity of the HPA (Thase et al., 2002). Reviews of sleep studies in depressed children and adolescents have suggested that adolescents display more similar patterns to adults than do children (Birmaher, Ryan, Williamson, Brent, Kaufman, Dahl, et al., 1996; Kaufman et al., 2001). Reduced rapid eye movement (REM) latency is an especially consistent finding in adolescents, and increased REM density also is observed. However, younger depressives have more normal sleep profiles than do older depressives, suggesting important developmental differences in the nature and function of sleep occurring across the life cycle.

Structural and Functional Brain Findings

Studies of the anatomy and neural circuitry of the brains of adult depressed patients have been the focus of considerable research using various neuroimaging techniques. A well-established finding is reduced blood flow and metabolism in the frontal/prefrontal cortex of depressed adults, with some studies also indicating reductions in amygdala volume. Hippocampal abnormalities also have been reported, with a suggestive link to hypercortisolemia (for a review, see Davidson, Pizzagalli, & Nitschke, 2002). However, the direction of causality between such abnormalities and depression is unclear. Moreover, limited research has been conducted with adolescent samples. Kaufman and colleagues (2001) note that neuroimaging studies of youth could help to detail developmental differences in both nondepressed and depressed samples.

Moreover, Davidson and colleagues (2002) have suggested that the neural circuitry underlying representation and regulation of emotion (such as prefrontal cortex, amygdala, and hippocampus) may be especially important in understanding depression—although the model has not been applied specifically to adolescent depression. Electrophysiological research has resulted in a promising model of emotional reactivity in adults that implicates atypical frontal brain activity as a vulnerability factor for negative emotional states such as depression (e.g., Davidson, 2000). Davidson and colleagues observed that depressed patients, and even previously depressed but remitted patients, showed relative left frontal hypoactivation. Davidson proposed that decreased left prefrontal activation represents an underactivation of the approach system, associated with reductions in the experience of pleasure and positive engagement with the environment. Investigators have speculated that these patterns may be genetically transmitted—or acquired prenatally or in early stressful interactions with a depressed mother—and may represent a mechanism of risk for the development of depression.

Commentary

Rapid developments in genetic and neurobiological research methods have yielded considerable new understanding of the brain and possible mechanisms of depression in recent years. Studies specifically of adolescent depressed samples have been relatively sparse, and findings have been somewhat unclear due to developmental changes in neuroendocrine and brain functioning during adolescence and puberty. Nevertheless, three conclusions seem possible. First, childhood and adolescent depressive disorders may not necessarily result from the same etiological processes. Second, genetic factors appear to be important in adolescent depression but do not account for as much explained variance as do personal environmental factors. The elaboration of genetic mechanisms is eagerly awaited and will certainly supply greater refinement in the search for both biological and psychosocial predictors of depression. Third, investigations of stress processes present a potentially fruitful but challenging arena for integrating various genetic, biological, psychological, and contextual factors that influence the development of depression in adolescence. Truly integrative research based on advances in research methods and growing insight into brain functioning likely will promote fuller understanding, as well as treatment and prevention, of youth depression in the foreseeable future.

Biological Transitions in Adolescence

The transition to adolescence presents biological challenges that may increase vulnerability to depression during this stage. Specifically, hormonal and physical changes associated with puberty have been investigated as potential risk factors for depression, particularly in girls. The role of pubertal maturation in explaining increases in depression in adolescent girls is supported by research demonstrating that pubertal status is a better predictor of sex differences in depression than is chronological age (Angold, Costello, & Worthman, 1998; Hayward et al., 1999). However, the extent to which differences in puberty-related hormones account for sex differences in adolescent depression remains unclear. Although some research suggests that higher levels of female pubertal hormones are linked to negative affect in girls (Angold, Costello, Erkanli, & Worthman, 1999; Susman, Dorn, & Chrousos, 1991), these effects are not consistent (e.g., Susman et al., 1987; for a review, see Nolen-Hoeksema, 2002). Other aspects of puberty must therefore be considered as potential vulnerability factors for depression. In particular, pubertal development is associated not only with biological transitions but also with a package of physical, psychological, and interpersonal changes that may enhance susceptibility to depression in adolescent girls (Petersen et al., 1993; Susman et al., 1985). The integral role of psychological and social influences in determining the impact of puberty is most clearly reflected in evidence that the *timing* of puberty, rather than status *per se*, is the best predictor of affective and behavioral outcomes, with early maturation placing adolescent girls at particular risk (Graber, Lewinsohn, Seeley, & Brooks-Gunn, 1997; Susman et al., 1985). Moreover, dissatisfaction with body image and physical appearance in adolescent girls, which often is linked to pubertal changes and may be exacerbated in early-maturing girls, seems to partly account for sex differences in adolescent depression (for a review, see Hankin & Abramson, 2001). Thus, developmentally sensitive models of adolescent depression must take into account both the biological and psychosocial influences of puberty.

Pubertal changes also may interact with other biological systems involved in depression, resulting in differences across development in the biological correlates of depression. Interestingly, cortisol response to social separation in male monkeys is blunted relative to females during puberty (Suomi, 1991), suggesting that HPA activation may be heightened in females relative to males during this developmental stage. Further investigation is necessary to determine whether sex differences in neuroendocrine functioning, specifically HPA dysregulation, or in other biological markers of depression (e.g., sleep abnormalities and left prefrontal hypoactivation), may contribute to girls' increased vulnerability to depression during adolescence.

Cognitive Models

Cognitive theories propose that negative belief systems and maladaptive thought processes confer a vulnerability to depression. The majority of cognitive theories are framed in terms of a diathesis–stress perspective, wherein maladaptive cognitive appraisals about the self and the world heighten susceptibility to depression when individuals are faced with stressful life experiences. Several variants of these models are discussed, along with relevant empirical evidence in adolescents (for a comprehensive review of cognitive theories of youth depression, see Kaslow et al., 2000). Importantly, although many aspects of these theories are relevant to adolescents, cognitive-developmental changes (e.g., changes in the basis for self-evaluation and advances in abstract thinking) likely influence the strength and nature of cognitive vulnerability during this time, as is discussed later.

Information-Processing/Cognitive Schemas

According to Beck's (1967) information-processing model, depression occurs as a result of systematic biases in thinking and negative interpretations of events. These maladaptive thought patterns are believed to result from the operation of negative cognitive schemas, or internal structures that guide information processing in the form of attention, interpretation, and memory. Consistent with this theory, depression in adolescents has been linked to self-critical beliefs and negative thoughts about the world, including diminished self-worth, irrational beliefs, dysfunctional attitudes, and negative automatic thoughts (Garber, Weiss, & Shanley, 1993; Gotlib, Lewinsohn, Seeley, Rohde, & Redner, 1993; Hops, Lewinsohn, Andrews, & Roberts, 1990; for reviews, see Garber & Hilsman, 1992; Kaslow et al., 2000; Weisz, Rudolph, Granger, & Sweeney, 1992). Direct investigations of information processing using laboratory paradigms have yielded mixed

evidence for depressive biases (for a review, see Garber & Kaminski, 2000). Studies of attentional processes usually have not revealed a significant bias toward negative information in depressed youth. In contrast, studies of memory biases (in mixed samples of children and adolescents) have revealed idiosyncratic processing of self-referent adjectives. Consistent with an information-processing perspective, depressed youth (mixed preadolescents and adolescents) also tend to seek out negative feedback that verifies their negative self-views more than nondepressed youth (Joiner, Katz, & Lew, 1997).

Attributional Style/Control-Related Beliefs

A second set of cognitive theories focuses on the role of maladaptive inferences about the causes, consequences, and self-implications of negative events and one's ability to control such events. The helplessness/hopelessness model (Abramson, Metalsky, & Alloy, 1989; Abramson, Seligman, & Teasdale, 1978) proposes that depression results from a depressive inferential style, which involves a tendency to make internal, global, and stable attributions for negative experiences, to assume that negative consequences will occur as a result of stressful events, and to interpret negative events in ways that compromise one's self-worth. For instance, depressed adolescents may believe that being turned down for a date means that they are socially incompetent and undesirable, they will never find a romantic partner, and they are unworthy of love from others. In a similar vein, self-regulation perspectives on depression (Cole, Martin, & Powers, 1997; Harter & Whitesell, 1996; Rehm, 1977; Weisz, Southam-Gerow, & McCarty, 2001) suggest that depression results from negative expectations about outcomes (e.g., low perceptions of control and competence) and high personal investment in successful outcomes. For example, depressed adolescents may believe that any efforts to achieve their goals will be futile and may possess a strong investment in meeting unrealistic and perfectionistic standards. In general, research has supported these theories. Specifically, adolescent depression has been linked to negative attributional style, hopelessness, and maladaptive control-related beliefs and self-regulatory processes (e.g., negative self-evaluation, high standard-setting, and perfectionism; Abela, 2001; Hankin, Roberts, &

Gotlib, 1997; Weisz et al., 2001; for reviews, see Garber & Hilsman, 1992; Kaslow et al., 2000).

Cognitive–Interpersonal Models

In recent years, cognitive theories of depression have been extended beyond a focus on self-representation to consider the role of cognitive representations in the context of relationships (Cummings & Cicchetti, 1990; Hammen, 1992; Rudolph, Hammen, & Burge, 1997). Research examining these elaborated cognitive-interpersonal theories has supported links between depressive symptoms in adolescents and negative interpersonal perceptions, biased processing of interpersonal information, and maladaptive beliefs about relationships (e.g., Hammen et al., 1995; Rudolph & Clark, 2001). This preliminary evidence suggests the importance of considering the intersection between cognitive and interpersonal theories of depression.

Commentary

Although research consistently supports a link between various types of dysfunctional thought patterns and adolescent depression, many of the early studies failed to test certain essential components of these theories. Whereas cognitive theories emphasize that maladaptive cognitive processes confer a vulnerability to future depression, particularly when activated by a negative mood state or stressful circumstances, investigators often have failed to use prospective designs and have overlooked the contextual element of these theories. In support of these two assumptions of cognitive theories, more recent investigations have demonstrated that dysfunctional cognitions predict future depression in adolescents (Hankin, Abramson, & Siler, 2001; Lewinsohn, Allen, Seeley, & Gotlib, 1999; Rudolph, Kurlakowsky, & Conley, 2001; Rudolph, Lambert, Clark, & Kurlakowsky, 2001), and have supported diathesis–stress models (see "Socioenvironmental Models" section), although these findings have been inconsistent across studies (for reviews, see Garber & Horowitz, 2002; Hammen & Rudolph, 2003; Kaslow et al., 2002). The priming of depressive cognitions with negative mood has not been examined in depressed adolescents. Thus, additional research is needed to confirm the premise that depressogenic cognitive styles are triggered by negative mood and stressful life experiences.

Cognitive Transitions in Adolescence

Although investigations of adolescent depression generally support the application of cognitive theories developed for adults to this age group, it is important to consider possible differences in cognitive vulnerability across development. These differences may account in part for the rise in depression during adolescence, particularly in girls. Specifically, several cognitive-developmental changes occur during late childhood and the transition to adolescence that may influence both the type of cognitive vulnerability expressed during this stage, as well as the strength of the link between cognitive vulnerability and depression. For example, in contrast to earlier childhood, adolescents form judgments about the self in comparison to others rather than in relation to absolute standards, construct self-concepts that are focused on abstract and stable attributes and competencies rather than superficial and unstable behaviors, and have a greater sense of personal responsibility for events (Cicchetti, Rogosch, & Toth, 1994; Garber, 1984; Kaslow et al., 2000). These changes in self-evaluative processes can in turn foster heightened self-focus, concerns about negative social judgments, self-consciousness, self-critical thinking, and excessive guilt (Garber, 1984; Zahn-Waxler, Kochanska, Krupnick, & McKnew, 1990). Views of the self and the world also may be more consolidated in adolescents than preadolescents, leading to more rigid schemas that are less flexible to feedback. Thus, adolescents may become more susceptible to depression linked to negative self-evaluation and negative beliefs about the world. Moreover, advances in cognitive abilities during adolescence foster an increased capacity for generalization across situations and time. Consequently, negative affect associated with maladaptive social-cognitive processes may become pervasive and chronic, leaving adolescents at risk for more severe and recurrent depressive episodes. In general, girls are more susceptible to such negative self-evaluative processes and ruminative concerns than boys, and these sex differences may intensify during adolescence (Broderick, 1998; Ruble, Greulich, Pomerantz, & Gochberg, 1993), perhaps explaining why rates of depression increase more dramatically in girls during the transition to adolescence.

The proposal that changes in social-cognitive processes during adolescence may create differential vulnerability to depression across development is supported by evidence of age differences in the cognition–depression association. Several studies have revealed that the link between particular cognitive diatheses and depression becomes stronger across age, with certain associations not emerging until adolescence (Abela, 2001; Turner & Cole, 1994; Weisz et al., 2001). These findings are consistent with the idea that cognitive styles stabilize during the adolescent years and therefore become more potent contributors to depression than in early and middle childhood.

Specific domains of cognitive vulnerability to depression also may emerge during adolescence. For example, adolescent girls are particularly likely to demonstrate cognitive vulnerability in the form of negative beliefs about their physical appearance and body image, and these concerns may account in part for sex differences in adolescent depression (Wichstrom, 1999).

Developmentally grounded cognitive theories of depression also benefit from a consideration of the origins of cognitive vulnerability. Although cognitive styles may be quite resistant to change by adulthood, they are still under construction during earlier developmental stages. It is therefore important to determine how and when these styles become fully formed. Recent theory and research have begun to consider the processes through which cognitive vulnerability emerges over time. These models suggest that negative views of the self and the world are influenced by social learning, parent socialization practices, exposure to stress, and negative environmental feedback. Several studies have provided preliminary support for these models (Alloy et al., 2001; Garber & Flynn, 2001; Rudolph, Kurlakowsky, & Conley, 2001; for a review, see Garber & Martin, 2002). Moreover, research in younger children indicates that depressive symptoms may themselves undermine subsequent beliefs, leaving a cognitive "scar" (Cole, Martin, Peeke, Seroczynski, & Hoffman, 1998; Nolen-Hoeksema, Girgus, & Seligman, 1992; Pomerantz & Rudolph, 2003). These findings highlight the ongoing transactions between vulnerability and depression over time. Indeed, research in adolescents supports a reciprocal process in which an increase in negative cognitive styles predicts growth in depressive symptoms over time, and growth in depressive symptoms predicts an increase in negative cognitive styles over time (Garber, Keiley, & Martin, 2002). It remains unclear, however, at what point in development children's beliefs become more resistant to change or which influences remain active in shaping depressive cognitions over the course of adolescence.

Behavioral/Interpersonal Models

Original behavioral theories conceptualized depression as a consequence of skill deficits and a consequent inability to elicit positive feedback and reinforcement from the environment (Lewinsohn, 1974). Although traditional behavioral models of depression have received little empirical attention, they have formed the basis for more elaborate theories that consider how the reciprocal transactions between individuals and their environments play a role in depression. For example, Cole's competence-based model of depression (Cole, Martin, Powers, & Truglio, 1996; Cole et al., 1997) proposes that negative competence-related feedback from significant others (e.g., parents, peers, and teachers) is internalized by children in the form of negative self-perceptions, which act as a vulnerability for future depression. Focusing more specifically on social interactions, interpersonal theories of depression propose that depressed individuals both *react* and *contribute* to interpersonal disruption (Gotlib & Hammen, 1992; Joiner, Coyne, & Blalock, 1999). That is, depressive symptoms and associated behaviors are presumed to elicit negative reactions from others; these aversive interpersonal experiences then foster the persistence or exacerbation of depression. The many changes and disruptions that occur within relationships during adolescence, coupled with the strong emphasis placed on developing social networks outside the family at this time, likely create a context in which interpersonal influences on depression are particularly salient.

Interpersonal Relationships

Consistent with interpersonal models, depressed adolescents demonstrate significant difficulties in many aspects of their close friendships and more general peer relationships (for reviews, see Gotlib & Hammen, 1992; Weisz et al., 1992). For instance, depressed adolescents report decreased support and negative relationship qualities (e.g., higher levels of conflict and hostility) in their close friendships (Hops et al., 1990; Lewinsohn, Roberts, et al., 1994; Puig-Antich et al., 1993; Windle, 1994) and less secure attachment to their peers (Armsden, McCauley, Greenberg, Burke, & Mitchell, 1990). Information from others confirms that the negative self-perceptions of depressed youth are, at least in part, accurate appraisals of difficulties in their relationships. For example, depression in early adolescents has been linked to teacher-reported deficits in interpersonal behavior, such as decreased prosocial engagement and heightened aggression (Rudolph & Clark, 2001). During late adolescence, both depressed women and their romantic partners perceive these women as less interpersonally competent; these perceptions are consistent with interviewer ratings of increased chronic stress in friendships and romantic relationships (Daley & Hammen, 2002). Although little evidence is available from direct observations, one study demonstrated that depressed adolescents elicit negative reactions from peers during dyadic transactions (Connolly, Geller, Marton, & Kutcher, 1992). This negative impact of depressed adolescents on their peers also is reflected in lower levels of peer popularity and higher levels of social rejection and isolation (Connolly et al., 1992; Rudolph & Clark, 2001).

Specific Behavioral Deficits

Interpersonal difficulties in depressed individuals are likely fueled by deficits in behavioral and emotional processes related to problem solving, coping, and emotion regulation in social contexts. Such deficits may lead adolescents to engage in behaviors that interfere with the formation or maintenance of positive social relationships. Depressed youngsters may experience particular difficulty regulating their emotions and behavior in arousing situations (Zahn-Waxler, Klimes-Dougan, & Slattery, 2000). For example, when depressed adolescents experience conflict with their peers, they may become emotionally overaroused and thus attempt to avoid future social encounters, creating feelings of isolation, as well as active rejection by others.

Indeed, depressed adolescents have been found to engage in less active, assertive, and problem-focused coping, and more passive, avoidant, ruminative, and helpless responses to challenges, including interpersonal problems and conflict (Herman-Stahl & Petersen, 1999; Kobak & Ferenz-Gillies, 1995; Rudolph, Kurlakowsky, & Conley, 2001). Applying a multidimensional model of responses to stress that distinguishes between voluntary versus involuntary responses, and engagement versus disengagement responses, Compas and colleagues (Compas, Connor-Smith, Saltzman, Thomsen, & Wadsworth, 2001) have linked internalizing symptoms, including depression, in adolescents to lower levels of engagement coping (e.g., problem solving and positive thinking) and higher levels of disengagement coping (e.g., avoidance and denial) and involuntary responses to stress (e.g., rumination, emotional arousal, and inaction). These findings are consistent with Nolen-Hoeksema's (2002) response styles theory of depression, which suggests that a passive, ruminative style involving excessive focus on depressive symptoms and their potential causes and consequences heightens risk for depression.

Depressed adolescents also seem to demonstrate a ruminative style in their interpersonal interactions. For example, depressed adolescents have been found to engage in excessive reassurance seeking in an effort to elicit confirmation of acceptance and self-worth from others (for a review, see Joiner, Metalsky, Katz, & Beach, 1999). Interestingly, the friends of depressed adolescents report that they provide more emotional support in their friendships than do the friends of nondepressed adolescents, perhaps suggesting that they make efforts to provide reassurance to these individuals (Daley & Hammen, 2002). These types of maladaptive behaviors displayed by depressed youth are likely to explain in part the interpersonal disruption that characterizes their peer relationships and friendships.

Commentary

Despite ample evidence indicating problematic peer relationships and friendships in depressed adolescents, much of the research to date has involved cross-sectional designs that fail to examine the transactional component of interpersonal models—that is, the hypothesized reciprocal association between interpersonal impairment and depression (Gotlib & Hammen, 1992; Joiner et al., 1999; Rudolph & Hammen, 1999). However, some longitudinal research confirms that interpersonal difficulties represent both an antecedent and a consequence of depression. On the one hand, decreased closeness with friends, lower levels of social competence, and increased rejection by the peer group predict increases in adolescent depressive symptoms over time (Cole et al., 1996; Vernberg, 1990). Moreover, many of the interpersonal difficulties displayed by depressed adolescents remain even after symptom remission (Lewinsohn, Roberts, et al., 1994). On the other hand, depression has been found to disrupt social relationships. For instance, depressive symptoms in adolescents predict subsequent increases in peer rejection (Little & Garber, 1995), and depressed adolescents tend to evoke negative responses from unfamiliar peers (Connolly et al. 1992). Together, these findings illustrate the importance of interpersonal models that emphasize the ongoing transactions between depressed adolescents and their interpersonal environments over time.

Interpersonal Transitions in Adolescence

Developmental transitions in interpersonal relationships are important to consider when evaluating the applicability of interpersonal models developed in adults to adolescent depression. During adolescence, many changes occur in the peer system that may heighten risk for depression. The peer group becomes an increasingly important socialization context at this time, as adolescents spend more time with peers and rely more on peers for emotional support (Furman & Buhrmester, 1992; Laursen, 1996). Moreover, interpersonal roles and relationships often change significantly, resulting in alienation from familiar peer networks and the formation of new relationships and friendships (Rudolph, 2002; Simmons, Burgeson, Carlton-Ford, & Blyth, 1987). At the same time, adolescents, particularly girls, begin to place a greater emphasis on intimacy, loyalty, and closeness in their friendships (Furman & Buhrmester, 1992; Laursen, 1996). This tension between the desire for intimacy with peers and the insecurity created by significant changes in peer relationships during adolescence may create an interpersonal backdrop that increases risk for depression onset or exacerbation.

Because of the value placed by adolescent girls on maintaining close relationships, they may show a particularly strong interpersonal vulnerability to depression (Gore, Aseltine, & Colton, 1993; Rudolph, 2002). In addition, adolescent girls experience more disruption in their peer relationships than do adolescent boys (Rudolph & Hammen, 1999; Wagner & Compas, 1990), and they may cope in less adaptive ways with these problems (Broderick, 1998). Thus, a heightened risk for depression in adolescent girls may result both from the experience of higher levels of interpersonal disruption and from stronger links between interpersonal difficulties and depression. Indeed, research demonstrates that sex differences in exposure and reactions to interpersonal problems partly account for higher rates of depressive symptoms in adolescent girls than boys (Gore et al., 1993; Rudolph, 2002).

Adolescents also begin to develop more extensive platonic heterosexual relationships and engage in more frequent dating and romantic relationships than do preadolescents. Such experiences may present additional interpersonal challenges, as adolescents learn how to negotiate a new set of roles, relationships, and interaction styles (Leaper & Anderson, 1997). Moreover, the frequent instability of early romantic relationships may set the stage for depression. Indeed, one study demonstrated that adolescent girls (especially those in advanced stages of puberty) who were romantically involved with boys experienced particularly high levels of depressive symptoms (Hayward & Sanborn, 2002). Moreover, breakups of romantic relationships predict the onset of MDEs during late adolescence (Monroe, Rohde, Seeley, & Lewinsohn, 1999). Participation in both platonic and romantic heterosexual relationships may be more difficult for girls than for boys because girls are less able to exert an influence in these relationships (Maccoby, 1990). Negotiating the transition to heterosexual relationships may be particularly stressful for early-maturing girls who often begin dating earlier than their peers, before they are fully prepared to cope with these changes (Susman et al., 1985). Overall, therefore, interpersonal models can contribute significantly toward understanding why girls may be especially vulnerable to increases in depression during adolescence.

Family Models

Several theories of depression emphasize family influences on the development of psychopathology. These theories hold that the family not only contributes a genetic predisposition to depression, as discussed earlier, but also may transmit a psychosocial vulnerability. Disturbances in the family that disrupt early social bonds and create unhealthy learning environments may interfere with the mastery of a variety of developmental tasks (e.g., development of secure attachment relationships, emergence of a healthy sense of self, and acquisition of adaptive coping and emotion-regulation skills); difficulties in these areas may in turn confer a heightened risk for depression. Understanding the family context of risk for depression during adolescence therefore requires a consideration of which developmental tasks are most likely to be disrupted by an adverse family environment at this stage. Moreover, normative changes in family relationships during adolescence also may create heightened risk during this time.

Psychodynamic Theories

Early conceptualizations of depression, as reflected in psychoanalytic and object relations theories, focused on disruptions in caregiving relationships as a primary vulnerability factor for depression. Depression was believed to result from either physical loss of a caregiver due to death or separation or symbolic loss due to emotional deprivation, rejection, or inadequate parenting (Fairbairn, 1952; Freud, 1917/1951). These theories posited that depression resulted from anger or hostility that initially was felt toward the lost object but then was directed inward in the form of guilt and self-criticism. Because children were believed to lack the level of superego development necessary to produce guilt, these theories presumed that early loss was not reflected in depression until adulthood.

Attachment Theory

In contrast to early psychodynamic theories, attachment theory holds that disruption of caregiver–child attachment bonds creates a risk for psychopathology throughout childhood and adulthood (Bowlby, 1969). In particular, depression and other forms of psychopatholo-gy are believed to result from conditions that undermine the development of a secure attachment relationship (e.g., a lack of caregiver accessibility, contingent responsivity, and emotional supportiveness). When these conditions are compromised, the child presumably fails to develop a sense of security and trust that lays the foundation for healthy adjustment. Although attachment theory originally was applied primarily to understanding adjustment problems during early childhood, elaborations of this theory provide a basis for understanding the etiology of depression during adolescence. Specifically, early attachment experiences are believed to be represented in the form of "internal working models," which encompass beliefs about the self and relationships that may be carried throughout development (Bowlby, 1969; Main, Kaplan, & Cassidy, 1985). These internalized processes may emerge as risk factors for depression in later years, particularly when triggered by adverse experiences in relationships (Cummings & Cicchetti, 1990; Hammen, 1992; Rudolph et al., 1997).

Two approaches have been employed to investigate the links between family influences and depression. The first approach involves studies of the families of depressed youth; the second approach involves studies of depressed parents and their offspring (high-risk studies), who themselves often are at risk for depression. These investigations have yielded substantial support for family models of depression (for reviews, see Goodman & Gotlib, 1999; Gotlib & Hammen, 1992).

Parent–Child Relationships and Family Context

Parents of Depressed Adolescents. Research examining family influences on adolescent depression has revealed significant difficulties in both specific aspects of parent–child relationships and interactions and in the broader family environment, including significant family, marital, and sibling discord and stress, decreased family support, and abuse and neglect (for reviews, see Goodman & Gotlib, 1999; Gotlib & Hammen, 1992). Using self-report questionnaires, a large database suggests that adolescent depression is associated with perceived parent–child relationship disturbances and a compromised family environment. For example, adolescent depression has been linked to decreased intimacy and satisfaction in parent–child relationships (Herman-Stahl & Petersen, 1999), lower levels of parental acceptance and higher levels of parental psychological control (Garber, Robinson, & Valentiner, 1997), insecure parent–child attachment (Armsden et al., 1990; Pavlidis & McCauley, 2001), and perceptions of the family as less cohesive and adaptable, less open to emotional expressiveness, more hostile and rejecting, more conflictual and disorganized, and less likely to engage in pleasant activities (e.g., Hops et al., 1990; Sheeber & Sorenson, 1998).

Interviews with depressed adolescents and their parents similarly suggest that parent–child relationships are characterized by poorer communication, decreased warmth, and increased hostility compared to those of nondepressed groups (Puig-Antich et al., 1993). Studies also reveal that parental descriptions of their depressed offspring are marked by higher levels of criticism and emotional overinvolvement than are those of nondepressed offspring (Asarnow, Tompson, Hamilton, Goldstein, & Guthrie, 1994).

Although less information is available from direct observations of parent–adolescent interactions, findings from these studies generally are consistent with self-report and interview data. Specifically, mothers of depressed adolescents have been found to show more dominance (Kobak, Sudler, & Gamble, 1991) and less support, validation, and positive behavior (e.g., smiling and approving) toward their offspring (Sheeber & Sorenson, 1998). Depressed youth also demonstrate less effective interactional styles with their parents than do nondepressed youth, as reflected in poorer communication and problem solving, decreased support, and fewer displays of assertiveness (Kobak & Ferenz-Gillies, 1995; Sheeber & Sorenson, 1998). Observations of depressed adolescents and their parents have not, however, provided substantial support for the presence of overt conflict (Sheeber & Sorenson, 1998).

Offspring/High-Risk Studies. High-risk studies indicate high rates of depression in the offspring of depressed parents. Because many of the high-risk investigations involve offspring from a large age range, we include in our discussion studies of mixed samples of preadolescents and adolescents but focus wherever possible on studies of adolescent offspring.

Although genetic factors likely play a role in the transmission of depression, studies of depressed mothers and their offspring have revealed a variety of difficulties in parenting and parent–child interactions that may contribute to youth depression (for reviews, see Cummings & Davies, 1999; Goodman & Gotlib, 1999; Hammen, 1991). A meta-analytic summary of these studies (Lovejoy, Graczyk, O'Hare, & Neuman, 2000) revealed that depressed mothers (particularly those with current depression) display more negative behavior (e.g., negative affect and criticism) and disengagement (e.g., ignoring, withdrawal, and silence), and less positive behavior (e.g., pleasant affect, praise, and affectionate contact) than do nondepressed mothers. Offspring of depressed mothers in turn demonstrate more passive and disengaged behavior and negativity during interactions with their mothers (Hammen, 1991).

A few recent studies have examined family influences in adolescent samples of high-risk families. Consistent with earlier studies of younger and mixed-aged groups of children, these investigations have revealed a variety of dysfunctional family characteristics and interactions that may place adolescents at risk for future depression. Several of these studies also have identified mediational pathways linking maternal psychopathology and family disruption with symptoms in adolescent offspring. For instance, Fergusson, Horwood, and Lynskey (1995) found that adverse family factors mediated the impact of maternal depressive symptoms on adolescent girls' depression. Similarly, Garber and Little (2001) found that family dysfunction predicted adolescent symptoms in the offspring of depressed mothers; moreover, this effect was mediated by youth perceptions of emotional autonomy. Elaborating further on such pathways, Hammen, Shih, and Brennan (2004) demonstrated that the impact of maternal depression on youth depression was mediated by family discord and perceptions of negative parenting; these family influences had a direct influence on the youth's own stressors and social competence, which in turn were the proximal predictors of depression.

Microanalytic behavioral observation techniques also have been used to examine the impact of specific parental depressive behaviors on their adolescent offspring. This research has revealed that distinct patterns of responses to interparental depressive behaviors (behaviors expressed by one parent toward another parent) predict increases in depression in adolescent girls and boys. Specifically, adolescent girls who displayed facilitative and depressive behavior and who suppressed aggressive behavior in response to interparental depressive behavior showed increases in their own depressive symptoms over time; risk for subsequent depression in adolescent boys, in contrast, was associated with aggressive and depressive responses to interparental depressive behavior (Davis, Sheeber, Hops, & Tildesley, 2000). These findings complement those of high-risk studies to support the role of family interactions in the intergenerational transmission of depression.

Commentary

Research from a variety of perspectives and using multiple methodologies has established a clear link between family dysfunction and adolescent depression. Although additional research is needed to elaborate on the nature of this link, some preliminary data support a transactional model whereby family disruption contributes to adolescent depression, which further exacerbates family difficulties. On the one hand, family disturbances may contribute to the onset, persistence, or recurrence of depression. Indeed, some research reveals that family disturbances predict higher levels of adolescent depression over time (Herman-Stahl & Petersen, 1999; Hops et al., 1990). On the other hand, depressive symptoms in adolescents may interfere with the formation of healthy family relationships. Consistent with a transactional framework, Hammen and colleagues found that depressed mothers and their offspring exerted mutual negative influences on each other (Hammen, Burge, & Stansbury, 1990). Future research therefore would benefit from attention to the reciprocal interactions between depressed adolescents and their families.

Recent elaborations of family models of depression also have begun to consider the *processes* through which parental depression, maladaptive parenting, and family stress contribute to risk for depression (for reviews, see Garber & Martin, 2002; Goodman & Gotlib, 2002). Disturbances in the family may interfere with the acquisition of a variety of competencies essential for healthy develop-

ment. Psychological unavailability or rejection by parents may be translated into insecure attachment. These problematic relationship experiences may then be internalized in the form of negative beliefs and expectancies about the self and relationships and impaired social skills. Family dysfunction also may foster maladaptive patterns of coping and emotion regulation, either through modeling of parents or through explicit parental socialization practices, and may induce a sense of helplessness.

Preliminary research has implicated several pathways through which parental depression and family dysfunction may confer vulnerability to depression. For example, depression in parents, family disruption, and dysfunctional styles of parent–child interaction have been linked to insecure attachment, depressogenic cognitions (e.g., low self-worth, negative attributional styles, hopelessness, and decreased perceptions of control), biased information processing, and maladaptive social skills and problem-solving deficits (e.g., Garber & Flynn, 2001; Goodman, Brogan, Lynch, & Fielding, 1993; Hammen & Brennan, 2001; Rudolph, Kurlakowsky, et al., 2001; Taylor & Ingram, 1999; Teti, Gelfand, Messinger, & Isabella, 1995). Early mother–child interactions associated with maternal depression also may alter the development of neural circuits that guide emotion expression and regulation (e.g., Dawson, Frey, Panagiotides, Osterling, & Hessl, 1997; Goodman & Gotlib, 1999). Although this research provides a promising starting point for understanding family processes associated with depression vulnerability, much of this work has been conducted in younger children. Far less is known about whether these processes generalize to adolescent depression.

Family Transitions in Adolescence

Adolescence is marked by many changes in family relationships that may contribute to an increased risk for depression during this period. For example, this transition period often is characterized by heightened conflict with parents (for a review, see Laursen, 1996). Adolescent girls may experience particularly high levels of parent–child conflict due to a discrepancy between their perceptions of emotional autonomy from parents (Steinberg & Silverberg, 1986) and parental tendencies to grant less autonomy to girls than boys

(Pomerantz & Ruble, 1998). A developmental mismatch (Eccles & Midgley, 1989) may occur between adolescents' needs and desires for more autonomy and parents' attempts to protect their offspring from negative experiences often associated with adolescence, such as drops in school performance or detrimental peer influences. This mismatch and the ensuing conflict may increase risk for depression.

In addition to these normative changes at adolescence, developmentally sensitive models of depression must consider the stage-specific consequences of non-normative family disruption, such as parental depression or problematic parenting. Family dysfunction may confer risk for depression through different pathways across development, depending on the particular developmental tasks associated with various stages. Critical developmental tasks during adolescence include establishing autonomy from the family while maintaining relatedness (Allen, Hauser, Bell, & O'Connor, 1994), establishing a sense of personal identity (Arnett, 2000), and establishing a network of social relationships outside the family (Laursen, 1996). Consequently, significant disruptions in family processes during this time may lead to problems associated with a failure to successfully complete these tasks. Of course, many forms of family dysfunction are likely to start early in life and continue through adolescence. Deficits during adolescence may therefore reflect the cumulative effects of disruption over many different stages of development, resulting in compromised functioning across a variety of domains.

Socioenvironmental Models

Integral to many models of depression is the impact of environmental influences on depression onset, exacerbation, and recurrence. A range of environmental stressors has been implicated, including severe stressful life events, chronic stressful circumstances, daily hassles, social disadvantage, and normative environmental transitions. In light of the increases in stress often associated with adolescence, many explanations of adolescent risk for depression incorporate the role of environmental stressors.

Stress-Exposure and Diathesis–Stress Models

Original life-stress theories viewed depression as a reaction to negative life events, particularly "fateful" events that are beyond an individual's control, such as the death of a close family member or an illness (Brown & Harris, 1978). Both concurrent and prospective studies link negative life events, as well as chronic stressful circumstances and daily hassles, to depression in adolescents (e.g., Compas, Howell, Phares, Williams, & Giunta, 1989; Ge et al., 1994; Goodyer et al., 2000b; Hops et al., 1990). Adolescent depression also is associated with broader stressful conditions, such as socioeconomic disadvantage, family structure (e.g., living in a single-parent household), parental unemployment, and low levels of parental education (Gore et al., 1992; for a review, see Kaslow, Deering, & Racusin, 1994).

Advancing beyond theories that predict links between cumulative life stress and depression, researchers have begun to investigate whether specific types of stress play a particularly prominent role in risk for depression. Because interpersonal relationships influence the formation of self-perceptions, emotion regulation, social competencies, and other processes integral to depression, it has been suggested that exposure to stress within close relationships may be especially likely to foster depression (Cicchetti & Toth, 1998; Hammen, 1992; Rudolph, 2002; see earlier section "Behavior/Interpersonal Models"). Interference with such processes may become particularly relevant during adolescence when demands increase for self-regulation of emotion and independent problem-solving skills. Consistent with this perspective, interpersonal stress and disruption (e.g., interpersonal conflict, loss of significant others, and romantic relationship breakups) have been found to be strongly associated with depression (Goodyer & Altham, 1991; Eley & Stevenson, 2000; Monroe et al., 1999; Rudolph & Hammen, 1999; Rudolph et al., 2000). Because many of these studies linking interpersonal stress and depression have been conducted with mixed preadolescent and adolescent samples, additional research is needed that distinguishes among different domains of stress as precursors of adolescent depression.

Although stress clearly plays a role in adolescent depression, individuals vary in their responses to stress. Diathesis–stress models propose that depression results from the interaction between personal vulnerability and stressful events or circumstances. The majority of research testing diathesis–stress models of adolescent depression has construed vulnerability in terms of maladaptive appraisals of events. Several studies have discovered significant interactions between cognitive styles (e.g., negative attributional style and low perceived self-efficacy) and life stress in the prediction of adolescent depression (e.g., Herman-Stahl & Petersen, 1999; Hilsman & Garber, 1995; Lewinsohn, Joiner, & Rohde, 2001; Robinson, Garber, & Hilsman, 1995). Refining these theories even further, researchers have speculated that a key determinant of depression may be the *match* between a particular cognitive vulnerability (e.g., a tendency to base one's self-worth on success in interpersonal relationships) and the nature of the stressful experience (e.g., an interpersonal conflict). Supporting these theories, diathesis–stress interactions seem to be most powerful when there is a match between the type of cognitive vulnerability and the type of stress experienced (e.g., Turner & Cole, 1994). Interestingly, consistent with the idea discussed earlier that cognitive styles may not yet be consolidated in younger children, cognition–stress interactions have been found to predict depression in adolescents but not in preadolescents (Abela, 2001; Turner & Cole, 1994).

Stress-Generation Models

Although stress-exposure models have been useful for understanding the etiology of depression, developmental models of psychopathology need to consider the transactional relations that emerge between children and their social contexts across development (Cicchetti & Schneider-Rosen, 1984; Rudolph & Hammen, 1999). Consistent with this transactional perspective, Hammen (1992) has proposed a stress-generation model of depression, which focuses on the role that depressed individuals play in the creation of stressful circumstances that contribute to psychopathology. A stress-generation model may be particularly important to understanding depression during childhood and adolescence because a self-perpetuating cycle may develop early in life, whereby depressive symptoms and associated impairment lead to the generation of stressful circumstances that interrupt normative developmental trajectories and increase risk for future psychopathology.

In support of stress-generation models, preliminary empirical investigations have linked depression to self-generated stress, particularly within interpersonal relationships (Rudolph & Hammen, 1999; Rudolph et al., 2000; Williamson, Birmaher, Anderson, Al-Shabbout, & Ryan, 1995). Although these findings confirm that life stress may at times result from characteristics or behaviors of depression-prone individuals, the concurrent nature of the data prevents conclusions about the nature of the stress–depression association. However, two longitudinal studies have confirmed that depressive symptoms in adolescents predict the occurrence of subsequent dependent negative events (Cohen, Burt, & Bjorck, 1987; Daley et al., 1997). Additional prospective research is needed to understand the transactional linkages between stress and depression over the course of development.

Commentary

A great deal of progress has been made in expanding life-stress conceptualizations of depression to account for the many complexities that characterize individuals' interactions with their environments. However, several issues remain to be resolved in the next generation of research on life-stress models.

Although research supports cognition × stress interactions as predictors of depression, additional research is needed to identify other types of personal vulnerability that exacerbate depressive responses to stress. Other likely candidates include genetic and biological predispositions, behavioral styles, coping repertoires and problem-solving skills, and sociodemographic variables. For example, a negative problem-solving orientation has been found to moderate the association between stress and depression in adolescents (Spence, Sheffield, & Donovan, 2002). Moreover, research suggests that a behavioral style characterized by extreme levels of anxious solitude predicts a maintenance or increase in depressive symptoms over time in early adolescents who experience interpersonal stress in the form of exclusion from their peer group (Gazelle & Rudolph, 2004). Sensitivity to stress also may be influenced by external risks and resources, such as the presence of family strain, parental psychopathology, or social support.

Stress-generation models of depression would benefit from an expanded understanding of the processes that drive the generation of stressful events and circumstances. Beyond depressive symptoms themselves, other attributes of adolescents may cause them to create stress in their lives. To date, several attributes have been found to predict stress generation, including demographic variables such as age and sex (Rudolph & Hammen, 1999; Rudolph et al., 2000), personality styles (Daley, Hammen, Davila, & Burge, 1998; Nelson, Hammen, Daley, Burge, & Davila, 2001), negative conceptions of relationships (Caldwell, Rudolph, Troop-Gordon, & Kim, 2004), low social competence (Herzberg et al., 1998), and problematic interpersonal problem-solving styles (Davila, Hammen, Burge, Paley, & Daley, 1995).

Another exciting direction for future research concerns the integration of genetic and life-stress models of depression (for reviews, see Goodyer, 2001; Silberg, Rutter, Neale, & Eaves, 2001; Wallace et al., 2002). Preliminary research has documented the influence of genetic liability on both exposure and reactions to stressful environments (Kendler, 1995; Kendler, Neale, Kessler, Heath, & Eaves, 1993). Moreover, genetic liability to major depression in females has been linked to increased exposure to certain types of life events (Kendler & Karkowki-Shuman, 1997). However, the mechanisms through which genetic liability is translated into exposure to stress and consequent vulnerability to depression have not yet been delineated. One suggestion has been that genetically linked exposure to high-risk environments reflects a self-selection process, whereby individuals with certain genetically transmitted personality traits or behaviors (e.g., impulsivity) seek out risky environments that heighten their exposure to stress (Kendler & Karkowski-Shuman, 1997; Kendler et al., 1993). Another possibility is that genetic factors contribute to personal attributes that promote stress-generating behaviors, such that genetically prone individuals actually create the stressful environments in which they live (Rudolph et al., 2000). Integrating genetic and life-stress models therefore presents several interesting possibilities for more comprehensive models of depression.

Socioenvironmental Transitions in Adolescence

Although stressful events and circumstances create a risk for depression throughout development, the transition into adolescence is likely to be a time of intensified stress and challenge as adolescents are confronted with many new experiences and demands. Adolescents may be especially likely to experience higher levels of dependent stress due to experimentation or peer pressure that leads to stress-inducing behaviors, such as engaging in truancy from school or conflict with authority figures, and to the greater responsibility and control that adolescents exert over certain aspects of their lives, such as friendship selection. Indeed, research has demonstrated higher levels of life events during adolescence than preadolescence (Ge et al., 1994; Rudolph & Hammen, 1999).

Several theoretical models of depression propose that sex differences in stress exposure and stress generation during adolescence, particularly within relationships, contribute to heightened vulnerability to depression in adolescent girls (e.g., Gore et al., 1993; Hankin & Abramson, 2001; Nolen-Hoeksema & Girgus, 1994; Rudolph, 2002). Consistent with these models, environmental risks seem to be particularly prevalent in adolescent girls (Compas & Wagner, 1991; Simmons et al., 1987; Wagner & Compas, 1990), especially in the context of interpersonal relationships (Davies & Windle, 1997; Rudolph & Hammen, 1999). Moreover, some evidence suggests that increased exposure to interpersonal stress contributes to sex differences in depression during adolescence (Rudolph, 2002), and a genetic liability to experiencing high levels of stress may account in part for the increased rates of depression in adolescent girls (Silberg et al., 1999). Adolescent girls' increased exposure to traumatic sexual abuse experiences also may increase their risk for depression and affect their biological and psychological reactivity to other social stressors (Nolen-Hoeksema, 2002).

Adolescent girls also may possess characteristics that make them more vulnerable to depression when faced with stress (Hankin & Abramson, 2001; Nolen-Hoeksema & Girgus, 1994; Rudolph, 2002). Although evidence is mixed, some studies have documented stronger links between stress (Ge et al., 1994; Schraedley, Gotlib, & Hayward, 1999), especially interpersonal stress (Goodyer & Altham, 1991; Rudolph, 2002; Rudolph & Hammen, 1999), and depression in girls than in boys. Researchers have suggested that vulnerability to stress in adolescent girls may be linked to a variety of factors, including hormonal influences (Brooks-Gunn & Warren, 1989), maladaptive coping styles (Nolen-Hoeksema, 2002), and heightened investment in relationships (Gore et al., 1993; Rudolph, 2002), but little research actually has demonstrated direct links between these characteristics and stress reactivity in girls.

In addition to considering the influence of specific stressful events and circumstances during adolescence, socioenvironmental models of adolescent depression need to take into account normative transitions that may create a developmental context of risk during adolescence. Adolescents experience many changes in their daily ecology, which in some cases may contribute to depression. One such challenge that has received a great deal of attention in terms of understanding adolescent adjustment is the experience of school transitions (i.e., entering middle school or high school). Ecological transitions such as a change of schools involve novel experiences, disruptions in familiar roles, and new demands that may overwhelm adolescents (Eccles, Wigfield, & Schiefele, 1998; Rudolph, Lambert, et al., 2001). For example, school transitions are associated with significant shifts in educational climate, academic expectations, and teacher–student relationships, as well as disruptions in peer networks. The stress associated with such changes is reflected in a variety of adjustment difficulties, including decreases in self-esteem, declines in academic performance and motivation, and negative emotions related to school (for a review, see Eccles et al., 1998). Such changes may place adolescents at risk for depression.

Consistent with diathesis–stress models, however, some adolescents may experience greater difficulties negotiating stressful transitions than others. Specifically, individual differences in preexisting vulnerabilities, such as maladaptive social-cognitive processes or compromised coping resources, may be activated by the challenges of adolescence, leading to risk for depression. In support of this perspective, research has demonstrated that personal vulnerability, in the form of maladaptive self-regulatory beliefs (e.g., low perceptions of control), predicted higher levels of subsequent depression in adolescents who experienced a school transition but not those who remained in a stable school environment (Rudolph, Lambert, et al., 2001). More research is needed to determine characteristics of adolescents that increase vulnerability to depression during normative developmental transitions.

AN INTEGRATIVE MODEL OF ADOLESCENT DEPRESSION

Figure 8.1 presents an integrative model of adolescent depression that considers the complex interplay among genetic, biological, cognitive, interpersonal, family, and environmental factors and developmental challenges. This model draws from an earlier model of childhood depression (Hammen & Rudolph, 1996, 2003) but incorporates the special attributes of adolescents and their environments that may enhance risk for depression during this developmental stage.

According to the model, family disruption resulting from parent psychopathology and stressful circumstances interferes with the development of nurturing and supportive parent–child relationships. These adverse experiences in the family are internalized in the form of maladaptive conceptions about the self and interpersonal relationships, such as views of the self as unworthy of love and relationships as unpredictable and unrewarding. Family dysfunction also likely fosters maladaptive emotion- and behavior-regulation styles through modeling or explicit socialization of ineffective strategies, or by creating a general sense of helplessness. Moreover, family risk may be transmitted in the form of a genetic predisposition to disorder, or to temperamental characteristics that increase susceptibility to disorder or even promote the generation of stress. Maladaptive conceptions of relationships, ineffective coping and emotion regulation, and biological vulnerability in turn may cause adolescents to create difficulties in their relationships, resulting in depression, or may augment adolescents' vulnerability to depression in the face of high levels of stress.

Sensitivity to stress may be highest during normative developmental transitions marked by physical maturational changes (e.g., the onset of puberty) or social–contextual changes (e.g., school transitions). Specifically, the disruption, novelty, and uncertainty that mark the adolescent transition period may activate the processes underlying depression and thereby intensify the association between prior vulnerability and depression. Girls are expected to be at particular risk during this time due to personal characteristics that make them more vulnerable to the effects of transitions (e.g., a tendency toward negative self-evaluation, less adaptive responses to

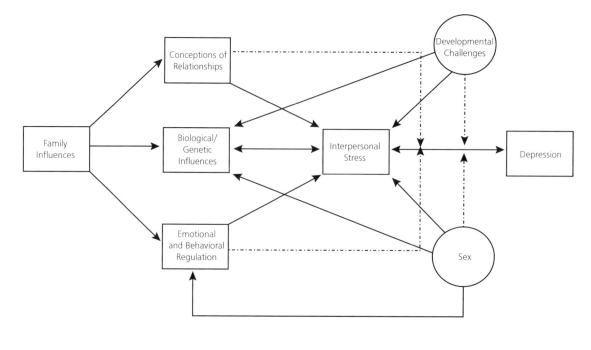

FIGURE 8.1. Theoretical model of adolescent depression. From Hammen and Rudolph (2003). Copyright 2003 by the Guilford Press. Adapted by permission.

stress, and investment in maintaining close relationships), as well as their increased exposure to stress during the adolescent transition. Early pubertal maturation is expected to put girls at particularly high risk as they may be faced with a variety of additional challenges (e.g., heightened parental expectations and concerns and earlier onset of dating and romantic relationships) before they have the psychological resources to cope with these challenges. Thus, the proposed model accounts for why adolescence represents a period of increased vulnerability to depression, particularly in girls.

Depression in adolescence is likely to further compromise development by interfering with the achievement of key developmental tasks (e.g., negotiating changes in family relationships and establishing close friendship networks), resulting in the generation of additional stress, and perhaps even contributing to compromised neurobiological development and sensitization to future stress and depres-

sion. These processes may account in part for why adolescent-onset depression tends to be recurrent throughout the lifespan.

ASSESSMENT OF ADOLESCENT DEPRESSION

The availability and use of reliable and valid assessment tools are critical for both the researcher and the clinician interested in adolescent depression. Without evidence of reliability, validity, and developmental appropriateness of depression measures, the foundation of both research and clinical enterprises is compromised. A comprehensive discussion of every tool to assess adolescent depression is well beyond the scope of this section. Instead, major issues and methods are highlighted (for recent extensive reviews of traditional assessment measures, see Brooks & Kutcher, 2001; Myers & Winters, 2002; for a comprehensive review of performance-based approaches to assessment, see Garber & Kaminski, 2000).

Targets of Assessment

The targets of tools for assessing depression include depressed mood, a depressive syndrome (encompassing a cluster of depressive symptoms and other empirically related emotions and behaviors), or a diagnosis of major depression or dysthymia, typically based on DSM-IV criteria (see Compas, Ey, & Grant, 1993). The choice of a target should be determined by the goal of the researcher or clinician. If the goal is to assess whether or not an adolescent meets formal diagnostic criteria for a depressive disorder, the use of a structured or semistructured interview typically is required. In contrast, if the goal is to evaluate the severity of depressive symptoms, both at clinical and subclinical levels, depression rating scales (self-report, informant report, or clinician rated) may be more useful.

Appropriateness of Current Measures for Adolescents

More than one-third of recently published studies on adolescent depression used measures that were designed for use with adults (Brooks & Kutcher, 2001). As previously described, there are few alterations to the standard diagnostic criteria for depression when evaluating adolescents. Given that the only major changes are the addition of irritability as a substitute for depressed mood or anhedonia, and the 1-year, rather than 2-year, duration criterion for dysthymia, measures designed for adults require only minor modifications to encompass the symptoms defining depressive disorders in adolescents. However, the language of adult measures may be too sophisticated for many adolescents. This is particularly an issue for self-report measures that are completed independently by adolescents, especially for those at a lower reading level (Reynolds, 1994). Furthermore, the context in which adults and adolescents function is different: Items that reflect impairment in work and sexual domains will be less relevant for teenagers than those that address, for instance, school performance. Moreover, more thorough assessment may be needed of symptoms found to typify depression in adolescence, as discussed earlier. Accordingly, researchers and clinicians should con-

sider the wording and range of items in addition to the age and the reading level of their population before opting for a measure originally designed for adults.

Decision-Making Strategies for Assessment of Adolescents

One key general issue in assessing adolescent psychopathology is the selection of informants and the problem of integrating reports from different sources of information. Unlike very young children, adolescents certainly possess the cognitive and linguistic ability to report on their internal feelings and perceptions, and they may be more sensitive than their parents to their own depressive symptoms (e.g., Angold et al., 1987), making self-reports of these internal experiences important targets of assessment. However, adolescents may have limited cognitive ability to reflect on their functioning in the context of their own prior history and what is typical of other teens. Because diagnostic criteria require such judgments (e.g., a diminished interest or pleasure in activities and psychomotor agitation or retardation), adults, who may possess a broader perspective, may provide valuable input.

A central dilemma, however, is that adolescents, their parents, and their teachers often hold discrepant views of symptoms (Achenbach, McConaughy, & Howell, 1987). If multiple informants are reliably rating a single construct, one might expect that their agreement would be high. Unfortunately, for ratings of childhood and adolescent depression, inter-informant agreement often is low (for a thorough discussion, see Kazdin, 1994). One potential source of these observed discrepancies is rater effects, wherein some characteristic of the informant introduces a separate source of variance. For instance, maternal depression is associated with lower parent–child concordance in ratings of children's depression; mothers who are currently depressed appear to overestimate the level of their children's depressive symptoms (Renouf & Kovacs, 1994). However, discrepancies also may result from true differences in behavior observed in diverse settings, for instance, at school versus at home (see Clarizio, 1994). At present, there is little clarity in how best to integrate data from different informants, and data on the predictive validity of different sources of information are especially needed (Kazdin, 1994).

Methods of Assessment

Self-Report Rating Scales

Several rating scales exist and are commonly used to assess adolescent depression. The three most commonly used self-report measures of depressive symptoms are, in order of frequency (Brooks & Kutcher, 2001), the Children's Depression Inventory (CDI; Kovacs, 1992), the Beck Depression Inventory (BDI; Beck, Ward, Mendelsohn, Mock, & Erbaugh, 1961), and the Center for Epidemiologic Studies—Depression Scale (CES-D; Radloff, 1977). All of these measures have adequate internal consistency, generally moderate stability (with substantial variation among studies), and evidence of concurrent validity (correlations with other depression measures, self-esteem scales, etc.; Myers & Winters, 2002). None of these was designed as a diagnostic instrument, although they have some utility as screening tools (see Dierker et al., 2001, for recent data on the CES-D; Roberts et al., 1991 for the BDI; Craighead, Curry, & Ilardi, 1995, for the CDI). In addition, the specificity of each of these measures has been questioned, particularly with regard to their relation to symptoms of anxiety disorders, and it may be prudent to view them as measures of general distress or dysphoria (Brooks & Kutcher, 2001).

A less widely used measure to date, but one with strong psychometric properties and extensive normative information, is the Reynolds Adolescent Depression Scale (RADS; Reynolds, 1986). The RADS was designed specifically for adolescents, and normative data are available based on a sample of 2,460 ethnically diverse adolescents. Internal consistency and stability have been found to be high in diverse samples of adolescents, and scores correlate substantially with other self-report and clinician-rated measures of depression (Reynolds, 1994). Similar to the other rating scales, the RADS was not developed as a diagnostic tool, but a cutoff score may be used to screen for adolescents likely to have a depressive disorder (Reynolds & Mazza, 1998).

Clinician Rating Scales

Two clinician rating scales for quantifying the severity of depressive symptoms, the Hamilton Rating Scale for Depression (HRSD; Hamilton, 1960) and the Children's Depression Rating Scale—Revised (CDRS-R; Poznanski & Mokros, 1999), have been used extensively in investigations of adolescents, particularly in treatment studies. The HRSD was originally designed for use with adults, and the CDRS-R is a downward extension of the HRSD, adapted particularly for use with preadolescents (ages 6–12), although it has been used widely with adolescents. Both require trained clinicians to conduct interviews and make judgments about the severity of symptoms. The CDRS-R has been shown to have adequate internal consistency and good interrater reliability, and there is some evidence of concurrent validity. Less data are available on the reliability, and particularly the validity, of the HRSD in adolescent samples, making the CDRS-R the preferred clinician rating scale for teens (Myers & Winters, 2002).

Diagnostic Interviews

Several structured and semistructured interviews are available for assessing diagnostic status in adolescents. These include interviews that require the administration and interpretation of responses by a trained clinician, such as the Schedule for Affective Disorders and Schizophrenia in School-Age Children (K-SADS; Puig-Antich & Chambers, 1978), several versions of which exist, and the Child and Adolescent Psychiatric Assessment (CAPA; Angold et al., 1995). Both interviews have been shown to have acceptable test–retest and interrater reliability (see Angold & Costello, 1995, for the CAPA; Kaufman et al., 1997, for a recent version of the K-SADS). Other interviews are designed to be respondent based and may be administered by lay interviewers. These include the Diagnostic Interview Schedule for Children (the most recent version of which is the DISC-IV; Shaffer, Fisher, Lucas, Dulcan, & Schwab-Stone, 2000) and the Diagnostic Interview for Children and Adolescents (the most recent version of which is the DICA-IV; Reich, 2000). Both of these have demonstrated adequate test–retest reliability for major depression diagnoses in mixed child/adolescent samples, and both have some evidence of concurrent validity (see Reich, 2000; Shaffer et al., 2000). However, for diagnostic interviews in general, rates of parent–child agreement often are low. Typically a combination of information derived from parent and child interviews is used to generate a consensus diagnosis, but there is little empirical basis for particular decision rules. Until more basic research addresses the issue of informant variability, researchers have few concrete guidelines with which to merge and weight the different perspectives of adolescents and their parents (McClellan & Werry, 2000).

Commentary

Many options exist for the researcher or clinician seeking to assess the severity of depressive symptoms and diagnostic status in adolescents. Many of these measures have adequate psychometric properties in terms of test–retest reliability, internal consistency, and interrater reliability. Self-report measures, in particular, have received some criticism in terms of their nonspecificity to depression versus other forms of psychopathology, but this issue is difficult to disentangle from that of comorbidity, given that multiple symptoms frequently do coexist. A fundamental unresolved issue is how to integrate the different perspectives of parents, teachers, peers, and adolescents themselves. Unfortunately, same-informant ratings of different traits in child/adolescent samples (e.g., depression and anger; see Saylor, Finch, Baskin, Furey, & Kelly 1984) often are more substantially correlated than different informants' ratings of the same trait. Accordingly, further basic work on the concurrent and especially the predictive validity of data from different informants is necessary to clarify what should be asked of whom and how discrepancies should be resolved.

TREATMENT AND PREVENTION OF ADOLESCENT DEPRESSION

Psychological Interventions

Cognitive-Behavioral Therapy

Psychosocial approaches have shown promise in the treatment of adolescent depression, with substantial overall effects seen collapsing across various psychotherapeutic approaches (see Michael & Crowley, 2002). Of the psychosocial interventions, cognitive-behavioral therapy (CBT) has received the most empirical attention in adolescent samples. Focusing specifically on adolescents, a meta-analysis of six controlled studies found moderate to large effects of CBT (Reinecke, Ryan, & Dubois, 1998). Reinecke and colleagues (1998) noted several limitations to the extant data at that time, including a substantial reliance on school-based samples, group-based interventions, and self-report measures. However, since that review, several studies have addressed these concerns, demonstrating, for instance, the efficacy of CBT in an individual, rather than group-based, format (e.g., Rossello & Bernal, 1999) and in clinical samples of adolescents, using clinician ratings of depressive symptoms (e.g., Brent et al., 1997). Considerable rates of remission also have been observed in clinical (65% in Brent et al., 1997) and nonclinical (67% in Clarke, Rohde, Lewinsohn, Hops, & Seeley, 1999) samples of adolescents meeting diagnostic criteria for major depression or dysthymia. Thus, in the available studies, CBT has yielded consistent effects in reducing acute depressive symptoms and promoting remission in a range of adolescent samples.

Interpersonal Approaches

Although they have received less attention to date, interpersonal approaches also show promise in the treatment of adolescent depression. In assessing the effect of interpersonal therapy (IPT) in a clinic sample of adolescents, Mufson, Weissman, Moreau, and Garfinkel (1999) demonstrated that adolescents treated with IPT experienced a greater decrease in clinician-rated depressive symptoms than those in a clinical monitoring control group, and that 75% of treated patients met criteria for "recovery" on a joint index of clinician-rated and self-reported symptoms. Likewise, Rossello and Bernal (1999) showed significantly greater reductions in self-reported depressive symptoms for school-referred adolescents treated with IPT than for those placed on a wait list. Finally, in a test of a newer therapeutic approach, Diamond, Reis, Diamond, Siqueland, and Isaacs (2002) found support for their attachment-based family therapy (ABFT) in a sample of school-referred adolescents. Subjects meeting criteria for major depression were randomly assigned either to 12 weeks of ABFT or to a 6-week wait list. Those in the treatment group were significantly less likely to meet criteria for major depression on a clinical interview, were less likely to have self-reported depression scores in the clinical range, and had lower clini-cian-rated depressive symptoms at the end of the study than those on the wait list. Thus, these preliminary results suggest promise for a family-based interpersonal approach, in addi-tion to individual and group treatments.

Psychopharmacological Interventions

Biological approaches to the treatment of ado-lescent depression center primarily on psycho-pharmacology. Although electroconvulsive therapy is used in treatment-refractory adoles-cents, and available data (predominantly based on case studies) suggest efficacy comparable to what is seen in adults, no controlled trials of the treatment have been performed in adoles-cent samples (Rey & Walter, 1997). In terms of pharmacological approaches, the two groups of medications that have received considerable systematic empirical investigation are the tricyclic antidepressants and the selective sero-tonin reuptake inhibitors.

Tricyclic Antidepressants

In contrast to findings with adults, tricyclic an-tidepressants (TCAs) generally have not been found to be effective in the treatment of depres-sion among adolescents (Birmaher, Ryan, Wil-liamson, Brent, & Kaufman, 1996). Most con-trolled trials have failed to demonstrate a statistically significant response to TCAs (e.g., Boulous et al., 1991; Geller, Cooper, Graham, Marsteller, & Bryant, 1990; Kutcher et al., 1994; Kye et al., 1996) (for an exception, using intravenous administration of clomipramine in a small sample of adolescents, see Sallee, Vrindavanam, Deas-Nesmith, Carson, & Sethuraman, 1997). Although adolescents tak-ing TCAs may show a substantial improvement in symptoms, most double-blind trials indicate that such improvement is not greater than that associated with a placebo (e.g., Birmaher et al., 1998). This lack of efficacy may be a function of the less developed noradrenergic system in adolescents than in adults (Ryan, 1990). Fur-thermore, children and adolescents may be at greater risk than adults for serious medical complications when taking TCAs, including se-vere cardiovascular side effects (Geller, Reising, Leonard, Riddle, & Walsh, 1999). Accordingly, TCAs are not recommended as a first-line treatment of adolescent depression (Birmaher, 1998).

Selective Serotonin Reuptake Inhibitors

In contrast, the selective serotonin reuptake in-hibitors (SSRIs) have garnered greater support in controlled trials with youngsters. In a sample of 98 youngsters with major depression (Emslie et al., 1997), fluoxetine was associated with significantly better response in terms of clini-cians' blind ratings of improvement and level of depressive symptoms, and effects were simi-lar across age groups (comparing adolescents 13 or older to children 12 and younger). How-ever, only a minority of patients (31% of the fluoxetine group and 23% of the placebo group) achieved the designation of "minimal symptoms" by the end of the study, and the two groups did not differ in terms of self-re-ported depressive symptoms.

In a second controlled trial of fluoxetine in 219 children and adolescents (Emslie et al., 2002), clinician ratings of depressive symptoms again decreased more in the medication than in the placebo group, and no age effects (compar-ing children and adolescents) were found. Once again, there were no differences between the groups in terms of change in self-reported de-pressive symptoms.

Finally, in a third controlled study, an 8-week trial in a sample of 190 adolescents with major depression (Keller et al., 2001), paroxetine was found to be associated with sig-nificantly greater improvement than placebo (or imipramine) in terms of certain measures of clinician-rated symptoms (e.g., the HRSD de-pressed mood item and total score of 8 or be-low; clinical global impression of "improved or "much improved"). Mean scores on the K-SADS depression scale, the HRSD total score, and the mean clinician global impression scale were not different for the paroxetine and pla-cebo groups, although there were trends in sup-port of paroxetine.

Thus, in three controlled, double-blind trials of SSRIs, antidepressant medications have been associated with greater improvement than pla-cebo on most, if not all, clinician-rated mea-sures of depression. The positive findings for SSRIs, coupled with their lower risk of serious side effects than the TCAs, have made them the favored first-line pharmacological approach for treating depressed youngsters (Hughes et al., 1999; Weller & Weller, 2000). However, the existing data do not suggest that the SSRIs yield greater improvement in self-reported de-pressive symptoms than do placebos, and only a minority of treated youngsters are considered to be in remission at the end of the medication trial.

Prevention of Relapse and Recurrence

Most of the aforementioned studies have focused on treatment of the acute depressive episode. As discussed earlier, adolescent depression often is recurrent. Unfortunately, very few studies have assessed long-term prevention of relapse and recurrence in treated adolescents. In a combined child/adolescent sample treated with fluoxetine, 39% of those who achieved remission had a recurrence during a 1-year naturalistic follow-up (Emslie et al., 1998). Likewise, in a sample of adolescents treated with CBT, systematic behavioral family therapy, or nondirective supportive therapy, 30% of those who recovered went on to experience a recurrence within 2 years (Birmaher, Brent, et al., 2000). Accordingly, further attention should be paid to the role of maintenance or booster treatment.

Promising results suggesting a protective effect of continuation CBT in adolescents were obtained in a pilot study by Kroll, Harrington, Jayson, Fraser, and Gowers (1996), although this was not a randomized, controlled trial. In contrast, booster sessions had no positive effect on the 2-year rate of recurrence in a controlled study of CBT by Clarke and colleagues (1999). Thus, further work is needed to determine what types of interventions will enhance long-term maintenance of treatment gains among depressed adolescents.

Prevention Programs

Given the recurrent nature of the disorder, more promising, perhaps, will be prevention efforts aimed at deterring youngsters from embarking on a pathway of repeated and continuing episodes and associated impairment. Two such programs have received empirical scrutiny. Clarke and colleagues (1995) implemented a prevention program in high school students who had elevated depressive symptoms but did not meet criteria for a diagnosis of depression. The teenagers were randomly assigned to either a 15-session after-school, group-based program with an emphasis on cognitive techniques or to a "usual care" condition. During the 12-month follow-up period, teenagers in the treatment group were signifi-

cantly less likely than controls to develop a diagnosis of unipolar depression. Likewise, Gillham, Reivich, Jaycox, and Seligman (1995) implemented a 12-week group cognitive and social problem-solving intervention program in preadolescents at risk by virtue of elevated self-reported depression scores. As compared to the no-treatment group, the youngsters in the prevention program had significantly fewer depressive symptoms at 18 and 24 months posttreatment, as they transitioned into adolescence. Those who did not receive treatment were twice as likely as those in the prevention group to have symptoms in the moderate to severe range at the 2-year follow-up. The effect of the program grew larger over time, suggesting that early targeted prevention can have effects that become even more pronounced during the critical years in which depressive symptoms sharply increase.

Commentary

Overall, the data indicate that SSRIs, CBT, and interpersonal approaches all result to some degree in the reduction of acute depressive symptoms in adolescents. However, many, and sometimes most, of the adolescents in treated samples do not achieve full remission during the acute treatment phase, and a substantial rate of recurrence has been observed. In addition, few comparisons of these approaches have been conducted. To date, no controlled trials exist comparing psychosocial approaches to the SSRIs in adolescents. In terms of psychotherapies, although CBT has shown an edge over nonspecific therapeutic approaches in speed of symptom remission, longer-term follow-ups have not shown clear differences between treatments (see Curry, 2001). Thus, although several available treatments do indeed appear to result in at least the reduction of immediate depressive symptoms in adolescents, much work remains to be done in terms of evaluating aspects of patient–treatment match, improving remission rates, and evaluating the role of maintenance or booster treatment. Interventions for adolescent depression also would benefit from increased emphasis on prevention programs that target at-risk youth before they enter into a downward cycle of depression and associated impairment. Finally, public policy efforts to increase education about the dangers of adolescent depression are needed.

DESCRIPTION OF ADOLESCENT BIPOLAR DISORDER

A key consideration with regard to adolescent bipolar disorder is whether the *onset* was in childhood or adolescence. Generally speaking, adolescent-onset bipolar disorder is similar to adult-onset bipolar disorder and is largely the focus here. However, adolescent bipolar disorder with apparent onset in childhood may reflect many of the confusing and controversial issues presently surrounding the topic of childhood bipolar disorder. To clarify the distinction, a brief digression is in order.

Childhood-Onset Bipolar Disorder

The major source of controversy in this field stems from the difficulties associated with valid diagnosis of bipolar disorder in children. Although some have suggested that the syndrome exists in children, although rare, and can be identified by similar criteria as those used in adults, others have argued that it is far more common than previously suspected and often is "masked" by ADHD or other forms of severe disruptive behavior disorders (e.g., Biederman et al., 1996; Faraone, Biederman, Wozniak, et al., 1997). Thus, proponents of the latter perspective have suggested that a substantial minority of children with such diagnoses may, in fact, have a bipolar disorder.

The diagnosis of bipolarity in children becomes further complicated by the fact that it rarely follows an episodic course with clear and distinct periods of depression and mania. Children suspected of having bipolar disorder may have chronic symptoms, "mixed states" of manic and depressive symptoms, and very rapid mood swings even within the same day (Geller & Luby, 1997; Geller et al., 1998). To date, there are insufficient longitudinal data to determine whether those who are diagnosed with childhood-onset bipolar disorder actually continue to display bipolar disorder at later ages and whether their disorders mark an especially malignant form of illness with continuing chronicity, mixed states, and ultradian cycling. It is likely that a significant number of adolescents who first receive a diagnosis of bipolar disorder in adolescence had previous severe symptoms that were unrecognized as bipolar. Possibly, such youth have a different course and outcome from those whose onset of symptoms actually occurs in adolescence, and whose clinical presentation may resemble more "classic" bipolar I or bipolar II disorder.

Adolescent-Onset Bipolar Disorder

The diagnosis of bipolar I (with mania) or bipolar II (with hypomania) disorder is based on the same criteria as for adults. Key to the diagnosis is the presence of manic (or hypomanic) symptoms, but with developmental consideration given to the nature of the symptoms. For example, Geller and Luby (1997) note that grandiose beliefs may show themselves in an adolescent who, despite lack of talent, believes that he or she will become a rock star, or whose reduced need for sleep might take the form of sneaking out and partying all night. Engagement in high-risk pleasurable activities may involve heightened interest in sex and high-risk sexual experiences, excessive spending through use of parents' credit cards, taking dares, or driving wildly (Geller & Luby, 1997).

The first presentation of bipolar disorder often is depression rather than mania, which may obscure the true diagnosis in the absence of longitudinal follow-up. Kutcher, Robertson, and Bird (1998) found that depressions were the first affective episodes in 75% of their sample of adolescents with bipolar I disorder, with a mean age of onset of depression at 15.8 years. In the Oregon community sample of adolescents with bipolar-spectrum disorders, 61% had an initial depressive episode before the occurrence of mania or hypomania (Lewinsohn, Klein, & Seeley, 1995). Obviously, however, depression may be misidentified as unipolar rather than bipolar, and "switch rates" of up to 25% in child and adolescent samples (Faedda et al., 1995; Kovacs, 1996) indicate that the presence of severe depression may herald eventual bipolarity in a significant number of cases. Unfortunately, few studies have identified potential markers of bipolarity in depression. Strober and Carlson (1982) suggested that rapid onset of depression, psychotic features, family history of mood disorders (especially bipolar), psychomotor retardation, and antidepressant-induced manic symptoms may predict bipolar course. However, this vital question requires further study.

A further challenge to accurate diagnosis of bipolar disorder in youth is the presence of comorbid symptoms. Teenage bipolar disorder with psychotic symptoms was often likely misdiagnosed as schizophrenia in past years before the syndromes were defined clearly in current terms. Also, severe behavioral dysregulation and substance abuse may make the diagnosis difficult, given that mood swings and excessive, impulsive, or dangerous behaviors also are affected by drugs, alcohol, and poor judgment.

EPIDEMIOLOGY OF ADOLESCENT BIPOLAR DISORDER

Few community surveys of bipolar disorder have been conducted with adolescent samples, but existing data as well as retrospective reports of adult bipolar patients indicate two trends: overall similar rates (approximately 1%) in adolescents as adults and apparent increases in rates of bipolar disorder in birth cohorts born more recently (e.g., Kessler et al., 2001; Thomsen, Moller, Dehlholm, & Brask, 1992; Verhulst, van der Ende, Ferdinand, & Kasius, 1997). For example, the Oregon Adolescent Depression Project reported a lifetime prevalence of about 1%, including bipolar II and cyclothymia. An additional 5.7% of adolescents had significant subsyndromal symptoms of bipolar disorder with functional impairment. Elevated levels of hypomanic personality traits also were associated with various indices of impaired functioning (Klein, Lewinsohn, & Seeley, 1996). It is unclear whether hypomanic traits predict eventual Axis I bipolar disorder or whether they reflect stable, personality traits. Longitudinal studies of behavioral and offspring high-risk groups are needed to help clarify the outcomes of early subclinical forms of bipolar disorder.

DEVELOPMENTAL COURSE AND OUTCOMES OF ADOLESCENT BIPOLAR DISORDER

Psychotic symptoms may occur in one-third to one-half of adolescent bipolar patients (e.g., Kafantaris, Coletti, Dicker, Padula, & Pollack, 1998). Kafantaris and colleagues (1998) found that half of the bipolar youth in their study who presented with psychotic mania had no prior psychiatric history and seemed to have an acute onset after functioning well. They suggested that this subgroup may represent "classic" bipolar disorder, characterized by discrete episodes of depression and mania interspersed

with well periods (a subtype often responsive to lithium).

A significant proportion of bipolar adolescents display mixed states and rapid cycling (Faraone et al., 1997; Kutcher et al., 1998; McElroy, Strakowski, West, Keck, & McConville, 1997). It has been speculated that such courses may result in part from antidepressant-induced cycles before the underlying bipolar nature of depression is detected. Relatively few studies have followed bipolar youth for substantial periods of time to observe course features. However, indications point to relatively similar patterns as those observed in adults: probable recovery from episodes but high rates of recurrence of major episodes with substantial percentages of adolescents who show chronic symptoms and impairment (McClellan, McCurry, Snell, & DuBose, 1999; Strober et al., 1995).

ETIOLOGICAL HYPOTHESES AND IMPLICATIONS OF EARLY IDENTIFICATION OF BIPOLAR DISORDER

Bipolar disorder is considered to be one of the most genetically determined forms of major mental illness, and increasingly sophisticated genetic analyses are underway to identify potential gene loci. The mechanisms of the disorder are as yet unknown, although various neural circuits and cellular mechanisms of neurotransmitter systems are under investigation (e.g., Blumberg et al., 2000; Goodwin & Ghaemi, 1999). Imperfect concordance between monozygotic twins, however, makes it clear that interactions among genetic vulnerability and environmental factors play a role in expression of the disorder. Identification of markers of risk for eventual bipolar disorder is viewed as a high priority in the field.

The high-risk methodology (studying children of depressed parents) has been employed relatively less in bipolar than unipolar families. Lapalme, Hodgins, and LaRoche (1997) conducted a meta-analysis of high-risk studies, and concluded that 52% of the offspring of bipolar parents met criteria for some diagnosis, compared with 29% of the offspring of parents with no disorders. In total, 26.5% of the offspring of bipolar parents had an *affective* disorder (including major, minor, or intermittent depression and dysthymia, as well as mania, hypomania, cyclothymia, and hyperthymic states) compared with 8.3% of children of non-ill parents. *Bipolar* disorder occurred in 5.4% of the offspring of bipolar parents, whereas none of the children of non-ill parents were bipolar. Several investigations of high-risk samples have included subsyndromal and temperament measures thought to reflect the bipolar spectrum (e.g., Grigoroiu-Serbanescu et al., 1989; Grigoroiu-Serbanescu, Christodorescu, Totoescu, & Jipescu, 1991; Klein, Depue, & Slater, 1985). It is an intriguing question whether such traits reflect prodromal signs of later bipolarity or indicate stable subclinical states with heritable components. Investigations of neurocognitive characteristics of high-risk youth are a research direction to pursue in future studies.

The prevalent "kindling" model of bipolar disorder (e.g., Post, 1992) suggests that bipolar episodes have a progressive effect on the brain, "sensitizing" the organism to react with episodes to increasingly milder triggering events. Therefore, one important implication is that fewer early episodes might predict a more benign course of disorder. Some investigators and clinicians have urged rapid institution of mood stabilizer treatment of presumed bipolar disorder in the hope of improving the eventual course. Thus, early diagnosis or detection of youngsters at apparent risk for bipolar disorder is an important research priority with considerable consequences.

TREATMENT OF BIPOLAR DISORDER IN ADOLESCENTS

An accumulating body of research suggests that the treatment of adolescent bipolar disorder with lithium and anticonvulsant mood stabilizers results in relatively comparable rates of symptom reduction and functional improvement as seen in adults (for a review, see Pavuluri, Naylor, & Janicak, 2002). In general, however, large-scale double-blind placebo-controlled clinical trials have not been conducted, and evidence of prophylactic effects is sparse. Similarly, the concern that ADHD-masked bipolar disorder treated with stimulant medication might complicate the course of illness has not been empirically tested in sufficiently controlled studies. In reviewing treatment issues, State, Altshuler, and Frye (2002) suggest that the efficacy and safety of combining mood stabilizers and ADHD treatments

need to be investigated. Also, psychotherapy and family interventions for bipolar youth are increasingly recommended as an adjunct to medication (Pavuluri et al., 2002), and a few studies assessing the efficacy of these treatments are presently underway.

CURRENT NEEDS AND FUTURE DIRECTIONS

Conceptualizing and Understanding Depression in Adolescents

Throughout the chapter, we have underscored many areas in need of further inquiry to extend our understanding of adolescent depression. Here we focus on three general issues that deserve additional attention.

First, remarkably little is known about the distinction between childhood-onset and adolescent-onset depression. Although depression tends to follow a chronic and recurring course, some youth show an onset early in life, whereas others do not show signs of a clinical depression until mid to late adolescence. The vast majority of studies of adolescent depression do not distinguish between symptoms or disorders with an initial onset during adolescence and disorders that are continuing or recurring episodes following an onset in childhood. As discussed earlier, however, preliminary research suggests that these courses may be associated with different clinical characteristics and outcomes; less is known about differing etiologies, with the exception of a possibly stronger genetic basis to adolescent-onset depression. A similar distinction is likely needed between childhood-onset and adolescent-onset bipolar disorder. It will therefore be critical in future research to determine whether mood disorders with varying developmental timelines reflect different subtypes.

Second, a controversial issue in theory and research on mood disorders concerns the continuity among mood, syndromes, and disorders. As previously noted, data increasingly suggest that even subclinical levels of depressive and manic symptoms are associated with significant functional impairment, and they often forecast future clinical depression and bipolar disorder. However, research is needed to determine under what circumstances subsyndromal symptoms dissipate over time or crystallize into more significant clinical disorders later in life.

Third, an ongoing challenge facing depression researchers is the development of theories that clearly distinguish vulnerability to depression versus other types of psychopathology. Whereas some risk factors for depression appear specific, others have been found to heighten risk for many other types of disorders as well. Moreover, given the high rates of comorbidity between depression and other forms of psychopathology, understanding depression requires theory and research that distinguish between adolescents with and without co-occurring symptoms.

Assessment and Treatment

Although several treatments have been shown to reduce depressive symptoms, full remission often is not achieved, and recurrence is common. Accordingly, further work is necessary to refine existing therapeutic approaches, to identify characteristics of individuals that may moderate the effectiveness of particular treatments, and to clarify the role of prevention and maintenance treatment. Moreover, remarkably little is known about the processes that account for treatment success; a great deal more work is therefore needed to understand the active ingredients and mechanisms of change associated with psychological interventions. Finally, resolving discrepancies between treatment outcomes associated with different symptom measures will require further work on fundamental questions in the assessment of adolescent depression, particularly issues of informant variability and predictive validity.

ACKNOWLEDGMENTS

Preparation of this chapter was supported in part by a William T. Grant Foundation Faculty Scholars Award and NIMH Grant No. R01 MH59711 awarded to Karen D. Rudolph, and by NIMH Grant No. R01 MH52239 awarded to Constance Hammen. We would like to express our thanks to Alison J. Dupre, Sarah Quinlan, and Tanya Juarez for their assistance in preparation of this chapter.

REFERENCES

Abela, J. R. Z. (2001). The hopelessness theory of depression: A test of the diathesis–stress and causal mediation components in third and seventh grade children. *Journal of Abnormal Child Psychology, 29,* 241–254.

Abramson, L. Y., Metalsky, G. I., & Alloy, L. B. (1989). Hopelessness depression: A theory-based subtype of depression. *Psychological Review, 96,* 358–372.

Abramson, L. Y., Seligman, M. E. P., & Teasdale, J. D. (1978). Learned helplessness in humans: Critique and reformulation. *Journal of Abnormal Psychology, 37,* 49–74.

Achenbach, T. M., McConaughy, S. H., & Howell, C. T. (1987). Child/adolescent behavioral and emotional problems: Implications of cross-informant correlations for situation specificity. *Psychological Bulletin, 101,* 213–232.

Allen, J. P., Hauser, S. T., Bell, K. L., & O'Connor, T. G. (1994). Longitudinal assessment of autonomy and relatedness in adolescent–family interactions as predictors of adolescent ego development and self-esteem. *Child Development, 65,* 179–194.

Alloy, L. B., Abramson, L. Y., Tashman, N. A., Berrebbi, D. S., Hogan, M. E., Whitehouse, W. G., et al. (2001). Developmental origins of cognitive vulnerability to depression: Parenting, cognitive, and inferential feedback styles of the parents of individuals at high and low cognitive risk for depression. *Cognitive Therapy and Research, 25,* 397–423.

American Psychiatric Association. (2000). *Diagnostic and statistical manual of mental disorders* (4th ed., text rev.). Washington, DC: Author.

Angold, A., & Costello, E. (1995). A test–retest reliability study of child-reported psychiatric symptoms and diagnoses using the Child and Adolescent Psychiatric Assessment. *Psychological Medicine, 25,* 755–762.

Angold, A., Costello, E. J., & Erkanli, A. (1999). Comorbidity. *Journal of Child Psychology and Psychiatry, 40,* 57–87.

Angold, A., Costello, E. J., Erkanli, A., & Worthman, C. M. (1999). Pubertal changes in hormones of adolescent girls. *Psychological Medicine, 29,* 1043–1053.

Angold, A., Costello, E. J., & Worthman, C. M. (1998). Puberty and depression: The roles of age, pubertal status and pubertal timing. *Psychological Medicine, 28,* 51–61.

Angold, A., Prendergast, M., Cox, A., Harrington, R., Simonoff, E., & Rutter, M. (1995). The Child and Adolescent Psychiatric Assessment (CAPA). *Psychological Medicine 25,* 739–753.

Angold, A., & Rutter, M. (1992). Effects of age and pubertal status on depression in a large clinical sample. *Development and Psychopathology, 4,* 5–28.

Angold, A., Weissman, M., John, K., Merikangas, K. R., Prusoff, B. A., Wickramaratne, P., et al. (1987). Parent and child reports of depressive symptoms in children at low and high risk of depression. *Journal of Child Psychology and Psychiatry, 28,* 901–915.

Angst, J., Sellaro, R., & Merikangas, K. R. (2000). Depressive spectrum diagnoses. *Comprehensive Psychiatry, 41,* 39–47.

Armsden, G. C., McCauley, E., Greenberg, M. T., Burke, P. M., & Mitchell, J. R. (1990). Parent and peer attachment in early adolescent depression. *Journal of Abnormal Child Psychology, 18,* 683–697.

Arnett, J. J. (1999). Adolescent storm and stress, reconsidered. *American Psychologist, 54,* 317–326.

Arnett, J. J. (2000). Emerging adulthood: A theory of development from the late teens through the twenties. *American Psychologist, 55,* 469–480.

Asarnow, J. R., Tompson, M., Hamilton, E. B., Goldstein, M. J., & Guthrie, D. (1994). Family-expressed emotion, childhood-onset depression, and childhood-onset schizophrenia spectrum disorders: Is expressed emotion a nonspecific correlate of child psychopathology or a specific risk factor for depression? *Journal of Abnormal Child Psychology, 22,* 129–146.

Avenevoli, S., & Steinberg, L. (2001). The continuity of depression across the adolescent transition. *Advances in Child Development and Behavior, 28,* 139–173.

Avenevoli, S., Stolar, M., Li, J., Dierker, L., & Merikangas, K. R. (2001). Comorbidity of depression in children and adolescents: Models and evidence from a prospective high-risk family study. *Biological Psychiatry, 49,* 1071–1081.

Bardone, A., Moffitt, T., Caspi, A., Dickson, N., & Silva, P. (1996). Adult mental health and social outcomes of adolescent girls with depression and conduct disorder. *Development and Psychopathology, 8,* 811–829.

Beardslee, W. R., Versage, E. M., & Gladstone, T. R. (1998). Children of affectively ill parents: A review of the past 10 years. *Journal of the American Academy of Child and Adolescent Psychiatry, 37,* 1134–1141.

Beck, A. T. (1967). *Depression: Clinical, experimental, and theoretical aspects.* New York: Harper & Row.

Beck, A. T., Ward, C. H., Mendelsohn, M., Mock, J., & Erbaugh, J. (1961). An inventory for measuring depression. *Archives of General Psychiatry, 4,* 561–571.

Biederman, J., Faraone, S., Mick, E., Wozniak, J., Chen, L., Ouellette, C., et al. (1996). Attention-deficit hyperactivity disorder and juvenile mania: An overlooked comorbidity? *Journal of the American Academy of Child and Adolescent Psychiatry, 35,* 997–1008.

Bird, H. R., Canino, G., Rubio-Stipec, M., Gould, M. S., Ribera, J., Sesman, M., et al. (1988). Estimates of the prevalence of childhood maladjustment in a community survey in Puerto Rico. *Archives of General Psychiatry, 45,* 1120–1126.

Birmaher, B. (1998). Should we use antidepressant medications for children and adolescents with depressive disorders? *Psychopharmacology Bulletin, 34,* 35–39.

Birmaher, B., Brent, D. A., Kolko, D., Baugher, M., Bridge, J., Holder, D., et al. (2000). Clinical outcome after short-term psychotherapy for adolescents with major depressive disorder. *Archives of General Psychiatry, 57,* 29–36.

Birmaher, B., Dahl, R. E., Williamson, D. E., Perel, J. M., Brent, D. A., Axelson, D. A., et al. (2000). Growth hormone secretion in children and adolescents at high risk for major depressive disorder. *Archives of General Psychiatry, 57,* 867–872.

Birmaher, B., Ryan, N. D., Williamson, D. E., Brent, D. A., & Kaufman, J. (1996). Childhood and adolescent depression: A review of the past 10 years. Part II. *Journal of the American Academy of Child and Adolescent Psychiatry, 35,* 1575–1583.

Birmaher, B., Ryan, N. D., Williamson, D. E., Brent, D. A., Kaufman, J., Dahl, R. E., et al. (1996). Childhood and adolescent depression: A review of the past 10 years. Part I. *Journal of the American Academy of Child and Adolescent Psychiatry, 35,* 1427–1439.

Birmaher, B., Waterman, G. S., Ryan, N. D., Perel, J., McNabb, J., Balach, L., et al. (1998). Randomized, controlled trial of amitriptyline versus placebo for adolescents with "treatment-resistant" major depression. *Journal of the American Academy of Child and Adolescent Psychiatry, 37,* 527–535.

Blumberg, H. P., Stern, E., Martinez, D., Ricketts, S., de Asis, J., White, T., et al. (2000). Increased anterior cingulate and caudate activity in bipolar mania. *Biological Psychiatry, 48,* 1045–1052.

Boulous, C., Kutcher, S., Marton, P., Simeon, J., Ferguson, B., & Roberts, N. (1991). Response to desipramine treatment in adolescent major depression. *Psychopharmacology Bulletin, 27,* 59–65.

Bowlby, J. (1969). *Attachment and loss: Vol. I. Attachment.* New York: Basic Books.

Brent, D. A., Holder, D., Kolko, D., Birmaher, B., Baugher, M., Roth, C., et al. (1997). A clinical psychotherapy trial for adolescent depression comparing cognitive, family, and supportive therapy. *Archives of General Psychiatry, 54,* 877–885.

Broderick, P. C. (1998). Early adolescent gender differences in the use of ruminative and distracting coping strategies. *Journal of Early Adolescence, 18,* 173–191.

Brooks, S. J., & Kutcher, S. (2001). Diagnosis and measurement of adolescent depression: A review of commonly utilized instruments. *Journal of Child and Adolescent Psychopharmacology, 11,* 341–376.

Brooks-Gunn, J., & Warren, M. P. (1989). Biological and social contributions to negative affect in young adolescent girls. *Child Development, 60,* 40–55.

Brown, G. W., & Harris, T. (1978). *Social origins of depression: A study of psychiatric disorders in women.* New York: Free Press.

Caldwell, M. S., Rudolph, K. D., Troop-Gordon, W., & Kim, D. (2004). Reciprocal influences among relational self-views, social disengagement, and peer stress during early adolescence. *Child Development, 75,* 1140–1154.

Cicchetti, D., Rogosch, F. A., & Toth, S. L. (1994). A developmental psychopathology perspective on depression in children and adolescents. In W. M. Reynolds & H. F. Johnston (Eds.), *Handbook of depression in children and adolescents. Issues in clinical child psychology* (pp. 123–141). New York: Plenum Press.

Cicchetti, D., & Schneider-Rosen, K. (1984). Toward a transactional model of childhood depression. *New Directions for Child Development, 26,* 5–27.

Cicchetti, D., & Toth, S. L. (1998). The development of

depression in children and adolescents. *American Psychologist, 53,* 221–241.

Clarizio, H. F. (1994). Assessment of depression in children and adolescents by parents, teachers, and peers. In W. M. Reynolds & H. F. Johnston (Eds.), *Handbook of depression in children and adolescents* (pp. 235–248). New York: Plenum Press.

Clarke, G. N., Hawkins, W., Murphy, M., Sheeber, L. B., Lewinsohn, P. M., & Seeley, J. R. (1995). Targeted prevention of unipolar depressive disorder in an at-risk sample of high school adolescents. *Journal of the American Academy of Child and Adolescent Psychiatry, 34,* 312–321.

Clarke, G. N., Rohde, P., Lewinsohn, P. M., Hops, H., & Seeley, J. R. (1999). Cognitive behavioral treatment of adolescent depression: Efficacy of acute group treatment and booster sessions. *Journal of the American Academy of Child and Adolescent Psychiatry, 38,* 272–279.

Cohen, L. H., Burt, C. E., & Bjorck, J. P. (1987). Life stress and adjustment: Effects of life events experienced by young adolescents and their parents. *Developmental Psychology, 23,* 583–592.

Cohen, P., Cohen, J., Kasen, S., Velez, C. N., Hartmark, C., Johnson, J., et al. (1993). An epidemiological study of disorders in late childhood and adolescence: I. Age and gender-specific prevalence. *Journal of Child Psychology and Psychiatry, 34,* 851–867.

Cole, D. A., Martin, J. M., Peeke, L. G., Seroczynski, A. D., & Hoffman, K. (1998). Are cognitive errors of underestimation predictive or reflective of depressive symptoms in children: A longitudinal study. *Journal of Abnormal Psychology, 107,* 481–496.

Cole, D. A., Martin, J. M., & Powers, B. (1997). A competency-based model of child depression: A longitudinal study of peer, parent, teacher, and self-evaluations. *Journal of Child Psychology and Psychiatry and Allied Disciplines, 38,* 505–514.

Cole, D. A., Martin, J. M., Powers, B., & Truglio, R. (1996). Modeling causal relations between academic and social competence and depression: A multitrait–multimethod longitudinal study of children. *Journal of Abnormal Psychology, 105,* 258–270.

Compas, B. E., Connor-Smith, J. K., Saltzman, H., Thomsen, A. H., & Wadsworth, M. E. (2001). Coping with stress during childhood and adolescence: Problems, progress, and potential in theory and research. *Psychological Bulletin, 127,* 87–127.

Compas, B. E., Ey, S., & Grant, K. E. (1993). Taxonomy, assessment, and diagnosis of depression during adolescence. *Psychological Bulletin, 114,* 323–344.

Compas, B. E., Howell, D. C., Phares, V., Williams, R. A., & Giunta, C. T. (1989). Risk factors for emotional/behavioral problems in young adolescents: A prospective analysis of adolescent and parental stress and symptoms. *Journal of Consulting and Clinical Psychology, 57,* 732–740.

Compas, B. E., & Wagner, B. M. (1991). Psychosocial stress during adolescence: Intrapersonal and interpersonal processes. In M. E. Colten & S. Gore (Eds.), *Adolescent stress: Causes and consequences. Social institutions and social change* (pp. 67–85). New York: Aldine de Gruyter.

Connolly, J., Geller, S., Marton, P., & Kutcher, S. (1992). Peer responses to social interaction with depressed adolescents. *Journal of Clinical Child Psychology, 21,* 365–370.

Cooper, P. J., & Goodyer, I. (1993). A community study of depression in adolescent girls I: Estimates of symptom and syndrome prevalence. *British Journal of Psychiatry, 163,* 369–374.

Coryell, W., Akiskal, H., Leon, A., Winokur, G., Maser, J., Mueller, T., & Keller, M. B. (1994). The time course of nonchronic major depressive disorder: Uniformity across episodes and samples. *Archives of General Psychiatry, 51,* 405–410.

Costello, E. J., Angold, A., Burns, B. J., Stangl, D. K., Tweed, D. L., Erkanli, A., & Worthman, C. M. (1996). The Great Smoky Mountains Study of Youth: Goals, design, methods, and the prevalence of DSM-III-R disorders. *Archives of General Psychiatry, 53,* 1129–1136.

Craighead, W. E., Curry, J. F., & Ilardi, S. S. (1995). Relationship of Children's Depression Inventory factors to major depression among adolescents. *Psychological Assessment, 7,* 171–176.

Cross-National Collaborative Group. (1992). The changing rate of major depression: Cross-national comparisons. *Journal of the American Medical Association, 268,* 3098–3105.

Cummings, E. M., & Cicchetti, D. (1990). Toward a transactional model of relations between attachment and depression. In M. T. Greenberg, D. Cicchetti, & E. M. Cummings (Eds.), *Attachment in the preschool years: Theory, research, and intervention* (pp. 339–372). Chicago: University of Chicago Press.

Cummings, E. M., & Davies, P. T. (1999). Depressed parents and family functioning: Interpersonal effects and children's functioning and development. In T. E. Joiner & J. C. Coyne (Eds.), *The interactional nature of depression: Advances in interpersonal approaches* (pp. 299–327). Washington, DC: American Psychological Association.

Curry, J. F. (2001). Specific psychotherapies for childhood and adolescent depression. *Biological Psychiatry, 49,* 1091–1100.

Cyranowski, J. M., Frank, E., Young, E., & Shear, M. K. (2000). Adolescent onset of the gender difference in lifetime rates of major depression. *Archives of General Psychiatry, 57,* 21–27.

Daley, S. E., & Hammen, C. (2002). Depressive symptoms and close relationships during the transition to adulthood: Perspectives from dysphoric women, their best friends, and their romantic partners. *Journal of Consulting and Clinical Psychology, 70,* 129–141.

Daley, S. E., Hammen, C., Burge, D., Davila, J., Paley, B., Lindberg, N., & Herzberg, D. S. (1997). Predictors of the generation of episodic stress: A longitudinal study of late adolescent women. *Journal of Abnormal Psychology, 106,* 251–259.

Daley, S. E., Hammen, C., Davila, J., & Burge, D. (1998). Axis II symptomatology, depression, and life stress during the transition from adolescence to adulthood. *Journal of Consulting and Clinical Psychology, 66,* 595–603.

Davidson, R. J. (2000). Affective style, psychopathology, and resilience: Brain mechanisms and plasticity. *American Psychologist, 55,* 1196–1214.

Davidson, R. J., Pizzagalli, D., & Nitschke, J. (2002). The representation and regulation of emotion in depression: Perspectives from affective neuroscience. In I. H. Gotlib & C. L. Hammen (Eds.), *Handbook of depression* (pp. 219–244). New York: Guilford Press.

Davies, P. T., & Windle, M. (1997). Gender-specific pathways between maternal depressive symptoms, family discord, and adolescent adjustment. *Developmental Psychology, 33,* 657–668.

Davila, J., Hammen, C., Burge, D., Paley, B., & Daley, S. E. (1995). Poor interpersonal problem solving as a mechanism of stress generation in depression among adolescent women. *Journal of Abnormal Psychology, 104,* 592–600.

Davis, B., Sheeber, L., Hops, H., & Tildesley, E. (2000). Adolescent responses to depressive parental behaviors in problem-solving interactions: Implications for depressive symptoms. *Journal of Abnormal Child Psychology, 28,* 451–465.

Dawson, G., Frey, K., Panagiotides, H., Osterling, J., & Hessl, D. (1997). Infants of depressed mothers exhibit atypical frontal brain activity: A replication and extension of previous findings. *Journal of Child Psychology and Psychiatry, 38,* 179–186.

Diamond, G. S., Reis, B. F., Diamond, G. M., Siqueland, L., & Isaacs, L. (2002). Attachment-based family therapy for depressed adolescents: A treatment development study. *Journal of the American Academy of Child and Adolescent Psychiatry, 41,* 1190–1196.

Dierker, L. C., Albano, A. M., Clarke, G. N., Heimberg, R. G., Kendall, P. C. Merikangas, K. R., et al. (2001). Screening for anxiety and depression in early adolescence. *Journal of the American Academy of Child and Adolescent Psychiatry, 40,* 929–936.

Dinan, T. G. (1998). Psychoneuroendocrinology of depression: Growth hormone. *Psychoneuroendocrinology, 21,* 325–339.

Eaves, L. J., Silberg, J. L., Meyer, J. M., Maes, H. H., Simonoff, E., Pickles, A., Rutter, M., et. al. (1997). Genetics and developmental psychopathology: 2. The main effects of genes and environment on behavioral problems in the Virginia Twin Study of Adolescent Behavioral Development. *Journal of Child Psychology and Psychiatry and Allied Disciplines, 38,* 965–980.

Eccles, J. S., & Midgley, C. (1989). Stage-environment fit: Developmentally appropriate classrooms for young adolescents. In R. E. Ames & C. Ames (Eds.), *Research on motivation in education* (Vol. 3, pp. 139–181). New York: Academic Press.

Eccles, J. S., Wigfield, A., & Schiefele, U. (1998). Motivation to succeed. In N. Eisenberg (Ed.) & W.

Damon (Series Ed.), *Handbook of child psychology: Vol. 3. Social, emotional, and personality development* (5th ed., 1017–1095). New York: Wiley.

Eley, T. C., & Stevenson, J. (2000). Specific life events and chronic experiences differentially associated with depression and anxiety in young twins. *Journal of Abnormal Child Psychology, 28,* 383–394.

Emslie, G. J., Heiligenstein, J. H., Wagner, K. D., Hoog, S. L., Ernest, D. E., Brown, E., et al. (2002). Fluoxetine for acute treatment of depression in children and adolescents: A placebo-controlled randomized clinical trial. *Journal of the American Academy of Child and Adolescent Psychiatry, 41,* 1205–1215.

Emslie, G. J., Rush, A. J., Weinberg, W. A., Kowatch, R. A., Carmody, T., & Mayes, T. L. (1998). Fluoxetine in child and adolescent depression: Acute and maintenance treatment. *Depression and Anxiety, 7,* 32–39.

Emslie, G. J., Rush, A. J., Weinberg, W. A., Kowatch, R. A., Hughes, C. W., Carmody, T., et al. (1997). A double-blind, randomized, placebo-controlled trial of fluoxetine in children and adolescents with depression. *Archives of General Psychiatry, 54,* 1031–1037.

Faedda, G., Baldessarini, R., Suppes, T., Tondo, L., Becker, I., & Lipschitz, D. (1995). Pediatric-onset bipolar disorder: A neglected clinical and public health problem. *Harvard Review of Psychiatry, 3,* 171–195.

Fairbairn, W. (1952). *An object relations theory of personality.* New York: Basic Books.

Faraone, S. V., Biederman, J., Wozniak, J., Mundy, E., Mennin, D., & O'Donnell, D. (1997). Is comorbidity with ADHD a marker for juvenile-onset mania? *Journal of the American Academy of Child and Adolescent Psychiatry, 36,* 1046–1055.

Fergusson, D. M., Horwood, J., & Lynskey, M. T. (1995). Maternal depressive symptoms and depressive symptoms in adolescents. *Journal of Child Psychology and Psychiatry, 7,* 1161–1178.

Fleming, J. E., Boyle, M. H., & Offord, D. R. (1993). The outcome of adolescent depression in the Ontario child health study follow-up. *Journal of the American Academy of Child and Adolescent Psychiatry, 32,* 28–33.

Freud, S. (1951). Mourning and melancholia. In J. Strachey (Ed. and Trans.), *The standard edition of the complete works of Sigmund Freud* (Vol. 14, pp. 237–260). London: Hogarth Press. (Original work published 1917)

Furman, W., & Buhrmester, D. (1992). Age and sex differences in perceptions of networks of personal relationships. *Child Development, 63,* 103–115.

Garber, J. (1984). Classification of childhood psychopathology: A developmental perspective. *Child Development, 55,* 30–48.

Garber, J., & Flynn, C. A. (2001). Predictors of depressive cognitions in young adolescents. *Cognitive Therapy and Research, 25,* 353–376.

Garber, J., & Hilsman, R. (1992). Cognitions, stress, and depression in children and adolescents. *Child and Adolescent Psychiatric Clinics of North America, 1,* 129–167.

Garber, J., & Horowitz, J. L. (2002). Depression in children. In I. H. Gotlib & C. L. Hammen (Eds.), *Handbook of depression* (pp. 510–540). New York: Guilford Press.

Garber, J., & Kaminski, K. M. (2000). Laboratory and performance-based measures of depression in children and adolescents. *Journal of Clinical Child Psychology, 29,* 509–525.

Garber, J., Keiley, M. K., & Martin, N. C. (2002). Developmental trajectories of adolescents' depressive symptoms: Predictors of change. *Journal of Consulting and Clinical Psychology, 70,* 79–95.

Garber, J., & Little, S. (2001). Emotional autonomy and adolescent adjustment. *Journal of Adolescent Research, 16,* 355–371.

Garber, J., & Martin, N. C. (2002). Negative cognitions in offspring of depressed parents: Mechanisms of risk. In S. H. Goodman & I. H. Gotlib (Eds.), *Children of depressed parents: Mechanisms of risk and implications for treatment* (pp. 121–153). Washington, DC: American Psychological Association.

Garber, J., Robinson, N. S., & Valentiner, D. (1997). The relation between parenting and adolescent depression: Self-worth as a mediator. *Journal of Adolescent Research, 12,* 12–33.

Garber, J., Weiss, B., & Shanley, N. (1993). Cognitions, depressive symptoms, and development in adolescents. *Journal of Abnormal Psychology, 102,* 47–57.

Gazelle, H., & Rudolph, K. D. (2004). Moving toward and away from the world: Social approach and avoidance trajectories in anxious solitary youth. *Child Development, 75,* 829–849.

Ge, X., Lorenz, F. O., Conger, R. D., Elder, G. G., & Simons, R. L. (1994). Trajectories of stressful life events and depressive symptoms during adolescence. *Developmental Psychology, 30,* 467–483.

Geller, B., Cooper, T. B., Graham, D. L., Marsteller, F. A., & Bryant, M. (1990). Double-blind placebo-controlled study of nortriptyline in depressed adolescents using a "fixed plasma level" design. *Psychopharmacology Bulletin, 26,* 85–90.

Geller, B., & Luby, J. (1997). Child and adolescent bipolar disorder: Review of the past 10 years. *Journal of the American Academy of Child and Adolescent Psychiatry, 36,* 1168–1176.

Geller, B., Reising, D., Leonard, H. L., Riddle, M. A., & Walsh, B. T. (1999). Critical review of tricyclic antidepressant use in children and adolescents. *Journal of the American Academy of Child and Adolescent Psychiatry, 38,* 513–516.

Geller, B., Williams, M., Zimerman, B., Frazier, J., Beringer, L., & Warner, K. (1998). Prepubertal and early adolescent bipolarity differentiate from ADHD by manic symptoms, grandiose delusions, ultra-rapid or ultradian cycling. *Journal of Affective Disorders, 51,* 81–91.

Gillham, J. E., Reivich, K. J., Jaycox, L. H., & Seligman, M. E. P. (1995). Prevention of depressive symptoms in schoolchildren: Two-year follow-up. *Psychological Science, 6,* 343–351.

Goodman, S. (2002). Depression and early adverse experiences. In I. H. Gotlib & C. L. Hammen (Eds.), *Handbook of depression* (pp. 245–267). New York: Guilford Press.

Goodman, S. H., Brogan, D., Lynch, M. E., & Fielding, B. (1993). Social and emotional competence in children of depressed mothers. *Child Development, 64,* 516–531.

Goodman, S. H., & Gotlib, I. H. (1999). Risk for psychopathology in the children of depressed mothers: A developmental model for understanding mechanisms of transmission. *Psychological Review, 106,* 458–490.

Goodman, S. H., & Gotlib, I. H. (2002). Transmission of risk to children of depressed parents: Integration and conclusions. In S. H. Goodman & I. H. Gotlib (Eds.), *Children of depressed parents: Mechanisms of risk and implications for treatment* (pp. 307–326). Washington, DC: American Psychological Association.

Goodman, S. H., Schwab-Stone, M., Lahey, B., Shaffer, D., & Jensen, P. (2000). Major depression and dysthymia in children and adolescents: Discriminant validity and differential consequences in a community sample. *Journal of the American Academy of Child and Adolescent Psychiatry, 39,* 761–770.

Goodwin, F., & Ghaemi, N. (1999). Bipolar disorder: State of the art. *Dialogues in Clinical Neuroscience, 1,* 41–51.

Goodyer, I. M. (2001). Life events: Their nature and effects. In I. M. Goodyer (Ed.), *The depressed child and adolescent. Cambridge child and adolescent psychiatry* (2nd ed., pp. 204–232). New York: Cambridge University Press.

Goodyer, I. M., & Altham, P. M. E. (1991). Lifetime exit events and recent social and family adversities in anxious and depressed school-age children and adolescents: I. *Journal of Affective Disorders, 21,* 219–228.

Goodyer, I., & Cooper, P. (1993). A community study of depression in adolescent girls: II. The clinical features of identified disorder. *British Journal of Psychiatry, 163,* 374–380.

Goodyer, I. M., Herbert, J., Tamplin, A., & Altham, P. M. E. (2000a). First-episode major depression in adolescents: Affective, cognitive and endocrine characteristics of risk status and predictors of onset. *British Journal of Psychiatry, 176,* 142–149.

Goodyer, I. M., Herbert, J., Tamplin, A., & Altham, P. M. E. (2000b). Recent life events, cortisol, dehydroepiandrosterone and the onset of major depression in high-risk adolescents. *British Journal of Psychiatry, 177,* 499–504.

Gore, S., Aseltine, R. H., & Colton, M. E. (1992). Social structure, life stress and depressive symptoms in a high school-aged population. *Journal of Health and Social Behavior, 33,* 97–113.

Gore, S., Aseltine, R. H., & Colton, M. E. (1993). Gender, social–relational involvement, and depression. *Journal of Research on Adolescence, 3,* 101–125.

Gotlib, I. H., & Hammen, C. (1992). *Psychological as-*

pects of depression: Toward a cognitive-interpersonal integration. London: Wiley.

Gotlib, I. H., Lewinsohn, P. M., & Seeley, J. R. (1995). Symptoms versus a diagnosis of depression: Differences in psychosocial functioning. *Journal of Consulting and Clinical Psychology, 63,* 90–100.

Gotlib, I. H., Lewinsohn, P. M., & Seeley, J. R. (1998). Consequences of depression during adolescence: Marital status and marital functioning in early adulthood. *Journal of Abnormal Psychology, 107,* 686–690.

Gotlib, I. H., Lewinsohn, P. M., Seeley, J. R., Rohde, P., & Redner, J. E. (1993). Negative cognitions and attributional style in depressed adolescents: An examination of stability and specificity. *Journal of Abnormal Psychology, 102,* 607–615.

Graber, J. A., Lewinsohn, P. M., Seeley, J. R., & Brooks-Gunn, J. (1997). Is psychopathology associated with the timing of pubertal development? *Journal of the American Academy of Child and Adolescent Psychiatry, 36,* 1768–1776.

Grigoroiu-Serbanescu, M., Christodorescu, D., Jipescu, I., Totoescu, A., Marinescu, E., & Ardelean, V. (1989). Psychopathology in children aged 10–17 of bipolar parents: Psychopathology rate and correlates of the severity of the psychopathology. *Journal of Affective Disorders, 16,* 167–179.

Grigoroiu-Serbanescu, M., Christodorescu, D., Totoescu, A., & Jipescu, I. (1991). Depressive disorders and depressive personality traits in offspring aged 10–17 of bipolar and of normal parents. *Journal of Youth and Adolescence, 20,* 135–148.

Hamilton, M. (1960). A rating scale for depression. *Journal of Neurological and Neurosurgical Psychiatry, 23,* 56–62.

Hammen, C. (1991). *Depression runs in families: The social context of risk and resilience in children of depressed mothers.* New York: Springer-Verlag.

Hammen, C. (1992). Cognitive, life stress, and interpersonal approaches to a developmental psychopathology model of depression. *Development and Psychopathology, 4,* 191–208.

Hammen, C., & Brennan, P. A. (2001). Depressed adolescents of depressed and nondepressed mothers: Tests of an interpersonal impairment hypothesis. *Journal of Consulting and Clinical Psychology, 69,* 284–294.

Hammen, C., Burge, D., Burney, E., & Adrian, C. (1990). Longitudinal study of diagnoses in children of women with unipolar and bipolar affective disorder. *Archives of General Psychiatry, 47,* 1112–1117.

Hammen, C., Burge, D., Daley, S. E., Davila, J., Paley, B., & Rudolph, K. D. (1995). Interpersonal attachment cognitions and prediction of symptomatic responses to interpersonal stress. *Journal of Abnormal Psychology, 104,* 436–443.

Hammen, C., Burge, D., & Stansbury, K. (1990). Relationship of mother and child variables to child outcomes in a high-risk sample: A causal modeling analysis. *Developmental Psychology, 26,* 24–30.

Hammen, C., & Rudolph, K. D. (1996). Childhood mood disorders. In E. J. Mash & R. A. Barkley (Eds.), *Child psychopathology.* New York: Guilford Press.

Hammen, C., & Rudolph, K. D. (2003). Childhood mood disorders. In E. J. Mash & R. A. Barkley (Eds.), *Child psychopathology* (2nd ed., pp. 233–278). New York: Guilford Press.

Hammen, C., Shih, J., & Brennan, P. (2004). Intergenerational transmission of depression: Test of an interpersonal stress model in a community sample. *Journal of Consulting and Clinical Psychology, 72,* 511–522.

Hankin, B. L., & Abramson, L. Y. (2001). Development of gender differences in depression: An elaborated cognitive vulnerability-transactional stress theory. *Psychological Bulletin, 127,* 773–796.

Hankin, B. L., Abramson, L. Y., Moffitt, T. E., Silva, P. A., McGee, R., & Angell, K. E. (1998). Development of depression from preadolescence to young adulthood: Emerging gender differences in a 10–year longitudinal study. *Journal of Abnormal Psychology, 107,* 128–140.

Hankin, B. L., Abramson, L. Y., & Siler, M. (2001). A prospective test of the hopelessness theory of depression in adolescence. *Cognitive Therapy and Research, 25,* 607–632.

Hankin, B. L., Roberts, J., & Gotlib, I. H. (1997). Elevated self-standards and emotional distress during adolescence: Emotional specificity and gender differences. *Cognitive Therapy and Research, 21,* 663–679.

Harrington, R., Fudge, H., Rutter, M., Pickles, A., & Hill, J. (1990). Adult outcomes of childhood and adolescent depression: Psychiatric status. *Archives of General Psychiatry, 47,* 465–473.

Harrington, R., & Vostanis, P. (1995). Longitudinal perspectives and affective disorder in children and adolescents. In I. M. Goodyer (Ed.), *The depressed child and adolescent: Developmental and clinical perspectives* (pp. 311–341). New York: Cambridge University Press.

Harter, S., & Whitesell, N. R. (1996). Multiple pathways to self-reported depression and psychological adjustment among adolescents. *Development and Psychopathology, 8,* 761–777.

Hayward, C., Gotlib, I. H., Schraedley, P. K., & Litt, I. F. (1999). Ethnic differences in the association between pubertal status and symptoms of depression in adolescent girls. *Journal of Adolescent Health, 25,* 143–149.

Hayward, C., & Sanborn, K. (2002). Puberty and the emergence of gender differences in psychopathology. *Journal of Adolescent Health, 30,* 49–58.

Heim, C., & Nemeroff, C. B. (2001). The role of childhood trauma in the neurobiology of mood and anxiety disorders: Preclinical and clinical studies. *Biological Psychiatry, 49,* 1023–1039.

Herman-Stahl, M., & Petersen, A. C (1999). Depressive symptoms during adolescence: Direct and stress-buffering effects of coping, control beliefs, and family relationships. *Journal of Applied Developmental Psychology, 20,* 45–62.

Herzberg, D. S., Hammen, C., Burge, D., Daley, S. E., Davila, J., & Lindberg, N. (1998). Social competence as a predictor of chronic interpersonal stress. *Personal Relationships, 5,* 207–218.

Hilsman, R., & Garber, J. (1995). A test of the cognitive diathesis–stress model of depression in children: Academic stressors, attributional style, perceived competence, and control. *Journal of Personality and Social Psychology, 69,* 370–380.

Hofstra, M. B., van der Ende, J., & Verhulst, F. C. (2000). Continuity and change of psychopathology from childhood into adulthood: A 14–year follow-up study. *Journal of the Academy of Child and Adolescent Psychiatry, 39,* 850–858.

Hops, H., Lewinsohn, P. M., Andrews, J. A., & Roberts, R. E. (1990). Psychosocial correlates of depressive symptomatology among high school students. *Journal of Clinical Child Psychology, 3,* 211–220.

Hughes, C. W., Emslie, G. J., Crismon, M. L., Wagner, K. D., Birmaher, B., Geller, B., et al. (1999). The Texas Children's Medication Algorithm Project: Report of the Texas consensus conference panel on medication treatment of childhood major depressive disorder. *Journal of the American Academy of Child and Adolescent Psychiatry, 38,* 1442–1454.

Joiner, T. E., Coyne, J. C., & Blalock, J. (1999). On the interpersonal nature of depression: Overview and synthesis. In T. E. Joiner & J. C. Coyne (Eds.), *The interactional nature of depression.* Washington, DC: American Psychological Association.

Joiner, T. E., Katz, J., & Lew, A. S. (1997). Self-verification and depression among youth psychiatric inpatients. *Journal of Abnormal Psychology, 106,* 608–618.

Joiner, T. E., Metalsky, G. I., Katz, J., & Beach, S. R. H. (1999). Depression and excessive reassurance-seeking. *Psychological Inquiry, 10,* 269–278.

Kafantaris, V., Coletti, D. J., Dicker, R., Padula, G., & Pollack, S. (1998). Are childhood psychiatric histories of bipolar adolescents associated with family history, psychosis, and response to lithium treatment? *Journal of Affective Disorders, 51,* 153–164.

Kaminski, K. M., & Garber, J. (2002). Depressive spectrum disorders in adolescents: Episode duration and predictors of time to recovery. *Journal of the American Academy of Child and Adolescent Psychiatry, 41,* 410–418.

Kaslow, N. J., Adamson, L. B., & Collins, M. H. (2000). A developmental psychopathology perspective on the cognitive components of child and adolescent depression. In A. J. Sameroff, M. Lewis, & S. M. Miller (Eds.), *Handbook of developmental psychopathology* (2nd ed., pp. 491–510). New York: Kluwer/Plenum Press.

Kaslow, N. J., Deering, C. G., & Racusin, G. R. (1994). Depressed children and their families. *Clinical Psychology Review, 14,* 39–59.

Kaslow, N. J., McClure, E. B., & Connell, A. M. (2002). Treatment of depression in children and adolescents. In I. H. Gotlib & C. L. Hammen (Eds.), *Handbook of depression* (pp. 441–464). New York: Guilford Press.

Kaufman, J., Birmaher, B., Brent, D., Rao, U., Flynn, C., Moreci, P., et al. (1997). Schedule for Affective Disorders and Schizophrenia for School-Age Children—Present and Lifetime Version (K-SADS-PL): Initial reliability and validity data. *Journal of the American Academy of Child and Adolescent Psychiatry, 36,* 980–988.

Kaufman, J., Martin, A., King, R. A., & Charney, D. (2001). Are child-, adolescent-, and adult-onset depression one and the same disorder? *Biological Psychiatry, 49,* 980–1001.

Kazdin, A. E. (1994). Informant variability in the assessment of childhood depression. In W. M. Reynolds & H. F. Johnston (Eds.), *Handbook of depression in children and adolescents* (pp. 249–271). New York: Plenum Press.

Keller, M. B., Ryan, N. D., Strober, M., Klein, R. G., Kutcher, S. P., Birmaher, B., et al. (2001). Efficacy of paroxetine in the treatment of adolescent major depression: A randomized, controlled trial. *Journal of the American Academy of Child and Adolescent Psychiatry, 40,* 762–772.

Kendler, K. S. (1995). Adversity, stress and psychopathology: A psychiatric genetic perspective. *International Journal of Methods in Psychiatric Research, 5,* 163–170.

Kendler, K. S., & Gardner, C. (2001). Monozygotic twins discordant for major depression: A preliminary exploration of the role of environmental experiences in the aetiology and course of illness. *Psychological Medicine, 31,* 411–423.

Kendler, K. S., & Karkowski-Shuman, L. (1997). Stressful life events and genetic liability to major depression: Genetic control of exposure to the environment? *Psychological Medicine, 27,* 539–547.

Kendler, K. S., Neale, M. C., Kessler, R. C., Heath, A. C., & Eaves, L. J. (1993). A twin study of recent life events and difficulties. *Archives of General Psychiatry, 50,* 789–796.

Kessler, R. C., Avenevoli, S., & Merikangas, K. R. (2001). Mood disorders in children and adolescents: An epidemiologic perspective. *Biological Psychiatry, 49,* 1002–1014.

Kessler, R. C., McGonagle, K. A., Swartz, M., Blazer, D. G., & Nelson, C. B. (1993). Sex and depression in the National Comorbidity Survey: I. Lifetime prevalence, chronicity and recurrence. *Journal of Affective Disorders, 29,* 85–96.

Kessler, R. C., & Walters, E. E. (1998). Epidemiology of DSM-III-R major depression and minor depression among adolescents and young adults in the National Comorbidity Survey. *Depression and Anxiety, 7,* 3–14.

Klein, D. N., Depue, R. A., & Slater, J. F. (1985). Cyclothymia in the adolescent offspring of parents with bipolar affective disorder. *Journal of Abnormal Psychology, 94,* 115–127.

Klein, D. N., Lewinsohn, P. M., Rohde, P., Seeley, J. R., & Durbin, C. E. (2002). Clinical features of major depressive disorder in adolescents and their relatives: Impact on familial aggregation, implications for phenotype definition and specificity of transmission. *Journal of Abnormal Psychology, 111,* 98–106.

Klein, D. N., Lewinsohn, P. M., & Seeley, J. R. (1996). Hypomanic personality traits in a community sample of adolescents. *Journal of Affective Disorders, 38,* 135–143.

Klein, D. N., Lewinsohn, P. M., Seeley, J. R., & Rohde, P. (2001). A family study of major depressive disorder in a community sample of adolescents. *Archives of General Psychiatry, 58,* 13–20.

Kobak, R. R., & Ferenz-Gillies, R. (1995). Emotion regulation and depressive symptoms during adolescence: A functionalist perspective. *Development and Psychopathology, 7,* 183–192.

Kobak, R. R., Sudler, N., & Gamble, W. (1991). Attachment and depressive symptoms during adolescence: A developmental pathways analysis. *Development and Psychopathology, 3,* 461–474.

Kovacs, M. (1990). Comorbid anxiety disorders in childhood-onset depressions. In J. D. Maser & C. R. Cloninger (Eds.), *Comorbidity of mood and anxiety disorders* (pp. 272–281). Washington, DC: American Psychiatric Press.

Kovacs, M. (1992). *Children's Depression Inventory Manual.* North Tonawanda, NY: Multi-Health Systems.

Kovacs, M. (1996). Presentation and course of major depressive disorder during childhood and later years of the life span. *Journal of the American Academy of Child and Adolescent Psychiatry, 35,* 705–715.

Kroll, L., Harrington, R., Jayson, D., Fraser, J., & Gowers, S. (1996). Pilot study of continuation cognitive-behavioral therapy for major depression in adolescent psychiatric patients. *Journal of the American Academy of Child and Adolescent Psychiatry, 35,* 1156–1161.

Kutcher, S. P., Boulos, C., Ward, B., Marton, P., Simeon, J., Ferguson, H. B., et al. (1994). Response to desipramine treatment in adolescent depression: A fixed-dose, placebo-controlled trial. *Journal of the American Academy of Child and Adolescent Psychiatry, 33,* 686–694.

Kutcher, S. P., Robertson, H. A., & Bird, D. (1998). Premorbid functioning in adolescent onset bipolar I disorder: A preliminary report from an ongoing study. *Journal of Affective Disorders, 51,* 137–144.

Kye, C. H., Waterman, S. G., Ryan, N. D., Birmaher, B., Williamson, D. E., Iyengar, S., & Dachille, S. (1996). A randomized, controlled trial of amitriptyline in the acute treatment of adolescent major depression. *Journal of the American Academy of Child and Adolescent Psychiatry, 35,* 1139–1144.

Lapalme, M., Hodgins, S., & LaRoche, C. (1997). Children of parents with bipolar disorder: A meta-analysis of risk for mental disorders. *Canadian Journal of Psychiatry, 42,* 623–631.

Laursen, B. (1996). Closeness and conflict in adolescent peer relationships: Interdependence with friends and romantic partners. In W. M. Bukowski, A. F. Newcomb, & W. W. Hartup (Eds.), *The company they keep: Friendship in childhood and adolescence* (pp. 186–210). New York: Cambridge University Press.

Leaper, C., & Anderson, K. J. (1997). Gender development and heterosexual romantic relationships during adolescence. In S. Shulman & W. A. Collins (Eds.), *Romantic relationships in adolescence: Developmental perspectives* (New Directions for Child Development, No. 78, pp. 85–103). San Francisco: Jossey-Bass.

Lewinsohn, P. M. (1974). A behavioral approach to depression. In R. Friedman & M. Katz (Eds.), *The psychology of depression: Contemporary theory and research* (pp. 157–185). Washington, DC: Winston-Wiley.

Lewinsohn, P. M., Allen, N. B., Seeley, J. R., & Gotlib, I. H. (1999). First onset versus recurrence of depression: Differential processes of psychosocial risk. *Journal of Abnormal Psychology, 108,* 483–489.

Lewinsohn, P. M., Clarke, G. N., Seeley, J. R., & Rohde, P. (1994). Major depression in community adolescents: Age at onset, episode duration, and time to recurrence. *Journal of the American Academy of Child and Adolescent Psychiatry, 33,* 809–818.

Lewinsohn, P. M., & Essau, C. A. (2002). Depression in adolescents. In I. H. Gotlib & C. L. Hammen (Eds.), *Handbook of depression* (pp. 541–559). New York: Guilford Press.

Lewinsohn, P. M., Hops, H., Roberts, R. E., Seeley, J. R., & Andrews, J. A. (1993). Adolescent psychopathology: I. Prevalence and incidence of depression and other DSM-III-R disorders in high school students. *Journal of Abnormal Psychology, 102,* 133–144.

Lewinsohn, P. M., Joiner, T. E., & Rohde, P. (2001). Evaluation of cognitive diathesis–stress models in predicting major depressive disorder in adolescents. *Journal of Abnormal Psychology, 110,* 203–215.

Lewinsohn, P. M., Klein, D. N., & Seeley, J. R. (1995). Bipolar disorders in a community sample of older adolescents: Prevalence, phenomenology, comorbidity, and course. *Journal of the American Academy of Child and Adolescent Psychiatry, 34,* 454–463.

Lewinsohn, P. M., Roberts, R. E., Seeley, J. R., Rohde, P., Gotlib, I. H., & Hops, H. (1994). Adolescent psychopathology: II. Psychosocial risk factors for depression. *Journal of Abnormal Psychology, 103,* 302–315.

Lewinsohn, P. M., Rohde, P., Klein, D. N., & Seeley, J. R. (1999). Natural course of adolescent major depressive disorder: I. Continuity into young adulthood. *Journal of the American Academy of Child and Adolescent Psychiatry, 38,* 56–63.

Lewinsohn, P. M., Rohde, P., & Seeley, J. R. (1994). Psychosocial risk factors for future adolescent suicide attempts. *Journal of Consulting and Clinical Psychology, 62,* 297–305.

Lewinsohn, P. M., Rohde, P., & Seeley, J. R. (1995). Adolescent psychopathology: III. The clinical consequences of comorbidity. *Journal of the Academy of Child and Adolescent Psychiatry, 34,* 510–519.

Lewinsohn, P. M., Rohde, P., & Seeley, J. R. (1996). Adolescent suicidal ideation and attempts: Prevalence, risk factors, and clinical implications. *Clinical Psychology: Science and Practice, 3,* 25–46.

Lewinsohn, P. M., Rohde, P., & Seeley, J. R. (1998). Major depressive disorder in older adolescents: Prevalence, risk factors, and clinical implications. *Clinical Psychology Review, 18,* 765–794.

Lewinsohn, P. M., Rohde, P., Seeley, J. R., & Baldwin, C. L. (2001). Gender differences in suicide attempts from adolescence to young adulthood. *Journal of the Academy of Child and Adolescent Psychiatry, 40,* 427–434.

Lewinsohn, P. M., Striegel-Moore, R. H., & Seeley, J. R. (2000). Epidemiology and natural course of eating disorders in young women from adolescence to young adulthood. *Journal of the American Academy of Child and Adolescent Psychiatry, 39,* 1284–1292.

Little, S. A., & Garber, J. (1995). Aggression, depression, and stressful life events predicting peer rejection in children. *Development and Psychopathology, 7,* 845–856.

Lovejoy, C. M., Graczyk, P. A., O'Hare, E., & Neuman, G. (2000). Maternal depression and parenting behavior: A meta-analytic review. *Clinical Psychology Review, 20,* 561–592.

Maccoby, E. E. (1990). Gender and relationships: A developmental account. *American Psychologist, 45,* 513–520.

Main, M., Kaplan, N., & Cassidy, J. (1985). Security in infancy, childhood, and adulthood: A move to the level of representation. *Monographs of the Society for Research in Child Development, 50,* 66–104.

McClellan, J., McCurry, C., Snell, J., & DuBose, A. (1999). Early-onset psychotic disorders: Course and outcome over a 2–year period. *Journal of the Academy of Child and Adolescent Psychiatry, 38,* 1380–1388.

McClellan, J. M., & Werry, J. S. (2000). Introduction: Special section: Research psychiatric diagnostic interviews for children and adolescents. *Journal of the American Academy of Child and Adolescent Psychiatry, 39,* 19–27.

McElroy, S. L., Strakowski, S. M., West, S. A., Keck, P. E., & McConville, B. J. (1997). Phenomenology of adolescent and adult mania in hospitalized patients with bipolar disorder. *American Journal of Psychiatry, 154,* 44–49.

Michael, K. D., & Crowley, S. L. (2002). How effective are treatments for child and adolescent depression? A meta-analytic review. *Clinical Psychology Review, 22,* 247–269.

Monroe, S. M., Rohde, P., Seeley, J. R., & Lewinsohn, P. M. (1999). Life events and depression in adolescence: Relationship loss as a prospective risk factor for first onset of major depressive disorder. *Journal of Abnormal Psychology, 108,* 606–614.

Mufson, L., Weissman, M. M., Moreau, D., & Garfinkel, R. (1999). Efficacy of interpersonal psychotherapy for depressed adolescents. *Archives of General Psychiatry, 56,* 573–579.

Murphy, J. M., Laird, N. M., Monson, R. R., Sobol, A. M., & Leighton, A. H. (2000). A 40–year perspective on the prevalence of depression: The Stirling County Study. *Archives of General Psychiatry, 57,* 209–215.

Myers K., & Winters, N. C. (2002). Ten-year review of rating scales. II: Scales for internalizing disorders. *Journal of the American Academy of Child and Adolescent Psychiatry, 41,* 634–59.

Nelson, D. R., Hammen, C., Daley, S. E., Burge, D., & Davila, J. (2001). Sociotropic and autonomous personality styles: Contributions to chronic life stress. *Cognitive Therapy and Research, 25,* 61–76.

Nolen-Hoeksema, S. (2002). Gender differences in depression. In I. H. Gotlib & C. L. Hammen (Eds.), *Handbook of depression* (pp. 492–509). New York: Guilford Press.

Nolen-Hoeksema, S., & Girgus, J. S. (1994). The emergence of gender differences in depression during adolescence. *Psychological Bulletin, 115,* 424–443.

Nolen-Hoeksema, S., Girgus, J. S., & Seligman, M. E. P. (1992). Predictors and consequences of childhood depressive symptoms: A 5–year longitudinal study. *Journal of Abnormal Psychology, 101,* 405–422.

Pavlidis, K., & McCauley, E. (2001). Autonomy and relatedness in family interactions with depressed adolescents. *Journal of Abnormal Child Psychology, 29,* 11–21.

Pavuluri, N., Naylor, M., & Janicak, P. (2002). Recognition and treatment of pediatric bipolar disorder. *Contemporary Psychiatry, 7,* 2–10.

Petersen, A. C., Compas, B. E., Brooks-Gunn, J., Stemmler, M., Ey, S., & Grant, K. E. (1993). Depression in adolescence. *American Psychologist, 48,* 155–168.

Petersen, A. C., Sarigiani, P. A., & Kennedy, R. E. (1991). Adolescent depression: Why more girls? *Journal of Youth and Adolescence, 20,* 247–271.

Pine, D. S., Cohen, E., Cohen, P., & Brook, J. (1999). Adolescent depressive symptoms as predictors of adult depression: Moodiness or mood disorder? *American Journal of Psychiatry, 156,* 133–135.

Pine, D. S., Cohen, P., Gurley, D., Brook, J. S., & Ma, Y. (1998). The risk for early-adulthood anxiety and depressive disorders in adolescents with anxiety and depressive disorders. *Archives of General Psychiatry, 55,* 56–64.

Plotsky, P. M., Owens, M. J., & Nemeroff, C. B. (1998). Psychoneuroendocrinology of depression. *Psychoneuroendocrinology, 21,* 293–307.

Pomerantz, E. M., & Ruble, D. N. (1998). The role of maternal control in the development of sex differences in child self-evaluative factors. *Child Development, 69,* 458–478.

Pomerantz, E. M., & Rudolph, K. D. (2003). What ensues from emotional distress? Implications for competence estimation. *Child Development, 74,* 329–345.

Post, R. M. (1992). Transduction of psychosocial stress into the neurobiology of recurrent affective disorder. *American Journal of Psychiatry, 149,* 999–1010.

Poznanski, E. O., & Mokros, H. B. (1999). *Children's Depression Rating Scale—Revised (CDRS-R).* Los Angeles: Western Psychological Services.

Puig-Antich, J., & Chambers, W. (1978). *The Schedule for Affective Disorders and Schizophrenia for School-Age Children (Kiddie-SADS).* New York: State Psychiatric Institute.

Puig-Antich, J., Kaufman, J., Ryan, N. D., Williamson, D. E., Dahl, R. E., Lukens, E., et al. (1993). The psychosocial functioning and family environment of depressed adolescents. *Journal of the American Academy of Child and Adolescent Psychiatry, 32,* 244–253.

Radloff, L. S. (1977). The CES-D Scale: A self-report depression scale for research in the general population. *Applied Psychological Measurement, 1,* 385–401.

Rao, U., Hammen, C., & Daley, S. (1999). Continuity of depression during the transition to adulthood: A 5-year longitudinal study of young women. *Journal of the American Academy of Child and Adolescent Psychiatry, 38,* 908–915.

Rao, U., Ryan, N. D., Birmaher, B., Dahl, R. E., Williamson, D. E., Kaufman, J., et al. (1995). Unipolar depression in adolescents: Clinical outcomes in adulthood. *Journal of the American Academy of Child and Adolescent Psychiatry, 34,* 566–578.

Rehm, L. P. (1977). A self-control model of depression. *Behavior Therapy, 8,* 787–804.

Reich, W. (2000). Diagnostic Interview for Children and Adolescents (DICA). *Journal of the American Academy of Child and Adolescent Psychiatry, 39,* 59–66.

Reinecke, M. A., Ryan, N. E., & Dubois, D. L. (1998). Cognitive-behavioral therapy of depression and depressive symptoms during adolescence: A review and meta-analysis. *Journal of the American Academy of Child and Adolescent Psychiatry, 37,* 26–34.

Renouf, A. G., & Kovacs, M. (1994). Concordance between mothers' reports and children's self-reports of depressive symptoms: A longitudinal study. *Journal of the American Academy of Child and Adolescent Psychiatry, 33,* 208–216.

Rey, J. M., & Walter, G. (1997). Half a century of ECT use in young people. *American Journal of Psychiatry, 154,* 595–602.

Reynolds, W. M. (1986). *Reynolds Adolescent Depression Scale.* Odessa, FL: Psychological Assessment Resources.

Reynolds, W. M. (1994). Assessment of depression in children and adolescents by self-report questionnaires. In W. M. Reynolds & H. F. Johnston (Eds.), *Handbook of depression in children and adolescents* (pp. 209–234). New York: Plenum Press.

Reynolds, W. M., & Mazza, J. J. (1998). Reliability and validity of the Reynolds Adolescent Depression Scale with young adolescents. *Journal of School Psychology, 36,* 295–312.

Roberts, R. E., Lewinsohn, P. M., & Seeley, J. R. (1991). Screening for adolescent depression: A comparison of depression scales. *Journal of the American Academy of Child and Adolescent Psychiatry, 30,* 58–66.

Roberts, R. E., Roberts, C. R., & Chen, Y. R. (1997). Ethnocultural differences in prevalence of adolescent depression. *American Journal of Community Psychology, 25,* 95–110.

Robinson, N. S., Garber, J., & Hilsman, R. (1995). Cognitions and stress: Direct and moderating effects on depressive versus externalizing symptoms during the junior high school transition. *Journal of Abnormal Psychology, 104,* 453–463.

Rohde, P., Lewinsohn, P. M., & Seeley, J. R. (1990). Are people changed by the experience of having an episode of depression? A further test of the scar hypothesis. *Journal of Abnormal Psychology, 99,* 264–271.

Rossello, J., & Bernal, G. (1999). The efficacy of cognitive-behavioral and interpersonal treatments for depression in Puerto Rican adolescents. *Journal of Consulting and Clinical Psychology, 67,* 734–745.

Ruble, D. N., Greulich, F., Pomerantz, E. M., & Gochberg, B. (1993). The role of gender-related processes in the development of sex differences in self-evaluation and depression. *Journal of Affective Disorders, 29,* 97–128.

Rudolph, K. D. (2002). Gender differences in emotional responses to interpersonal stress during adolescence. *Journal of Adolescent Health, 30,* 3–13.

Rudolph, K. D., & Clark, A. G. (2001). Conceptions of relationships in children with depressive and aggressive symptoms: Social-cognitive distortion or reality? *Journal of Abnormal Child Psychology, 29,* 41–56.

Rudolph, K. D., & Hammen, C. (1999). Age and gender as determinants of stress exposure, generation, and reactions in youngsters: A transactional perspective. *Child Development, 70,* 660–677.

Rudolph, K. D., Hammen, C., & Burge, D. (1997). A cognitive-interpersonal approach to depressive symptoms in preadolescent children. *Journal of Abnormal Child Psychology, 25,* 33–45.

Rudolph, K. D., Hammen, C., Burge, D., Lindberg, N., Herzberg, D. S., & Daley, S. E. (2000). Toward an interpersonal life-stress model of depression: The developmental context of stress generation. *Development and Psychopathology, 12,* 215–234.

Rudolph, K. D., Kurlakowsky, K. D., & Conley, C. S. (2001). Developmental and social-contextual origins of depressive control-related beliefs and behavior. *Cognitive Therapy and Research, 25,* 447–475.

Rudolph, K. D., Lambert, S. F., Clark, A. G., & Kurlakowsky, K. D. (2001). Negotiating the transition to middle school: The role of self-regulatory processes. *Child Development, 72,* 929–946.

Rudolph, K. D., Laurent, J., Joiner, T. E., Catanzaro, S. J., Lambert, S. F., Osborne, L., et al. (2005). *Developmental considerations in anxiety and depression:*

The emergence of sex differences across early adolescence. Manuscript in preparation.

Rushton, J. L., Forcier, M., & Schectman, R. M. (2002). Epidemiology of depressive symptoms in the National Longitudinal Study of Adolescent Health. *Journal of the Academy of Child and Adolescent Psychiatry, 41,* 199–205.

Ryan, N. D. (1990). New research: Pharmacological treatment of adolescent depression. *Psychopharmacology Bulletin, 26,* 75–79.

Sallee, F. R., Vrindavanam, N. S., Deas-Nesmith, D., Carson, S. W., & Sethuraman, G. (1997). Pulse intravenous clomipramine for depressed adolescents: Double-blind, controlled trial. *American Journal of Psychiatry, 154,* 668–673.

Saylor, C. F., Finch, A. J., Baskin, C. H., Furey, W., & Kelly, M. M. (1984). Construct validity for measures of childhood depression: Application of multitrait–multimethod methodology. *Journal of Consulting and Clinical Psychology, 52, 977–985.*

Schraedley, P. K., Gotlib, I. H., & Hayward, C. (1999). Gender differences in correlates of depressive symptoms in adolescents. *Journal of Adolescent Health, 25,* 98–108.

Shaffer D., Fisher P., Lucas C. P., Dulcan M. K., & Schwab-Stone M. E. (2000). NIMH Diagnostic Interview Schedule for Children Version IV (NIMH DISC-IV): Description, differences from previous versions, and reliability of some common diagnoses. *Journal of the American Academy of Child and Adolescent Psychiatry 39,* 28–38.

Sheeber, L., & Sorenson, E. (1998). Family relationships of depressed adolescents: A multimethod assessment. *Journal of Clinical Child Psychology, 27,* 268–277.

Silberg, J. L., Pickles, A., Rutter, M., Hewitt, J., Simonoff, E., & Maes, H., et al. (1999). The influence of genetic factors and life stress on depression among adolescent girls. *Archives of General Psychiatry, 56,* 225–232.

Silberg, J. L., Rutter, M., Neale, M., & Eaves, L. (2001). Genetic moderation of environmental risk for depression and anxiety in adolescent girls. *British Journal of Psychiatry, 179,* 116–121.

Simmons, R. G., Burgeson, R., Carlton-Ford, S., & Blyth, D. A. (1987). The impact of cumulative change in early adolescence. *Child Development, 58,* 1220–1234.

Solomon, D. A., Keller, M. B., Leon, A. C., Mueller, T. I., Lavori, P. W., Shea, T., et al. (2000). Multiple recurrences of major depressive disorder. *American Journal of Psychiatry, 157,* 229–233.

Spence, S. H., Sheffield, J., & Donovan, C. (2002). Problem-solving orientation and attributional style: Moderators of the impact of negative life events on the development of depressive symptoms in adolescence? *Journal of Clinical Child and Adolescent Psychology, 31,* 219–229.

State, R. C., Altshuler, L. L., & Frye, M. A. (2002). Mania and attention deficit hyperactivity disorder in a prepubertal child: Diagnostic and treatment challenges. *American Journal of Psychiatry, 159,* 918–925.

Steinberg, L., & Silverberg, S. B. (1986). The vicissitudes of autonomy in early adolescence. *Child Development, 57,* 841–851.

Strober, M., & Carlson, G. (1982). Bipolar illness in adolescents with major depression: Clinical, genetic, and psychopharmacologic predictors in a three- to four-year prospective follow-up investigation. *Archives of General Psychiatry, 39,* 549–555.

Strober, M., Lampert, C., Schmidt, S., & Morrell, W. (1993). The course of major depressive disorder in adolescents: Recovery and risk of manic switching in a 24–month prospective, naturalistic follow-up of psychotic and non_psychotic subtypes. *Journal of the American Academy of Child and Adolescent Psychiatry, 32,* 34–42.

Strober, M., Schmidt-Lackner, S., Freeman, R., Bower, S., Lampert, C., & DeAntonio, M. (1995). Recovery and relapse in adolescents with bipolar affective illness: A five-year naturalistic, prospective follow-up. *Journal of the American Academy of Child and Adolescent Psychiatry, 34,* 724–731.

Sullivan, P. F., Neale, M. C., & Kendler, K. S. (2000). Genetic epidemiology of major depression: Review and meta-analysis. *American Journal of Psychiatry, 157,* 1552–1562.

Suomi, S. J. (1991). Adolescent depression and depressive symptoms: Insights from longitudinal studies with rhesus monkeys. *Journal of Youth and Adolescence, 20,* 273–287.

Susman, E. J., Dorn, L. D., & Chrousos, G. P. (1991). Negative affect and hormone levels in young adolescents: Concurrent and predictive perspectives. *Journal of Youth and Adolescence, 20,* 167–190.

Susman, E. J., Inoff-Germain, G. E., Nottelmann, E. D., Cutler, G. B., Loriaux, D. L., & Chrousos, G. P. (1987). Hormones, emotional dispositions and aggressive attributes in young adolescents. *Child Development, 58,* 1114–1134.

Susman, E. J., Nottelmann, E. D., Inoff, G. E., Dorn, L. D., Cutler, G. B., Loriaux, D. L., et al. (1985). The relation of relative hormone levels and physical development and social–emotional behavior in young adolescents. *Journal of Youth and Adolescence, 14,* 245–264.

Taylor, L., & Ingram, R. E. (1999). Cognitive reactivity and depressotypic information processing in children of depressed mothers. *Journal of Abnormal Psychology, 108,* 202–210.

Teti, D. M., Gelfand, D. M., Messinger, D. S., & Isabella, R. (1995). Maternal depression and the quality of early attachment: An examination of infants, preschoolers, and their mothers. *Developmental Psychology, 31,* 364–376.

Thapar, A., & McGuffin, P. (1994). A twin study of depressive symptoms in childhood. *British Journal of Psychiatry, 165,* 259–265.

Thase, M. E., Jindal, R., & Howland, R. H. (2002). Biological aspects of depression. In I. H. Gotlib & C. L.

Hammen (Eds.), *Handbook of depression* (pp. 192–218). New York: Guilford Press.

Thomsen, P. H., Moller, L. L., Dehlholm, B., & Brask, B. H. (1992). Manic-depressive psychosis in children younger than 15 years: A register-based investigation of 39 cases in Denmark. *Acta Psychiatrica Scandinavica, 85*, 401–406.

Turner, J. E., & Cole, D. A. (1994). Developmental differences in cognitive diatheses for child depression. *Journal of Abnormal Child Psychology, 22*, 15–32.

Verhulst, F. C., van der Ende, J., Ferdinand, R. F., & Kasius, M. C. (1997). The prevalence of DSM-III-R diagnoses in a national sample of Dutch adolescents. *Archives of General Psychiatry, 54*, 329–336.

Vernberg, E. M. (1990). Psychological adjustment and experiences with peers during early adolescence: Reciprocal, incidental, or unidirectional relationships? *Journal of Abnormal Child Psychology, 18*, 187–198.

Wade, T. J., Cairney, J., & Pevalin, D. J. (2002). Emergence of gender differences in depression during adolescence: National panel results from three countries. *Journal of the Academy of Child and Adolescent Psychiatry, 41*, 190–198.

Wagner, B. M., & Compas, B. E. (1990). Gender, instrumentality, and expressivity: Moderators of the relation between stress and psychological symptoms during adolescence. *American Journal of Community Psychology, 18*, 383–406.

Wallace, J., Schneider, T., & McGuffin, P. (2002). Genetics of depression. In I. H. Gotlib & C. L. Hammen (Eds.), *Handbook of depression* (pp. 169–191). New York: Guilford Press.

Weissman, M. M., Wolk, S., Goldstein, R. B., Moreau, D., Adams, P., & Greenwald, S., et al. (1999). Depressed adolescents grown up. *Journal of the American Medical Association, 281*, 1707–1713.

Weissman, M. M., Wolk, S., Wickramaratne, P. J., Goldstein, R., Adams, P., Greenwald, S., et al. (1999). Children with prepubertal-onset major depressive disorder and anxiety grown up. *Archives of General Psychiatry, 56*, 794–801.

Weisz, J. R., Rudolph, K. D., Granger, D. A., & Sweeney, L. (1992). Cognition, competence, and coping in child and adolescent depression: Research findings, developmental concerns, therapeutic implications. *Development and Psychopathology, 4*, 627–653.

Weisz, J. R., Southam-Gerow, M. A., & McCarty, C. A. (2001). Control-related beliefs and depressive symptoms in clinic-referred children and adolescents: Developmental differences and model specificity. *Journal of Abnormal Psychology, 110*, 97–109.

Weller, E. B., & Weller, R. A. (2000). Treatment options in the management of adolescent depression. *Journal of Affect Disorders, 61*(Suppl.), 23–28.

Wichstrom, L. (1999). The emergence of gender difference in depressed mood during adolescence: The role of intensified gender socialization. *Developmental Psychology, 35*, 232–245.

Williamson, D. E., Birmaher, B., Anderson, B. P., Al-Shabbout, M., & Ryan, N. D. (1995). Stressful life events in depressed adolescents: The role of dependent events during the depressive episode. *Journal of the American Academy of Child and Adolescent Psychiatry, 34*, 591–598.

Windle, M. (1994). A study of friendship characteristics and problem behaviors among middle adolescents. *Child Development, 65*, 1764–1777.

Zahn-Waxler, C., Klimes-Dougan, B., & Slattery, M. (2000). Internalizing problems of childhood and adolescence: Prospects, pitfalls, and progress in understanding the development of anxiety and depression. *Development and Psychopathology, 12*, 443–466.

Zahn-Waxler, C., Kochanska, G., Krupnick, J., & McKnew, D. (1990). Patterns of guilt in children of depressed and well mothers. *Developmental Psychology, 26*, 51–59.

9

Suicidal and Nonsuicidal Self-Harm Behaviors

David B. Goldston
Stephanie Sergent Daniel
Elizabeth Mayfield Arnold

Suicidal behaviors and nonsuicidal self-harm behaviors have been the focus of much attention as they have been identified as serious but preventable health problems. After accidents and homicides, suicide is the third leading cause of death among 15- to 24-year-olds (Anderson, 2002). Adolescent suicide attempts are considerably more common than deaths by suicide and are associated with high risk for psychiatric disorder (Gould et al., 1998; Kovacs, Goldston, & Gatsonis, 1993) as well as other risk behaviors (Burge, Felts, Chenier, & Parrillo, 1995; DuRant, Krowchuk, Kreiter, Sinal, & Woods, 1999). Not only are suicide attempts associated with increased likelihood of eventual death by suicide (Lonnqvist & Ostano, 1991), increased risk of repeat suicidal behavior (Goldston et al., 1999; Leon, Friedman, Sweeney, Brown, & Mann, 1989), and risk of physical injury, but suicidality is also one of primary reasons for child psychiatric emergencies and psychiatric hospitalizations (Peterson, Zhang, Santa Lucia, King, & Lewis, 1996). The importance of trying to better understand, prevent, and offer treatment for suicidal behaviors has been emphasized in the Sur-

geon General's *Call to Action to Prevent Suicide* (U.S. Public Health Service, 1999), the National Strategy for Suicide Prevention (U.S. Public Health Service, 2001), and the Institute of Medicine report, *Reducing Suicide: A National Imperative* (Goldsmith, Pellmar, Kleinman, & Bunney, 2002). Recent research has focused more on adolescent suicidal behavior than on adolescent nonsuicidal self-harm behavior, but available data do tend to indicate that nonsuicidal self-harm behavior is associated with high rates of psychological distress as well (Nixon, Cloutier, & Aggarwal, 2002).

BRIEF HISTORICAL CONTEXT

Suicidal behavior, of course, has not always been considered treatable or preventable, and, indeed, attitudes about suicide have changed markedly over the centuries. Historical attitudes and approaches to dealing with the phenomenon of suicide and suicidal behavior have been richly described by Alvarez (1971) in *The Savage God: A Study of Suicide* and Minois (1995/1999) in *History of Suicide: Voluntary*

Death in Western Culture. The ancient Greeks considered suicide to be acceptable in specific circumstances, such as in the context of grief or to avoid dishonor (Alvarez, 1971). However, suicide was not tolerated when it was thought to be disrespectful to the gods, and Aristotle argued against suicide on the grounds that it resulted in the loss of a potentially productive citizen (Alvarez, 1971). In some parts of ancient Greece, individuals could ask permission of the officials to attempt suicide, and stores of poison were actually kept on hand for such occurrences (Alvarez, 1971).

The Romans considered suicide to be reflective of honor and principle (Alvarez, 1971). Suicide was not treated as something to be feared and was not punished in cases such as illness or "lunacy" (Alvarez, 1971). Nonetheless, not all cases of suicide were acceptable to the Romans (Alvarez, 1971). For example, a slave who attempted to kill himself was punished because the act was interpreted as potentially depriving the owner of property (Alvarez, 1971).

Early Christians valued martyrdom and, by extension, suicide, as a way to achieve eternal life (Alvarez, 1971; Minois, 1995/1999). However, later Christians focused on suicide as contrary to the prohibition against murder in the Old Testament (Alvarez, 1971; Minois, 1995/1999). Individuals who were not Christian during the Middle Ages were noted to kill themselves to avoid persecution during the Crusades (Minois, 1995/1999).

From the time of the Renaissance through the 19th century, attitudes about suicide were mixed. On the one hand, during the Renaissance, there was greater recognition and discussion of suicide, as eloquently evidenced in Shakespeare's passage in *Hamlet*, "To be or not to be" (Minois, 1995/1999). In the 17th and 18th centuries, there was greater tolerance regarding suicide among the aristocracy in England and Europe and greater recognition of the association of suicide with psychiatric or physical problems (Minois, 1995/1999). During the late 18th century, there also were increased descriptions and reports of romantic suicides, particularly among young people (Minois, 1995/1999). On the other hand, except for a period of decriminalization in the late 18th century, suicide often was still considered sinful and against the law, and it was associated with punishment such as desecration of the bodies of suicide victims (Minois, 1995/1999).

In the 19th century, there also was some consideration of whether publicity about suicide in the press had any effect on individuals thought to be vulnerable to suicidal behavior (Minois, 1995/1999). Durkheim (1897/1951) also published the book *Suicide*, which described, from a sociological and statistical analysis, the phenomenon of suicide and the role that various facets of society play in suicidal behavior.

In the early 20th century, Freud described suicide as a manifestation of anger or aggression that was directed inwardly, and he wrote about the death instinct (Minois, 1995/1999). In the latter half of the 20th century, there was greater consideration of fact that suicide and suicidal behaviors often occurred in the context of treatable psychiatric problems, primarily, but not exclusively, depression. Attention began to be focused on the biological substrates or correlates of suicidal behavior. The possibilities of suicide prevention and treatment, familial risk of suicidal behavior, and suicide contagion all received increased attention as well.

CONCEPTUALIZING THE DISORDER IN ADOLESCENTS

Suicidal behavior in adolescents can be considered at several different levels. For example, suicidal behavior can be viewed as a poor outcome in and of itself, with increased risk for repeat suicide attempts and death by suicide. In this regard, Lewinsohn, Rohde, and Seeley (1996) have noted that suicidality can be conceptualized as a continuum ranging from thoughts of death and dying to attempted suicide and death by suicide. Suicidal behavior also can be viewed as a symptom of other psychiatric disorders and psychiatric distress, or as one of a constellation of risk taking and impulsive, or potentially self-destructive, behaviors. In this context, Lewinsohn and colleagues (1995) have described the theoretical interrelationship between different life-affirming and life-threatening behaviors.

As described later, adolescent suicidal and nonsuicidal self-harm behavior also often occurs in the context of both proximal and distal risk factors (Moscicki, 1999). Proximal risk factors for suicidal behavior are often of a legal/disciplinary or interpersonal nature (Beautrais, Joyce, & Mulder, 1997). Volatility in interpersonal relationships can be particularly marked for some adolescents engaging in their first sexual or serious relationships (or facing the loss of these relationships) and may pose particular risk when there are few other positive or few adequate sources of social support, or a perception of lack of control over various aspects of one's life. Family difficulties also are associated with suicidal behavior among preadolescents and adolescents (Asarnow, 1992; Asarnow, Carlson, & Guthrie, 1987; Hollis, 1996), an issue that is compounded by the fact that younger youth in particular are still dependent on their parents. Adolescence also is a period in which youth are at higher risk for sexual abuse and/or may be grappling with issues regarding sexual orientation. Sexual abuse has been noted to be a risk factor for both suicidal behavior and nonsuicidal self-harm behavior (Briere & Gil, 1998; Wagner, 1997), and suicidal behavior has been noted to be more common among youth who are gay, lesbian, and bisexual (Garofalo, Wolf, Wissow, Woods, & Goodman, 1999).

NEED FOR DEVELOPMENTAL PSYCHOPATHOLOGY FRAMEWORK

There are several reasons for conceptualizing adolescent suicidal behavior in a developmental psychopathology framework. First, suicide attempts are relatively rare prior to early adolescence, but rates of suicide attempts increase rapidly thereafter (Lewinsohn, Rohde, Seeley, & Baldwin, 2001). There is some evidence that gender differences emerge over time, with rates for female adolescents increasing more than for male adolescents during early to midadolescence, and then decreasing more rapidly than male adolescents in late adolescence, with the net result that the rates for males and females converge as individuals enter young adulthood (Lewinsohn et al., 2001). There also are developmental trends in the rates of suicide. For example, suicide is very rare prior to the age of 15 but increases, particularly for males, in the 15–19-year-old age range; moreover, the yearly prevalence of suicide is approximately 55% higher for 20- to 24-year-olds than for 15- to 19-year-olds (Anderson, 2002).

The second reason for conceptualizing adolescent suicidal behavior in a developmental psychopathology framework is the fact that a substantial number of suicide attempts and suicide deaths occur in the context of diagnosable affective disorders (Gould et al., 1998; Kovacs et al., 1993; Shaffer et al., 1996). These diagnosable affective disorders, in turn, have increased prevalence from childhood to adolescence to young adulthood (Lewinsohn et al., 2001). In addition, it is possible that the relationship between various psychiatric disorders (or the course of those disorders) and suicidal behavior may change (i.e., strengthen or diminish) as youth grow older.

A third reason for invoking a developmental psychopathology framework for suicidal behavior is that suicidal behavior is not only a problem in its own right but also portends risk for subsequent suicidal behavior and other poor nonsuicidal outcomes (Spirito, Boergers, & Donaldson, 2000). As described later in the chapter, nonsuicidal self-harm behavior has been noted to have addictive qualities (Nixon et al., 2002), and suicidal behaviors have been suggested to increase the likelihood of recurrent suicidal behavior (Goldston et al., 1999). Behavioral contingencies and sensitization processes that occur over time may account for increasing risk for future suicidal behavior as a function of prior experience with suicidal behavior.

One last reason to consider adolescent suicide behavior in a developmental psychopathology framework is that impulsivity is often noted to be associated with suicidal behavior (Horesh, Gothelf, Ofek, Weizman, & Apter, 1999; Pfeffer, Hurt, Peskin, & Siefker, 1995). Although no empirical data of which we are aware suggest that adolescent suicide attempts or suicides are any more impulsive than those of adults, there are suggestions that impulsivity is at its highest point during early adolescence among high-risk youth (Tiet, Wasserman, Loeber, McReynolds, & Miller, 2001), and at least a subset of adolescents often engage impulsively in a number of other high-risk (and potentially lethal) behaviors.

Other purported risk and protective factors for suicidal behavior may change in their influence over the course of development as well. For example, suicidal behavior among adolescents is often precipitated by conflict in the family. Particularly for younger adolescents, these family stresses may be associated with a degree of "role captivity" (Pearlin, 1983) in which there may be little opportunity to escape sources of distress, particularly those associated with family dynamics (Haggerty, Sherrod, Garmezy, & Rutter, 1994). As adolescents grow older, however, they broaden their network of supportive relationships outside the family, often have greater mobility, and eventually may move out of the home, all of which may afford some protection against the stresses of family conflict and therein buffer against psychiatric problems and suicidal behavior.

DESCRIPTION OF THE PHENOMENON IN ADOLESCENTS, CORE FEATURES, AND ASSOCIATED CHARACTERISTICS

The primary methods for making suicide attempts are ingestion and cutting (Brent, 1987; Lewinsohn et al., 1996; Spirito, Stark, Fristad, Hart, & Owens-Stively, 1987). However, Lewinsohn et al. (1996) also found that more than half of adolescent male's suicide attempts were made by methods other than overdose and cutting, such as gun use, hanging, and other means. In contrast to methods of nonlethal suicide attempts, data from the Centers for Disease Control (CDC; 2002) indicate that 57% of suicides in the year 2000 by individuals 15–24 were by firearms, 28.4% were by hanging or suffocation, 7.6% were by poisoning or overdose, 2.7% were by falls or jumping, and the remaining 4.5% were by other means. There has been an increase in the proportion of suicides by young people by hanging or suffocation (from 18.7%) and a decrease in the proportion of suicides by firearms (from 65.0%) since 1990 (CDC, 2002). Suicides by females ages 15–24 involve less use of firearms than those by males (39.3% vs. 59.7%), and more use of poisoning (18.6% vs. 5.8%; CDC, 2002). Despite these differences, firearms are still the leading method for suicide-related deaths among both genders.

Particularly for adolescents living with family members, who are often at home, suicide attempts may be interrupted while they are in progress. In adult patients, it has been found that such interrupted suicidal behavior actually is associated with a higher risk of eventual death by suicide than nonlethal suicide attempts that were not interrupted (Steer, Beck, Garrison, & Lester, 1988). There are a variety of possible explanations for such findings (e.g., clinicians taking less seriously the interrupted suicide attempts; Steer et al., 1988), but at the very least, these findings underscore the fact that interrupted suicidal behavior should be treated very seriously by clinicians.

There are some suggestions that suicidal tendencies also may be manifested indirectly as risk-taking behavior or refusal to take the steps necessary for taking care of one's health. For example, among youth with insulin-dependent diabetes mellitus, suicidal thoughts have been noted to be associated with serious noncompliance with the medical regimen (Goldston, Kovacs, Ho, Parrone, & Stiffler, 1994; Goldston et al., 1997). Victim-precipitated homicides—that is, instances in which someone provokes actions (e.g., by a policeman or gang member) to bring an end to their lives (Wolfgang, 1959)—also have been suggested to be a manifestation of suicidality (Klinger, 2001).

Suicide attempts by definition are associated with at least some desire to die, but most suicidal behavior is associated with mixed motives and ambivalence. Other motivations sometimes associated with suicidal behavior include "to get relief," "to escape," or "to make people sorry" or "get back at them" (Boergers, Spirito, & Donaldson, 1998; Hawton, Cole, O'Grady, & Osborn, 1982; Kienhorst, De Wilde, Diekstra, & Wolters, 1995).

The most common method of nonsuicidal self-harm behavior is cutting on oneself (Ross & Heath, 2002). Other methods associated with nonsuicidal self-harm include hitting, pinching, scratching, or biting oneself (Ross & Heath, 2002). Motivations associated with nonsuicidal behavior among adolescents include to "cope with feelings of depression," "release unbearable tension," "cope with nervousness or fear," "express frustration," "express anger/revenge," "feel pain in one area when other pain . . . is unbearable," "distract (oneself) from unpleasant memories," "punish self," "stop suicidal ideation or attempt," "stop feeling alone and empty," "have control," and "stop feeling numb/out of touch" (Nixon et al., 2002).

DIAGNOSTIC CRITERIA AND CONSIDERATIONS

In terms of classification, suicidal behavior and nonsuicidal self-harm behavior are typically considered to be symptoms of other diagnoses or psychiatric disorders (the fact that some suicides appear to occur without preexisting psychopathology notwithstanding; Brent, Perper, Moritz, & Allman, 1993). According to DSM-

IV-TR (American Psychiatric Association [APA], 2000), one of the criteria for a major depressive episode is the presence of recurring thoughts of death, recurrent suicidal ideation without a plan, suicidal ideation with a plan, or suicide attempt. Despite the fact that suicide attempts and suicidal ideation also often occur in the context of dysthymic disorder, suicidal ideation or attempts are not part of the diagnostic criteria for dysthymic disorder. Rather, hopelessness, the psychological state that often is persistent and associated with suicidal ideation or attempts, is considered one of the criteria for dysthymia. Suicidal behavior or threats or nonsuicidal self-harm behavior also are among the criteria for borderline personality disorder.

DSM-IV does not provide operational definitions for suicidal behavior. According to the nomenclature recommended by O'Carroll, Berman, Maris, and Moscicki (1996), suicide is defined as "death from injury, poisoning, or suffocation where there is evidence (either explicit or implicit) that the injury was self-inflicted and that the decedent intended to kill himself/herself" (pp. 246–247). A suicide attempt is defined as "a potentially self-injurious behavior with a nonfatal outcome, for which there is evidence (either explicit or implicit) that the person intended at some non-zero level to kill himself/herself. A suicide attempt may or may not result in injuries" (p. 247). Suicidal ideation is defined as "any self-reported thoughts of engaging in suicide related behavior" (p. 247). By extension, self-harm or self-injurious behaviors not associated with any desire to kill oneself (e.g., behaviors engaged in solely for the purpose of relieving stress or pain) are not considered suicidal.

Occasionally, in the past, the term "suicidal gesture" has been used to describe particular forms of suicidal behavior. This term has been used to refer to behavior of low suicide intent or of low medical lethality, suicidal behavior thought to be manipulative or instrumental in intent, behavior thought to "resemble" or be part of a threat to engage in suicidal behavior, and nonsuicidal self-harm behavior (Goldston, 2003). Unfortunately, this term also is sometimes used in a dismissive manner to refer to suicidal behaviors (Goldston, 2003). Because of the multiple and often imprecise ways in which the term "suicide gesture" has been used in the past, the term is not a recommended descriptor referring to suicidal behavior (Berman, Jobes, & Silverman, 2005; Goldston, 2003).

EPIDEMIOLOGY

Prevalence

Suicide has been noted to be a major health care and mental health problem in society for most age groups. As mentioned at the beginning of this chapter, suicide is the third leading cause of death among persons between the ages of 10 and 24 in the United States (Anderson, 2002). The prevalence of suicide increases from childhood to adolescence, with rates of 1.5, 8.2, and 12.8 per 100,000 for 10- to 14-year-olds, 15- to 19-year-olds, and 20- to 24-year-olds, respectively. It should be noted that estimates of the prevalence of suicide may be conservative insofar as suicide is sometimes misclassified as accidental death or undetermined death (Mohler & Earls, 2001).

Since 1995, there has been an overall decrease in the rate of suicide deaths among young people, primarily among males (National Center for Health Statistics [NCHS], 2002). Specifically, the rates of suicide among males ages 15–24 declined from 22.5/100,000 to 17.4/100,000 from 1995 to 2000, whereas the rates for females declined from 3.7/100,000 to 3.0/100,000 (NCHS, 2002). Nonetheless, contemporary rates of suicide among 15- to 24-year-olds in the United States are still considerably higher than they were in the 1950s (NCHS, 2002). There has been considerable speculation about the possible explanations for the recent decrease in rates of suicide, including the greater recognition of depression and prescription of medications (specifically, selective serotonin reuptake inhibitors) for depression, decreases in substance use among young people, proportionately decreased use of firearms in suicide attempts, and socioeconomic factors such as the favorable economic climate of the United States during the aforementioned period of time (Berman, 2003; Shaffer, Pfeffer, & Workgroup on Quality Issues, 2001).

Despite much publicity and concern about school-related violence in the aftermath of the Columbine shootings, homicide–suicide initiated by young people is uncommon, particularly in school settings. Indeed, the annual rate of school-related violent deaths in the United States is .068/100,000 (Anderson et al., 2001). Of the school-related violent death events in the United States identified between 1994 and 1999, 11 of the 220 (5%) were homicide–suicides (Anderson et al., 2001). Most joint instances of homicide and suicide tend to occur in the family (Barraclough & Harris, 2002) and are not initiated by young people.

Rates of suicidal ideation and attempts are also sometimes difficult to determine because of differences in definitions of key terms (Meehan, Lamb, Saltzman, & O'Carroll, 1992). In addition, parents often are unaware of the suicidal behavior of their offspring (Breton, Tousignant, Bergeron, & Berthiaume, 2002; Klimes-Dougan, 1998; Velez & Cohen, 1988; Walker, Moreau, & Weissman, 1990). Prior to adolescence, suicide attempts are relatively uncommon, with a prevalence of less than 1% for 5- to 11-year-olds (Lewinsohn et al., 2001). Self-report data from adolescents collected via the Youth Risk Behavior Survey by the CDC indicated that 8.8% of high school students in the United States attempted suicide in the last year, 14.8% made a specific plan to attempt suicide, and 19% reported that they "seriously considered" attempting suicide (Grunbaum et al., 2002).

There have been few investigations of the prevalence of nonsuicidal self-harm behavior (not associated with developmental disabilities or psychosis) in adolescents in the general population. In an adult sample, Briere and Gil (1998) estimated that approximately 4% of their adult community sample had engaged in self-mutilation in the last half year. Garrison, Addy, McKeown, and Cuffe (1993) found that approximately 2–3% of adolescents engaged in nonsuicidal self-harm behavior. Rates of cutting have been noted to be considerably higher among adolescents in clinically ascertained samples, up to 61% in adolescent inpatient psychiatric settings (DiClemente, Ponton, & Hartley, 1991). The degree of overlap between nonsuicidal self-harm behaviors and suicidal behavior among adolescents in the community has not yet been well documented.

Sex Differences

Sex differences have been consistently noted in suicide and suicidal behavior. The ratio of male to female suicide deaths is 3.8:1 for 10- to 14-year-olds, and 4.7:1 for 15- to 19-year-olds (Anderson, 2002). The ratio increases to 6.7:1 for individuals between the ages of 20 and 24 years (Anderson, 2002). The increase in suicide among young people from the 1950s through the 1990s was primarily attributable to increases in suicides among males. Specifically, the rate of suicide among males ages 15–24 was 6.5/100,000 in 1950 but was 18.5/100,000 in 1998 (NCHS, 2002). By contrast, the rate for females in the same age range was 2.6/100,000 in 1950 and 3.3/100,000 in 1998 (NCHS, 2002).

Sex differences emerge in the opposite direction for attempted suicide. In the nationwide survey using the Youth Risk Behavior Survey, it was found for grades 9–11 that girls were more likely than boys to have felt sad or hopeless for at least 2 weeks, to have seriously considered suicide, and to have made a suicide plan in the last year (Grunbaum et al., 2002). Among white non-Hispanic and Hispanic populations, girls also attempted suicide more than boys; the same trend was more modest and not statistically reliable for black individuals (Grunbaum et al., 2002).

Complementary findings have been reported from a large community-based longitudinal study. Prior to age 12, there are few gender differences in attempted suicide (Lewinsohn et al., 2001). From age 12 through mid- to late adolescence, girls tend to attempt suicide for the first time more than boys (Lewinsohn et al., 2001). Lewinsohn and colleagues (2001) found that as of young adulthood, gender differences in incidence of suicide attempts tend to dissipate. When focusing on the prevalence in three different age groups (5–11, 12–18, 19–23), Lewinsohn and colleagues reported that females consistently had higher rates of attempts at all age groups than boys, but the differences were found to be statistically reliable only for the 12- to 18-year-olds (i.e., the group with the highest number of attempts). Other sources of data from community studies (including the Epidemiologic Catchment Area and National Comorbidity Studies in the United States) have indicated that by adulthood, women tend to attempt suicide more than men (Weissman et al., 1999).

In clinical samples of adolescents, females tend to engage in nonsuicidal self-harm behavior at considerably higher rates than males; for example, in one study of self-harm patients recruited from inpatient and partial hospitalization settings, 36 of 42 subjects were female (Nixon et al., 2002). However, it should be noted that at least one study of self-mutilation among adults in the community has failed to document sex differences (Briere & Gil, 1998).

Social Class and Family Structure

Multiple studies have demonstrated that lethal and nonlethal suicidal behavior among young people is more common when youth have lost a parent or do not live in two-parent households, although the effect is sometimes modest (Agerbo, Nordentoft, & Mortensen, 2002; Blum et al., 2000; Weitoft, Hjern, Haglund, & Rosen, 2003). Based on data from a Swedish sample, Weitoft and colleagues (2003) found that the effects of single- versus two-parent households were in part a function of socioeconomic differences between the two groups. Indeed, Blum and colleagues (2000) also found a modest relationship between income and suicidal behavior in younger but not older adolescents. Kerfoot, Dyer, Harrington, and Woodham (1996) similarly found that adolescents who overdosed were more likely to be receiving public benefits than psychiatric outpatients and community controls. In a Danish sample, Agerbo and colleagues (2002) found that the effects of socioeconomic status dissipated after controlling for parental psychiatric history.

A clear relationship between socioeconomic status and nonsuicidal self-harm among children and adolescents has not yet been demonstrated. Unfortunately, many of the potentially informative studies have focused on deliberate self-harm without consideration of whether the behavior was nonsuicidal or associated with suicidal intentions (e.g., Gunnell, Shepherd, & Evans, 2000).

Ethnicity and Culture

In the United States, the rate of suicide is highest for American Indians and lowest for individuals of Asian descent and Pacific Islanders (Anderson, 2002). Specifically, for 15- to 19-year-olds, the rates of suicide (per 100,000) for different racial/ethnic groups are as follows: white, non-Hispanic: 8.9, black, non-Hispanic: 5.9, Hispanic: 6.2, Asian/Pacific Islander: 6.1, American Indian: 18.4 (Anderson, 2002). However, it should be noted that suicide rates among American Indians differ depending on tribal affiliation.

Although suicide has historically been more common among white relative to black adolescents, from 1980 to 1995, rates of suicide deaths among black youth increased 114%, more than the increase in rates for white youth (CDC, 1998). The great majority of this increase was due to suicide by males. In addition, suicides due to firearms were linked to 96% of this increase. Over the last several years, the increasing trends in suicide have reversed some-

what, with a 21% decrease in suicide rates among black males from 1995 to 2000 (NCHS, 2002). There is a need to examine whether risk factors are different for black as compared to white youths (CDC, 1998), and to better understand the various factors associated with these secular trends.

Using a school survey with middle school (grades 6–8) students, Roberts, Chen, and Roberts (1997) compared differences for nine different ethnic groups in the rates of suicidal ideation, thoughts about suicide occurring in the past 2 weeks, previous suicide plans, and suicide attempts. Pakistani American, Mexican American, Vietnamese American, and mixed ancestry adolescents had higher rates of suicidal behaviors on at least one of the outcome variables under study relative to Anglo Americans. Chinese youths were reported to be at lower risk for all of the outcome variables under study. By contrast, in the National Longitudinal Study of Adolescent Health, Blum and colleagues (2000) did not find racial/ethnic differences in suicidal thoughts or attempts at grades 7–8. However, such differences were found for grades 9–12; specifically, white and Hispanic youths were more likely to report suicidal thoughts or attempts than black youths. Data from the nationwide Youth Risk Behavior Survey have indicated that Hispanic females have higher rates of suicide attempts than either black or white (non-Hispanic) females (Grunbaum et al., 2002).

Some of the differences in rates of suicidal behaviors among different ethnic groups may be due to factors such as socioeconomic status, willingness to admit to or report suicidal behavior, acculturation, recency of immigration, conflicting role expectations in different cultures, and use of language. There also may be differences in the classification of suicide deaths (vs. accidental deaths or undetermined deaths) among different race/ethnicity and age groups (Mohler & Earls, 2001).

The research has consistently shown that those who engage in nonsuicidal self-harm are most typically white. For example, in two samples, one clinical and one of self-identified self-mutilators from the general population, studied by Briere and Gil (1998), both groups were predominantly white (81% and 91% respectively). The reasons for high rates of nonsuicidal self-harm among whites and, conversely, the underrepresentation of nonwhites in clinical samples of self-harming individuals are not clear.

DEVELOPMENTAL COURSE AND OUTCOME

There has been considerable interest in the developmental course for suicidal behavior among youths. Pfeffer and colleagues have noted that children who demonstrate suicidal behavior prior to puberty are at increased risk for suicidal behavior in adolescence (Pfeffer et al., 1991, 1993). Goldston and colleagues (1999) similarly have found that suicidal behavior prior to or during adolescence is associated with increased risk of repeat suicide attempts. A relationship between early-onset depressive disorders and both contemporaneous and subsequent suicidal behavior also has been noted (Harrington et al., 1994; Kovacs et al., 1993; Rao, Weissman, Martin, & Hammond, 1993). It is possible that depression is linked to later suicidal behaviors because of the high rates of recurrence of depressive disorders. However, not all adolescents who attempt suicide are depressed; indeed, there is considerable heterogeneity in the population of suicide attempters (Goldston et al., 1996, 1998; Walrath et al., 2001). Little is known about the trajectories of different groups of suicidal youth, including those with and without depressive disorders, and those who become more chronically or repeatedly suicidal as contrasted with those who do not.

As mentioned in the section on epidemiology, youth at different ages may be at different risks for suicidal and nonsuicidal self-harm behaviors. For example, in clinical and community samples, youth have been noted to have an increase in nonlethal suicidal behaviors from early to midadolescence (Angle, O'Brian, & McIntire, 1983; Kovacs et al., 1993; Lewinsohn et al., 2001). Rates of nonlethal suicidal behavior may decline thereafter, particularly for females (Lewinsohn et al., 2001), but because of a dearth of longitudinal repeated assessment studies, it is unclear whether there are recurrent periods of heightened risk.

In addition, at least some youth who engage in suicidal behaviors also have been noted to have a number of other poor outcomes (Spirito et al., 2000). For example, some suicidal youth continue to have poor relationships with peers and family members (Granboulan, Rabain, & Basquin, 1995; Spirito et al., 1992). Suicidal youth may also continue to have difficulties in school (Spirito et al., 1992), behavioral problems, or legal difficulties (Kerfoot & McHugh, 1992; Laurant, Foussard, David, Boucharlat,

& Bost, 1998; Spirito et al., 1992), and substance abuse (Kerfoot & McHugh, 1992). Many of these nonsuicidal "outcomes" may be stresses in and of themselves, which may in turn increase the likelihood of recurrent suicidal behavior.

THEORIES

Theories to Explain Adolescent Suicide

There are a variety of theories used to explain suicide among adolescents. However, few are specific to adolescents. Furthermore, there is no one theory that is believed to provide the best explanation of the nature of suicidal behaviors among this population. The existing theories are diverse in their perspectives, and most have not been subject to empirical testing. The most commonly accepted theories used to explain suicidal behavior among this population are described in this section.

Social Causes

Durkheim (1897/1951) is responsible for perhaps the most well-known theory of suicide. He theorized that there are social causes of and social groups at risk for suicide, and that these social factors are more important than individual (e.g., rates of disorder or genetics) or other factors in explaining suicide. While acknowledging that there are combined types, he classified suicides into three main categories based on their relationship to society. *Egoistic suicides* are characterized by "excessive individualism" and detachment from society. These individuals are isolated from others and are not well integrated into religious society, families, or communities. Because of their detachment from others, they may have difficulty perceiving a reason for existence. *Altruistic suicides,* in contrast, are motivated to engage in suicide by a sense of duty or obligation, or self-sacrifice (e.g., because they are a burden to others in some way). Altruistic suicides have characteristics that are very dissimilar to those of egoistic suicides insofar as they kill themselves because of their bonds with others rather than because of their disengagement. *Anomic suicides* occur in the context of changes in social conditions such as changes in economic situation or loss of relationships that make it difficult to fulfill needs or maintain roles or standards of living. Because of difficulties engendered by these changes, these individuals may feel angry, disillusioned, or disappointed with life; may feel that life has deceived them; or may blame others or him- or herself for the current situation that precipitates the suicide.

Psychoanalytic Theory

In contrast to sociological theory, psychoanalytic theory focuses on causation at the level of individual development and resulting conscious and unconscious processes. In this vein, Menninger (1933/1996) suggested that suicidal wishes were associated with three elements in varying degrees. First, suicidal individuals at some level evidence a wish to kill. This wish to kill may be manifested as aggression toward the introjected love object, or as an indirect means of aggressing against others (e.g., in the case of killing oneself to hurt someone else), and has its origins in the ego. Second, the suicidal wish may be associated with a wish to be killed (e.g., the case of guilt because of forbidden impulses). This guilt and the resulting wish to be killed arise from the superego. Finally, individuals with suicidal wishes may have a wish to die, consistent with Freud's speculation about the death instinct (arising from the *id*).

Behavioral Theory

Lester (1987) asserts that suicidal behavior in part has its roots in learning experiences and occurs in the context of environmental influences. Although not dismissing the contributions of other factors, he asserts that other factors are insufficient in helping us understand why some individuals engage in suicidal behaviors. For example, suicidal behaviors can be learned through social learning (i.e., by observation and modeling) and maintained through operant conditioning via positive and negative reinforcement. Reinforcing consequences for suicidal behavior include increased attention, being removed from stresses, and tension relief. Lester also describes cultural and familial learning experiences that may affect the likelihood of individuals engaging in suicidal behavior. Given that much suicidal behavior occurs in the context of depression, Lester also acknowledges notions regarding lack of reinforcement (Lewinsohn, 1974) and learned helplessness (Seligman, 1975) in the etiology of depression. Although learning theory is not intrinsically developmental, individuals may have more opportunities for experiencing the consequences of their behaviors, more opportunities for observing others, or more accumulated learning experiences in the community or family or social groups as they have lived longer.

Cognitive Conceptualizations

According to Beck's cognitive model of depression (Beck, Rush, Shaw, & Emery, 1979), individuals are vulnerable to depression by virtue of their "depressive schemas" (which in turn are based in part on past experiences). These depressive schemas can be revealed by a set of negatively biased attitudes about oneself, the world, and the future, which color the perception of one's experiences. When negative thoughts about the future are extreme, individuals lose hope of their circumstances ever changing, and they become preoccupied with the futility of their lives. The cognitive state of hopelessness, in turn, has been found to be associated with suicide intent (Nock & Kazdin, 2002; Spirito, Sterling, Donaldson, & Arrigan, 1996) and to be predictive of repeat suicidal behavior among adolescents (Goldston et al., 2001).

In 1996, Beck extended his cognitive theory to encompass associative notions that can help to explain the repetition of suicidal behavior. According to this conceptualization, the hopeless–suicidal mode and other psychological modes are characterized by interrelated cognitive, affective, and motivational–behavioral schemas and associated physiological patterns of activation. With repeated exposure to events that may activate or "build up the charge" in these modes, increasingly minor events or cues can trigger or activate these modes or networks. Therein, individuals are more likely to respond in certain ways to their environments (e.g., with hopelessness or suicidality) because of their past experiences which have sensitized them to such cues.

Locus of Control

Another theory of suicidal behavior that is applicable to adolescents relates to one's locus of control. There have been suggestions that suicidal adolescents see themselves as more often controlled by external matters or people than nonsuicidal, nondepressed adolescents (De Wilde, Kienhorst, Diekstra, & Wolters, 1993).

A lack of sense of control over one's circumstances and mood may result in feelings of hopelessness, and eventual consideration of suicide. Goldney (1982) found that young women who attempted suicide had a more external locus of control than did nonsuicidal women in a community health center. In a study of Australian adolescents (Pearce & Martin, 1993), those who were categorized as having an external locus of control reported statistically significant higher rates of suicidal ideation, plans to commit suicide, and suicidal behavior. The authors suggest the possibility that those youth with an external locus of control may have been indicating through a suicide attempt that they need help but were leaving their fate to others.

Psychological Pain

One commonly accepted theory is based on the assertion that suicide is driven by intense emotional pain. Shneidman (1996) asserts that suicide is driven by a desire to escape psychological pain for which the individual sees no other option. This pain ("psychache") arises from psychological needs that remain unsatisfied over time and the resulting unbearable negative emotions. There are five primary clusters of thwarted psychological needs that are associated with the intense psychological pain that lead to suicide: (1) needs associated with affiliation, love, and acceptance; (2) needs associated with control, predictability, and order; (3) needs related to maintenance of self-image and the avoidance of shame or defeat; (4) needs related to the maintenance of key and nurturing relationships; and (5) needs associated with dominance or aggression (p. 25).

Shneidman (1996) also described several commonalities associated with most suicides. Most suicides arise out of frustrated needs and the resulting psychological pain. Most suicides are attempts to seek solutions, to seek an end to pain (i.e., the cessation of consciousness), and to escape. Most suicides occur in the context of feelings of hopelessness or helplessness, and most suicidal individuals are operating from a vantage of perceptual constriction (i.e., they have difficulties recognizing any acceptable alternatives to their actions). Most suicides are associated with ambivalence, but they tend to represent consistent patterns of frustrated needs or difficulties with coping within individuals over time.

Integrative Models

Rather than examine risk of suicide from one particular theoretical model, others have posited that such behavior is the result of a variety of factors that lead one to consider suicide as an option. Drawing on the work of Shaffer (1994), Harrington (2001) presents a model of adolescent pathways to suicide that posits that three contributing factors contribute to suicide:

1. Individual disposition, including substance abuse, mental disorders, and personality;
2. Triggering factors, including stressful events, an altered state of mind, and opportunity; and
3. The social milieu of the youth, including role models in the community, taboos, and media coverage.

Research has underscored the importance of each of these sets of risks or contextual factors. However, implicit in this model is the fact that suicide is multiply determined and that various risk and contextual factors may interact to raise the risk or increase the likelihood of suicidal behavior. In addition, because different adolescents are not identical in terms of their dispositions, milieu, and precipitating factors for suicidal behavior, there is implicit recognition that there are multiple pathways or trajectories that culminate in suicidal behavior.

Current Theories of Nonsuicidal Self-Harm Behavior

In contrast to the numerous theories that seek to explain suicidal behavior, relatively few theoretical notions have been proposed for understanding of nonsuicidal self-harm behavior. For example, it has been noted that nonsuicidal self-harm behavior is very strongly linked to childhood experiences of trauma, but surprisingly little has been written about the processes underlying such an association. One theory that does consider the role of past history and is relevant to our understanding of nonsuicidal self-harm behavior is Linehan's biosocial model of borderline personality disorder.

Linehan's Biosocial Theory of Borderline Personality Disorder

Linehan (1993) has described a developmental and transactional model for explaining the etiology of borderline personality disorder (BPD; of which suicidality and nonsuicidal self-harm behaviors are symptoms). Because this model is both developmental and transactional, it has implications not only for effective treatment with older individuals but also for prevention with high-risk youths and families before patterns of nonsuicidal self-harm behavior are well entrenched. Briefly, individuals with BPD are posited to have high emotional vulnerability and difficulties with emotional modulation that are thought to have biological correlates. Unfortunately, this often results in intense emotionality that is extremely painful for both the individual and his or her family members. Thus, the transactions that occur between individuals with BPD and their family members often result in emotional expressions that are punished or invalidated. In the case of sexual abuse, individuals with BPD are often not believed when they describe what has happened to them, which is an extreme form of invalidation.

Because of emphasis in these families on controlling or punishing rather than recognizing emotional states, individuals with BPD often do not learn skills necessary for emotional regulation. Rather, they learn that in order for their distress to be noticed or dealt with, they need to escalate their behavior or evidence more extreme or demanding displays. Individuals with BPD may engage in suicidal and nonsuicidal self-harm behavior partially as a means of trying to elicit validation from the environment, and also as a way of relieving pain or communicating the need for help or treatment. However, their families typically respond with additional invalidation, which results in individuals with BPD escalating their behavior further in a transactional cycle. To the extent that self-harm behaviors are effective in eliciting help or validation from the environment, or in reducing negative affect, the behaviors will be reinforced and more likely to occur.

In this context, it is noteworthy that the most common function cited in the literature for self-mutilation is affect regulation (Briere & Gil, 1998). Tension-reducing behaviors may be used to draw the person away from emotional distress and help them cope with distressing dissociation (Briere, 1992). There is a biological basis for this relief with self-harm behaviors often resulting in the release of endorphins (Richardson & Zaleski, 1986). Similar to Linehan (1993), Briere and Gil (1998) note

that through negative reinforcement that brings temporary distress reduction, these behaviors tend to be repeated.

ETIOLOGY

Although examination of the etiology of suicidal and self-harm behaviors is important, Hawton (1987) notes some of the limitations of reliance on risk factors as they relate to suicide risk. Risk factors may help us to understand which groups are at increased risk for suicide but are less helpful in predicting individual risk. In addition, risk factors are different for various groups and certain factors that may put an individual at risk may change over time or in the course of development. Factors associated with short-term risk (typically the concern of the clinician) may not be the same as long-term risk factors (typically studied by researchers). Furthermore, given the low base rate of suicide, even among those at high risk, it is difficult to accurately predict such behavior.

Despite the difficulty in assessing and predicting risk, there are a variety of risk factors that appear to impact the likelihood that a youth will engage in suicide or self-harm behavior. Moscicki (1999) has distinguished between distal risk factors (those factors that increase long-term risk) and proximal risk factors (those factors that act as precipitants or triggers) for suicidal behavior. In this section, we review both the distal and the proximal risk factors for suicidal behavior and self-harm, including the risk factors for repeat behaviors.

Biological/Genetic

It is commonly accepted that both biological and genetic factors play a role in suicidal behavior and deliberate self-harm. In terms of biological risk factors, those who engage in suicidal behavior are believed to have biochemical changes or abnormalities in the brain. For example, Placidi and colleagues (2001) found that lower cerebrospinal fluid levels of 5-HIAA (a serotonin metabolite) in hospitalized depressed adults were associated with both suicide attempts of greater intent and aggression. In addition, in postmortem analyses, Mann and colleagues (2000) described altered serotonin binding in the prefrontal cortex of individuals who died by suicide relative to those who had nonsuicidal deaths. Differences in serotonin binding, in turn, were related to lifetime history of major depression. Mann and colleagues suggested that this altered serotonin functioning may be associated with impulsivity, or propensity to act on suicidal thoughts when they are present. Tryptophan is a serotonin precursor, and Clark (2003) found that lower concentrations of tryptophan relative to other amino acids was predictive of later suicide attempts in adolescents, independent of the presence of major depressive disorder (although the number of adolescents who attempted suicide during the follow-up was low). Fawcett, Busch, Jacobs, Kravitz, and Fogg (1997) examined serum cholesterol among suicidal inpatients and found that subjects had significantly lower levels than documented in other population studies. However, cholesterol levels were not correlated with body mass index or recent weight loss—possible depression-related symptoms. The authors hypothesized that low serum cholesterol levels may be an indicator of serotonin function but that more research is needed to better understand this possible relationship.

Self-harm behavior may also be linked to brain chemistry changes that result from trauma. Sansone, Sansone, and Wiederman (1995) suggest that the relationship between trauma early in one's life and self-destructive behaviors are complex and likely involve neurobiological changes that affect one's ability to manage emotions and learn adaptive skills.

For youth who attempt suicide, a family history of psychiatric problems and/or suicidal and self-harm behaviors is common. In a sample of children under 16 years of age who had engaged in deliberate self-poisoning, Kerfoot (1988) reported that 41% had someone with a previous psychiatric disorder in their family, most commonly a mother. In particular, there are strong family histories of affective disorders among adolescents who commit suicide (Brent et al., 1988).

Twin and adoption studies have implicated familial transmission of suicidal behavior (Roy, Nielsen, Rylander, Sarchiapone, & Segal, 1999). In addition, higher rates of suicidal ideation, suicide attempts, and suicide deaths have been found among first-degree and second-degree relatives of suicidal youth as compared to community controls (Brent, Bridge, Johnson & Connolly, 1996). Brent et al. (2002) also reported that offspring of suicide attempters are six times more likely to attempt suicide as compared to offspring of nonattempters.

With this evidence of familial association, there has been much work trying to elucidate the genetic linkages associated with suicide and suicidal behavior. Most of this work has focused on genetic loci that are known to be associated with serotonin action. Thus far, however, research has failed to identify the genetic linkages with suicide (e.g., Mann et al., 2000; Nishiguchi et al., 2002; Turecki et al., 2003).

Psychological/Psychosocial

Depression

Not surprisingly, the most consistent finding from the research on suicidal behavior among adolescents is that adolescents who attempt suicide have higher rates of affective disorders. Among adolescent suicide victims, high rates of affective disorders have been noted (Brent et al., 1988; Shaffer et al., 1996). Brent and colleagues (1988), in particular, noted that bipolar disorder and affective disorder with nonaffective comorbidity were more common among suicide victims than among hospitalized suicide attempters. High rates of depressive disorders similarly have been noted among youth who make suicide attempts (Beautrais, Joyce, & Mulder, 1998; Brent et al., 1988; Gould et al., 1998; Kovacs et al., 1993), particularly those who make repeat suicide attempts (Goldston et. al., 1998). A greater amount of depressive symptomatology also has been noted among youth and young adults making nearly lethal suicide attempts that are not impulsive (defined as considered more than 5 minutes) relative to individuals making impulsive attempts (Simon et al., 2001).

Kienhorst, De Wilde, Diekstra, and Wolters (1992) found that severity of depression did not distinguish between depressed youth and youth who attempted suicide but found that the two groups did report different types of depressive symptoms. Those who had not attempted suicide reported more fatigue, whereas suicide attempters reported more social withdrawal, anhedonia, episodes of tearfulness or crying, and hopelessness. Others have similarly documented the problem of social withdrawal among youth with depressive symptoms who commit suicide (Rich, Sherman, & Fowler, 1990). Hence, whereas depression is a risk factor for adolescent suicide, the presence of depression alone may be insufficient to predict individual risk.

For those who engage in nonsuicidal self-harm, depression also is typically present. For example, Garrison and colleagues (1993) found nonsuicidal self-harm behaviors, suicidal ideation, and depression to be interrelated among adolescents. Guertin, Lloyd-Richardson, Spirito, Donaldson, and Boergers (2001) found that adolescent suicide attempts with a history of self-mutilation had higher rates of the diagnoses of major depression and dysthmic disorder than adolescent suicide attempters without such a history.

Anxiety

Anxiety also is common among youth who engage in suicidal behaviors. Suicidal adolescents also have been reported to have higher levels of state and trait anxiety than normal adolescents (De Wilde et al., 1993). In a case control study, Beautrais and colleagues (1998) documented that 14.7% of young people who made suicide attempts had an anxiety disorder, and Shaffer and colleagues (1996) reported that 27% of adolescents who committed suicide had anxiety diagnoses. Similarly, Gould and colleagues (1998) found higher rates of anxiety disorders among youth with suicidal ideation and attempts, and higher rates of separation anxiety among youth with attempts relative to ideation only. Similar to findings with adult populations (e.g., Weissman, Klerman, Markowitz, & Ouellette, 1989), Gould and colleagues (1998) found that panic attacks were related to increased risk of suicidal ideation and attempts, particularly for girls. Repeat suicide attempters report high levels of trait anxiety (Goldston et al., 1996), and trait anxiety is predictive of suicide attempts following discharge from the hospital (Goldston et al., 1999). Others (Fawcett et al., 1997) have posited a pathway to suicide associated with anxiety, agitation and hypothalamic–pituitary–adrenal activation. For adults who engage in deliberate self-mutilation, there appears to be a high likelihood of anxiety disorder associated with exposure to trauma (i.e., posttraumatic stress disorder) (Briere & Gil, 1998).

Substance Abuse

Substance abuse also has been found to be associated with lethal and nonlethal suicide attempts (Beautrais et al., 1998; Garrison et al., 1993; Gould et al., 1998; Shaffer et al., 1996).

For example, Gould and colleagues (1998) found that substance abuse or dependence was more common among adolescent suicide attempters than among either suicide ideators or nonsuicidal youth. Shaffer and colleagues (1996) found that older adolescent males who died by suicide, but not younger adolescent males or females, evidenced higher rates of substance use disorders (SUDs) than adolescents chosen from the community. Indeed, a greater proportion of older adolescent males had SUDs than major depression. Guertin and colleagues (2001) found that adolescent suicide attempters with a history of self-mutilation had higher rates of alcohol use than adolescent suicide attempters without self-mutilation.

Other studies have yielded findings suggesting the possibility that it is the comorbidity between depression and SUDs, rather than the substance abuse or SUDs in and of themselves, that increases the risk of suicidal behavior (Brent et al., 1993, Bukstein, Brent, Perper, & Mortitz, 1993). For example, in a case control study, Brent and colleagues (1993) found that substance use disorders without affective disorders increased the risk of suicide threefold but, when in the presence of affective disorder, increased the risk of suicide seventeenfold.

A significant number of youth who attempt or die by suicide engage in alcohol or other substance use at the time of the suicidal behavior. Hoberman and Garfinkel (1988) found that 28% of children and adolescents who committed suicide had ingested alcohol within 12 hours of their suicide. In addition, suicide after earlier suicidal or nonsuicidal self-harm behavior is also associated with substance misuse (Hawton, Fagg, Platt & Hawkins, 1993).

Behavior Disorders and Problems

In addition to substance abuse, behavior problems are also frequently documented in youth who commit or attempt suicide. In their research and a review of 11 earlier studies of suicide, Rich and colleagues (1990) found that behavior problems were reported for 68% of youth who died by suicide. In a case-control study of 119 adolescent suicides, Shaffer and colleagues (1996) similarly found that 50% of adolescent boys and 32% of adolescent girls who died by suicide had diagnoses of conduct disorder. Over and beyond the psychiatric diagnoses, aggressiveness also was found to be related to suicide (Shaffer et al., 1996). Relevant to the issue of joint homicide–suicide, it is noteworthy that perpetrators of homicide in the schools have been noted to have criminal charges and problems with authority, to be gang members, and to associate with other "high-risk" peers more often than homicide victims (Anderson et al., 2001).

As for nonlethal suicide attempts, Gould and colleagues (1998) found that adolescents who reported either suicidal ideation or attempts had higher rates of both oppositional defiant disorder and conduct disorder than did nonsuicidal adolescents. Kerfoot and colleagues (1996) similarly noted that oppositional defiant disorder was the second most common diagnosis (after major depression) found in a sample of adolescents who attempted suicide via overdose, and Simon and colleagues (2001) found that being in a physical fight within the last 12 months was associated with impulsive suicide attempts among adolescents and young adults. Guertin and colleagues (2001) found that adolescent suicide attempters with histories of self-mutilation had higher rates of oppositional defiant disorder than did adolescent suicide attempters without such a history.

Nonetheless, there have been some inconsistencies in findings between suicidality and externalizing behaviors or disorders. For example, Goldston and colleagues (1998) found that hospitalized adolescents with first-time or repeat suicide attempts actually evidenced a lower rate of externalizing disorders (oppositional defiant and conduct disorder) than did nonsuicidal hospitalized adolescents. In addition, Goldston and colleagues (1999) found that conduct and oppositional defiant disorder by themselves were not predictive of either first-time or repeat suicide attempts in a clinically ascertained sample of adolescents. Others have suggested that it is the combination of depression and externalizing disorders rather than the externalizing disorders per se that is related to higher risk of attempted suicide and death by suicide (Brent et al., 1988; Kovacs et al., 1993).

Impulsivity

Impulsivity is a known risk factor for adolescent suicide. Hoberman and Garfinkel (1988) have reported that suicides in children and adolescents often are impulsive and related to re-

cent stressors or crises. Similarly, Pfeffer and colleagues (1995) found that suicidal children had poorer impulse control than non-patients. In a 6- to 8-year follow-up, children with histories of suicide attempts were rated as having less impulse control than youth who did not attempt suicide (Pfeffer et al., 1995). In addition, Brown, Overholser, Spirito, and Fritz (1991) reported that a higher proportion of adolescents who make impulsive suicide attempts tend to be of low socioeconomic status as compared to adolescents who have made nonimpulsive attempts. There is also believed to be a genetic component to this behavior (Mann, Brent, & Arango, 2001). Fawcett and colleagues (1997) hypothesized that the impulsivity may be linked to suicidal behavior due to low serotonin function, which may in turn be related to low serum cholesterol. Impulsivity may be the characteristic via which substance abuse and conduct disorders are linked to increased risk of suicidality.

Sexual Abuse

A history of sexual abuse is a risk factor for suicidal behavior among adolescents (Beautrais, Joyce, & Mulder, 1996). Data from a nonclinical sample of adolescents revealed that youth with histories of sexual abuse were more than three times likely to attempt suicide (Riggs, Alario, McHorney, 1990). Sexual abuse in childhood is linked to increased risk for suicide attempts in adolescence and adulthood, as well as repeat attempts during both time periods (Brown, Cohen, Johnson, & Smailes, 1999). In addition, youth with histories of sexual abuse report higher numbers of previous suicide attempts as compared to hospitalized youth without such histories (Shaunesey, Cohen, Plummer, & Berman, 1993).

Briere and Gil (1998) assert that a history of sexual and physical abuse has emerged from the existing research as the strongest predictor of the development of self-mutilation behavior. Similarly, in a review of the literature on childhood abuse and adult deliberate self-harm and suicidal behavior, Santa Mina and Gallop (1998) reported that although there are methodological differences in the existing research, the research consistently has documented high rates of these behaviors among individuals who have reported sexual and/or physical abuse. In addition to sexual and physical abuse, witnessing violence and the number of types of abuse reported are also related to self-destructive be-haviors among adult females (Sansone et al., 1995).

Lesbian, Gay, or Bisexual Orientation

Youths who identify as being lesbian, gay, or bisexual (LGB) appear to be at increased risk for suicidal behavior. For example, using data from the Youth Risk Behavior Survey, Garofalo and colleagues (1999) reported that adolescents who were LGB or unsure of their sexual orientation were more likely to report a suicide attempt than heterosexual youth. According to data from the National Longitudinal Study of Adolescent Health, adolescent same-sex sexual orientation was found to be a risk factor for suicidality; however, some of this increased risk seemed to be a function of other known risk factors for suicidal behavior among the general population of adolescents, such as depression and hopelessness (Russell & Joyner, 2001).

Among LGB youth, Hershberger, Pilkington and D'Augelli (1997) found that those who at-tempted suicide had lost more friends and ex-perienced more victimization because of their sexual orientation as compared to those with-out a history of a suicide attempt. More-over, among this population, suicide attempts tend to follow recognition of same-sex feel-ings and take place prior to disclosure by the youth of their sexual orientation (D'Augelli, Hershberger, & Pilkington, 2001). In addition, negative parental reactions to disclosure of sex-ual orientation are also associated with at-tempts (D'Augelli et al., 2001).

Despite these findings, evidence from at least one case-control study of suicide does not indi-cate that a significant number of adolescents who died by suicide were LGB (Shaffer, Fisher, Parides, & Gould, 1995). However, it should be noted that in this psychological autopsy study, the information was gathered by infor-mants such as parents, teachers, and peers who might not have known about the issues of sexu-ality with which the adolescents were strug-gling.

School Problems

Youth who engage in suicidal behaviors are likely to have experienced problems in school. Gould, Fisher, Parides, Flery, and Shaffer (1996) reported that adolescents who commit-ted suicide were 6.1 times more likely to have

been suspended from school and 3.3 times more likely to have failed a grade than commu-nity controls. Arnold, Walsh, and Goldston (2003) found higher rates of suicidal thoughts and attempts among adolescents with poor reading relative to those with normal reading skills. Adolescents with suicidal thoughts/behavior were more likely to eventually drop out of school. With reference to the issue of joint homicide–suicide, it is of note that homi-cide-related events are more likely to occur at the beginning of the school semesters (CDC, 2001), a time that may be associated with a va-riety of new or increased academic and social pressures.

Family Environment

Youth who have experienced family conflict or stress are at high risk for committing suicide and engaging in self-harm. In their review of the most common stressors experienced by ad-olescent suicide victims across studies, Rich and colleagues (1990) found that 40% had ex-perienced family discord. In a more recent re-view, Wagner (1997) noted that although the literature on this topic is not extensive and the direction of effect is sometimes unclear, there is support for the notion that family stress is asso-ciated with suicidal behavior among adoles-cents. Kienhorst and colleagues (1992) re-ported that youth who attempted suicide had higher rates of family dysfunction, including changes in their living situation, conflict be-tween their parents, conflict with their mother, family financial problems, and sexual abuse than depressed youth who did not attempt sui-cide. Others have similarly found that adoles-cents who overdosed were more likely than psychiatric outpatients and community con-trols to come from a home without both bio-logical parents or to have family dysfunction (Kerfoot et al., 1996).

Stressful Life Events

Distal risk factors may provide information about who is at risk for suicidal or nonsuicidal self-harm behavior, but they do not provide in-formation about when those individuals are at risk. Proximal risk factors such as precipitating life stresses, in turn, provide information about when individuals are at risk for suicidal or self-harm behavior but not necessarily who is at risk (given that the experience of various life stresses is normative, but most individuals do not engage in suicidal or self-harm behavior).

In a nationwide study of suicide among adolescents and adults in Finland (Heikkinen, Aro, & Lonnqvist, 1994), 80% of subjects had experienced one or more stressful life events in the 3 months prior to their suicide attempt (mean = 2.6 events). The authors note, though, that some events may have been critical to the suicidal act whereas others may have not played a significant role. Other research similarly has noted increased rates of life events in the 3 months, and particularly, in the week prior to death by suicide among adolescents and young adults (Cooper, Appleby, & Amos, 2002). In a community study, youth who attempt suicide were found to have experienced more life stresses than those reporting suicide ideation (King et al., 2001).

A number of studies have noted that relationship and interpersonal difficulties and losses commonly precede suicidal behavior (Adams, Overholser, & Spirito, 1994; Beautrais et al., 1997; Rich et al., 1990). For females, pregnancy and abortions appear to be more common among attempters than among depressed adolescents (Kienhorst et al., 1992). Other life stresses noted across studies include family discord, school problems, job or financial difficulties, and legal or disciplinary problems (Beautrais et al., 1997; Gould et al., 1996; Heikkinen et al., 1994; Rich et al., 1990). With reference to homicide–suicides, perpetrators of homicides in the schools have more often been noted to be bullied by peers or be socially isolated, have criminal charges, or have problems with authority than have homicide victims (Anderson et al., 2001).

Nonetheless, it is worth noting that some life events may be normative for a particular developmental stage or caused directly or indirectly by an individual's own behavior or poor problem-solving ability (Davila, Hammen, Burge, Paley, & Daley, 1995; Hammen, 1991; Heikkinen et al., 1994). Moreover, it is of note that Beautrais and colleagues (1997) found that approximately one-third of suicide attempters could not name a precipitating life event for their suicidal behavior.

There is little research on life stressors and nonsuicidal self-harm. However, Garrison and colleagues (1993) did note a relationship between nonsuicidal physically self-damaging behaviors and undesirable life events. Anecdotal reports have noted difficulties in relationships and/or losses of important relationships among adolescents with self-cutting behaviors. Clinicians who work with youth who have histories of self-harm should examine the possible relationship between upsetting life events or relationship turmoil and these behaviors.

Access to Firearms

A documented risk factor for suicide among adolescents is the presence of firearms in the home (Brent et al., 1988). Furthermore, studies of adolescent suicide victims have found that the most common method of suicide is the use of a firearm, particularly for males (CDC, 2002). Unfortunately, families are often noncompliant in removing guns from the home as recommended by clinicians (Brent, Baugher, Birmaher, Kolko, & Bridge, 2000).

Other Environmental Factors

One of the concerns for persons at risk for suicide and self-harm, particularly for adolescents who are in a difficult developmental period of their lives, is the impact of environmental factors. At the community level, one's neighborhood is believed to have an impact on suicidal behavior for some youth—perhaps through the relationship of neighborhood to other known risk factors. Perez-Smith, Spirito, and Boergers (2002) found that after controlling for depression and family socioeconomic status (SES), the neighborhood context of adolescent suicide attempters contributed to their level of hopelessness. Hopelessness was higher among youth who lived in neighborhoods with a greater concentration of males and adults as compared to females and children. Thus, they conclude that neighborhood social networks are an important factor to consider in understanding hopelessness that can contribute to suicidal behavior. In addition, given the transient nature of families today, it can be difficult to build meaningful relationships if one is not assimilated into the community.

When one or more youth in a community commit suicide, there is cause for immediate concern for the well-being of other youth who may be considering suicide. The media commonly focuses on clusters of suicide in communities. The CDC (1988) notes that although the definition of a "suicide cluster" is complex, one must consider both the number of suicides and the relationships between the individuals. In many cases, suicides or attempts have been preceded by one or more traumatic deaths, either intentional or unintentional acts, among the young people in the area (CDC, 1988). In a national study of attempted suicide in New Zealand, Gould, Petrie, Kleinman, and Wallenstein (1994) found support for the clustering of suicide attempts among those of younger age, particularly among 15–19-year-olds and 20–24-year-olds.

Through proactive means to address the issue, it is hoped that additional suicides can be prevented. To encourage responsible reporting of suicide and discourage reporting that might inadvertently increase the likelihood of suicide imitation or contagion, the American Foundation for Suicide Prevention (AFSP) and the Annenberg Public Policy Center cosponsored a workshop (attended by multiple government and prevention organizations) in which guidelines for responsible media coverage of suicide were drafted (AFSP, 2001). In these guidelines, it was suggested that the media avoid dramatizing or romanticizing suicides, or idealizing suicide victims, and avoid using the word "suicide" or referring to the cause of death in headlines (AFSP, 2001). It was suggested that media be cautious about describing suicides as inexplicable and in the reporting of interviews with grieving family members who still may be shocked and may not have recognized warning signs (AFSP, 2001). The media were encouraged to ask questions such as whether suicide victims may have had problems with depression or substance use, to present a balanced picture of the decedent's life and not oversimplify the precipitants of suicides, and to provide information about the availability of effective treatments.

In addition to concerns that the suicide or traumatic death of a youth in the community can precipitate other such actions, the portrayal of suicide in the popular media has raised concerns. The most well-known theory that addresses the issue of suicides and environmental factors is the "Werther effect." As described by Phillips (1974), the Werther effect, based on the hero in Goethe's novel, *The Sorrow of the Young Werther*, who commits suicide, is the notion that suicides increase after publicity about suicide. Phillips asserts that the more publicity, the greater the effect on suicidal behavior, even among those who may not have been considering suicide. In addition, the type of publicity is important, including whether alternatives to suicide are presented in the media. The assertion is also that the more famous the person, the more the person feels that the circumstances are similar to his or her life, or the more the person has in common with the deceased (e.g., race and gender), the more likely the individual is to imitate the behavior and attempt suicide. Bollen and Philips (1982) suggest that imitative effects following television news stories about suicide appear to wane after approximately 10 days.

Fictionalized accounts of suicide in the media also may influence someone considering suicide to act on these thoughts. In one example (Hawton, Kingsbury, Steinhardt, James, & Fagg, 1999), after viewing a British television drama that involved a storyline on an individual overdosing on paracetamol (acetaminophen), there was no increase in mortality immediately after the broadcast. However, the rate of self-poisoning increased 17% the first week after the broadcast, and 9% in the second week. Eighteen percent of overdose patients in the week after the broadcast stated that they had watched the episode, and of this group, 15% reported that seeing the show had impacted their decision to overdose.

It is not clear whether there are any media effects associated with higher likelihood of nonsuicidal self-harm behavior. However, two studies that did not differentiate suicidal from nonsuicidal self-harm behavior did demonstrate clustering effects in self-harm behavior (primarily cutting) among psychiatrically treated adolescents (Walsh & Rosen, 1985; Taiminen, Kallio-Soukianen, Nokso-Koivisto, Kaljonen, & Helenius, 1998).

Risk for Repetition of Suicidal and Self-Harm Behaviors

One of the obvious concerns for youth who engage in suicidal and self-harm behaviors is that these acts will be repeated and will ultimately lead to serious injury or death. Previous research on repetition of self-harm among adults suggests that the probability of repeating the behavior increases with the number of previous episodes (Leon et al., 1989). Similarly, in adolescent samples, the number of prior suicide attempts has been found to be a strong predictor of future suicidal behavior (Goldston et al., 1999).

However, other factors may also play a role in repetition of behaviors. In early research,

Morgan, Barton, Pottle, Pocock, and Burns-Cox (1976) reported that previous psychiatric treatment was highly associated with repeat self-harm. However, such relationships could be artifactual and reflective of the fact that the individuals with the most psychiatric problems both are at highest risk for suicidal behavior and are most likely to present for treatment. With that consideration, Goldston and colleagues (1999) found that the first 6 months to 1 year following psychiatric hospitalization was a particularly high-risk period of time for suicide attempts.

Other factors differentiating repeat and one-time suicide attempters may provide clues as to which youth are at highest risk for repeat suicide attempters. Esposito, Spirito, Boergers, and Donaldson (2003) found that adolescents who were hospitalized or seen in the emergency department after making a repeat suicide attempt had more affective disorders, more severe depressive symptoms and anger, more disruptive behavior disorders, more hopelessness, and more self-mutilation than adolescents with single attempts. Among children and adolescents presenting for outpatient services, Walrath and colleagues (2001) found that repeat attempters had higher rates of sexual abuse, runaway behavior, and drug and alcohol use than first-time attempters. Others have reported that adolescents who repeat self-harm have less effective problem-solving skills as compared to those who do not repeat; however, the differences were not significant after controlling for depression, another major factor in repeat self-harm behavior (Hawton et al., 1999). In a prospective study of previously psychiatrically hospitalized adolescents, Goldston and colleagues (1999, 2001) found that affective disorders, more severe depressive symptoms, hopelessness, and lower survival and coping beliefs were all more predictive of repeat suicide attempts than they were of first-time suicide attempts.

ASSESSMENT

As mentioned previously, prior suicidal behavior is one of the best predictors of future suicidal behavior. Therein, it is incumbent upon the clinician to ask about history of suicidal behavior even in those circumstances in which suicidal behavior risk is not the primary complaint. Clinical interviewing is the most common means of inquiring about history of recurrent suicidal ideation or behavior. Nonetheless, clinicians sometimes are apprehensive or reluctant to ask about suicidal behavior. Some may fear, for instance, that by asking about suicidal behavior, they may give vulnerable individuals "ideas" that they may act on. Nonetheless, suicidal ideation and behavior are common among individuals identified as depressed, and suicidal individuals may be relieved to be able to talk about this topic (Fremouw, Perczel, & Ellis, 1990).

Children and adolescents are typically better reporters of their suicidal behaviors than adults. Indeed, a number of studies (Breton et al., 2002; Klimes-Dougan, 1998; Velez & Cohen, 1988; Walker et al., 1990) suggest that adolescents often report suicidal behaviors of which their parents are unaware. Also, unfortunately, it is sometimes the case that parents may misinterpret or not take their offspring's self-destructive behavior seriously, refusing to recognize it as suicidal in intent. Such an attitude, of course, does not recognize the reality that most suicidal behavior occurs in the context of ambivalence and is associated with mixed motives.

There also may be occasions in which the adolescent's report of suicidality is inaccurate. Establishing sufficient rapport with adolescents can help to minimize these occurrences. (Goldston, 2003). When adolescents overreport suicidality, it may be because the reports of suicidal behavior are in part instrumental (e.g., a cry for help or an effort to prevent a relationship from dissolving) (Goldston, 2003). There also may be occasions in which adolescents underreport suicidal ideation or behavior. In these occasions, the adolescent may be embarrassed to admit that he or she has been feeling suicidal (Goldston, 2003). Alternatively, adolescents also may be attempting to forestall telling their parents or other loved ones that they tried to end their lives, or they may deny suicidality in an effort to avoid treatment, either because they are uncomfortable talking about their feelings or thoughts or because they do not like the idea of the restrictiveness of some treatment options such as hospitalization (Goldston, 2003). Child and adolescent report is certainly very important, but it should never preempt the judgment of a clinician. Clinicians should always err on the side of caution in making judgments about the risk of suicidal behavior; conversely, clinicians should be extraordinarily careful not to be dismissive of adolescent self-reports of suicidal ideation or behavior (Goldston, 2003). To assist the clinician in making informed judgments, a number of instruments have been developed for measuring suicidal behavior and risk. These instruments are described in the next sections.

Normative Information

As described earlier in the section on epidemiology, there are age trends in suicidal behaviors. In particular, suicidal ideation seems to be very prevalent during the period of adolescence, and suicide attempts per se seem to be increasingly more common from the period from early adolescence through midadolescence. Nonetheless, despite the fact that adolescence is a period during which adolescents are faced with numerous difficulties, including family problems, struggles for autonomy, and often emotionally intense peer and relationship problems, most adolescents do not seriously consider suicide, and only a minority actually make suicide attempts. Although some instruments for severity of suicidal ideation or risk have been developed specifically for use with children or adolescents, no instruments of which we are aware have been age-normed with consideration of developmental differences. There are also no age-normed instruments of which we are aware for assessing nonsuicidal self-harm behaviors.

Appropriateness of Current Measures for Adolescents

Among the currently available instruments for assessing self-harm behaviors and risks, several were developed specifically for use with adolescents, and a number of other instruments were initially developed for adults that have been used with adolescents. Examples of instruments developed specifically for assessing the presence or severity of suicidality in adolescents include Suicidal Ideation Questionnaire (Reynolds, 1988), Suicidal Behaviors Interview (Reynolds, 1989, 1990), the Spectrum of Suicidal Behavior Scale of the Child Suicide Potential Scales (Pfeffer, Conte, Plutchik, & Jerrett, 1979), and the Evaluation of Suicide Risk among Adolescents and Imminent Danger Assessment (Bradley & Rotheram-Borus, 1990; Rotheram-Borus, 1987, 1989). Instruments developed for assessing risk of suicidal behaviors

specifically among children and/or adolescents include the Child Suicide Potential Scales (Pfeffer et al., 1979), the Columbia Suicide Screen (Shaffer et al., 2004), the Measure of Adolescent Potential for Suicide (Eggert, Thompson, & Herting, 1994), the Hopelessness Scale for Children (Kazdin, Rodgers, & Colbus, 1986), and the Reasons for Living Inventory—Adolescent Version (Osman et al., 1998). A number of scales developed for use with adults also have been used widely with adolescent populations. Adult instruments for assessing the presence/absence, severity, or risk of suicidal behavior that have been used with adolescents include the Lifetime Parasuicide Count (Linehan & Comtois, 1997), the Beck Scale for Suicide Ideation (Beck & Steer, 1991), the Beck Hopelessness Scale (Beck, Schuyler, & Herman, 1974; Beck & Steer, 1988; Steer & Beck, 1988), and the Reasons for Living Inventory (Linehan, Goodstein, Nielsen, & Chiles, 1983).

Targets and Assessment

There are several different types of instruments for assessing self-harm behaviors, and the purpose of the assessment should help drive the decision about which assessment instruments are used. For example, if one is primarily interested in assessing the presence or severity of self-harm behavior, the most appropriate types of instruments are detection instruments (Goldston, 2003). There a number of different types of detection instruments. These range from psychiatric diagnostic interviews with items assessing suicidal ideation and attempts, to interviews specifically developed for assessing self-harm behaviors, to self-report questionnaires assessing suicidality, to behavior checklists and rating scales that can be used (or have items that can be used) for assessing suicidal ideation and/or behaviors. Detection instruments are most appropriate for determining whether or not someone has engaged in self-harm behaviors recently or in the past, or has evidenced suicidal ideation. Detection instruments also can be used for assessing self-harm behaviors when trying to assess the relationship between self-harm and other variables, or they can be used to describe the course of self-harm behaviors over time if used in repeated assessments. Last but not least, detection instruments can be used to assess the effects of interventions in reducing self-harm behaviors.

If one is interested in assessing the risk of future suicidal behavior, a number of risk assessment instruments have been developed (Goldston, 2003). Risk assessment instruments include self-report questionnaires or rating scales as well as multitiered screening systems. The instruments can potentially be used for helping to estimate or gauge the risk of suicidal behavior (although it should be noted that only a limited number of risk assessment instruments have demonstrated predictive validity). In addition, risk assessment instruments can be used as outcome measures for interventions to the extent that such interventions have attempted to focus on reducing various risk factors for suicidal behavior.

A third group of instruments is used for describing the clinical characteristics of suicidal behavior such as method of attempt, intent associated with suicidal behavior, or medical lethality (Goldston, 2003). Despite the fact that clinical characteristics of suicidal behavior are often used in formulating clinical decisions about the risk of future suicidal behavior (Peruzzi & Bongar, 1999), there is little evidence to document the usefulness of clinical characteristics of current suicidal behavior in predicting either the intent or the lethality of future suicidal behavior or the occurrence of future suicidal behavior per se among adolescents (Goldston, 2003). Hence, at this time, these instruments are primarily useful in describing or characterizing suicidal behavior for other clinicians and in research studies. It should be noted that medical lethality and intent of suicidal behavior have inconsistently been found to be interrelated in adolescent samples (DeMaso, Ross, & Beardslee, 1994; Lewinsohn et al., 1996; Nasser & Overholser, 1999; Plutchik, Van Praag, Picard, Conte, & Korn, 1989).

In addition to the decision about whether or not a detection instrument, risk assessment instrument, or instrument for assessing clinical characteristics of suicidal behavior is to be used, there are a number of other considerations in the choice of assessment instruments. For example, some instruments such as the Columbia Teen Screen were developed for use in larger-scale school screenings, although they can easily be on an individual basis as well. A second consideration is the population(s) in which the instruments were developed and have prior demonstrated use. Instruments may not have the same predictive validity or clinical utility in different populations with differing base rates of risk factors for suicidal behaviors and/or differing base rates of suicidal behaviors. A third consideration in regard to the choice of detection instruments is the definitions of self-harm behaviors that are used. For example, because of inconsistencies in how various terms regarding suicidal behaviors are used, O'Carroll and colleagues (1996) have recommended standard operational definitions for basic terms such as suicide attempts and suicide ideation. However, instruments vary in the degree to which they are consistent with this recommended nomenclature. As previously described, a fourth consideration specifically pertinent to risk assessment instruments is that of predictive validity. Risk assessment instruments conceptually should be of use primarily in ascertaining the risk of *future* self-harm behavior. If an instrument has to be administered repeatedly, as in a treatment study, a fifth consideration is whether or not there is any evidence of attenuation in responding with needed assessments. There has been scant research to explore this issue of self-harm assessment instruments, but sensitivity to this issue is particularly important when one interprets findings, for example, suggesting that there is a reduction in suicidal behavior over time. Other considerations, of course, include the cost involved of assessment and the time involved in the administration of the assessments.

Almost all structured and semistructured psychiatric diagnostic interviews that assess depressive disorders include questions assessing suicidal ideation or behavior. There are four instruments in particular for which both the reliability of the queries regarding suicidal ideation and behavior has been demonstrated and for which the predictive validity of responses has also been demonstrated. Two of these instruments are structured interviews—the Diagnostic Interview Scale for Children and Adolescents (Shaffer, Fisher, Lucas, Dulcan, & Schwab-Stone, 2000) and the Diagnostic Interview for Children and Adolescents (Reich, 2000). The other two instruments are semistructured in nature—the Interview Schedule for Children and Adolescents (Sherrill & Kovacs, 2000) and the Schedule for Affective Disorder and Schizophrenia—School Age—Epidemiologic Version (Orvaschel, 1994).

Other suicide detection instruments include clinician rating scales and interviews developed specifically for assessing suicidality. For example, the Children's Depression Rating Scale (Poznanski & Mokros, 1999) is a rating scale for symptoms of depression and includes an item that is appropriate for assessing suicidality. The Spectrum of Suicidal Behavior Scale (Pfeffer et al., 1979) is a clinician-rated item that was developed specifically for rating the severity of suicidal behavior. The Suicidal Behaviors Interview is often used as a follow-up to the Suicidal Ideation Questionnaire but provides a more comprehensive assessment of suicidality including communications about suicidal ideation and behavior and recency of prior attempts (Reynolds, 1989, 1990). The Lifetime Parasuicide Count (Linehan & Comtois, 1997) was originally developed for use with adults but can be used with adolescents for assessing both suicidal and nonsuicidal self-harm behavior (but does not include items focusing specifically on suicidal ideation).

There are several different self-report questionnaires and behavior checklists that can be used for assessing the presence or absence or severity of suicidal ideation or behavior. Some of these instruments, such as the Adolescent Psychopathology Scale (Reynolds, 1998) assess a variety of psychiatric problems but also include specific items or a specific scale related to suicidality. There are also a number of instruments more narrowly focused on suicidality or depressive symptoms. Some of these scales, such as the Beck Depression Inventory (Beck & Steer, 1987) and the Children's Depression Inventory (Kovacs, 1985, 1992), include single items that assess suicidality in the context of assessment of other depressive symptoms. Other self-report instruments focus specifically on severity of suicidality. The two most widely used self-report instruments for assessing suicidality among adolescents are the Beck Scale for Suicidal Ideation (Beck & Steer, 1991) and the Suicidal Ideation Questionnaire (Reynolds, 1989). These instruments have been found to have adequate test–retest reliability and have both been used as outcome measures in treatment research (Goldston, 2003). The Suicidal Ideation Questionnaire has been used with both clinically referred and community samples, but the Beck Scale has been used primarily in clinical settings (Goldston, 2003).

Few self-report instruments have been developed for the identification of nonsuicidal self-harm behaviors in adolescents. One such instrument is the Self-Injury Inventory (Zlotnick,

Donaldson, Spirito, & Pearlstein, 1997), which can be used to assess a variety of nonsuicidal self-harm behaviors as well as other risk-taking behaviors.

There also are a large number of clinician rating scales and self-report questionnaires for assessing the risk of suicidal behaviors. Unfortunately, as previously described, the predictive validity of most of these instruments has not yet been demonstrated. The Beck Hopelessness Scale (Beck & Steer, 1988) has been found to be associated with increased likelihood of recurrent suicidal behavior in a formally psychiatrically hospitalized sample (Goldston et al., 2001). The Hopelessness Scale for Children (Kazdin et al., 1986) and the Suicide Probability Scale (Cull & Gill, 1988) also have been found to have some evidence of predictive validity, although in the latter case, the scale was still unable to identify most of the individuals who eventually engaged in suicidal behavior (Shaffer, 1996).

In addition to focusing on risk for suicidal behavior, several instruments have been developed for assessing protective factors or resilience to suicidal behavior. These include the Reasons for Living Inventory (Linehan et al., 1983), the Reasons for Living Inventory—Adolescent Version (Osman et al., 1998), the Suicide Resilience Inventory (Gutierrez et al., 2002), and the Positive and Negative Suicide Ideation Scale (Osman et al., 2002). The Survival and Coping Beliefs scale of the Reasons for Living Inventory, in particular, has been found to be associated with decreased likelihood of recurrent suicidal behavior (Goldston et al., 2001).

There are also several different assessment procedures that have been developed for multistage screening procedures with adolescents. These include the Columbia Suicide Screen followed by the Diagnostic Interview Schedule for Children and Adolescents (Shaffer & Craft, 1999; Shaffer et al., 2004), the Suicide Ideation Questionnaire followed by the Suicide Behaviors Inventory (Reynolds, 1991), the High School Questionnaire followed by the Measure of Adolescent Potential for Suicide (Eggert et al., 1994), and the Evaluation of Suicide Risk Among Adolescents and Imminent Danger Assessment (Bradley & Rotheram-Borus, 1990; Rotheram-Borus, 1987, 1989). The first three of these multitiered assessment procedures were developed for use in the schools, and the last two assessment procedures were designed to be administered to youth identified as potentially high risk. Each of these multitiered assessments offer the advantage of more comprehensive and careful assessment of youth identified as potentially at risk in initial screenings.

In addition, there may be therapeutic benefits from participating in comprehensive assessments. For example, in the procedure developed by Rotheram-Borus (1987, 1989), youth initially identified as at risk for suicidal behavior are then asked to complete several tasks that are thought to be incompatible with suicide. These tasks include being able to articulate the precipitant of their distress, being able to name good things about themselves, being able to name possible support individuals, and being able to agree with a safety plan. Youth who cannot do these tasks are considered to be in imminent danger of engaging in suicidal behavior and are referred for more intensive evaluation and possible psychiatric treatment on an emergency basis. These youth who are able to complete the tasks may actually benefit from the exercise.

Finally, instruments have been developed for describing the clinical characteristics of suicidal behaviors. Among instruments for assessing suicide intent is the Beck Suicide Intent Scale (Beck et al., 1974). Two instruments appear to have particular utility in assessing medical lethality of suicidal behavior—the Lethality of Suicide Attempt Rating Scale (Smith, Conroy, & Ehler, 1984) and the Self-Inflicted Injury Severity Form (Potter et al., 1998). Although these instruments have been demonstrated to yield reliable assessments, their predictive validity (i.e., their ability to predict later suicidal behavior) has not yet been demonstrated (Goldston, 2003).

PREVENTION OF SELF-HARM

As reviewed by Gould and Kramer (2001), the most common type of prevention interventions are suicide awareness programs in the schools. These interventions typically focus on providing education about the problem of suicide and also often include efforts to encourage adolescents to tell others if they know of someone who is feeling suicidal (Gould & Kramer, 2001). There are some data suggesting that these awareness programs may be useful in increasing the knowledge or changing attitudes

about suicidal behaviors among adolescents (Kalafat & Elias, 1994). There have even been some indications that suicide prevention programs that include a focus on suicide awareness may be associated with the decrease in the rates of suicide deaths among students (Kalafat & Ryerson, 1999; Zenere & Lazarus, 1997). However, despite the well-intended nature of these programs, some of the programs have also been found to be associated with some deleterious effects (Shaffer et al., 1990). For example, some adolescents participating in such programs find the programs to be upsetting and report being less likely to refer a suicidal peer to a mental health center after participating in some suicidal awareness programs (Kalafat & Elias, 1994; Shaffer et al., 1990).

Additional suicide prevention efforts have included efforts to reduce access to methods of suicide such as firearms. As mentioned in a previous section, access to firearms has been found to be one of the factors that distinguish between suicidal adolescents who are psychiatrically hospitalized and adolescents who die by suicide (Brent et al., 1988). There have been some indications that communities that have more restricted access to firearms may have lower rates of suicide deaths among young people, particularly by firearms, than similar communities with less restrictive access to firearms (Sloan, Rivara, Reay, Ferris, & Kellerman, 1990). In some states, there recently have been efforts to require gun locks or otherwise restrict unsupervised access to firearms by young people. Emerging evidence suggests that the introduction of laws requiring minimum age for purchase or possession of firearms has not reduced suicide rates, but that child access prevention laws (e.g., requiring gun locks or adequate gun storage) have resulted in an approximately 11% reduction in firearm suicides among 14- to 17-year-olds (Webster, Vernick, Zeoli, & Manganello, 2004).

Gatekeeper training is another form of prevention intervention. A basic presumption of gatekeeper training is that various adults have contact with adolescents and potentially should be in a position to help or at least recognize youth who are having crises and, therein, need intervention (Gould & Kramer, 2001). Such gatekeepers include schoolteachers, coaches, religious leaders, and primary care physicians among others. As described by Gould and Kramer (2001), gatekeeper training efforts have generally focused on providing education and raising awareness about the problem of suicide, helping gatekeepers to better recognize or identify and refer youth thought to be a risk for suicidal behavior. In some instances, gatekeepers have been provided training regarding how to intervene with suicidal individuals. Results from gatekeeper training programs have indicated increased awareness, knowledge about suicide, and improved referral practices for at-risk individuals (Reisman & Scharfman, 1991; Shaffer, Garland, Whittle, & Underwood, 1988). It is not clear whether gatekeeper training yields reductions in suicidal behaviors among youth.

There have been several multitiered screening systems that have been developed for identifying at-risk youth in need of intervention (Eggert et al., 1994; Reynolds, 1991; Shaffer & Craft, 1999; Shaffer et al., 2004). Each of these screening and identification prevention approaches is predicated on the notion that it is more efficient to target resources and prevention efforts to high-risk groups or individuals than it is to direct such efforts at the general population of adolescents. When used in school settings, such prevention efforts may begin with large-scale screenings of youth or they may focus on identified groups of high-risk youth (e.g., those at risk for dropping out of school). Based on the results of the initial screening, youth considered to be potentially at risk are typically interviewed individually to determine risk and need for intervention (therein reducing the number of false positives identified with the first screening). Although such prevention efforts often take place in the schools, they can take place in any setting in which high-risk youth can be identified (Goldston, 2003). For example, some prevention efforts and screenings have focused on youth presenting for treatment, or settings in which homeless or runaway youth, or LGB adolescents can be identified (Bradley & Rotheram-Borus, 1990; Rotheram-Borus, 1987, 1989).

Data from these multilevel screenings suggest that the approach can be used very successfully in identifying adolescents who are in need of treatment or thought to be at risk for suicidal behavior (Goldston, 2003). Whether or not such multitiered screening systems actually reduce the rates of suicide deaths, or even suicide attempts, remains to be seen. An occasionally voiced concern about using such multitiered screening systems, particularly in the schools, is that the schools may not have the resources to fill the need, and the mental health system may not be able to accommodate the number of youth who are identified.

Crisis hotlines represent another type of prevention intervention effort for suicidality among adolescents. Gould and Kramer (2001) described a number of potential advantages of crisis hotlines in the prevention of suicide. For example, much suicidal behavior occurs in the context of crisis and crisis hotlines provide adolescents with the opportunity to call, ventilate, problem-solve, and potentially defuse the crisis situation. In addition, individuals who make suicide attempts and who die by suicide often have expressed ambivalence about their suicidal acts. In this context, the crisis hotlines provide potential opportunity for highlighting this ambivalence and focusing on the reasons for not completing suicides. Moreover, suicide hotlines offer the advantage of anonymity, and therein, adolescents may call the crisis hotline who might not reach out for other services from mental health professionals or other adults. This, of course, also is a disadvantage as the crisis line workers may be limited in the degree to which they can immediately intervene when an individual is thought to be making a suicide attempt.

Some limited data suggest that teenage females are the most likely individuals to use crisis hotlines (Boehm & Campbell, 1995), and that crisis hotlines have been most successful in reducing suicide among white females age 24 or younger (Miller, Coombs, Leeper, & Burton, 1984). Teenage males do not appear to use crisis hotlines as much as females, nor do younger males appear to benefit as much as younger females (Boehm & Campbell, 1995; Miller et al., 1984). In general, however, the effectiveness of crisis hotlines in reducing suicidal behavior has not been well evaluated.

Finally, there are various skills-building approaches that have been developed for youth potentially at risk for high-risk behaviors. A potential advantage of such programs is that they often do not focus specifically on suicide but, rather, focus on enhancing or improving skills relevant to mental health and life choices more generally (Gould & Kramer, 2001). Hence, such programs may be less likely to be associated with possible deleterious effects among at-risk individuals than the more narrowly focused suicide awareness prevention programs. One such program is the Reconnecting Youth intervention developed for youth at risk for dropping out of school (Thompson, Eggert, Randell, & Pike, 2001). This group-based intervention consists of skills building and social support and has been found to be efficacious at reducing suicidality and depression and improving problem-solving ability (Thompson et al., 2001).

Unlike the proliferation of different prevention approaches for suicidal youth, no prevention efforts to our knowledge have been developed for reducing nonsuicidal self-harm behaviors among adolescents.

INTERVENTIONS FOR SUICIDAL AND SELF-HARMING ADOLESCENTS

Recent reviews have reported few empirical studies of treatments for suicidal behavior among adults (Hawton et al., 1998; Linehan, 1997; Rudd, 2000). There are even fewer reports of controlled clinical trials addressing suicidal or self-harming behaviors with youth. The lack of research on treatments for suicidal behavior is disconcerting given the prevalence of suicidal ideation and behaviors among adolescents. Research progress in this area has likely been delayed for several clinical reasons, including the realities that suicidal patients are often difficult to treat, do not follow through with treatment recommendations, and drop out of therapy. The research progress in this area has also likely been delayed for several research and methodological reasons, including a focus in some studies on treating the primary diagnosis (most typically depression) without specifically targeting suicidal ideation and behavior, the exclusion of individuals who are at high risk for suicide from research protocols, inadequate power to determine the efficacy of various interventions, and the liabilities to researchers and research sponsors associated with research in this area (Pearson, Stanley, King, & Fisher, 2001).

The American Academy of Child and Adolescent Psychiatry (AACAP) has published guidelines intended as a standard of care for treating suicidal behavior (Shaffer et al., 2001). These guidelines include but are not limited to information on how to respond to the initial crisis, safety precautions, and inpatient hospitalization and medication therapy options.

Psychological Interventions

Very few empirical studies have assessed whether psychosocial interventions reduce suicidality or self-harm behaviors among youth. These interventions include group therapy (Ross & Motto, 1984; Wood, Trainor, Rothwell, Moore, & Harrington, 2001); social work outreach (reminding families of appointments, providing transportation, serving as liaison, etc.) and health care provider education (Deykin, Hsieh, Joshi, & McNamarra, 1986); motivational–educational intervention to improve adherence with aftercare recommendations (Rotheram-Borus, Piancentini, Cantwell, Belin, & Song, 2000; Spirito, Boergers, Donaldson, Bishop, & Lewander, 2002); provision of a token allowing readmission to a hospital in the event of a crisis (Cotgrove, Zirinksi, Black, & Weston, 1995); social problem solving (Lerner & Clum, 1990); cognitive-behavioral therapy (Rotheram-Borus, Piacentini, Miller, Graae, & Castro-Blanco, 1994); family-based problem solving (Harrington et al., 1998; Harrington et al., 2000) and multisystemic family therapy (Huey et al., 2004); adaptations of dialectical behavioral therapy (DBT; Katz, Cox, Gunasekara, & Miller, 2004; Rathus & Miller, 2002); and a social networking intervention (King, 2000). In another controlled intervention targeting depression but assessing suicidality, adolescents received either cognitive-behavioral therapy, systemic behavior family therapy, or nondirective supportive therapy (Birmaher et al., 2000; Brent et al., 1997; Brent, Kolko, Birmaher, Baugher, & Bridge, 1999).

Only a portion of these studies have published results and included a comparison or control group against which to gauge the effects of the intervention under study (Birmaher et al., 2000; Brent et al., 1997, 1999; Cotgrove et al., 1995; Deykin et al., 1986; Harrington et al., 1998, 2000; Huey et al., 2004; Katz et al., 2004; Lerner & Clum, 1990; Rathus & Miller, 2002; Spirito et al., 2002; Wood et al., 2001). Overall, results have been mixed. In the study of social work outreach and health care provider education (Deykin et al., 1986), there were no reported effects on the frequency of repeat suicide attempts. However, this study did report a slight decrease in emergency room admissions for suicidal behaviors. The motivational–educational interventions both improved number of sessions attended

(Rotheram-Borus et al., 2000; Spirito et al., 2002). However, in one case (Spirito et al., 2002), the difference was statistically significant only after considering and controlling for baseline characteristics, and in the one study in which the outcome was measured, the intervention did not result in a significantly different rate of suicidality (Rotheram-Borus et al., 2000). In the study in which youth were allowed access to hospitalization via a token, there was a trend for youth in the intervention group to have fewer suicide attempts than youth without access to the hospital (Cotgrove et al., 1995). In a randomized trial of group therapy of eclectic orientation (cognitive-behavioral, problem-solving, psychodynamic), adolescents who received the intervention were less likely to engage in repeat self-harm behavior (both suicidal and nonsuicidal) than youth receiving treatment as usual but without the group therapy (Wood et al., 2001). Youth receiving an outpatient adaptation of dialectical behavioral intervention had fewer suicide attempts than youth receiving treatment as usual, but this finding failed to reach statistical significance (Rathus & Miller, 2002). Within the DBT group, reductions in suicidal ideation also were noted (Rathus & Miller, 2002). Nonetheless, in this study, it should be noted that patients were not randomly assigned to interventions and pretreatment differences existed between the groups. In another study of DBT, at 1-year follow-up, there were no statistically significant differences in rates of suicide attempts, suicidal ideation, or depression between adolescents who received an inpatient adaptation of DBT and adolescents in the hospital who did not receive DBT (Katz et al., 2004). One of the home-based family interventions reduced suicidal ideation, but only among youth without major depression (Harrington et al., 1998, 2000). In contrast, at a 1-year follow-up, youth treated with multisystemic family therapy had greater reductions in youth-reported suicide attempts than comparable youth who were hospitalized and then treated in the community (Huey et al., 2004). Interestingly in this study, multisystemic therapy did not result in a greater reduction in risk factors for suicidal behavior, including suicidal ideation, hopelessness, and depression (Huey et al., 2004). The study focusing on depression but assessing suicidal behavior found no differences across conditions in reductions in

suicidality (Birmaher et al., 2000; Brent et al., 1997, 1999), but did find that suicidal youth were more likely to drop out of treatment and benefited more (in terms of reduced likelihood of continued depression) from either the cognitive-behavioral or family therapy than they did from the nondirective supportive therapy (Barbe, Bridge, Birmaher, Kolko, & Brent, 2001). It should be noted, however, that the most seriously suicidal patients were excluded from participating in this study.

In summary, there have not been a sufficient number of clinical trials with comparison groups to reach any definitive conclusions about the efficacy of psychosocial interventions in reducing suicidal ideation or behavior. There has been much discussion of the potential utility of cognitive-behavioral interventions with suicidal individuals, as these individuals often are described as having a despairing view of their future and a constricted vision of the potential alternatives available to them in solving problems in life. Nonetheless, at this juncture, the empirical evidence neither supports nor refutes the utility of these approaches with suicidal adolescents. Moreover, no published study to date has examined the utility of cognitive-behavioral therapy in augmenting the effects of pharmacotherapy in the treatment of suicidal adolescents.

Most treatment outcome studies for youth with suicidal behavior have focused on treatment of the primary diagnosis, which is often a depressive disorder. It is not clear whether or not interventions should focus on the primary diagnosis, comorbid diagnoses, the symptom of suicidal behavior in and of itself, or some combination of these. It also is not known which interventions are most efficacious or effective with suicidal youth who are not suffering from depressive disorders or experiencing depressive disorders that are comorbid with other conditions such as conduct or substance use disorders. Furthermore, it is unknown whether or not treatment approaches should be different for repeat suicide attempters, single attempters, or youth with suicidal ideation but no history of attempts. It is clear that interventions that focus on individuals who have made suicide attempts almost by definition include elements of relapse prevention; that is, these youth have already made suicide attempts and therefore are at risk, and efforts should be made to help prevent the youth from engaging in this behavior again.

Psychopharmacological Interventions

Pharmacotherapy often is employed clinically with persons who are depressed and/or at risk for harming themselves in an effort to effect symptom change quickly. Several medications that have been used effectively in the treatment of depression among adults have been prescribed clinically in the treatment of depression among children and adolescents (Arnold, 1993; Kye & Ryan, 1995; Popper, 1995; Vitiello & Jensen, 1997). Although clinicians have prescribed tricyclic antidepressants for depression in children and adolescents, the results of clinical trials conducted with tricyclic antidepressants in this population have been mixed at best (Kutcher et al., 1994; Kye et al., 1996; Ryan et al., 1986; Strober, Freeman, & Rigali, 1990; Thurber, Ensign, Punnett & Welter, 1995). The use of tricyclic antidepressants may be especially contraindicated for depressed, suicidal children and adolescents due to the potential for drug overdose and subsequent cardiotoxicity with the tricyclic antidepressants (Birmaher, Brent & Benson, 1998). In addition, there have been some cases of sudden death reported in children and adolescents who were prescribed one of the tricyclic antidepressants (Biederman, 1991).

More recently, clinicians have begun to prescribe another class of antidepressant medications (i.e., selective serotonin reuptake inhibitors, or SSRIs) commonly used in the treatment of adults for the treatment of depression among children and adolescents (Leonard, March, Rickler, & Allen, 1997). Although the number of studies is small, there are emerging data regarding the efficacy of fluoxetine in particular for adolescent depression. In two double-blind randomized controlled trials of fluoxetine in depressed children and adolescents, fluoxetine was associated with greater reduction in depressive symptom severity relative to placebo, but many youth did not experience a complete remission of depressive symptoms (Emslie et al., 1997, 2002). Results of another trial indicated that fluoxetine treatment produced significant decreases in depression among most subjects and decreases of over 50% in self-reported suicidal ideation in seven of nine subjects (Colle, Belair, DiFeo, & Weiss, 1994). Results of a large randomized controlled trial indicated that rates of response (defined as ratings of "much improved" or "very much improved") to combined fluoxetine and cognitive-behavioral therapy, fluoxetine alone, cognitive-behavioral therapy alone, and placebo were 71%, 61%, 43%, and 35%, respectively (Treatment of Adolescent Depression Study [TADS] Team, 2004). All groups evidenced a reduction in suicidal ideation, although the adolescents receiving a combination of fluoxetine and cognitive-behavioral therapy had the greatest reductions in suicidal thoughts (TADS Team, 2004).

In many cases, the SSRIs have been preferred clinically over the tricyclic antidepressants because of the presumption of fewer severe side effects reported and less risk for medication overdose with these agents (Leonard et al., 1997). Nonetheless, there also have been concerns raised about the risk of agitation and suicidal behavior among a subset of individuals treated with these agents. Specifically, in the aforementioned randomized controlled trial of treatments for depressed adolescents, it was found that fluoxetine-treated adolescents had a twofold increased risk of "harm-related adverse events" (e.g., nonsuicidal cutting, suicide attempts, worsening of suicidal ideation, and harm to others) relative to depressed adolescents not treated with medication (TADS Team, 2004). No adolescents in the study died by suicide, and 1.6% attempted suicide (TADS Team, 2004). Similarly, the Food and Drug Administration (FDA) reviewed the evidence regarding adverse events associated with SSRI medication in clinical trials with children and adolescents and found roughly a two-fold increase in suicidality (FDA, 2004). Specifically, there was a 4% rate of increased suicidal ideation and behavior among SSRI-treated youth, and a 2% rate of increased suicidality among placebo-treated patients (FDA, 2004). Jick, Kaye, and Jick (2004) suggested that the increased risk for adverse events with antidepressant medications occurs primarily in the early stages of treatment.

Hence, the use of SSRI medication for depressed and suicidal adolescents presents the possibility for both costs and benefits. Fluoxetine appears to be effective in reducing a major risk factor for suicidality, depression, and together with cognitive-behavioral therapy, it may reduce suicidal thoughts. Nonetheless, a small proportion of youth treated with such agents actually appear to have increases in harm-related behaviors, particularly early in the course of treatment. These findings suggest that if SSRI agents are used with youth, they should be carefully monitored, particularly in the early stages of treatment (FDA, 2004). In addition, a proportion of depressed adolescents may not have complete symptom remission in response to pharmacotherapy interventions. The lack of complete remission of some depressed adolescents treated with medication alone and the possible protective effects of cognitive-behavioral therapy in counteracting the increased risk for harm-related adverse events associated with pharmacotherapy (TADS Team, 2004) highlight the potential utility of combined psychosocial and pharmacological treatments for depressed adolescents with suicidal and nonsuicidal self-harming behavior.

SPECIAL PROBLEMS AND NEEDS

There are several identifiable problems and needs to be considered in providing treatment to suicidal adolescents. First, investigators have documented that youth who have made suicide attempts often do not remain in treatment as long as recommended or have poor adherence to treatment subsequent to the attempt (Trautman, Stewart, & Morishima, 1993). For example, Trautman and colleagues (1993) estimated that adolescent suicide attempters remained in treatment a median of 3 sessions, whereas nonsuicidal adolescents remained in treatment a median of 11 sessions prior to discontinuing treatment. It is of note that adolescents in psychiatric hospital settings have notably higher rates of aftercare follow-through than the rates reported for suicidal adolescents presenting in emergency room settings (Spirito et al., 2002).

Given the documented poor rates of adherence to treatment recommendations for youth who are not hospitalized, interventions with suicidal youth need to include efforts to maximize compliance and adherence with recommended treatments and follow-through with scheduled appointments for treatment. As described in the overview of results, Rotheram-Borus and colleagues (1996) and Spirito and colleagues (2002) have suggested that emergency room interventions can be improved to enhance treatment adherence for adolescent suicide attempters and their families. Rotheram-Borus and colleagues recommended that emergency room personnel be trained in how to respond to adolescent suicide attempters in order to improve the quality of interac-

tions between staff, the youth, and the youth's family. The authors also recommended that it is important to assist patients and their families in developing realistic treatment goals and a contract for time-limited therapy that includes the patient and his or her family. Spirito and colleagues also emphasized the importance of reviewing (and modifying as needed) expectations about treatment and removing barriers to treatment, and they also suggested the potential utility of contracting with families for initial treatment adherence.

Second, treatments for youth need to address the significant interpersonal difficulties and family problems that are common among suicidal adolescents. Investigators have attempted to do this in different ways. Some have suggested that inclusion of the family in the intervention or treatment sessions is very important (Rotheram-Borus et al., 1994). Others have suggested that assisting youth in developing or improving social support within the family, the community, and among peers may be key to preventing future suicidal behaviors (King, 2000).

Third, many adolescents with suicidal behavior receive services from multiple community agencies and mental health specialty services at any given time. Interventions with this population need to make every effort to coordinate services for better continuity of care and to prevent excessive burden on the patient and family.

Fourth, treatments for adolescents with suicidal behaviors need to take into consideration ethnic and cultural differences. Specifically, special consideration should be given to attitudes, customs, or mores that may increase resistance to treatment or be perceived as a barrier to treatment. Depending on the geographic region, language may be a barrier to treatment for some minority populations. In addition, other special populations (such as youth with chronic or life-threatening medical illnesses, in residential treatment settings or in detention centers, or LGB, homeless, or runaway youth) may have additional treatment needs to be considered and included in treatment planning. Although it remains an unanswered empirical question, consideration of these needs in treatment may enhance treatment adherence among suicidal youth.

Fifth, religion and spiritual factors may play a role in protecting youth from suicidal behavior (Shaffer et al., 2001). Treatment efforts should take into consideration the religious and spiritual beliefs of youth and should capitalize on the youth's existing support network within a particular religious community.

EVALUATING TREATMENT OUTCOMES

One must first identify the goals of treatment in evaluating treatment outcomes for suicidal youth. Specifically, some might suggest the goal of treatment with suicidal youth is to reduce the risk for future suicidal behaviors or to decrease suicidal ideation or self-harm behaviors (Pearson et al., 2001). Others might suggest that a more immediate goal of treatment with suicidal youth is to reduce current distress and to ensure the safety of the patient (Pearson et al., 2001). The specific outcomes evaluated are determined, at least in part, by the treatment goals specified.

There are several additional factors that complicate evaluation of treatment outcomes in adolescents. First, as previously described, treatment compliance and follow-through with treatment are sometimes difficult, as many youth drop out of treatment prematurely or after the initial crisis has passed. Parents may not realize the seriousness of their child's actions, or they may deny that a suicide attempt was actually an attempt, and in this context, they may not recognize the need for treatment of their son or daughter beyond the initial crisis. Second, treatment compliance and follow-through with treatment may be further complicated by diagnostic comorbidities or factors. In particular, individuals with substance use disorders and/or personality disorder features may have poor follow-through with treatment. This issue is important to address, as comorbid diagnoses and substance abuse have been identified as risk factors for lethal and nonlethal suicide attempts. To the extent that suicide attempters have various psychiatric diagnoses, different treatment outcomes may need to be evaluated or measured. Third, there are other barriers to treatment that may have an impact on the accurate evaluation of treatment outcomes in adolescents. For example, youth from rural communities may not have access to services for suicidal behavior and may have transportation problems that prevent travel to obtain treatment for such behaviors. Fourth, although there are accepted guidelines for the evaluation

and treatment of suicidal behavior published by the AACAP (Shaffer et al., 2001), there are no empirically validated approaches to treatment and there are likely multiple approaches to the treatment of suicidal behavior in use in the community and clinical settings. Indeed, Spirito and colleagues (2002) recently documented the variability in length and types of "treatment as usual" received by suicidal adolescents in the community. Evaluating treatment outcomes in some standard fashion with such variability in treatment approaches would be difficult at best.

CURRENT NEEDS AND FUTURE DIRECTIONS

Conceptualizing and Understanding Suicidal and Self-Harm Behaviors in Adolescents

An increasing amount is known about the prevalence and risk factors for suicidal behaviors. Perhaps the greatest need in understanding suicidal behaviors is the recognition of the fact that there is potentially great heterogeneity in the population of suicide attempters. Not all who contemplate suicide actually attempt suicide, and only a portion of those who attempt suicide go on to make multiple attempts or eventually die by suicide. There are likely different developmental trajectories associated with suicidal behaviors among youth; some youth may remain persistently at high risk for suicidal behavior, others may make suicide attempts in crisis and then never make additional attempts again, some youth may never attempt despite the presence of multiple risk factors, and some youth may experience increasing risk over time. Youth with different developmental trajectories likely have different outcomes in multiple areas, and the different developmental trajectories may be associated with differing patterns of individual, family, and environmental risk and protective factors.

Nonsuicidal self-harm behavior is very much understudied among adolescents. It is striking that estimates from epidemiological or community studies of nonsuicidal self-harm behaviors are rare. Such estimates are essential in better delineating the extent and course of this problem, as well as its correlates. Similar to suicidal behaviors, there are likely different subgroups of youth with nonsuicidal self-harm behaviors, and we need more information about the heterogeneity within this population, and the associated developmental trajectories of these youth. Finally, with increasing media accounts of nonsuicidal self-harm behavior, and preliminary reports from treatment settings about possible contagion, we need to know more about the extent to which nonsuicidal self-harm behavior occurs in clusters or is influenced by the popular media.

Assessment and Treatment

There is a need for additional research regarding the validation of assessment instruments for suicidal and self-harm behaviors, and the utility of assessment instruments with populations or in settings other than those for which the instruments were originally developed. Although there already are a number of risk assessment instruments for suicidal behaviors available, greater attention in particular needs to be given to the issue of whether or not these instruments actually have demonstrated predictive validity. "Risk factors" for suicidal behavior that are associated or correlated at a single point in time with suicidality may not necessarily be predictive of future suicidality. The primary purpose for administering a risk assessment instrument is to help make judgments about the extent of future risk of suicidal behavior, and longitudinal studies are necessary for evaluating such issues. However, for the great majority of risk assessment instruments, the requisite longitudinal studies have not been undertaken.

Clinicians also often weigh heavily the clinical characteristics of prior suicidal behavior when making judgments about future risk. However, the predictive validity of these clinical characteristics has not been clearly demonstrated for adolescents. Future work is needed to examine, for example, whether suicidal behavior associated with greater medical lethality or greater stated intent is associated with increased risk for future suicidal behavior or greater likelihood of very "serious" suicidal behavior.

In addition, the appropriateness or clinical utility of some of our existing assessment instruments for special populations (such as youth with chronic health problems and newly immigrant youth) or specific settings (such as juvenile detention facilities or primary care physicians' offices) has not been demonstrated. Differing factors may be relevant or predictive of suicidal behavior in groups of youth or in different settings. Attention to the development of instruments (or demonstration of the clinical utility of existing instruments) which are sensitive to and specific to the needs of differing high-risk groups and particular settings is needed. Moreover, advances are being made in our understanding of the biological correlates of suicidal behavior and risk for completed suicide. There is a need for developing assessment tools that are informed by what we have learned about the biological underpinnings of suicidal behavior. It also is apparent that much greater attention has been placed on the assessment of suicidal behavior than on the assessment and risk on nonsuicidal self-harm behavior. Additional work in this area is greatly needed.

Currently, a greater amount of research has focused on prevention of adolescent suicidal behavior than on intervention with suicidal youth. In addition, considerable efforts have been made to develop methods for screening for youth at risk for engaging in suicidal behavior, but we know little about whether the efforts to intervene with such identified youth are effective. Moreover, there have been relatively few controlled treatment studies of suicidal behaviors among adolescents, and the literature regarding the best ways of treating adolescent nonsuicidal self-harm behavior is especially lacking. Given the heterogeneity and differing patterns of psychiatric comorbidity among youth, it is unlikely that a "one size fits all" approach will be effective for all suicidal adolescents. Specifically, the needs of youth with both suicidal and nonsuicidal self-harm behavior may differ from those of suicidal youth without nonsuicidal self-harm behavior, just as the needs of suicidal youth with comorbid conduct or SUDs differ from those of suicidal youth without such problems. Given the high dropout rates of suicidal individuals from treatment, there is a need for new interventions that include a focus on engagement and reduction of ambivalence regarding change. Particularly when relatively low base rate behaviors such as suicide attempts are involved, large multisite studies may be needed to demonstrate definite treatment effects. Treatment studies with high-risk populations such as suicidal and self-harming adolescents are difficult and face numerous challenges but are especially needed, given the public health importance of suicidal and self-harm behaviors in young people.

ACKNOWLEDGMENTS

Preparation of this chapter was supported in part by NIH Grant Nos. MH66252 and MH48762 to David B. Goldston, No. MH63433 to Stephanie Sergent Daniel, and No. DA16742 to Elizabeth Mayfield Arnold. We thank Drs. Alan Berman, Jill Compton, David Jobes, and Joel Sherrill for their comments and suggestions on this chapter.

REFERENCES

Adams, J., Overholser, J., & Spirito, A. (1994). Stressful life events associated with adolescent suicide attempts. *Canadian Journal of Psychiatry, 39,* 43–48.

Agerbo, E., Nordentoft, M., & Mortensen, P. (2002). Familial, psychiatric, and socioeconomic risk factors for suicide in young people: nested case-control study. *British Medical Journal, 325*(7355), 74.

Alvarez, A. (1971). *The savage God: A study of suicide.* New York: Random House.

American Foundation for Suicide Prevention. (2001). *Reporting on suicide: Recommendations for the media* [Online]. Available: http://www.afsp.org/education/recommendations/index.html

American Psychiatric Association. (2000). *Diagnostic and statistical manual of mental disorders* (4th ed., text rev.). Washington, DC: Author.

Anderson, M., Kaufman, J., Simon, T., Barrios, L., Paulozzi, L., Ryan, G., et al. (2001). School-associated violent deaths in the United States, 1994–1999. *Journal of the American Medical Association, 286,* 2695–2702.

Anderson, R. (2002). Deaths: Leading causes for 2000. *National Vital Statistics Reports, 50*(16), 1–86.

Angle, C., O'Brian, T., & McIntire, M. (1983). Adolescent self-poisoning: A nine-year follow-up. *Development and Behavioral Pediatrics, 4,* 83–87.

Arnold, E., Walsh, A., & Goldston, D. (2003, January). *Reading disabilities and suicidal behavior among adolescents.* Paper presented at the meeting of the Society on Social Work Research, Washington, DC.

Arnold, L. (1993). A comparative overview of treatment research methodology: Adult vs. child and adolescent, psychopharmacological vs. psychosocial treatments. *Psychopharmacology Bulletin, 29,* 5–17.

Asarnow, J. (1992). Suicidal ideation and attempts during middle childhood: Associations with perceived family stress and depression among child psychiatric inpatients. *Journal of Clinical Child Psychology, 21,* 35–40.

Asarnow, J., Carlson, G., & Guthrie, D. (1987). Coping strategies, self-perceptions, hopelessness, and perceived family environments in depressed and suicidal children. *Journal of Consulting and Clinical Psychology, 55,* 361–366.

Barbe, R., Bridge, J., Birmaher, B., Kolko, D., & Brent, D. (2001). *Outcome of a psychotherapy treatment in a population of suicidal depressed adolescents.* Paper presented at the Congress on Suicide and Suicide Prevention in Youth, Geneva, Switzerland.

Barraclough, B., & Harris, C. (2002). Suicide preceded by murder: The epidemiology of homicide–suicide in England and Wales 1988–1992. *Psychological Medicine, 32,* 577–584.

Beautrais, A., Joyce, P., & Mulder, R. (1996). Risk factors for serious suicide attempts among youth aged 13 through 24 years. *Journal of the American Academy of Child and Adolescent Psychiatry, 35,* 1174–1182.

Beautrais, A., Joyce, P., & Mulder, R. (1997). Precipitating factors and life events in serious suicide attempts among youth aged 13 through 24 years. *Journal of the American Academy of Child and Adolescent Psychiatry, 36,* 1543–1551.

Beautrais, A., Joyce, P., & Mulder, R. (1998). Psychiatric illness in a New Zealand sample of young people making serious suicide attempts. *New Zealand Medical Journal, 111,* 44–48.

Beck, A. (1996). Beyond belief: A theory of modes, personality, and psychopathology. In P. Salkovskis (Ed.), *Frontiers of cognitive therapy* (pp. 1–25). New York: Guilford Press.

Beck, A. T., Rush, A. J., Shaw, B. F., & Emery, G. (1979). *Cognitive therapy of depression.* New York: Guilford Press.

Beck, A., Schuyler, D., & Herman, I. (1974). Development of suicidal intent scales. In A. Beck, H. Resnik, & D. Lettieri (Eds.), *The prediction of suicide* (pp. 45–56). Bowie, MD: Charles Press.

Beck, A., & Steer, R. (1987). *Manual for the Beck Depression Inventory.* San Antonio, TX: Psychological Corporation.

Beck, A., & Steer, R. (1988). *Beck Hopelessness Scale Manual.* San Antonio, TX: Psychological Corporation.

Beck, A., & Steer, R. (1991). *Manual for the Beck Scale for Suicidal Ideation.* San Antonio, TX: Psychological Corporation.

Berman, A. (2003, April). *Why are suicide rates declining? A panel discussion.* Paper presented at the meeting of the American Association of Suicidology, Santa Fe, NM.

Berman, A., Jobes, D., & Silverman, M. (2005). *Adolescent suicide: Assessment and intervention.* Washington, DC: American Psychological Association Press.

Biederman, J. (1991). Clinical comment: Sudden death in children treated with a tricyclic antidepressant. *Journal of the American Academy of Child and Adolescent Psychiatry, 30,* 495–498.

Birmaher, B., Brent, D., & Benson, R. (1998). Summary of the practice parameters for the assessment and treatment of adolescent major depression. *Journal of the American Academy of Child and Adolescent Psychiatry, 37,* 1234–1238.

Birmaher, B., Brent, D., Kolko, D., Baugher, M., Bridge, J., Holder, D., et al. (2000). Clinical outcome after short-term psychotherapy for adolescents with major depressive disorder. *Archives of General Psychiatry, 57*, 29–36.

Blum, R., Beuhring, T., Shew, M., Bearinger, L., Sieving, R., & Resnik, M. (2000). The effects of race/ethnicity, income, and family structure on adolescent risk behavior. *American Journal of Public Health, 90*, 1879–1884.

Boehm, K., & Campbell, N. (1995). Suicide: A review of calls to an adolescent peer listening phone service. *Child Psychiatry and Human Development, 26*, 61–66.

Boergers, J., Spirito, A., & Donaldson, D. (1998). Reasons for adolescent suicide attempts: Associations with psychological functioning. *Journal of the American Academy of Child and Adolescent Psychiatry, 37*, 1287–1293.

Bollen, K., & Phillips, D. (1982). Imitative suicides: A national study of the effects of televised news stories. *American Sociological Review, 47*, 802–809.

Bradley, J., & Rotheram-Borus, M. (1990). *Evaluation of imminent danger for suicide: A training manual.* Tulsa, OK: National Resource Center for Youth Services.

Brent, D. (1987). Correlates of the medical lethality of suicide attempts in children and adolescents. *Journal of the American Academy of Child and Adolescent Psychiatry, 26*, 87–91.

Brent, D., Baugher, M., Birmaher, B., Kolko, D., & Bridge, J. (2000). Compliance with recommendations to remove firearms in families participating in a clinical trial for adolescent depression. *Journal of the American Academy of Child and Adolescent Psychiatry, 39*, 1220–1226.

Brent, D., Bridge, J., Johnson, B., & Connolly, J. (1996). Suicidal behavior runs in families. A controlled family study of adolescent suicide victims. *Archives of General Psychiatry, 53*, 1145–1152.

Brent, D., Holder, D., Kolko, D., Birmaher, B., Baugher, M., Roth, C., et al. (1997). A clinical psychotherapy trial for adolescent depression comparing cognitive, family, and supportive therapy. *Archives of General Psychiatry, 54*, 877–885.

Brent, D., Kolko, D., Birmaher, B., Baugher, M., & Bridge, J. (1999). A clinical trial for adolescent depression: Predictors of additional treatment in the acute and follow-up phases of the trial. *Journal of the American Academy of Child and Adolescent Psychiatry, 38*, 263–271.

Brent, D., Oquendo, M., Birmaher, B., Greenhill, L., Kolko, D., Stanley, B., et al. (2002). Familial pathways to early-onset suicide attempt—Risk for suicidal behavior in offspring of mood-disordered suicide attempters. *Archives of General Psychiatry, 59*, 801–807.

Brent, D., Perper, J., Goldstein, C., Kolko, D., Allan, M., Allman, C., & Zelenak, J. (1988). Risk factors for adolescent suicide: A comparison of adolescent suicide victims with suicidal inpatients. *Archives of General Psychiatry, 45*, 581–588.

Brent, D., Perper, J., Moritz, G., & Allman, C. (1993).

Psychiatric risk factors for adolescent suicide: A case-control study. *Journal of the American Academy of Child and Adolescent Psychiatry, 32*, 521–529.

Breton, J., Tousignant, M., Bergeron, L., & Berthiaume, C. (2002). Informant-specific correlates of suicidal behavior in a community survey of 12– to 14–year-olds. *Journal of the American Academy of Child and Adolescent Psychiatry, 41*, 723–730.

Briere, J. (1992). *Child abuse trauma: Theory and treatment of the lasting effects.* Newbury Park, CA: Sage.

Briere, J., & Gil, E. (1998). Self-mutilation in clinical and general population samples: Prevalence, correlates, and functions. *American Journal of Orthopsychiatry, 68*, 609–620.

Brown, J., Cohen, P., Johnson, J., & Smailes, E. (1999). Childhood abuse and neglect: Specificity of effects on adolescent and young adult depression and suicidality. *Journal of the American Academy of Child and Adolescent Psychiatry, 38*, 1490–1496.

Brown, L., Overholser, J., Spirito, A., & Fritz, G. (1991). The correlates of planning in adolescent suicide attempts. *Journal of the American Academy of Child and Adolescent Psychiatry, 30*, 95–99.

Bukstein, O., Brent, D., Perper, J., & Moritz, G. (1993). Risk factors for completed suicide among adolescents with a lifetime history of substance abuse: A case-control study. *Acta Psychiatrica Scandinavica, 88*, 403–408.

Burge, V., Felts, M., Chenier, T., & Parrillo, A. (1995). Drug use, sexual activity, and suicidal behavior in U.S. high school students. *Journal of School Health, 65*, 222–227.

Centers for Disease Control and Prevention. (1988). CDC recommendations for a community plan for the prevention and containment of suicide clusters. *Morbidity and Mortality Weekly Report, 27*(S-6), 1–12.

Centers for Disease Control and Prevention. (1998). Suicide among black youths—United States, 1980–1995. *Morbidity and Mortality Weekly Report, 47*, 193–196.

Centers for Disease Control and Prevention. (2001). Temporal variations in school-associated student homicide and suicide events—United States, 1992–1999. *Morbidity and Mortality Weekly Report, 50*, 657–660.

Centers for Disease Control and Prevention. (2002). Centers for Disease Control and Prevention Web-based Injury Statistics Query and Reporting System (WISQARS) [Online]. Available: http://www.cdc.gov/ncipc/wisqars

Clark, D. (2003). Serum tryptophan ratio and suicidal behavior in adolescents: A prospective study. *Biological Psychiatry, 119*, 199–204.

Colle, L., Belair, J., DiFeo, M., & Weiss, J. (1994). Extended open-label fluoxetine treatment of adolescents with major depression. *Journal of Child and Adolescent Psychopharmacology, 4*, 225–232.

Cooper, J., Appleby, L., & Amos, T. (2002). Life events preceding suicide by young people. *Social Psychiatry & Epidemiology, 37*, 271–275.

Cotgrove, A., Zirinsky, L., Black, D., & Weston, D. (1995). Secondary prevention of attempted suicide in adolescence. *Journal of Adolescence, 18,* 569–577.

Cull, J., & Gill, W. (1988). *Suicide Probability Scale (SPS) Manual.* Los Angeles: Western Psychological Services.

D'Augelli, A., Hershberger, S., & Pilkington, N. (2001). Suicidality patterns and sexual orientation-related factors among lesbian, gay, and bisexual youths. *Suicide and Life-Threatening Behavior, 31,* 250–264.

Davila, J., Hammen, C., Burge, D., Paley, B., & Daley, S. (1995). Poor interpersonal problem-solving as a mechanism of stress generation in depression among adolescent women. *Journal of Abnormal Psychology, 104,* 592–600.

DeMaso, D., Ross, L., & Beardslee, W. (1994). Depressive disorders and suicidal intent in adolescent suicide attempters. *Developmental and Behavioral Pediatrics, 15,* 74–77.

De Wilde, E., Kienhorst, I., Diekstra, R., & Wolters, W. (1993). The specificity of psychological characteristics of adolescent suicide attempters. *Journal of the American Academy of Child and Adolescent Psychiatry, 32,* 51–59.

Deykin, E., Hsieh, C., Joshi, N., & McNamarra, J. (1986). Adolescent suicidal and self- destructive behavior: Results of an intervention study. *Journal of Adolescent Health Care, 7,* 88–95.

DiClimente, R., Ponton, L., & Hartley, D. (1991). Prevalence and correlates of cutting behavior: Risk for HIV transmission. *Journal of the American Academy of Child and Adolescent Psychiatry, 30,* 735–739.

DuRant, R. H., Krowchuk, D., Kreiter, S., Sinal, S., & Woods, C. (1999). Weapon carrying on school property among middle school students. *Archives of Pediatrics and Adolescent Medicine, 153,* 21–26.

Durkheim, E. (1951). *Suicide: A study in sociology.* New York: Free Press. (Original work published 1897)

Eggert, L., Thompson, E., & Herting, J. (1994). A measure of adolescent potential for suicide (MAPS): Development and preliminary findings. *Suicide and Life-Threatening Behavior, 24,* 359–381.

Emslie, G., Heiligenstein, J., Wagner, K., Hoog, S., Ernest, D., Brown, E., et al. (2002). Fluoxetine for acute treatment of depression in children and adolescents: A placebo-controlled randomized clinical trial. *Journal of the American Academy of Child and Adolescent Psychiatry, 41,* 1205–1215.

Emslie, G., Rush, A., Weinberg, W., Kowatch, R., Hughes, C., Carmody, T., & Rintelmann, J. (1997). A double-blind, randomized placebo-controlled trial of fluoxetine in depressed children and adolescents. *Archives of General Psychiatry, 54,* 1031–1037.

Esposito, C., Spirito, A., Boergers, J., & Donaldson, D. (2003). Affective, behavioral, and cognitive functioning in adolescents with multiple suicide attempts. *Suicide and Life-Threatening Behavior, 33,* 389–399.

Fawcett, J., Busch, K., Jacobs, D., Kravitz, H., & Fogg, L. (1997). Suicide: A four pathway clinical–biochemical model. *Annals of the New York Academy of Sciences, 836,* 288–301.

Food and Drug Administration. (2004). *FDA Public Health Advisory. Suicidality in children and adolescents being treated with antidepressant medications* [Online]. Available: http://www.fda.gov/cder/drug/antidepressantss/SSRIPHA200410.htm

Fremouw, W., Perczel, M & Ellis, T. (1990). *Suicide risk: Assessment and response guidelines.* New York: Pergamon Press.

Garland, A., & Zigler, E. (1993). Adolescent suicide prevention: Current research and social policy implications. *American Psychologist, 48,* 169–182.

Garofalo, R., Wolf, R., Wissow, L., Woods, E., & Goodman, E. (1999). Sexual orientation and risk of suicide attempts among a representative sample of youth. *Archives of Pediatrics and Adolescent Medicine, 153,* 487–493.

Garrison, C., Addy, C., McKeown, R., & Cuffe, S. (1993). Nonsuicidal physically self-damaging acts in adolescents. *Journal of Child and Family Studies, 2,* 339–352.

Goldney, R. (1982). Locus of control in young women who have attempted suicide. *Journal of Nervous and Mental Disease, 170,* 198–201.

Goldsmith, S., Pellmar, T., Kleinman, A., & Bunney, W. (2002). *Reducing suicide: A national imperative.* Washington, DC: National Academy Press.

Goldston, D. (2003). *Measuring suicidal behaviors and risk among children and adolescents.* Washington, DC: American Psychological Press.

Goldston, D., Daniel, S, Melton, B., Reboussin, D, Kelley, A., & Frazier P. (1998). Psychiatric disorders among previous suicide attempters, first-time, and repeat attempters on an adolescent inpatient psychiatry unit. *Journal of the American Academy of Child and Adolescent Psychiatry, 37,* 924–932.

Goldston, D., Daniel, S., Reboussin, D., Kelley, A., Ievers, C., & Brunstetter, R. (1996). First-time suicide attempters, repeat attempters, and previous attempters on an adolescent inpatient psychiatry unit. *Journal of the American Academy of Child and Adolescent Psychiatry, 35,* 631–639.

Goldston, D., Daniel, S., Reboussin, D., Melton, B., Frazier, P., & Kelley, A. (1999). Suicide attempts among formerly hospitalized adolescents: A prospective naturalistic study of risk during the first five years following discharge. *Journal of the American Academy of Child and Adolescent Psychiatry, 38,* 660–671.

Goldston, D., Daniel, S., Reboussin, B., Reboussin, D., Frazier, P., & Harris, A. (2001). Cognitive risk factors and suicide attempts among formerly hospitalized adolescents: A prospective naturalistic study. *Journal of the American Academy of Child and Adolescent Psychiatry, 40,* 91–99.

Goldston, D., Kelley, A., Reboussin, D., Daniel, S., Smith, J., Schwartz, R., et al. (1997). Suicidal ideation and behavior and noncompliance with the medical regimen among diabetic adolescents. *Journal of* the American Academy of Child and Adolescent Psychiatry, 36, 1528–1536.

Goldston, D., Kovacs, M., Ho, V., Parrone, P., & Stiffler, L. (1994). Suicidal ideation and suicide attempts among youth with insulin-dependent diabetes mellitus. *Journal of the American Academy of Child and Adolescent Psychiatry, 33,* 240–246.

Gould, M., Fisher, P., Parides, M., Flory, M., & Shaffer, D. (1996). Psychosocial risk factors of child and adolescent completed suicide. *Archives of General Psychiatry, 53,* 1155–1162.

Gould, M., King, R., Greenwald, S., Fisher, P. Schwab-Stone, M., Kramer, R., et al. (1998). Psychopathology associated with suicidal ideation and attempts among children and adolescents. *Journal of the American Academy of Child and Adolescent Psychiatry, 37,* 915–923.

Gould, M., & Kramer, R. (2001). Youth suicide prevention. *Suicide and Life-Threatening Behavior, 31,* 6–31.

Gould, M., Petrie, K., Kleinman, M., & Wallenstein, S. (1994). Clustering of attempted suicide: New Zealand national data. *International Journal of Epidemiology, 23,* 1185–1189.

Granboulan, V., Rabain, D., & Basquin, M. (1995). The outcome of adolescent suicide attempts. *Acta Psychiatrica Scandinavica, 91,* 265–270.

Grunbaum, J., Kann, L., Kinchen, S., Williams, B., Ross, J., Lowry, R., & Kolby, L. (2002). Youth Risk Behavior Surveillance—United States, 2001. *Morbidity and Mortality Weekly Report, 51*(No. SS-4), 1–68.

Guertin, T., Lloyd-Richardson, E., Spirito, A., Donaldson, D., & Boergers, J. (2001). Self-mutilative behavior in adolescents who attempt suicide by overdose. *Journal of the American Academy of Child and Adolescent Psychiatry, 40,* 1062–2069.

Gunnell, D., Shepherd, M., & Evans, M. (2000). Are recent increases in deliberate self-harm associated with changes in socio-economic conditions? An ecological analysis of patterns of deliberate self-harm in Bristol 1972–3 and 1995–6. *Psychological Medicine, 2000,* 1197–1203.

Gutierrez, P., Osman, A., Watkins, R., Konick, L., Muehlenkamp, J., & Brausch, M. (2002, October). *Development and validation of the Suicide Resilience Inventory—25 (SRI-25) in clinical and non-clinical samples.* Paper presented at the Kansas Conference in Clinical Child and Adolescent Psychology, Lawrence.

Haggerty, R., Sherrod, L., Garmezy, N., & Rutter, M. (1994). *Stress, risk, and resilience in children and adolescents: Processes, mechanisms, and interventions.* New York: Cambridge University Press.

Hammen, C. (1991). Generation of stress in the course of unipolar depression. *Journal of Abnormal Psychology, 100,* 555–561.

Harrington, R. (2001). Depression, suicide and deliberate self-harm in adolescence. *British Medical Bulletin, 57,* 47–60.

Harrington, R., Bredenkamp, D., Gromhues, C., Rutter, M., Fudge, H., & Pickles, A. (1994). Adult outcomes of childhood and adolescent depression, III; Links with suicidal behaviours. *Journal of Child Psychology and Psychiatry, 35,* 512–518.

Harrington, R., Kerfoot, M., Dyer, E., McNiven, F., Gill, J., Harrington, V., & Woodham, A. (2000). Deliberate self-poisoning in adolescence: Why does a brief family intervention work in some cases and not others? *Journal of Adolescence, 23,* 13–20.

Harrington, R., Kerfoot, M., Dyer, E., McNiven, F., Gill, J., Harrington, V., et al. (1998). Randomized trial of a home-based family intervention for children who have deliberately poisoned themselves. *Journal of the American Academy of Child and Adolescent Psychiatry, 37,* 512–518.

Hawton, K. (1987). Assessment of suicide risk. *British Journal of Psychiatry, 150,* 145–153.

Hawton, K., Arensman, E., Townsend, E., Bremner, S., Feldman, E., Goldney, R., et al. (1998). Deliberate self harm: Systematic review of efficacy of psychosocial and pharmacological treatments in preventing repetition. *British Medical Journal, 317,* 441–447.

Hawton, K., Cole, D., O'Grady, J., & Osborn, M. (1982). Motivational aspects of deliberate self-poisoning in adolescents. *British Journal of Psychiatry, 141,* 286–291.

Hawton, K., Fagg, J., Platt, S., & Hawkins, M. (1993). Factors associated with suicide after parasuicide in young people. *British Medical Journal, 306,* 1641–1644.

Hawton, K., Kingsbury, S., Steinhardt, K., James, A., & Fagg, J. (1999). Repetition of deliberate self-harm by adolescents: The role of psychological factors. *Journal of Adolescence, 22,* 369–378.

Heikkinen, M., Aro, H., & Lonnqvist, J. (1994). Recent life events, social support and suicide. *Acta Psychiatrica Scandinavica, 377*(Suppl.), 65–72.

Hershberger, S., Pilkington, N., & D'Augelli, A. (1997). Predictors of suicide attempts among gay, lesbian, and bisexual youth. *Journal of Adolescent Research, 12,* 477–497.

Hoberman, H., & Garfinkel, B. (1988). Completed suicide in children and adolescents. *Journal of the American Academy of Child and Adolescent Psychiatry, 27,* 689–695.

Hollis, C. (1996). Depression, family environment, and adolescent suicidal behavior. *Journal of the American Academy of Child and Adolescent Psychiatry, 35,* 622–630.

Horesh, N., Gothelf, D., Ofek, H., Weizman, T., & Apter, A. (1999). Impulsivity as a correlate of suicidal behavior in adolescent psychiatric inpatients. *Crisis, 20,* 8–14.

Huey, S., Henggeler, S., Rowland, M., Halliday-Boykins, C., Cunningham, P., Pickrel, S., & Edwards, J. (2004). Multisystemic therapy effects on attempted suicide by youths presenting psychiatric emergencies. *Journal of the American Academy of Child and Adolescent Psychiatry, 43,* 183–190.

Jick, H., Kaye, J., & Jick, S. (2004). Antidepressants

and the risk of suicidal behaviors. *Journal of the American Medical Association, 292,* 338–343.

Kalafat, J., & Elias, M. (1994). An evaluation of a school-based suicide awareness intervention. *Suicide and Life-Threatening Behavior, 24,* 224–233.

Kalafat, J., & Ryerson, D. (1999). The implementation and institutionalization of a school-based youth suicide prevention program. *Journal of Primary Prevention, 19,* 157–175.

Katz, L., Cox, B., Gunasekara, S., & Miller, A. (2004). Feasibility of dialectical behavior therapy for suicidal adolescent inpatients. *Journal of the American Academy of Child and Adolescent Psychiatry, 43,* 276–282.

Kazdin, A., Rodgers, A., & Colbus, D. (1986). The Hopelessness Scale for Children: Psychometric characteristics and concurrent validity. *Journal of Consulting and Clinical Psychology, 54,* 241–245.

Kerfoot, M. (1988). Deliberate self-poisoning in childhood and early adolescence. *Journal of Child Psychology and Psychiatry, 29,* 335–343.

Kerfoot, M., Dyer, E., Harrington, V., & Woodham, A. (1996). Correlates and short-term course of self-poisoning in adolescents. *British Journal of Psychiatry, 168,* 38–42.

Kerfoot, M., & McHugh, G. (1992). The outcome of childhood suicidal behavior. *Acta Paedopsychiatrica, 55,* 141–154.

Kienhorst, C., De Wilde, E., Diekstra, R., & Wolters, W. (1992). Differences between adolescent suicide attempters and depressed adolescents. *Acta Psychiatrica Scandinavica, 85,* 222–228.

Kienhorst, I., De Wilde, E., Diekstra, R., & Wolters, W. (1995). Adolescents' image of their suicide attempt. *Journal of the American Academy of Child and Adolescent Psychiatry, 34,* 623–628.

King, C. (2000, April). Connect Five: A youth suicide prevention strategy. In B. Wagner (Moderator), *Coping efforts of suicidal adolescents: Basic research, treatment, and preventive intervention.* Panel presentation at the meeting of the American Association of Suicidology, Los Angeles.

King, R., Schwab-Stone, M., Flisher, A., Greenwald, S., Kramer, R., Goodman, S., et al. (2001). Psychosocial and risk behavior correlates of youth suicide attempts and suicidal ideation. *Journal of the American Academy of Child and Adolescent Psychiatry, 40,* 837–846.

Klimes-Dougan, B. (1998). Screening for suicidal ideation in children and adolescents: Methodological considerations. *Journal of Adolescence, 21,* 435–444.

Klinger, D. (2001). Suicidal intent in victim-precipitated homicide: Insights from the study of "suicide-by-cop." *Homicide Studies: An Interdisciplinary and International Journal, 5,* 206–226.

Kovacs, M. (1985). The Children's Depression Inventory (CDI). *Psychopharmacology Bulletin, 21,* 995–998.

Kovacs, M. (1992). *Children's Depression Inventory manual.* North Tonawanda, NY: Multi-Health Systems.

Kovacs, M., Goldston, D., & Gatsonis, C. (1993). Suicidal behaviors and childhood-onset depressive disorders: A longitudinal study. *Journal of the American Academy of Child and Adolescent Psychiatry, 32,* 8–20.

Kutcher, S., Boulos, C., Ward, B., Marton, P., Simeon, J., Ferguson, H., et al. (1994). Response to desipramine treatment in adolescent depression: A fixed-dose, placebo-controlled trial. *Journal of the American Academy of Child and Adolescent Psychiatry, 33,* 686–694.

Kye, C., & Ryan, N. (1995). Pharmacologic treatment of child and adolescent depression. *Child and Adolescent Psychiatric Clinics of North America, 4,* 261–281.

Kye, C., Waterman, G., Ryan, N., Birmaher, B., Williamson, D., Iyengar, S., & Dachille, S. (1996). A randomized, controlled trial of amitriptyline in the acute treatment of adolescent major depression. *Journal of the American Academy of Child and Adolescent Psychiatry, 35,* 1139–1144.

Laurent, A., Foussard, N., David, M., Boucharlat, J., & Bost, M. (1998). A 5–year follow-up study of suicide attempts among French adolescents. *Journal of Adolescent Health, 22,* 424–430.

Leon, A., Friedman, R., Sweeney, J., Brown, R., & Mann, J. (1989). Statistical issues in the identification of risk factors for suicidal behavior: The application of survival analysis. *Psychiatry Research, 31,* 99–108.

Leonard, H., March, J., Rickler, K., & Allen, A. (1997). Pharmacology of the selective serotonin reuptake inhibitors in children and adolescents. *Journal of the American Academy of Child and Adolescent Psychiatry, 36,* 725–736.

Lerner, M., & Clum, G. (1990). Treatment of suicidal ideators: A problem-solving approach. *Behavior Therapy, 21,* 403–411.

Lester, D. (1987). *Suicide as a learned behavior.* Springfield, IL: Charles C Thomas.

Lewinsohn, P. (1974). The behavioral study and treatment of depression. In N. Hersen, R. Eisler, & P. Miller (Eds.), *Progress in behavior modification.* New York: Academic Press.

Lewinsohn, P., Langhinrichsen-Rohling, J., Langford, R., Rohde, P., Seeley, J., & Chapman, J. (1995). The Life Attitudes Schedule: A scale to assess adolescent life-enhancing and life-threatening behaviors. *Suicide and Life-Threatening Behavior, 25,* 458–478.

Lewinsohn, P., Rohde, P., & Seeley, J. (1996). Adolescent suicidal ideation and attempts: Prevalence, risk factors, and clinical implications. *Clinical Psychology: Science and Practice, 3,* 25–46.

Lewinsohn, P., Rohde, P., Seeley, J., & Baldwin, C. (2001). Gender differences in suicide attempts from adolescence to young adulthood. *Journal of the American Academy of Child and Adolescent Psychiatry, 40,* 427–434.

Linehan, M. M. (1993). *Cognitive-behavioral treatment of borderline personality disorder.* New York: Guilford Press.

Linehan, M. M. (1997). Behavioral treatments of suicidal behavior: Definitional obfuscation and treatment outcomes. *Annals of the New York Academy of Sciences, 836,* 302–328.

Linehan, M. M., & Comtois, K. (1997). *Lifetime Parasuicide Count.* Unpublished instrument, University of Washington, Seattle.

Linehan, M. M., Goodstein, J., Nielsen, S., & Chiles, J. (1983). Reasons for staying alive when you are thinking of killing yourself: The Reasons for Living Inventory. *Journal of Consulting and Clinical Psychology, 51,* 276–286.

Lonnqvist, J., & Ostano, A. (1991). Suicide following the first suicide attempt: A five-year follow-up using a survival analysis. *Psychiatria Fennica, 22,* 171–179.

Mann, J., Brent, D., & Arango, V. (2001). The neurobiology and genetics of suicide and attempted suicide: A focus on the serotonergic system. *Neuropsychopharmacology, 24,* 467–477.

Mann, J., Huang, Y., Underwood, M., Kassir, S., Openheim, S., Kelly, T., et al. (2000). A serotonin transporter gene promoter polymorphism (5–HTTLPR) and prefrontal cortical binding in major depression and suicide. *Archives of General Psychiatry, 57,* 729–738.

Meehan, P., Lamb, J., Saltzman, L., & O'Carroll, P. (1992). Attempted suicide among young adults: Progress toward a meaningful estimate of prevalence. *American Journal of Psychiatry, 149,* 41–44.

Menninger, K. (1996). Psychoanalytic aspects of suicide. In J. Maltsburger & M. Goldblatt (Eds.), Essential papers on suicide. New York: New York University Press. (Original work published 1933)

Miller, H., Coombs, D., Leeper, J., & Barton, S. (1984). An analysis of the effects of suicide prevention facilities on suicide rates in the United States. *American Journal of Public Health, 74,* 340–343.

Minois, G. (1995/1999). *History of suicide: Voluntary death in Western culture.* Baltimore: Johns Hopkins University Press.

Mohler, B., & Earls, F. (2001). Trends in adolescent suicide: Misclassification bias? *American Journal of Public Health, 91,* 150–153.

Morgan, H. G., Barton, J., Pottle, S., Pocock, H., & Burns-Cox, C. (1976). Deliberate self-harm: A follow-up study of 279 patients. *British Journal of Psychiatry, 128,* 361–368.

Moscicki, E. (1999). Epidemiology of suicide. In D. Jacobs (Ed.), *The Harvard Medical School guide to suicide assessment and intervention* (pp. 40–51). San Francisco: Jossey-Bass/Pfeiffer.

Nasser, E., & Overholser, J. (1999). Assessing varying degrees of lethality in depressed adolescent suicide attempters. *Acta Psychiatrica Scandinavica, 99,* 423–431.

National Center for Health Statistics. (2002). *Health,* United States, 2002. With chartbook on trends in the health of Americans. Hyattsville, MD: Author.

Nishiguchi, N., Shirakawa, O., Ono, H., Nishimura, A., Nushida, H., Ueno, Y., & Maeda, K. (2002). Lack of an association between 5–HAT1A receptor gene structural polymorphisms and suicide victims. *American Journal of Medical Genetics, 114,* 423–425.

Nixon, M., Cloutier, P., & Aggarwal, S. (2002). Affective regulation and addictive aspects of repetitive self-injury in hospitalized adolescents. *Journal of the American Academy of Child and Adolescent Psychiatry, 41,* 1333–1341.

Nock, M., & Kazdin, A. (2002). Examination of affective, cognitive, and behavioral factors and suicide-related outcomes in children and young adolescents. *Journal of Clinical Child and Adolescent Psychology, 31,* 48–58.

O'Carroll, P., Berman, A., Maris, R., & Moscicki, E. (1996). Beyond the Tower of Babel: A nomenclature for suicidology. *Suicide and Life-Threatening Behavior, 26,* 237–252.

Orvaschel, H. (1994). *Schedule for Affective Disorders and Schizophrenia for School-Aged Children—Epidemiologic Version 5 (K-SADS-E).* Unpublished instrument, Nova Southeastern University, Ft. Lauderdale, FL.

Osman, A., Barrios, F., Gutierrez, P., Wrangham, J., Kopper, B., Truelove, R., et al. (2002). The Positive and Negative Suicide Ideation (PANSI) Inventory: Psychometric evaluation with adolescent psychiatric inpatient samples. *Journal of Personality Assessment, 79,* 522–540.

Osman, A., Downs, W., Kopper, B., Barrios, F., Baker, M., Osman, J., et al. (1998). The Reasons for Living Inventory for Adolescents (RFL-A): Development and psychometric properties. *Journal of Clinical Psychology, 54,* 1063–1078.

Pearce, C. M., & Martin, G. (1993). Locus of control as an indicator of risk for suicidal behaviour among adolescents. *Acta Psychiatrica Scandinavica, 88,* 409–414.

Pearlin, L. (1983). Role strains and personal stress. In H. B. Kaplan (Ed.), *Psychosocial stress* (pp. 3–32). New York: Academic Press.

Pearson, J., Stanley, B., King, C., & Fisher, C. (2001). Intervention research with persons at high risk for suicidality: Safety and ethical considerations. *Journal of Clinical Psychiatry, 62*(Suppl. 125), 17–26.

Perez-Smith, A., Spirito, A., & Boergers, J. (2002). Neighborhood predictors of hopelessness among adolescent suicide attempters: Preliminary investigation *Suicide and Life-Threatening Behavior, 32,* 139–145.

Peruzzi, N., & Bongar, B. (1999). Assessing risk for completed suicide in patients with major depression: Psychologists' view of critical factors. *Professional Psychology, Research and Practice, 30,* 576–580.

Peterson, B., Zhang, H., Santa Lucia, R., King, R., & Lewis, M. (1996). Risk factors for presenting problems in child psychiatric emergencies. *Journal of the*

American Academy of Child and Adolescent Psychiatry, 35, 1162–1173.

Pfeffer, C., Conte, H., Plutchik, R., & Jerrett, I. (1979). Suicidal behavior in latency age children: An empirical study. *Journal of the American Academy of Child Psychiatry, 18,* 679–692.

Pfeffer, C., Hurt, S., Peskin, J., & Siefker, C. (1995). Suicidal children grow up: Ego functions associated with suicide attempts. *Journal of the American Academy of Child and Adolescent Psychiatry, 34,* 1318–1325.

Pfeffer, C., Klerman, G., Hurt, S., Kakuna, T., Peskin, J., & Siefker, C. (1993). Suicidal children grow up: Rates and psychological risk factors for suicide attempts during follow-up. *Journal of the American Academy of Child and Adolescent Psychiatry, 32,* 609–616.

Pfeffer, C., Klerman, G., Hurt, S., Lesser, M., Peskin, J., & Siefker, C. (1991). Suicidal children grow up: Demographic and clinical risk factors for adolescent suicide attempts. *Journal of the American Academy of Child and Adolescent Psychiatry, 32,* 106–113.

Phillips, D. (1974). The influence of suggestion on suicide: Substantive and theoretical implication of the Werther effect. *American Sociological Review, 39,* 340–354.

Placidi, G., Oquendo, M., Malone, K., Huang, Y., Ellis, S., & Mann, J. (2001). Aggressivity, suicide attempts, and depression: Relationship to cerebrospinal fluid monoamine metabolite levels. *Biological Psychiatry, 50,* 783–391.

Plutchik, R., Van Praag, H., Picard, S., Conte, H., & Korn, M. (1989). Is there a relationship between the seriousness of suicidal intent and the lethality of the suicide attempt? *Psychiatry Research, 27,* 71–79.

Popper, C. (1995). Balancing knowledge and judgment: A clinician looks at new developments in child and adolescent psychopharmacology. *Child and Adolescent Psychiatric Clinics of North America, 4,* 483–513.

Potter, L., Kresnow, M., Powell, K., O'Carroll, P., Lee, R., Frankowski, R., et al. (1998). Identification of nearly fatal suicide attempts: Self-Inflicted Injury Severity Form. *Suicide and Life-Threatening Behavior, 28,* 174–186.

Poznanski, E., & Mokros, H. (1999). *Children's Depression Rating Scale Revised (CDRS-R)—Manual.* Los Angeles: Western Psychological Services.

Rao, U., Weissman, M., Martin, J., & Hammond, R. (1993). Childhood depression and risk of suicide: A preliminary report of a longitudinal study. *Journal of the American Academy of Child and Adolescent Psychiatry, 32,* 21–27.

Rathus, J., & Miller, A. (2002). Dialectical behavioral therapy adapted for suicidal adolescents. *Suicide and Life-Threatening Behavior, 32,* 146–157.

Reich, W. (2000). Diagnostic Interview for Children and Adolescents (DICA). *Journal of the American Academy of Child and Adolescent Psychiatry, 39,* 59–66.

Reisman, B., & Scharfman, M. (1991). *Teenage suicide prevention workshops for guidance counselors.*

Douglaston, NY: Pride of Judea Mental Health Center.

Reynolds, W. (1988). *Suicidal Ideation Questionnaire: Professional Manual.* Odessa, FL: Psychological Assessment Resources.

Reynolds, W. (1989). *Suicidal Behaviors Inventory (SBI).* Unpublished instrument, University of Wisconsin, Madison.

Reynolds, W. (1990). Development of a semistructured clinical interview for suicidal behaviors in adolescents. *Psychological Assessment, 2,* 382–393.

Reynolds, W. (1991). A school-based procedure for the identification of adolescents at risk for suicidal behaviors. *Family and Community Health, 14,* 64–75.

Reynolds, W. (1998). *Adolescent Psychopathology Scale: Psychometric and technical manual.* Odessa, FL: Psychological Assessment Resources.

Rich, C. L., Sherman, M., & Fowler, R. C. (1990). San Diego suicide study: The adolescents. *Adolescence, 25,* 855–865.

Richardson, J., & Zaleski, W. (1986). Endogenous opiates and self-mutilation. *American Journal of Psychiatry, 143,* 938–939.

Riggs, S., Alario, A., & McHorney, C. (1990). Health risk behaviors and attempted suicide in adolescents who report prior maltreatment. *Journal of Pediatrics, 116,* 815–821.

Roberts, R., Chen, Y., & Roberts, C. (1997). Ethnocultural differences in prevalence of adolescent suicidal behaviors. *Suicide and Life-Threatening Behavior, 27,* 208–217.

Ross, C., & Motto, J. (1984). Group counseling for suicidal adolescents. In H. Sudak, A. Ford, & N. Rushforth (Eds.), *Suicide in the young* (pp. 367–392). Boston: John Wright—PSG.

Ross, S., & Heath, N. (2002). A study of the frequency of self-mutilation in a community sample of adolescents. *Journal of Youth and Adolescence, 31,* 67–77.

Rotheram-Borus, M. (1987). Evaluation of imminent danger for suicide among youth. *American Journal of Orthopsychiatry, 57,* 102–110.

Rotheram-Borus, M. (1989). Evaluation of suicide risk among youths in community settings. *Suicide and Life-Threatening Behavior, 19,* 108–119.

Rotheram-Borus, M., Piacentini, J., Cantwell, C., Belin, T., & Song, J. (2000). The 18–month impact of an emergency room intervention for adolescent female suicide attempters. *Journal of Consulting and Clinical Psychology, 68,* 1081–1093.

Rotheram-Borus, M., Piacentini, J., Miller, S., Graae, F., & Castro-Blanco, D. (1994). Brief cognitive-behavioral treatment for adolescent suicide attempters and their families. *Journal of the American Academy of Child and Adolescent Psychiatry, 33,* 508–517.

Rotheram-Borus, M., Piacentini, J., Miller, S., Graae, F., Dunne, E., & Cantwell, C. (1996). Toward improving treatment adherence among adolescent suicide attempters. *Clinical Child Psychology and Psychiatry, 1,* 99–108.

Roy, A., Nielsen, D., Rylander, G., Sarchiapone, M., &

Segal, N. (1999). Genetics of suicide in depression. *Journal of Clinical Psychiatry, 60S*, 12–17.

Rudd, M. D. (2000). Integrating science into the practice of clinical suicidology: A review of the psychotherapy literature and a research agenda for the future. In R. W. Maris, S. S. Cannetto, J. L. McIntosh, & M. M. Silverman (Eds.), *Review of suicidology, 2000* (pp. 47–83). New York: Guilford Press.

Russell, S., & Joyner, K. (2001). Adolescent sexual orientation and suicide risk: Evidence from a national study. *American Journal of Public Health, 91*, 1276–1281.

Ryan, N., Puig-Antich, J., Cooper, T., Rabinovich, H., Ambrosini, P., Davies, M., et al. (1986). Imipramine in adolescent major depression: Plasma level and clinical response. *Acta Psychiatrica Scandinavica, 73*, 275–288.

Sansone, R. A., Sansone, L. A., & Wiederman, M. (1995). The prevalence of trauma and its relationship to borderline personality symptoms and self-destructive behaviors in a primary care setting. *Archives of Family Medicine, 4*, 439–442.

Santa Mina, E., & Gallop, R. (1998). Childhood sexual and physical abuse and adult self-harm and suicidal behaviour: A literature review. *Canadian Journal of Psychiatry, 43*, 793–800.

Seligman, M. (1975). *Helplessness: On depression, development, and death.* Oxford, UK: Freeman.

Shaffer, D. (1994). Suicide and attempted suicide. In M. Rutter, E. Taylor, & L. Hersov (Eds.), *Child and adolescent psychiatry: Modern approaches* (3rd ed., pp. 407–424). Oxford, UK: Blackwell Scientific.

Shaffer, D. (1996). Discussion of "Predictive validity of the Suicide Probability Scale among adolescents in group home treatment." *Journal of the Academy of Child and Adolescent Psychiatry, 35*, 172–174.

Shaffer, D., & Craft, L. (1999). Methods of adolescent suicide prevention. *Journal of Clinical Psychiatry, 60*, 70–74.

Shaffer, D., Fisher, P., Lucas, C., Dulcan, M., & Schwab-Stone, M. (2000). NIMH Diagnostic Interview Schedule for Children, Version IV (NIMH DISC-IV): Description, differences from previous versions, and reliability of some common diagnoses. *Journal of the American Academy of Child and Adolescent Psychiatry, 39*, 28–38.

Shaffer, D., Fisher, P., Parides, M., & Gould, M. (1995). Sexual orientation in adolescents who commit suicide. *Suicide and Life-Threatening Behavior, 25*(Suppl.), 64–71.

Shaffer, D., Garland, A., Whittle, B., & Underwood, M. (1988). *An evaluation of the adolescent suicide prevention programs (Contract No. 50013).* Trenton, NJ: Governor's Council on Adolescent Suicide.

Shaffer, D., Gould, M., Fisher, P., Trautman, P., Moreau, D., Kleinman, M., & Flory, M. (1996). Psychiatric diagnoses in child and adolescent suicide. *Archives of General Psychiatry, 53*, 339–348.

Shaffer, D., Pfeffer, C., & Workgroup on Quality Issues. (2001). Practice parameters for the assessment and treatment of children and adolescents with suicidal behavior. *Journal of the American Academy of Child and Adolescent Psychiatry, 40*, 24S–51S.

Shaffer, D., Scott, M., Wilcox, H., Maslow, C., Hicks, R., Lucas, C., et al. (2004). The Columbia Suicide Screen: Validity and reliability of a screen for youth suicide and depression. *Journal of the American Academy of Child and Adolescent Psychiatry, 43*, 71–79.

Shaffer, D., Vieland, V., Garland, A., Roias, M., Underwood, M., & Busner, C. (1990). Adolescent suicide attempters: Response to suicide prevention programs. *Journal of the American Medical Association, 264*, 3151–3155.

Shaunesey, K., Cohen, J., Plummer, B., & Berman, A. (1993). Suicidality in hospitalized adolescents: Relationship to prior abuse. *American Journal of Psychiatry, 63*, 113–119.

Sherrill, J., & Kovacs, M. (2000). The Interview Schedule for Children and Adolescents (ISCA). *Journal of the American Academy of Child and Adolescent Psychiatry, 39*, 67–75.

Shneidman, E. (1996). The suicidal mind. New York: Oxford University Press.

Simon, T., Swann, A., Powell, K., Potter, L., Kresnow, M., & O'Carroll, P. (2001). Characteristics of impulsive suicide attempts and attempters. *Suicide and Life-Threatening Behavior, 32*(Suppl.), 49–59.

Sloan, J., Rivara, F., Reay, D., Ferris, J., & Kellermann, A. (1990). Firearm regulations and rates of suicide. A comparison of two metropolitan areas. *New England Journal of Medicine, 322*, 369–373.

Smith, K., Conroy, R., & Ehler, B. (1984). Lethality of Suicide Attempt Rating Scale. *Suicide and Life-Threatening Behavior, 14*, 215–242.

Spirito, A., Boergers, J., & Donaldson, D. (2000). Adolescent suicide attempters: Post-attempt course and implications for treatment. *Clinical Psychology and Psychotherapy, 7*, 161–173.

Spirito, A., Boergers, J., Donaldson, D., Bishop, D., & Lewander, W. (2002). An intervention trial to improve adherence to community treatment by adolescents after a suicide attempt. *Journal of the American Academy of Child and Adolescent Psychiatry, 41*, 435–442.

Spirito, A., Plummer, B., Gispert, M., Levy, S., Kurkjian, J., Lewander, W., et al. (1992). Adolescent suicide attempts: Outcomes at follow-up. *American Journal of Orthopsychiatry, 62*, 464–468.

Spirito, A., Stark, L., Fristad, M., Hart, K., & Owens-Stively, J. (1987). Adolescent suicide attempters hospitalized on a pediatric unit. *Journal of Pediatric Psychology, 12*, 171–189.

Spirito, A., Sterling, C., Donaldson, D., & Arrigan, M. (1996). Factor analysis of the Suicide Intent Scale with adolescent suicide attempters. *Journal of Personality Assessment, 67*, 90–101.

Steer, R., & Beck, A. (1988). Use of the Beck Depression Inventory, Hopelessness Scale, Scale for Suicidal Ideation, and Suicidal Intent Scale with adolescents. *Advances in Adolescent Mental Health, 3*, 219–231.

Steer, R., Beck, A., Garrison, B., & Lester, D. (1988). Eventual suicide in interrupted and uninterrupted attempters: A challenge to the cry-for-help hypothesis. *Suicide and Life-Threatening Behavior, 18,* 119–128.

Strober, M., Freeman, R., & Rigali, J. (1990). The pharmacotherapy of depressive illness in adolescence: An open label trial of imipramine. *Psychopharmacology Bulletin, 26,* 80–84.

Taiminen, T., Kallio-Soukianen, K., Nokso-Koivisto, H., Kaljonen, A., & Helenius, H. (1998). Contagion of deliberate self-harm among adolescent inpatients. *Journal of the American Academy of Child and Adolescent Psychiatry, 37,* 211–217.

Thompson, E., Eggert, E., Randell, B.., & Pike, K. (2001). Evaluation of indicated suicide risk prevention approaches for potential high school dropouts. *American Journal of Public Health, 91,* 742–752.

Thurber, S., Ensign, J., Punnett, A., & Welter, K. (1995). A meta-analysis of antidepressant outcome studies that involved children and adolescents. *Journal of Clinical Psychology, 51,* 340–345.

Tiet, Q., Wasserman, G., Loeber, R., McReynolds, L., & Miller, L. (2001). Developmental and sex differences in types of conduct problems. *Journal of Child and Family Studies, 10,* 181–197.

Trautman, P., Stewart, M., & Morishima, A. (1993). Are adolescent suicide attempters noncompliant with outcome care? *Journal of the American Academy of Child and Adolescent Psychiatry, 32,* 89–94.

Treatment of Adolescent Depression Study Team. (2004). Fluoxetine, cognitive-behavioral therapy, and their combination for adolescents with depression. *Journal of the American Medical Association, 292,* 807–820.

Turecki, G., Sequeira, A., Gingras, Y., Seguin, M., LeSage, A., Tousignant, M., et al. (2003). Suicide and serotonin: Study of variation at seven serotonin receptor genes in suicide completers. *American Journal of Medical Genetics, 118B,* 36–40.

U.S. Public Health Service. (1999). *The Surgeon General's call to action to prevent suicide.* Washington, DC: U.S. Government Printing Office.

U.S. Public Health Service. (2001). *National strategy for suicide prevention: Goals and objectives for action.* Washington, DC: U.S. Government Printing Office.

Velez, C., & Cohen, P. (1988). Suicidal behavior and ideation in a community sample of children: Maternal and youth reports. *Journal of the American Academy of Child and Adolescent Psychiatry, 27,* 349–356.

Vitiello, B., & Jensen, P. (1997). Medication development and testing in children and adolescents: Current problems, future directions. *Archives of General Psychiatry, 54,* 871–876.

Wagner, B. (1997). Family risk factors for child and adolescent suicidal behavior. *Psychological Bulletin, 121,* 246–298.

Walker, M., Moreau, D., & Weissman, M. (1990). Parents' awareness of children's suicide attempts. *American Journal of Psychiatry, 147,* 1364–1366.

Walrath, C., Mandell, D., Liao, Q., Holden, E. W., DeCarolis, G., Santiago, R., & Leaf, P. (2001). Suicidal behaviors among children in the Comprehensive Community Mental Health Services for Children and Their Families program. *Journal of the American Academy of Child and Adolescent Psychiatry, 40,* 1197–1205.

Walsh, B., & Rosen, P. (1985). Self-mutilation and contagion: an empirical test. *American Journal of Psychiatry, 142,* 119–120.

Webster, D., Vernick, J., Zeoli, A., & Manganello, J. (2004). Association between youth-focused firearm laws and youth suicides. *Journal of the American Medical Association, 292,* 594–601.

Weissman, M., Bland, R., Canino, G., Greenwald, S., Hwu, H., Joyce, P., et al. (1999). Prevalence of suicide ideation and suicide attempts in nine countries. *Psychological Medicine, 29,* 9–17.

Weissman, M., Klerman, G., Markowitz, J., & Ouellette, R. (1989). Suicidal ideation and attempts in panic disorder and attacks. *New England Journal of Medicine, 321,* 1209–1214.

Weitoft, G., Hjern, A., Haglund, B., & Rosen, M. (2003). Mortality, severe morbidity, and injury in children living with single parents in Sweden: A population-based study. *Lancet, 361(9354),* 289–295.

Wolfgang, M. (1959). Suicide by means of victim-precipitated homicide. *Journal of Clinical and Experimental Psychopathology, 20,* 335–349.

Wood, A., Trainor, G., Rothwell, J., Moore, A., & Harrington, R. (2001). Randomized trial of group therapy for repeated deliberate self-harm in adolescents. *Journal of the American Academy of Child and Adolescent Psychiatry, 40,* 1246–1253.

Zenere, F., & Lazarus, P. (1997). The decline of youth suicidal behavior in an urban, multicultural, public school system following the introduction of a suicide prevention and intervention program. *Suicide and Life-Threatening Behavior, 24,* 387–403.

Zlotnick, C., Donaldson, D., Spirito, A., & Pearlstein, T. (1997). Affect regulation and suicide attempts in adolescent inpatients. *Journal of the American Academy of Child and Adolescent Psychiatry, 36,* 793–798.

IV

DEVELOPMENTAL DISORDERS

10

Mental Retardation

Robert M. Hodapp
Ellie Kazemi
Beth A. Rosner
Elisabeth M. Dykens

The study of adolescents with mental retardation is reminiscent of the study of adolescents in general. As an area once ignored in child development, clinical child psychology, and child psychiatry, adolescence as a stage of life has received increasing attention only in recent years. For example, after the appearance of a separate chapter in its 1946 edition (Dennis, 1946), the *Handbook of Child Psychology* did not feature any sustained discussions of adolescence until its 1983 edition (Mussen, 1983). Similarly, although the journal *Adolescence* first appeared in 1966, the *Journal of Adolescence* and the *Journal of Research on Adolescence* only began in 1978 and 1991, respectively. In the field of child psychiatry, the salience of adolescence was officially recognized in 1987, when the main American journal (and organization) changed its name from the *Journal of the American Academy of Child Psychiatry* to the *Journal of the American Academy of Child and Adolescent Psychiatry*. A similar change in name, from the *Journal of Clinical Child Psychology* to the *Journal of Clinical Child and Adolescent Psychology*, oc-

curred in 2001. Even as it concerns typically developing children, then, the field of adolescence has come of age relatively recently.

In many ways, the status of adolescents with mental retardation is similar. Although various researchers study children during the adolescent years, no real subdiscipline of adolescence currently exists within the mental retardation field. In the most recent third edition of the *Handbook of Mental Deficiency, Psychological Theory, and Research* (MacLean, 1997), no chapter or even entry within the index mentions adolescence, even as many chapters cite studies of adolescent-age individuals. Other examples could also be provided, but the study of adolescents with mental retardation parallels that of typically developing adolescents a decade or so ago.

Such a state of general neglect may, however, be changing. Many studies are beginning to explore various aspects of adolescence and adolescent problems in individuals with mental retardation, and a full-fledged field of adolescents with mental retardation seems imminent. Before beginning our review of the problems of adolescents with mental retardation, we briefly review three main influences that are leading toward a formal field of the psychology of adolescents with mental retardation.

THE GROWTH AND LEGITIMACY OF THE FIELD OF DUAL DIAGNOSIS

Over the past two decades, a burgeoning field of dual diagnosis has arisen. This field emphasizes that persons with mental retardation can—and often do—have additional psychiatric problems. Such a seemingly obvious conclusion has, unfortunately, not always been so obvious. Part of the reason for the historical disregard for psychiatric problems pertains to politics, especially the need by advocates, researchers, and even policymakers to differentiate the problems of persons with mental retardation from those with psychiatric disorders (Scheerenberger, 1983, 1987). Other influences concerned the tendency on the part of many professionals to consider any behavior problems as part and parcel of mental retardation per se, the so-called diagnostic overshadowing of mental illness by the "mental retardation" diagnosis (Reiss & Szyszko, 1983). Finally, many professionals earlier considered the effects of large, impersonal institutions as the sole reason for any emotional–behavioral problems found in individuals who had recently begun to reside in community residences (see Jacobson, 1999, for a review).

Fortunately, many such issues have now been addressed and there is currently a thriving field of "dual diagnosis," which has begun to examine the age, gender, living status, familial, and etiological causes and correlates of maladaptive behavior in individuals with mental retardation (e.g., Bouras, 1999). Although many of these areas are still in their infancy, studies are accumulating at a rapid rate. As we note here, studies particularly focused on adolescents are now beginning to appear, and more will undoubtedly be performed in the coming years.

INTEREST AND ADVANCES IN GENE–BRAIN–BEHAVIOR CONNECTIONS

Within the mental retardation field, researchers are becoming increasingly excited by possible connections between specific genetic disorders, brain correlates, and behavioral outcomes (State, King, & Dykens, 1997). Numerous articles tout the possibility that a specific disorder might serve as a model for one or another gene–brain–behavior pathway, and magnetic resonance imaging (MRI), electroencephalographic (EEG), pharmacological, and other brain-related studies have proliferated at a dizzying pace.

Within the mental retardation field, many of these advances relate to specific genetic disorders. As we note herein, particular genetic disorders predispose affected individuals to show specific maladaptive behaviors and psychiatric conditions (Dykens, Hodapp, & Finucane, 2000). Recent work has begun to add developmental, age-related changes to this story. Thus, different groups show etiology-related maladaptive behaviors, but it is also the case that the presence, nature, and course of these behaviors might all change with age.

To date, such work has been influenced only slightly by the many studies showing brain and behavioral changes among typically developing adolescents. But as adolescence researchers are well aware, many brain changes occur in typically developing children over the adolescent years, some of which make adolescents more susceptible to a variety of psychiatric conditions (Walker, 2002). It remains unknown to what extent such brain changes also occur in adolescents with mental retardation or in those who have particular genetic syndromes. As we delve more deeply into different types of psychopathology in specific syndromes, it becomes necessary to explore whether brain changes that occur in typically developing adolescents mirror brain changes in individuals with mental retardation, and whether brain–behavior links are similar.

ADDITIONAL ISSUES WITHIN MENTAL RETARDATION THAT SPECIFICALLY PERTAIN TO ADOLESCENCE

A third influence leading to an adolescent specialty concerns issues specific to mental retardation. Such issues either do not apply when discussing adolescents of normal intelligence or, if they are present, they play themselves out very differently.

To give a few examples, for over a century professionals have debated the degree to which persons with mental retardation are responsible for their actions. At one point Walter Fernald (1912), one of the field's great figures, proclaimed that "The feebleminded are a parasitic, predatory class, never capable of self-support or of managing their own affairs. . . . Every feebleminded person, especially [those with mild mental retardation], is a potential criminal, needing only the proper environment and opportunity for the development and expression of his criminal tendencies" (from Davies & Ecob, 1959, pp. 47–48).

Such concerns continue to this day. In a recent high-profile case, the U.S. Supreme Court ruled, by a 6–3 vote, that defendants with mental retardation can be tried and sentenced but not given the death penalty (*Atkins v. Virginia*, 2002). The degree to which adolescents or young adults with mental retardation are suggestible or gullible (Greenspan, Loughlin, & Black, 2001); when and how someone can be considered to know right from wrong; the appropriate punishment for a person who may have a diminished cognitive-moral capacity—are all issues that remain intriguing, unresolved, and important to society.

Other issues could also be cited. Among these are the high prevalence rates of abuse of adolescents with mental retardation (Sullivan & Knutson, 2000) and the interactions between parents–families and their offspring during the adolescent years (Zetlin & Morrison, 1998). A final issue involves transition, the subfield tackling questions related to work and living situations for adolescents with mental retardation as they enter adulthood. Such concerns relate to how schools and adult-service systems provide transition services, and to how parents and families intersect with the adolescent or young adult's decision-making process, as well as with schools, state agencies, and other service providers (Miner & Bates, 1997).

Given that a field of dual diagnosis in adolescence seems imminent, this chapter reviews the state of the art for such a field. We begin by examining basic issues such as the definition, classification, and etiology of mental retardation, as well as its status within DSM. We then tackle issues more germane to adolescence, including the epidemiology, description, course, and assessment of maladaptive behavior–psychopathology in adolescents with mental retardation in general and in several genetic disorders more specifically. After discussing assessment, treatment, and several "special issues" that mostly pertain only to adolescents

with mental retardation, we end this chapter by discussing five issues for future work.

MENTAL RETARDATION: BASIC ISSUES

Three issues—definition, causes, and status within DSM—seem necessary as background to appreciating the emotional and behavioral problems of adolescents with mental retardation.

Definition and Classification

Although the definition of mental retardation has been hotly debated in recent years, most would agree that mental retardation involves subaverage intellectual functioning, with concurrent deficits in adaptive behavior, that begin during the childhood or adolescent years. Thus, DSM-IV (American Psychiatric Association, 1994, p. 46) proposes the following three criteria of mental retardation:

A. Significantly subaverage intellectual functioning: an IQ of approximately 70 or below on an individually administered IQ test.
B. Concurrent deficits or impairment in present adaptive functioning (i.e., the person's effectiveness in meeting the standards expected for his or her age by his or her cultural group) in at least two of the following skill areas: communication, self-care, home living, social/interpersonal skills, use of community resources, self-direction, functional academic skills, work, leisure, health, and safety.
C. Onset is before age 18 years.

An additional issue concerns classification within the population with mental retardation itself. Historically, persons with mental retardation have been categorized based on their levels of intellectual impairment. Specifically, individuals have been classified as having mild, moderate, severe, and profound levels of mental retardation. Table 10.1 provides general descriptions for individuals at each level of functioning.

Before describing the causes of mental retardation, we should acknowledge that both definitional and classificatory issues are extremely controversial within the field of mental retardation–developmental disabilities. Indeed, with two recent definitional–classificatory manuals, the main professional organization in mental retardation—the American Association on

TABLE 10.1. Levels of Functioning

1. *Mild mental retardation* (IQ 55–70) constitutes the largest group of persons with mental retardation, possibly as many as 90% of all persons with mental retardation (DSM-IV; American Psychiatric Association, 1994). These individuals appear similar to nonretarded individuals, and often blend into the nonretarded population in the years before and after formal schooling. As adults, some of these individuals hold jobs, marry, raise families and are indistinguishable from nonretarded people—they may simply appear slow or need extra help in negotiating life's problems and tasks. More persons with mild mental retardation come from minority and low socioeconomic backgrounds than would be expected from their numbers in the general population (Hodapp, 1994; Stromme & Magnus, 2000).

2. *Moderate mental retardation* (IQ 40–54), the second most common level of impairment, refers to those individuals who are more impaired intellectually and adaptively. More of these individuals are diagnosed as having mental retardation during the preschool years. Many individuals with moderate mental retardation show one or more clear organic causes for their mental retardation. For example, many persons with Down syndrome and with fragile X syndrome are at moderate levels of mental retardation. Although some persons with moderate mental retardation require few supportive services, most continue to require some help throughout life.

3. *Severe mental retardation* (IQ 25–39) refers to persons with more severe impairments. The majority of these individuals suffer from one or more organic causes of mental retardation. Many persons with severe mental retardation show concurrent physical or ambulatory problems, while others have respiratory, heart, or other co-occurring conditions. Most persons with severe mental retardation require some special assistance throughout their lives. Many live in supervised group homes or small regional facilities, and most work in either workshop or "preworkshop" settings.

4. *Profound mental retardation* (IQ below 25 or 20) involves persons with the most severe levels of intellectual and adaptive impairments. These persons generally learn only the rudiments of communicative skills, and intensive training is required to teach basic eating, grooming, toileting, and dressing behaviors. Persons with profound mental retardation require lifelong care and assistance. Almost all show organic causes for their mental retardation, and many have severe co-occurring conditions that sometimes lead to death during childhood or early adulthood. Some persons with profound mental retardation can perform preworkshop tasks, and most live in supervised group homes or small, specialized facilities.

Note. From Hodapp and Dykens (2003). Copyright 2003 by The Guilford Press. Adapted by permission.

Mental Retardation (AAMR)—has attempted to deemphasize the importance of IQ tests, and to increase the weight given to "social competence." In addition, starting with the 1992 definitional manual (AAMR, 1992), the AAMR committee has attempted to do away with the levels-of-impairment classification scheme, preferring instead to speak of intermittent, limited, extensive, and pervasive levels of support needed by the individual. To date, such proposed changes have been ignored by almost all researchers (Polloway, Smith, Chamberlain, Denning, & Smith, 1999), as well as by the majority of state disability guidelines (Denning, Chamberlain, & Polloway, 2000). Still, definition and classification continue to be hotly debated within the mental retardation field.

Etiology

A second issue concerns the etiology or causes of mental retardation. Historically, researchers have noted that mental retardation could generally be divided into two types. In the first, or "organic," form, the individual showed a clear organic cause for his or her mental retardation. In the second type, the cause of the person's disabilities was unknown. Even the names for this second group have ranged wildly, from familial, cultural–familial, or sociocultural–familial mental retardation to retardation due to environmental deprivation to "nonspecific" or "undifferentiated" mental retardation. In the past, roughly 25% of individuals were thought to have a clear organic cause for their mental retardation, whereas 75% were thought to show no clear organic cause.

Although this two-group approach to mental retardation has been around for many years (Zigler, 1967; see Hodapp & Zigler, 1995, for a review), the approach has currently been updated in several respects. First, with the increased ability to diagnose persons with any number of organic problems, the percentage of individuals with a clear organic cause has increased and the percentage in the second, nonspecific, group has declined. Although numbers remain imprecise, approximately one-third to one-half of all persons with mental retardation show a clear organic cause (Dykens et al., 2000).

A related issue concerns the breakdown of organic versus nonspecific mental retardation at various levels of impairment. Although persons with certain genetic conditions comprise some (and possibly, an increasing) percentage of persons with mild mental retardation (Rutter, Simonoff, & Plomin, 1996), virtually all persons with more severe levels of mental retardation show organic impairments. Using the latest genetic tests and other tests for organicity, Stromme and Hagberg (2000) reported that a full 96% of their group with severe mental retardation showed one or more "biopathological" causes (only 4% of these children showed unspecified causes). In contrast, only 68% of children with mild mental retardation showed one or another organic cause, with 32% having unspecified causes. Thus, the large majority of persons at more severe levels show a clear etiology for the mental retardation, whereas some sizable percentage at more mild levels do not.

Second, advances have now been made in specifying some of the factors influencing the "unknown" group. Given that approximately 50% of the variation in IQ scores is due to the environment and that there is an association of family socioeconomic status (SES) with mild mental retardation (Broman, Nichols, Shaughnessy, & Kennedy, 1987; Stromme & Magnus, 2000), a portion of the unspecified group is likely caused by poor environments, particularly the most impoverished. Finally, behavior geneticists have now identified at least one of the many "polygenes" responsible for the 50% of IQ variation due to genetic factors. This gene is located on chromosome 6. One variant of that gene was found much more often in high-IQ children in two independent samples and seems to account for approximately 2% of the variance in IQ (Chorney et al., 1998). Many different environmental and genetic factors—operating separately or together—probably account for the intellectual disabilities in children with nonspecific mental retardation.

Third, recent years have also seen major advances in understanding the organic group as well. The main advance has been in differentiating that group, in terms of both the number of such causes and their effects on behavior. It is now estimated that over 1,000 genetic disorders are associated with mental retardation (King, Hodapp, & Dykens, 2005). Granted, many of these disorders occur only rarely, but more and more genetic forms of mental retardation have recently been discovered.

More important than numbers per se, however, are the effects on behavior shown by many of these syndromes. Over the past 10 years, an entire field of "behavioral phenotypes" has arisen, with the express purpose of exploring etiology-related differences in behaviors (Dykens & Hodapp, 2001; Hodapp & Dykens, 2004). Such etiology-related behaviors have now been noted in emotional–behavioral problems, in cognitive–linguistic–adaptive profiles, and even in changing rates (i.e., trajectories) of development at different ages. Although so far most etiology-related studies have focused on only a few genetic syndromes, the numbers of studies devoted to such disorders as Down syndrome, fragile X syndrome, Prader–Willi syndrome, and Williams syndrome have increased exponentially from the 1980s to the 1990s and beyond (Hodapp & Dykens, 2004). As a result, we increasingly appreciate the ways that different genetic disorders affect behavior. In future years, we should be able to design interventions based on such emotional–behavioral problems, cognitive–linguistic–adaptive profiles, or changing trajectories of development.

Status within DSM

Within all the diagnostic–classificatory manuals in psychiatry and child psychiatry, mental retardation is considered a psychiatric disorder. In DSM-IV, for example, mental retardation is the first disorder examined in the section "Disorders usually first diagnosed in infancy, childhood, or adolescence." As an Axis II disorder, its listing "on a separate axis ensures that consideration will be given to the possible presence of Personality Disorders and Mental Retardation that might otherwise be overlooked when attention is directed to the usually more florid Axis I disorders" (American Psychiatric Association, 1994, p. 26).

But as it involves lower IQ, impaired adaptive behavior, and onset during the childhood and adolescent years, mental retardation is not synonymous with emotional–behavioral problems. Although many adolescents with mental retardation do have (other) psychiatric disorders or significant levels of behavioral dysfunction, the majority do not. Thus, our discussion that follows looks at those who are dually diagnosed—that is, those who are diagnosed with both mental retardation and with one or more additional DSM diagnoses.

Second, in line with the work on mental retardation in general and on specific etiologies of mental retardation more specifically, we distinguish between studies of adolescents with mental retardation in general versus those that examine particular genetic syndromes. Given the current state of mental retardation behavioral research, more studies examine maladaptive behavior and psychopathology in "mixed groups" of persons with mental retardation compared to those examining individuals with any of the estimated 1,000+ genetic mental retardation disorders (Dykens, 1996). As we noted previously, this situation may be changing, as over the past decade the numbers of behavioral studies on several syndromes have increased exponentially. We therefore begin by discussing studies of adolescents with mental retardation in general (i.e., the "mixed group" studies), and only later examine studies of those with several genetic syndromes.

BEHAVIOR PROBLEMS–PSYCHOPATHOLOGY IN ADOLESCENTS WITH MENTAL RETARDATION IN GENERAL

Epidemiology

Three epidemiological issues—prevalence, type of psychiatric disorder, and correlates—have generally been discussed concerning dual diagnosis in adolescents with mental retardation.

The first issue concerns *prevalence rates*. How often do adolescents with mental retardation show psychopathology? Are their rates higher than those found among nonretarded adolescents?

Although more research is needed, epidemiological studies over the years converge on the finding that clinical levels of psychopathology occur fairly often among adolescents with mental retardation. In the classic Isle of Wight study, Rutter, Graham, and Yule (1970) reported that children and adolescents with mental retardation show high levels of maladaptive behaviors three to four times more often than do their nonretarded age-mates. Following up on the Isle of Wight study, Gillberg, Persson, Grufman, and Themner (1986) examined 149 adolescents—ages 13–17 years—from Goteborg, Sweden. These adolescents comprised all children with mental retardation (i.e., IQ < 70) born over a 4-year period. Using psychiatrist's diagnoses based on a structured interview of the mother, Gillberg and colleagues reported major psychiatric disorders in 64% of children with severe mental retardation, 57% of those

with mild mental retardation. More recently, Einfeld and Tonge (1996) found a psychiatric prevalence rate of 40.7% from among children and adolescents from New South Wales (Australia), whereas Cormack, Brown, and Hastings (2000) reported that 50.4% of children and adolescents attending schools for those with severe intellectual disability scored above clinical cutoff levels. Using data from the nationwide survey of the National Health of Children and Adolescents in Great Britain, Emerson (2003) has recently found that 39.0% of 5–15-year-olds with mental retardation also have one or more ICD-10 diagnoses. Whatever the exact percentages, extremely high rates of psychopathology—rates much higher than those found among nonretarded adolescents—seem evident among adolescents with mental retardation.

A second issue concerns which *specific psychiatric disorders* are displayed by adolescents with mental retardation. Do adolescents with mental retardation (like those without mental retardation) suffer from the entire gamut of psychiatric disorders? At earlier points, several researchers had argued that certain disorders were less likely to occur in populations with mental retardation. Depression, for example, might occur less often in groups with mental retardation (vs. those without) because depression involves higher-level tendencies to "turn against the self" (as opposed to "turning against others") and revolves around symptoms connected with thinking (higher level) as opposed to action (lower level). In this sense, then, depression might be considered a disorder that is of a higher level developmentally (e.g., Glick, 1998). Given their lower levels of cognitive functioning, adolescents with mental retardation might be expected to experience clinical depression less frequently.

Such thinking receives some, but not total, support. Within the group with mental retardation, adolescents at more mild (as opposed to severe) levels of intellectual impairment are more likely to be formally diagnosed with depression. In Hardan and Shal's (1997) examination of in- and outpatient medical records from 298 children and adolescents, depression was found in 28% of those with mild mental retardation, and in 6% and 4.5% of those with moderate and profound mental retardation, respectively. Borthwick-Duffy, Lane, and Widaman (1997) also found a negative relationship between Child Behavior Checklist

(CBCL; Achenbach, 1991) Internalizing problems and IQ levels. Using the Children's Depression Inventory (CDI), Reynolds Adolescent Depression Scale (RADS), and the Bellevue Index of Depression (BID-R), Manikam, Matson, Coe, and Hillman (1995) also reported higher levels of depression in adolescents with mild mental retardation (IQs = 55–69) compared to those with moderate mental retardation (IQs 40–54). It remains unclear, however, whether more severely delayed adolescents cannot suffer from clinical depression, or if instead depression in these individuals might manifest itself differently (e.g., irritability and declines in adaptive functioning). Such considerations have given rise to alternative diagnostic criteria for depression in those with moderate to severe mental retardation (Szymanski et al., 1998).

But in another sense, predictions from classical–developmental views toward psychopathology (Zigler & Glick, 1986) have not been supported. Specifically, adolescents with mental retardation do suffer from clinical depression reasonably often. In Meyers's (1987) study of 10–21-year-olds seen for a psychiatric consultation, 9.7% of patients had primary diagnoses of depression, a figure almost identical to Hardan and Shal's (1997) record review of 233 children and adolescents participating in various programs for persons with disabilities. Although other studies report lower percentages (e.g., Emerson, 2003; 1.5% overall, though somewhat higher during adolescence), depression still seems reasonably common among adolescents with mental retardation.

In addition to experiencing depression, adolescents with mental retardation can suffer as well from all other psychiatric disorders. Among the most commonly noted disorders are conduct and oppositional defiant disorder, attention-deficit/hyperactivity disorder (ADHD), and autism and pervasive developmental disorder—not otherwise specified (PDD-NOS). Aggressive and self-injurious behaviors are also commonly noted. Adolescents with mental retardation, like those of average intelligence, can suffer from any psychiatric disorder.

A third epidemiological issue concerns *correlates of psychopathology*. As noted previously, intellectual level may be a correlate of different types of problem behavior. For example, Einfeld and Tonge (1996) noted that disruptive and antisocial behaviors were more prominent among children and adolescents functioning at the more mild levels of delay, whereas self-absorbed and autistic behaviors more commonly occurred among children–adolescents who were more severely delayed.

The presence of associated epilepsy and other physical disabilities also influences the amount and type of psychopathology in adolescents with mental retardation. In examining 98 children–adolescents with mental retardation and epilepsy, Steffenburg, Gillberg, and Steffenburg (1996) noted at least one psychiatric diagnosis in 59% of subjects. The most common diagnosis was autism, occurring in 27% of those with a psychiatric diagnosis (another 11% had an autistic-like condition). A similar connection between epilepsy and increased psychopathology was earlier noted by Meyers (1987), who found that "major pathology" (bipolar disorder, schizophrenia, and organic mental disorder) occurred more often in those with (vs. without) epilepsy.

In contrast, physical problems apart from epilepsy may lead to lesser degrees of maladaptive behaviors–psychopathology. Cormack and colleagues (2000) examined children and adolescents (4–18 years) with more severe physical problems—meaning issues with physical mobility, medical conditions impairing everyday functioning, greater dependence in personal care, and lessened abilities to manipulate one's hands. In correlational analyses, those with mental retardation and greater levels of physical problems were less likely to show behavior problems; ratings of emotional and behavioral problems also tended to decrease with age over the 4–18-year period.

Description and Course

With the few exceptions described later, neither the description nor the course of psychiatric disorders in adolescents with mental retardation has received adequate research attention. The general sense, however, is that psychiatric disorders are essentially the same in adolescents with versus without mental retardation. In a recent summary of psychiatric practice parameters, Szymanski and King (1999) concluded "the disorders themselves are essentially the same" (p. 1606). In a review of psychiatric disorders in adolescents with mental retardation, Masi (1998) also concludes that similar symptoms occur in the two groups for most disorders.

The sole exception to this general conclusion involves adolescents at more severe and profound levels of mental retardation. As these individuals are less able to verbally report about their thoughts or emotions, diagnosis becomes more problematic. In diagnosing mood disorders among children and adolescents with severe–profound mental retardation, Szymanski and King (1999) emphasize obtaining detailed information from caregivers and more heavily weighing neurovegetative signs for help in determining mood change. Masi (1998) as well notes that often clinical features are more vague. She further adds that clinicians might make use of symptoms mimicking a depressive state (apathy, crying); vegetative symptoms (loss of appetite or weight); psychomotor agitation with tantrums; and self-injurious or other behaviors.

In the few studies that examine such issues, this "same but (slightly) different" pattern does seem to be supported. Johnson, Handen, Lubetsky, and Sacco (1995) studied the presenting problems and the total array of symptoms appearing in depressed children and adolescents with mental retardation (average age = 13 years). Although aggression was the most common referral problem, the behavioral symptoms of these children and adolescents (mostly boys) were similar to those commonly identified in children and adolescents without mental retardation. Depressed children and adolescents with mental retardation showed suicidal ideation or gestures, crying, irritability, sleep problems, agitation, mood lability, and social withdrawal/isolation. In another study, Masi, Pfanner, and Marcheschi (1998) examined 15 adolescents diagnosed with depression according to both DSM-IV criteria and the Montgomery Asberg Depression Rating Scale (Montgomery & Asberg, 1979). Both cognitive symptoms (e.g., depressed ideation) and functioning symptoms (disturbed sleep, appetite) occurred less often than did emotional symptoms (sadness, inner tension) and psychomotor symptoms.

The clinical course of various disorders is also not well described for the large majority of psychiatric conditions for adolescents with mental retardation. As before, the consensus is that the course of various psychiatric conditions is similar among adolescents with and without mental retardation. Masi (1998), however, notes from her clinical experience that the onset of schizophrenia "occurs frequently in late adolescence" and that "It is less reversible, and prognosis is considerably worse"

(pp. 427–428) than for those without mental retardation. Szymanski and King (1999), however, make no such observations, and the relevant studies that might decide the question do not exist.

Recently, however, there have been a few follow-up studies of children and adolescents who also have ADHD. In one study, Aman, Armstrong, Buican, and Sillick (2002) followed 20 children with ADHD and low IQs 4.5 years after their initial assessments (these children had been enrolled in a longitudinal drug study). Children averaged 8.5 years at the beginning of the study (range from 5–14 years), and 12.5 years at the follow-up. As rated by parents, 70% of subjects screened positive for ADHD at the first contact, with 45% of these subjects subsequently screening positive again at the second contact. It was also found that, whereas 45% of children were rated positively by parents for oppositional defiant disorder or conduct disorder at the first contact, the prevalence rate rose to 55% at the 4-year follow-up.

BEHAVIOR PROBLEMS–PSYCHOPATHOLOGY IN ADOLESCENTS WITH SPECIFIC GENETIC DISORDERS OF MENTAL RETARDATION

The foregoing discussions all pertain to psychiatric problems of adolescents with mental retardation in general. Thus, when speaking of adolescents with, for example, moderate mental retardation, we have been concerned only about adolescents whose IQs ranged from 40 to 54. The cause of the person's disability has not been considered, even though groups with moderate degrees of impairment are comprised of individuals with different etiologies. Such "mixed group" approaches continue to characterize the majority of behavioral studies in individuals with mental retardation (Dykens & Hodapp, 2001).

But over the past two decades, a gradual shift has occurred in mental retardation behavioral work. Increasing numbers of genetic causes of mental retardation have now been identified, and research has exploded in documenting various aspects of behavior in these groups. Comparing the 1980s to the 1990s, the numbers of behavioral research articles increased from 10 to 81 in Williams syndrome, from 24 to 86 in Prader–Willi syndrome, and from 60 to 149 in fragile X syndrome. Even in Down syndrome, the single syndrome featuring a longstanding history of behavioral research, the numbers of articles almost doubled—from 607 to 1,140—from the 1980s to the 1990s (Hodapp & Dykens, 2004).

Such increases also reflect increasing knowledge about many behaviors in each of these disorders. Behavioral work now focuses on cognitive, linguistic, and adaptive strengths and weaknesses, and on how such strengths–weaknesses change as children develop. In addition, growing numbers of studies examine the families of children with different syndromes, with the aim of discovering how the behaviors of children and adolescents with particular disorders might influence their parents, siblings, and families (Hodapp, 2002). Finally, many studies examine the nature and changes with age in maladaptive behavior–psychopathology in several different genetic disorders.

Before discussing issues specific to the emotional and behavioral problems of adolescents with three specific syndromes, we first tackle the issue of how genetic disorders influence behavior, or the general topic of "behavioral phenotypes." Although there remains no consensus definition of this term, probably the most agreed-on definition notes that behavioral phenotypes involve "the heightened probability or likelihood that people with a given syndrome will exhibit certain behavioral or developmental sequelae relative to those without the syndrome" (Dykens, 1995, p. 523). This definition highlights several issues, each of which is essential to understand emotional-behavioral problems in adolescents with different genetic syndromes:

1. *Many, but not all, individuals with a given syndrome will show the syndrome's "characteristic" behaviors.* The effects of any genetic disorder are best viewed in probabilistic terms. Thus, although many persons with a particular genetic syndrome show that disorder's "characteristic" behavior (or behaviors), rarely does every single person show the behavior(s) in question. Nor will each individual show that behavior to the same extent or to the same level of severity, or even at the same point during development. Some within-syndrome variability exists within every genetic syndrome.

In this sense, genetic disorders do not determine outcomes for all individuals, but they *predispose* the person to have one or another etiology-related behavior. Thus, a particular

behavior or set of behaviors will occur more often (or more intensely) in a specific genetic disorder, but a disorder will rarely result in a particular behavior in all affected persons.

2. *Some etiology-related behaviors will be unique to a single syndrome, whereas others are common to two or more syndromes.* A probabilistic view of behavioral phenotypes holds only that the behavior in question occurs more commonly in a specific genetic syndrome than in groups with mental retardation per se. Left unclear is the degree to which that behavior or behaviors is found in a single syndrome or in several syndromes.

To date, some connections between genetic syndromes and specific outcomes seem unique, whereas others do not (Hodapp, 1997). In the first, unique pattern, a genetic syndrome sometimes results in a particular outcome that is not seen in other genetic disorders. The extreme hyperphagia (i.e., overeating) in Prader–Willi syndrome is one of these unique outcomes. No other genetic syndrome has been found to display hyperphagia as often or as severely as occurs in Prader–Willi syndrome.

In contrast, most etiology-related behaviors are shared by two or more genetic disorders. For example, compared to groups with mental retardation in general, hyperactivity is more frequently found in children with 5p- syndrome (Dykens & Clarke, 1997) and in boys with fragile X syndrome (Baumgardner, Reiss, Freund, & Abrams, 1995). In both syndromes, hyperactivity is found in higher percentages of individuals than is commonly noted among others with mental retardation, but hyperactivity is unique to neither syndrome. As clinical geneticist John Opitz (1985) concludes, "The causes are many, but the common developmental pathways are few" (p. 9).

3. *Behavioral phenotypes change as the child gets older.* Behavioral phenotypes are not static. When one examines closer, many of these behaviors or strengths–weaknesses are limited to—or first appear when—children are of a particular age.

Such age-related changes have so far mainly been noted in cognitive–linguistic profiles. In Down syndrome, for example, most children show advantages in visual versus auditory short-term memory. But this profile becomes more pronounced as children get older. Across three age groups, Hodapp and Ricci (2002) compared performance on one task involving visual and one of auditory short-term memory

(Bead Memory and Sentence Memory on the Stanford–Binet IV, respectively). Among 5–10-year-olds, the average difference of visual-over-auditory memory was about 4 months (0.31 years), and only 36% of subjects showed a 6-or-more month advantage on the visual subtest. By 10–15 years, discrepancies averaged 8 months (0.66 years), with 60% of subjects showing 6+ month visual advantages. By 15–21 years, "visual over auditory" differences averaged 18 months (1.52 years), and 75% of subjects showed 6+ month discrepancies. Other syndromes also display patterns of relative strengths becoming stronger and weaknesses weaker with increasing age (Hodapp, Dykens, Ort, Zelinsky, & Leckman, 1991; Jarrold, Baddeley, Hewes, & Phillips, 2001).

Given these three issues, we now discuss emotional and behavioral problems in adolescents with Down syndrome, Prader–Willi syndrome, and Williams syndrome. We focus on these three because they are reasonably common, feature intriguing new findings, and exemplify syndrome-specific understandings of psychopathology. For each disorder, we first briefly describe the cause, prevalence rates, and interesting cognitive–linguistic behaviors before turning to maladaptive behavior–psychopathology. We end by describing how emotional–behavioral problems might change during adolescence.

Down Syndrome

As the most common genetic (chromosomal) cause of intellectual disabilities, Down syndrome occurs in about 1 in 800 births. Down syndrome has been the recipient of almost as much behavioral research as all other genetic mental retardation syndromes combined (Hodapp, 1996).

In addition to the relative strengths in visual—and weaknesses in auditory—short-term memory tasks, language has been identified as an area of particular weakness for these individuals. Children and adolescents with Down syndrome have particular (i.e., greater than mental age-level) difficulties in linguistic grammar (Fowler, 1990), articulation (Kumin, 1994), and expressive as opposed to receptive language (Miller, 1999).

Persistent personality descriptions depict persons with Down syndrome as cheerful, friendly, eager to please, and affectionate. It remains unclear whether this personality description is or is not accurate. Many mothers describe their children with Down syndrome as having a wide range of personality features (Rogers, 1987), and the temperaments of some children with Down syndrome are active, distractible, and difficult (Ganiban, Wagner, & Cicchetti, 1990). Further, some studies find that children with Down syndrome are no easier to rear than children with other types of disabilities (Cahill & Glidden, 1996). At the same time, however, mothers generally do report that their children with the syndrome (compared to children with other types of mental retardation) are more reinforcing and more acceptable (Hodapp, Ly, Fidler, & Ricci, 2001). In addition, compared to mothers of children with mental retardation in general, mothers of these children rate their children higher on a questionnaire of "Down syndrome personality" (Hodapp, Ricci, Ly, & Fidler, 2003). Apart from findings either way, the personality stereotype persists, with parents and researchers alike often remarking that children and adults with Down syndrome are charming and eager to please.

Yet these endearing features do not necessarily protect these same individuals from showing such behavioral problems as stubbornness, defiance, aggressive behavior, and psychopathology. About 13–15% of children with Down syndrome appear to have significant behavioral difficulties, with prevalence estimates higher and more variable in studies of children and adolescents, ranging from 18–38% (Gath & Gumley, 1986; Meyers & Pueschel, 1991). Primary problems include disruptive disorders such as ADHD, oppositional and conduct disorders, and occasionally, anxiety disorders.

In contrast to the "externalizing" disorders of childhood, a particular vulnerability to depressive disorders occurs in adults (Collacott, Cooper, & McGrother, 1992; Meyers & Pueschel, 1991). During adulthood, depression in Down syndrome is often characterized by passivity, apathy, withdrawal, and mutism, and several cases of major depressive disorder have now been well described (e.g., Dosen & Petry, 1993). Prevalence estimates of affective disorders among adults with Down syndrome range from 6% to 11% (Collacott et al., 1992; Meyers & Pueschel, 1991).

Recently, adolescence has been suggested as the entrypoint into adult depression in many individuals with Down syndrome. Although changes during adolescence have not been noted in all studies (e.g., Einfeld, Tonge, Turner, Parmenter, & Smith, 1999), one recent study found increases in a variety of internalizing symptoms beginning during adolescence. Dykens, Shah, Sagun, Beck, and King (2002) cross-sectionally examined 211 children and adolescents across four age groups: 4–6 years (*n* = 61), 7–9 years (62); 10–13 years (51); and 14–19 years (37). Using the CBCL (Achenbach, 1991), Dykens and colleagues noted that mean Internalizing scores almost doubled from the two younger groups compared to the adolescent years. In contrast to parents' reporting that the child "Prefers to be alone" in 28% and 45% of 4–6- and 7–9-year-olds, 66% and 63% of parents endorse this behavior when children reach 10–13 and 14–19 years of age, respectively. Such behaviors as secretive, underactive, and overweight also increased into and through the teen years. Although the reasons for such changes remain unclear, many adolescents with Down syndrome are gradually changing in their sociable, upbeat personalities, and withdrawal, depression, and internalizing behaviors seem to be increasing.

Prader–Willi Syndrome

First identified in 1956, Prader–Willi syndrome affects about 1 in 15,000 births. About 70% of Prader–Willi syndrome cases are caused by a deletion on the long arm of chromosome 15 contributed from the father. Remaining cases are attributed to maternal uniparental disomy (UPD) of chromosome 15, in which both members of the chromosome 15 pair come from the mother. In either variant of Prader–Willi syndrome, there is an absence of the paternally derived contribution to this specific region of the genome (Dykens, & Cassidy, 1996).

Although children and adults with Prader–Willi syndrome display distinct cognitive strengths and weaknesses and IQs average about 70, most work on this syndrome has addressed hyperphagia, or extreme overeating. Somewhere during the 2–6-year period, most children with this syndrome develop hyperphagia and such food-seeking behavior as foraging and hoarding. These food preoccupations are lifelong, and without prolonged dietary management, affected individuals invariably become obese. Indeed, complications of obesity remain the leading cause of death in this syndrome (Butler et al., 2002).

Even compared to others with mental retardation, children and adults with Prader–Willi syndrome also show high rates of many behavior problems. Most—but not all—individuals show temper tantrums, aggression, stubbornness, underactivity, excessive daytime sleepiness, and emotional lability (Dykens & Kasari, 1997). Coupled with food seeking, these impulsive behaviors often lead people with Prader–Willi syndrome to need more restrictive levels of care than would be predicted by their mild levels of disability.

Although persons with Prader–Willi syndrome show high rates of many maladaptive behaviors, several researchers have recently focused on obsessions and compulsions. Although individuals with Prader–Willi syndrome obsess about food, a remarkably high proportion of persons also show nonfood obsessions and compulsive behaviors. Dykens, Leckman, and Cassidy (1996) compared 43 adults with Prader–Willi syndrome to 43 individuals without mental retardation but who had been diagnosed as having obsessive–compulsive disorder (OCD). The two subject groups did not differ in their mean number of compulsions, nor in the mean severity level of the compulsions that they did have. For example, whereas 33% of individuals with Prader–Willi syndrome reported the need to clean excessively, the percentage was 37% among the OCD subjects. For some symptoms—for example, hoarding objects—higher percentages were shown in the Prader–Willi syndrome group (PWS = 79%; OCD = 7%); for others—performing checking rituals—the OCD group was higher (PWS = 16%; OCD = 55%). But overall, the two groups were remarkably similar. In addition, just as in the OCD group, often these symptoms were associated with distress or adaptive impairment, suggesting marked risks of OCD in this population (Dykens et al., 1996).

Recent work also describes the course of such maladaptive behaviors throughout the childhood, adolescent, and adult years. To date, the main studies of change over time have identified the preschool period as important. Along with the beginnings of hyperphagia, Dimitropoulus, Feurer, Butler, and Thompson (2001) found that obsessions and compulsions begin during the preschool years. These symptoms, however, intensify from the childhood into the adolescent and adult years. In ongoing work, Dykens (2004) cross-sectionally examined 245 individuals with Prader–Willi syndrome ranging from 3 to 50 years. Examining scores on the CBCL (Achenbach, 1991), children ages 3–10 years showed relatively low levels of maladaptive behavior compared to adolescents (10–19 years) and young adults (20–30), before a decline set in for adults ages 30 and older. Thus, children in the 3–9-year-old group showed an average Externalizing raw score of 15.37, compared to a score of 20.00 among the 10–20-year group ($n = 80$) (scores of 15+ and 12+ are above the 95th percentile for 4–11 and 12–18-year-old nonretarded children, respectively). Similar findings occurred in Internalizing behaviors, where the pre-10-year-old group averaged 8.52, compared to the adolescent average of 14.33 (95th percentile scores for Internalizing are 12+ for 4–11 years and 14+ for 12–18 years). Although adolescence has so far received little attention among researchers—and the reasons for such adolescence-related changes remain unclear—the adolescent period nevertheless seems one in which maladaptive behavior increases markedly in Prader–Willi syndrome.

Williams Syndrome

Williams syndrome is caused by a microdeletion on one of the chromosome 7s that includes the gene for elastin, a protein that provides strength and elasticity to certain tissues such as the heart, skin, blood vessels, and lungs (Ewart et al., 1994). Affecting about 1 in 20,000 births, persons with Williams syndrome often show hyperacusis, hypercalcemia, neuromuskeletal and renal abnormalities, and characteristic facial features described as elfin-like, cute, and appealing (Pober & Dykens, 1996). People with Williams syndrome also typically show cardiovascular disease, especially supravalvular aortic stenosis, and these problems are likely associated with elastin insufficiency.

Williams syndrome is best known for its cognitive–linguistic profile. Many people with Williams syndrome show pronounced weaknesses in perceptual and visual–spatial functioning. Despite these difficulties, however, they often do well on facial recognition tasks. Relative strengths are often seen in expressive language, including vocabulary, syntax, semantics, and prosody (e.g., Reilly, Klima, & Bellugi, 1990; Udwin & Yule, 1991).

In contrast to work on cognitive–linguistic profiles, studies have only begun to examine the personality and psychiatric features of people with Williams syndrome. Early descriptions of people with Williams syndrome included such descriptors as pleasant, unusually friendly, affectionate, loquacious, engaging, and interpersonally sensitive and charming (Dilts, Morris, & Leonard, 1990). Using the Reiss Personality Profiles (Reiss & Havercamp, 1998), Dykens and Rosner (1999) also found that relative to controls, adolescents and adults with Williams syndrome are more likely to initiate interactions with others (87% of sample), to enjoy social activities (83%), to be kindspirited (100%) and caring (94%), and to empathize with others' positive feelings (75%) or when others are in pain (87%) (Dykens & Rosner, 1999). At the same time, however, these subjects did not fare well in making or keeping friends and were often dangerously indiscriminate in their relating to others.

Indeed, although sociability in Williams syndrome has generally been viewed as a strength, these features also seem to reflect the type of social disinhibition that characterizes people who are anxious, impulsive, and overly aroused. Not surprisingly, salient problems in Williams syndrome include hyperactivity and inattentiveness and a proneness for ADHD that may diminish with age (Gosch & Pankau, 1997; Pober & Dykens, 1996).

Attention has also begun to focus on anxieties and fears in this population. Generalized anxiety, worry, and perseverative thinking are commonly seen in Williams syndrome (Einfeld, Tonge, & Florio, 1997), and people with the syndrome appear to show unusually high levels of fears and phobias. Similarly, compared to others with mental retardation, fears in this syndrome are more frequent, wide-ranging, severe, and associated with impaired social–adaptive adjustment. In one recent study, Dykens (2003) compared fears in 120 people with Williams syndrome (ages 6–48 years) to those with mixed etiologies. Only two fears—getting a shot and going to the dentist—were mentioned by over 50% of the comparison group. In contrast, 50 different fears were mentioned by over 60% of subjects with Williams syndrome. Such fears ran the gamut. Some involved interpersonal issues like being teased, getting punished, or getting into arguments with others. Others involved such physical issues as shots-injections, being in a fire or getting burned, or getting stung by a bee. Still others related to these children's hyperacusis or clumsiness (loud noises–sirens; falling from high places; thunderstorms).

As in Down syndrome and Prader–Willi syndrome, in Williams syndrome age-related changes appear during adolescence. In this particular syndrome, certain fears and anxieties went up with age for both boys and girls, whereas others increased only among adolescent girls and young adult women (Dykens, 2003). For both genders, fears relating to failure and criticism from others increased from 6–12 years to the adolescent (13–18) and adult (19–48) years. In contrast to preadolescent children, adolescent girls and adult women became more fearful about minor injury and small animals, as well as about danger and death (these are two subscales of Ollendick, King, and Frary's [1989] Fear Survey for Children—Revised). Although it remains unclear why specific fears increase beginning during the adolescent years for both genders or for girls alone, adolescents with William syndrome do seem especially fearful, and certain age-related changes begin in adolescence.

In summarizing research on Down syndrome, Prader–Willi syndrome, and Williams syndrome, these disorders predispose affected individuals to specific problem behaviors. Researchers are also identifying how such behaviors change with age, often beginning in adolescence. Future work will undoubtedly elaborate on both the nature and causes of such adolescent age changes, as well as expand to other genetic etiologies of mental retardation.

ASSESSMENT

Assessment of psychopathology remains an important—maybe even *the* important—challenge to the study of psychopathology in adolescents with mental retardation. Recently, however, several lines of work are appearing concerning measurement of psychopathology in individuals with mental retardation. The first involves a set of behavioral surveys and rating scales. Most such measures are specifically geared for individuals with mental retardation, including items and factors of items that seem common to persons with mental retardation who display associated psychiatric disorders. These include the Aberrant Behavior Checklist (Aman & Singh, 1994), Reiss Screen (Reiss, 1988), and Developmental Behaviour Checklist (Einfeld & Tonge, 1992). Each in-

strument shows excellent psychometric properties (see Aman, 1991, for a review).

The strength (and problem) of these measures is their direct applicability to individuals with mental retardation. Though these scales are sensitive to the unique concerns of those with mental retardation, they are not always compatible with DSM- or ICD-based psychiatric diagnoses. In addition, each scale was designed for a slightly different purpose, and each has slightly different sets of items and factor structures. As a result, any inconsistent findings across studies remain difficult to reconcile (Dykens, 2000).

In a similar vein, other researchers have raised concerns about the applicability of traditional DSM or ICD diagnoses for those with mental retardation (Sovner, 1986). Many problems relate to the psychiatric interview itself, including acquiescence bias, and the more limited abilities of persons with mental retardation to express abstract thoughts and feelings, or to answer questions about the onset, duration, frequency, and severity of symptoms (see Moss, 1999, for a review). In response to these challenges, some researchers have adapted traditional DSM or ICD criteria for those with delay (King DeAntonio, McCracken, Forness, & Ackerland, 1994; Szymanski et al., 1998). Others shy away from formal diagnoses and embrace a more functional analysis of challenging behavior (Sturmey, 1999), while still others have designed interview schedules specifically for those with mental retardation, including the Psychiatric Assessment Schedule for Adults with Developmental Disability (PASS-ADD; Moss et al., 1997). When using these options, direct interviews with both respondents and informants seem best, resulting in fewer cases of missed diagnoses (Moss, Prossner, Ibbotson, & Goldenberg, 1996).

In addition to the various assessment instruments designed for children and adolescents with mental retardation in general, recent years have seen increased interest in assessments for children–adolescents with different genetic syndromes of mental retardation. In many studies, the instruments normed either on (nonretarded) clinical populations or on children-adolescents with mental retardation have sufficed. Witness, for example, Dykens and colleagues' (2002) use of the CBCL with persons with Down syndrome from the childhood into the adult years, and a similar use of the Yale–Brown Obsessive Compulsive Scales (Y-BOCS) for obsessions and compulsions in Prader–Willi syndrome (Dykens et al., 1996). For some other syndromes, however, specific observations or checklists have been needed. For example, Finucane, Konar, Haas-Givler, Kurtz, and Scott (1994) examined the proneness of intense "self-hugging" behavior in children and adolescents with Smith Magenis syndrome by observing individuals for 1-hour periods in classrooms, recreational activities, and at home and counting the number of self-hugging behaviors. Similarly, Holland, Treasure, Coskeran, and Dallow (1995) examined eating behavior and satiety in Prader–Willi syndrome by allowing individuals to eat as much as they wanted in a situation in which individuals had free access to food. In short, although assessments of adolescents with different genetic syndromes have often been possible using instruments normed on either nonretarded individuals or on mixed groups with mental retardation, examining certain issues has sometimes required more etiology-specific assessment techniques.

TREATMENT

A wide variety of treatments have been tried with individuals with mental retardation (Moss, 2001). Although few studies focus on adolescents per se, several expert and consensus reports now list therapies that are useful for dually diagnosed persons (e.g., Rush & Frances, 2000; Szymanski & King, 1999).

Pharmacotherapy

Pharmacological treatments for adolescents with mental retardation focus either on the diagnosed DSM disorder or, instead, on specific symptoms. Based on Kalachnick and colleagues' (1998) guidelines for pharmacological interventions, drug treatments should be considered only after in-depth assessments of the individual's medical pathology; psychosocial and environmental conditions; health status; current medications; presence of a psychiatric disorder; history of previous interventions; and a functional analysis of behavior. Similarly cautious approaches should be taken for dosing strategies, evaluating treatment effects, and watching for side effects.

The larger question of "do drug regimens work" is more difficult to answer. As might be expected, most treatments for adolescents—

both drug and otherwise—adopt a "follow the problem" approach (Hodapp & Dykens, 2001). Just as one uses a particular drug (or nondrug) therapy when confronted with a specific problem in nonretarded individuals, so too should one generally adopt the same drug when the problem is observed in adolescents with mental retardation. Beyond this overarching statement, a wide variety of specific drugs have been tried over the years for dually diagnosed individuals. For specific information, readers should refer to Reiss and Aman's (1998) *Psychotropic Medication and Developmental Disabilities: International Consensus Handbook.*

More generally, though, two issues often arise. The first involves the lack of proper diagnosis for the psychiatric disorders of many children and adolescents with mental retardation. Historically, professionals have tended to allow the diagnosis of mental retardation to "overshadow" other, associated psychiatric diagnoses (Reiss & Szyszko, 1983). Faced with the person with mental retardation who is depressed, or shows attentional or conduct disorder or other problems, professionals often feel that such disorders are simply inherent to mental retardation. The many difficult assessment issues with this population further complicate the problem of diagnostic overshadowing.

A second, almost opposite concern relates to inappropriate medication. With few exceptions, most mental health professionals have not received formal training in mental retardation and persons with mental retardation constitute only a small portion of their caseloads. As a result, these professionals generally have little experience in prescribing drugs for dually diagnosed persons. Such professionals often do not know which drugs (or their dosage levels) work best for different problems, and the problem of polypharmacy—the inappropriate use of multiple drugs—also arises.

Several studies from the United Kingdom show the extent to which either drugs are overprescribed or the dosage levels are too high in the population with mental retardation. Branford (1996) examined a drug review program of patients under the care of the National Health Service who were being treated with antipsychotic drugs. Of 198 patients examined, reviewers agreed that treatment should be amended for 123 patients (= 62.1%). Of the 43 patients who were totally withdrawn from drugs, 31 were able to be maintained off drugs over the next year. Of the remaining 80 for whom doses were lowered, 40 suffered deteriorating behavior to an extent that doses had to be increased again. A similar study by Branford (1997)—examining formerly institutionalized individuals after 6 years of community living—again showed that the prevalence of prescribing many psychotropic drugs was high (and went up over the 6 years) in the community setting.

Behavioral and Cognitive Therapies

As in the general population, pharmacotherapies work best in adolescents with mental retardation when they are coupled with other appropriate therapeutic interventions. These interventions are diverse and may include a wide array of behavioral and cognitive therapies, supportive counseling, expressive therapies, social skills and activities, and family support. Often, a blending of these approaches is used, although studies have yet to examine their combined efficacy in adolescents.

Treatment approaches in adolescents with mental retardation should follow a thorough, multidisciplinary evaluation of presenting problems and behaviors. Curry and colleagues (1997) recently presented a consensus report with recommended clinical evaluations for persons with mental retardation. These evaluations should include the following:

- A history (prenatal, birth, developmental);
- A family pedigree (learning, psychiatric problems);
- A physical examination (neurological, growth, physical and facial anomalies); and
- Other evaluations as needed (dermatologic, audiologic, metabolic, chromosomal, psychological studies).

In addition to providing a more focused evaluation of behavioral or psychiatric problems, these data are often necessary for clinicians to rule in or out particular diagnoses and to establish a treatment plan. It would help to know, for example, if aggressive or acting-out behavior from an adolescent with Down syndrome might be associated with persistent communication problems and hearing loss. Similarly, as detailed later in the chapter, knowing the etiology of the adolescent's mental retardation helps inform treatment planning (Dykens et al., 2000). Thus, although social skills groups might be highly recommended for an adolescent with Williams syndrome, such groups would be counterindicated for an adolescent male with fragile X syndrome (who often show various types of gaze avoidance and social anxiety; Dykens et al., 2000).

Most treatment plans for behavioral or psychiatric difficulties in adolescents with mental retardation include a functional analysis of the problem behavior or symptom (e.g., antecedents, consequences, duration, onset, and severity). Ideally, such analyses should be conducted across home, school, and recreational/vocational settings. As with adolescents without mental retardation, treatment outcomes are optimized when the same approaches to problem behaviors or symptoms are used by parents, teachers, speech and recreational therapists, job coaches, and so on.

Behavioral and cognitive-behavioral therapies have been widely used in persons with mental retardation. In recent years, there has been an increased emphasis on teaching persons self-management skills and self-control as opposed to external management techniques (see Benson & Valenti-Hein, 2001; Gardner, Graeber-Whalen, & Ford, 2001, for reviews). Controlled studies generally support the success of a wide variety of behavioral therapies, including operant-based learning, systematic desensitization, stimulus exposure procedures, skills training, modeling, relaxation, anger management, and assertiveness training. These approaches have been used to target such problems as self-injurious behaviors, aggression, fears, and inappropriate social relating. These approaches have also helped individuals develop more adaptive communication, personal, and social skills.

Due to the adolescent with mental retardation's cognitive limitations, many clinicians assume that these adolescents cannot readily take advantage of such therapies as supportive counseling, or verbal, insight-oriented psychotherapies (Hollins, 1997). Yet although less researched than behavioral techniques, many persons with mental retardation do benefit from psychotherapies, especially when they are altered to address the unique concerns of those with mental retardation. Thus, some clinicians emphasize the need for shorter, more frequent sessions and the use of easily attained goals (Hurley, 1989). The use of alternative techniques may also be helpful, including expressive therapies such as music, art, movement, drama, and role playing. While the flexible, multimodal approaches that clinicians rely on in therapy with children are often helpful in treating those with mental retardation, play therapies per se are generally inappropriate for these older adolescents or adults.

Once they leave the school setting, older adolescents and young adults with mental retardation are at risk for social isolation, especially if they are not enrolled in a formal job training or recreational program. Parents and clinicians thus need to ensure that the treatment plans for these young adults include a vocational training component or a life skills or social skills program. Joining groups such as the Special Olympics may also boost socially competent skills and self-esteem (Dykens & Cohen, 1996).

Finally, treatment plans for adolescents with mental retardation often include a family support component. Over the past few decades, such support has changed dramatically to reflect more up-to-date conceptualizations of families of offspring with mental retardation. While early writings conceptualized parents as pathologically stressed, contemporary views hold that stress levels often change over the course of the family life cycle, and that many families derive positive benefits from having a child with mental retardation (see Hodapp, 2002, for a review.) Family support thus needs to be tailored over time and may include family counseling, help with a specific parenting technique, or obtaining short- or long-term respite care (to provide a break from full-time care).

In addition, the field currently emphasizes family advocacy and techniques to empower families to successfully negotiate educational, state, and other systems to obtain services for their offspring. Parent groups are often available for families of offspring with specific types of disabilities, and these groups provide formal and informal ways for parents to meet and advocate for their children. Finally, family support has recently included increased attention to siblings, especially for brothers and sisters who have a sibling with mental retardation and behavioral or psychiatric problems. Sibling workshops, groups, and newsletters are all currently available.

Etiology

A final consideration concerns the adolescent's type of mental retardation. As noted previously, individuals with several genetic disorders seem to show higher levels of maladaptive behaviors during the adolescent years. Adolescents with Down syndrome show increased amounts of internalizing problems (Dykens et al., 2002), while externalizing and internalizing behaviors increase during adolescence in Prader–Willi syndrome (Dykens, 2004). In Williams syndrome, certain fears–anxieties went up both during the adolescent and early adult years (Dykens, 2003).

As noted earlier for adolescents with mental retardation in general, treating such problems has generally followed an approach of following the symptom, as well as using etiology-related cognitive–linguistic profiles when appropriate (Hodapp & Dykens, 2001). One might, for example, capitalize on the relatively high-level verbal skills and sociability (almost hypersociability) of adolescents with Williams syndrome to recommend talk and group therapies (Dykens & Hodapp, 1997). In Prader–Willi syndrome, food and weight control are obviously critical, but so might be extra warnings about upcoming changes in routine, thereby allowing adolescents with this disorder to become "unstuck."

Although many of these recommendations make sense, most to date have not been formally evaluated. In addition to evaluating treatments that might make sense of the basis of symptoms alone, there is also a movement in some genetic disorders to tie treatments to underlying brain dysfunction. Thus, in fragile X syndrome, Galvez, Gopal, and Greenough (2003) have recently used animal models to understand the development of brain mechanisms underlying the hyperactivity and social anxieties shown by many of these individuals. The goal, as yet unrealized, is to tie pharmacological agents with underlying brain pathology. As in the wider fields of psychiatry and child psychiatry, then, so too is there a version of pharmacogenetics within the fields that examine maladaptive behavior–psychopathology in adolescents with genetic mental retardation syndromes.

SPECIAL PROBLEMS FOR ADOLESCENTS WITH MENTAL RETARDATION

Besides maladaptive behavior–psychopathology, five other issues pertain mainly to adolescents with mental retardation. We now turn to these issues.

Criminality

Although controversial for over 100 years, prevalence rates of criminal behavior remain undetermined for adolescents and young adults with mental retardation. Difficulties relate to a wide variety of issues. Did a particular study define mental retardation based on IQ, or on whether the defendant attended a special school or had difficulties in academic tasks? How, exactly, did the study identify its subjects (through court records, jails, hospitals)? How careful was the study in ensuring that all criminal defendants with possible mental retardation were screened? Did the study limit itself to individuals with IQs below 70, or did it also include individuals with IQs in the "borderline" range (from IQ 70–84)? Because few studies are immune from such problems, overall prevalence rates of criminality become difficult to ascertain.

Still, in a recent paper summarizing the available research, Simpson and Hogg (2001a) concluded that no credible evidence exists that persons with mental retardation show a higher prevalence of criminal offending than do their nonretarded peers. Although records studies often show higher rates (e.g., Crocker & Hodgins, 1997), studies do not show high rates when researchers directly examine all persons leaving or entering custody over a set period of time. In Winter, Holland, and Collins's (1997) examination of all offenders leaving or entering custody over a 33-day period, 212 offenders (for 240 offenses) were identified. Of these, 47 (22%) indicated that they had previously experienced difficulties in school, but only two (1%) had Full-Scale IQs below 70.

A further issue concerns the level of IQ among those adolescents or adults who commit crimes. Though several studies report IQ ranges of criminal subjects ranging into borderline levels, few report any criminals whose IQs are below 50. Among those criminal defendants with borderline IQs, sexual offenses, as well as criminal damage and burglary, seem more common as compared to those with IQs below 70.

Other predisposing factors also seem at play in criminals who have mental retardation (Simpson & Hogg, 2001a, 2001b). These include being male as opposed to female, lower versus higher SES, parental history of criminality, personal history of offending or behavior problems, and homelessness. It also seems that criminals with mental retardation are likely to be older. Thus, Kearns and O'Connor (1988) found that 40% of offenders with mental retardation were between 21 and 35 years, with 29% between 35 and 50 years. Similarly, Hodgins (1992) found a higher percentage of first offending occurring later among persons with mental retardation—later in the teen years as opposed to the 15 or so age of first offending found among nonretarded offenders.

Child Abuse

The flip side of the perpetrator–victim coin concerns child abuse. For many years, social service providers have sensed that compared to typically developing children and adolescents, children–adolescents with mental retardation and other disabilities were more often the objects of abuse. In reviewing the research literature, Westcott and Jones (1999) also concluded that children and adolescents with disabilities experience abuse more often than do typically developing children. Although prevalence rates vary depending on the study's methodology and its definition of disability, most studies nevertheless find that children with disabilities are more often abused than are typically developing children.

To give a recent example, Sullivan and Knutson (2000) dovetailed records from schools, social service agencies, and the police to examine the prevalence and correlates of child abuse for all 50,000 school-age children from Omaha, Nebraska. The authors further broke down their findings by four different disability groups and different types of abuse and neglect (neglect, physical abuse, emotional abuse, and sexual abuse). Children with disabilities were 3.4 times more likely—and children with mental retardation 4 times more likely—to be abused than were their nondisabled peers. For children with mental retardation, maltreatment risks were close to four times those of nonretarded children across all four types of abuse–neglect. In addition, within the group with mental retardation, the first instances of maltreatment most often occurred during the preschool or elementary school period (both 31.5%), as compared to either the middle school (23.4%) or high school (14.5%) periods.

Recent studies have also examined the presence of sexual abuse among adolescents with mental retardation. Using a retrospective case-record review, Balogh and colleagues (2001) examined 43 young participants between the ages of 9 and 21 who were involved with sexual abuse either as victims or as perpetrators. Half of the victims (50%) had been abused by a member of their close or extended family. Most victims (62%) were adolescents and the authors found support for gender differences in sexual abuse patterns. Most victims were abused by male perpetrators, and most were adolescents with mild or moderate mental retardation (very few—7%—of abused adolescents had severe impairments).

An additional issue concerns the connections between specific etiologies and child abuse. As noted earlier, children and adolescents with Williams syndrome show high levels of language and social disinhibition. As such, these adolescents may be at particularly high risk for sexual exploitation and abuse. In Davies, Udwin, and Howlin's (1998) study of adults with Williams syndrome, 10% of their sample had reported sexual assaults to police, and an additional 10% made allegations of assault that had not been reported. In studies of nonretarded children, the rates for girls of childhood sexual abuse are generally about double the rates for boys (Cutler & Nolen-Hoeksema, 1991), even though the female:male ratio of sexual abuse may differ somewhat for adolescents with mental retardation (Sobsey, Randall, & Parrila, 1997). Girls with Williams syndrome may therefore be at higher risk compared to boys with this syndrome, or compared to girls or boys with other types of mental retardation.

Relationships with Peers

Adolescence is also a time marked by the increasing importance of social groups and peers. But adolescents with mental retardation often have difficulty making and maintaining friends. Using observational measures and self-reports from interviews, Zetlin and Murtaugh (1988) compared adolescents with and without mental retardation on friendship patterns. As a whole, adolescents with mental retardation had fewer friends, and their friendships tended to be less intimate, less empathetic, and with same-sex relatives. For the adolescents with mental retardation, contact with peers often occurred mostly during school hours. Friendships of adolescents with mental retardation were also less stable and more conflict-ridden.

Larger studies using more standardized measures report similar findings. Heiman (2000) compared the friendship patterns of 265 non-disabled students to two groups with mental retardation: 121 students who attended special schools, 189 who attended self-contained classrooms in general education schools. Students and their teachers were asked to complete Friendship Quality Questionnaires. Just as in Zetlin and Murtaugh (1988), Heiman found nonretarded students (as opposed to those with mental retardation) more often characterized a friend as "one who helps," and such help concerned other-than-school-related issues. As before, friends in different groups met in different places: Whereas 63% of students without disability reported meeting their friends in their home, such home meetings occurred in only 41% and 8% of students with mental retardation in self-contained classrooms and in special schools, respectively. In addition, 21% of nonretarded adolescents reported feeling "alone," compared to 76% and 87% of students from special schools or self-contained classrooms (respectively; see also Heiman & Margalit, 1998).

Relationships with Family

In American society, most children leave home sometime after high school, either by getting a job and apartment or by attending college. This long anticipated movement produces changes for both adolescents and for their parents, who are now faced with an "empty nest." Indeed, adolescence in general and "launching children and moving on" have been considered two of the most important stages in the family life cycle (Carter & McGoldrick, 1988).

When an adolescent has mental retardation, the situation often differs. Whereas the adolescent with mild levels of mental retardation may mostly act as a typical adolescent, such may not be the case for adolescents with more severe intellectual impairments. Seltzer and Ryff (1994) refer to such parenting as "nonnormative," and they focus on the adolescent's continuing need to rely on parents. Indeed, the entire process of disengaging from parents may be absent in this case, as adolescents with mental retardation may be unable to separate themselves from their families during the late teen and early adult years.

This general sense of delayed—or even abandoned—launching has now been substantiated by several studies. Murtaugh and Zetlin (1988) compared adolescents with and without mental retardation on issues of autonomy and found that adolescents with mental retardation were more likely to stay close to home during their free times and less likely to challenge their parents' restrictions. Furthermore, patterns of parental controls established during childhood did not change as these children became adolescents and graduated from high school.

And yet, although they may act differently, adolescents with mental retardation have many of the same desires as typically developing adolescents. Zetlin and Morrison (1998) reported that adolescents with and without mental retardation express similar desires to disengage or separate from their families, to become more autonomous, and to escape from parental controls. But whereas the parents of nonretarded adolescents acknowledged the need for developmental change, parents of adolescents with mental retardation stressed the need for family continuity and supervision at home.

Transition

Given the many difficulties experienced by adolescents with mental retardation as they consider assuming adult roles, the social service systems serving this population have developed a series of transition services. Beginning in 1990, the main federal law mandating school services, the Individuals with Disabilities Education Act (IDEA), mandated that schools prepare students for the transition to adult life. IDEA mandated that schools include transition plans in the individualized education program (IEP) of students by the age of 14 years, no later than age 16. Thus, from 14–16 years until leaving school (usually at 21), adolescents with mental retardation are being taught skills thought necessary for their successful functioning as adults.

To simplify slightly, all transition services focus on skills needed for independent living and working. The goal is that, upon graduation, young adults with mental retardation might be able to live either on their own or in a community group home and to be competitively employed in the community. To live independently, students are taught to shop for clothes or food within a budget, to use the post office, to understand schedules and take public buses or trains, and to visit a doctor or dentist. To be able to be hired by community businesses (i.e., to be "competitively employed"), students are trained in a variety of vocational skills. Such training addresses more general issues as being punctual, courteous, and "on task," as well as providing actual practice in working in un-

skilled or semiskilled jobs within the community.

As might be expected, the transition to adulthood brings up difficult challenges for the adolescents themselves, for social service agencies, and for families. Studies show that, when young adults with mental retardation fail at jobs, such failures are generally not caused by their intellectual limitations. Instead, young adults with mental retardation fail at jobs mainly due to social reasons: they too often arrive late or are absent from work; they cannot stay "on task" because of attentional problems, depression, or overfriendliness; or they get into conflicts and do not comply with the wishes of supervisors (Granat & Granat, 1978). For success in the work setting, then, young adults with mental retardation need effective social skills training to promote generalization and maintenance of appropriate social behaviors (Black & Lagone, 1997; Greenspan & Granfield, 1992).

A second, related problem involves navigating the social service system that is currently in place for adults. During the school years, many services for the child are handled by the school and within the child's IEP. In this sense, schools might be considered "one-stop shopping," a coordinated system of services. In contrast, adult services are usually under the control of the state's department of disabilities or mental retardation but contracted out to individual service providers. An adult with mental retardation may therefore go to one site for vocational services; another for speech–language therapy; yet others for medical, dental, occupational, or physical therapies. In addition, such adult services are in most cases not mandated by federal law, and regional centers or state-level agencies have difficulties meeting the needs of all adults in the system.

A successful transition thus requires good communication from one agency to another, good coordination of services, the collaboration of community-based agencies, and social support (Elliott, Alberto, Arnold, Taber, & Bryar, 1996). In addition, case managers and other social service providers must provide information about the wide variety of services that young adults with mental retardation may receive. Many young adults do not know about all the job opportunities available (Betz, 1998), and many do not know that they can have job coaches and trainers to help them in keeping and progressing in their jobs.

A final issue concerns the connections between transition services and families. In a qualitative study of adolescents with one of four separate disabilities, Morningstar, Turnbull, and Turnbull (1995) asked students their perspectives of the importance of family involvement in the transition from school to adult life. Students found family input and support very important in their decision making and their families influenced their career aspirations. But students also identified conflicts between parents and service providers or school personnel as a major barrier families face in helping their adolescents plan for their future. As such, some providers have begun IEP "preplanning" meetings. Miner and Bates (1997) found that when parents and families were involved in premeetings, they then participated more during the actual meeting, perhaps because they were more comfortable and aware of their potential contributions to the transition planning process. As services move from a focus on families during the childhood years ("family-centered planning") to the individuals themselves during the adult years ("person-centered planning"), parents must encourage their young adults with mental retardation to be as independent as possible and to advocate for themselves.

FUTURE DIRECTIONS

We end this chapter by discussing five directions for future research. As we detail below, each area requires a more fully fledged, explicit research area devoted exclusively to the problems of adolescents with mental retardation.

Differentiation of "Biopsychosocial" Models of Psychopathology during Adolescence

As in many fields that examine psychopathology, mental retardation researchers have considered it important to consider the problems of adolescents with mental retardation within a "biopsychosocial" perspective (Matson, 1985). Thus, biological, psychological, and social influences are all considered important.

Although such a perspective makes sense, it remains unhelpful if it also remains unspecified. One must first coordinate the biopsychosocial model with developmental issues. Consider the various adolescent-related changes in psychopathology in adolescents with Down syndrome, Prader–Willi syndrome, and Williams syndrome. Although a few studies have

examined when puberty occurs in each syndrome, so far none have attempted to link changes in either the prevalence or course of such maladaptive behaviors to any biological changes. In short, we need to dovetail what we know behaviorally with brain changes that may be occurring during adolescence.

Similar issues relate to the "psychological" and to the "social" within this model. We know, for example, that although peers are important during adolescence, adolescents with mental retardation have difficulties with friendships. How might such difficulties relate to, for example, increased withdrawal in Down syndrome during the early and later adolescent periods? How do adolescents with mental retardation think about friendships and how might such thinking relate to emotional or behavioral problems? Although some work has addressed these issues in mental retardation (Heiman, 2000; Zetlin & Murtaugh, 1988) and in autism (Bauminger & Kasari, 2000), no studies have yet linked such psychological processes to changes in prevalence rates of psychopathology or to changes in the course of psychopathology within particular individuals. From the opposite perspective, no studies have yet examined the entire issue of protective factors—whether particular biological characteristics (e.g., early vs. later puberty), social characteristics (more or closer friendships), or psychological characteristics (certain personality traits) might serve as protective factors against psychopathology for adolescents with mental retardation.

Attention to Gender during Adolescence

A related issue concerns gender and possible gender differences beginning during the adolescent years. On average in the nonretarded population, girls and women seem about twice as likely as boys and men to become clinically depressed sometime during their lives (Wolk & Weissman, 1995). Such sex differences in prevalence rates mainly begin during the 10–15-year period, as do marked increases in female (as opposed to male) depressive symptoms not associated with full-blown depression (Garber, Keiley, & Martin, 2002).

Are such gender differences in depression found among adolescents with mental retardation in general or among adolescents with specific genetic syndromes? In most studies, gender differences are not reported, but it remains unclear whether gender differences in problems during adolescence are really not present or, instead, whether the researchers have not looked. In a review of the emotional–behavioral problems of girls with mental retardation, Hodapp and Dykens (2005) note that only about one-quarter of articles in the two main mental retardation journals report how many boys and girls participated in the study *and* whether gender differences occurred. Thus, we simply do not know whether the "usual" gender differences in susceptibility to depression are found in adolescent girls versus boys with mental retardation.

Attention to Families and Transition during and out of Adolescence

For reasons that are not always clear, family work in mental retardation has generally bypassed the adolescent years. Much work exists on families of young children, and a few studies have even begun to longitudinally examine family issues of children with disabilities from early intervention into the school-age years (Hauser-Cram, Warfield, Shonkoff, & Krauss, 2001). Other studies examine children with mental retardation in general or with specific genetic syndromes throughout the childhood years, with no special attention to adolescence (see Hodapp, 2002, for a review). Finally, over the past decade, several research groups have begun to examine the many issues–problems facing families of adults with mental retardation (e.g., Seltzer & Krauss, 2002).

Lost in this "before and after" picture is a specific focus on adolescence per se. Indeed, with the exception of the few studies mentioned earlier, we know little about the role families play in the lives of adolescents with mental retardation, or the interplay of families with the adolescent's anticipated launching, mental health, or other concerns. To the extent that families have been of interest during the adolescent period, much of the focus has revolved around transition issues and the role families play in advocacy and provision of social services. Researchers and practitioners argue about the degree to which services should be person-centered versus family-centered, and about whether adolescents–young adults with mental retardation can be informed about and advocate for their own services. From the opposite perspective, professionals debate the circumstances under which young adults with mental retardation should not be considered legally responsible, and how parents can (or should) assume the legal rights that generally would go to their young adult offspring ("conservatorship"). Although such issues are obviously important, they are not enough.

Attention to Issues of Culture and Socioeconomic Status during Adolescence

As in many areas of mental retardation behavioral research, adolescent work has generally been limited to a Caucasian, middle-class perspective. Although some attempts have recently been made to examine children with mental retardation—and their families—in terms of cultural and socioeconomic issues, such attempts are still fairly rare.

In discussing issues related to the transition from late adolescence into the adult years, Blacher (2001) notes that such issues often concern acculturation. Acculturation refers to the degree to which a family of a particular ethnic group has or has not adopted the values, practices, and perspectives of the wider, mainstream culture. To give one example, in Latino cultures it is fairly common for families to have a strong sense of "familism," or interdependence among family members that provides support, loyalty, and solidarity. In addition to such support helping Latino mothers to adapt—partly by helping to take care of the adult with mental retardation (Magana, 1999)—a familist perspective may even account for where adults with mental retardation live. In one study, Russell (1999; cited in Blacher, 2001) compared the percentages of Latino versus Anglo or African American families that had adults with mental retardation still living within the home. Compared to a home-living rate of 63% in the Latino families, only 50% and 46% of Anglo and of African American families (respectively) had their adults with mental retardation living within the family home. Clearly, such attention to ethnic differences is an area of badly needed study in the future.

Ties to Service Delivery during and out of Adolescence

Finally, as might be expected, neglecting adolescence as a period of life hurts service delivery. If we do not focus on the specific problems of adolescents with mental retardation—if we do not even know whether such problems are specific to adolescence—then we cannot hope to provide services that are better tailored to this group's needs.

The problems here arise on many levels. Beyond the difficulty of addressing a problem that one does not know about, other issues are specific to mental retardation. The first issue concerns the very prevalence rates of mental retardation. Across a wide variety of studies, one finds that prevalence rates of mental retardation are fairly low in the preschool years, increase over the school years, then decline thereafter. In short, the movement from school into adulthood is a critical time, a time of "losing" individuals with mental retardation. One suspects that such lost individuals are probably losing needed services as well.

A second issue concerns the ways that service delivery occurs. Unlike school services, services after the school years are neither mandated nor in a single physical location. As a result, one finds that families that insist on services, and know how to mobilize their own and friendly professionals' resources, are able to receive services for their soon-to-be-adult offspring. In contrast, those families that are less able to mobilize have adolescents who receive fewer and less effective services upon entering adulthood.

Obviously, such issues involve policy matters beyond the scope of this chapter. But if our society truly wants to support adolescents and young adults with mental retardation, it needs to find the appropriate resources. Even so, the lack of a clearly defined research base is problematic. With no research backup, it becomes impossible to use scientific studies to highlight the needs of this group, leaving unclear just what better services might look like.

We began this chapter with a prediction. We noted that although it may not currently exist, a formal subdiscipline concerning adolescents with mental retardation is imminent. The time seems ripe to take that next step, to mirror the fields of child development and of child and adolescent psychiatry and make adolescence a clearly defined subfield within mental retardation.

REFERENCES

Achenbach, T. M. (1991). *Manual for the Child Behavior Checklist—4–18—and 1991 profiles*. Burlington, VT.

Aman, M. G., Armstrong, S., Buican, B., & Sillick, T. (2002). Four-year follow-up of children with low intelligence and ADHD: A replication. *Research in Developmental Disabilities, 23*, 119–134.

Aman, M. G., & Singh, N. N. (1994). *Aberrant behavior checklist–community supplementary manual*. East Aurora, NY: Slosson.

American Association on Mental Retardation. (1992). *Mental retardation: Definition, classification, and systems of supports* (9th ed.). Washington, DC: Author.

American Psychiatric Association. (1994). *Diagnostic and statistical manual of mental disorders* (4th ed.). Washington, DC: Author.

Atkins v. Virginia. (U.S., June, 2002).

Balogh, R., Bretherton, K., Whibley, S., Berney, T., Graham, S., Richhold, P., et al. (2001). Sexual abuse in children and adolescents with intellectual disability. *Journal of Intellectual Disability Research, 45*, 194–201.

Baumgardner, T. L., Reiss, A. L., Freund, L. S., & Abrams, M. T. (1995). Specification of the neurobehavioral phenotype in males with fragile X syndrome. *Pediatrics, 95*, 744–752.

Bauminger, N., & Kasari, C. (2000). Loneliness and friendship in high-functioning children with autism. *Child Development, 71*, 447–456.

Benson, B., & Valenti-Hein, D. (2001). Cognitive and social learning treatments. In A. Dosen & K. Day (Eds.), *Treatment of mental illness and behavior disorders in children and adults with mental retardation* (pp. 101–118). Washington, DC: American Psychiatric Press.

Betz, C. L. (1998). Adolescent transitions: A nursing concern. *Pediatric Nursing, 24*, 23–28.

Blacher, J. (2001). Transition to adulthood: Mental retardation, families, and culture. *American Journal on Mental Retardation, 106*, 173–188.

Black, R. S., & Lagone, J. (1997). Social awareness and transitions to employment for adolescents with mental retardation. *Remedial and Special Education, 18*(4), 214–222.

Borthwick-Duffy, S. A., Lane, K. L., & Widaman, K. F. (1997). Measuring problem behaviors in children with mental retardation: Dimensions and predictors. *Research in Developmental Disabilities, 18*, 415–433.

Bouras, N. (Ed.). (1999). *Psychiatric and behavioural disorders in developmental disabilities and mental retardation*. Cambridge, UK: Cambridge University Press.

Branford, D. (1996). A review of antipsychotic drugs prescribed for people with learning disabilities who live in Leicestershire. *Journal of Intellectual Disability Research, 40*, 358–368.

Branford, D. (1997). A follow-up study of prescribing for people with learning disabilities previously in National Health Service care in Leicestershire, England. *Journal of Intellectual Disability Research, 41*, 339–345.

Broman, S., Nichols, P. L., Shaughnessy, P., & Kennedy,

W. (1987). *Retardation in young children: A developmental study of cognitive deficit.* Hillsdale, NJ: Erlbaum.

Butler, J. V., Whittington, J. E., Holland, A. J., Boer, H., Clarke, D., & Webb, T. (2002). Prevalence of, and risk factors for, physical ill-health in people with Prader–Willi syndrome: A population-based study. *Developmental Medicine and Child Neurology, 44,* 248–255.

Cahill, B. M., & Glidden, L. M. (1996). Influence of child diagnosis on family and parent functioning: Down syndrome versus other disabilities. *American Journal on Mental Retardation, 101,* 149–160.

Carter, B., & McGoldrick, M. (1988). The changing family life cycle: A framework for family therapy. In B. Carter & M. McGoldrick (Eds.), *The changing family life cycle* (2nd ed., pp. 3–28). New York: Gardner Press.

Chorney, M. J., Chorney, K., Seese, N., Owen, M. J., Daniels,J., McGuffin, P., et al. (1998). A quantitative trait locus associated with cognitive ability in children. *Psychological Science, 9,* 159–166.

Collacutt, R. A., Cooper, S. A., & McGrother, C. (1992). Differential rates of psychiatric disorders in adults with Down's syndrome compared with other mentally handicapped adults. *British Journal of Psychiatry, 161,* 671–674.

Cormack, K. F. M., Brown, A. C., & Hastings, R. P. (2000). Behavioral and emotional difficulties in students attending schools for children and adolescents with severe intellectual disability, *Journal of Intellectual Disability Research, 44,* 124–129.

Crocker, A. G., & Hodgins, S. (1997). The criminality of noninstitutionalized mentally retarded persons: Evidence from a birth cohort followed to age 30. *Criminal Justice and Behavior, 24,* 432–454.

Curry, C. I., Stevenson, R. E., Aughton, D., Byrne, J., Carey, J. C., Cassidy, S. B., et al. (1997). Evaluation of mental retardation: Recommendations of a consensus conference. *American Journal of Medical Genetics, 72,* 468–477.

Cutler, S. E., & Nolen-Hoeksema, S. (1991). Accounting for sex differences in depression through female victimization: Childhood sexual abuse. *Sex Roles, 24,* 425–438.

Davies, M., Udwin, O., & Howlin, P. (1998). Adults with Williams syndrome. *British Journal of Psychiatry, 172,* 273–276.

Davies, S. P., & Ecob, K. C. (1959). The challenge to the schools. In S. P. Davies (Ed.), *The mentally retarded in society* (pp. 173–191). New York: Columbia University Press.

Denning, C. B., Chamberlain, J. A., & Polloway, E. A. (2000). An evaluation of state guidelines for mental retardation: Focus on definition and classification practices. *Education and Training in Mental Retardation, 35,* 226–232.

Dennis, W. (1946). The adolescent. In L. Carmichael (Ed.), *Manual of child psychology* (pp. 633–666). Oxford, UK: Wiley.

Dilts, C. V., Morris, C. A., & Leonard, C. O. (1990).

Hypothesis for development of a behavioral phenotype in Williams syndrome. *American Journal of Medical Genetics, 6,* 126–131.

Dimitropoulos, A., Feurer, I. D., Butler, M. G., & Thompson, T. (2001). Emergence of compulsive behavior and tantrums in children with Prader–Willi syndrome. *American Journal on Mental Retardation, 106,* 39–51.

Dosen, A., & Petry, D. (1993). Treatment of depression in persons with mental retardation. In R. J. Fletcher & A. Dosen (Eds.), *Mental health aspects of mental retardation: Progress in assessment and treatment* (pp. 242–260). New York: Lexington.

Dykens, E. M. (1995). Measuring behavioral phenotypes: Provocations from the "new genetics. " *American Journal on Mental Retardation, 99,* 522–532.

Dykens, E. M. (1996). DNA meets DSM: The growing importance of genetic syndromes in dual diagnosis. *Mental Retardation, 34,* 125–127.

Dykens, E. M. (2000). Psychopathology in children with intellectual disabilities. *Journal of Child Psychology and Psychiatry, 41,* 407–417.

Dykens, E. M. (2003). Anxiety, fears, and phobias in persons with Williams syndrome. *Developmental Neuropsychology, 23,* 291–316.

Dykens, E. M. (2004). Maladaptive and compulsive behavior in Prader–Willi syndrome: New insights from older adults. *American Journal on Mental Retardation, 109,* 142–153.

Dykens, E. M., & Cassidy, S. B. (1996). Prader–Willi syndrome: Genetic, behavioral and treatment issues. *Child and Adolescent Psychiatric Clinics of North America, 5,* 913–928.

Dykens, E. M., & Clarke, D. J. (1997). Correlates of maladaptive behavior in individuals with 5p- (cri du chat) syndrome. *Developmental Medicine and Child Neurology, 39,* 752–756.

Dykens, E. M., & Cohen, D. J. (1996). Effects of Special Olympics International on social competence in persons with mental retardation. *Journal of the American Academy of Child and Adolescent Psychiatry, 35,* 223–229.

Dykens, E. M., & Hodapp, R. M. (1997). Treatment issues in genetic mental retardation syndromes. *Professional Psychology: Research and Practice, 28,* 263–270.

Dykens, E. M., & Hodapp, R. M. (2001). Research in mental retardation: Toward an etiologic approach. *Journal of Child Psychology and Psychiatry, 42,* 49–71.

Dykens, E. M., Hodapp, R. M., & Finucane, B. M. (2000). *Genetics and mental retardation syndromes: A new look at behavior and interventions.* Baltimore: Brookes.

Dykens, E. M., & Kasari, C. (1997). Maladaptive behaviors in children with Prader–Willi syndrome, Down syndrome, and non-specific mental retardation. *American Journal on Mental Retardation, 102,* 228–237.

Dykens, E. M., Leckman, J. F., & Cassidy, S. B. (1996). Obsessions and compulsions in Prader–Willi syndrome. *Journal of Child Psychology and Psychiatry*, 37, 995–1002.

Dykens, E. M., & Rosner, B. A. (1999). Refining behavioral phenotypes: Personality–motivation in Williams and Prader–Willi syndromes. *American Journal on Mental Retardation*, 104, 158–169.

Dykens, E. M., Shah, B., Sagun, J., Beck, T., & King, B. Y. (2002). Maladaptive behavior in children and adolescents with Down syndrome. *Journal of Intellectual Disability Research*, 46, 484–492.

Einfeld, S. L., & Tonge, B. J. (1992). *Manual for the developmental behavioral checklist: Primary care version*. Sydney: School of Psychiatry, University of New South Wales.

Einfeld, S. L., & Tonge, B. J. (1996). Population prevalence of psychopathology in children and adolescents with intellectual disability: Epidemiological findings, *Journal of Intellectual Disability Research*, 40, 99–109.

Einfeld, S. L., Tonge, B. J., & Florio, T. (1997). Behavioral and emotional disturbance in individuals with Williams syndrome. *American Journal on Mental Retardation*, 102, 45–53.

Einfeld, S. L., Tonge, B., Turner, G., Parmenter, T., & Smith, A. (1999). Longitudinal course of behavioural and emotional problems of young persons with Prader–Willi, fragile X, and Down syndromes. *Journal of Intellectual and Developmental Disability*, 24, 349–354.

Elliott, N. E., Alberto, P. A., Arnold, S. E., Taber, T. A., & Bryar, M. R. (1996). The role of school district interagency transition committees within an overall collaborative structure, *Journal of Applied Rehabilitation Counseling*, 27, 63–68.

Emerson, E. (2003). Prevalence of psychiatric disorders in children and adolescents with and without intellectual disability. *Journal of Intellectual Disability Research*, 47, 51–58.

Ewart A. K., Morris, C. A., Atkinson, D., Jin, W., Sternes, K., Spallone, P., et al. (1993). Hemizygosity at the elastin locus in a developmental disorder, Williams syndrome. *Nature Genetics*, 5, 11–16.

Fernald, W. (1912). The burden of feeblemindedness. *Journal of Psycho-Aesthetics*, 17, 87–111.

Finucane, B. M., Konar, D., Haas-Givler, B., Kurtz, & M. B., & Scott, C. I., Jr. (1994). The spasmodic upper-body squeeze: A characteristic behavior in Smith–Magenis syndrome. *Developmental Medicine and Child Neurology*, 36, 78–83.

Fowler, A. (1990). The development of language structure in children with Down syndrome. In D. Cicchetti & M. Beeghly (Eds.), *Children with Down syndrome: A developmental perspective* (pp. 302–328). New York: Cambridge University Press.

Galvez, R., Gopal, A. R., & Greenough, W. T. (2003). Somatosensory cortical barrel dendritic abnormalities in a mouse model of the fragile X mental retardation syndrome. *Brain Research*, 971, 83–89.

Ganiban, J., Wagner, S., & Cicchetti, D. (1990). Temperament and Down syndrome. In D. Cicchetti & M.

Beeghly (Eds.), *Children with Down syndrome: A developmental perspective* (pp. 63–100). New York: Cambridge University Press.

Garber, J., Keiley, M. K., & Martin, N. C. (2002). Developmental trajectories of adolescents' depressive symptoms: Predictors of change. *Journal of Consulting and Clinical Psychology*, 70, 79–95.

Gardner, W. I., Graeber-Whalen, J. L., & Ford, D. R. (2001). Behavioral therapies. In A. Dosen & K. Day (Eds.), *Treatment of mental illness and behavior disorders in children and adults with mental retardation* (pp. 69–100). Washington, DC: American Psychiatric Press.

Gath, A., & Gumley, D. (1986). Behavior problems in retarded children with special reference to Down's syndrome. *British Journal of Psychiatry*, 149, 156–151.

Gillberg, C., Persson, E., Grufman, M., & Themner, U. (1986). Psychiatric disorders in mildly and severely mentally retarded urban children and adolescents: Epidemiological aspects. *British Journal of Psychiatry*, 149, 68–74.

Glick, M. (1998). A developmental approach to psychopathology in people with mild mental retardation. In J. A. Burack, R. M. Hodapp, & E. Zigler (Eds.), *Handbook of mental retardation and development* (pp. 563–580). New York: Cambridge University Press.

Gosch, A., & Pankau, R. (1997). Personality characteristics and behavior problems in individuals of different ages with Williams syndrome. *Developmental Medicine and Child Neurology*, 39, 527–533.

Granat, K., & Granat, S. (1978). Adjustment of intellectually below-average men not identified as mentally retarded. *Scandinavian Journal of Psychology*, 19, 41–51.

Greenspan, S., & Granfield, J. M. (1992). Reconsidering the construct of mental retardation: Implications for a model of social competence. *American Journal of Mental Retardation*, 96, 442–453.

Greenspan, S., Loughlin, G., & Black, R. S. (2001). Credulity and gullibility in people with developmental disorders: A framework for future research. *International Review of Research in Mental Retardation*, 24, 101–135.

Hardan, A., & Shal, R. (1997). Psychopathology in children and adolescents with developmental disorders. *Research in Developmental Disabilities*, 18, 369–382.

Hauser-Cram, P., Warfield, M. E., Shonkoff, J. P., & Krauss, M. W. (2001). Children with disabilities. *Monographs of the Society for Research in Child Development*, 66(3, Serial No. 266).

Heiman, T. (2000). Quality and quantity of friendship. *School Psychology International*, 21, 265–281.

Heiman, T., & Margalit, M. (1998). Loneliness, depression, and social skills among students with mild mental retardation in different educational settings. *Journal of Special Education*, 32, 154–163.

Hodapp, R. M. (1994). Cultural–familial mental retardation. In R. Sternberg (Ed.), *Encyclopedia of intelligence* (pp. 711–717). New York: Macmillan.

Hodapp, R. M. (1996). Down syndrome: Developmental, psychiatric, and management issues. *Child and Adolescent Psychiatric Clinics of North America, 5,* 881–894.

Hodapp, R. M. (1997). Direct and indirect behavioral effects of different genetic disorders of mental retardation. *American Journal on Mental Retardation, 102,* 67–79.

Hodapp, R. M. (2002). Parenting children with mental retardation. In M. Bornstein (Ed.), *Handbook of parenting. Volume 1: How children influence parents* (2nd ed., pp. 355–381). Hillsdale, NJ: Erlbaum.

Hodapp, R. M., & Dykens, E. M. (2001). Strengthening behavioral research on genetic mental retardation syndromes. *American Journal on Mental Retardation, 106,* 4–15.

Hodapp, R. M., & Dykens, E. M. (2003). Mental retardation (intellectual disabilities). In E. J. Mash & R. A. Barkley (Eds.), *Child psychopathology* (2nd ed., pp. 486–519). New York: Guilford Press.

Hodapp, R. M., & Dykens, E. M. (2004). Studying behavioural phenotypes: Issues, benefits, challenges. In E. Emerson, C. Hatton, T. Parmenter, & T. Thompson (Eds.), *International handbook of applied research in intellectual disabilities* (pp. 203–220). Sussex, UK: Wiley.

Hodapp, R. M., & Dykens, E. M. (2005). Problems of girls and young women with mental retardation (intellectual disabilities). In D. Bell-Dolan, S. Foster, & E. Mash (Eds.), *Handbook of behavioral and emotional disorders in girls* (pp. 239–262). New York: Kluwer/Plenum Press.

Hodapp, R. M., Dykens, E. M., Ort, S. I., Zelinsky, D. G., & Leckman, J. F. (1991). Changing patterns of intellectual strengths and weaknesses in males with fragile X syndrome. *Journal of Autism and Developmental Disorders, 21,* 503–516.

Hodapp, R. M., Ly, T. M., Fidler, D. J., & Ricci, L. A. (2001). Less stress, more rewarding: Parenting children with Down syndrome. *Parenting: Science and Practice, 1,* 317–337.

Hodapp, R. M., & Ricci, L. A. (2002). Behavioural phenotypes and educational practice: The unrealized connection. In G. O'Brien & O. Udwin (Eds.), *Behavioural phenotypes in clinical practice* (pp. 137–151). London: Mac Keith Press.

Hodapp, R. M., Ricci, L. A., Ly, T. M., & Fidler, D. J. (2003). The effects of the child with Down syndrome on maternal stress. *British Journal of Developmental Psychology, 21,* 137–151.

Hodapp, R. M., & Zigler, E. (1995). Past, present, and future issues in the developmental approach to mental retardation and developmental disabilities. In D. Cicchetti & D. Cohen (Eds.), *Manual of developmental psychopathology. Vol. 2: Risk, disorder, and adaptation* (pp. 299–331). New York: Wiley.

Hodgins, S. (1992). Mental disorder, intellectual disabil-

ity, and crime: Evidence from a birth cohort. *Archives of General Psychiatry, 49,* 476–483.

Holland, A. J., Treasure, J., Coskeran, P., & Dallow, J. (1995). Characteristics of the eating disorder in Prader–Willi syndrome: Implications for treatment. *Journal of Intellectual Disability, 39,* 373–381.

Hollins, S. (1997). Counselling and psychotherapy. In O. Russell (Ed.), *Seminars in the psychiatry of learning disabilities* (pp. 245–258). London: Gaskell, The Royal College of Psychiatrists.

Hurley, A. D. (1989). Individual psychotherapy with mentally retarded individuals: A review and call for research. *Research in Developmental Disabilities, 10,* 261–275.

Jacobson, J. W. (1999). Dual diagnosis services: History, progress, and perspectives. In N. Bouras (Ed.), *Psychiatric and behavioural disorders in developmental disabilities and mental retardation* (pp. 329–358). Cambridge, UK: Cambridge University Press.

Jarrold, C., Baddeley, A. D., Hewes, A. K., & Phillips, C. (2001). A longitudinal assessment of diverging verbal and non-verbal abilities in the Williams syndrome phenotype. *Cortex, 37,* 423–431.

Johnson, C. R., Handen, B. L., Lubetsky, M. J., & Sacco, K. A. (1995). Affective disorders in hospitalized children and adolescents with mental retardation: A retrospective study. *Research in Developmental Disabilities, 16,* 221–231.

Kalachnik, J. E., Levanthal, B. L., James, D. H., Sovner, R., Kastner, T. A., Walsh, K. K., et al. (1998). Guidelines for the use of psychotropic medication. In S. Reiss & M. G. Aman (Eds.), *Psychotropic medication and developmental disabilities: International consensus handbook* (pp. 45–72). Columbus: Ohio State University, Nisonger Center.

Kearns, A., & O'Connor, A. (1988). The mentally handicapped criminal offender: A 10-year study of two hospitals. *British Journal of Psychiatry, 152,* 848–851.

King, B. H., DeAntonio, C., McCracken, J. T., Forness, S. R., & Ackerland, V. (1994). Psychiatric consultation in severe and profound mental retardation. *American Journal of Psychiatry, 151,* 1802–1808.

King, B. H., Hodapp, R. M., & Dykens, E. M. (2005). Mental retardation. In H. I. Kaplan & B. J. Sadock (Eds.), *Comprehensive textbook of psychiatry* (8th ed., pp. 3076–3106). Baltimore: Williams & Wilkins.

Kumin, L. (1994). Intelligibility of speech in children with Down syndrome in natural settings: Parents' perspective. *Perceptual and Motor Skills, 78,* 307–313.

MacLean, W. E., Jr. (Ed.). (1997). *Ellis' handbook of mental deficiency, psychological theory and research* (3rd ed.). Mahwah, NJ: Erlbaum.

Magana, S. M. (1999). Puerto Rican families caring for an adult with mental retardation: Role of familism. *American Journal on Mental Retardation, 104,* 456–482.

Manikam, R., Matson, J. L., Coe, D. A., & Hillman, N. (1995). Adolescent depression: Relationships of self-report to intellectual and adaptive functioning. - *Research in Developmental Disabilities, 16,* 349–364.

Masi, G. (1998). Psychiatric illness in mentally retarded adolescents: Clinical features, *Adolescence, 33,* 425–434.

Masi, G., Pfanner, P., & Marcheschi, M. (1998). Depression in adolescents with mental retardation: A clinical study. *British Journal of Developmental Disabilities, 44,* 112–118.

Matson, J. (1985). Biosocial theory of psychopathology: A three by three factor model. *Applied Research in Mental retardation, 6,* 199–227.

Meyers, B. A. (1987). Psychiatric problems in adolescents with developmental disabilities. *Journal of the American Academy of Child and Adolescent Psychiatry, 26,* 74–79.

Meyers, B. A., & Pueschel, S. M. (1991). Psychiatric disorders in persons with Down syndrome. *Journal of Nervous and Mental Disease, 179,* 609–613.

Miller, J. (1999). Profiles of language development in children with Down syndrome. In J. F. Miller, M. Leddy, & L. A. Leavitt (Eds.), *Improving the communication of people with Down syndrome* (pp. 11–39). Baltimore: Brookes.

Miner, C. A., & Bates, P. E. (1997). The effects of person centered planning activities on the IEP/Transition planning process. *Education and Training in Mental Retardation and Developmental Disabilities, 32,* 105–112.

Montgomery, S. A., & Asberg, M. (1979). A new depression scale designed to be sensitive to change. *British Journal of Psychiatry, 134,* 382–389.

Morningstar, M. E., Turnbull, A. P., & Turnbull, H. R. (1995). What students with disabilities tell us about the importance of family involvement in the transition from school to adult life? *Exceptional Children, 62,* 249–260.

Moss, S. (1999). Assessment: conceptual issues. In N. Bouras (Ed.), *Psychiatric and behavioural disorders in developmental disabilities and mental retardation* (pp. 18–37). Cambridge, UK: Cambridge University Press.

Moss, S. (2001). Psychiatric disorders in adults with mental retardation. *International Review of Research in Mental Retardation, 24,* 211–243.

Moss, S., Ibbotson, B., Prosser, H., Godgerb, D. P., Patel, P., & Simpson, N. (1997). Validity of the PAS-ADD for detecting psychiatric symptoms in adults with learning disability. *Social Psychiatry and Psychiatric Epidemiology, 32,* 344–354.

Moss, S. C., Prossner, H., Ibbotson, B., & Goldenberg, D. P. (1996). Respondent and informant accounts of psychiatric symptoms in a sample of patients with learning disability. *Journal of Intellectual Disability Research, 40,* 457–465.

Murtaugh, M., & Zetlin, A. G. (1988). Achievement of autonomy by non-handicapped and mildly handicapped adolescents. *Journal of Youth and Adolescents, 17,* 445–460.

Mussen, P. (Ed.). (1983). *Handbook of child psychology* (4th ed.). New York: Wiley.

Ollendick, T. H., King, N. J., & Frary, R. B. (1989). Fears in children and adolescents: Reliability and generalizability across age, gender, and nationality. *Behaviour Research and Therapy, 27,* 19–26.

Opitz, J. M. (1985). Editorial comment: The developmental field concept. *American Journal of Medical Genetics, 21,* 1–11.

Pober, B. R., & Dykens, E. M . (1996). Williams syndrome: An overview of medical, cognitive, and behavioral features. *Child and Adolescent Psychiatric Clinics of North America, 5,* 929–943.

Polloway, E. A., Smith, J. D., Chamberlain, J., Denning, C. B., & Smith, T. E. C. (1999). Levels of deficits or supports in the classification of mental retardation: Implementation practices. *Education and Training in Mental Retardation, 34,* 200–206.

Reilly, J. S., Klima, E., & Bellugi, U. (1990). Once more with feeling: Affect and language in atypical populations. *Development and Psychopathology, 2,* 367–391.

Reiss, S. (1988). *The Reiss screen for maladaptive behavior.* Worthington, OH: IDS.

Reiss, S., & Aman, M. G. (Eds.). (1998) *Psychotropic medication and developmental disabilities: International consensus handbook.* Columbus: Ohio State University, Nisonger Center.

Reiss, S., & Havercamp, S. H. (1998). Toward a comprehensive assessment of functional motivation: Factor structure of the Reiss profiles. *Psychological Assessment, 10,* 97–106.

Reiss, S., & Szyszko, J. (1983). Diagnostic overshadowing and professional experience with mentally retarded persons. *American Journal of Mental Deficiency, 87,* 396–402.

Rogers, C. (1987). Maternal support for the Down's syndrome personality stereotype: The effect of direct experience on the condition. *Journal of Mental deficiency Research, 31,* 271–278.

Rush, A. J., & Frances, A. (Eds.). (2000). Special issue: Expert consensus guideline series: Treatment of psychiatric and behavioral problems in mental retardation. *American Journal on Mental Retardation, 105* (Whole No. 3), 159–228.

Rutter, M., Graham, P., & Yule, W. (1970). A neuropsychiatric study in childhood. *Clinics in Developmental Medicine.* London: SIM with Heinemann Medical.

Rutter, M., Simonoff, E., & Plomin, R. (1996). Genetic influences on mild mental retardation: Concepts, findings, and research implications. *Journal of Biosocial Science, 28,* 509–526.

Scheerenberger, R. C. (1983). *A history of mental retardation.* Baltimore: Brookes.

Scheerenberger, R. C. (1987). *A history of mental retardation: A quarter century of progress.* Baltimore: Brookes.

Seltzer, M. M., & Krauss, M. W. (2002). Quality of life of adults with mental retardation who live with their families. *Mental Retardation and Developmental Disabilities Research Reviews, 7,* 105–114,

Seltzer, M. M., & Ryff, C. D. (1994). Parenting across the life span: The normative and nonnormative case. *Life-Span Development and Behavior, 12,* 1–40.

Simpson, M. K., & Hogg, J. (2001a). Patterns of offending among people with intellectual disability: A systematic review. Part I: Methodology and prevalence data. *Journal of Intellectual Disability Research, 45,* 383–396.

Simpson, M. K., & Hogg, J. (2001b). Patterns of offending among people with intellectual disability: A systematic review. Part II: Predisposing factors. *Journal of Intellectual Disability Research, 45,* 397–406.

Sobsey, D., Randall, W., & Parrila, R. K. (1997). Gender differences in abused children with and without disabilities. *Child Abuse and Neglect, 21,* 707–720.

Sovner, R. (1986). Limiting factors in the use of DSM-III with mentally ill/mentally retarded persons. *Psychopharmacology Bulletin, 22,* 1055–1059.

State, M. W., King, B. H., & Dykens, E. M. (1997). Mental retardation: A review of the past 10 years. II. *Journal of the American Academy of Child and Adolescent Psychiatry, 36,* 1664–1671.

Steffenburg, S., Gillberg, C., & Steffenburg, U. (1996). Psychiatric disorders in children and adolescents with mental retardation and active epilepsy. *Archives of Neurology, 53,* 904–912.

Stromme, P., & Hagberg, G. (2000). Aetiology in severe and mild mental retardation: A population-based study of Norwegian children. *Developmental Medicine and Child Neurology, 42,* 76–86.

Stromme, P., & Magnus, P. (2000). Correlations between socioeconomic status, IQ, and aetiology in mental retardation: A population-based study of Norwegian children. *Social Psychiatry and Psychiatric Epidemiology, 35,* 12–18.

Sturmey, P. (1999). Classification: concepts, progress, and future. In N. Bouras (Ed.), *Psychiatric and behavioural disorders in developmental disabilities and mental retardation* (pp. 3–17). Cambridge, UK: Cambridge University Press.

Sullivan, P. M., & Knutson, J. F. (2000). Maltreatment and disabilities: A population-based epidemiological study. *Child Abuse and Neglect, 24,* 1257–1273.

Szymanski, L., & King, B. H. (1999). Summary of the practice parameters for assessment and treatment of children, adolescents, and adults with mental retardation and comorbid mental disorders. *Journal of the American Academy of Child and Adolescent Psychiatry, 38,* 1606–1610.

Szymanski, L. S., King, B., Goldberg, B., Reid, A. H., Tonge, B. J., & Cain, N. (1998). Diagnosis of mental disorders in people with mental retardation. In S. Reiss & M. G. Aman (Eds.), *The international consensus handbook: Psychotropic medications and developmental disabilities* (pp. 3–18). Columbus: Ohio State University, Nisonger Center.

Udwin, O., & Yule, W. (1991). A cognitive and behavioral phenotype in Williams syndrome. *Journal of Clinical and Experimental Neuropsychology, 13,* 232–244.

Walker, E. F. (2002). Adolescent neurodevelopment and psychopathology. *Current Directions in Psychological Sciences, 11,* 24–28.

Westcott, H. L., & Jones, D. P. H. (1999). The abuse of disabled children. *Journal of Child Psychology and Psychiatry, 40,* 497–506.

Winter, N., Holland, A. J., & Collins, S. (1997). Factors predisposing to suspected offending by adults with self-reported learning disabilities. *Psychological Medicine, 27,* 595–607.

Wolk, S. I., & Weissman, M. M. (1995). Women and depression: An update. In J. Oldham & M. Riba (Eds.), *American Psychiatric Press review of psychiatry* (Vol. 14, pp. 227–259). Washington, DC: American Psychiatric Press.

Zetlin, A. G., & Morrison, G. M. (1998). Adaptation through the life span. In J. A. Burack, R. M. Hodapp, & E. Zigler (Eds.), *Handbook of mental retardation and development* (pp. 481–503). New York: Cambridge University Press.

Zetlin, A. G., & Murtaugh, M. (1988). Friendship patterns of mildly learning handicapped and nonhandicapped high school students. *American Journal on Mental Retardation, 92,* 447–454.

Zigler, E. (1967). Familial mental retardation: A continuing dilemma. *Science, 155,* 292–298.

Zigler, E., & Glick, M. (1986). *A developmental approach to adult psychopathology.* New York: Wiley.

11

Learning Disabilities

Orly Lipka
Linda S. Siegel

Denise had difficulties with reading from the beginning of school. She has always performed below grade level and has had difficulty with sounding words out. However, she was energetic, motivated, and popular with her elementary school classmates. Now, in grade 11, Denise still has difficulties with reading. On a standardized reading test, her score was still below average and she had a low score on a spelling test.

Denise has been unable to keep up with grade-level academic work since the fourth grade. In her adolescent years, upon entering high school in grade 8, she had major difficulties and did not pass. By the end of grade 10, she had an emotional breakdown and was hospitalized for several weeks. She is now completing 11th-grade work in an alternative program after changing schools three times in 2 years. She is in an alternative grade 11 program, not because she passed 9th and 10th grades after all but, rather, because there is no other option for her at her age.

According to a school assessment battery completed in grade 4, Denise showed no evidence of a learning disability, although the assessment did not test for some important skills and processes that were relevant to

reading. Throughout Denise's schooling, her difficulties have been addressed as though they were behavioral in nature and not a result of a learning disability. In elementary school, she saw the school counselor once a week for disruptive behavior, whereas in high school, the visits to the counselor occurred when she misbehaved. She received no help for her reading.

With the onset of adolescence, Denise's behavior has become increasingly depressive and aggressive. She has become extremely frustrated and angry with school and has often dealt with her frustrations in anger and rage or becoming very depressed and quiet. She was aggressive toward her younger brother and sister and she developed suicidal and very paranoid behaviors. She ran away from home several times. She has become so marginalized in the system that the types of friends she had for a while were street youth and drug addicts. According to Denise, she turned to heavy drug use "because it is the only thing that makes me feel better!" In her parents' words, "A once very sweet child has become a monster."

Denise's present and future looks grim right now. Although she is attending an alternative schooling program, it is geared more toward supporting students with behavioral difficulties rather than students with learning disabilities. Denise continues to search for relief through drugs; however, the effects are nothing other than increased depressive behavior and poor judgment.

When asked about Denise's future, her mother says, "Denise was a kind, happy and very sensitive person before her academic downfall in schools. She was a happy girl. She is no longer that young girl. I hope that with help, including rehab, she will be able to regain some of the strengths she once had. She is very creative. I think she could use her creative talents to build on for her future. However, she is often very negative about her abilities probably because she has had so much failure."

Denise is a real person and this is her story; thus identifying details about her life were changed. Denise has a learning disability—unfortunately, one that was never identified but should have been.

Learning difficulties, in most cases, are a persistent problem throughout an individual's lifetime. The transition from the requirements in elementary school to demands in high school may place additional pressure on individuals with learning difficulties. For example, reading requirements, length of texts, and the level of comprehension coupled with extensive writing may put adolescents with learning disabilities at a disadvantage. In addition, the emotional "storm and stress" that characterizes the adolescent years may also influence the performance of adolescents with learning disabilities (LDs).

Denise's case study is a true story about a student who was not identified with LDs in her childhood. In her adolescent life she is at greater risk for social, emotional, and academic risk. In fact, this case study illustrates several of the most critical questions in the field of LDs and, in particular, questions related to adolescents with LDs:

- How do you define learning disabilities?
- What are the characteristics of individuals with LD?
- How should adolescents be assessed for LD?
- What are the risk factors associated with LD in adolescence?
- What accommodations and interventions should be provided to adolescents with LD?

This chapter addresses these five questions.

DEFINITION OF LD

It is difficult to decide when the history of "learning disabilities" begins, whether it should be related to the terminology, or to the recognition of the difficulties. Many have chronicled the identification of the difficulties, including Pringle-Morgan (1896) and Hinshelwood (1917). More than 85 years ago Burt (1927) (later discredited for apparent research irregularities) recognized the need to differentiate between those with "congenital word-blindness" from one who is in every respect mentally defective" (p. 265). Burt suggested that (1) the reading process involves many different cognitive abilities, (2) any one of those abilities may fail independently, (3) the failure of one of those abilities will adversely affect the reading process, and (4) these children can be taught, provided the teaching styles match the child's learning styles.

The term "learning disability" came from "prepared but informal remarks" (Cruickshank, 1981, p. 81) made in 1963 by Samuel A. Kirk at a dinner for concerned parents of children with learning problems in Chicago, Illinois. Kirk (1966) provided one of the first formal definitions of LD: "A learning disability refers to a specific retardation or disorder in one or more of the processes of speech, language, perception, behavior, reading, spelling, or arithmetic" (pp. 1–2). In addition, Kirk described who should be excluded from the definition of LD. Not all children who show retardation in school can be considered children with LDs. A deaf child, for example, has a language disability and speech disability, yet he cannot be classified as having an LD because his retardation in language and speech is the result of his inability to hear.

This problem of terminology is complicated by the confusion in terms used to describe some or all of LD populations. Since Kirk's first attempt to define LD, Cruickshank (1972) observed that more than 40 English terms have been used in the literature to refer to some or all of the children and adolescents subsumed under the LD label. Hammill, Leigh, McNutt, and Larsen (1981) also noted that a variety of terms such as minimal brain dysfunction/injury, psychoneurological learning disorders, dyslexia, or perceptual handicap, to name a few, have been used to refer to LD populations. Furthermore, at least 11 definitions have been accepted as the "official" definition of LD (Hammill, 1990).

Since Kirk's attempt to define LD, the definition has been used as a label to describe many individuals with diverse difficulties. In response to the confusion within the definitional issues, the National Joint Committee on Learning Disabilities (NJCLD, 1981) adopted the following definition:

> Learning disabilities is a generic term that refers to a heterogeneous group of disorders manifested by significant difficulties in the acquisition and use of listening, speaking, reading, writing, reasoning, or mathematical abilities. These disorders are intrinsic to the individual and are presumed to be due to central nervous system dysfunction. Even though a learning disability may occur concomitantly with other handicapping conditions (e.g., sensory impairment, mental retardation, social or emotional disturbance) or environmental influences (e.g., cultural differences, insufficient/inappropriate instruction, psychogenic factors), it is not the direct result of these conditions or influences. (Hammill et al., 1981, p. 336)

As a number of investigators have suggested (e.g., Fletcher & Morris, 1986; Siegel & Heaven, 1986; Wong, 1986), this definition is also difficult to operationalize because it is vague and unspecific. Wong (1986) and Keogh (1986, 1987) note that in spite of this definition and the rules and regulations for implementing Public Law 94-142 (Federal Register, 1977), special education categories still differ from state to state and from district to district. To complicate matters further, Epps, Ysseldyke, and Algozzine (1985) found that states may be using different category names but using the same criteria to identify LD children, while others use the same category names (LD) but different criteria.

Unfortunately, there are many different ways that learning disabilities have been defined. That is, there are different operational definitions that exist for the definition of the concept of LD. Problems are revealed when investigators use different operational definitions to diagnose or determine who is actually suffering from an LD.

These definitions use a variety of components, which are an integral part of determining whether an individual has an LD. Four components of the definition that are frequently used are (Durrant, 1994; Kavale & Nye, 1981) (1) ex-clusion of other conditions and/or factors, (2) the actual formula or quantification for identifying LD, (3) IQ, and (4) achievement tests. Each of these components has a historic, well-established background as one of the basic criteria in the definition of LD.

Exclusionary Criteria

There are usually four common exclusion components:

1. A learning disability is not the result of an inadequate education.
2. The LD is not caused by sensory deficits, such as hearing or visual impairment.
3. The LD is not caused any serious neurological disorders that may interfere with learning.
4. The LD is not caused major social and/or emotional difficulties that might interfere with learning.

However, these exclusions have not been defined on a systematic basis, nor substantiated by research.

The exclusion component was necessary to establish LD as a separate and discrete category of special education for funding and legislative reasons (Kavale & Forness, 2000).

As well as comorbidity issues (e.g., the LD component of those with LD and another difficulty such as deafness being largely ignored), there was considerable concern with the social and emotional components. Clinical evidence suggests that emotional difficulties may frequently be a consequence of the LD, particularly when they only start to appear during adolescence. Although we can never be certain of cause and effect, case studies such as Denise's, where emotional difficulties increase with age, provide strong indicators that the probable cause of the emotional difficulties is LD. However, longitudinal research will not be able to confirm the clinical observations, as this would involve unethical methods (i.e., early identification of individuals for whom support and intervention are not provided). However, a comparison between those with and without early identification and intervention using historical data shows significantly fewer emotional difficulties, particularly those manifesting during adolescence, when early intervention is provided.

Formulas and Quantification Systems for Identifying LDs

According to some definitions, there has to be a "discrepancy" in order for provision of service to be given. If there is no "discrepancy," the individual is functioning at an appropriate level. The difficulties in the area of LD arise due to the problems of determining what "test" results should be compared, what level of difference constitutes a discrepancy, and whether the comparison should be "within child," with the local population, or with a state provincial or national norm. One of the difficulties in assessing the adolescent individual is a shortage of appropriate tests. Fundamental cognitive processing tests (e.g., phonological manipulation skills and auditory short-term memory) are abundant and frequently used with children for identification in the early years. However, the transition from primary school to middle and high school includes a transition of underlying cognitive demands. Unfortunately, although we have the basic cognitive tests for older children, there is shortage of adequate tasks to measure higher skills such as reading comprehension, the ability to put thoughts on paper, and the interference of emotional issues, all of which are necessary for academic performance, and all of which have a severe impact on the functioning of the adolescent with LD.

One common formula that is used to define LD is the discrepancy between actual achievement and measured "intelligence" or measured "potential." The definition offered by Bateman (1965) is an example of this discrepancy concept:

> Children who have learning disorders are those who manifest an educationally significant discrepancy between their estimated intellectual potential and actual level of performance related to basic disorders in the learning process, which may or may not be accomplished by demonstrable central nervous system dysfunction, and which are not secondary to generalized mental retardation, educational or cultural deprivation, severe emotional disturbance, or sensory loss. (p. 220)

Since then, various investigators have attempted to operationize the definition. Many of the states in the United States are still using the discrepancy between ability and achievement as the definition of LDs (Frankenberger & Franzaglio, 1991; Mercer, Jordan, Allsop, & Mercer, 1996), but their criteria vary considerably. Hence, Bowen (2004) reiterates the joke that "in the United States is that the best way to fix a learning disability is to cross a state line" (p. 236)

Another common formula used to define LD is the achievement formula, which assumes ideas that students with LD are at the low end of the achievement distribution. Based on this definition, students will be identified as having an LD if their achievement on norm-referenced achievement tests is below age level. The idea of this formula is that if there is significant discrepancy between a student's reading, spelling, and/or arithmetic skills and his or her age, that student will be considered to have an LD.

One issue in the calculation of the IQ–achievement discrepancy is the specific cutoff that is used in the formula to identify who has an LD. Most of the studies that used the IQ–achievement discrepancy to identify LD did not require that the achievement scores be below average. The implication of this is that "gifted students" with average IQ scores and also above-average achievement test results can demonstrate a significant discrepancy between the IQ score and achievement score. According to the definition of LD, this student will be included as having a reading disability (RD), even though his or her reading ability is above average. These students do not have the same deficit as the students with low reading scores (e.g., O'Malley, Francis, Foorman, Fletcher & Swank, 2002).

Rivers and Smith (1988) examined a frequently used criteria, the discrepancy between Verbal and Performance IQ, for 200 elementary school children labeled as having a specific LD. The purpose was to determine whether the differences between the Verbal and Performance and achievement levels identified different numbers of students as eligible for service (Rivers & Smith, 1988). The results indicated that 60% of the students showed no significant Verbal–Performance discrepancy, although they had significantly low scores on achievement tests. Most of the students did not have severe discrepancies between IQ and achievement, as well as differences between the Wechsler Intelligence Scale for Children—Revised (WISC-R) subtests. The results of this and other studies questioned the validity of those formulas and suggested that more uniform criteria were needed to determine LD (e.g., D'Angiulli & Siegel, 2003; Rivers & Smith, 1988).

Furthermore, there is inconsistency in the type of achievement tests that are used in the research as well as in schools to assess achievement in both the IQ–achievement discrepancy formula and in achievement and grade formulas. This situation was noted in a study by Perlmutter and Parus (1986). Their study examined the use of different diagnostic criteria and tests to assess LD using a discrepancy between IQ and achievement as their definition. They found that schools used a different number of tests (using between 2 and 13 subtests) and different types of tests in the assessment process. The problem with a large variety of tests is that different tests of the same apparent skill may yield very different scores (e.g., Siegel, 1999).

In 1994, Durrant reviewed 208 studies of LD published in 10 major journals between 1988 and 1990, and over two-thirds of the studies used a discrepancy between ability and achievement as the criteria to identify LD (Durrant, 1994). Despite research evidence of the difficulties with this method, there seems to be a growing trend in the use of the discrepancy between ability and achievement formula.

Studies that used the achievement and grade formula to define LD rely on low achievement performance of two grades below the actual child's actual grade for it to be considered that they have an LD. The problem with these scores is that the same amount of discrepancy between actual achievement and expected grade does not mean the same degree of disability at all ages. Younger children with RD may not be detected, whereas older children may be defined as having an RD (Gaddes, 1976; Siegel & Linder, 1984; Siegel & Ryan, 1984). For instance, in a sample of children with RD, there were 45 younger children (ages 7–10) who were not two grades behind in achievement but who had percentile scores on the Wide Range Achievement Test (WRAT) of < 25, and 33 children who were not one and a half grades behind but who had percentiles of < 25. Conversely, there were eight older children (ages 10–14) who had scores above the 25th percentile but who were delayed two or more grades according to grade level; as well, there were 21 children who were 10–14 years old who had scores above the 25th percentile but who were one and a half or more grades

delayed in reading (Siegel & Linder, 1984; Siegel & Ryan, 1984). Therefore, grade level represents unequal units of measurement at different ages (Siegel & Heaven, 1986). That is, children who are, for example, 2 years below grade level when they are in the third grade are very far behind, but those who are two grades below in the 10th grade may not be as far behind. Percentile or standard scores will reflect an actual reading level in a more accurate way. Unfortunately, grade levels are still widely used in studies and assessment in spite of their lack of psychometric validity.

IQ Tests

It has been argued that the use of the IQ test has come about as due to a lack of any alternative. Following the Education for All Handicapped Children Act (EAHCA) of 1975, there was a concern that a lack of measurable criteria made identification difficult. As a consequence, the Office of Education attempted to provide more explicit guidelines for identification that included a discrepancy between IQ and achievement.

The use of IQ tests as part of the formula to define LD is problematic. Many studies have provided evidence that standard IQ tests are not valid in the measurement of potential learning ability for individuals with RD (e.g., Fletcher et al., 1989; Fletcher, Francis, Rourke, Shaywitz, & Shaywitz, 1992; Siegel, 1988a, 1988b, 1989, 1992). Because IQ tests measure expressive language skills, short-term memory, speed of information processing, speed of responding, and knowledge of specific facts (Siegel, 1990), and studies indicate that these functions are deficient in many individuals with LDs (Siegel, 1985; Siegel & Feldman, 1983; Siegel & Linder, 1984; Siegel & Ryan, 1984, 1988; Swanson, 1993, 1994; Vellutino, 1978, 1979), the use of the IQ test cannot be regarded as a valid measure of the intelligence of individuals with LD/RD.

Some researchers have suggested that IQ is not an accurate measure of intellectual ability and have provided alternate ways to conceptualize ability (e.g., Gardner, 1983; Goleman, 1995; Lazear, 1994). Gardner (1983) suggested the concept of multiple intelligences, claiming that there is not only one type of intelligence that correlates with success in life but several kinds of intelligences. He defined intelligence as a multidimensional phenomenon that is present at multiple levels of our brain/mind/body system and noted that IQ tests are based on a very limited idea of intelligence. Research demonstrates that the use of the IQ component as part of the LD definition to prove discrepancies between so-called potential measured by IQ test and actual performance is not tenable. For example, Siegel (1988a) conducted a study to determine whether or not children with RDs and those without RDs with different IQ scores would show distinctive patterns of performance on cognitive tasks. The surprising result was that IQ scores did not appear to be predictors of the cognitive processes involved in reading, spelling, language skills, and memory tasks. Siegel (1989) concluded that there is a need to abandon the IQ test in the analysis of children with LDs.

Another challenge to the validity of the IQ measure is the "Matthew effect" (Stanovich, 1986). Stanovich (1993) suggested that reading itself develops related cognitive abilities. That is, not only do the cognitive skills influence the reading ability, but also the quantity of reading will affect the cognitive skills, which in turn will affect the performance on an IQ test.

In terms of intervention programs, IQ scores did not predict an ability to benefit from a remediation program. The IQ scores did not differentiate between poor readers who were found to be easily remediated and poor readers who were difficult to remediate (Vellutino, Scanlon, & Lyon, 2000; Vellutino, Scanlon, & Sipay, 1996). Overall, it seems clear that IQ is irrelevant to the definition of LD, except for a possible use to define the border between LD and retardation. Most of the claimed use of the IQ test has been clearly demonstrated to be based on false premises. This is not to say that individual subtests in some of the IQ tests cannot provide useful information but that an overall score, or subscore, provides no useful information in the identification and intervention in LD.

Achievement Tests

Achievement refers to the basic skills taught in school, including reading, writing, spelling, and arithmetic. School curricula are designed in such a way as to gradually build on the complexity of these skills during the school years. In each grade, there are certain skills that a student needs to master. These skills can be measured by achievement tests that compare the performance of the individual to norms from a population of the same age or grade.

There are several problems with the use of the achievement tests in the identification of LD. For instance, investigators do not report on achievement tests used, assess different skills under the title "achievement," and use informal instead of standardized achievement tests. Frequently investigators do not describe fully how specific skills were assessed, apparently failing to appreciate the influence of assessment methods and criteria on the results. For example, a test of reading comprehension using a cloze task will produce a different result from that using a multiple-choice task, because they measure different components of what some may describe as comprehension. Some researchers measure not only reading but also spelling and occasionally mathematics to describe the LD cohort. However, using different criteria will affect the result and, as a consequence, will produce a cohort that has a very different type of LD from those evaluated only using reading. There is no right or wrong, but it is important to appreciate the distinction when making comparisons based on achievement measures.

A Resolution of Definitional Issues

The question of how to diagnose LDs is one of the most critical for the field. Without a valid and reliable operational definition, individuals who need assistance may not receive it and thus may not be able to achieve their full potential. The ability to identify and assist individuals with LD is even more essential in the secondary and postsecondary educational systems, where the academic demands are higher. One recent illustration of this problematic situation was provided by the *Guckenberger v. Boston University* case. In this case, Boston University argued that sufficient evidence had not been presented for some students who claimed to be learning disabled; the plaintiffs claimed that they did. This case illustrated the chaotic situation in the field, where "each evaluation used different tests, different terminology, and different labels for LD" (Siegel, 1999, p. 314). Clearly the field of special education continues to have problems defining and classifying children with LD. Current discrepancy definitions are problematic and should be reconsidered, as they cannot be justified in light of their illogical nature. But where does that leave us and where can we go from here?

Recognizing that there are problems inherent in operational definitions, we suggest that LDs should refer to a significant difficulty in a school-related area. For example, after appropriate consultation, the Health Council of the Netherlands produced a series of criteria that they would use to determine the acceptability of a definition of dyslexia (Gersons-Wolfensberger & Ruijssenaars, 1997). It should be noted that dyslexia is only one possible LD, but these definitions can serve as a model for other disabilities. The criteria used were that it should (1) be descriptive with no explanatory elements; (2) be specific enough to identify dyslexia within the whole of reading and spelling problems; (3) be general enough to allow for various scientific explanatory models and any developments those models might undergo; (4) be capable of being operationalized for the purposes of research into people and groups; (5) inform the intervention process; and (6) be applicable in a wide range of circumstances.

With these criteria in mind, the committee produced the following "working definition": Dyslexia is present when the automatization of word identification (reading) and/or spelling does not develop or does so very incompletely or with great difficulty. This leads to the question of what tests should be used to actually define a reading disability. Stanovich (1986, 1989) has suggested that the core deficits in an RD are problems in phonological processing, at least in the English language. Although reading is more than simply decoding and recognizing words (one has to remember what was read, put it into context, and so on), current tests to measure reading comprehension have many difficulties (for a complete discussion of this issue, see Siegel, 1999; Siegel & Heaven, 1986; Tal & Siegel, 1996). Further empirical evidence suggests that when a difficulty with phonological processing and/or word recognition is used as the basis of the definition of a reading problem, those with an RD in English appear to have reasonably homogeneous cognitive profiles and, in particular, deficits in the language areas (e.g., Fletcher, 1985a, 1985b; Rourke & Finlayson, 1978; Rourke & Strang, 1978; Siegel & Ryan, 1984, 1988, 1989a; Strang & Rourke, 1983). Therefore, we and others (e.g., Siegel & Heaven 1986; Siegel & Ryan, 1989a; Vellutino, 1978, 1979) argue that single-word or pseudo word reading constitutes the purest measures of reading. Pseudowords are pronounceable combinations of English letters that can be sounded out with basic rules of grapheme–phoneme correspondences. This type of test assesses awareness of the phonological aspects of a language, which is the key to decoding words in an alphabetic language such as English. Therefore, an operational definition of an RD should be based on pseudoword tests to measure phonological skills and/or single-word tests to measure word recognition skills.

TYPES OF LDs

Given the heterogeneity of LD groups, Siegel (1988b) contends that if all children with LDs are grouped together, inaccurate conclusions may be reached. Evidence in support of this position has been found by many investigators (e.g., Fletcher, 1985a, 1985b; McKinney, Short, & Feagans, 1985; Siegel, 1999; Siegel & Linder, 1984; Siegel & Ryan, 1984, 1988, 1989a).

Because of this heterogeneity of LD groups, considerable effort has been made to identify specific subgroups of children with LD who share common attributes that distinguish them from other subtypes. Not only do subtypes exist, but they seem to take several forms in terms of achievement patterns and/or associated cognitive information-processing abilities.

The most commonly known LD is an RD, sometimes called dyslexia. Another equally prevalent but less commonly known disability is an arithmetic (mathematics) disability, sometimes called "nonverbal learning disability," "developmental output failure," or "writing–arithmetic disability" or "visual–spatial disability." Although there is, admittedly, some heterogeneity within the two major clusters, they do share enough common characteristics to be considered specific entities.

Reading Disabilities (Dyslexia)

Depending on the theoretical biases of the particular investigator, the country, the circumstances, and so on, the word "dyslexia" may be used instead of "reading disability." However, there is no difference between dyslexia and an RD; they are exactly the same.

In the LD literature it is often reported that males are more likely to be identified than females as LD, with ratio ranges from 3:1 to 15:1 (for review, see Finucci & Childs, 1981). Several explanations for this gender difference have been suggested. Part of the researchers suggested genetic reasons (Geschwind & Galaburda, 1985; Tallal, Ross, & Curtiss, 1989). Other reasons for gender differences are referral biases—for example, teachers tend to refer more boys for assessment for LD than girls (e, g., Shaywitz, Shaywitz, Fletcher & Escobar, 1990; Wadsworth, DeFries, Stevenson, Gilger & Pennington, 1992). Another reason is statistical artifacts (Share, McGee, McKenzie, Williams & Silva, 1987; Van der Wissel & Zegers, 1985). However, several studies indicated that the actual ratio is similar to the gender ratio within the population (DeFries & Gillis, 1991; Shaywitz et al., 1990).

In the RD category, some clinic and school-identified samples have a ratio of two or three boys to each girl (Naiden, 1976; Vogel, 1990; Wadsworth et al., 1992). A recent study conducted by Share and Silva (2003) has suggested another explanation as the source for gender bias. They found that when the general distribution of reading scores for boys was lower on average than the distribution for girls, the IQ discrepancy regression formula produced a preponderance of boys with RD because the reading scores were systematically overestimated for boys and thus were inflating the discrepancies. The converse occurred for girls. The bias arose from general differences between boys and girls in the reading score distributions (lower means and greater variance for boys) and not from differences in IQ scores. Thus, what is the conclusion regarding sex differences in RD? There is no strong evidence for a gender bias. When studies found a bias, it may be a referral one meaning that children with behavioral problems are more likely to be referred and boys are more likely to have behavior problems so more boys will be found to have RDs, but this is an artifact of the referral bias.

RD involves difficulties with phonological processing, including such abilities as knowing the relationship between letters and sounds and phonological awareness—that is, the ability to segment the speech stream into separate elements. Over the years, a consensus has emerged that one core deficit in RD is a severe difficulty with phonological processing (e.g.,

Rack, Snowling, & Olson, 1992; Siegel, 1993a, 1993b; Snowling, 1980; Stanovich, 1988a, 1988b; Rayner, Foorman, Perfetti, Pesetsky, & Seidenberg, 2002). Children with an RD have a core deficit in phonological processing. The evidence that is available clearly demonstrates that adults with RD have deficits in phonological processing (e.g., Bruck, 1990, 1992; Felton, Naylor, & Wood, 1990; Gottardo, Siegel, & Stanovich, 1997; Greenberg, Ehri, & Perin, 1997; Pennington, Van Orden, Smith, Green, & Haith, 1990; Pratt & Brady, 1988; Read & Ruyter, 1985; Russell, 1982; Scarborough, 1984; Shafrir & Siegel, 1994a, 1994b; Siegel, 1998). Most individuals with RD show problems in the area of memory and language (Siegel & Ryan, 1984, 1988; Snowling, 1980; Stanovich, 1988b, 1988c; Vellutino, 1978). Usually individuals with RD have spelling problems, but the presence of spelling difficulties without reading difficulties does not indicate RD. Padget, Knight, and Sawyer (1996) provide a definition of RD that captures the other problems that often co-occur with it:

> Dyslexia is a language-based learning disorder that is biological in origin and primarily interferes with the acquisition of print literacy (reading, writing, and spelling). Dyslexia is characterized by poor decoding and spelling abilities as well as a deficit in phonological awareness and/or phonological manipulation. These primary characteristics may co-occur with spoken language difficulties and deficits in short-term memory. Secondary characteristics may include poor reading comprehension (due to the decoding and memory difficulties) and poor written expression, as well as difficulty organizing information for study and retrieval. (p. 55)

Current theories in the development of reading skills in English stress that phonological processing is the most significant underlying cognitive process (Stanovich 1988a, 1988b, 1988c). Children and adults with an RD have difficulty with phonological processing. Phonological processing involves a variety of functions, but in the context of the development of reading skills, the most significant is the association of sounds with letters or combinations of letters. This function is referred to as the understanding of grapheme–phoneme conversion rules, and because of the irregular nature of the correspondences in English, the learning of these rules is a very complex process. The child who is learning to read must map oral language onto written language by decomposing the word into phonemes and associating each letter (or combination of letters) with these phonemes.

The task of the beginning reader is to extract these grapheme–phoneme conversion rules. The alternative is simply to memorize each word as a visual configuration and to associate a meaning with it. This kind of learning may occur, but it is inefficient and makes tremendous demands on visual memory. In English, no one-to-one correspondence exists between a letter (or letters) and a sound. The same letter represents different sounds and the same sound may be represented by different letters.

In an alphabetic language such as English, the best measure of phonological processing skills is the reading of pseudowords, that is, pronounceable combinations of letters that can be read by the application of grapheme–phoneme conversion rules, but that are, of course, not real words in English. Examples include such pseudowords as "shum," "laip," and "cigbet." Pseudowords can be read by anyone who is familiar with the grapheme–phoneme conversion rules of English even though they are not real words and have not been encountered in print or in spoken language before.

The development of the ability to read pseudowords has been studied extensively (e.g., Calfee, Lindamood, & Lindamood, 1973; Hogaboam, & Perfetti, 1978; Siegel & Ryan, 1988; Venezky & Johnson, 1973). Ample evidence indicates that children with dyslexia have a great deal of difficulty reading pseudowords. Studies such as those of Ehri and Wilce (1983), Snowling (1980), Siegel and Ryan (1988), and Waters, Bruck, and Seidenberg (1985) have shown that those with RD have more difficulty reading pseudowords than do normal readers matched on either chronological age or reading level. For example, Siegel and Ryan (1988) studied the development of the ability to read pseudowords in normal readers and those with RD ages 7–14 years. By the age of 9, the normal readers were quite proficient and performed at almost a perfect level for even the most difficult pseudowords, with, in some cases, as many as three syllables. Similarly, Backman, Bruck, Hebert, and Seidenberg (1984) showed that 10-year-olds perform as well as adults on tasks involving the reading of pseudowords; however, Siegel and Ryan found that the perfor-

mance of the children with RD was quite different. These children appear to acquire these reading skills very late in development and even children with RD at the age of 14 were performing no better than normal readers at the age of 7.

To control, at least partially, for experience with print, Siegel and Ryan (1988) used a comparison of normal readers and those with RD matched on reading grade level. Even when the children with RD and the normal readers were matched on reading level (hence the children with RD were considerably older than the normal readers), the performance of the children with RD on a task involving the reading of pseudowords was significantly poorer than that of the normal readers.

Thus, difficulties with phonological processing seem to be the fundamental problem of children with an RD, and this problem continues into adulthood. Many adults with an RD become reasonably fluent readers but still have difficulty reading pseudowords or read them very slowly (e.g., Barwick & Siegel, 1996; Bruck, 1990; Shafrir & Siegel 1994a, 1994b).

For children learning to read English, the learning of grapheme–phoneme conversion rules is a result of systematic instruction and the extraction of the rules is a result of repeated encounters with print. No evidence is available as to how much of the development of decoding skills is a result of specific instruction in the grapheme–phoneme conversion rules and how much is a result of experience with print. In any case, the understanding of the grapheme–phoneme conversion rules develops rapidly in the first years of experience with print under normal conditions.

Some individuals have difficulties only with writing and/or spelling. As these written language problems usually occur in the context of problems with reading and/or arithmetic and mathematics problems, the existence of a separate written language disability is not clearly established, nor is there a clear definition of it, especially in the adult population. Spelling difficulties can occur in the absence of severe RDs (e.g., Bruck & Waters, 1988; Lennox & Siegel, 1993). There also may be problems with understanding or producing language. These problems have not been documented as distinct LDs and are often components of dyslexia. If LDs are to be treated as measurable entities and if individuals are to receive educational services based on the presence of a single or multiple LDs, then, obviously, it is important to determine what these LDs are.

The majority of the research on reading difficulties has focused on those children who demonstrate difficulties in the initial stages of reading acquisition. Although there are studies on university students, a very limited number of studies examined the cognitive and reading skills of students with LD. One explanation may be that since a common difficulty of LD is with reading and decoding, the assumption is that in the early years of school this difficulty will occur. However, adolescents with LD also experience difficulties with reading skills (e.g., reading comprehension), and therefore future research should focus on this age group as well.

Arithmetic Disabilities

Individuals with "developmental output failure" or "writing–arithmetic disability" have difficulty with computational arithmetic and written language, typically in the absence of reading difficulties, although, this disability can co-occur with dyslexia. They often have difficulties with spelling and have problems with fine-motor coordination, visual–spatial processing, short- and long-term memory (e.g., multiplication tables) but usually have good oral-language skills (Fletcher, 1985a, 1985b; Johnson & Mykelbust, 1967; Kinsbourne & Warrington, 1963; Kosc, 1974; Levine, Oberklaid, & Meltzer, 1981; Morrison & Siegel, 1991; Rourke, 1991; Rourke & Finlayson, 1978; Shafrir & Siegel, 1994b; Siegel & Feldman, 1983; Siegel & Linder, 1984; Spellacy & Peter, 1978). Rourke and his associates (e.g., Rourke, Del Dotto, Rourke, & Casey, 1990; Rourke & Tsatsanis, 1996) have described a syndrome called "nonverbal learning disabilities" that is similar to "writing–arithmetic disability." However, the operational definition of this LD is problematic; it is not clear how a diagnosis can be made. Often, these individuals have verbal IQ scores significantly higher than performance IQ, but this discrepancy is neither necessary nor sufficient to make the diagnosis. Often, they have arithmetic scores lower than reading scores but the differences between these scores are not always significant (e.g., Rourke et al., 1990). (For an extended discussion of the definitional issue and conceptualization of this disability, see Morrison & Siegel, 1991.)

A number of deficits have been found in these individuals. Children identified as having mathematics disabilities have been found to be less skilled than their academically normal peers in detecting counting errors, in computational arithmetic ability and in the implementation of appropriate counting strategies (Geary, 1990, 1993; Geary, Bow-Thomas, & Yao, 1992; Geary, Brown, & Samaranayake, 1991; Geary, Hoard, & Hamson, 1999; Russell & Ginsburg, 1984). They perform more poorly on story problems and number fact problems (Russell & Ginsburg, 1984), especially under timed conditions (Jordan & Montani, 1997); they exhibit deficits in visual–spatial organizational measures (Harnadek & Rourke, 1994); and there appears to be a specific working memory deficit in relation to the processing of numerical information (Passolunghi & Siegel, 2001; Siegel & Ryan, 1989a; Swanson & Cooney, 1996; Wilson & Swanson, 2001).

Investigators (e.g., Fletcher, 1985b; Rourke & Finlayson, 1978; Rourke & Strang, 1978; Siegel & Feldman, 1983; Siegel & Ryan, 1984, 1988, 1989a) have found evidence that children with specific arithmetic deficits and average or above-average word recognition scores on the WRAT appear to have a variety of cognitive and neuropsychological deficits that differentiate them from children with at least reading deficits as defined by depressed scores on the Reading subtest on the WRAT. The cognitive and neuropsychological profiles of children identified as having specific arithmetic disabilities (AD) are also different from normally achieving children.

Evidence (Fletcher, 1985a; Siegel & Linder, 1984; Siegel & Ryan, 1984, 1988, 1989a) suggests that those children meeting the criteria of the specific arithmetic-disabled subtype have deficits in short-term and working memory that are dependent on the type of stimulus and the aspect of memory assessed. Specifically, Siegel and Linder (1984), in a study of the role of phonemic coding in short-term memory, compared three groups of children, one with RDs (as defined by scores on the WRAT Reading subtest of equal to or below the 25th percentile and no cutoff on the other two WRAT subtests), a second with arithmetic disabilities (as defined by scores on the WRAT Arithmetic subtest of equal to or above the 30th percentile), and a normally achieving group (as defined by scores of greater than or equal to the 30th percentile on all three WRAT subtests).

The children, ages 7–13, were administered a series of tasks that involved the visual or auditory presentation of rhyming and nonrhyming letters and either an oral or written response. Patterns and levels of performance were compared statistically across three age groups (7–8, 9–11, 12–13) and between each subtype and normally achieving children.The results indicated that both older disabled groups, like their normal counterparts, had significantly poorer recall of rhyming as opposed to nonrhyming letters (except for the oldest—12–13 years—group with AD, where the authors suggest that the children may be functioning at the upper limit of their visual, short-term memory). For stimuli presented visually, the overall performance levels of both groups with LD were significantly lower than the normally achieving group. For the auditory stimuli, only the group with RD but not the other disabilities differed significantly from the normally achieving peers. The group with AD was distinguished from the group with RD in terms of the type of stimulus.

Fletcher (1985a) found differences in memory tasks between groups with LD as defined by WRAT scores. He compared four groups of children with LDs (a reading–spelling-disabled group, a reading–spelling–arithmetic-disabled group, a spelling–arithmetic-disabled group, and an arithmetic-disabled group) and a normally achieving group of children on storage and retrieval aspects of memory for verbal and nonverbal stimuli. He found that relative to the normally achieving controls, both the arithmetic- and the arithmetic–spelling-disabled subgroups had significantly lower storage and retrieval scores on the nonverbal task but did not differ from each other; the reading–spelling subgroup differed only on retrieval scores on the verbal task; while the reading–spelling–arithmetic subgroup differed on the retrieval scores on the verbal task and storage and retrieval scores on the nonverbal task. As with Siegel and Linder (1984), the differences between subgroups depended on the type of stimulus (verbal vs. nonverbal) and the aspect of memory (storage or retrieval) being assessed. The results demonstrated the ability to assess different LD subtypes.

Siegel and Ryan (1988) also compared children with RD (as defined by WRAT subtest scores), specific children with AD (as defined by WRAT subtest scores), and normally achieving children on a variety of skills involving grammatical sensitivity, phonology, and short-term memory. In general, it was found that older children with specific AD performed in a manner similar to the normally achieving group in grammatical sensitivity and phonological tasks. Some exceptions were found in that the children with AD in the 7–10 age group performed more poorly on a sentence repetition task. This difficulty was attributed to the short-term memory component of the task. As well, this age group performed more poorly than normally achieving children on the pseudoword spelling sections (a writing task) of the phonics task. However, in tasks that measure short-term memory (phonological coding), the group with specific AD performed in a manner similar to the group with RD and significantly more poorly than the normally achieving group. The authors conclude that compared to normally achieving children, both of the two disabled groups have deficits in short-term memory; however, only the group with RD had deficits in tasks said to represent a language disorder.

Siegel and Ryan (1989a) examined the same types of groups, using two working memory tasks, one involving sentences and the other involving numbers. Again the disabled groups differed from each other on the types of memory deficits observed. The group with RD differed from the normally achieving children on both tasks while the children with AD differed from their normally achieving peers only on the numbers task. It would appear from the research (Fletcher, 1985a; Siegel & Linder, 1984; Siegel & Ryan, 1988, 1989a) that although both subtypes of children with LD have deficits in short-term and working memory, those children with reading deficits are more generalized involving both verbal and nonverbal aspects of memory and those with arithmetic deficits and normal or above-normal reading are more limited to visual, nonverbal, and numerical material.

Evidence from a number of sources (Fletcher, 1985b; Rourke & Finlayson, 1978; Share, Moffitt, & Silva, 1988; Siegel & Feldman, 1983; Spellacy & Peter, 1978; Webster, 1979) indicates that children with specific AD (as defined by deficient scores on the WRAT Arithmetic subtest and the age-appropriate scores on the WRAT Reading and Spelling subtests—Group 3) had age-appropriate auditory–perceptual and verbal abilities but are deficient on measures of visual–perception and visual–

spatial abilities. However, children with RD (as defined by being relatively proficient at arithmetic as compared with their WRAT Reading and Spelling subtest scores—Group 2) had age-appropriate visual–perception and visual–spatial abilities but were deficient on measures of auditory–perceptual and verbal abilities (Rourke & Finlayson, 1978). Also, children with AD exhibited difficulty with tasks such as the Halstead Category Test, which require "higher order" visual–spatial analysis and visual–perceptual organization (Strang & Rourke, 1983). They also exhibited deficits in measures of psychomotor abilities and on tests such as the Tactile Performance Tests (Reitan & Davison, 1974), the Grooved Pegboard Test (Klove, 1963), and the Maze Test (Klove, 1963), designed to identify tactile–perceptual impairment (Rourke & Strang, 1978; Siegel & Feldman, 1983; Spellacy & Peter, 1978). On the other hand, Rourke and Strang (1978) and Strang and Rourke (1983) found that Group 2 children (relatively proficient in arithmetic, compared to their reading and spelling) were proficient at these tasks.

Passolunghi and Siegel (2001) compared children who were poor in arithmetic problem solving to children who were good problem solvers. The results corroborate the hypothesis of poor problem solvers' general deficit in inhibitory processes. The poor arithmetic problem solvers had lower scores and made more intrusion errors in a series of working memory tasks requiring inhibition of irrelevant information. Span tasks that imply passive storage of information showed that poor problem solvers were impaired when they have to retain numerical information but did not differ from children who did not have difficulty with mathematics when the material included words (Passolunghi & Siegel, 2001).

As with the research with memory deficits cited earlier, Rourke and Finlayson (1978), Rourke and Strang (1978), and Strang and Rourke (1983) suggest that the characteristics described are different from those of other students with LDs (who showed deficits on all the WRAT subtests—Group 1, or just on the reading and spelling subtests, compared with the arithmetic subtest—Group 2). This has led Rourke and colleagues (Rourke, 1982, 1983, 1985, 1987; Rourke & Finlayson, 1978; Rourke & Fisk, 1988) to hypothesize that those children with arithmetic deficits belong to the larger nonverbal group with LD with

right-hemisphere processing problems, while those children with deficits in reading as well as arithmetic belong to the larger linguistic group with LD with left-hemisphere processing problems. Clearly, children who only have severe deficits in arithmetic can be differentiated from children with reading difficulties. The children with LD can be also differentiated from normally achieving children on cognitive and neuropsychological profiles.

Subtypes of LD have validity in research. Most of the research that examined the classification of LDs has concentrated on children in the elementary school years, or combined a wide range of ages in their classification including children from early childhood to adolescence. Very few researchers have conducted studies to extend the classification to adolescence because so far there is no research that provides evidence that there are differences in subtypes between children and adolescents. Shafrir and Siegel (1994b) investigated a classification scheme that was developed for the subtyping of children with LD on a population of adolescents and adults. They compared three groups: individuals with AD, RD, and both reading and arithmetic disabilities (RADs), with a comparison group with normal achievement (NA), on a variety of cognitive and achievement measures. Individuals in the RD group performed at or below the 25th percentile on the reading subtest, and at or above the 30th percentile on the Arithmetic subtest of the WRAT-R. Individuals in the RAD group performed at or below the level of the 25th percentile on both the Reading and Arithmetic subtests of the WRAT-R. Individuals in the AD group performed at or below the 25th percentile on the Arithmetic subtest of the WRAT-R and at or above the 30th percentile on the Reading subtest of the WRAT-R.

The NA group differed significantly from the other groups on reading, spelling, memory, and other cognitive abilities. The reading disability groups (RD and RAD) were characterized by deficits in phonological processing, reading, spelling, and short-term memory. A visual reading deficit involving the correct recognition of the visual form of a word was present only in the RAD group. Unlike the RD and the RAD groups, the AD group did not have a deficit in reading, spelling, or phonological processing. The performance of this group was similar to that of the control group on the measures of pseudoword reading and phonological processing. This group was characterized by poor performance compared to the NA group on word reading and vocabulary measures, even though their scores were in the normal range. The results also indicated a deficit in visual–spatial functioning in the AD group on the Space Relations and the Block Design tasks. The space relations is a timed test that consists of 60 visual patterns that can be folded into figures. To the right of each pattern are four figures, and the subject has to decide which one of the figures can be made by folding the pattern. In the Block Design task, the subject is asked to reproduce a design with the aid of four or nine blocks with red, white, and half-red, half-white sides. Another purpose was to test the hypothesis that, within adolescents and adults with LDs, using an additional criterion based on the educational level (postsecondary vs. below that level, regardless of age) results in a further refinement, or increase in the degree of homogeneity, of the subtypes. However, when educational level was added to the classification scheme, there was a deficit in visual–spatial functioning in the AD group at the postsecondary level but not at the nonpostsecondary levels, whereas only the RAD group showed a generalized deficit in visual–spatial processing across both educational levels. It therefore appears that the distinction between the NA group and the AD group is greater at the postsecondary level than at the nonpostsecondary level. On most of the tasks, the RAD group performed more poorly than the control group and the group with AD. On some tasks, the RAD group performed more poorly than the RD group. This group was considered to have the most severe LDs of the three (Shafrir & Siegel, 1994).

Recently, an alternate approach to the classification of dyslexic students has been suggested by Wolf and Bowers (1999). According to their approach, the double-deficit hypothesis stemmed from observations that there are dyslexic students with adequate decoding but poor comprehension for whom the phonological hypothesis is unable to provide appropriate identification and remedial assistance. Therefore, they propose that dyslexic children may have a naming speed deficit and/or a phonological deficit (Lovett, Steinbach, & Frijters, 2000; Manis, Doi, & Bhadha, 2000; Schatschneider, Carlson, Francis, Foorman, & Fletcher, 2002; Sunseth & Bowers, 2002; Wolf et al., 2002). For instance, Sunseth and Bowers (2002) were able to classify their cross-sectional sample of grade 3 children into three groups based on the double-deficit hypothesis; however, the authors selected children who were below average in naming speed and phonological processing without considering reading ability. This consideration had serious implications on the design of the study as their double-deficit group had an average standard score of 100 on measures of reading ability. This means that it is vital to first identify a dyslexic group based on below-average reading scores and then attempt to classify the dyslexic students based on the double-deficit hypothesis. A recent review of the literature has found little evidence for the existence of a naming speed deficit independent of a phonological deficit (Vukovic, Lesaux, & Siegel, in press).

Another attempt to characterize subgroups of RD was based on different brain functioning, using functional magnetic resonance images (fMRI). In fMRI, MRIs are acquired rapidly, so that they can capture the change in blood flow associated with cognitive activity (Shaywitz et al., 2000). Shaywitz and colleagues (2003) conducted a recent study on young adults, ages 18.5–22.5 years, in order to examine whether and how two groups of young adults who were poor readers as children differed from nonimpaired readers and if there are any factors that distinguishing the two RD groups. Two RD groups were examined: in the first RD group—persistently poor readers—the subjects met the criteria for poor reading in grade 2 and grade 4 and again in grade 9 or 10. In the second RD group—the compensated readers—met the criteria for poor reading in grade 2 and grade 4 but not in grade 9 or 10. In the third group there were nonimpaired readers who did not meet the criteria for poor reading in grades 2–10 and had reading score above the 40th percentile and had average Full Scale IQ. Poor reading was defined by one of the two definitions: the discrepancy definition or low achievement definition. The investigators used fMRI to examine brain activation patterns while the subjects engaged in two visually presented tasks: (1) deciding whether two pseudowords rhymed, and (2) judging whether two real words were in the same semantic category. The results demonstrated that the compensated readers had a relative underactivation in posterior neural systems for reading located in left parietotemporal and occipitotemporal regions. Persistently poor readers activated posterior reading systems but engaged them differently from the nonimpaired readers, appearing to rely more on memory-based rather than analytic word identification strategies. The two groups of RD began school with comparable reading skills and family socioeconomic status, but the compensated readers exhibited better cognitive ability that minimizes, in part, the consequence of their phonologic deficit. These cognitive abilities probably provided some degree of compensation for RD. The authors concluded that the findings suggest a neural basis for reading outcomes of the two RD groups: compensation and persistence in adults with childhood dyslexia (Shaywitz et al., 2003). However, the poor readers in this study were identified by two different RD definitions, and the readers do not know the number of students in each RD group who were identified as such by one of the definitions. The different definitions may have influenced the results of this study.

Spelling Problems

Problems with spelling do exist, but they can co-occur with either reading and or arithmetic difficulties, and it is rare to find a child who has difficulties with spelling and no problems in any other areas of functioning. There are children who may have specific difficulties with spelling when they are required to write the word from memory rather than when they are required to recognize the correct spelling of a word. In addition, English words are characterized by both regular spelling (e.g., signing and print)—that is, words in which the letter–sound correspondences are predictable—and irregular spelling—that is, spelling that is not predicted from the rules of spelling–sound correspondence (e.g., island and knight). The possibility exists that children may be able to spell regular words but have more difficulty with the irregular words. In any case, spelling difficulties do occur but, as we noted earlier, usually in combination with other problems. Furthermore, studies, for example, by Bruck and Waters (1988), Jorm (1981), and Lennox and Siegel (1996) have found significant differences in the understanding of letter–sound correspondence rules and the orthographic awareness between children who were poor readers and spellers and children who were only poor spellers. On the basis of findings such as these,

and for the reasons discussed previously, reading and spelling need to be treated as separate variables.

ASSESSMENT OF ADOLESCENTS WITH LDs

Determining who has LDs requires careful and systematic assessment. The two following questions address the assessment of LDs:

1. How should achievement be measured and with what tests?
2. What cutoff scores should be used to identify an LD?

The assessment should be consistent with the principles described above

Measures of Achievement

Standardized achievement tests use norms that offer the opportunity to compare the performance of the student to the level of achievement of his or her age or grade peers from the normal population. These tests appear to be the best way to compare an individual to others of the same age in order to determine a significant problem.

A general assessment battery to identify LD from kindergarten age to adulthood should include at least three measures: phonological processing, word reading, and arithmetic measures. Specifically, to assess the possibility of an LD in adolescence, an assessment battery should include six essential measures. Particular tests should be selected on the basis of available information regarding the validity of the test. The following are suggested skills that should be assessed.

Word Recognition Skills

Assessment should include a measure of word recognition skills. Word recognition is one of the critical building blocks in gaining meaning from print, and it is important to know whether the basic skills in this area are significantly below average. Tests of reading single real words typically require the individual to read a set of words aloud. These words may vary on several dimensions such as regular words that follow the letter–sound correspondence rules to irregular words that involve unpredictable letter–sound correspondences. Another dimension is reading of familiar words, such as "book" or "cat" or less familiar words such as "predatory" or "terpsichorean." The WRAT-3: Reading subtest (WRAT3; Wilkinson, 1993) and the Woodcock Johnson III (WJ III; Woodcock, McGrew, & Mather, 2001) Letter–Word Identification can both assess word recognition skill.

Phonological Processing

Another critical skill that is the basis of an RD is phonological processing (e.g., Bruck, 1990; Felton et al., 1990; Shafrir & Siegel, 1994a). This is a key skill necessary for decoding words in an alphabetic language and can be assessed by reading pseudowords. When an individual reads a particular word correctly, there is no indication if she or he has merely memorized this word; this is not the case in the reading of pseudowords. Therefore, the assessment of reading pseudowords is essential to identify phonological awareness difficulties. Reading of pseudowords can be assessed by the Word Attack subtest in the WJ III (Woodcock et al., 2001).

Reading Comprehension

Especially for adolescents and adults, it is necessary to include a reading comprehension test. An example of a reading comprehension test is the Stanford Diagnostic Reading Test (Karlsen & Gardner, 1995). Another test to assess reading comprehension of adolescents is the Nelson–Denny Reading Test (Brown, Vick Fishco & Hanna, 1993).

Reading comprehension is a relevant measure for higher education in which there are significant demands on reading of long texts. Unlike the assessment of reading single words or pseudowords, the assessment of reading comprehension is more complex. Text processing is usually measured by reading sentences and paragraphs. In both cases, there are clues to the meaning of words from the surrounding context. In this case, it is difficult to assess whether an individual read the word or made a good guess based on the context. Sentences or paragraphs can be read silently or aloud. If we were to assess silent reading, there would be no way of assessing what the individual is actually reading.

Another dimension of text reading tests is that there is usually a time limit on the test. Most of the variance among individuals is caused by differences in reading rate or speed of task completion and not by a differential in understanding of the material. However, a text assessment should differentiate between individuals who are merely slow readers and those with poor word reading and decoding skills. The first type will be able to decode the words and answer the questions but will need more time, whereas the poor decoding type will have problems decoding the words and extra time may not improve their performance. On a timed text comprehension task, both types may perform poorly for different reasons.

Another concern that is relevant to the issue of time is that different strategies/abilities in information may influence reading time. For instance, an individual who can recall information about a story may have a faster time than someone who cannot recall the target information but can remember its spatial location and look back quickly. The individual who can recall information will have a faster time than a person who cannot remember anything about the target information and has to search throughout the passage.

There are also differences in the required output or responses in text reading tests. Some tests require expressive output while others require written language. Furthermore, the comprehension questions themselves may vary. Text comprehension questions may involve inferences, memory for details, or the general idea of the passage. Sometimes, reading comprehension ability consists of memory skills (e.g., Tal & Siegel, 1996), especially when recall of exact wording or details is not essential. Another dimension that may influence individual performances on text comprehension is an individual's familiarity with the material in the text (e.g., Drum, Calfee, & Cook, 1981; Marr & Gormley, 1982). Sometimes, an individual need not be familiar with the text; rather, some questions can be answered with a reasonable amount of accuracy without reading or comprehending the text (e.g., Tal & Siegel, 1996). When so many dimensions exist in text comprehension, different skills can be assessed, and poor performance on text comprehension may be a result of different causes. Therefore, it is important to be familiar with the text reading tests and the different requirements of each type of test.

Spelling

Spelling is another required skill in an academic setting. Therefore, a test of dictation words should be included in the assessment battery, such as the WRAT3: spelling subtest (Wilkinson, 1993) and the Spelling subtest of the WJ III (Woodcock et al., 2001).

Computational Arithmetic

There should be a test of computational arithmetic skills to determine what the individual understands about the fundamental arithmetic operations. The WRAT3: Arithmetic subtest (Wilkinson, 1993) is a timed test that assessed this skill. Also the WJ III: Calculation subtest assessed written arithmetic computation (Woodcock et al., 2001).

Another mathematical skill that should be included is problem solving. This skill can be assessed by the Applied Problem subtest from the WJ III. This subtest administered orally to assess math "word problems," solved with paper and pencil (Woodcock et al., 2001).

Writing

Writing is also a necessary skill in higher education; however, this type of assessment is complicated. There is a need for extensive time to allow for planning as well as writing. One option is to ask the individual to bring in a sample of his or her writing; in this case, some type of brief assessment in the context of the assessment session is useful. The scoring of written products is subjective, and currently there is no agreement on an accepted scoring system. One system that has potential for becoming an evaluative tool for writing was suggested by Berninger (1994) and contains six dimensions: (1) handwriting quality (legibility), (2) handwriting fluency (number of words copied within time limits), (3) single-word spelling from dictation (on standardized lists of increasing difficulty), (4) spelling in composition (percentage of correctly spelled words), (5) composition fluency (number of words produced within time limits), and (6) composition quality (content and organization of paragraph construction). Writing is complicated to assess, but the WJ III has some subtests that may be useful. For example, the Writing Sample subtest (Woodcock et al., 2001) assesses the ability to write sentences according to directions; many items include pictures. Another is the Writing Fluency subtest, which assesses the ability to compose simple sentences as quickly as possible (Woodcock et al., 2001).

The Cutoff Scores to Identify an LD

The question arises as to how low a score should be in order to identify an LD. One of the aspects of the definitional issues is that we are not dealing with a clearly identifiable entity when we speak of an LD. It is not clear at what point or how low the score should be for the person to be considered learning disabled. Deciding on the appropriate cutoff score that will identify an LD is problematic. As a guideline, many have typically used scores below the 25th percentile (e.g., Fletcher, 1985; Rourke, 1991). This cutoff is arbitrary, but there is some evidence of the validity of this score. First, a number of studies have found that this percentile separates individuals with an LD from normally achieving individuals on a variety of tasks (e.g., Fletcher, 1985a; Rourke & Finlayson, 1978; Shaywitz et al., 1990; Siegel & Ryan, 1988). Does that mean that 25% of the population will be called learning disabled? In reality, this is not the case and this cutoff identifies about 7–8% of the population as learning disabled on the basis of a word reading test such as the WRAT3 Reading subtest (Fletcher et al., 1994; Rourke & Finlayson, 1978; Shaywitz et al., 1990).

There is no way of knowing what a valid cutoff score is; there is no magic number to separate those with an LD from those without LDs. An argument could just as easily be made for the 20th percentile or the 15th percentile, instead of the 25th percentile. No blood test, x-ray, or magnetic imaging technique can be used to diagnose an LD. However, for the educational system to identify who will receive the accommodations and remediation, we must take a continuous variable (e.g., reading performance) and make it a dichotomous one.

A Model for Assessment

In this field there are issues of what constitutes appropriate assessment for LDs. It certainly is the tradition to do extensive additional testing besides achievement testing. However, the usefulness of additional testing for the identification of learning disabilities is not clear. It is likely that the primary reasons for doing assessments are to document the existence of an LD and to recommend appropriate remediation and accommodations. To accomplish these aims, the achievement testing described previously is clearly needed. Typically, tests of cognitive processes and intelligence tests are included in many assessments. Do we really need tests of "auditory memory," "visual memory," "language," and "visual closure"? Is there such an entity as "auditory memory"? Suppose the stimuli for an "auditory memory" task are words and the individual is asked to repeat them, or suppose they are musical phrases or melodies and the person is asked to discriminate them. Would conclusions about auditory memory be the same if these diverse stimuli were used? The question should always be, How does the task or test being used in the assessment relate to the determination of the LD and/or, perhaps more important, the provision of remediation or accommodations? Of course, the individual may be interested in learning more about his or her strengths and weaknesses. An extended assessment may also be valid for these reasons. However, it is not necessary to define the LD to propose accommodations or remedial strategies.

There were a number of problems with the assessments of LD. In one review of the evaluations to assess possible LDs (Siegel, 1999), each evaluation used different tests, different terminology, and different labels for the LD. Here are some examples of the types of LDs that were reported to exist: "Language based learning disability," "subtle verbal processing," "attentional and long-term memory limitations," difficulty in "visual processing speed," "statistically significant disparity between relative conceptual language strengths compared with mathematics and written output," "slow processing speed," "visuoperceptual processing inefficiencies," problems with the "ability to process auditory and visual information," "mild frontal lobe disorder," and "poor auditory processing." There is little empirical validation for this terminology research on LD.

The process of assessing whether or not there is an LD has been made unnecessarily complex. Standardized tests of reading, spelling, arithmetic calculation, and mathematical problem solving as described earlier are essential. Obtaining a sample of writing is important. Other tests may be done for interest and/or research, but they are not essential to the diagnosis of an LD.

In addition to the achievement tests discussed earlier, an important part of any assessment is the use of analyses of errors. Systematic analyses of errors may provide useful information about an individual's level of functioning in reading, spelling, and arithmetic and may provide information about appropriate accommodations. Numerous studies such as those of Barwick and Siegel (1996), Bruck and Waters (1988), Werker, Bryson, and Wassenberg (1989), and Lennox and Siegel (1993, 1996) have used analyses of errors as a means to understanding the nature of the difficulties in individuals with LDs. Error analyses also provide some information about the types of questions the individual was able to answer correctly. For example, are the spelling errors good phonological equivalents of the word to be spelled (e.g., "nature" spelled as "nachure")? Or, are they good visual errors—that is, a close match to the visual form of the word—for example, nature written as natur (this is a close visual but not a close phonological match) (e.g., Lennox & Siegel, 1993, 1996)? Analyses such as these help us understand the strategies that the individual is using and can provide guidelines for remediation.

Finally, an assessment should include a direct interview with the student to analyze strengths as well as weaknesses not detected by achievement tests. Many individuals with LDs have talents in the areas of art, dancing, mechanics, music, and/or sports. For example, both Agatha Christie and W. B. Yeats had LDs (Miner & Siegel, 1992; Siegel, 1988a) that can be documented, but, obviously, they were individuals with considerable talent. The recognition of these strengths is important to the development of educational strategies and to the self-esteem of the individual with LDs (e.g., Vail, 1990).

RISK FACTORS FOR ADOLESCENTS WITH LDs

Risk factors are associated with the increased likelihood of an individual developing an emotional or behavioral disorder in comparison to a randomly selected person from the general population (Garmezy, 1983). Therefore, there is an increased risk for adolescents with LD to develop social, emotional, and academic problems.

Social Risk Factors

Students with LD experience social difficulties. Studies that have investigated social skills in students with LD suggested that the difficulty in achieving social acceptance may be related to their deficient perception and interpretation of social and emotional cues in social situations. Social difficulties can be manifested in different ways, starting with the ability, or inability, to recognize emotional expression, social problem solving, and friendship.

Wiig and Harris (1974) conducted one of the earliest studies that examined how adolescents with LD perceived nonverbal behavior. They found that adolescents with LD were significantly less accurate than adolescents without LD at labeling the emotion expressed by young women's videotaped nonverbal expressions of anger, embarrassment, fear, frustration, joy, and love.

Social skills are also manifested in the ability to make friends. Parents of early adolescents with LD reported that their children more often chose younger playmates than did children without LD (Wiener & Sunohara, 1998). Wiener and Schneider (2002) examined the friendship patterns of children in grades 4–8 with and without LDs. They found that the friendships of children with LD in grades 4–6 were less stable than the friendships of children without LD. However, adolescents with LD in grades 7 and 8 were as likely as children without LD to have stable friendships. The authors concluded that the acquisition of a pattern of having more stable friendships appears to be delayed in children with LD.

Another aspect of friendship is loneliness. Loneliness is an unpleasant experience when individuals perceive a discrepancy between the desire and accomplished patterns of their social networks (Peplau & Perlman, 1982). A comparison between adolescents with and without LD in grades 6 and 7 demonstrated that the former reported higher levels of loneliness as compared to their matched peers (Sabornie, 1994).

Emotional Risk Factors

Adolescents with LD may be at risk for emotional problems such as depression, self-concept, juvenile delinquency, and substance use and abuse. One of the risk factors for adolescents with LD is depression. Depression is characterized by a negative patterns of thinking or attitudes' regarding one's self, the future, and the environment (Beck, 1976). Many adolescents with LD are characterized by this negative pattern of thinking. Although some studies report high levels of depression among adolescents with LD (e.g., Gregg, Hoy, King, Moreland & Jagota, 1992; Maag & Behrens, 1989), other studies report no differences in the prevalence of depression between adolescents with LD and adolescents without LD (e.g., Navarrete, 1999). The differences in the results may be due to the different definitions that studies used in order to identify LD, as well as different assessment tools to assess depression and different levels of depression.

Another emotional factor that may place adolescents with LD at greater risk for emotional difficulties than adolescents who are normal achievers is problems with their self-concept. The rationale is that individuals with LD most often experience academic failure that may influence their global self-concept (Cooley & Ayres, 1988). There are different types of self-concept: global self-concept refers to the general view that one has of oneself; academic self-concept refers to one's perception of him- or herself as a student. Huntington and Bender (1993), in their review of studies on adolescents with LD, reported inconsistent results among studies, especially during the first decade of research on self-concept in the 1980s. They noted that the inconsistent findings were a result of inconsistent use of the term "self-concept": "this confusion began to clear somewhat when a more refined understanding of self-concept was developed and explored" (Huntington & Bender, 1993, p. 160). It was only when investigators began to compare adolescents with LD to adolescents who were nondisabled on academic self-concept that serious deficits were demonstrated more consistently (e.g., Boetsch, Green, & Pennington, 1996; Chapman, 1988; Harter, Whitesell, & Junkin, 1998). For instance, 71 adolescents with LD in junior high school were compared to adolescents who were normally achieving on an academic self-concept over 3 academic years (Chapman, 1988). The Perception of Ability Scale measured academic self-concept of students (Boersma & Chapman, 1990). Adolescents with LD scored significantly lower than adolescents who were nondisabled on the academic self-concept, and there were no significant changes in the academic self-concept of the LD group over the 3 years. Gans, Kenny, and Ghany (2003) compared adolescents in grades 6, 7, and 8, primarily Hispanic, to their typically normal achieving peers to determine whether students with LD have different self concepts, both global and specific such as academically and behaviorally. Adolescents with LD in this study were identified as having a discrepancy of 1.5 standard deviations or more between their IQ standard score and their achievement standard score in math, reading, or written expression. Adolescents with LD scored significantly lower on the Piers–Harris Children's Self-Concept Scale (Piers, 1994) subscale of intellectual and school status, confirming that adolescents with LD have a negative self-concept on their abilities and academic skills than their peers. However, the adolescents with LD did not demonstrate a lower global self-concept than their peers. The investigator suggested that the LD group did not generalize their feelings of academic weakness to more generalized self-concept perceptions, such as physical appearance and academic skills (Gans et al., 2003). Another interesting finding in this study was that adolescents with LD scored lower than their peers on the self-concept subscale of behavior. The meanings of these results are that adolescents with LD either were more willing to acknowledge their behavioral difficulties or had more behavioral difficulties than their peers (Gans et al., 2003).

Delinquency is an extreme consequence of social emotional difficulties. Some of the current studies in the field of LD have indicated a connection between delinquency and LD, while others have not provided support for the idea that the presence of LDs increases the risk of becoming a juvenile delinquent. There are some hypotheses that postulate a link between LD and juvenile delinquency, specifically, the school failure rationale and the susceptibility theory. The school failure hypothesis is that LD produces academic failure, which leads to a negative self-image, in turn resulting in school dropout and delinquent behavior. In this model, there are several possible causes for the delinquent behavior: First, adults perceive the child as a disciplinary problem; second, children with LD are labeled negatively by others and themselves and become hostile to school and teachers in relation; third, as a result of the preceding factors, the youth with LD drops out or is suspended from school, which leads to increased opportunities for delinquent behavior

through involvement with antisocial peers. There is support for the correlation between low achievement and delinquent behaviors (Grande, 1988) and remedial programs that support improvement in academic skills reducing the delinquency of youth with LD who had been officially adjudicated (Keilitz & Dunivant, 1986).

The susceptibility hypothesis postulates that individuals with LD possess certain personality characteristics that make them more susceptible to opportunities for engaging in delinquent activities. These characteristics may be unrelated to the LD or may be separate components of the LD—for example, lack of impulse control, inability to anticipate consequences of actions, irritability, suggestibility, and the tendency to act out (Murray, 1976). Waldie and Spreen (1993) examined the relationship between LD and continuing delinquency based on these two models. The students were first assessed between the ages of 8 and 12. An LD in this study was indicated by school records, achievement testing (2 standard deviations below the mean for age), and parent report. The participants were reexamined at a mean age of 18.9 and only the subjects who reported any contact with police were included. In the second follow-up, at age 25, the population was divided into two groups: subjects who had no further police contact ($n = 25$) and subjects with persisting police contacts ($n = 40$). The investigators conducted discriminant analyses and found that overall the susceptibility theory was supported in that "LD may be linked to certain underdeveloped personality skills, such as general impulsiveness and poor judgment. A deficiency in these skills may lead to increased susceptibility to delinquent behavior through unwise social choices. Supports for the school failure theory was weak" (Waldie & Spreen, 1993, p. 422), because the selected variables, except for drinking behavior, were not significant predictors of persistent delinquency, with only 64% of cases that were correctly classified.

Another study reported contradictory results. This longitudinal study from a 7-year perspective, examined whether the presence of LDs increases the adolescent's risk of becoming a juvenile delinquent (Malmgren, Abbott, & Hawkins, 1999). Adolescents with LD were identified mainly by severe discrepancy between intellectual ability and achievement in one or more academic areas. The results demonstrated that after controlling for gender, ethnicity, and socioeconomic status (SES), there was not a direct relationship between LD and delinquency (Malmgren et al., 1999). However, the identification of individuals with LD in this study required only a discrepancy and not low achievement, and it may be the case that some of the adolescents may not have had an LD or did have an LD but were not diagnosed.

Substance use and abuse is another serious emotional risk factor for adolescents with LD. Adolescents with LD are at increased risk for the development of substance use disorder (SUD), particularly when they continue to manifest LD in young adulthood (Beitchman, Wilson, Douglas, Young, & Adlaf, 2001). Specifically, participants with LD at ages 12 and 19 were more likely to develop a SUD or a psychiatric disorder compared to participants without LD (Beitchman et al., 2001). Cosden (2001) reviewed the research on substance abuse for adolescents and adults with LD and concluded that potential risk factors for individuals with LD include a poor understanding of one's disability, a lack of skills for developing peer relationships, and the need for prolonged family support.

Academic Risk Factors

Adolescents with LD are especially at risk for various academic problems in their secondary school years. By definition, adolescents with LD will have difficulties with schoolwork, whether in reading, writing, or math, but we are referring to more extreme difficulties. Here we consider academic risk factors as grade retention, dropout rates, and the difficulties with transition from one school setting to another.

The number of students who were retained a grade has increased over the past decades (e.g., Larrabee, 1984; Shepard & Smith, 1989). However, there is no evidence for the benefit of grade retention for students of any age and research has demonstrated that there are negative consequences for retention in both the short and in the long term. For instance, children who were retained a grade exhibited lower self-concept and poorer attitude toward school and achieved a lower level than students who were promoted, during a follow-up year to the starting of the retention period (Holmes & Matthews, 1984). In the long term, students who were retained a grade had lower achievement and self-concept (Holmes, 1989). Another long-term effect is the increase in dropout rates among students who were retained (Hahn, 1987).

McLeskey and Grizzle (1992) examined grade retention of students with LDs. They collected data on 689 students who were identified as having an LD during the 1987–1988 school year in Indiana. They found that 58% of the students had been retained before being identified as learning disabled. From this group, 45% of the students were identified as learning disabled in the primary grades (kindergarten to grade 2), 34% of the students were identified as learning disabled in grades 3–5 and 22% of the students were only identified as learning disabled in the secondary level (grades 6–12). The investigators found that students with LD who were retained tended to have IQ and achievement levels significantly below students who were identified as learning disabled but not retained.

School dropout is another serious academic risk factor that adolescents with LD confront. Dropping out of the school system is a major consequence in itself: The students can find themselves isolated from their social friends, and not attending an educational system leads to further isolation. Furthermore, it also influences future employment opportunities. Individuals with a mild disability were at a disadvantage, even among employment opportunities that are suitable for individuals without high school credentials (e.g., Schwartz, 1995)

There is some inconsistency in the reports of the dropout rates among adolescents with LD, but most of the studies report higher rates than the general population, placing the adolescents with LD at higher risk for dropout from secondary school. The dropout rate for specific handicapping conditions ranges from a low of approximately 19% for students with orthopedic impairments to a high of 37% for students with LDs (Lichtenstein, 1987). Another study found that the dropout rate for students in Pittsburgh with LD approached 51%, while the dropout rate in the general population had been reported at 36% in that period (Levin, Zigmond, & Birch, 1985). In an overall national comparison, the dropout rate was 12%, while dropout rates for students with LD were estimated as ranging from 17% to 42% (Lichtenstein & Zantol-Wiener, 1988; National Center for Education Statistics, 1993, 1997, 1999).

Another academic challenge that adolescents face is the transition from elementary school to secondary school (Eccles & Midgley, 1989). In general, the transition from elementary to middle-level schools affects the achievement and motivation of early adolescents (e.g., Anderman & Maehr, 1994; Anderman & Midgley, 1997; Eccles & Midgley, 1989). The period of school transition often leads to a decline in student's self–perceptions, academic performance, and school-related behaviors (Eccles, Lord, & Midgley, 1991). Adolescents with LD will obviously experience even more difficulties through this transition. For instance, Anderman (1998) examined the relation between middle school transition and achievement gaps in math and science between adolescents with and without LD. Overall, there was a strong gap in achievement between the two groups at early adolescence. Anderman investigated whether there was any effect on the school type on the achievement in math and science. When hierarchical linear modeling was used to examine school effects on these achievement gaps, it was found that although there were achievement gaps in math and science between adolescents with LD and without LD, this gap was greatly reduced for adolescents who did not make a school transition until the ninth grade. The investigator concluded that the transition from the elementary school environment to the more impersonal middle school is difficult for all adolescents; however, results of the present study demonstrated that it may be a particularly difficult period for students with LD (Anderman, 1998).

Contradictory results were found in a study conducted by Forgan and Vaughn (2000). This study followed seven Hispanic students with LD and seven Hispanic students without LD over a 2-year period during their transition from a sixth-grade inclusive elementary classroom to seventh grade in middle school (Forgan & Vaughn, 2000). The adolescents were classified as learning disabled if their IQ score was the normal range; having one or more standard scores on the WISC-III below 1 standard deviation on either the Verbal or the Performance IQ; and having an evidence of existing difficulties in processing. It was not clear if the students had low achievement. This study examined the academic and social aspects during the transition time. Overall, the students with LDs and the students without LDs experienced the transition similarly in both academic and social aspects (Forgan & Vaughn, 2000). However, it is not clear if the adolescents with LD in this study had low achievement scores. It may be that some of the adolescents did not

have LDs. Also the study examined a very small number of students and as a result, the statistical power was low.

Some individuals were not identified as learning disabled in their elementary school years, when the academic demands were not as high. Undetected and unremediated learning problems constitute a significant problem for society. For example, adolescent homeless street youth are very likely to have an LD; Barwick and Siegel (1996) found that 82% of street youth living on the streets of downtown Toronto had an LD. In addition, McBride and Siegel (1997) found that all the adolescent suicides in a 3-year period in Ontario, Canada, showed evidence of an LD. For a variety of reasons, many LDs are not detected, and even if they are, appropriate remediation is not provided for them. Unfortunately, this can result in substantial emotional and social consequences to the individual as well as to society.

In summary, there is strong evidence that adolescents with LD are at a greater risk for developing academic, emotional, and social problems. However, there are inconsistent results and sometimes even contradictory ones. One explanation for these results is that each study defines LDs using a different definition, different tests, and different cutoffs. And, sometimes, it is not clear if the adolescents with LD had low achievement scores, which is one of the basic elements in the LD definition. This causes a problem with the validity of the results as well as the ability to generalize them. Furthermore, it is difficult to establish a consistent connection between LD and academic, emotional, and social risk factors and to provide support to these needed adolescents. When the field agrees on one operational definition, more consistent and relevant results will emerge. Having strong evidence concerning the risk factors of adolescents with LDs will bring the field one step forward in designing intervention programs to this most needed population, as well as will help in preventing the social, emotional, and academic consequences of an LD.

INTERVENTION FOR ADOLESCENTS WITH LDs

Once students experience difficulties in reading, writing, and math in the elementary grades, they usually will not catch up with their grade level in the upper grades (Lyon, 1996;

Torgesen, Wagner, Rashotte, Alexander, & Conway, 1997). In their longitudinal study, Fletcher and colleagues (1994) found that of those children diagnosed as reading disabled in third grade, 74% remained disabled in ninth grade. Children who fall behind in kindergarten and grade 1 fall further and further behind over time (Lyon, 1995). Therefore, it is necessary to support adolescents with LD with the appropriate intervention program. The literature about intervention programs has three aspects: (1) studies that describe intervention programs but do not test the efficacy; (2) studies that examined intervention programs; and (3) meta-analytic studies of intervention programs.

Adolescents with LD are a heterogeneous group. There are many intervention programs that were designed to address academic, emotional, and social difficulties. Ellis and Larkin (1998) reviewed key instructional principles, tools, and procedures that currently hold promise for teaching adolescents with LD. The principles of strategic instruction are providing explicit instruction, making covert processing more explicit, modeling procedures and processes, mediating and scaffolding procedures and processes, promoting verbal elaboration on to-be learned material and to require mastery of instructional objectives from the students. Ellis and Larkin indicate that one of the highest priorities for teachers of students with LD is the creation of an atmosphere that reinforces students to take responsibility for their lives, gaining independence, and being in control. The specific techniques for creating such an atmosphere include clarifying who is in control and the role of a special education teacher, creating an atmosphere that permeates student goal setting and self-reinforcement orientation, communication and teaching confidence, and emphasizing the role of personal effort.

Some of the studies examined specific intervention programs and their effect on adolescents with LD. For instance, Hock, Pulvers, Deshler, and Schumaker (2001) examined the effect of an after-school tutoring program on the academic performance of at-risk students and students with LD. The ultimate goal of strategic tutoring was to develop independent and proficient learners. In this intervention program, each student met individually after school with his or her assigned tutor, two or three times a week, for approximately 30 minutes. The tutoring lasted for 4–12 weeks. In the

strategic model, strategies for learning how to learn and perform are taught to the students while they receive help with current class assignments. Two studies were conducted: the first designed to test the overall viability of the strategic tutoring intervention and the second study broader in scope and including additional research questions. Counselors and special education teachers identified at-risk students. Students were considered at risk if they were currently failing two or more academic courses. There were three students in study one, and only one student in the second study who was identified as learning disabled in math and written language based on adequate IQ scores and low performance on the Woodcock–Johnson Achievement Test—Revised (40th percentile in reading comprehension, 6th percentile in basic math, 10th percentile in math concept, and 39th percentile in written expression). The students improved their semester grade in algebra and in some cases maintained their performance. In the second study, there were six students at risk who were identified by the school's counselor and teaching staff members. These students had low or failing grades. One student was diagnosed as having an LD in math based on achievement tests and adequate IQ scores (41st percentile in reading comprehension, 38th percentile in basic mathematics, 29th percentile in mathematics concepts, and 20th percentile in written expression). Five of the six students improved their academic performance on quizzes and tests from failing and below average to average and above average. The students were also able to increase their course grade and to increase their knowledge of specific strategies. Although this article also refers to LDs, the two students with LD who were included in this study were not necessarily learning disabled based on different cutoff scores, and the conclusion that can be drawn from such narrow cases is very limited.

Overall, there are various intervention programs that are being offered to adolescents with LD. Swanson and Hoskyn (2001) conducted a meta-analysis of the intervention programs for adolescents with LD. In their analysis, they examined the instructional components that positively influence performance of adolescents with LDs. In their comprehensive meta-analysis of intervention studies for students with LDs, they included 93 experimental intervention programs that were published between 1963 and 1997, where the mean sample age was above 10 years and below 19 years. Other criteria for selecting studies were at least one between instruction comparison, meaning having a control group, sufficient quantitative information to permit calculation of effect size, and that the treatment group received instruction, assistance, or therapy that was over and above what they would have received during typical classroom experiences. Another criterion for including studies in this meta-analysis was that the recipients of the intervention were adolescents with average intelligence who had problems in particular academic, social, and/or related behavior domains. The cutoff score for inclusion in the synthesis was a mean IQ above 84. Studies that did not report on specific IQ score but stated that the IQ scores were in the average range were included in the analysis.

Overall, there were 45 instructional activities that were grouped into 18 instructional components. From these 18 instructional components, there were eight instructional programs that captured the majority of intervention programs for adolescents with LD. The eight programs were Questioning, Sequencing and Segmentation, Explicit Skill Modeling, Organization and Explicit Practice, Small-Group Setting, Indirect Teacher Activities, Technology, and Scaffolding. However, only the Organization and Explicit factor contributed significant variance (16%) to effect size. This factor includes advanced organization and explicit practice. In advanced organization the adolescents are being directed to look over material before instruction. The adolescents directed to focus on particular information, providing prior information about task and/or the teacher stating objectives of instruction. It provided students with a "mental scaffold" on which to build new understandings of information. This scaffolding may consist of helping students access information already in their mind and new concepts or principles that can organize this information in a form that will aid in new learning. In explicit practice there is distributed review and practice, repeated practice, sequenced reviews, daily feedback, and/or weekly reviews. The retention of many types of knowledge is increased by practice at different time periods. Finally, the single instructional component that was related to large effect sizes was explicit practice. This component includes

treatment activities that are related to distributed review and practice, repeated practice, sequenced review, daily feedback, and/or weekly review. Further discussion about the organization/explicit factor and practical guidelines to direct instructional practice are provided by Swanson and Deshler (2003).

Elbaum and Vaughn (2001) conducted a meta-analytic review to examine the effectiveness of school-based interventions aimed at enhancing the self-concept of students with LD. This study focused on students' self-perception (because it can influence their school performance), motivation for academic tasks, career orientation, and expectations for future success. However, negative self-perceptions can be extremely resistant to change. Students with LD experience severe academic difficulty at school and, therefore, are considered to be particularly at risk for poor self-concept. This concern regarding the self-concept of students with LD has led researchers and educators to design and implement intervention programs to enhance the self-concept of these students. This meta-analysis was conducted in order to provide teachers, researchers, and parents with guidance regarding the efficacy of intervention designed to enhance the self-concept of students with LD. The criteria for the inclusion of studies in this meta-analysis were (1) studies that employed a group design, contrasting a treatment group with intervention group; (2) the participants consisted entirely or primarily of students with LD (students who in the primary research were identified as students with LD or mildly academically handicapped (in the normal range of intelligence or having IQ > 85); (3) if participants were a combination of students with and without LD, either the data for students with LD were analyzed separately or the students with LD were at least two-thirds of the participants; (4) the intervention took place in school or did not require any special facilities; (5) the study included a measure of self-concept; and (6) the data reported in the study were sufficient for calculation of an effect size.

The 82 interventions that were examined had a mean weighted effect size of 0.19. This small effect size means that the validity of self-concept interventions for this population is questionable; however, the investigators reported that the intervention effects were moderated by a number of variables. Self-concept interventions were more effective for young adolescents than for elementary school children or older adolescents. Furthermore, the type of intervention that was most effective appeared to differ by grade level; academic interventions were the most reliably effective for elementary students, where counseling interventions were the most consistently effective for middle and high school students. Although this study demonstrated the effectiveness of particular intervention programs for adolescents with LD, the authors acknowledge the fact that students with LD are not a homogeneous group in terms of the social functioning. However, none of the reviewed studies provided information on the social functioning of the students prior to the intervention. This may influence the low effect size across the interventions, because it might be that many of the students who participated in the interventions were not in need of intervention. Another problematic issue that the authors of this meta-analysis did not address is the different definitions of LD. Not only might it be that the students with LD had adequate self-perceptions, but, rather, it might be that some of them did not have an LD.

Accommodations for Students with LDs

It is important that adolescents with LDs be provided with the appropriate accommodations. One of the problems in evaluating effective accommodations in students is that in many cases there is little research evidence of their relative effectiveness. This is because the accommodations are usually based on a combination of good teaching practice and experience, and failure to implement them would be seen as detrimental to the individual. Put another way, in research it would be difficult to argue that it would be ethical to not use these accommodations as practitioners see their advantage on a day-to-day basis.

The issues are further complicated due to the divergence of individual strengths and weaknesses, as well as academic context. Thus it would be difficult to have a sufficient cohort to confirm that one method was more effective than another. Many of the accommodations listed below are developed by practitioners, though some are research based. However, experience has demonstrated that the student with LD is better off using these methods than no methods.

Recommendation for accommodations for the individual with LD may be categorized as follows:

- Training the individual for self-help,
- Creating an LD-friendly environment, and
- Providing support resources.

It is important that individuals with LDs do not feel they are alone, working against the system. Primary to support is an understanding of the issues, by the individual, the teachers, and the peer group.

Training the Individual for Self-Help

- Teach metacognitive strategies to help individuals with LDs enhance their learning (for a detailed discussion, see Butler, 1995; Montague, 1997; Schumaker & Deshler, 1992).
- Provide basic skills training in reading and arithmetic for some individuals with very low-level skills. However, there should be no assumptions about prior knowledge. Establishing a baseline to use as a foundation for learning must be the starting point, and failure to create a firm foundation is a common cause of academic failure (Chinn & Ashcroft, 1998).
- Encourage self-monitoring strategies to organize information and to avoid confusion when doing more than one activity. Strategies could include drawing plans or making lists to follow sequential steps from manual or verbal instructions (Ostler & Ward, 2002).
- Ensure that students with LDs understand that it is important to interrupt when they do not understand important concepts. They need to understand that if they do not understand current information, they will not have the foundation for future work.
- Teach study skills, including how to take note, how to revise for examinations, and how to plan an essay. These skills are not automatic for many individuals (Hornsby, 1996; Ostler & Ward, 2002).
- When computers are allowed or encouraged, ensure full training is provided, including keyboard skills (Crivelli, Thomson, & Andersson, 2004).
- Set realistic targets, which are pupil led (Ott, 1997).
- Practice proofreading (Ostler & Ward, 2002; Ott, 1997).

Creating an LD-Friendly Environment

• Make sure a full assessment of strengths and weaknesses has been carried out, with particular reference to the learning environment. This assessment should lead to an individual education plan, including outcomes and time scales (Smythe & Siegel, 2004).

• Individuals who experience difficulties with written output should be given sufficient time to complete written work and examinations and this accommodation may involve additional time.

• Ensure examinations evaluate ability and not disability. For example, consider accepting concept maps or tapes (audio or video) as examination responses. Spelling should only be assessed when it is integral to the context. Extra time should be provided whenever appropriate (see, e.g., DfEE, 2000; Hong Kong Disability Discrimination Ordinance, 2002).

• Ensure that teachers and support staff understand the difficulties of students with LDs (e.g., reading aloud in class) and ensure that they do not ridicule the individual. Teachers should be aware of their moral as well as legislative obligations with respect to all disabilities (see, e.g., Hong Kong Disability Discrimination Ordinance, 2002; see also Peer & Reid, 2001).

• Ensure that teachers and pupils do not see accommodations as an unfair advantage, particularly with the use of computers (Svensson, Jacobson, Björkman, & Sandell, 2000).

• Tape recording of lessons and lectures should be allowed and encouraged if the instructor is willing to give permission (Hornsby, 1996).

• Provided the principles of the examination are not compromised, answers to essay questions and class assignments should be completed in bullet-point form, concept maps, or other "alternative" formats.

• Copying from the blackboard is difficult for many students with LDs. Alternatives such as class handouts, photocopying other students' notes, or tape recording oral lessons should be considered (Hornsby, 1996).

• Do not assume that one set of strategies will work for all individuals. Strategies need to be developed for the specific individual and topic (Mackay, 2001; Peer & Reid, 2001).

• Do not assume all students learn in the same way. Every student with an LD has unique characteristics and learning abilities and should be treated as such (Chinn et al., 2001; UNESCO, 1994).

• Ensure that all students understand what it means to have reading difficulties and that teachers recognize strengths as well as weaknesses, in the same way they would with a deaf individual or somebody confined to a wheelchair.

• Ensure that good school/parent dialogues exist (Peer & Reid, 2001).

• Do not ignore the emotional aspects, including the need to provide praise and encouragement (Biggar & Barr, 1996).

Providing Support Resources

The student with LD may also require resources to ensure they can work effectively and, as far as possible, independently. Above all, the computer will provide an invaluable support (Keates, 2000). However, others should also be considered.

Learning keyboarding skills is important. Adolescents with LDs can use their keyboarding skills in class to take notes by using the class computer or personal laptop, as well as typing papers and work that needs to be submitted in writing. Especially in secondary school, when written work is usually required, adolescents with LDs may not be able to communicate their ideas in writing effectively. For such individuals, oral assessments may be appropriate. However, if they have alternative ways to express ideas, they will not be penalized for their writing difficulties. Laptop computers for use in the normal classroom environment increase confidence by providing a means for the student with LD to work in an alternative manner that may be better for him or her, as well as hide errors that cause embarrassment (e.g., reading and spelling) (Crivelli et al., 2004).

• Some individuals will have difficulties with written output. Copying from the blackboard is difficult and alternatives should be considered: class handouts, photocopying assignments, or other students' notes.

• Some adolescents with LDs will have difficulties in spelling. It is recommended that these adolescents use a computer (word processor) for written work. This may help improve the quality of written work. Using a computer spell-check often and early in the writing process will ensure correct spellings of words and can contribute to an enhanced knowledge of common word patterns. Because of spelling difficulties, consideration should be given to not reducing grades for spelling errors. If acceptable to the instructor, answers to essay questions should be completed in point form. Consideration should be given to a similar format for class assignments.

• The tape recorder is another alternative that provides an efficient way to record a lecture. Tape recording of lectures should be allowed and encouraged if the instructor is willing to give permission.

• Especially in the secondary schools, there is an increasing demand for intensive reading. Adolescents with reading difficulties will find it very frustrating to try to comprehend a text when they need to spend most of their time trying to read and decode words. Textbooks on tape can provide adolescents with the ability to concentrate on the comprehension of the text, as well as a more enjoyable experience of reading. Another advantage of using textbooks on tape is that the adolescents can be more independent as opposed to having an adult or tutor reading the required text to them.

• Text-to-speech computer software will translate the text on the screen into a spoken output and thus decrease the reading content of courses, allowing the student with LD to concentrate on the content and information processing (Crivelli et al., 2004).

• Some individuals with LD will be very slow in writing and will experience difficulties when written work is required. An alternative method to produce a written work will be the use of voice recognition software. This software translates the individual's voice to a written typed output. After a short training period, the individual with LD can use voice recognition software to produce most of his or her written output. Speech to text will offer the chance to decrease the writing components without affecting the amount of work submitted (Crivelli et al., 2004).

• Spelling and grammar checkers and word prediction software can be beneficial but should be used with caution. Choose the most suitable spell-checker (some produce a large list of alternatives, confusing the individual who is unable to choose the right word), and use word prediction with caution (Crivelli et al., 2004).

• Arithmetic knowledge should be judged in terms of both written knowledge and conceptual abilities. It is recommended that individuals with arithmetic difficulties use a calculator. These individuals usually have short-term memory problems, and they often arrive at an incorrect answer even though they used the correct operation. The use of the calculator provides these individuals with the ability to show their conceptual skills without errors due to short-term memory lapses.

• Provide a tutor who understands how best to support students with LDs. This should preferably be somebody who does not normally teach the individual (European Dyslexia Association, 1997).

• Develop a buddy system whereby students support each other, with weak students being helped by stronger students. Research clearly shows that in the mentoring context, both students gain (Fuchs & Fuchs, 2002).

FUTURE DIRECTIONS

Until the field of LDs resolves the definitional issues, significant progress will not be made in identification, remediation, and research. We must examine our basic concepts about the nature of LDs and our current practices. Specific and clear operational definitions are necessary to help the field advance. Without agreement on the definition of LDs, the field will not move forward.

Much of the research in the field of LD focused on the elementary school age children. Although it is clear that adolescents with LD have significant challenges, there is very limited research on LDs and adolescence. There is a need to examine the reading and mathematical development in adolescents with particular focus at the reading comprehension skills. Such investigation should focus on the development of reading comprehension at the sentence, paragraph, and text level. Also, it is necessary to examine different texts and different types of questions. This information can help in identifying specific difficulties for adolescents with LD.

There is a need to evaluate interventions and accommodations for the adolescent. There is a need to examine models of early identification and interventions, such as that of Lesaux and Siegel (2003), to prevent tragedies like those illustrated by the case of Denise, with which we began this chapter. Another factor is that educators do not know enough about LDs. Teacher education programs should remedy this state of affairs. Denise was not diagnosed with RD in elementary school; her present and, presumably, future are greatly influenced by this misidentification. One of the contributing factors was the insistence of the use of the IQ test, which delayed the identification because of the long waiting list to get tested. We know that the IQ test is unnecessary, so Denise should not have had to wait. Now, as an adolescent, it is not "just" her reading disability that Denise is facing but other serious emotional, and social difficulties. Unfortunately, Denise is not an isolated case (e.g., Barwick & Siegel, 1996; McBride & Siegel, 1997). It is critical for investigators and society as a whole to address this serious problem.

ACKNOWLEDGMENTS

This research was supported by a grant from the Natural Sciences and Engineering Research Council of Canada to Linda Siegel. We would like to acknowledge the valuable input provided by Ian Smythe on the section on accommodations.

REFERENCES

Anderman, E. M. (1998). The middle school experience: Effects on the math and science achievement of adolescents with LD. *Journal of Learning Disabilities, 31*, 128–138.

Anderman, E. M., & Maehr, M. L. (1994). Motivation and schooling in the middle grades. *Review of Educational Research, 64*, 287–309.

Anderman, E. M., & Midgley, C. (1997). Changes in achievement goal orientations, perceived academic competence, and grades across the transition to middle-level schools. *Contemporary Educational Psychology, 22*, 269–298.

Backman, J., Bruck, M., Hebert, M., & Seidenberg, M. (1984). Acquisition and use of spelling-sound correspondences in reading. *Journal of Experimental Child Psychology, 38*, 114–133.

Barwick, M., & Siegel, L. S. (1996). Learning difficulties in adolescent client of a shelter for runaway and homeless street youth. *Journal of Research on Adolescence, 6*, 649–670.

Bateman, B. D. (1965). An educational view of a diagnostic approach to learning disorders. In J. Hellmuth (Ed.), *Learning disorders* (pp. 219–239). Seattle, WA: Special Child.

Beck. A. T. (1976). *Cognitive therapy and the emotional disorders*. New York: International Universities Press.

Beitchman, J. H., Wilson, B., Douglas, L., Young, A., & Adlaf, E. (2001). Substance use disorders in young adults with and without LD: Predictive and concurrent relationships. *Journal of Learning Disabilities, 34*, 317–332.

Berninger, V. (1994). Future directions for research on writing disabilities: Integrating endogenous and exogenous variables. In G. R. Lyon (Ed.), *Frames of reference for the assessment of learning disabilities: New views on measurement issues* (pp. 419–440). Baltimore: Brookes.

Biggar, S., & Barr, J. (1996). The emotional world of specific learning difficulties. In G. Reid (Ed.), *Dimensions of dyslexia*. Edinburgh, Scotland: Moray House.

Boersma, F. L., & Chapman, J. W. (1990). *Perception of ability for students*. Los Angeles: Western Psychological Services.

Boetsch, E. A., Green, P. A., & Pennington, B. F. (1996). Psychosocial correlates of dyslexia across the life span. *Development and Psychopathology, 8*, 536–539.

Brown, J. I., Vick Fishco, V., & Hanna, G. (1993). *Nelson–Denny Reading Test*. Chicago: Riverside.

Bruck, M. (1990). Word-recognition skills of adults with childhood diagnosis of dyslexia. *Developmental Psychology, 26*, 439–454.

Bruck, M. (1992). Persistence of dyslexics' phonological awareness deficits. *Developmental Psychology, 28*, 874–886.

Bruck, M., & Waters, G. (1988). An analysis of the spelling errors of children who differ in their reading and spelling skills. *Applied Psycholinguistics, 9*, 77–92.

Burt, C. (1927). *Mental and scholastic tests*. London: P.S. King and Son.

Butler, D. L. (1995). Promoting strategic learning by post secondary students with learning disabilities. *Journal of Learning Disabilities, 28*, 170–190.

Calfee, R., Lindamood, C., & Lindamood, P. (1973). Acoustic–phonetic skills and reading—kindergarten through twelfth grade. *Journal of Educational Psychology, 64*, 293–298.

Chapman, J. W. (1988). Cognitive motivational characteristics and academic achievement of learning disabled children: A longitudinal study. *Journal of Educational Psychology, 80*, 357–365.

Chinn, S. J., & Ashcroft, J. R. (1998). *Mathematics for dyslexics: A teaching handbook* (2nd ed.). London: Whurr.

Chinn, S. J., McDonnagh, D., van Elswijk, R., Harmsen, H., Kay, J., McPhillips, T., et al. (2001). Classroom studies into cognitive style in mathematics for pupils with dyslexia in special education in the Netherlands, Ireland and the UK. *British Journal of Special Education, 28*, 80–85.

Cooley, E. J., & Ayres, J. (1988). Self-concept and the mildly handicapped: The role of social comparisons. *Journal of Special Education, 17,* 37–45.

Cosden, M. (2001). Risk and resilience for substance abuse among adolescents and adults with LD. *Journal of Learning Disabilities, 34,* 352–359.

Crivelli, V., Thomson, M., & Andersson, B. (2004). Using information and communication technology. In G. Reid & A. Fawcett (Eds.), *Dyslexia in context: Research, policy and practice.* Chichester, UK: Whurr.

Cruickshank, W. M. (1972). Some issues facing the field of learning disability. *Journal of Learning Disabilities, 5,* 380–388.

Cruickshank, W. M. (1981). Learning disabilities: A definitional statement. In W. M. Cruickshank (Ed.), *Concepts in learning disabilities.* Syracuse, NY: Syracuse University Press.

D'Angiulli, A., & Siegel, L. S. (2003). Cognitive functioning as measured by the WISC-R. *Journal of Learning Disabilities, 36,* 48–58.

DeFries, J. C., & Gillis, J. J. (1991). Etiology of reading deficit in learning disabilities: Quantitative genetic analyses. In J. E. Obrzut & G. W. Hynd (Eds.), *Neuropsychological foundations of learning disabilities: A handbook of issues, methods, and practice* (pp. 29–48). San Diego, CA: Academic Press.

DfEE. (2000). *Code of practice, 2000.* London: HMSO.

Drum, P. A., Calfee, R. C., & Cook, L. K. (1981). The effects of sentence structure variables on performance in reading comprehension tests. *Reading Research Quarterly, 16,* 486–514.

Durrant. J. E. (1994). A decade of research on learning disabilities: A report card on the state of the literature. *Journal of Learning Disabilities, 27,* 25–33.

Eccles, J. S., Lord, S., & Midgley, C. (1991). What are we doing to early adolescents? The impact of educational context on early adolescents. *American Journal of Education, 91,* 521–594.

Eccles, J. S., & Midgley, C. (1989). Stage/environment fit: Developmentally appropriate classrooms for early adolescents. In R. E. Ames & C. Ames (Eds.), *Research on motivation in education* (pp. 139–186). New York: Academic Press.

Ehri, L. C., & Wilce, L. S. (1983). Development of word identification speed in skilled and less-skilled beginning readers. *Journal of Educational Psychology, 75,* 3–18.

Elbaum, B., & Vaughn, S. (2001). School-based interventions to enhance the self-concept of students with learning disabilities: A meat-analysis. *Elementary School Journal, 101,* 303–329.

Ellis, E. S., & Larkin, M. J. (1998). Strategic instruction for adolescents with learning disabilities. In B. Y. L. Wong (Ed.), *Learning about learning disabilities* (pp. 585–656). San Diego, CA: Academic Press.

Epps, S., Ysseldyke, J., & Algozzine, B. (1985). An analysis of the conceptual Framework underlying definitions of learning disabilities. *Journal of School Psychology, 23,* 133–144.

European Dyslexia Association. (1997). *Guidance criteria for training teachers of dyslexic students.* Brussels: Author.

Federal Register. (1977). *The rules and regulations for implementing Public Law 94-142.* Washington, DC: U.S. Government Printing Office.

Felton, R. H., Naylor, C. E., & Wood, F. B. (1990). Neuropsychological profile of adult dyslexics. *Brain and Language, 39,* 485–497.

Finucci, J. M., & Childs, B. (1981). Are there really more dyslexic boys than girls? In A. Ansara, N. Geschwind, A. Galaburda, M. Albert, & N. Gartreli (Eds.), *Sex differences in dyslexia* (pp. 1–9). Baltimore: Orton Dyslexia Society.

Fletcher, J. M. (1985a). External validity of learning disability subtypes. In B. P. Rourke (Ed.), *Neuropsychology of learning disabilities: Essentials of subtype analysis.* (pp. 187–211). New York: Guilford Press.

Fletcher, J. M. (1985b). Memory for verbal and nonverbal stimuli in learning disability subgroups: Analysis by selective reminders. *Journal of Educational Child Psychology, 40,* 244–259.

Fletcher, J. M., Epsy, K. A., Francis, D. J., Davidson, K. C., Rourke, B. P., & Shaywitz, S. E. (1989). Comparison of cutoff score and regression-based definitions of reading disabilities. *Journal of Learning Disabilities, 22,* 334–338.

Fletcher, J. M., Francies, D. J., Rourke, B. P., Shaywitz, S. E., & Shaywitz, B. A. (1992). The validity of discrepancy-based definitions of reading disabilities. *Journal of Learning Disabilities, 25,* 555–561.

Fletcher, J. M., & Morris, R. (1986). Classification of disabled learners: Beyond exclusionary definitions. In S. J. Ceci (Ed.), *Handbook of cognitive, social, and neuropsychological aspects of learning disabilities* (pp. 55–80). Hillsdale, NJ: Erlbaum.

Fletcher, J., Shaywitz, S., Shankweiler, D., Katz, L., Liberman, I., Stuebing, K., et al. (1994). Cognitive profiles of reading disability: Comparisons of discrepancy and low achievement definitions. *Journal of Educational Psychology, 86,* 6–23.

Forgan, J. W., & Vaughn, S. (2000). Adolescents with and without LD make the transition to middle school. *Journal of Learning Disabilities, 33,* 33–43.

Frankenberger, W., & Franzaglio, K. (1991). A review of states' criteria and procedures for identifying children with learning disabilities. *Journal of Learning Disabilities, 24,* 495–500.

Gaddes, H. (1976). Prevalence estimates and the need for the definition of learning disabilities. In R. M. Knights & D. J. Bakker (Eds.), *The neuropsychology of learning disorders: Theoretical approaches* (p. 3024). Baltimore: Baltimore University Park Press.

Gans, A. M., Kenny, M. C., & Ghany, D. L. (2003). Comparing the self concept of students with and without learning disabilities. *Journal of Learning Disabilities, 36,* 287–296.

Gardner, H. (1983). *Frames of mind: The theory of multiple intelligences*. New York: Basic Books.

Garmezy, N. (1983). Stressors in childhood. In N. Garmezy & M. Rutter (Eds.), *Stress, coping and development in children* (pp. 42–84). Minneapolis: McGraw-Hill.

Geary, D. C. (1990). A componential analysis of an early learning deficit in mathematics. *Journal of Experimental Child Psychology, 49*, 363–383.

Geary, D. C. (1993). Mathematical disabilities: Cognitive, neuropsychological, and genetic components. *Psychological Bulletin, 114*, 345–362.

Geary, D. C., Bow-Thomas, C., & Yao, Y. (1992). Counting knowledge and skill in cognitive addition: A comparison of normal and mathematically disabled children. *Journal of Experimental Child Psychology, 54*, 372–391.

Geary, D. C., Brown, S. C., & Samaranayake, V. A. (1991). Cognitive addition: A short longitudinal study of strategy choice and speed-of-processing differences in normal and mathematically disabled children. *Developmental Psychology, 27*, 787–797.

Geary, D. C., Hoard, M. K., & Hamson, C. O. (1999). Numerical and arithmetical cognition: Patterns of functions and deficits in children at risk for a mathematical disability. *Journal of Experimental Child Psychology, 74*, 213–229.

Gersons-Wolfensberger, D. C., & Ruijssenaars, W. A. (1997). Definition and treatment of dyslexia: A report by the Committee on Dyslexia of the Health Council of The Netherlands. *Journal of Learning Disabilities, 30*, 209–213.

Geschwind, N., & Galaburda, A. M. (1985). Cerebral lateralisation, biological mechanism, associations and pathology. II: A Hypothesis and a programme for research. *Archives of Neurology, 42*, 521–552.

Goleman, D. (1995). *Emotional intelligence*. New York: Bantam Books.

Gottardo, A., Siegel, L. S., & Stanovich, K. E. (1997). The assessment of adults with reading disabilities: What can we learn from experimental tasks? *Journal of Research in Reading, 20*, 42–54.

Grande, C. G. (1988). Delinquency: The learning disabled student's reaction to academic school failure. *Adolescence, 23*, 209–219.

Greenberg, D., Ehri, L. C., & Perin, D. (1997). Are word-reading processes the same or different in adult literacy students and third–fifth graders matched for reading level? *Journal of Educational Psychology, 89*, 262–275.

Gregg, N., Hoy, C., King, M., Moreland, C., & Jagota, M. (1992). The MMPI-2 profiles of adults with learning disabilities in university and rehabilitation settings. *Journal of Learning Disabilities, 25*, 386–395.

Hahn, A. (1987). Reaching out to America's dropouts: What to do? *Phi Delta Kappan, 69*, 256–263.

Hammill, D. D. (1990). On defining learning disabilities: An emerging consensus. *Journal of Learning Disabilities, 23*, 74–84.

Hammill, D. D., Leigh, J. E., McNutt, G., & Larsen, S. C. (1981). A new definition of learning disabilities. *Learning Disability Quarterly, 4*, 336–342.

Harnadek, M., & Rourke, B. P. (1994). Principal identifying features of the syndrome of nonverbal learning disabilities. *Journal of Learning Disabilities, 27*, 144–154.

Harter, S., Whitesell, N. R., & Junkin, L. J. (1998). Similarities and differences in domain-specific and global self-evaluations of learning-disabled, behaviorally disordered, and normally achieving adolescents. *American Education Research Journal, 35*, 653–680.

Hinshelwood, J. (1917). *Congenital word-blindness*. London: H.K. Lewis.

Hock, M. F., Pulvers, K. A., Deshler, D. D., & Schumaker, J. B. (2001). The effects of an after-school tutoring program on the academic performance of at-risk students and students with LD. *Remedial and Special Education, 22*, 172–186.

Hogaboam, T. W., & Perfetti, C. A. (1978). Reading skill and their role of verbal experience in decoding. *Journal of Educational Psychology, 5*, 717–729.

Holmes, C. T. (1989). Grade level retention effects: A meta-analysis of research studies. In L. A. Shepard & M. L. Smith (Eds.), *Flunking grades: Research and policies on retention* (pp. 16–63). London: Falmer Press.

Holmes, C. T., & Matthews, K. M. (1984). The effects of nonpromotion on elementary and junior high school pupils: A meta-analysis. *Review of Educational Research, 54*, 225–236.

Hong Kong Disability Discrimination Ordinance. (2002). Hong Kong Government.

Hornsby, B. (1996). *Overcoming dyslexia: A straightforward guide for families and teachers*. London: Vermilion.

Huntington, D. D., & Bender, W. N. (1993). Adolescents with learning disabilities at risk? Emotional well being, depression, suicide. *Journal of Learning Disabilities, 26*, 159–166.

Johnson, D. J., & Mykelbust, H. R. (1967). *Learning disabilities: Education principles and practice*. New York: Grune & Stratton.

Jordan, N. C., & Montani, T. O. (1997). Cognitive arithmetic and problem solving: A comparison of children with specific and general mathematics difficulties. *Journal of Learning Disabilities, 30*, 624–635.

Jorm, A. F. (1981). Children with reading and spelling retardation. Functioning of whole-word and correspondence rule mechanisms. *Journal of Child Psychology and Psychiatry, 22*, 171–178.

Karlsen, B., & Gardner, E. F. (1995). *Stanford Diagnostic Reading Test* (4th ed.). New York: Harcourt Brace.

Kavale, K. A., & Forness, S. R. (2000). What definition of learning disability say and don't say. *Journal of Learning Disabilities, 33*, 239–256.

Kavale, K., & Nye, C. (1981). Identification criteria for learning disabilities: A survey of the research literature. *Learning Disability Quarterly, 4*, 383–388.

Keates, A. (2000). *Dyslexia and information and communications technology: A guide for teachers and parents.* London: David Fulton.

Keilitz, I., & Dunivant, N. (1986). The relationship between learning disability and juvenile delinquency: Current state of knowledge. *Remedial and Special Education, 7,* 18–26.

Keogh, B. K. (1986). Future of the LD field: Research and practice. *Journal of Learning Disabilities, 19,* 455–460.

Keogh, B. K. (1987). Learning disabilities: In defense of a construct. *Learning Disabilities Research, 3,* 4–9.

Kinsbourne, M., & Warrington, E. K. (1963). The developmental Gerstmann Syndrome. *Archives of Neurology, 8,* 490–501.

Kirk, S. A. (1966). *The diagnosis and remediation of psycholinguistic disabilities.* Chicago: University of Illinois.

Klove, H. (1963). Clinical neuropsychology. In F. M. Forster (Ed.), *The medical clinics of North America.* New York: Saunders.

Kosc, L. (1974). Developmental dyscalculia. *Journal of Learning Disabilities, 7,* 164–177.

Larrabee, D. G. (1984). Setting the standard: Alternative policies for student promotion. *Harvard Educational Review, 54,* 67–87.

Lazear, D. (1994). *Multiple intelligence approaches to assessment.* Tucson, AZ: Zephyr Press.

Lennox, C., & Siegel, L. S. (1993). Visual and phonological spelling errors in subtypes of children with learning disabilities. *Applied Psycholinguistics, 14,* 473–488.

Lennox, C., & Siegel, L. S. (1996). The development of phonological rules and visual strategies in average and poor spellers. *Journal of Experimental Child Psychology, 62,* 60–83.

Levin, E., Zigmond, N., & Birch, J. (1985). A follow-up study of 52 learning disabled adolescents. *Journal of Learning Disabilities, 18,* 2–7.

Levine, M. D., Oberklaid, F., & Meltzer, L. (1981). Developmental output failure: A study of low productivity in school-aged children. *Pediatrics, 67,* 18–25.

Lichtenstein, S. A. (1987). *A study of the post-school employment patterns of handicapped and nonhandicapped graduates and dropouts.* Unpublished doctoral dissertation, University of Illinois at Champaign-Urbana.

Lichtenstein, S., & Zantol-Wiener, K. (1988). *Special education dropouts* (Eric Digest No. 451). Reston, VA: ERIC Clearinghouse on Handicapped and Gifted Children. (ERIC Documentation Service No. ED 295 395)

Lovett, M. W., Steinbach, K. A., & Frijters, J. C. (2000). Remediating the core deficits of developmental reading disability: A double-deficit perspective. *Journal of Learning Disabilities, 33,* 334–358.

Lyon, G. R. (1995). Research initiatives in learning disabilities: Contributions from scientists supported by the National Institute of Child Health and Human Development. *Journal of Child Neurology, 10,* 120–126.

Lyon, G. R. (1996). Learning disabilities. *The Future of Children: Special Education for Students with Disabilities, 6,* 54–76.

Maag, J. W., & Behrens, J. T. (1989). Depression and cognitive self-statements of learning disabled and seriously emotionally disturbed adolescents. *Journal of Special Education, 23,* 17–27.

Mackay, N. (2001). Whole school approach—special section. In I. Smythe (Ed.), *The dyslexia handbook 2001.* Reading, UK: British Dyslexia Association.

Malmgrem, K., Abbott, R. D., & Hawkins, J. D. (1999). LD and delinquency: Rethinking the "link." *Journal of Learning Disabilities, 32,* 194–200.

Manis, F. R., Doi, L. M., & Bhadha, B. (2000). Naming speed, phonological awareness, and orthographic knowledge in second graders. *Journal of Learning Disabilities, 33,* 325–333.

Marr, M. B., & Gormley, K. (1982). Children's recall familiar and unfamiliar text. *Reading Research Quarterly, 18,* 89–104.

McBride, H., & Siegel, L. S. (1997). Learning disabilities and adolescent suicide. *Journal of Learning Disabilities, 30,* 652–659.

McKinney, J. D., Short, E. J., & Feagans, L. (1985). Academic consequences of perceptual–linguistic subtypes of learning disabled children. *Learning Disabilities Research, 1,* 6–17.

McLeskey, J., & Grizzle, K. L. (1992). Grade retention rates among students with learning disabilities. *Exceptional Children, 58,* 548–554.

Mercer, C. D., Jordan, L., Allsop, D. H., & Mercer, A. R. (1996). Learning disabilities definitions and criteria used by state education departments. *Learning Disability Quarterly, 19,* 217–232.

Miner, M., & Siegel, L. (1992). William Butler Yeats: Dyslexic? *Journal of Learning Disabilities, 25,* 372–375.

Montague, M. (1997). Cognitive strategy instruction in mathematics for students with learning disabilities. *Journal of Learning Disabilities, 30,* 164–177.

Morrison, S. R., & Siegel, L. S. (1991). Arithmetic disability: Theoretical considerations and empirical evidence for this subtype. In L. V. Feagans, E. J. Short, & L. Meltzer (Eds.). *Subtypes of learning disabilities: Theoretical perspectives and research* (pp. 189–208). Hillsdale, NJ: Erlbaum.

Murray, C. A. (1976). *The link between learning disabilities and juvenile delinquency: Current theory and knowledge.* Washington, DC: U.S. Government Printing Office.

Naiden, N. (1976). Ratio of boys to girls among disabled readers. *The Reading Teacher, 29,* 439–442.

National Center for Education Statistics. (1993). *Adult Literacy in America.* Washington, DC: Office of Educational Research and Improvement, U.S. Department of Education.

National Center for Education Statistics. (1997). *Profiles of Students with disabilities as identified in NELS: 88.* Washington, DC: Office of Educational

Research and Improvement, U.S. Department of Education.

National Center for Education Statistics. (1999). *Digest of education statistics*. Washington, DC: U.S. Department of Education.

National Joint Committee on Learning Disabilities. (1981). *Learning disabilities: Issues on definition*. Unpublished manuscript. (Available from the Orton Dyslexia Society, 724 York Road, Baltimore, MD 21204) (ERIC Document Service Reproduction No. ED 235 639)

Navarrete, L. A. (1999). Melancholy in the millennium: A study of depression among adolescents with and without learning disabilities. *High School Journal, 82,* 137–149.

O'Malley, K. J., Francis, D. J., Foorman, B. R., Fletcher, J. M., & Swank, P. R. (2002). Growth in precursor and reading-related skills: Do low-achieving and IQ-discrepant readers develop differently? *Learning Disabilities Research and Practice, 17,* 19–34.

Ostler, C., & Ward, F. (2002). *Advanced study skills*. Wakefield, UK: SEN Marketing.

Ott, P. (1997). *How to manage and detect dyslexia*. London: Heinemann.

Padget, S. Y., Knight, D. F., & Sawyer, D. J. (1996). Tennessee meets the challenge of dyslexia. *Annals of Dyslexia, 46,* 51–72.

Passolunghi, M. C., & Siegel, L. S. (2001). Short-term memory, working memory, and inhibitory control in children with difficulties in arithmetic problem solving. *Journal of Experimental Child Psychology, 80,* 44–57.

Peer, L., & Reid, G. (2001). *Dyslexia—Successful inclusion in the secondary school*. London: Fulton.

Pennington, B. F., Van Orden, G. C., Smith, S. D., Green, P. A., & Haith, M. M. (1990). Phonological processing skills and deficits in adult dyslexics. *Child Development, 61,* 1753–1778.

Peplau, L. A., & Perlman, D. (1982). Perspectives on loneliness. In L. A. Peplau & D. Perlman (Eds.), *Loneliness: A sourcebook of current theory, research and therapy* (pp. 1–18). New York: Wiley.

Perlmutter, B. F., & Parus, M. V. (1986). Identifying children with learning disabilities: A comparison of diagnostic procedures across school district. *Learning Disability Quarterly, 6,* 321–328.

Piers, E. V. (1994). *Revised manual for Piers–Harris children's Self-Concept Scale*. Los Angeles: Western Psychological Services.

Pratt, A. C., & Brady, S. (1988). Relations of phonological awareness to reading disability in children and adults. *Journal of Educational Psychology, 80,* 319–323.

Pringle-Morgan, W. (1896). A case study of congenital word blindness. *British Medical Journal, 2,* 1378.

Rack, J. P., Snowling, M., & Olson, R. (1992). The nonword reading deficit in developmental dyslexia: A review. *Reading Research Quarterly, 27,* 28–53.

Rayner, K., Foorman, B. R., Perfetti, C. A., Pesetsky, D., & Seidenberg, M. S. (2001). How psychological science informs the teaching of reading. *Psychological Science in the Public Interest, 2,* 31–74.

Read, C., & Ruyter, L. (1985). Reading and spelling skills in adults of low literacy. *Remedial and Special Education, 6,* 43–52.

Reitan, R. M., & Davidson, L. A. (1974). *Clinical neuropsychology: Current status and applications*. Washington, DC: Winston & Sons.

Rivers, D., & Smith, T. E. C. (1988). Traditional eligibility criteria for identifying students as specific learning disabled. *Journal of Learning Disabilities, 10,* 642–644.

Rourke, B. P. (1982). Central processing deficiencies in children: Toward a developmental neuropsychological model. *Journal of Clinical Neuropsychology, 4,* 1–18.

Rourke, B. P. (1983). Outstanding issues in learning disabilities research. In M. Rutter (Ed.), *Developmental neuropsychiatry* (pp. 1–25). New York: Guilford Press.

Rourke, B. P. (1985). *Neuropsychology of learning disabilities: Essentials of subtype analysis*. New York: Guilford Press.

Rourke, B. P. (1987). Syndrome of nonverbal learning disabilities: The final common pathway of white-matter disease/dysfunction? *Clinical Neuropsychologist, 1,* 209–234.

Rourke, B. P. (1991). Validation of learning disabilities subtypes: An overview. In B. P. Rourke (Ed.), *Neuropsychological validation of learning disability subtypes* (pp. 3–11). New York: Guilford Press.

Rourke, B. P., Del Dotto, J. E., Rourke, S. B., & Casey, J. E. (1990). Nonverbal learning disabilities: The syndrome and a case study. *Journal of School Psychology, 28,* 361–385.

Rourke, B. P., & Finlayson, M. A. J. (1978). Neuropsychological significance of variations in patterns of academic performance: Verbal and visual–spatial abilities. *Journal of Abnormal Child Psychology, 6,* 121–133.

Rourke, B. P., & Fisk, J. L. (1988). Subtypes of learning-disabled children: Implications for a neurodevelopmental model of differential hemispheric processing. In D. L. Molfese & S. J. Segalowitz (Eds.), *Brain lateralization in children: Developmental implications* (pp. 547–566). New York: Guilford Press.

Rourke, B. P., & Strang, J. D. (1978). Neuropsychological significance of variations in patterns of academic performance: Motor, psychomotor, and tactile–perceptual abilities. *Journal of Pediatric Psychology, 2,* 62–66.

Rourke, B. P., & Tsatsanis, K. D. (1996). Syndrome of nonverbal learning disabilities: Psycholinguistic assets and deficits. *Topics in Language Disorders, 16,* 30–34.

Russell, G. (1982). Impairment of phonetic reading in dyslexia and its persistence beyond childhood—Research note. *Journal of Child Psychology and Psychiatry, 23,* 459–475.

Russell, R. L., & Ginsburg, H. P. (1984). Cognitive

analysis of children's mathematics difficulties. *Cognition and Instruction, 1,* 217–244.

Sabornie, E. J. (1994). Social–affective characteristics in early adolescents identified as learning disabled and nondisabled. *Learning Disabilities Quarterly, 17,* 268–279.

Scarborough, H. (1984). Continuity between childhood dyslexia and adult reading. *British Journal of Psychology, 75,* 329–348.

Schatschneider, C., Carlson, C. D., Francis, D. J., Foorman, B. R., & Fletcher, J. M. (2002). Relationship of rapid automatized naming and phonological awareness in early reading development: Implications for the double-deficit hypothesis. *Journal of Learning Disabilities, 35,* 245–256.

Schumaker, J. B., & Deshler, D. D. (1992). Validation of learning strategy interventions for students with learning disabilities: Results of a programmatic research effort. In B. Y. L. Wong (Ed.), *Contemporary intervention research in learning disabilities: An international perspective* (pp. 22–46). New York: Springer-Verlag.

Schwartz, W. (1995). *New information on youth who drop out: Why they leave and what happens to them. For parents/about parents.* Washington, DC: U.S. Department of Education. Office of Educational Research and Improvement. (ERIC document Reproduction Service No. ED 396006)

Shafrir, U., & Siegel, L. S. (1994a). Preference for visual scanning strategies versus phonological rehearsal in university students with reading disabilities. *Journal of Learning Disabilities, 27,* 583–588.

Shafrir, U., & Siegel, L. S. (1994b). Subtypes of learning disabilities in adolescents and adults. *Journal of Learning Disabilities, 27,* 123–134.

Share, D. L., McGee, R. O., McKenzie, D., Williams, S. M., & Silva, P. A. (1987). Further evidence relating to the distinction between specific reading retardation and general reading backwardness. *British Journal of Developmental Psychology, 5,* 35–44.

Share, D. L., Moffitt, T. E., & Silva, P. A. (1988). Factors associated with arithmetic-and-reading disability and specific arithmetic disability. *Journal of Learning Disabilities, 21,* 313–321.

Share, D. L., & Silva, P. A. (2003). Gender bias in IQ-discrepancy and post-discrepancy definitions of reading disability. *Journal of Learning Disabilities, 26,* 4–14.

Shaywitz, S. E., Pugh, K. R., Jenner, A. R., Flubright, R. K., Fletcher, J. M., Gore, J. C., & Shaywitz, B. A. (2000). The neurobiology of reading and reading disability (dyslexia). In M. L. Kamil, P. B. Mosenthal, P. D. Pearson, & R. Barr (Eds.), *Handbook of reading research* (Vol. III, pp. 229–249). Mahwah, NJ: Erlbaum.

Shaywitz, S. E., Shaywitz, B. A., Fletcher, J. M., & Escobar, M. D. (1990). Prevalence of reading disability in boys and girls. *Journal of the American Medical Association, 264,* 998–1002.

Shaywitz, S. E., Shaywitz, B. A., Flubright, R. K.,

Skudlarski, P., Mencl, W. E., Constable, R. T., et al. (2003). Neural systems for compensation and persistence: Young adult outcome of childhood reading disability. *Biological Psychiatry, 54,* 23–33.

Shepard, L. A., & Smith, M. L. (1989). *Flunking grades: Research and policies on retention.* London: Falmer Press.

Siegel, L. S. (1985). Psycholinguistic aspects of reading disabilities. In L. S. Siegel & F. J. Morrison (Eds.), *Cognitive development in atypical children* (pp. 45–66). New York: Springer-Verlag.

Siegel, L. S. (1988a). Definitional and theoretical issues and research on learning disabilities. *Journal of Learning Disabilities, 21,* 264–270.

Siegel, L. S. (1988b). Evidence that IQ scores are irrelevant to the definition and analysis of reading disability. *Canadian Journal of Psychology, 42,* 202–215.

Siegel, L. S. (1989). IQ is irrelevant to the definition of learning disability. *Journal of Learning Disabilities, 22,* 469–478.

Siegel, L. S. (1990). IQ and learning disabilities: R. I. P. In H. L. Swanson & B. Keogh (Eds.), *Learning disabilities: Theoretical and research issues* (pp. 111–128). Hillsdale, NJ: Erlbaum.

Siegel, L. S. (1992). An evaluation of the discrepancy definition of dyslexia. *Journal of Learning Disabilities, 25,* 618–629.

Siegel, L. S. (1993a). Alice in IQ land or why IQ is still irrelevant to learning disabilities. In R. M. Joshi & C. K. Leong (Eds.), *Reading disabilities: Diagnosis and component processes* (pp. 71–84). Dordrecht, The Netherlands: Kluwer.

Siegel, L. S. (1993b). Phonological processing deficits as the basis of a reading disability. *Developmental Review, 13,* 246–257.

Siegel, L. S. (1998). Phonological processing deficits and reading disabilities. In L. Ehri & J. Metsala (Eds.), *Word recognition in beginning literacy* (pp. 141–160). Mahwah, NJ: Erlbaum.

Siegel, L. S. (1999). Issues in the definition and diagnosis of learning disabilities: A perspective on *Guckenberger v. Boston University. Journal of Learning Disabilities, 32,* 304–319.

Siegel, L. S., & Feldman, W. (1983). Non-dyslexic children with combined writing and arithmetic difficulties. *Clinical Pediatrics, 22,* 241–244.

Siegel, L. S., & Heaven, R. (1986). Categorization of learning disabilities. In S. J. Ceci (Ed.), *Handbook of cognitive, social, and neuropsychological aspects of learning disabilities* (Vol. 1, pp. 95–121). Hillsdale, NJ: Erlbaum.

Siegel, L. S., & Linder, B. A. (1984). Short-term memory process in children with reading and arithmetic learning disabilities. *Developmental Psychology, 20,* 200–207.

Siegel, L. S., & Ryan, E. B. (1984). Reading disability as a language disorder. *Remedial and Special Education, 5,* 28–33.

Siegel. L. S., & Ryan, E. B. (1988). Development of grammatical-sensitivity, phonological, and short-term memory skills in normally achieving and learning disabled children. *Developmental Psychology, 24,* 28–37.

Siegel, L. S., & Ryan, E. B. (1989a). The development of working memory in normally achieving and subtypes of learning disabled children. *Child Development, 60,* 973–980.

Smythe, I., & Siegel, L. S. (2004). Assessment of the dyslexic adult: A framework for Europe. In I. Smythe (Ed.), *Provision and use of information technology with adult dyslexic students in university in Europe.* Cardiff: WDP.

Snowling, M. J. (1980). The development of grapheme–phoneme correspondence in normal and dyslexic readers. *Journal of Experimental Child Psychology, 29,* 294–305.

Spellacy, F., & Peter, B. (1978). Dyscalculia and elements of the developmental Gerstmann Syndrome in school children. *Cortex, 14,*197–206.

Stanovich, K. E. (1986). Matthew effects in reading: Some consequences of individual differences in the acquisition of literacy. *Reading Research Quarterly, 21,* 360–407.

Stanovich, K. E. (1988a). The dyslexic and the garden-variety poor reader: The phonological–core variable difference model. *Journal of Learning Disabilities, 21,* 590–604.

Stanovich, K. E. (1988b). Explaining the differences between the dyslexic and garden variety poor reader: The phonological–core variance–difference model. *Journal of Learning Disabilities, 21,* 590–604, 612.

Stanovich, K. E. (1988c). The right and wrong places to look for the cognitive locus of reading disability. *Annals of Dyslexia, 38,* 154–177.

Stanovich, K. E. (1989). Has the learning disabilities field lost its intelligence? *Journal of Learning Disabilities, 22,* 487–492.

Stanovich, K. E. (1993). The construct validity of discrepancy definitions of reading disability. In G. R. Lyon, D. B. Gray, J. F. Kavanagh, & N. A. Krasemgor (Eds.), *Better understanding learning disabilities.* Baltimore: Brookes.

Strang, J. D., & Rourke, B. P. (1983). Concept-formation/non-verbal reasoning abilities of children who exhibit specific academic problems with arithmetic. *Journal of Clinical Child Psychology, 12,* 33–39.

Sunseth, K., & Bowers, P. G. (2002). Rapid naming and phonemic awareness: Contributions to reading, spelling and orthographic knowledge. *Scientific Studies of Reading, 6,* 401–429.

Svensson, I., Jacobson, C., Björkman, R., & Sandell, A. (2002). *Kan man ha kompensatoriska hjälpmedel för yngre skolbarn? [Can young pupils benefit from using compensatory ICT].* Retrieved May 2004, from http://www.fmls.nu/sprakaloss/jacobssonhjalpmedel.htm

Swanson, H. L. (1993). Individual differences in working memory: A model testing and subgroup analysis of learning-disabled and skilled readers. *Intelligence, 17,* 285–332.

Swanson, H. L. (1994). Short-term memory and working memory: Do both contribute to our understanding of academic achievement in children and adults with learning disabilities? *Journal of Learning Disabilities, 27,* 34–50.

Swanson, H. L., & Cooney, J. B. (1996). Learning disabilities and memory. In K. D. Redi, W. P. Hresko, & H. L. Swanson (Eds.), *Cognitive approaches to learning disabilities* (pp. 287–314). Austin, TX: Pro-ed.

Swanson, H. L., & Deshler, D. (2003). Instructing adolescents with learning disabilities: Converting a meta-analysis to practice. *Journal of Learning Disabilities, 36,* 124–135.

Swanson, H. L., & Hoskyn, M. (2001). Instructing adolescents with learning disabilities: A component and composite analysis. *Learning Disabilities Research and Practice, 16,* 109–119.

Tal, N. F., & Siegel, L. S. (1996). Pseudowords reading errors of poor, dyslexic and normally achieving readers on multi-syllable pseudowords. *Applied Psycholinguistics, 17,* 215–232.

Tallal, P., Ross, R., & Curtiss, S. (1989). Unexpected gender ratios in families of language/learning-impaired children. *Neuropsychologia, 27,* 987–998.

Torgesen, J. K. Wagner, R. K., & Rashotte, C. A., Alexander, A. W., & Conway, T. (1997). Preventive and remedial interventions for children with severe reading disabilities. *Learning Disabilities: A Multidisciplinary Journal, 8,* 51–61.

UNESCO. (1994). *The Salamanca statement and framework for action.* Paris: Author.

Vail, P. (1990). Gifts, talents, and the dyslexias: Wellsprings, Springboards and finding Foley's rocks. *Annals of Dyslexia, 40,* 3–17.

Van der Wissel, A., & Zegers, F. C. (1985). Reading retardation revisited. *British Journal of Developmental Psychology, 44,* 1–12.

Vellutino, F. R. (1978). Toward an understanding of dyslexia: Psychological factors in specific reading disability. In A. L. Benton & D. Pearl (Eds.), *Dyslexia: An appraisal of current knowledge* (pp. 61–112). New York: Oxford University Press.

Vellutino, F. R. (1979). *Dyslexia theory and research.* Cambridge, MA: MIT Press.

Vellutino, F. R., Scanlon, D. M., & Lyon, G. R. (2000). Differentiating between difficult-to-remediate and readily remediated poor readers: More evidence against the IQ–achievement discrepancy definition of reading disability. *Journal of Learning Disabilities, 33,* 223–238.

Vellutino, F. R., Scanlon, M., & Sipay, E. R. (1996). Cognitive profiles of difficult-to-remediate and readily remediated poor readers: Early intervention as a vehicle for distinguishing between cognitive and experiential deficits as basic causes of specific reading disability. *Journal of Educational Psychology, 88,* 601–638.

Venezky, R. L., & Johnson, D. (1973). Development of two letter-sound patterns in grades one through three. *Journal of Educational Psychology, 64,* 109–115.

Vogel, A. (1990). Gender differences in intelligence, language, visual–motor abilities, and academic achievement in males and females with learning disabilities: A review of the literature. *Journal of Learning Disabilities, 23,* 44–52.

Vukovic, R. K., Lesaux, N. K., & Siegel, L. S. (in press). *The double-deficit hypothesis: A critical analysis of the evidence.* Manuscript submitted for publication.

Wadsworth, S. J., DeFries, J. C., Stevenson, J., Gilger, J. W., & Pennington, B. F. (1992). Gender ratios among reading-disabled children and their siblings as a function of parental impairment. *Journal of Child Psychology and Psychiatry, 33,* 1229–1239.

Waldie, K., & Spreen, O. (1993). The relationship between learning disabilities and persisting delinquency. *Journal of Learning Disabilities, 6,* 417–423.

Waters, G. S., Bruck, M., & Seidenberg, M. (1985). Do children use similar processes to read and spell words? *Journal of Experimental Child Psychology, 39,* 511–530.

Webster, R. E. (1979). Visual and aural short-term memory capacity deficits in mathematics disabled students. *Journal of Educational Research, 72,* 272–283.

Werker, J. F., Bryson, S. E., & Wassenberg, K. (1989). Toward understanding the problem in severely disabled readers. Part II: Consonant errors. *Applied Psycholinguistics, 10,* 13–30.

Wiener, J., & Schneider, B. H. (2002). A multisource exploration of the friendship patterns of children with and without learning disabilities. *Journal of Abnormal Child Psychology, 30,* 127–141.

Wiener, J., & Sunohara, G. (1998). Parents' perception of the quality of friendship of their children with learning disabilities. *Learning Disabilities Research and Practice, 13,* 242–257.

Wiig, E. H., & Harris, S. P. (1974). Perception and interpretation of non-verbally expressed emotions by adolescents with learning disabilities. *Perceptual and Motor Skills, 38,* 239–245.

Wilkinson, G. S. (1993). *The Wide Range Achievement Test—3.* Wilmington, DE: Jastak Associates.

Wilson, K. M., & Swanson, H. L. (2001). Are mathematics disability due to a domain-general or a domain-specific working memory deficit? *Journal of Learning Disabilities, 34,* 237–248.

Wolf, M., & Bowers, P. G. (1999). The double-deficit hypothesis for the developmental dyslexias. *Journal of Educational Psychology, 91,* 415–438.

Wolf, M., O'Rourke, A. G., Gidney, C., Lovett, M., Cirino, P., & Morris, R. (2002). The second deficit: An investigation of the independence of phonological and naming-speed deficits in developmental dyslexia. *Reading and Writing: An Interdisciplinary Journal, 15,* 43–72.

Wong, B. (1986). Problems and issues in the definitions of learning disabilities. In J. K. Torgesen & B. Wong (Eds.), *Psychological and educational perspectives on learning disabilities* (pp. 3–26). New York: Academic Press.

Woodcock, R., McGrew, K., & Mather, N. (2001). *Woodcock–Johnson III.* Itasca, IL: Riverside.

12

Autism Spectrum Disorders

Steven G. Spector
Fred R. Volkmar

The interest in adolescents with autism began as the children, first described by Kanner in 1943, were followed by him over time. In 1971, Kanner noted the considerable variability in adolescent outcome. Although knowledge about autism and related conditions has increased dramatically in recent years comparatively much less has been written on these conditions as they are expressed in adolescents and, in some respects, we have not advanced tremendously since Kanner's 1971 follow-up.

Searches of standard databases yield about 6,500 articles on autism or related conditions published from 1943 to 2003; of these, perhaps 200 have focused on adolescents. Much of the available information is in the form of case reports—for example, follow-up studies of individuals first seen as children (e.g., Kanner, 1971; Sperry, 2001; Tantam, 2000a; Wolf & Goldberg, 1986). Furthermore, much of the available group data on developmental aspects of autism and related conditions is cross-sectional in nature. This poses difficulties for several reasons (e.g., there have been changes in diagnostic practices; Fombonne, 2001), and as criteria for autism have become somewhat less restrictive it is quite possible that what seems to be an apparent improvement in ado-

lescent outcome might really be a function of broadened definitions. Yet another problem with interpreting the cross-sectional data is that with the increased focus on early detection and intervention (National Research Council, 2001) there likely has been improved long-term outcome (Howlin, 2000). Again what might at first blush appear to be developmental changes in cross-sectional data may actually be the result of earlier detection and more effective interventions.

An additional obstacle for studies of adolescents with autistic disorder is that current diagnostic approaches, particularly categorical ones such as DSM-IV-TR (American Psychiatric Association [APA], 2000), may include or emphasize early history and development (i.e., for diagnostic purposes historical information rather than contemporaneous examination has been more important); this tends, in turn, to focus research on younger groups. To some extent this is less of an issue when using dimensionally based diagnostic approaches such as the Childhood Autism Rating Scale (CARS), although even for these the issue of how early development and developmental change are addressed can be a challenge (Lord & Corsello, 2005). For example, using the

CARS (Schopler, Reichler, DeVellis, & Daly, 1980), Mesibov and colleagues reported that, in general, levels of symptoms decreased as individuals became older (Mesibov, Schopler, & Caison, 1989). On the other hand it is clear that in some cases behavior does significantly worsen (e.g., with the onset of seizure disorder; Volkmar & Nelson, 1990).

The absence of a large body of work on autism in adolescence also results from earlier, sometimes continuing, diagnostic controversies. For example, autism was not officially recognized as a diagnostic category until 1980 (American Psychiatric Association, 1980). In addition, much of the more recent work has focused on younger children, and when adolescents are included in studies their responses may not be reported apart from other age groups. This is particularly unfortunate as information on life course may inform research, clinical work, and social policy (Schroeder, LeBlanc, & Mayo, 1996) and there is some suggestion of important developmental changes in response to such treatments as, for example, drug therapy (Martin, Koenig, Anderson, & Scahill, 2003).

This situation is now starting to change as interest in both adolescents and adults with autism spectrum disorders has increased following growing public awareness and better methods of diagnosis and detection. In this chapter we review information on diagnosis, associated features, epidemiology, assessment, and treatment with autism and related areas; we note some areas of agreement and many areas in which knowledge is lacking. Given the importance of issues of diagnosis and definition it is appropriate to begin the chapter with a discussion of relevant diagnostic concepts.

DIAGNOSTIC CONCEPTS AND CRITERIA

Autism and related disorders—officially referred to as the pervasive developmental disorders (PDDs) in DSM-IV-TR (APA, 2000) and unofficially as autism spectrum disorders (ASDs)—are a group of conditions characterized by difficulties in social interaction and communication and behavioral difficulties (Volkmar, Klin, & Cohen, 1997). Of these conditions autism is far and away the best known and most intensively studied, although information on related conditions such as Asperger disorder has increased dramatically in recent

years. Information on natural history, particularly follow-up into adolescence and adulthood, has been helpful in clarifying important aspects of developmental change in syndrome expression and will be discussed shortly.

Autistic Disorder

Any discussion of autistic disorder rightly begins with Kanner's (1943) classic initial description of 11 children "whose condition differ(ed) so markedly and uniquely" (p. 217) from other childhood disorders known at the time. Kanner used the term "autism" to describe the unusual self-centered quality exhibited by his first cases and emphasized that disordered social development was an essential feature of the condition. However, some aspects of Kanner's report proved misleading. For example, his initial report emphasized the very high levels of parental education and professional achievement in his original 11 cases; this, in part, led to much of the speculation in the 1950s and 1960s that psychological factors (i.e., poor parenting) might contribute to autism. It is now clear that a bias in case ascertainment accounted for the unusual levels of achievement seen in the parents of his first cases (Fombonne, 2003a; Wing, 1980). As children with autism were followed, various factors, including the high rate of seizure disorder, suggested that it was the brain of the child that was the locus of disorder (Volkmar & Nelson, 1990). Kanner's use of the word "autism" also suggested some potential overlap with schizophrenia and much of the research work conducted until the late 1970s assumed some basic continuity between autism and schizophrenia, which we no longer believe exists (Kolvin, 1971; Rutter, 1972). The available evidence supports the notion that adolescents and young adults with autism are not more likely than the general population to develop schizophrenia (Volkmar & Cohen, 1991).

In 1978, Rutter provided a new definition of autism that synthesized Kanner's original report and subsequent research; it emphasized the early onset of the condition (in the first years of life) and the centrality of social and language/communication problems (not solely due to any associated mental retardation) associated with unusual behavioral rigidity and "insistence on sameness" of the type described by Kanner. This definition was clear, practical, and highly influential in the decision to include autism in DSM-III (APA, 1987) where it was given official status for the first time (Volkmar et al., 1997) as a separate diagnostic category. The initial (DSM-III) definition focused very much on the *infantile* form of the disorder (i.e., criteria were proposed but most applicable to young children); a term "residual infantile autism" was available to describe the persistent difficulties of adolescents and adults with the disorder. The attempt to make the criteria more developmentally appropriate to adolescents and adults in DSM-III-R (APA, 1987) met with limited success and a major revision was undertaken for DSM-IV.

The current definition (DSM-IV-TR; APA, 2000) was derived based on a large body of empirical data; core symptoms are described in three critical areas: social development; communication and symbolic play; and restricted, repetitive, and stereotyped patterns of activity. This definition was developed based on a large, international field trial (Volkmar et al., 1994) with nearly 1,000 cases (including 144 children between the ages of 10 and 15 and 74 between the ages of 15 and 20 years as well as 95 adults) from over 20 sites around the world. Several considerations guided the final development of the final DSM-IV-TR definition—for example, that the criteria provided work well across both age and developmental level and that, if at all possible, there should be convergence with the definition then being developed for ICD-10 (World Health Organization, 1994).

Many potential criteria were evaluated before the final definition was produced. It is of interest that, as would be expected, criteria sometimes had strong developmental correlates (e.g., attachment to unusual objects was highly predictive of autism in younger children but not in adolescents or adults). Conversely, some criteria (e.g., those related to impaired conversational skills) are clearly more applicable to older individuals. Cross-sectional data with adolescents and young adults have, in general, suggested a general trend toward lower levels of symptom severity in adolescents (e.g., Boelte, Dickhut, & Poustka, 1999; Gilchrist et al., 2001; Piven, Harper, Palmter, & Arndt, 1996), although this is not a universal finding. For example, Gillberg and Steffenberg (1987) reported that puberty was associated with increased psychiatric and behavioral difficulties. In one recent study employing a very large sample Seltzer and colleagues (2003) used a structured diagnostic interview "keyed" to DSM-IV diagnostic criteria (Le Couteur et al., 1989) to assess patterns of symptomatology in adolescents and adults; they found that adolescents were more likely to improve in terms of symptom severity in the social domain while adults showed continued improvement in the area of restricted interests/unusual behaviors.

As Seltzer and colleagues (2003) note, various factors might account for differences in symptom presentation over the lifespan as well as the variability in cross-sectional studies. The issues posed by changes in diagnostic criteria and the inherent limitations of cross-sectional approaches have already been noted. Given that autism is a disorder of very early onset, maturational factors and development are presumed to interact with the basic core difficulties of autism and to have an impact on the acquisition of specific skills (Burack, Charman, Yirmiya, & Zelazo, 2001). This may, in part, account for some of the extreme variability of presentation in terms of cognitive and neuropsychological functioning seen in adolescents with the disorder (Klin et al., 1997).

Related Conditions

In addition to autism, several related conditions are now officially recognized in DSM-IV-TR; these include Asperger disorder (AD), Rett's disorder (RD), and childhood disintegrative disorder (CDD) as well the rather poorly defined "subthreshold" condition of pervasive developmental disorder not otherwise specified (PDD-NOS) or atypical autism. Given the recent recognition of these conditions, it is not surprising that information on adolescents with these conditions is not as extensive as that for strictly defined autism.

AD is a condition characterized by marked social problems (of the same type seen in autism) but with relatively good verbal abilities, motor difficulties, and unusual circumscribed interests. This condition was first described by Asperger (1944), who termed it "autistic psychopathy" (perhaps better translated as autistic personality disorder); like Kanner, he used the word "autism" to describe the unusual self-centered quality of social interaction. Interest in this condition was piqued in the 1980s by Wing's (1981) influential paper and the condition was eventually included in DSM-IV (APA, 1994), although its definition and relationship to autism remains controversial and the DSM-

IV definition problematic (Miller & Ozonoff, 1997).

A small body of work on adolescents with AD has appeared. In general, the suggestion is that those with AD have higher levels of cognitive and adaptive functioning but with persistent social difficulties and increased risk for certain psychiatric disorders, notably depression (Gilchrist et al., 2001; Tantam, 2000b, 2003). Several authors have noted unusual profiles on psychological testing often consistent with the nonverbal learning disability profile elaborated on by Rourke (Klin, Volkmar, Sparrow, Cicchetti, & Rourke, 1995; Rourke, 1989; Rourke & Tsatsanis, 2000). Although the data are limited, there is some suggestion that adolescents and young adults are at increased risk for difficulties with the law due to inappropriate behavior such as violence or social eccentricity (Baron-Cohen, 1988) and possibly for increased risk of developing psychosis (Klin, Volkmar, & Sparrow, 2000).

RD was described in 1966 by Rett who noted an unusual profile, in girls, of stereotyped hand movements, autistic behavior, deceleration of head growth, and a general decline in cognitive abilities (Rett, 1966). The condition was grouped with autism in DSM-IV because of the potential, at least briefly, for confusion with autism. Subsequent to its inclusion a gene, which appears to account for many cases of the disorder, has been identified. Adolescents with this condition are severely mentally retarded, have marked problems in movement and breathing, and have much worse outcomes than individuals with autism. Diagnostic criteria for the disorder focus on the initial manifestation of the condition, but the generally severe deterioration is well documented (Van Acker, 1997).

CDD was first described by Heller nearly 100 years ago; in this rare condition children develop normally for several years (usually 3 or 4) prior to marked developmental deterioration and the onset of what would, apart from the unusually late onset, be recognized as autism (Volkmar, 1997). The condition is quite rare; the main rational for its inclusion in DSM-IV has to do with its potential importance relative to research (e.g., in the search for genes that might then also be relevant to autism). The limited follow-up information available strongly suggests that outcome is worse than that for autism; most adolescents with the condition regain, at most, a limited capacity for speech (having once been fluent speakers) (Volkmar, 1997).

The most common, but least studied, is PDD-NOS (synonymous terms include atypical autism, atypical PDD, or PDD unspecified). Children with this condition fall short of meeting full criteria for autism or some other explicitly defined PDD and probably are two to three times more common than children who meet criteria for autism (Fombonne, 2003a, 2003b). The very limited available data suggest that long-term outcome, including in adolescence, is significantly better than that for strictly defined autism (Towbin, 1997). The lack of research on the condition has reflected the difficulties in securing support for research on an intrinsically poorly defined category. Fortunately, there is growing interest in this condition given the possibility, with current genetic work, that it represents a broader manifestation of the same genetic risk factors as for autism (Volkmar, Lord, Bailey, Schultz, & Klin, 2004). Some attempts have been made to defined subgroups/subtypes within this broad category (Towbin, 1997). It is likely that many adolescents with the condition go on to either lose this diagnosis or have other diagnoses as adults (e.g., personality disorders) (see Wolff, Townshend, McGuire, & Weeks, 1991).

Special Diagnostic Considerations in Adolescence

As noted previously, the diagnosis of autism and related conditions rests on both historical information and contemporaneous examination. Although diagnostic problems are occasionally noted, there has been general agreement on the utility of current categorical criteria for adolescents and young adults; the DSM-IV field trial validated the current definition in adolescents (Volkmar et al., 1994), showing a good balance of sensitivity and specificity. Although developmental changes do continue into adolescence, problems in social interaction, communication, and unusual responses to the environment do persist (Mesibov & Schaffer, 1986) and generally pose few problems for diagnosis. Problems may arise in some special circumstances—for example, when historical information is not available or when issues of diagnostic differentiation of the various subtypes of pervasive developmental disorders arise (Volkmar et al., 1997).

EPIDEMIOLOGY

Prevalence

In the earliest epidemiological study of autism by Lotter in 1966, the prevalence of autism was estimated to be 4 to 5 per 10,000 persons. Since that time more than 30 surveys have been completed with reported prevalence rates ranging from 0.7 per 10,000 to 21.1 per 10,000 individuals (Fombonne, 2003a, 2003b). At present an estimate of approximately 1 case of autism per 1,000 persons seems justified (Fombonne, 2003a, 2003b). There are some data suggesting a possible increase in autism over time (i.e., a secular increase); these data are, however, difficult to interpret given changes in the diagnostic criteria over time, the increased awareness of the disorder, earlier diagnosis, issues of study design, and "diagnostic substitution," for example, choosing to use a label of autism as opposed to a label of mental retardation for educational purposes (Fombonne, 2003a; Wing & Potter, 2002). In addition, current diagnostic approaches, as in DSM-IV-TR were specifically designed (Volkmar et al., 1994) to be applicable over the entire range of intellectual ability; that is, there was a deliberate attempt to be sure that criteria worked for adolescents and adults as well as for younger children, and as well for cognitively more able individuals.

Prevalence data for the other disorders in the PDD class are much more limited. It appears that rates of AD are lower than those of autism—probably about 1 case in 5,000 children. RD and CDD are clearly less common than DSM-IV autism (Fombone, 2003a), although, as noted earlier, it is clear that cases of PDD-NOS are more probably two to three times as common as strictly defined autism (Fombonne, 2003b; Towbin, 1997).

Sex Differences

Essentially all studies of sex differences show a higher incidence of autism in boys than in girls, with reported ratios averaging around 3.5 or 4.0 to 1.0 (Baron-Cohen & Hammer, 1997; Fombonne, 2003a; Lord, Schopler, & Revicki, 1982; Volkmar, Szatmari, & Sparrow, 1993). It is also the case that there is a strong association of mental handicap and sex ratio, with the males clearly outnumbering females among individuals functioning in the normal range of intelligence, but less so than for individuals with lower level of functioning. The nature of this gender difference is debated. Baron-Cohen (2003) has proposed a novel theory accounting for these differences suggesting that autism represents an extreme version of the "male brain" (Baron-Cohen & Hammer, 1997)—that is, a tendency toward systemizing versus empathizing; substantive data on this theory are, however, lacking. It is likely that as specific genes and vulnerability factors are identified, specific mechanisms that may account for the observed gender differences may be more robustly elucidated (Rutter, 1997).

Social Class

Kanner's (1943) original suggestion that children with autism were more likely to come from better educated and professionally successful families has not proven to be true and likely reflected an ascertainment bias (e.g., Fombonne, 2003a; Schopler, Andrews, & Strupp, 1979; Wing, 1980).

Ethnicity and Cultural Issues

Very little has been written about the impact of ethnicity or cultural factors on autism. In their recent review, Brown and Rogers (2003) note that in the context of a severely disabling condition such as autism, cultural factors can be readily overlooked. The limited information available on cultural issues has tended to focus either on differences in diagnostic assessment or, more commonly, on variations in service provision and treatment programs (Cohen & Volkmar, 1997). There has been a general assumption that diagnostic criteria work well across cultures, and the limited available data do suggest that this is probably the case (Cicchetti, Volkmar, Klin, & Showalter, 1995; Rutter & Schopler, 1993; Sponheim, 1996; Volkmar, Cicchetti, Bregman, & Cohen, 1992). On the other hand, it is also clear that there are marked variations in service provision within countries and, in the United States, sometimes even within states. The impact of cultural issues remains a critically important topic for future research (Schopler & Mesibov, 2000). At this point it appears that the greatest variations have to do with intervention and possibly models of family support (see Brown & Rogers, 2003, for review), while variations in diagnostic practices appear to generally be diminishing.

DEVELOPMENTAL COURSE AND OUTCOMES

Childhood Precursors

Autism and related conditions are chronic disorders with an onset in infancy and early childhood. Several reviews of autism and related conditions as manifest in infants and young children (Stone, 1997), as well as in school-age children, are available (Loveland & Tunali-Kotoski, 1997). Children with autism can profit significantly from intervention; even before intensive interventions were available a small number of children did well, although that number has now increased substantially (National Research Council, 2001). Prior to adolescence some children will have made substantial gains in degree of both social relatedness and communicative ability (Howlin, 2000).

Developmental Pathways

Various studies have documented the early developmental course of children with autism and related disorders in preschool and school-age children (Stone, 1997). With greater public awareness, better diagnostic methods, and increased research on younger children with autism spectrum disorders, the age at first diagnosis is decreasing and prolonged delays in providing service are much less common (Siegel, Pliner, Eschler, & Elliott, 1988; Volkmar et al., 2004). This is particularly important as a growing body of research has documented the potential for many children to exhibit very significant improvement if early, intensive intervention services are provided in a timely way (National Research Council, 2001); on the other hand, not all children make dramatic gains (Lord, 1995) and those factors that robustly predict treatment response remain to be elucidated.

Unfortunately, systematic research on adolescents with autism is relatively sparse (Mesibov & Handlan, 1997; Mesibov & Schaffer, 1986; Ousley & Mesibov, 1991; Volkmar & Wiesner, 2004). In addition there is a strong suggestion of a secular change in outcome with earlier detection and better service provision—accordingly, the available information should be viewed with some caution.

Puberty is not typically delayed in children with autism and related disorders; however, the changes associated with puberty can be much more difficult for several reasons (Gillberg & Schaumann, 1989). Some children with preexisting behavioral difficulties experience an exacerbation of these problems; such difficulties are even more difficult for parents to manage given the child's size and the level of severity of these problems. On the other hand, some children are reported to markedly improve in adolescence (Boelte et al., 1999; Gilchrist et al., 2001; Gillberg & Steffenburg, 1987; Piven et al., 1996). While speculation has centered on various factors (e.g., hormonal and neurochemical), definitive data are lacking.

Comorbid Disorders

Associations of autism with numerous medical conditions have been noted over the years (Fombonne, 2003a; Rutter, Bailey, Bolton, & Le Couteur, 1994). However, such impressions are often based on case reports and, in most instances, consistent, replicable causal associations have been hard to establish. Exceptions to this generalization include two strongly genetic conditions—fragile X syndrome and tuberous sclerosis—both of which appear more commonly in children with autism than would be expected based on chance alone (Rutter et al., 1994). These two conditions account, overall, for a small percentage of cases and usually are diagnosed before adolescence. The major medical complication encountered in adolescence is seizure disorder (Fombonne, 2003a, 2003b).

There appears to be a bimodal distribution of the onset of epilepsy in autism with one group of children developing seizures early in life while the other group is more likely to develop seizures in adolescence (Deykin & MacMahon, 1979; Rutter, 1970; Volkmar & Nelson, 1990). Relative to the onset of seizure disorder in the general population the risk for adolescents with autism to develop seizures is at least 20-fold increased over the general (typically developing) population; this risk continues, at a somewhat lower level, into young adult life.

Eventually about 20% of children with autistic disorder develop seizures; these are of various types. Unfortunately, the advent of seizures appears to further increase the adolescent's risk for additional behavioral and psychiatric difficulties; it remains unclear whether this is a direct result of the onset of the seizures, a side effect of the treatments for the seizures, or a function of whatever process(es) cause the seizures to occur in the first place. Although lower IQ appears to increase the risk for developing seizure disorder, even higher-functioning adolescents with autism sometimes develop seizures.

With the exception of RD, rather less is known regarding medical complications for other ASDs in adolescence (Volkmar & Wiesner, 2004). For individuals with AD no specific medical conditions appear to be specifically more common (psychiatric comorbidity is discussed subsequently). For children with RD there is an increased frequency of multiple medical complications including seizures, breathing problems (including sleep apnea), and scoliosis (Van Acker, 1997). Children with CDD appear to have about the same risk for developing seizures, as do children with autism. The health problems of adolescents with ASDs are, otherwise, not vastly different from those of typically developing adolescents, although issues of diagnosis and treatment can be complicated by the individual's social and communicative disabilities (Volkmar & Wiesner, 2004).

The issue of psychiatric comorbidity in adolescents with autism and related disorders is a complex one (Lord & Volkmar, 2002; Volkmar et al., 1997). On the one hand, it does appear that, as in work on mental retardation, a process of diagnostic overshadowing has tended to occur—that is, a tendency to overlook comorbid conditions given the significance of the individual's other developmental problems (Dykens, 2000). On the other hand it is also quite clear that, of itself, a condition such as autism will be associated with a range of additional symptoms that may not, necessarily, rise to the level of "disorder." For example, problems with attention are frequently seen in autism and AD, but it remains unclear whether such difficulties are sufficient to achieve an additional diagnosis of attention-deficit/hyperactivity disorder (ADHD), although some researchers have proposed that such a combination may prove to be a robust subtype (Landgren, Pettersson, Kjellman, & Gillberg, 1996; Towbin, 1997). This problem is further compounded when the issue is comorbid diagnosis of conditions, such as anxiety or depression, in lower-functioning adolescents (i.e., in individuals with little or no expressive language). In addition, much of the data on psychiatric comorbidity in adolescence rests largely on case reports. As noted elsewhere

(Kent, Evans, Paul, & Sharp, 1999; Slone, Durrheim, Kaminer, & Lachman, 1999; Volkmar & Woolston, 1997), this literature is difficult to interpret given the bias for positive associations to be published; the critical issue is whether rates of a given disorder in larger (ideally epidemiologically representative) samples can demonstrate significant elevations in the rates of comorbid conditions (Fombonne, 2003a). A final problem relates to some basic differences in approaches to comorbidity; for example, DSM-IV-TR tends, on balance, to encourage multiple diagnoses whereas the ICD-10 system, conversely, discourages this practice (Volkmar, Schwab-Stone, & First, 2002).

Interest in the problem of psychiatric comorbidity has centered particularly on AD—both for historical and practical reasons. Early interest focused on AD as a possible "transitional" condition between autism and schizophrenia (Klin & Volkmar, 2003). The verbal accessibility of individuals with AD also made it much easier to apply usual diagnostic models and criteria to them. To date, the strongest available data suggest that adolescents with AD are at increased risk for mood disorders—particularly depression (Ghaziuddin, Weidmer-Mikhail, & Ghaziuddin, 1998; Green, Gilchrist, Burton, & Cox, 2000; Kim, Szatmari, Bryson, Streiner, & Wilson, 2000; Klin & Volkmar, 1997; Volkmar, Klin, & Pauls, 1998). This observation is also consistent with the observation of Rourke and colleagues that adolescents with the nonverbal learning disability profile (commonly associated with AD) are at high risk for depression and suicidality (Rourke & Tsatsanis, 2000).

Some case reports have also suggested that adolescents with AD may be at higher risk for bipolar disorder (Duggal, 2003; Frazier, Doyle, Chiu, & Coyle, 2002; Kerbeshian, Burd, & Fisher, 1987; Kerbeshian, Burd, Randall, Martsolf, & Jalal, 1990). Despite early interest in the possible co-occurrence of AD and psychotic conditions the available evidence is quite limited and consists largely of case reports (Bejerot & Duvner 1995; Ghaziuddin, Leininger, & Tsai, 1995; Taiminen, 1994; Wolff, 1998).

For adolescents with autism, particularly for those more cognitively able, an increased risk for depression has also been noted (Kim et al., 2000). Despite the early impression that autism might represent a form of schizophrenia, it appears that rates of schizophrenia in adolescents with autism are not increased as compared to the general population (Volkmar & Cohen, 1991).

Sexuality

For adolescents with autism and related disorders, developing sexuality presents even more complex issues than those presented to typically developing children (Mesibov & Schaffer, 1986). Some individuals, particularly higher-functioning ones, may be very motivated to have a girl- or boyfriend; at times this extra motivation to "fit in" can help foster important developmental gains (Bemporad, 1979; Kanner, Rodriguez, & Ashenden, 1972; Volkmar & Cohen, 1985), particularly in the area of social interest and motivation to develop relationships. The impact of an ASD on social skills poses a major complication for relationship development and is a roadblock for the development of sustained sexual relationships. For those adolescents with good functional language the ability to discuss sexual feelings and issues and the ability to profit from the range of educational and other materials developed for other individuals with disabilities can be helpful (see Van Bourgondien, Reichle, & Palmer, 1997, and Volkmar & Wiesner, 2004, for reviews).

Although more and more clinical and teaching resources are available, research on sexuality in children with ASD is sparse. In one study (Ousley & Mesibov, 1991) groups of higher-functioning young adults with autism were compared to a group of individuals with mild to moderate mental retardation. Although levels of knowledge were rather similar across the two groups the individuals with autism were less likely to have had sexual experiences. In this study males generally had greater sexual interest than females and there was a positive correlation between intellectual level and knowledge.

Some cases of physical and/or sexual abuse in individuals with ASD have been reported, sometimes with important behavioral and psychiatric sequelae (Cook, Kieffer, Charak, & Leventhal, 1993). Individuals who are nonverbal are probably at greatest risk. For such adolescents, unusual changes in behavior, increased anxiety, agitation, depression, or avoidance of specific people or situations can be warning signs of physical or sexual abuse.

Adult Outcomes

Kanner (1971; Kanner et al., 1972) was one of the first to note that some children with autism exhibit marked gains in adolescence while others seem to lose ground developmentally. Recent reviews of outcomes have tended to support the notion that increasingly early case detection and rededication have improved the overall outcome for many adolescents (Howlin, 2000). For example, one early outcome study (DeMyer, Hingtgen, & Jackson, 1981) reported that only 1–2% of individuals with autism were able, as adults, to live independently and self-sufficiently as adults while more recent studies would suggest that perhaps 20% of individuals are now capable to do so (Howlin, 2000). One important limitation of the currently available outcome research has been the tendency to focus on a limited number of outcome measures (e.g., overall intelligence, adult placement, or the presence of specific behaviors; Howlin & Goode, 1998); other measures (e.g., of quality of life and associated psychiatric/behavioral disabilities in adolescence and adulthood) remain to be systematically studied.

In general, intelligence and academic skills are reasonably stable in adolescence, although higher-functioning individuals may continue to make gains (Ando, Yoshimura, & Wakabayahsi, 1980; Bartak & Rutter, 1973). Predictors of adult outcome include verbal abilities and overall intelligence (Lord & Venter, 1992; Venter, Lord, & Schopler, 1992). For the adolescent whose behavior deteriorates, recovery occurs in at least some instances (Gillberg, 1984). There is some suggestion that girls may be more likely to show behavioral regression; also, additional risk for psychiatric difficulties (because of life circumstances or family history) may increase such risk (Gillberg & Schaumann, 1981; Gillberg & Steffenburg, 1987).

THEORIES

During the 1950s and 1960s there was much speculation that autism was caused by early experience; this notion arose partly because of Kanner's (1943) initial report of higher than expected levels of parent education and because of the marked interest in the effects of early experience. As a result many parents were essentially blamed for their child's difficulties. As children with autism were followed the high rates of seizure disorder, persistence of unusual neurological signs and symptoms (e.g., persistent "primitive" reflexes), and other indicators of central nervous system abnormality convinced investigators that autism was a brain-based condition (Rutter, 1970). Early attempts were made to associate autism with a number of specific medical conditions, although as time went on it became apparent that the strongest associations were with a small number of strongly genetic conditions; furthermore, as studies of siblings, particularly twins, were conducted it became clear that autism and related conditions have a very strong genetic basis (Rutter, 1997; Volkmar et al., 2004). Having had one child with autism the chance of a couple having a second child with the condition is increased at least 50-fold (Rutter, 1997).

Efforts are currently underway to identify specific susceptibility genes for autism; it appears likely that multiple interacting genes are involved (Rutter, 1997). Research on the "autistic-like" conditions is generally not as advanced as that for autism (with the exception of RD for which a gene has now been identified); however, there does appear to be a strong genetic component to these conditions as well. For example, AD appears to have a strong genetic basis—possibly one even stronger than that for autism (Volkmar et al., 1998). Specification of the genetics of autism will likely lead to a greater understanding of the role of specific genetic and brain mechanisms in the broader range of "autistic-like" conditions as well.

Interest in possible environmental factors and autism has been stimulated, in part, by reports in the lay press about clusters of cases. Earlier reports of associations of autism with other (nongenetic) conditions (e.g., in relation to congenital infections or exposure to specific drugs or toxins and an awareness that even among identical twins discordance for autism is observed) have all led to interest in potential environmental factors. However, the currently available evidence for such etiologies is weak (Wing & Potter, 2002).

An increasingly sophisticated body of research, much of it conducted using adolescents and young adults, has been concerned with identifying potential brain mechanisms in autism. For example, Schultz and colleagues

(2000) used functional magnetic resonance imaging to demonstrate differences in processing of faces versus objects with individuals with autism not demonstrating expected activity in that area of the brain (the fusiform gyrus) usually involved in face processing; in contrast, their high-functioning group of adolescents without autism activated a brain region that typically is mobilized for viewing objects.

Various psychological models for autism have been proposed. This interesting literature has often tended to focus on cognitive processes and models (rather than on the social disability as such). Such models have centered on the constructs of "theory of mind" skills, a cognitive drive for central coherence, and a group of neuropsychological skills clustered together by the term "executive functions" (see Volkmar et al., 2004, for a review). Findings from neuroimaging and neuropsychology, however, increasingly point to involvement of broader and developmentally interrelated neural systems and are less suggestive of a single core deficit. New models that attempt to integrate recent neurobiological findings and focus on the autistic aspect of autism (i.e., the social difficulties) are now beginning to appear (Klin, Jones, Schultz, & Volkmar, 2003). Unfortunately, none of the developing models and theories has focused specifically on adolescents as such.

ASSESSMENT

Adolescents with ASDs typically exhibit problems in multiple areas of functioning, complicating the task of assessment. Other challenges for assessment can include highly variable cooperation and engagement as well as the need for involvement of a range of professionals (with attendant issues of coordination and communication). Guidelines for assessment of individuals with autism have been published (e.g., Volkmar, Cook, Pomeroy, Realmuto, & Tanguay, 1999) and emphasize the importance of a systematic process and careful coordination between the various individuals often involved in it. Psychological assessments should include the administration of any of a number of standard tests of intelligence or development; it is important that the examiner be aware of the particular patterns of strength/ weakness likely to be obtained on any specific instruments (see Klin et al., 1997, for a discussion). Adolescents with autistic disorder may, for example, exhibit a pattern in which nonverbal skills are less impaired than verbal ones, but the opposite pattern may be observed in AD (Klin, Volkmar, & Sparrow, 2000). Occasionally, greater degrees of intellectual handicap require the use of tests developed either for younger children or where verbal requirements are minimized. Assessment of adaptive behavior (Sparrow, Balla, & Cicchetti, 1984) is critical. Speech and communication assessments should not be limited simply to an evaluation of vocabulary but should include other aspects of communicative functioning, including prosody, pragmatic language skills, understanding of humorous or figurative language, and so forth (Klin et al., 1997). Various rating scales, checklists, and direct assessment instruments have been developed for use in individuals with autism (see Lord & Corsello, 2005, for a review); some of these are designed to be applicable to adolescents and young adults (e.g., the Psychoeducational Profile; Mesibov, Schopler, & Caison, 1989). Such instruments approach issues of development, historical information, and developmental change in different ways. Typically a thorough assessment includes both direct observation and consultation with parents and schools as well as direct work with the adolescent. With few exceptions (notably testing for fragile X in individuals with autism), the role of specific medical/laboratory tests is limited unless specific clinical indicators are present, for example, the onset of staring spells suggestive of epilepsy should prompt an EEG and/or neurological consultation (Volkmar & Wiesner, 2004).

TREATMENT

Educational and Behavioral Interventions

Numerous studies have supported the importance of carefully designed behavioral and educational interventions in adolescents with autism and related disorders (National Research Council, 2001). Gains in communication skills can be observed even for persons who are not speaking, for example, through use of sign, augmentative communication systems, and picture exchange (Paul, 1997). For individuals with severe communication problems, an emphasis on meaningful and functional activities is particularly important (Beisler & Tsai, 1983; Lord, 1988). Behavioral methods may also be used to facilitate communication skills and deal with behavioral difficulties during adolescence (Bregman, 1997). The North Carolina TEAACH program has developed comprehensive programs for adolescents including both prevocational and vocational training (Keel, Mesibov & Woods, 1997; Mesibov & Handlan, 1997; Schopler, Mesibov, & Hearsey, 1995).

Although many adolescents with ASDs display higher levels of social interest and motivation than they did as children, significant social difficulties persist. The severity of these persistent problems in interaction is vividly illustrated in work with higher-functioning individuals with autism and AD; clinicians who work with this population have countless examples of problematic social interactions (Mesibov & Handlan, 1997; Wing, 1981). For example, a rigid adherence to the "rules" can lead to unfortunate difficulty as there is no appreciation of the myriad exceptions to the rules (e.g., stopping when crossing the street when the light changes to don't walk or yelling at people in the grocery store if they have 11 rather than the posted maximum of 10 items in their shopping cart in the express line). An increasing body of work has focused on developing social skills in adolescents at all cognitive levels. Methods proposed can be primarily peer based (mentoring) or teacher/therapist based (direct social skills training) or combinations of the two (social skills groups) (see Paul, 2003, for a comprehensive review). Although a number of social skills curricula and teaching models are now available, research has tended to focus primarily on much younger children (Paul, 2003). This is unfortunate because, as Rutter (1970) and Kanner (1971) noted, social interest often increases in adolescence.

Programs for adolescents with ASDs typically have a strong emphasis on acquisition of basic adaptive skills (i.e., in helping the adolescent transfer knowledge into "real-world" settings); this is crucial given the major difficulties with generalization exhibited and given the centrality of adaptive skills for adult independence and self-sufficiency (Fredericks & Williams, 1998; Volkmar, 2003). Use of structured assessment instruments, such as the Vineland (Sparrow et al., 1984), can be used to outline skills that can be explicitly taught. Such teaching can include the entire range of needed abilities—for example, appropriate use of leisure time (Mesibov, 1984), understanding humor

(Van Bourgondien & Mesibov, 1987; Van Bourgondien & Schopler, 1990), and negotiation and social problem solving (McGee, Krantz, & McClannahan, 1984; Mesibov & Handlan, 1997).

Parents may find adolescence a particularly stressful time given both concerns about behavioral changes in adolescence and longer-term outcomes (Bristol & Schopler, 1983; Seltzer, Kraus, Orsmon, & Verstal, 2001). In one recent study Gray (2002) found that over half of parents of adolescents reported significant levels of stress, anxiety, and/or depression. Family support of the parents and siblings of the adolescent with ASDs is critical (Marcus, Kunce, & Schopler, 1997).

College, Vocational, and Residential Programs

For an increasing number of adolescents, college and ultimately independent or semi-independent living is possible (Howlin, 2000). For those adolescents able to attend college, support from the learning disabilities office is essential; for many students, smaller colleges prove less challenging (Harpur, Lawlor, & Fitzgerald, 2004). Those working with college students with autism or AD should also be aware of the entire range of potential resources available to the student (peer mentoring or support, mental health services, etc.). Sometimes special accommodation for the student is appropriate (e.g., untimed tests or use of laptops in the classroom). A few specialized college programs have been developed and likely more will be available in the future (Harper et al., 2004).

For less able adolescents, parents and the adolescent must cope with decisions about adult placements—both occupational and residential. Although marked regional disparities exist in terms of range of services, a number of different models have been developed; these range from supported apartments and supported employment to more traditional group homes and sheltered employment settings (Gerhardt & Holmes, 1997; Simonson, Simonson, & Volkmar, 1990). It is important that planning for adulthood begins during early adolescence (Morgan, 1996). In general, efforts should be made to base vocational planning on the adolescent's profile of strengths and weaknesses.

Pharmacological treatments are relatively common in adolescents with ASDs. Typical targets of treatment include agitation, behavioral rigidity, anxiety, depression, aggression, and attentional difficulties. Unfortunately, well-designed, placebo-controlled studies, have been not been common, although more are now being conducted (Martin, Scahill, Klin, & Volkmar, 1999; McCracken et al., 2002; McDougle et al., 1996, 1997, 2000). Drug treatments have not, at least to date, appeared to have a major impact on core social difficulties, but they can be of great benefit to adolescents in terms of symptom reduction and in making the individual more available to educational interventions (Volkmar 2001). Commonly used agents have included the neuroleptics, particularly the newer "second-generation" atypical neuroleptics (McCracken et al., 2002) and the selective serotonin reuptake inhibitors (McDougle et al., 1996; see Towbin, 2003, for a helpful summary). One limitation of the available literature has been a relative lack of attention to changes in drug efficacy (and adverse effects) with respect to adolescence (i.e., often children and adolescents have been grouped together). There is at least some suggestion that both gender and puberty may have a significant effect on drug efficacy and that gender differences in drug response may vary depending on pubertal status (Martin et al., 2003).

A host of nonestablished (alternative or complementary) treatments are available for adolescents with autism and related conditions. Although dramatic claims for remarkable gains or "cures" are often made, substantive data usually are quite limited; an additional complexity in evaluating such treatments is that families that seek and use them often are engaged in many such treatments at the same time (see Volkmar & Wiesner, 2004, for a review of alternative treatments).

CURRENT NEEDS AND FUTURE DIRECTIONS

As has been repeatedly noted in this chapter, adolescents with autism and related conditions have, in their own right, been the focus of relatively little research. This unfortunate state of affairs has reflected several factors. Given that these are conditions with an onset early in life, there has been a diagnostic focus on younger children and a similar emphasis on younger children in treatment studies. Although a few diagnostic and assessment tools have been developed specifically for adolescents (e.g.,

Mesibov, Schopler, Schaffer, & Michal, 1989), most of the time, when they have been studied at all, adolescents have often been grouped either with younger children or with adults rather than being studied in their own right. This is unfortunate as the available research clearly indicates that many individuals have considerable developmental change during adolescence; our knowledge of the factors that might be responsible for such change remains highly limited. Better assessment tools and outcome measures are needed. The specificity of interventions and their applicability to adolescents remains an important area for investigation, particularly in terms of social skills intervention. Factors responsible for good and poor outcome must be more clearly identified. The complex problem of psychiatric comorbidity and potential issues in drug response differences must also be addressed.

ACKNOWLEDGMENTS

We gratefully acknowledge the support of the National Institute of Child Health and Human Development (CPEA Program Project Grant No. 1PO1HD35482-01), the National Institute of Mental Health (STAART Grant No. U54-MH066494), and the National Alliance of Autism Research, Cure Autism Now, and the Doris Duke Foundation.

REFERENCES

Ando, H., Yoshimura, I., & Wakabayashi, S. (1980). Effects of age on adaptive behavior levels and academic skill levels in autistic and mentally retarded children. *Journal of Autism and Developmental Disorders, 10*(2), 173–184.

Asperger, H. (1944). Die "autistichen Psychopathen" im Kindersalter. *Archive fur psychiatrie und Nervenkrankheiten, 117,* 76–136.

American Psychiatric Association. (1980). *Diagnostic and statistical manual of mental disorders.* Washington, DC: Author.

American Psychiatric Association. (1987). *Diagnostic and statistical manual of mental disorders* (3rd ed., rev.). Washington, DC: Author.

American Psychiatric Association. (1994). *Diagnostic and statistical manual of mental disorders* (4th ed.). Washington, DC: Author.

American Psychiatric Association. (2000). *Diagnostic and statistical manual of mental disorders* (4th ed., text rev.). Washington, DC: Author.

Baron-Cohen, S. (1988). An assessment of violence in a young man with Asperger's syndrome. *Journal of Child Psychology and Psychiatry, 29*(3), 351–360.

Baron-Cohen, S. (2003). *The essential difference the truth about the male and female brain.* New York: Basic Books.

Baron-Cohen, S., & Hammer, J. (1997). Is autism an extreme form of the "male brain"? *Advances in Infancy Research, 11,* 193–217.

Bartak, L., & Rutter, M. (1973). Special educational treatment of autistic children: a comparative study. 1. Design of study and characteristics of units. *Journal of Child Psychology and Psychiatry, 14*(3), 161–179.

Beisler, J. M., & Tsai, L. Y. (1983). A pragmatic approach to increase expressive language skills in young autistic children. *Journal of Autism and Developmental Disorders, 13*(3), 287–303.

Bejerot, S., & Duvner, T. (1995). Asperger's syndrome or schizophrenia? *Nordic Journal of Psychiatry, 49*(2), 145.

Bemporad, J. R. (1979). Adult recollections of a formerly autistic child. *Journal of Autism and Developmental Disorders, 9*(2), 179–197.

Boelte, S., Dickhut, H., & Poustka, F. (1999). Patterns of parent-reported problems indicative in autism. *Psychopathology, 32*(2), 93–97.

Bregman, J. (1997). Behavioral interventions. In D. J. Cohen & F. R. Volkmar (Eds.), *Handbook of autism and pervasive developmental disorders* (2nd ed., pp. 606–630). New York: Wiley.

Bristol, M. M., & Schopler, E. (1983). Family resources and successful adaptation in autistic children. In E. Schopler & G. B. Mesibov (Eds.), *Autism in adolescents and adults* (pp. 251–279). New York: Plenum Press.

Brown, J. R., & Rogers, S. J. (2003). Cultural issues in autism. In R. L. Hendren, S. Ozonoff, & S. Rogers (Eds.), *Autism spectrum disorders* (pp. 209–226). Washington, DC: American Psychiatric Press.

Burack, J. A., Charman, T., Yirmiya, N., & Zelazo, P. R. (Eds.). (2001). *The development of autism: Perspectives from theory and research.* Mahwah, NJ: Erlbaum.

Cicchetti, D. V., Volkmar, F., Klin, A., & Showalter, D. (1995). Diagnosing autism using ICD-10 criteria: A comparison of neural networks and standard multivariate procedures. *Child Neuropsychology, 1*(1), 26–37.

Cohen, D. J., & Volkmar, F. R. (Eds.). (1997). *Handbook of autism and pervasive developmental disorders* (2nd ed.). New York: Wiley.

Cook, E. H., Jr., Kieffer, J. E., Charak, D. A., & Leventhal, B. L. (1993). Autistic disorder and posttraumatic stress disorder. *Journal of the American Academy of Child and Adolescent Psychiatry, 32*(6), 1292–1294.

DeMyer, M. K., Hingtgen, J. N., & Jackson, R. K. (1981). Infantile autism reviewed: A decade of research. *Schizophrenia Bulletin, 7*(3), 388–451.

Deykin, E. Y., & MacMahon, B. (1979). The incidence of seizures among children with autistic symptoms. *American Journal of Psychiatry, 136*(10), 1310–1312.

Duggal, H. S. (2003). Bipolar disorder with Asperger's disorder [Comment]. *American Journal of Psychiatry, 160*(1), 184–185.

Dykens, E. M. (2000). Psychopathology in children with intellectual disability. *Journal of Child Psychology and Psychiatry and Allied Disciplines, 41*(4), 407–417.

Fombonne, E. (2001). Is there an epidemic of autism? *Pediatrics, 107*(2), 411–412.

Fombonne, E. (2003a). Epidemiological surveys of autism and other pervasive developmental disorders: An update. *Journal of Autism and Developmental Disorders, 33*(4), 365–382.

Fombonne, E. (2003b). The prevalence of autism. *Journal of the American Medical Association, 289*(1), 87–89.

Frazier, J. A., Doyle, R., Chiu, S., & Coyle, J. T. (2002). Treating a child with Asperger's disorder and comorbid bipolar disorder. *American Journal of Psychiatry, 159*(1), 13–21.

Fredericks, D. W., & Williams, W. L. (1998). New definition of mental retardation for the American Association of Mental Retardation. *Image—The Journal of Nursing Scholarship, 30*(1), 53–56.

Gerhardt, P. F., & Holmes, D. L. (1997). Employment: Options and issues for adolescents and adults with autism. In D. J. Cohen & F. R. Volkmar (Eds.), *Handbook of autism and pervasive developmental disorders* (2nd ed., pp. 650–664). New York: Wiley.

Ghaziuddin, M., Leininger, L., & Tsai, L. (1995). Brief report: Thought disorder in Asperger syndrome: Comparison with high-functioning autism. *Journal of Autism and Developmental Disorders, 25*(3), 311–317.

Ghaziuddin, M., Weidmer-Mikhail, E., & Ghaziuddin, N. (1998). Comorbidity of Asperger syndrome: A preliminary report. *Journal of Intellectual Disability Research, 42*(4), 279–283.

Gilchrist, A., Green, J., Cox, A., Burton, D., Rutter, M., & Le Couteur, A. (2001). Development and current functioning in adolescents with Asperger syndrome: A comparative study. *Journal of Child Psychology and Psychiatry and Allied Disciplines, 42*(2), 227–240.

Gillberg, C. (1984). Autistic children growing up: problems during puberty and adolescence. *Developmental Medicine in Child Neurology, 26*(1), 125–129.

Gillberg, C., & Schaumann, H. (1981). Infantile autism and puberty. *Journal of Autism and Developmental Disorders, 11*(4), 365–371.

Gillberg, C., & Schaumann, H. (1989). *Autism: Specific problems of adolescence.* In C. Gillberg (Ed.), *Diagnosis and treatment of autism* (pp. 375–382). New York: Plenum Press.

Gillberg, C., & Steffenburg, S. (1987). Outcome and prognostic factors in infantile autism and similar conditions: A population-based study of 46 cases followed through puberty. *Journal of Autism and Developmental Disorders, 17*(2), 273–287.

Gray, D. E. (2002). Ten years on: A longitudinal study of families of children with autism. *Journal of Intellectual and Developmental Disability, 27*, 215–222.

Green, J., Gilchrist, A., Burton, D., & Cox, A. (2000). Social and psychiatric functioning in adolescents with Asperger syndrome compared with conduct disorder. *Journal of Autism and Developmental Disorders, 30*(4), 279–293.

Harpur, J., Lawlor, M., & Fitzgerald, M. (2004). *Succeeding in college with Asperger Syndrome.* London: Jessica Kingsley.

Howlin, P. (2000). Outcome in adult life for more able individuals with autism or Asperger syndrome. *Autism, 4*(1), 63–83.

Howlin, P., & Goode, S. (1998). Outcome in adult life for people with autism and Asperger's syndrome. In F. R. Volkmar (Ed.), *Autism and pervasive developmental disorders. Cambridge monographs in child and adolescent psychiatry* (pp. 209–241). New York: Cambridge University Press.

Kanner, L. (1943). Autistic disturbances of affective contact. *Nervous Child, 2*, 217–250.

Kanner, L. (1971). Follow-up study of eleven autistic children originally reported in 1943. *Journal of Autism and Childhood Schizophrenia, 1*(2), 119–145.

Kanner, L., Rodriguez, A., & Ashenden, B. (1972). How far can autistic children go in matters of social adaptation? *Journal of Autism and Childhood Schizophrenia, 2*(1), 9–33.

Keel, J. H., Mesibov, G. B., & Woods, A. V. (1997). TEACCH-supported employment program. *Journal of Autism and Developmental Disorders, 27*(1), 3–9.

Kent, L., Evans, J., Paul, M., & Sharp, M. (1999). Comorbidity of autistic spectrum disorders in children with Down syndrome. *Developmental Medicine and Child Neurology, 41*(3), 153–158.

Kerbeshian, J., Burd, L., & Fisher, W. (1987). Lithium carbonate in the treatment of two patients with infantile autism and atypical bipolar symptomatology. *Journal of Clinical Psychopharmacology, 7*(6), 401–405.

Kerbeshian, J., Burd, L., Randall, T., Martsolf, J., & Jalal, S. (1990). Autism, profound mental retardation and atypical bipolar disorder in a 33–year-old female with a deletion of 15q12. *Journal of Mental Deficiencies Research, 34*(Pt. 2), 205–210.

Kim, J. A., Szatmari, P., Bryson, S. E., Streiner, D. L., & Wilson, F. J. (2000). The prevalence of anxiety and mood problems among children with autism and Asperger syndrome. *Autism, 4*(2), 117–132.

Klin, A., Carter, A., Volkmar, F. R., Cohen, D. J., Marans, W. D., & Sparrow, S. S. (1997). Assessment issues in children with autism. In D. J. Cohen & F. R. Volkmar (Eds.), *Handbook of autism and pervasive developmental dIsorders* (2nd ed., pp. 411–418). New York: Wiley.

Klin, A., Jones, W., Schultz, R., & Volkmar, F. (2003). The enactive mind, or from actions to cognition: lessons from autism. *Philosophical Transactions of the*

Royal Society of London—Series B: Biological Sciences, 358, 345–360.

Klin, A., Volkmar, F. R., & Sparrow, S. S. (Eds.). (2000). *Asperger syndrome.* New York: Guilford Press.

Klin, A., Volkmar, F., Sparrow, S., Cicchetti, D., & Rourke, B. P. (1995). Validity and neuropsychological characterization of Asperger syndrome: Convergence with nonverbal learning disabilities syndrome. *Journal of Child Psychology and Psychiatry, 36,* 1127–1140.

Klin, A., & Volkmar, F. R. (1997). Asperger syndrome. In D. J. Cohen & F. R. Volkmar (Eds.), *Handbook of autism and pervasive developmental disorders* (2nd ed., pp. 94–122). New York: Wiley.

Klin, A., & Volkmar, F. R. (2003). Asperger syndrome: Diagnosis and external validity. *Child and Adolescent Psychiatric Clinics of North America, 12*(1), 1–13.

Klin, A., Volkmar, F. R., & Sparrow, S. S. (Eds.). (2000). *Asperger syndrome.* New York: Guilford Press.

Kolvin, I. (1971). Studies in the childhood psychoses. I. Diagnostic criteria and classification. *British Journal of Psychiatry, 118*(545), 381–384.

Landgren, M., Pettersson, R., Kjellman, B., & Gillberg, C. (1996). ADHD, DAMP and other neurodevelopmental/psychiatric disorders in 6–year-old children: Epidemiology and co-morbidity. *Developmental Medicine and Child Neurology, 38*(10), 891–906.

Le Couteur, A., Rutter, M., Lord, C., Rios, P., Robertson, S., Holdgrafer, M., & McLennan, J. (1989). Autism diagnostic interview: A standardized investigator-based instrument. *Journal of Autism and Developmental Disorders, 19*(3), 363–387.

Lord, C. (1988). Enhancing communication in adolescents with autism. *Topics in Language Disorders, 9*(1), 72–81.

Lord, C. (1995). Follow-up of two-year-olds referred for possible autism. *Journal of Child Psychology and Psychiatry, 36*(8), 1365–1382.

Lord, C., & Corsello, C. (2005). Diagnostic instruments in autism spectrum disorders. In F. Volkmar, R. Paul, A. Klin, & D. J. Cohen (Eds.), *Handbook of autism and pervasive developmental disorders* (3rd ed., Vol. 2, pp. 730–771). New York: Wiley.

Lord, C., Schopler, E., & Revicki, D. (1982). Sex differences in autism. *Journal of Autism and Developmental Disorders, 12,* 317–330.

Lord, C., & Venter, A. (1992). Outcome and follow-up studies of high-functioning autistic individuals. In E. Schopler & G. B. Mesibov (Eds.), *High-functioning individuals with autism: Current issues in autism* (pp. 187–199). New York: Plenum Press.

Lord, C., & Volkmar, F. (2002). Genetics of childhood disorders: XLII. Autism, part 1: Diagnosis and assessment in autistic spectrum disorders. *Journal of the American Academy of Child and Adolescent Psychiatry, 41*(9), 1134–1136.

Loveland, K. A., & Tunali-Kotoski, B. (1997). The school age child with autism. In D. J. Cohen & F. R. Volkmar (Eds.), *Handbook of autism and pervasive developmental disorders* (2nd ed., pp. 283–308). New York: Wiley.

Marcus, L. M., Kunce L. J., & Schopler. E. (1997). Working with families. In D. J. Cohen & F. R. Volkmar (Eds.), *Handbook of autism and pervasive developmental disorders* (pp. 631–649). New York: Wiley.

Martin, A., Koenig, K., Anderson, G. M., & Scahill, L. (2003). Low-dose fluvoxamine treatment of children and adolescents with pervasive developmental disorders: A prospective, open-label study. *Journal of Autism and Developmental Disorders, 33,* 77–85.

Martin, A., Scahill, L., Klin, A., & Volkmar, F. R. (1999). Higher-functioning pervasive developmental disorders: Rates and patterns of psychotropic drug use. *Journal of the American Academy of Child and Adolescent Psychiatry, 38*(7), 923–931.

McCracken, J. T., McGough, J., Shah, B., Cronin, P., Hong, D., Aman, M. G., et al. (2002). Risperidone in children with autism and serious behavioral problems. *New England Journal of Medicine, 347*(5), 314–321.

McDougle, C. J., Holmes, J. P., Bronson, M. R., Anderson, G. M., Volkmar, F. R., Price, L. H., & Cohen, D. J. (1997). Risperidone treatment of children and adolescents with pervasive developmental disorders: A prospective open-label study. *Journal of the American Academy of Child and Adolescent Psychiatry, 36*(5), 685–693.

McDougle, C. J., Naylor, S. T., Cohen, D. J., Volkmar, F. R., Heninger, G. R., & Price, L. H. (1996). A double-blind, placebo-controlled study of fluvoxamine in adults with autistic disorder. *Archives of General Psychiatry, 53*(11), 1001–1008.

McDougle, C. J., Scahill, L., McCracken, J. T., Aman, M. G., Tierney, E., Arnold, E., et al. (2000). Research Units on Pediatric Psychopharmacology (RUPP) Autism Network: Background and rationale for an initial controlled study of risperidone. *Child and Adolescent Psychiatric Clinics of North America, 9*(1), 201–224.

McGee, G. G., Krantz, P. J., & McClannahan, L. E. (1984). Conversational skills for autistic adolescents: Teaching assertiveness in naturalistic game settings. *Journal of Autism and Developmental Disorders, 14*(3), 319–330.

Mesibov, G. B. (1984). Social skills training with verbal autistic adolescents and adults: A program model. *Journal of Autism and Developmental Disorders, 14*(4), 395–404.

Mesibov, G., & Handlan, S. (1997). Adolescents and adults with autism. In D. J. Cohen & F. R. Volkmar (Eds.), *Handbook of autism and pervasive developmental disorders* (2nd ed., pp. 309–324). New York: Wiley.

Mesibov, G. B., & Schaffer, B. (1986). Autism in adolescents and adults. *Advances in Developmental and Behavioral Pediatrics, 7,* 313–343.

Mesibov, G. B., Schopler, E., & Caison, W. (1989). The Adolescent and Adult Psychoeducational Profile: Assessment of adolescents and adults with severe developmental handicaps. *Journal of Autism and Developmental Disorders, 19*(1), 33–40.

Mesibov, G. B., Schopler, E., Schaffer, B., & Michal, N. (1989). Use of the childhood autism rating scale with autistic adolescents and adults. *Journal of the American Academy of Child and Adolescent Psychiatry, 28*(4), 538–541.

Miller, J. N., & Ozonoff, S. (1997). Did Asperger's cases have Asperger disorder? A research note. *Journal of Child Psychology and Psychiatry, 38*(2), 247–251.

Morgan, H. (1996). *Adults with autism: A guide to theory and practice.* Cambridge, UK: Cambridge University Press.

National Research Council. (2001). *Educating young children with autism.* Washington, DC: National Academy Press.

Ousley, O. Y., & Mesibov, G. B. (1991). Sexual attitudes and knowledge of high-functioning adolescents and adults with autism. *Journal of Autism an Developmental Disorders, 21*(4), 471–481.

Paul, R. (1997). Facilitating transitions in language development for children using AAC. *Augmentative and Alternative Communication, 13*(3), 141–148.

Paul, R. (2003). Promoting social communication in high functioning individuals with autistic spectrum disorders. *Child and Adolescent Psychiatric Clinics of North America, 12*(1), 87–106.

Piven, J., Harper, J., Palmter, P., & Arndt, S. (1996). Course of behavioral change in autism: A retrospective study of high-IQ adolescents and adults. *Journal of the American Academy of Child and Adolescent Psychiatry, 35*(4), 523–529.

Rett, A. (1966). Uber ein eigenartiges hirntophisces Syndroem bei hyperammonie im Kindersalter. *Wein Medizinische Wochenschrift, 118,* 723–726.

Rourke, B. P. (1989). *Nonverbal learning disabilities: The syndrome and the model.* New York: Guilford Press.

Rourke, B. P., & Tsatsanis, K. D. (2000). Nonverbal learning disabilities and Asperger syndrome. In A. Klin & F. R. Volkmar (Eds.), *Asperger syndrome* (pp. 231–253). New York: Guilford Press.

Rutter, M. (1970). Autistic children: Infancy to adulthood. *Seminars in Psychiatry, 2*(4), 435–450.

Rutter, M. (1972). Childhood schizophrenia reconsidered. *Journal of Autism and Childhood Schizophrenia, 2*(4), 315–337.

Rutter, M. (1997). Implications of genetic research for child psychiatry. *Canadian Journal of Psychiatry, 42*(6), 569–576.

Rutter, M., Bailey, A., Bolton, P., & Le Couter, A. (1994). Autism and known medical conditions: Myth and substance. *Journal of Child Psychology and Psychiatry and Allied Disciplines, 35*(2), 311–322.

Rutter, M., & Schopler, E. (1993). "Diagnosis by DSM-III—R versus ICD-10 criteria": Response. *Journal of Autism and Developmental Disorders, 23*(3), 573–574.

Schopler, E., Andrews, C. E., & Strupp, K. (1979). Do autistic children come from upper-middle-class parents? *Journal of Autism and Developmental Disorders, 9*(2), 139–152.

Schopler, E., & Mesibov, G. B. (2000). Cross-cultural priorities in developing autism services. *International Journal of Mental Health. 29*(1), 3–21.

Schopler, E., Mesibov, G. B., & Hearsey, K. (1995). Structured teaching in the TEACCH system. In E. Schopler & G. B. Mesibov (Eds.), *Learning and cognition in autism: Current issues in autism* (pp. 243–268). New York: Plenum Press.

Schopler, E., Reichler, R. J., DeVellis, R. F., & Daly, K. (1980). Toward objective classification of childhood autism: Childhood autism. *Journal of Autism and Developmental Disorders, 10*(1), 91–103.

Schroeder, S. R., LeBlanc, J. M., & Mayo, L. (1996). Brief report: A life-span perspective on the development of individuals with autism. *Journal of Autism and Developmental Disorders, 26*(2), 251–255.

Schultz, R. T., Gauthier, I., Klin, A., Fulbright, R. K., Anderson, A. W., Volkmar, F., et al. (2000). Abnormal ventral temporal cortical activity during face discrimination among individuals with autism and Asperger syndrome. *Archives of General Psychiatry, 57*(4), 331–340.

Seltzer, M. M., Kraus, M. W., Orsmond, G. I., & Verstal., C. (2001). Families of adolescents and adults with autism—uncharted territory. *International Review of Research in Mental Retardation, 23,* 267–294.

Seltzer, M. M., Krauss, M. W., Shattuck, P. T., Orsmond, G., Swe, A., & Lord, C. (2003). The symptoms of autism spectrum disorders in adolescence and adulthood. *Journal of Autism and Developmental Disorders, 33*(6), 565–581.

Siegel, B., Pliner, C., Eschler, J., & Elliott, G. R. (1988). How children with autism are diagnosed: difficulties in identification of children with multiple developmental delays. *Journal of Developmental Behavior and Pediatrics, 9*(4), 199–204.

Simonson, L. R., Simonson, S. M., & Volkmar, F. R. (1990). Benhaven's residential program. Special issue: Residential services. *Journal of Autism and Developmental Disorders, 20*(3), 323–337.

Slone, M., Durrheim, K., Kaminer, D., & Lachman, P. (1999). Issues in the identification of comorbidity of mental retardation and psychopathology in a multicultural context. *Social Psychiatry and Psychiatric Epidemiology, 34*(4), 190–194.

Sparrow, S. S., Balla, D., & Cicchetti, D. V. (1984). *Vineland Adaptive Behavior Scales.* Circle Pines, MN: American Guidance Service.

Sperry, V. W. (2001). *Fragile success: Ten autistic children, childhood to adulthood.* Baltimore: Brookes.

Sponheim, E. (1996). Changing criteria of autistic disorders: A comparison of the ICD-10 research criteria and DSM-IV with DSM-III-R, CARS, and ABC. *Journal of Autism and Developmental Disorders, 26*(5), 513–525.

Stone, W. L. (1997). Autism in infancy and early childhood. In D. J. Cohen & F. R. Volkmar (Eds.), *Handbook of autism and pervasive developmental disorders* (2nd ed., pp. 266–282). New York: Wiley.

Taiminen, T. (1994). Asperger's syndrome or schizophrenia: Is differential diagnosis necessary for adult patients? *Nordic Journal of Psychiatry, 48*(5), 325–328.

Tantam, D. (2000a). Adolescence and adulthood of individuals with Asperger syndrome. In A. Klin & F. R. Volkmar (Eds.), *Asperger syndrome* (pp. 367–399). New York: Guilford Press.

Tantam, D. (2000b). Psychological disorder in adolescents and adults with Asperger syndrome. *Autism, 4*(1), 47–62.

Tantam, D. (2003). The challenge of adolescents and adults with Asperger syndrome. *Child and Adolescent Psychiatric Clinics of North America, 12*(1), 143–163.

Towbin, K. E. (1997). Pervasive developmental disorder not otherwise specified. In D. J. Cohen & F. R. Volkmar (Eds.), *Handbook of autism and pervasive developmental disorders* (2nd ed., pp. 123–147). New York: Wiley.

Towbin, K. E. (2003). Strategies for pharmacologic treatment of high functioning autism and Asperger syndrome. *Child and Adolescent Psychiatric Clinics of North America, 12*(1), 23–45.

Van Acker, R. (1997). Rett's syndrome: A pervasive developmental disorder. In D. J. Cohen & F. R. Volkmar (Eds.), *Handbook of autism and pervasive developmental disorders* (2nd ed., pp. 60–93). New York: Wiley.

Van Bourgondien, M. E., & Mesibov, G. B. (1987). Humor in high-functioning autistic adults. *Journal of Autism and Developmental Disorders, 17*(3), 417–424.

Van Bourgondien, M. E., Reichle, N. C., & Palmer, A. (1997). Sexual behavior in adults with autism. *Journal of Autism and Developmental Disorders, 27*(2), 113–125.

Van Bourgondien, M. E., & Schopler, E. (1990). Critical issues in the residential care of people with autism. *Journal of Autism and Developmental Disorders, 20*(3), 391–399.

Venter, A., Lord, C., & Schopler, E. (1992). A follow-up study of high-functioning autistic children. *Journal of Child Psychology and Psychiatry, 33*(3), 489–507.

Volkmar, F. (2003). Adaptive skills. *Journal of Autism and Developmental Disorders, 33*(1), 109–110.

Volkmar, F. R. (1997). Childhood disintegrative disorder. In T. A. Widiger, H. A. Pincus, R. Ross, M. B. First, & W. Davis (Eds.), *DSM-IV sourcebook* (Vol. 3, pp. 35–42). Washington, DC: American Psychiatric Association Press.

Volkmar, F. R. (2001). Pharmacological interventions in autism: Theoretical and practical issues. *Journal of Clinical Child Psychology, 30*(1), 80–87.

Volkmar, F. R., Cicchetti, D. V., Bregman, J., & Cohen, D. J. (1992). Three diagnostic systems for autism: DSM-III, DSM-III—R, and ICD-10. Special issue: Classification and diagnosis. *Journal of Autism and Developmental Disorders, 22*(4), 483–492.

Volkmar, F. R., & Cohen, D. J. (1985). The experience of infantile autism: A first-person account by Tony W. *Journal of Autism and Developmental Disorders, 15*(1), 47–54.

Volkmar, F. R., & Cohen, D. J. (1991). Comorbid association of autism and schizophrenia. *American Journal of Psychiatry, 148*(12), 1705–1707.

Volkmar, F. R., Cook, E., Pomeroy, J., Realmuto, G., & Tanguay, P. (1999). Practice parameters for the assessment and treatment of children and adolescents with autism and pervasive developmental disorders. *Journal of the American Academy of Child and Adolescent Psychiatry 38*(12), 32S–54S.

Volkmar, F. R., Klin, A., & Cohen, D. J. (1997). Diagnosis and classification of autism and related conditions: Consensus and issues. In D. J. Cohen & F. R. Volkmar (Eds.), *Handbook of autism and pervasive developmental disorders* (2nd ed., pp. 5–40). New York: Wiley.

Volkmar, F. R., Klin, A., & Pauls, D. (1998). Nosological and genetic aspects of Asperger syndrome. *Journal of Autism and Developmental Disorders, 28*(5), 457–463.

Volkmar, F. R., Klin, A., Siegel, B., Szatmari, P., Lord, C., Campbell, M., et al. (1994). Field trial for autistic disorder in DSM-IV. *American Journal of Psychiatry, 151*(9), 1361–1367.

Volkmar, F. R., Lord, C., Bailey, A., Schultz, R. T., & Klin, A. (2004). Autism and pervasive developmental disorders. *Journal of Child Psychology and Psychiatry and Allied Disciplines, 45*(1), 135–170.

Volkmar, F. R., & Nelson, D. S. (1990). Seizure disorders in autism. *Journal of the American Academy of Child and Adolescent Psychiatry, 29*(1), 127–129.

Volkmar, F. R., Scwab-Stone, M., & First, M. (2002). Classification in child psychiatry: Principles and issues. In M. Lewis (Ed.), *Child and adolescent psychiatry: A comprehensive textbook* (3rd ed., pp. 499–506). Baltimore: Williams & Wilkins.

Volkmar, F. R., Szatmari, P., & Sparrow, S. S. (1993). Sex differences in pervasive developmental disorders. *Journal of Autism and Developmental Disorders, 23*(4), 579–591.

Volkmar, F., & Wiesner, E. (2004). *Health care for children on the autism spectrum*. Bethesda, MD: Woodbine.

Volkmar, F. R., & Woolston, J. L. (1997). Comorbidity of psychiatric disorders in children and adolescents. In S. Wetzler & W. C. Sanderson (Eds.), *Treatment strategies for patients with psychiatric comorbidity* (pp. 307–322). New York: Wiley.

Wing, L. (1980). Childhood autism and social class: A question of selection? *British Journal of Psychiatry, 137*, 410–417.

Wing, L. (1981). Asperger's syndrome: A clinical account. *Psychological Medicine, 11*(1), 115–129.

Wing, L., & Potter, D. (2002). The epidemiology of autistic spectrum disorders: Is the prevalence rising? *Mental Retardation and Developmental Disabilities Research Reviews, 8*, 151–161.

Wolf, L., & Goldberg, B. (1986). Autistic children grow up: An eight to twenty-four year follow-up study. *Canadian Journal of Psychiatry, 31*(6), 550–556.

Wolff, S. (1998). Schizoid personality in childhood: The links with Asperger syndrome, schizophrenia spectrum disorders, and elective mutism. In E. Schopler & G. B. Mesibov (Eds.), *Asperger syndrome or high-functioning autism? Current issues in autism* (pp. 123–142). New York: Plenum Press.

Wolff, S., Townshend, R., McGuire, R. J., & Weeks, D. J. (1991). "Schizoid" personality in childhood and adult life. II: Adult adjustment and the continuity with schizotypal personality disorder. *British Journal of Psychiatry, 159*, 620–629.

World Health Organization, (1994). *Diagnostic criteria for research, International Classification of Diseases* (10th ed.). Geneva, Switzerland: Author.

V

PERSONALITY AND HEALTH-RELATED DISORDERS

13

Personality Disorders

Jeffrey G. Johnson
Elizabeth Bromley
Robert F. Bornstein
Joel R. Sneed

According to the *Diagnostic and Statistical Manual of Mental Disorders* (DSM-IV-TR; American Psychiatric Association [APA], 2000), "A Personality Disorder is an enduring pattern of inner experience and behavior that deviates markedly from the expectations of the individual's culture, is pervasive and inflexible, has an onset in adolescence or early adulthood, is stable over time, and leads to distress or impairment" (p. 685). Personality disorders (PDs) are widely recognized as being common, chronic psychiatric conditions that tend to be associated with considerable impairment and distress and poor long-term outcomes. There has been a substantial increase in research on PDs since 1980, when specific diagnostic criteria for personality disorders were introduced in DSM-III. PD research accelerated considerably following the development and validation of structured diagnostic interviews such as the Personality Disorder Examination (PDE; Loranger et al., 1994) and the Structured Clinical Interview for DSM-IV Personality Disorders (SCID-II; First, Spitzer, Gibbon, & Williams, 1995a).

Most of what is currently known about PDs is based on research conducted with adults. This research has indicated that PDs are relatively common in the general population. Prevalence estimates from studies of representative community samples, using DSM diagnostic criteria (DSM-III [APA, 1980]; DSM-III-R [APA, 1987]; and DSM-IV [APA, 1994]), have ranged from approximately 7–15% of the adult population, depending on the diagnostic procedures used and the range of PDs assessed (Klein et al., 1995; Maier, Lichtermann, Klingler, Heun, & Hallmayer, 1992; Moldin, Rice, Erlenmeyer-Kimling, & Squires-Wheeler, 1994; Samuels et al., 2002; Torgerson, Kringlen, & Cramer, 2001). Research has also indicated that PD symptoms tend to be moderately stable over time during early and middle adulthood (First, Spitzer, Gibbon, Williams, Davies, et al., 1995; Johnson et al., 1997; Ouimette & Klein, 1995; Perry, 1993; Ronningstam, Gunderson & Lyons, 1995; Vetter & Koller, 1993; Zimmerman, 1994), although many PD symptoms also become less prevalent or less evident with age (Farrington, 1991; Johnson, Williams, et al.,

1997; Johnson, Cohen, Kasen, et al., 2000; Lenzenweger, 1999; Robins & Regier, 1991; Samuels et al., 2002).

In this chapter, we summarize the research findings that are currently available regarding PDs during adolescence. Although there has been a major increase in the amount of research investigating adolescent PDs in recent years, many important questions remain unanswered. Despite long-standing uncertainties about the appropriateness of diagnosing PDs among adolescents (Bleiberg, 1994; Rey, 1996), most of the findings that are currently available regarding adolescent PDs are broadly similar to the findings obtained from studies of adults. Thus, although there are some differences in the procedures used to assess PDs among adolescents and adults, and although the symptoms may be expressed differently as a function of age,[1] PDs during adolescence and adulthood do not appear to be fundamentally different conditions.

We begin by describing the general diagnostic criteria for personality disorders, as set forth in DSM-IV-TR (APA, 2000) and then summarize the unique diagnostic considerations that have been stipulated for use in determining whether adolescents meet these diagnostic criteria. We then turn our attention to the interface between normal and pathological personality functioning. The remainder of the chapter summarizes research findings regarding the reliability and validity of adolescent PD diagnoses; impairment, distress, and outcomes associated with adolescent PDs; the stability and prevalence of adolescent PDs; risk factors associated with the development of adolescent PDs; gender differences in PD in adolescents; and treatment considerations with adolescents.

DSM-IV-TR DIAGNOSTIC CRITERIA AND SPECIAL CONSIDERATIONS FOR ASSESSMENT OF ADOLESCENTS

Although DSM-IV-TR states that PD traits may be evident during childhood, and that PDs can be diagnosed among both children and adolescents, it goes on to note that "the traits of a Personality Disorder that appear in childhood will often not persist unchanged into adult life" (p. 687). Similarly, DSM-II (APA, 1968), DSM-III (APA, 1980), and DSM-III-R (1987) stated that PDs are often recognizable by adolescence or earlier. Thus, although there have been on-

going concerns about diagnosing PDs among adolescents, it has long been considered appropriate to diagnose a PD among youth who clearly meet the diagnostic criteria.

In addition to the specific diagnostic criteria for particular types of PDs, the characteristic features of which are presented by cluster in Table 13.1, the following general criteria for a PD are listed (APA, 2000, p. 689):

A. An enduring pattern of inner experience and behavior that deviates markedly from the expectations of the individual's culture. This pattern is manifested in two (or more) of the following areas: (1) Cognition (i.e., ways of perceiving and interpreting self, other people, and events); (2) Affectivity (i.e., the range, intensity, lability, and appropriateness of emotional response); (3) Interpersonal functioning; (4) Impulse control.

B. The enduring pattern is inflexible and pervasive across a broad range of personal and social situations.

C. The enduring pattern leads to clinically significant distress or impairment in social, occupational, or other important areas of functioning.

D. The pattern is stable and of long duration, and its onset can be traced back at least to adolescence or early adulthood.

E. The enduring pattern is not better accounted for as a manifestation or consequence of another mental disorder.

F. The enduring pattern is not due to the direct physiological effects of a substance or a general medical condition.

In addition to these general diagnostic criteria, DSM-IV-TR stipulates that the following diagnostic considerations should also be used in assessing PDs among children and adolescents:

1. "Personality Disorder categories may be applied to children or adolescents in those relatively unusual instances in which the individual's particular maladaptive personality traits appear to be pervasive, persistent, and unlikely to be limited to a particular developmental stage or an episode of an Axis I disorder" (APA, 2000, p. 687).

2. "To diagnose a Personality Disorder in an individual under age 18 years, the features must have been present for at least 1 year" (APA, 2000, p. 687).

3. "The one exception to this is Antisocial Personality Disorder, which cannot be diagnosed in individuals under age 18 years

TABLE 13.1. Characteristic Features of DSM-IV Personality Disorders by Cluster

Cluster A (odd)

Paranoid	Pervasive mistrust of others where motives of others are interpreted as malevolent
Schizoid	Pervasive pattern of detachment from social and interpersonal relationships accompanied by a restricted range of affect and emotional expression in interpersonal situations
Schizotypal	Pervasive pattern of social and interpersonal deficits characterized by acute discomfort and diminished capacity for close relationships accompanied by cognitive and perceptual distortions and behavioral eccentricities

Cluster B (dramatic)

Antisocial	Pervasive pattern of disregard and violation of the rights of others characterized by deceit and manipulation beginning in childhood or adolescence and continuing into adulthood
Borderline	Pervasive pattern of interpersonal, affective, and identity instability accompanied by marked impulsivity
Histrionic	Pervasive pattern of excessive emotionality and attention seeking
Narcissistic	Pervasive pattern of grandiosity, need for admiration, and inability to empathize with others

Cluster C (anxious)

Avoidant	Pervasive pattern of social inhibition, feelings of inadequacy, and hypersensitivity to negative evaluation
Dependent	Pervasive pattern of clinging and submissive behavior motivated by the need to be taken care of and an intense fear of separation
Obsessive–compulsive	Intense preoccupation with orderliness, perfectionism, and mental and interpersonal control at the expense of flexibility, openness, and efficiency

(APA, 2000, p. 687)." The unique limitations associated with early diagnosis of antisocial personality disorder are due primarily to the fact that—alone among Axis II syndromes—antisocial personality disorder has a formally defined diagnostic precursor. Thus, an additional diagnostic criterion for diagnosis of antisocial personality disorder in adulthood is that "there is evidence of Conduct Disorder with onset before age 15 years" (APA, 2000, p. 706).

It is important to note several issues regarding the application of these general diagnostic criteria and special considerations for the identification of PDs among adolescents. First, some personality traits that may be regarded as being pathological when expressed during adulthood are considered relatively normal during adolescence (e.g., affective lability and impulsivity). Thus, as noted previously (Criterion A), it is particularly important to recognize that a personality trait must deviate markedly from cultural expectations in order to be considered symptomatic of a PD.

Second, as noted previously, DSM-IV-TR stipulates that "Personality Disorder categories may be applied to children or adolescents in those *relatively unusual instances* in which the individual's particular maladaptive personality traits appear to be pervasive, persistent, and unlikely to be limited to a particular developmental stage or an episode of an Axis I disorder" (APA, 2000, p. 687, emphasis added). However, the same basic conditions are required in order for a PD to be diagnosed in an adult, and DSM-IV-TR does not state unequivocally that the instances in which a PD is diagnosed must be more "unusual" when the subject is an adolescent than when the subject is an adult.

Due to the paucity of research on adolescent PDs, it is not yet clear whether PDs are more or less common among adolescents than they are among adults. However, the evidence that is currently available suggests that PDs may be as prevalent—or more prevalent—among adolescents as among adults (Farrington, 1991; Johnson, Cohen, Kasen, et al., 2000; Lenzenweger, 1999; Robins & Regier, 1991; Samuels et al., 2002). These and related findings are described more extensively in a later section of this chapter.

Third, with the exception of antisocial personality disorder (APD), which cannot be diagnosed until age 18, identical sets of diagnostic criteria are used to identify the other DSM-IV PDs (e.g., borderline personality disorder) among adolescents and adults. Most PDs are diagnosed based on these diagnostic criteria for specific types of PDs (Torgerson et al., 2001), although the diagnosis of personality disorder not otherwise specified (PD-NOS) is sometimes assigned. However, pathological personality traits, like many other types of psychiatric symptoms, tend to be more common among adolescents than they are among adults (Johnson, Cohen, Kasen, et al., 2000; see Derogatis, 1983). For this reason, and because the likelihood of a PD diagnosis increases with the number of PD traits identified as being present (APA, 2000), PDs are likely to be as prevalent, if not more prevalent, among adolescents as they are among adults.

ASSOCIATIONS OF PERSONALITY TRAITS WITH PD DIAGNOSES

One criticism of the DSM-IV diagnostic system is its conception of PDs as categorical (Livesley, Schroeder, Jackson, & Jang, 1994), which does not reflect the widespread belief among many researchers and clinicians that personality disorder symptoms are extreme expressions of normal personality characteristics (Costa & Widiger, 2002; Oldham & Skodol, 2000). According to this perspective, the difference between normal personality and PD is quantitative rather than qualitative; that is, a matter of degree. According to Widiger (1998), "Personality disorders are not qualitatively distinct from normal personality functioning, they are simply maladaptive, extreme variants of common personality traits" (p. 865). Supporting this position, O'Connor (2002) used factor analysis on published data of 37 personality and psychopathology inventories and observed that the dimensional universes of the normal and abnormal are the same. Similarly, Livesley, Jackson, and Schroeder (1992) found that the factor structures of 100 self-report measures of PD were highly similar in both clinical and nonclinical samples. Although it is clear that the "overwhelming majority favor a dimensional approach" (Oldham & Skodol, 2000, p. 24), it is unclear which dimensional model is most accurate.

There are many dimensional models of PD that depict PD as consisting of extreme variants of normal personality functioning. For example, Millon (1987) conceived of PD as consisting of extreme variants of two fundamental dimensions: reinforcement and coping style. Wiggins (1982) argued that PDs could be located on a circumplex consisting of two orthogonal dimensions defined as love–warmth–affiliation (nurturance) and dominance–status–control (dominance). Torgersen and Alnaes's (1989) created a decision tree model of PD based on the presence or absence of personality traits on four dimensions of personality labeled reality-weak, extroversion, oral, and obsessive. Cloninger and Svrakic's (1994) postulated a seven-factor model of PD that included the dimensions of novelty seeking, harm avoidance, reward dependence, persistence, self-directedness, cooperativeness, and self-transcendence. The five-factor model (FFM; Costa & McCrae, 1992; Costa & Widiger, 2002; Widiger, Trull, Clarkin, Sanderson, & Costa, 2002) conceptualizes personality as maladaptive, extreme variants of openness to experience, conscientiousness, extraversion, agreeableness, and neuroticism.

O'Connor and Dyce (1998) reviewed and empirically evaluated the foregoing models, and 10 additional models of PD, by conducting factors analyses on 12 previously published data sets and found the strongest support for a four-factor model based on the FFM (see Table 13.2). The trait dimensions of neuroticism (negative emotionality), extraversion (positive emotionality), conscientiousness, and agreeableness appear to be most relevant whereas the trait dimension openness to experience does not appear to play an important role in PD. This four-factor model of PD based on the FFM is consistent with the integrative hierarchical structure of personality and psychopathology proposed by Watson, Clark, and Harkness (1994) and arrived at empirically by Livesley, Jang, and Vernon (1998). Livesley and colleagues (1998) defined four factors through factor analysis of the Dimensional Assessment of Personality Disorder—Basic Questionnaire labeled as emotional dysregulation, dissocial (rejection, callousness, sensation seeking, and conduct problems), inhibition (intimacy problems, identity problems, and restricted emotional expression), and compulsivity, which are closely related to the four factors derived from the FFM (Widiger, 1998). This suggests that PDs conceived of as continua of normal personality traits might best be described in terms

**TABLE 13.2. The Four Factors
of Personality Most Implicated in the Personality
Trait-to-Disorder Interface**

Neuroticism or negative emotionality	Level of emotional adjustment and instability; facets include anxiety, angry hostility, depression, self-consciousness, impulsivity, and vulnerability.
Extraversion or positive emotionality	Quantity and intensity of interpersonal relationships, activity level, and capacity for positive feelings; facets include warmth, gregariousness, assertiveness, activity, excitement seeking, and positive emotions.
Conscientiousness	Extent of organization, persistence, control, and motivation in goal-directed behavior; facets include competence, order, dutifulness, achievement striving, self-discipline, and deliberation.
Agreeableness	Interpersonal interactions ranging from compassionate to antagonistic; facets include trust, straightforwardness, altruism, compliance modesty, and tender-mindedness.

of four higher-order traits reflecting the capacity for self-discipline, the ability to get along with others, and the tendency to experience positive and negative emotions.

RELIABILITY AND VALIDITY OF PD ASSESSMENT IN ADOLESCENT POPULATIONS

Most of the current research findings indicate that PDs can be diagnosed among adolescents in a reliable and valid manner. Numerous studies have demonstrated that when different clinicians provide independent ratings of diagnostic interviews, interrater agreement tends to be acceptable, ranging from moderate to high (Becker, Grilo, Edell, & McGlashan, 2002; Brent, Zelenak, Bukstein, & Brown, 1990; Daley et al., 1999; Grilo, McGlashan, et al., 1998; Guzder, Paris, Zelkowitz, & Marchessault, 1996; Lenzenwegger, 1999;

Ludolph et al., 1990; Westen, Ludolph, Block, Wixom, & Wiss, 1990; Westen, Shedler, Durrett, Glass, & Martens, 2003).

Findings regarding the retest reliability or temporal stability of PDs, which are summarized in greater detail later, indicate that PD traits tend to be moderately stable during adolescence, while PD diagnoses are somewhat less stable, due to fluctuations in personality traits above and below the diagnostic threshold (e.g., Barasch, Frances, Hurt, Clarkin, & Cohen, 1985; Bernstein et al., 1993; Daley et al., 1999; Johnson, Cohen, Kasen, et al., 2000; Korenblum, Marton, Golombek, & Stein, 1987, 1990; Lenzenwegger, 1999; Mattanah, Becker, Levy, Edell, & McGlashan, 1985). Similar findings regarding the temporal stability of PD diagnoses and traits have been obtained from adult samples when similar retest intervals and assessment procedures have been used (e.g., Ferro, Klein, Schwartz, Kasch, & Leader, 1998; Johnson, Williams, et al., 1997; Johnson, Cohen, Kasen, et al., 2000; Loranger et al., 1994; McDavid & Pilkonis, 1996; Paris, 1988; Perry, 1993; Pilkonis, Heape, Ruddy & Serrao, 1991; Trull et al., 1998; Vaglum, Friis, Karterud, Mehlum, & Vaglum, 1993; Vetter & Koller, 1993; Zimmerman, 1994).

Support for the concurrent, construct, and predictive validity of adolescent PD diagnoses has been provided by research indicating that adolescent PDs are associated with significant impairment and distress, maladaptive personality traits and defense styles, and elevated risk for Axis I disorders, interpersonal aggression, suicide, and other adverse outcomes (Bernstein et al., 1993; Brent et al., 1990, 1993, 1994; Daley, Hammen, Davila, & Burge, 1998; Daley et al., 1999; Grilo, Walker, Becker, Edell, & McGlashan, 1997; Guzder et al., 1996; Johnson, 1993; Johnson & Bornstein, 1991, 1992; Johnson, Bornstein, & Krukonis, 1992; Johnson, Cohen, Dohrenwend, Link, & Brook, 1999; Johnson, Cohen, Smailes, et al., 2000; Johnson, Hyler, Skodol, Bornstein, & Sherman, 1995; Johnson, Quigley, & Sherman, 1997; Lavan & Johnson, 2002; Levy et al., 1999; Pinto, Grapentine, Francis, & Picariello, 1996; Westen et al., 1990, 2003; Zaider, Johnson, & Cockell, 2000). These findings are summarized in greater detail later.

Further evidence in support of the reliability and validity of adolescent PD diagnoses has been provided by a number of other studies. Research has indicated that risk factors for borderline personality disorder (BPD) during childhood are similar to those associated with BPD during adulthood (Guzder et al., 1996), that adolescents with BPD have self-concept disturbances that are not accounted for solely by depressive traits (Pinto et al., 1996), and that—consistent with familial aggregation studies of adult PDs—first-degree adult relatives of adolescents with PDs are at elevated risk for having the same types of PDs (Johnson, Brent, et al., 1995). PD traits have been found to have similar correlates in adolescent and adult samples (DeClercq & Fruyt, 2003). Research has also indicated that when similar assessment procedures are used, the prevalence of PDs among adolescent inpatients is nearly identical to the prevalence of PDs among adult inpatients (Becker et al., 2002; Grilo, McGlashan, et al., 1998).

PREVALENCE OF PDs AMONG ADOLESCENTS IN THE GENERAL POPULATION

Because few community-based studies have investigated PDs among adolescents in the general population, and because different sampling and assessment procedures have been used, it is not yet possible to draw firm conclusions regarding the prevalence of adolescent PDs in the general population. However, the evidence that is currently available based on DSM-III-R and DSM-IV diagnostic criteria indicates that PDs are likely to be as prevalent, or slightly more prevalent, among adolescents than among adults in the general population.[2]

Estimates of the prevalence of DSM-III-R and DSM-IV PDs among adolescents in representative community or primary care settings have ranged from 6% to 17%, based on data from clinical interviews (Daley et al., 1999; Lenzenweger, Loranger, Korfine, & Neff, 1997; Zaider et al., 2000), interviews of multiple informants (Bernstein et al., 1993; Johnson, Cohen, Dohrenwend, et al., 1999), or self-report instruments that have been modified to correct for low questionnaire specificity (Johnson, Bornstein, & Sherman, 1996). The median of these PD prevalence estimates is 11.0%, based on studies that used representative samples and validated assessment procedures. The prevalence estimate based on the unweighted mean is 11.9% (SD = 4.1).[3] In comparison, it has been estimated that approximately 10%

of the adults in the general population are likely to have a current PD (Merikangas & Weissman, 1986; Oldham, 1994; Weissman, 1993).

Research has indicated that maladaptive PD traits may be more prevalent during early and middle adolescence than during late adolescence (Johnson, Cohen, Kasen, et al., 2000), perhaps because there tends to be more behavioral variability and emotional lability during early and middle adolescence than there is during late adolescence. In accordance with this hypothesis, the highest estimates of PD diagnostic prevalence have been obtained from studies of youth in early and middle adolescence (Bernstein et al., 1993; Johnson, Cohen, Dohrenwend, et al., 1999; Zaider et al., 2000). Studies of youth in late adolescence have yielded lower estimates, more closely approximating those based on data from adult samples (Daley et al., 1999; Johnson, Williams, et al., 1996; Lenzenwegger et al., 1997). With respect to specific Axis II diagnoses, Cluster B diagnoses (antisocial, borderline, histrionic, and narcissistic) have been found to be most common, followed by Cluster A (paranoid, schizoid, and schizotypal), and Cluster C (avoidant, dependent, and obsessive–compulsive) in one community-based, longitudinal study of adolescents (Johnson, Cohen, Kasen, et al., 2000).

These findings suggest that PDs are at least as prevalent among adolescents as they are among adults in the general population. This conclusion is consistent with findings indicating that when similar assessment procedures are used in clinical samples, PDs tend to be as prevalent among adolescents as among adults (Becker et al., 2002; Grilo et al., 1998). However, because data are only available from a comparatively small number of community-based studies, future epidemiological research will need to investigate the prevalence of adolescent PDs in a more definitive manner.

BEHAVIORAL, EMOTIONAL, AND PSYCHOSOCIAL PROBLEMS ASSOCIATED WITH ADOLESCENT PDs

Adolescent PDs tend to be associated with impairment and distress, with other maladaptive personality traits, and with co-occurring Axis I psychiatric disorders. Studies of adolescent inpatients and outpatients have indicated that patients with PDs tend to have more attitudinal, behavioral, and impulse-control problems and higher rates of psychiatric comorbidity than patients without PDs.

Like adult patients, adolescent patients with PDs have been found to experience high levels of functional impairment; interpersonal, educational, and occupational difficulties; distress; and psychiatric comorbidity (Guzder et al., 1996; Levy et al., 1999; Lofgren, Bemporad, King, Linden, & O'Driscoll, 1991; Westen et al., 1990, 2003). Youth with BPD have been found to have a poor self-concept, to have elevated scores on measures of assaultiveness, and to be more likely than patients without BPD to have a history of aggressive behavior and suicide attempts (e.g., Brent et al., 1994; Pinto et al., 1996). Adolescent patients with other types of PDs have also been found to have elevated rates of affective, anxiety, disruptive, eating, and substance use disorders; high-risk sexual behavior; and overall psychiatric symptom levels (e.g., Brent et al., 1990, 1994; Grilo et al., 1997; Guzder et al., 1996; Lavan & Johnson, 2002; Levy et al., 1999; Pinto et al., 1996; Westen et al., 2003; Zaider et al., 2000).

Although PDs in the general population tend to be less severe than those in clinical settings, adolescents in the community who have PDs have been found to experience elevated levels of psychosocial difficulties and psychiatric symptoms (e.g., Bernstein et al., 1993). Community-based studies have provided compelling evidence that adolescents in the general population who have PDs tend to experience a wide range of psychosocial difficulties. Findings of the Children in the Community Study (CICS), the largest and most comprehensive longitudinal study of PDs among adolescents in the general population, indicated that individuals with PDs during middle adolescence had significantly elevated scores on 12 measures of distress and functional impairment (Bernstein et al., 1993). Youth with PDs experienced shorter friendships, fewer social activities, less enjoyment of interpersonal interaction, more contact with police, and more educational and occupational difficulties than did youth without PDs. Adolescents with PDs were also more likely than those without PDs to have co-occurring Axis I disorders (Bernstein et al., 1993).

Other studies of nonclinical samples have yielded similar results, indicating that adolescent PDs tend to be associated with elevated levels of impairment and distress. Adolescent PDs have been found to be associated with increased psychoactive substance use among youth in both Europe and the United States. PDs have also been found to be associated with maladaptive and image-distorting defense styles, poor psychosocial development, and elevated levels of depression and substance abuse during late adolescence, even among ostensibly high-functioning populations such as college students (Daley et al., 1999; Johnson, 1993; Johnson, Hyler, et al., 1995; Johnson & Bornstein, 1992; Johnson et al., 1992).[4]

LONG-TERM OUTCOMES ASSOCIATED WITH ADOLESCENT PDs

Adolescent PDs are frequently associated with poor long-term outcomes, including aggressive behavior, criminal behavior, externalizing symptoms, psychiatric disorders, and suicide (Brent et al., 1993, 1994; Crawford, Cohen, & Brook, 2001b; Levy et al., 1999; Daley et al., 1998, 1999; Johnson & Bornstein, 1991; Johnson, Cohen, Skodol, et al., 1999; Johnson, Cohen, Smailes, et al., 2000; Johnson, Quigley, & Sherman, 1997; Marton et al., 1989; McManus, Lerner, Robbins, & Barbour, 1984; Pfeffer, Newcorn, & Kaplan, 1988; Runeson & Beskow, 1991; Westen et al., 2003). Adolescent inpatients with PDs have been found to be at elevated risk for substance use and rehospitalization (Levy et al., 1999). Adolescent patients with BPD tend to have poor long-term outcomes, including chronic PD, homelessness, interpersonal difficulties, occupational impairment, and substance abuse (Lofgren et al., 1991). In addition, young patients with PDs are at elevated risk for suicide attempts and completed suicide (Brent et al., 1993, 1994; Marton et al., 1989; McManus et al., 1984; Pfeffer et al., 1988; Runeson & Beskow, 1991; Westen et al., 2003).

Paralleling the results obtained in clinical samples, community-based research has indicated that adolescents with PDs in the general population are at elevated risk for a variety of adverse outcomes (Crawford, Cohen, Johnson, Sneed, & Brook, 2004; Daley et al., 1998, 1999; Johnson & Bornstein, 1991; Johnson, Cohen, Dohrwenend, et al., 1999; Johnson, Cohen, Smailes, et al., 2000; Johnson, Quigley, & Sherman, 1997), including aggressive and criminal behavior, Axis I disorders, and suicide attempts by early adulthood. This increase in risk does not appear to be attributable to co-occurring psychopathology (Johnson, Cohen, Dohrwenend, et al., 1999; Johnson, Cohen, Smailes, et al., 2000).

Similarly, adolescent PD symptoms have been found to predict increased levels of depression, interpersonal difficulties, and chronic stress over a 2-year follow-up period, even after baseline depressive symptoms are accounted for (Daley et al., 1998, 1989). In addition, PD symptoms during late adolescence predicted subsequent Axis I symptom levels after baseline Axis I symptoms were controlled statistically (Johnson & Bornstein, 1991). These findings are consistent with research indicating that maladaptive personality traits during childhood and adolescence tend to be associated with a variety of adverse outcomes including academic problems, behavior problems, interpersonal difficulties, and substance abuse during late adolescence or early adulthood (Brook, Brook, & Cohen, 1998; Cloninger, Sigvardsson, & Bohman, 1988; Cooper, Wood, Orcutt, & Albino, 2003; Hart, Hofmann, Edelstein, & Keller, 1997; Newman, Caspi, Moffitt, & Silva, 1997; Robins, 1966; Shiner, 2000).

STABILITY OF PD SYMPTOMS DURING ADOLESCENCE

Among both adolescents and adults, PD traits tend to be moderately stable over time. Studies of adolescents and adults have yielded similar findings regarding the temporal stability of PD diagnoses and traits when similar retest intervals and assessment and sampling procedures were used (e.g., Bernstein et al., 1993; Crawford, Cohen, & Brook, 2001a; Daley et al., 1999; Ferro et al., 1998; Grilo, Becker, Edell, & McGlashan, 2001; Johnson, Williams, et al., 1997; Johnson, Cohen, Kasen, et al., 2000; Korenblum et al., 1987, 1990; Lenzenwegger, 1999; Loranger et al., 1994; Mattanah et al., 1985; McDavid & Pilkonis, 1996; Perry, 1993; Trull et al., 1998; Vaglum et al., 1993; Vetter & Koller, 1993; Zimmerman, 1994). However, estimates of the stability of PD diagnoses among adolescents and adults have ranged from low to moderate. As in studies of normal personality traits, estimates of the stability of PD traits and diagnoses based on these studies have tended to be inversely associated with the length of the intertest interval.

Although research has indicated that PD diagnoses are not highly stable in either adolescents or adults, several methodological issues merit consideration. First, research has suggested that the temporary effects of mood states and stress on the assessment of maladaptive personality traits may contribute to artificially low estimates of the temporal stability of PD traits (Loranger et al., 1991; Ouimette & Klein, 1995). Second, despite their modest temporal stability, PDs during adolescence and adulthood have been found to predict a wide range of adverse long-term outcomes. Such findings, combined with the findings indicating that PD traits tend to be more stable than PD diagnoses, suggest that adolescents and adults with PDs may experience chronically elevated PD trait levels that account, in part, for their chronic or recurrent impairment and distress. This conclusion has been supported by research indicating that adolescents with PDs tend to have significantly elevated PD trait levels during early adulthood (Johnson, Cohen, Kasen, et al., 2000). Third, like some chronic or recurrent Axis I disorders (e.g., dysthymic disorder), PDs may remit or vary in severity as a function of life events and other changes in environmental or physical circumstances (Johnson, Cohen, Kasen, et al., 2000b).

THE DEVELOPMENT OF PDs BEFORE, DURING, AND AFTER ADOLESCENCE

PD traits tend to decrease in prevalence over time among children, adolescents, and adults in clinical and community settings (Bernstein et al., 1993; Black, Baumgard, & Bell, 1995; Farrington, 1991; Garnet, Levy, Mattanah, Edell, & McGlashan, 1994; Grilo et al., 2001; Johnson, Williams, et al., 1997; Johnson, Cohen, Kasen, et al., 2000; Korenblum et al., 1987; Lenzenweger, 1999; Mattanah et al., 1995; Orlandini et al., 1997; Ronningstam et al., 1995; Trull et al., 1998; Vaglum et al., 1993; Vetter & Koller, 1993). Cross-sectional findings have similarly indicated that the prevalence of PD traits tends to be inversely associated with age among adolescents and adults (e.g., Johnson, Cohen, Kasen, et al., 2000; Kessler et al., 1994; Robins & Regier, 1991; Samuels et al., 2002). These findings may indicate that most youth and adults eventually learn to inhibit the expression of maladaptive personality traits because these traits are associated with negative consequences (Black et al., 1995; Farrington, 1991; Johnson, Cohen, Kasen, et al., 2000; Korenblum et al., 1987; Robins, 1966).

It is likely that a variety of factors, including parenting, mentoring, biological maturation, societal enforcement of adult role expectations, and other normative socialization experiences contribute to declines in PD traits from childhood through early adulthood (Stein, Newcomb, & Bentler, 1986). According to this developmental hypothesis, expressed implicitly in DSM-II, DSM-III, DSM-III-R, DSM-IV, and DSM-IV-TR (APA, 1968, 1980, 1987, 1994, 2000), PD traits and other maladaptive personality traits should peak in prevalence during childhood or early adolescence and then diminish steadily among most individuals throughout adolescence and early adulthood. Although little longitudinal evidence is currently available regarding the prevalence of PDs from childhood through adulthood, research has supported the hypothesis that PD traits decline gradually in prevalence from late childhood through early adulthood (Johnson, Cohen, Kasen, et al., 2000). These findings are consistent with the assertion in DSM-II (APA, 1968) and DSM-III-R (APA, 1987) that personality disorders are often recognizable by adolescence or earlier. Such findings are also consistent with the statements in DSM-IV-TR that personality disorders "can be traced back at least to adolescence or early adulthood" (APA, 2000, p. 689), and that "the traits of a Personality Disorder that appear in childhood will often not persist unchanged into adult life" (APA, 2000, p. 687).[5]

In addition to the aforementioned studies cited, many other studies have yielded findings that are consistent with the hypothesis that PD traits tend to develop during childhood or early adolescence and then decline gradually throughout adolescence and adulthood. Community-based longitudinal studies indicate that many maladaptive personality traits originate during childhood and persist into adolescence and adulthood (Caspi & Roberts, 2001; Charles, Reynolds, & Gatz, 2001; Cohen, 1999; McGue, Bacon, & Lykken, 1993; Roberts & DelVecchio, 2000; Shiner, 2000; Shiner, Masten, & Tellegen, 2002). In addition, behavioral and emotional problems during childhood are often associated with PD traits during adolescence and adulthood (Bernstein, Cohen, Skodol, Bezirganian, & Brook, 1996; Cohen,

1999; Drake, Adler, & Vaillant, 1988; Hart et al., 1997; Newman et al., 1997). Indirect support for the hypothesis that PD traits tend to decline during adolescence and adulthood has been provided by cross-sectional studies indicating that overall psychiatric symptom levels tend to be higher among adolescents than among adults in the community (Derogatis, 1983; Pancoast & Archer, 1992).[6]

FACTORS ASSOCIATED WITH RISK FOR PD DURING ADOLESCENCE

Although a number of constitutional and environmental factors are associated with risk for PDs, maladaptive or traumatic interpersonal experiences during childhood and adolescence appear to play a particularly important role. This conclusion is suggested by studies that have used a wide range of methodologies to assess childhood experiences and PD symptoms. It has long been known that adolescents and adults with PDs are more likely than those without these disorders to report a history of childhood abuse, neglect, or maladaptive parenting (e.g., Brodsky, Cloitre, & Dulit, 1995; Goldman, D'Angelo, DeMaso, & Mezzacappa, 1992; Herman, Perry, & van der Kolk, 1989; Johnson, Quigley, & Sherman, 1997; Klonsky, Oltmanns, Turkheimer, & Fiedler, 2000; Ludolph et al., 1990; Norden, Klein, Donaldson, Pepper, & Klein, 1995; Raczek, 1992; Shearer, Peters, Quaytman, & Ogden, 1990; Weaver & Clum, 1993; Westen et al., 1990). Although such findings are not conclusive, given the possibility of biased recall of childhood adversities, there is abundant evidence from other studies confirming the association of adverse childhood experiences with risk for the development of PDs.

Prospective longitudinal studies and studies that obtained evidence of childhood maltreatment from official records have provided stronger evidence of a possible cause–effect association between childhood maltreatment and risk for PD. Such studies have indicated that childhood abuse, neglect, and maladaptive parenting tend to be associated with elevated risk for PDs during adolescence and adulthood (e.g., Cohen, 1996; Cohen, Brown, & Smailes, 2001; Drake et al., 1988; Guzder et al., 1996; Johnson, Smailes, et al., 2000; Johnson, Cohen, Brown, Smailes, & Bernstein, 1999; Johnson, Cohen, Kasen, et al., 2001; Johnson, Cohen,

Smailes, et al., 2001; Ludolph et al., 1990; Luntz & Widom, 1994). Several of these studies indicated that physical, sexual, and verbal or psychological abuse are independently associated with risk for PDs (Guzder et al., 1996; Ludolph et al., 1990; Johnson, Cohen, Brown, et al., 1999; Johnson, Cohen, Kasen, et al., 2001; Johnson, Cohen, Smailes, et al., 2001; Johnson, Smailes, et al., 2000). Childhood neglect and maladaptive parenting have been found to be independently associated with elevated risk for PDs even after childhood abuse and parental psychiatric disorders are accounted for (Guzder et al., 1996; Johnson, Cohen, Brown, et al., 1999; Johnson, Cohen, Kasen, et al., 2001; Johnson, Smailes, et al., 2000; Ludolph et al., 1990).

Chronic adversities, such as maladaptive parenting and childhood abuse and neglect are likely to have a particularly adverse impact on personality development because they interfere with or alter the trajectory of normative socialization processes during childhood and adolescence. Normal personality development requires continuous socialization throughout childhood and adolescence, as the child's behavior is molded and refined through day-to-day interactions with parents, other adults, and peers. Although every child has unique temperament characteristics that may be evident from early infancy (Thomas & Chess, 1984), and although these characteristics tend to have an enduring impact on personality development (Hart et al., 1997), socialization and other life experiences tend to modify these traits considerably (Cohen, 1999). Regardless of the child's temperament, parents, teachers, and other adults who are involved in childrearing typically devote extensive effort to teaching children how to interact appropriately with others, how to obey rules, how to control impulsive tendencies, and how to cope with unpleasant emotions and situations (Cohen, 1999).

Research has suggested that deficits in socialization during childhood may contribute to the development of enduring PD traits (Johnson, Cohen, Kasen, et al., 2001). For example, inadequate parental supervision or inconsistent discipline throughout childhood may undermine the development of impulse control skills, leading to the chronic impulsive behavior that tends to be associated with APD and BPD. Many other PD traits may also result from inadequate socialization. For example, although some borderline, dependent, histrionic, narcis-

sistic, and passive–aggressive traits tend to be considered normative or acceptable during childhood (e.g., labile affect, egocentricity, and separation anxiety), these are generally expected to diminish during the transition to adulthood. The persistence of these traits into late adolescence and adulthood is likely to result, at least in part, from a failure in the socialization process (Johnson, Cohen, Kasen, et al., 2000, 2001). In many cases, this may be partially attributable to factors such as the loss or death of a parent or chronic socioeconomic disadvantage beyond the parents' control (e.g., Brennan & Shaver, 1998; Johnson, Cohen, Dohrenwend, et al., 1999). In this respect, the onset of PDs during adolescence may stem in part from failure to inhibit certain maladaptive childhood responses and in part from the development of problematic behavior patterns that are associated with maladaptive socialization experiences (e.g., affiliation with troubled peers).

Another factor that may contribute to socialization deficits among many individuals is the presence of a dysfunctional attachment style in one or both parents. Most PDs are characterized by a pattern of maladaptive interpersonal behavior, and these patterns of interpersonal functioning may stem in part from the development of a dysfunctional attachment style during childhood (Fossati et al., 2003; Nakash-Eisikovits, Dutra, & Westen, 2002). It is noteworthy in this regard that parental attachment styles appear to influence the interpersonal and personality development of the offspring, and that the offspring of parents with dysfunctional attachment styles are at elevated risk for a broad array of psychiatric symptoms (Rosenstein & Horowitz, 1996; Sroufe, Carlson, Levy, & Egeland, 1999). For example, dependent personality disorder during adolescence and adulthood appears to stem in part from insecure attachment to the parents throughout childhood (Pincus & Wilson, 2001).

Traumatic experiences, including childhood abuse, excessively harsh punishment, and other forms of victimization such as assault, bullying, and intimidation (as well as more extreme and atypical experiences such as kidnapping, trafficking, and exposure to warfare), may also contribute to the onset of PD traits by promoting affective dysregulation, aggressive behavior, dissociative symptoms, interpersonal withdrawal, and profound mistrust of others

(Johnson, 1993; van der Kolk, Hostetler, Herron, & Fisler, 1994). Research has suggested that youth who are victims of aggressive or abusive behavior may be at elevated risk for the development of antisocial, avoidant, borderline, depressive, paranoid, passive–aggressive, schizoid, and schizotypal personality disorder traits (e.g., Johnson, Cohen, Brown, et al., 1999; Johnson, Cohen, Kasen, et al., 2001; Johnson, Cohen, Smailes, et al., 2001).

Findings suggesting that maladaptive parenting plays a significant role in the development of PDs may have important clinical and public health implications. It may be possible to prevent the onset of chronic PDs among some youth by providing high-risk parents with educational and social services that assist them in developing more adaptive parenting behaviors. Research has indicated that it is possible to reduce the likelihood that children will develop psychiatric symptoms by helping parents to learn more effective childrearing techniques (Irvine, Biglan, Smolkowski, Metzler, & Ary, 1999; Redmond, Spoth, Shin, & Lepper, 1999; Spoth, Lopez, Redmond, & Shin, 1999). In addition, because maladaptive parenting may be associated with parental psychiatric disorders, and because parents with psychiatric disorders who receive treatment may be less likely to engage in maladaptive parenting, it may be possible to reduce offspring risk for PDs by improving the recognition and treatment of psychiatric disorders among parents in the community (Chilcoat, Breslau, & Anthony, 1996; Johnson, Cohen, Kasen, et al., 2001; Johnson, Cohen, Kasen, & Brook, in press).

It is also important to note that parental behavior tends to be influenced by offspring temperament and psychiatric symptoms, and that parents and their offspring are typically involved in a complex, dynamic, and evolving interpersonal system (Kendler, 1996). Although parental behavior is likely to play an important role in offspring personality development, genetic and prenatal factors (e.g., prenatal malnutrition, stress, and substance use) also contribute to the development of temperament difficulties, which may be developmental precursors of some PD traits (Cohen, 1999; Johnson, Brent, et al., 1995; Livesley, Jang, Jackson, & Vernon, 1993; Neugebauer, Hoek, & Susser, 1999). Maladaptive personality traits such as antisocial behavior may also result, in part, from the interaction of genetic vulnerability factors with childhood maltreatment (Caspi et al., 2002). Because personality development is such a complex phenomenon, research based on a multifactorial approach that recognizes the importance of biological, psychological, social, and cultural factors will be needed in order for the field to develop a truly comprehensive understanding of the development of PDs.

GENDER DIFFERENCES IN PDs

If we return to the idea that PDs can be conceptualized as extreme variants of normal personality traits such as those list in Table 13.2, we would expect that gender differences observed in normal personality functioning would extend to gender differences in pathological or maladaptive personality functioning. Feingold (1994) conducted four meta-analyses and observed that men on average scored higher than women on assertiveness and self-esteem and women on average scored higher than men on extraversion, anxiety, trust, and tender-mindedness. These differences are consistent with Gilligan's (1982) argument that male personality development tends to be particularly characterized by separation, autonomy, and individuation whereas female development tends to be characterized by attachment, connectedness, and intimacy. For example, parents are more likely to discuss emotions with girls than boys, girls' childhood relationships are characterized by intimate friendships and cooperation whereas boys' groups are characterized by competitiveness and rough play, and parents are more likely to assign girls child-care responsibilities than boys (Cross & Madson, 1997). Cross and Madson (1997) have even argued that women's self-concepts are characterized by interdependence (self-definition based on one's relationships and group membership), which would be consistent with women scoring higher on extraversion, trust, and tender-mindedness, whereas men's self-concepts are characterized by independence (self-definition based on autonomy, uniqueness, distinction, and separateness from others), which would be consistent with men scoring higher on assertiveness and self-esteem.

One might expect to find on the basis of these gender differences in normal personality-analogous gender differences in PDs. In line with this expectation, according to DSM-IV, paranoid, schizoid, schizotypal, antisocial, obsessive–compulsive, and narcissistic PDs tend to occur more frequently in men than in women, whereas histrionic, borderline, and dependent PDs are expected to occur more frequently in women than in men. Linking differences in self-concept to PD diagnosis, Klein, Wonderlich, and Crosby (2001) found that autonomous self-concept ratings were associated with passive–aggressive, compulsive, antisocial, and schizoid PD, whereas affiliative self-concept ratings were associated with histrionic, narcissistic, borderline, and avoidant PDs.

However, despite the relatively straightforward connection between gender-related differences in normal personality and self-concept formation and PDs, empirical work is far from conclusive. The only consistent observation in which adolescent girls are diagnosed more frequently than adolescent boys is BPD. In one study of 17 female and 8 male adolescent hospitalized adolescents ranging in age from 14 to 17, Myers, Burket, and Otto (1993) found that BPD was more frequently diagnosed in girls than in boys whereas conduct disorder (APD) was not differentially diagnosed between genders. Examining the co-occurrence of PD and conduct disorder (CD) in 21 female and 79 male incarcerated youth ranging in age from 11 to 17, Eppright, Kashani, Robison, and Reid (1993) observed that BPD was more frequently observed in females with CD than in males with CD. In a study of gender differences in PD in a sample of 138 psychiatric adolescent inpatients (mean age = 15.5 years), Grilo and colleagues (1996) found that BPD was more frequently diagnosed in females and narcissistic PD was diagnosed only in males. BPD has also been found to be more frequently diagnosed in female than in male alcohol-abusing and dependent adolescent inpatients ranging in age from 12 to 18 (Grilo, Becker, et al., 1998). Sinha and Watson (2001) examined gender differences in PD symptoms in first-year college students and found that males scored higher on antisocial, schizoid, and schizotypal PDs whereas females scored higher on borderline, dependent, and histrionic PDs.

Adolescent boys are diagnosed more frequently with conduct disorder (APD after 18 years of age) than are adolescent girls (Lahey et al., 2000; Verhulst, van der Ende, Ferdinand, & Kasius, 1997). However, the gender differences observed for CD are partly explained by the weight given to aggressive behavior in the diagnosis. When the criteria for CD are broken down, research has indicated that adolescent boys tend to score higher on physical aggres-sion, but there is no evidence of a gender discrepancy for other criteria such as stealing, lying, relational aggression, or substance use (Tiet, Wasserman, Loeber, McReynolds, & Miller, 2001).

LIMITATIONS OF PREVIOUS RESEARCH AND RECOMMENDATIONS FOR FUTURE RESEARCH

There are a number of limitations in the empirical literature on adolescent PDs, leading to several recommendations for future research:

1. Although there has been a considerable expansion of interest in research on adolescent PDs in recent years, few studies have investigated the prevalence, correlates, and sequelae of PDs among adolescents in the community. Further epidemiological studies are needed to examine more definitively the prevalence, course, and sequelae of PDs during early, middle, and late adolescence.

2. Most studies of the temporal stability of PD traits among adolescents and adults have used relatively brief intertest intervals. Few studies have explored the development and course of PD symptoms from adolescence through early adulthood. More longitudinal research is needed in this area.

3. Most investigations of adolescent and adult PDs have been based exclusively on clinical interviews, archival records, and self-report instruments. Greater attention to the behavioral manifestations of PD traits and diagnoses—and the processes that mediate and moderate these behaviors—is needed. Observational, experimental, and multi-informant studies will be useful in this regard (see Bornstein, 2003).

Because culture plays a role in the development of normal and pathological interpersonal behavior (Alarcon, 1996), and is central to the DSM-IV definition of PD, greater attention to cultural and subcultural influences on PD onset and course is needed. Cross-cultural comparisons of epidemiological data have suggested that certain PDs may be more prevalent in some societies than in others (e.g., Torgerson et al., 2001). Further research in this area may lead to an improved understanding of the role of socialization and acculturation experiences in the development of normal and abnormal personality traits.

TREATMENT

In recent years there has been a substantial increase in the development and validation of clinical interventions designed specifically for treating PDs (e.g., Beck & Freeman, 1990; Linehan, 1987, 1993; Clarkin, Yeomans, & Kernberg, 1999). Although maladaptive personality traits may be difficult to manage, research has indicated that most PDs can be treated effectively with psychotherapy. In particular, a recent meta-analyses has supported the effectiveness of both cognitive-behavioral and psychodynamic psychotherapies for PDs (Leichsenring & Leibing, 2003).

Cognitive therapy of PDs (Beck, 1998; Beck & Freeman, 1990) conceives of PDs as consisting of a collection of automatic, maladaptive cognitions about the self, others, and their world with each distinct PD characterized by a distinctive set of core beliefs and assumptions as well as over- and underdeveloped behavioral strategies. According to Beck (1998), core beliefs represent the individual's schemas that act as templates for the interpretation of experience. These dysfunctional core beliefs serve to selectively filter information that is consistent with the self, and discard information or experiences that are inconsistent with one's core beliefs. These core beliefs lead to a restricted set of behavioral strategies that serve to maintain one's view of the world. For example, the core belief for an individual with dependent PD is "I'm helpless," the assumption is, "If I rely on myself, I'll fail" and "if I depend on others, I'll survive" (Beck, 1998). These beliefs and assumptions, in turn, lead to a predominant behavioral strategy of reliance of others (see Beck, 1998, for specific core beliefs, assumptions, and strategies for each specific PD).

According to Beck (1998), cognitive therapy of PD shares many components with the more standard treatment of depression (Beck, Rush, Shaw, & Emery, 1979). For example, cognitive treatment of both PD and depression focus on maladaptive cognitive schemas, collaborative therapist–client working relationship, structured therapy, problem solving, Socratic questioning of dysfunctional core beliefs, and homework. However, cognitive treatment of PD places greater emphasis on developmental history, consistent with the belief that maladaptive beliefs and dysfunctional automatic thoughts regarding the self, others, and the world form during childhood. In addition, it is believed that the course of treatment for PDs is longer and the process more complex.

Of the 22 studies listed in Leichsenring and Leibing's (2003) meta-analysis of the effectiveness of psychodynamic and cognitive-behavioral treatment of PD, over half (12) specifically concerned BPD. With most approaches that have received empirical support focusing on BPD, we limit our discussion here of therapeutic approaches for PD to those explicitly concerned with the treatment of BPD. In particular, we focus on dialectical behavior therapy (DBT; Linehan, 1987, 1993), a cognitive-behavioral treatment, and transference-focused psychotherapy (TFP; Clarkin et al., 1999), a psychodynamic approach.

DBT (Linehan, 1993) is an empirically validated, highly effective, protocol outpatient treatment for BPD (Koerner & Dimeff, 2000; Koerner & Linehan, 2000) DBT is a flexible treatment that has been successfully integrated into inpatient and residential program settings (Wolpow, 2000), and most recently extended to the psychiatric emergency room to enhance outpatient treatment compliance (Sneed, Balestri, & Belfi, 2003). The central focus of DBT is on the dialectical tension between accepting the patient and effecting change through the analysis of maladaptive cognitions and behavioral antecedents and consequences. As such, it is a cognitive-behavioral therapy rooted in the Eastern tradition of mindfulness and dialectical philosophy. It is cognitive in its focus on identifying maladaptive thinking styles and automatic thoughts through the use of chain analyses and self-monitoring diaries. It is behavioral in its focus on contingency management, particularly with respect to life-threatening and therapy interfering behaviors.

DBT distinguishes between three dimensions of behavior patterns along which borderline behavior can be characterized. The first dimension (emotional vulnerability vs. self-invalidation) reflects the high emotional arousal and sensitivity characteristic of BPD and the tendency to invalidate the experience of these emotions, which have been associated with shame and guilt developmentally. The second dimension (active passivity vs. apparent competence) reflects, on the one hand, the borderline patient's tendency to approach life's problems passively while actively demanding that other people solve problems for them. Simultaneously, these patients portray themselves as competent, which may in fact be the case in a particular area of life, when in actuality their competency will not generalize across life's conditions. The third dimension (unrelenting crises vs. inhibited grieving) refers to the patient's chronic inhibition or inability to fully experience grief most likely associated with trauma and, at the same time, the tendency to perpetuate crisis after crisis with the inability to recover fully from any one crisis.

According to DBT, the emotional dysregulation that typifies BPD has its etiology in the interaction between biology and environment. The biological underpinnings of emotional dysregulation are high sensitivity and high reactivity to painful affects, as well as a slow return to emotional baseline after arousal. As a result, borderline patients are primed for high emotional reactivity because the biological concomitants of negative affectivity are still active and have not returned to premorbid levels. In conjunction with the biological vulnerability, borderline patients are often subjected to invalidating environments. Typical features of the invalidating environment are being exposed to caregivers or significant others who (1) respond erratically and inappropriately to private emotional experiences, (2) are insensitive to people's emotional states, (3) have a tendency to over- or underreact to emotional experiences, (4) emphasize control over negative emotions, and (5) have a tendency to trivialize painful experiences and/or attribute such experiences to negative traits (e.g., lack of motivation or discipline). The interaction between emotional vulnerability and invalidating environments results in not being able to label and modulate emotions, tolerate emotional or interpersonal distress, and trust private experiences as valid (Linehan, 1993).

TFP (Clarkin et al., 1999) is a psychodynamic approach to BPD rooted in Kernberg's (1984) object relations theory of personality organization. According to this approach, personality organization is characterized by degree of reality testing (capacity to differentiate self from other and external reality from one's internal world), psychological defense (splitting and projection at the pathological end and repression and reaction formation at the more adjusted end), and identity development (integration of positive and negative concepts of self and other into a cohesive notion of self). Recently, Lezenweger, Clarkin, Kernberg, and Foelsch (2001) obtained empirical support for this view of personality by developing and validating the Inventory of Personality Organiza-

tion (IPO), a 155-item self-report instrument consisting of three primary scales measuring psychological defense, reality testing, and identity.

Treatment based on TFP is organized around the concept of transference, the reenactment or reactivation of early object relationships in the therapeutic relationship in the here-and-now. Patients at a borderline level of personality organization are unable to integrate positive and negative internal representations of self and other and, as a result, rely on primitive defensive operations such as splitting, which serves to keep separate disparate concepts of self and other that have connected to them unwanted and threatening negative affects. As a result, such unintegrated representations often become activated in the transference in caricatured form. One of the principle functions of the therapist in the treatment BPD is to be able to identify and label the internal object representations activated in the treatment situation and help the patient integrate these split-off, fragmented representations of self and other through the use of interpretation. Recent research has provided preliminary support for this approach. In a study of 23 female patients meeting criteria for BPD, twice-weekly TFP for a duration of 12 months reduced number of suicide attempts, severity of self-injurious behavior, number of hospitalizations, and number of days hospitalized (Clarkin et al., 2001).

Most psychotherapeutic treatment approaches used to treat personality-disordered adults can be modified for use with adolescents (see Bleiberg, 2001; Turkat, 1990), and the key considerations in adapting these strategies for younger patients include taking into account the increased impulsivity, elevated risk for substance use, and prominent identity issues that characterize this age period.

Because adolescents as a group tend to show greater impulsivity—and poorer long-term planning—than adults, treatment of personality-disordered adolescents must include an explicit focus on the risk of acting out. This is particularly true of PDs characterized by significant risk of self-destructive behavior even in adults (e.g., borderline and antisocial). Certain PD treatment strategies involve arousing affect or using paradoxical interventions to increase insight, alter long-standing thought patterns, or effect behavior change (e.g., Linehan, 1993). These strategies may involve increased risk in adolescents and may not always be warranted in younger patients with less effective coping and self-control skills.

Adolescent impulsivity may be exacerbated by substance use, which, when chronic, has been shown to have both short- and long-term disinhibitory effects (Hussong, Hicks, Levy, & Curran, 2001). Moreover, certain PDs (e.g., borderline) are associated with increased likelihood of suicidal gestures and attempts, and in many cases these same syndromes are also associated with increased risk for substance abuse. When significant personality pathology is coupled with the disinhibitory effects of alcohol or drug abuse, the risk of a negative outcome increases substantially.

A third consideration in adapting PD treatment strategies for use with adolescents concerns the confounding effect of identity instability. Although research suggests that the identity concerns frequently reported in adolescents are to some degree culture-specific, cross-cultural studies indicate that the transition from childhood dependence to adult autonomy creates identity challenges for adolescents and young adults in many different societies (Bleiberg, 2001; Bretherton, 1991). Because many PDs are characterized by identity confusion, it is imperative that the practitioner working with personality-disordered adolescents distinguish the expectable identity concerns of this developmental epoch from the more problematic identity problems resulting from personality pathology (Triandis, 1996).

Taken together, these considerations suggest that PD treatment strategies used in adults must be used with greater caution—and increased attention to the possibility of unintended negative effects—with adolescents. Of the approaches reviewed, only DBT has been specifically adapted for use with adolescents (Miller, 1999; Miller, Glinski, Woodberry, Mitchell, & Indik, 2002; Rathus & Miller, 2000; Woodberry, Miller, Glinski, Indik, & Mitchell, 2002). For example, the concomitant skills training group in which DBT patients participate, which focuses on mindfulness, emotion regulation, distress tolerance, and interpersonal effectiveness, is shortened and simplified (Miller, 1999). Also, there is greater focus on the family of origin in DBT treatment with adolescents, which makes sense given that the family of origin is not only a contributor to emotional dysregulation through the invalidating environment but also a potential source of support (Woodberry et al., 2002).

SUMMARY AND CONCLUSIONS

According to DSM-IV-TR, adolescents who meet the diagnostic criteria may be diagnosed with a PD, although special considerations are stipulated for assessing PDs among adolescents. Although there are many important questions that remain unanswered, a review of the extant literature on PDs during adolescence supports the following conclusions:

1. Numerous studies have indicated that adolescent PDs can be diagnosed in a reliable and valid manner.

2. Although few community-based studies have examined PD prevalence among adolescents, the available evidence indicates that PDs are likely to be as common, and perhaps somewhat more common among adolescents than they are among adults in the community.

3. Adolescent PDs are associated with significant impairment and distress, co-occurring Axis I disorders, and maladaptive personality traits.

4. Adolescent PDs have been found to be associated with elevated risk for a wide range of negative long-term outcomes, including aggressive behavior, Axis I disorders, and suicidal behavior during adulthood.

5. PD symptoms tend to be moderately stable during adolescence, and PD traits are nearly as stable among adolescents as they are among young and middle-age adults.

6. PD symptoms tend to decline in prevalence from adolescence through middle adulthood.

7. Most PD traits tend to originate during childhood or adolescence. Although many risk factors are associated with the development of PD traits, adverse socialization experiences including maladaptive parenting, and traumatic experiences such as childhood maltreatment and other forms of victimization may play a particularly important role in the development of enduring PD traits. Research findings in this area have important implications for treatment and prevention of PDs during adolescence.

8. Although PDs can be difficult to treat, most adolescents and adults with PDs can be treated effectively with psychotherapy. Improved recognition and treatment of PDs among adolescents and adults may help to alleviate current distress and impairment and to prevent adverse long-term outcomes.

NOTES

1. As described in greater detail later in this chapter, there is considerable evidence indicating that PD traits tend to decline with age during middle and later adulthood.

2. Studies that relied on self-report questionnaires to assess PD symptoms are not cited in this section unless additional procedures were used to correct for low questionnaire specificity, because such questionnaires are not generally recognized as providing valid diagnostic data regarding PDs. Community-based studies are cited if a representative sample was used. Community-based studies that have oversampled individuals with psychological problems, resulting in an elevated prevalence of PD, are not cited in this section (e.g., Korenblum et al., 1987, 1990).

3. When consideration is limited to studies that used structured clinical interviews to assess PDs, the median prevalence estimate is 11.0% and the estimate based on the unweighted mean is 11.3% (SD = 5.5).

4. Nearly all the studies, cited in this chapter that were conducted with samples of college students had a mean age of 18, 19, or 20. There are varying views about when adolescence ends and early adulthood begins. Further, the transition to adulthood is likely to depend more on the extent to which adult roles have been assumed, rather than on biological age. Most individuals who are 18–21 years of age may be considered to be in late adolescence, insofar as they remain partially dependent on their parents and do not yet have all the legal rights and responsibilities associated with adulthood.

5. Cluster B personality disorder symptoms (i.e., symptoms of antisocial, borderline, histrionic, and narcissistic personality disorders), such as impulsive or risky behavior, may be particularly likely to become less evident during late adolescence and early adulthood (Johnson, Cohen, Kasen, et al., 2000).

6. It is important to take into account the possibility that cross-sectional findings indicating that psychiatric symptoms are inversely associated with age may be attributable, at least in part, to cohort effects.

REFERENCES

Alarcon, R. D. (1996). Personality disorders and culture in DSM-IV: A critique. *Journal of Personality Disorders, 10*, 260–270.

American Psychiatric Association. (1968). *Diagnostic and statistical manual of mental disorders* (2nd ed.). Washington, DC: Author.

American Psychiatric Association. (1980). *Diagnostic and statistical manual of mental disorders* (3rd ed.). Washington, DC: Author.

American Psychiatric Association. (1987). *Diagnostic and statistical manual of mental disorders* (3rd ed., rev.). Washington, DC: Author.

American Psychiatric Association. (1994). *Diagnostic and statistical manual of mental disorders* (4th ed.). Washington, DC: Author.

American Psychiatric Association. (2000). *Diagnostic and statistical manual of mental disorders* (4th ed., text rev.). Washington, DC: Author.

Barasch, A., Frances, A., Hurt, S., Clarkin, J., & Cohen, S. (1985). Stability and distinctness of borderline personality disorder. *American Journal of Psychiatry, 12*, 1484–1486.

Beck, A. T., & Freeman, A. (1990). *Cognitive therapy of personality disorders.* New York: Guilford Press.

Beck, A. T., Rush, A. J., Shaw, B. F., & Emery, G. (1979). *Cognitive therapy of depression.* New York: Guilford Press.

Beck, J. S. (1998). Complex cognitive therapy treatment for personality disorder patients. *Bulletin of the Menninger Clinic, 62*, 170–194.

Becker, D. F., Grilo, C. M., Edell, W. S., & McGlashan, T. H. (2002). Diagnostic efficiency of borderline personality disorder criteria in hospitalized adolescents: Comparison with hospitalized adults. *American Journal of Psychiatry, 159*, 2042–2047.

Bernstein, D. P., Cohen, P., Skodol, A., Bezirganian, S., & Brook, J. S. (1996). Childhood antecedents of adolescent personality disorders. *American Journal of Psychiatry, 153*, 907–913.

Bernstein, D. P., Cohen, P., Velez, N., Schwab-Stone, M., Siever, L. J., & Shinsato L. (1993). Prevalence and stability of the DSM-III-R personality disorders in a community-based survey of adolescents. *American Journal of Psychiatry, 150*, 1237–1243.

Black, D. W., Baumgard, C. H., & Bell, S. E. (1995). A 16- to 45-year follow-up of men with antisocial personality disorder. *Comprehensive Psychiatry, 36*, 130–140.

Black, D. W., Bell, S., Hulbert, J., & Nasrallah, A. (1988). The importance of Axis II in patients with major depression: A controlled study. *Journal of Affective Disorders, 14*, 115–122.

Bleiberg, E. (1994). Borderline disorders in children and adolescents: The concept, the diagnosis, and the controversies. *Bulletin of the Menninger Clinic, 58*, 169–196.

Bleiberg, E. (2001). *Treating personality disorders in children and adolescents: A relational approach.* New York: Guilford Press.

Brennan, K. A., & Shaver, P. R. (1998). Attachment styles and personality disorders: Their connections to each other and to parental divorce, parental death, and perceptions of parental caregiving. *Journal of Personality, 66*, 835–878.

Brent, D. A., Johnson, B. A., Bartle, S., Bridge, J., Rather, C., Matta, J., et al. (1993). Personality disorder, tendency to impulsive violence, and suicidal behavior in adolescents. *Journal of the American Academy of Child and Adolescent Psychiatry, 32*, 69–75.

Brent, D. A., Johnson, B. A., Perper, Connolly, J., Bridge, J., Bartle, S., & Rather, C. (1994). Personality disorder, personality traits, impulsive violence, and completed suicide in adolescents. *Journal of the American Academy of Child and Adolescent Psychiatry, 33,* 1080–1086.

Brent, D. A., Zelenak, J. P., Bukstein, O., & Brown, R. V. (1990). Reliability and validity of the structured interview for personality disorders in adolescents. *Journal of the American Academy of Child and Adolescent Psychiatry, 29,* 349–354.

Bretherton, I. (1991). The social self as internal working model. *Minnesota Symposium on Child Psychology, 23,* 1–41.

Brodsky, B. S., Cloitre, M., & Dulit, R. A. (1995). Relationship of dissociation to self-mutilation and childhood abuse in borderline personality disorder. *American Journal of Psychiatry, 152,* 1788–1792.

Brook, J. S., Brook, D., & Cohen, P. (1998). Longitudinal study of co-occurring psychiatric disorders and substance use. *Journal of the American Academy of Child and Adolescent Psychiatry, 37*(3), 322–330.

Caspi, A., McClay, J., Moffitt, T. E., Mill, J., Martin, J., Craig, I. W. et al. (2002). Role of genotype in the cycle of violence in maltreated children. *Science, 297,* 851–854.

Caspi, A., & Roberts, B. W. (2001). Personality development across the life course: The argument for change and continuity. *Psychological Inquiry, 12,* 49–66.

Charles, S. T., Reynolds, C. A., & Gatz, M. (2001). Age-related differences and change in positive and negative affect over 23 years. *Journal of Personality and Social Psychology, 80,* 136–151.

Chilcoat, H. D., Breslau, N., & Anthony, J. C. (1996). Potential barriers to parent monitoring: Social disadvantage, marital status, and maternal psychiatric disorder. *Journal of the American Academy of Child and Adolescent Psychiatry, 35,* 1673–1682.

Clarkin, J. F., Foelsch, P. A., Levy, K., Hull, J. W., Delaney, J. C., & Kernberg, O. F. (2001). The development of a psychodynamic treatment for patients with borderline personality disorder: A preliminary study of behavioral change. *Journal of Personality Disorders, 15,* 487–495.

Clarkin, J. F., Yeomans, F. E., & Kernberg, O. F. (1999). *Psychotherapy for borderline personality.* New York: Wiley.

Cloninger, C. R., Sigvardsson, S., & Bohman, M. (1988). Childhood personality predicts alcohol abuse in young adults. *Alcoholism: Clinical and Experimental Research, 12,* 494–505.

Cloninger, C. R., & Svrakic, D. M. (1994). Differentiating normal and deviant personality by the seven-factor personality model. In S. Strack & M. Lorr (Eds.), *Differentiating normal and abnormal personality* (pp. 40–64). New York: Springer.

Cohen, P. (1996). Childhood risks for young adult symptoms of personality disorder: Method and substance. *Multivariate Behavioral Research, 31*(1), 121–148.

Cohen, P. (1999). Personality development in childhood: Old and new findings. In C. R. Cloninger (Ed.), *Personality and psychopathology* (pp. 101–127). Washington, DC: American Psychiatric Press.

Cohen, P., Brown, J., & Smailes, E. (2001). Child abuse and neglect and the development of mental disorders in the general population. *Development and Psychopathology, 13*(4), 981–999.

Cooper, M. L., Wood, P. K., Orcutt, H. K., & Albino, A. (2003). Personality and the predisposition to engage in risky or problem behaviors during adolescence. *Journal of Personality and Social Psychology, 84,* 390–410.

Costa, P. T., & McCrae, R. R. (1992). The five-factor model of personality and its relevance to personality disorders. *Journal of Personality Disorders, 6,* 343–359.

Costa, P. T., & Widiger, T. A. (Eds.). (2002). *Personality disorders and the five-factor model* (2nd ed.). Washington, DC: American Psychological Association.

Crawford, T. N., Cohen, P., & Brook, J. S. (2001a). Dramatic–erratic personality disorder symptoms: I. Continuity from early adolescence into adulthood. *Journal of Personality Disorders, 15*(4), 319–335.

Crawford, T. N., Cohen, P., & Brook, J. S. (2001b). Dramatic–erratic personality disorder symptoms: II. Developmental pathways from early adolescence to adulthood. *Journal of Personality Disorders, 15*(4), 336–350.

Crawford, T. N., Cohen, P., Johnson, J., G., Sneed, J. R., & Brook, J. S. (2004). The early course of personality disorder symptoms: Erikson's developmental theory revisited. *Journal of Youth and Adolescence, 33,* 373–387.

Cross, S. E., & Madson, L. (1997). Models of the self: Self-construals and gender. *Psychological Bulletin, 122,* 5–37.

Daley, S. E., Hammen, C., Burge, D., Davila, J., Paley, B., Lindberg, N., & Herzberg, D. S. (1999). Depression and axis II symptomatology in an adolescent community sample: Concurrent and longitudinal associations. *Journal of Personality Disorders, 13,* 47–59.

Daley, S. E., Hammen, C., Davila, J., & Burge, D. (1998). Axis II symptomatology, depression, and stress during the transition from adolescence to adulthood. *Journal of Consulting and Clinical Psychology, 66,* 595–603.

DeClercq, B. D., & De Fruyt, F. (2003). Personality disorder symptoms in adolescence: A five-factor model perspective. *Journal of Personality Disorders, 17,* 269–292.

Derogatis, L. R. (1983). *SCL-90-R administration, scoring, and procedures manual.* Towson, MD: Clinical Psychometric Research.

Drake R. E., Adler, D. A., & Vaillant, G. E. (1988). Antecedents of personality disorders in a community sample of men. *Journal of Personality Disorders, 2,* 60–68.

Eppright, T. D., Kashani, J. H., Robison, B. D., & Reid, J. C. (1993). Comorbidity of conduct disorder and personality disorders in an incarcerated juvenile population. *American Journal of Psychiatry, 150,* 1233–1236.

Farrington, D. P. (1991). Antisocial personality from childhood to adulthood. *The Psychologist: Bulletin of the British Psychological Society, 4,* 389–394.

Feingold, A. (1994). Gender differences in personality: A meta-analysis. *Psychological Bulletin, 116,* 429–456.

Ferro, T., Klein, D. N., Schwartz, J. E., Kasch, K. L., & Leader, J. B. (1998). 30-month stability of personality disorder diagnoses in depressed outpatients. *American Journal of Psychiatry, 155,* 653–659.

First, M. B., Spitzer, R. L., Gibbon, M., & Williams, J. B. W. (1995). The Structured Clinical Interview for DSM-III-R Personality Disorders (SCID-II), Part I: Description. *Journal of Personality Disorder, 9,* 83–91.

First, M. B., Spitzer, R. L., Gibbon, M., Williams, J. B. W., Davies, M., Borus, J., et al. (1995). The Structured Clinical Interview for DSM-III-R Personality Disorders (SCID-II). Part II: Multi-site test–retest reliability study. *Journal of Personality Disorders, 9,* 92–104.

Fossati, A., Feeney, J. A., Donati, D., Donini, M., Novella, L., Bagnato, M., et al. (2003). Personality disorders and adult attachment dimensions in a mixed psychiatric sample: A multivariate study. *Journal of Nervous and Mental Disease, 191,* 30–37.

Garnet, K. E., Levy, K. N., Mattanah, J. J. F., Edell, W. S., & McGlashan, T. H. (1994). Borderline personality disorder in adolescents: Ubiquitous or specific? *American Journal of Psychiatry 151,* 1380–1382.

Gilligan, C. (1982). *In a different voice: Psychological theory and women's development.* Cambridge, MA: Harvard University Press.

Goldman, S. J., D'Angelo, E. J., DeMaso, D. R., & Mezzacappa, E. (1992). Physical and sexual abuse histories among children with borderline personality disorder. *American Journal of Psychiatry, 149,* 1723–1726.

Grilo, C. M., Becker, D. F., Edell, W. S., & McGlashan, T. H. (2001). Stability and change of DSM-III-R personality disorder dimensions in adolescents followed up 2 years after psychiatric hospitalization. *Comprehensive Psychiatry, 42,* 364–368.

Grilo, C. M., Becker, D. F., Fehon, D. C., Walker, M. L., Edell, W. S., & McGlashman, T. H. (1996). Gender differences in personality disorders in psychiatrically hospitalized adolescents. *American Journal of Psychiatry, 153,* 1089–1091.

Grilo, C. M., Becker, D. F., Fehon, D. C., Walker, M. L., Edell, W. S., & McGlashan, T. H. (1998). Psychiatric morbidity differences in male and female adolescent inpatients with alcohol use disorders. *Journal of Youth and Adolescence, 27,* 29–41.

Grilo, C. M., McGlashan, T. H., Quinlan, D. M., Walker, M. L., Greenfeld, D., & Edell, W. S. (1998). Frequency of personality disorders in two age cohorts of psychiatric inpatients. *American Journal of Psychiatry 155,* 140–142.

Grilo, C. M., Walker, M. L., Becker, D. F., Edell, W. S., & McGlashan, T. H. (1997). Personality disorders in adolescents with major depression, substance use disorders, and coexisting major depression and substance use disorders. *Journal of Consulting and Clinical Psychology, 65,* 328–332.

Guzder, J., Paris, J., Zelkowitz, P., & Marchessault, K. (1996). Risk factors for borderline pathology in children. *Journal of the American Academy of Child and Adolescent Psychiatry, 35,* 26–33.

Hart, D., Hofmann, V., Edelstein, W., & Keller, M. (1997). The relation of childhood personality types to adolescent behavior and development: A longitudinal study of Icelandic children. *Developmental Psychology, 33,* 195–205.

Herman, J. L., Perry, J. C., & van der Kolk, B. A. (1989). Childhood trauma in borderline personality disorder. *American Journal of Psychiatry, 146,* 490–495.

Hussong, A. M., Hicks, R. E., Levy, S. A., & Curran, P. J. (2001). Specifying the relation between affect and heavy alcohol use among young adults. *Journal of Abnormal Psychology, 110,* 449–461.

Irvine, A. B., Biglan, A., Smolkowski, K., Metzler, C. W., & Ary, D. V. (1999). The effectiveness of a parenting skills program for parents of middle school students in small communities. *Journal of Consulting and Clinical Psychology, 67,* 811–825.

Johnson, B. A., Brent, D. A., Connolly, J., Bridge, J., Matt, J., Constantine, D., et al. (1995). Familial aggregation of adolescent personality disorders. *Journal of the American Academy of Child and Adolescent Psychiatry, 34,* 798–804.

Johnson, J. G. (1993). Relationships between psychosocial development and personality disorder symptomatology in late adolescents. *Journal of Youth and Adolescence, 22,* 33–42.

Johnson, J. G., & Bornstein, R. F. (1991). Personality Diagnostic Questionnaire-Revised (PDQ-R) personality disorder scores and negative life events independently predict changes in Hopkins Symptom Checklist (SCL-90) psychopathology scores. *Journal of Psychopathology and Behavioral Assessment, 13,* 61–72.

Johnson, J. G., & Bornstein, R. F. (1992). Utility of the Personality Diagnostic Questionnaire-Revised in a nonclinical population. *Journal of Personality Disorders, 6,* 450–457.

Johnson, J. G., Bornstein, R. F., & Krukonis, A. B. (1992). Defense styles as predictors of personality disorder symptomatology. *Journal of Personality Disorders, 6,* 408–416.

Johnson, J. G., Bornstein, R. F., & Sherman, M. F. (1996). A modified scoring algorithm for the PDQ-R: Psychiatric symptomatology and substance use in adolescents with personality disorders. *Educational and Psychological Measurement, 56,* 91–104.

Johnson, J. G., Cohen, P., Brown, J., Smailes, E. M., & Bernstein, D. P. (1999). Childhood maltreatment increases risk for personality disorders during early adulthood. *Archives of General Psychiatry, 56,* 600–606.

Johnson, J. G., Cohen, P., Dohrenwend, B. P., Link, B. G., & Brook, J. S. (1999). A longitudinal investigation of social causation and social selection processes involved in the association between socioeconomic status and psychiatric disorders. *Journal of Abnormal Psychology, 108,* 490–499.

Johnson, J. G., Cohen, P., Kasen, S., & Brook, J. S. (in press). Maternal psychiatric disorders, parenting, and maternal behavior in the home during the child rearing years. *Journal of Child and Family Studies.*

Johnson, J. G., Cohen, P., Kasen, S., Skodol, A. E., Hamagami, F., & Brook, J. S. (2000). Age-related changes in personality disorder trait levels between early adolescence and adulthood: A community-based longitudinal investigation. *Acta Psychiatrica Scandinavica, 102,* 265–275.

Johnson, J. G., Cohen, P., Kasen, S., Smailes, E., & Brook, J. S. (2001). Association of maladaptive parental behavior with psychiatric disorder among parents and their offspring. *Archives of General Psychiatry, 58,* 453– 460.

Johnson, J. G., Cohen, P., Smailes, E., Kasen, S., Oldham, J. M., Skodol, A. E., & Brook, J. S. (2000). Adolescent personality disorders associated with violence and criminal behavior during adolescence and early adulthood. *American Journal of Psychiatry, 157,* 1406–1412

Johnson, J. G., Cohen, P., Smailes, E. M., Skodol, A. E., Brown, J., & Oldham, J. M. (2001). Childhood verbal abuse and risk for personality disorders during adolescence and early adulthood. *Comprehensive Psychiatry, 42,* 16–23.

Johnson, J. G., Hyler, S. E., Skodol, A. E., Bornstein, R. F., & Sherman, M. (1995). Personality disorder symptomatology associated with adolescent depression and substance abuse. *Journal of Personality Disorders, 9,* 318–329.

Johnson, J. G., Quigley, J. F., & Sherman, M. F. (1997). Adolescent personality disorder symptoms mediate the relationship between perceived parental behavior and Axis I symptomatology. *Journal of Personality Disorders, 11,* 381–390.

Johnson, J. G., Smailes, E. M., Cohen, P., Brown, J., & Bernstein, D. P. (2000). Associations between four types of childhood neglect and personality disorder symptoms during adolescence and early adulthood: Findings of a community-based longitudinal study. *Journal of Personality Disorders, 14,* 171–187.

Johnson, J. G., Williams, J. B. W., Goetz, R. R., Rabkin, J. G., Lipsitz, J. D., & Remien, R. H. (1997). Stability and change in personality disorder symptomatology: Findings from a longitudinal study of HIV+ and HIV- men. *Journal of Abnormal Psychology, 106,* 154–58.

Johnson, J. G., Williams, J. B. W., Goetz, R. R., Rabkin, J. G., Remien, R. H., Lipsitz, J. D., & Gorman, J. M. (1996). Personality disorders predict onset of Axis I disorders and impaired functioning among homosex-ual men with and at risk for HIV infection. *Archives of General Psychiatry, 53,* 350–357.

Kernberg, O. F. (1984). *Severe personality disorders: Psychotherapeutic strategies.* New Haven, CT: Yale University Press.

Kessler, R. C., McGonagle, K. A., Zhao, S., Nelson, C. B., Hughes, M., Eshleman, S., et al. (1994). Lifetime and 12–month prevalence of DSM-III-R psychiatric disorders in the United States. Results from the National Comorbidity Survey. *Archives of General Psychiatry, 51,* 8–19.

Klein, D. N., Riso, L. P., Donaldson, S. K., Schwartz, J. E., Anderson, R. L., Ouimette, P. C., et al. (1995). Family study of early-onset dysthymia: Mood and personality disorders in relatives of outpatients with dysthymia and episodic major depression and normal controls. *Archives of General Psychiatry, 52,* 487–496.

Klein, M. H., Wonderlich, S. A., & Crosby, R. (2001). Self-concept correlates of the personality disorders. *Journal of Personality Disorders, 15,* 150–156.

Klonsky, E. D., Oltmanns, T. F., Turkheimer, E., & Fiedler, E. R. (2000). Recollections of conflict with parents and family support in the personality disorders. *Journal of Personality Disorders, 14,* 327–338.

Koerner, K., & Dimeff, L. A. (2000). Further data on dialectical behavior therapy. *Clinical Psychology: Science and Practice, 7,* 104–112.

Koerner, K., & Linehan, M. M. (2000). Research on dialectical behavior therapy for patients with borderline personality disorder. *Borderline Personality Journal, 23,* 151–165.

Korenblum, M., Marton, P., Golombek, H., & Stein, B. (1987). Disturbed personality functioning: Patterns of change from early to middle adolescence. *Adolescent Psychiatry, 14,* 407–416.

Korenblum, M., Marton, P., Golombek, H., & Stein, B. (1990). Personality status: Changes through adolescence. adolescence: Psychopathology, normality, and creativity. *Psychiatric Clinics of North America, 13,* 389–399.

Lahey, B. B., Schwab-Stone, M., Goodman, S. H., Waldman, I. R., Canino, G., Rathouz, P. J., et al. (2000). Age and gender differences in oppositional behavior and conduct problems: A cross-sectional household study of middle childhood and adolescence. *Journal of Abnormal Psychology, 109,* 488–503.

Lavan, H., & Johnson, J. G. (2002). The association between Axis I and II psychiatric symptoms and high-risk sexual behavior during adolescence. *Journal of Personality Disorders, 16,* 73–94.

Leichsenring, F., & Leibing, E. (2003). The effectiveness of psychodynamic therapy and cognitive behavior therapy in the treatment of personality disorders: A meta-analysis. *American Journal of Psychiatry, 160,* 1223–1232.

Lenzenweger, M. F. (1999). Stability and change in personality disorder features: the longitudinal study of personality disorders. *Archives of General Psychiatry, 56,* 1009–1015.

Lenzenweger, M. F., Clarkin, J. F., Kernberg, O. F., & Foelsch, P. A. (2001). The inventory of personality organization: Psychometric properties, factorial composition, and criterion relations with affect, aggressive dyscontrol, psychosis proneness, and self-domains in a non-clinical sample. *Psychological Assessment, 13,* 577–591.

Lenzenweger, M. F., Loranger, A. W., Korfine, L. & Neff, C. (1997). Detecting personality disorders in a nonclinical population. Application of a 2–stage procedure for case identification. *Archives of General Psychiatry, 54,* 345–351.

Levy, K. N., Becker, D. F., Grilo, C. M., Mattanah, J. J. F., Garnet, K. E., Quinlan, D. M., et al. (1999). Concurrent and predictive validity of the personality disorder diagnosis in adolescent inpatients. *American Journal of Psychiatry, 156,* 1522–1528.

Linehan, M. M. (1987). Dialectical behavior therapy for borderline personality disorder: Theory and method. *Bulletin of the Menninger Clinic, 51,* 261–276.

Linehan, M. M. (1993). *Cognitive-behavioral treatment of borderline personality disorder.* New York: Guilford Press.

Livesley, W. J., Jackson, D. N., & Schroeder, M. L. (1992). Factorial structure of traits delineating personality disorders in clinical and general population samples. *Journal of Abnormal Psychology, 101,* 432–440.

Livesley, W. J., Jang, K. L., Jackson, D. N., & Vernon, P. A. (1993). Genetic and environmental contributions to dimensions of personality disorder. *American Journal of Psychiatry, 150,* 1826–1831.

Livesley, W. J., Jang, K. L., & Vernon, P. A. (1998). Phenotypic and genetic structure of traits delineating personality disorder. *Archives of General Psychiatry, 55,* 941–948.

Livesley, W. J., Schroeder, M. L., Jackson, D. N., & Jang, K. L. (1994). Categorical distinctions in the study of personality disorder: Implications for classification. *Journal of Abnormal Psychology, 103,* 6–17.

Lofgren, D. P., Bemporad, J., King, J., Linden, K., & O'Driscoll, G. (1991). A prospective follow-up study of so-called borderline children. *American Journal of Psychiatry, 148,* 1541–1547.

Loranger, A. W., Lenzenweger, M. F., Gartner, A. F., Susman, V. L., Herzig, J., Zammit, G. K., et al. (1991). Trait-state artifacts and the diagnosis of personality disorders. *Archives of General Psychiatry, 48,* 720–728.

Loranger, A. W., Sartorius, N., Andreoli, A., Berger, P., Buchheim, P., Channabasavanna, S., et al. (1994). The International Personality Disorder Examination: The World Health Organization/Alcohol, Drug Abuse, and Mental Health Administration International pilot study of personality disorders. *Archives of General Psychiatry, 51,* 215–224.

Ludolph, P. S., Westen, D., Misle, B., Jackson, A.,

Wixom, J., & Wiss, F. C. (1990). The borderline diagnosis in adolescents: symptoms and developmental history. *American Journal of Psychiatry, 147,* 470–476.

Luntz, B. K., & Widom, C. S. (1994). Antisocial personality disorder in abused and neglected children grown up. *American Journal of Psychiatry, 151,* 670–674.

Maier, W., Lichtermann, D., Klingler, T., Heun, R., & Hallmayer, J. (1992). Prevalences of personality disorders (DSM-III—R) in the community. *Journal of Personality Disorders, 6,* 187–196.

Marton, P., Korenblum, M., Kutcher, S., Stein, B., Kennedy, B., & Pakes, J. (1989). Personality dysfunction in depressed adolescents. *Canadian Journal of Psychiatry, 34,* 810–813.

Mattanah, J. J. F., Becker, D. F., Levy, K. N., Edell, W. S., & McGlashan, T. H. (1995). Diagnostic stability in adolescents followed up 2 years after hospitalization. *American Journal of Psychiatry, 152,* 889–894.

McDavid, J. D., & Pilkonis, P. A. (1996). The stability of personality disorder diagnoses. *Journal of Personality Disorders, 10,* 1–15.

McGue, M., Bacon, S., & Lykken, D. T. (1993). Personality stability and change in early adulthood: A behavioral genetic analysis. *Developmental Psychology, 29,* 96–106.

McManus, M., Lerner, H., Robbins, D., & Barbour, C. (1984). Assessment of borderline symptomatology in hospitalized adolescents. *Canadian Journal of Psychiatry, 23,* 685–695.

Merikangas, K. R., & Weissman, M. M. (1986). Epidemiology of DSM-III Axis II personality disorders. In A. J. Frances & R. E. Hales (Eds.), *American Psychiatric Association annual review* (Vol. 5, pp. 58–79). Washington, DC: American Psychiatric Press.

Miller, A. L. (1999). Dialectical behavior therapy: A new treatment approach for suicidal adolescents. *American Journal of Psychotherapy, 53,* 413–417.

Miller, A. L., Glinski, J., Woodberry, K. A., Mitchell, A. G., & Indik, J. (2002). Family therapy and dialectical behavior therapy: Part I: Proposing a clinical synthesis. *American Journal of Psychotherapy, 56,* 568–584.

Moldin, S. O., Rice, J. P., Erlenmeyer-Kimling, L., & Squires-Wheeler, E. (1994). Latent structure of DSM-III-R Axis II psychopathology in a normal sample. *Journal of Abnormal Psychology, 103,* 259–266.

Myers, W. C., Burkett, R. C., & Otto, T. A. (1993). Conduct disorder and personality disorders in hospitalized adolescents. *Journal of Clinical Psychiatry, 54,* 21–26.

Nakash-Eisikovits, O., Dutra, L., & Westen, D. (2002). Relationship between attachment patterns and personality pathology in adolescents. *Journal of the American Academy of Child and Adolescent Psychiatry, 41,* 1111–1123.

Neugebauer, R., Hoek, H. W., & Susser E. (1999). Prenatal exposure to wartime famine and development of antisocial personality disorder in early adulthood. *Journal of the American Medical Association, 282,* 455–462.

Newman, D. L., Caspi, A., Moffitt, T. E., & Silva, P. A. (1997). Antecedents of adult interpersonal functioning: Effects of individual differences in age 3 temperament. *Developmental Psychology, 33,* 206–217.

Norden, K. A., Klein, D. N., Donaldson, S. K., Pepper, C. M., & Klein, L. M. (1995). Reports of the early home environment in DSM-III-R personality disorders. *Journal of Personality Disorders, 9,* 213–223.

O'Connor, B. P. (2002). The search for dimensional structure differences between normality and abnormality: A statistical review of published data on personality and psychopathology. *Journal of Personality and Social Psychology, 83,* 962–982.

Oldham, J. M. (1994). Personality disorders; current perspectives. *Journal of the American Medical Association, 272,* 1770–1776.

Oldham, J. M., & Skodol, A. E. (2000). Charting the future of Axis II. *Journal of Personality Disorders, 14,* 17–29.

Orlandini, A., Fontana, S., Clerici, S., Fossati, A., Fiorilli, M., Negri, G., & Muller, I. (1997). *Personality modifications in adolescence: A three-year follow-up study.* Paper presented at the 5th International Congress on the Disorders of Personality, Vancouver, Canada.

Ouimette, P. C., & Klein, D. N. (1995). Test–retest stability, mood–state dependence, and informant–subject concordance of the SCID-Axis II Questionnaire in a nonclinical sample. *Journal of Personality Disorders, 9,* 105–111.

Pancoast, D. L., & Archer, R. P. (1992). MMPI response patterns of college students: Comparisons to adolescents and adults. *Journal of Clinical Psychology, 48,* 47–53.

Paris, J. (1988). Follow-up studies of borderline personality disorder: A critical review. *Journal of Personality Disorders, 2,* 189–197.

Perry, J. C. (1993). Longitudinal studies of personality disorders. *Journal of Personality Disorders, 7*(Suppl.), 63–85.

Pfeffer, C. R., Newcorn, J., & Kaplan, G. (1988). Suicidal behavior in adolescent psychiatric inpatients. *Journal of the American Academy of Child and Adolescent Psychiatry, 27,* 357–361.

Pfohl, B., Coryell, W., Zimmerman, M., & Stangl, D. (1987). Prognostic validity of self-report and interview measures of personality disorder in depressed inpatients. *Journal of Clinical Psychiatry, 48,* 468–472.

Pilkonis, P. A., Heape, C. L., Ruddy, J., & Serrao, P. (1991). Validity in the diagnosis of personality disorders: The use of the LEAD standard. *Journal of Psychological Assessments, 3,* 45–54.

Pincus, A. L., & Wilson, K. R. (2001). Interpersonal variability in dependent personality. *Journal of Personality, 69,* 223–251.

Pinto, A., Grapentine, W. L., Francis, G., & Picariello, C. M. (1996). Borderline personality disorder in adolescents: Affective and cognitive features. *Journal of the American Academy of Child and Adolescent Psychiatry, 34,* 1338–1343.

Raczek, S. W. (1992). Childhood abuse and personality disorders. *Journal of Personality Disorders, 6,* 109–116.

Rathus, J. H., & Miller, A. L. (2000). DBT for adolescents: Dialectical dilemmas and secondary treatment targets. *Cognitive and Behavioral Practice, 7,* 425–234.

Redmond, C., Spoth, R., Shin, C., & Lepper, H. S. (1999). Modeling long-term parent outcomes of two universal family-focused preventive interventions: One-year follow-up results. *Journal of Consulting and Clinical Psychology, 67,* 975–984.

Reich, J. H., & Green, A. I. (1991). Effect of personality disorders on outcome of treatment. *Journal of Nervous and Mental Disease, 179,* 74–82.

Roberts, B. W., & DelVecchio, W. F. (2000). The rank-order consistency of personality traits from childhood to old age: A quantitative review of longitudinal studies. *Psychological Bulletin, 126,* 3–25.

Robins, L. N. (1966). *Deviant children grown up: A sociological and psychiatric study of sociopathic personality.* Baltimore: Williams & Wilkins.

Robins, L. N., & Regier, D. (1991). *Psychiatric disorders in America: The epidemiological catchment area study.* New York: Free Press.

Ronningstam, E., Gunderson, J., & Lyons, M. (1995). Changes in pathological narcissism. *American Journal of Psychiatry, 152,* 253–257.

Rosenstein, D. S., & Horowitz, H. A. (1996). Adolescent attachment and psychopathology. *Journal of Consulting and Clinical Psychology, 64,* 244–253.

Runeson, B., & Beskow, J. (1991). Borderline personality disorder in young Swedish suicides. *Journal of Nervous and Mental Disease, 179,* 153–156.

Samuels, J., Eaton, W. W., Bienvenu III, O. J., Brown, C. H., Costa, Jr., P. T., & Nestadt, G. (2002). Prevalence and correlates of personality disorders in a community sample. *British Journal of Psychiatry, 180,* 536–542.

Shearer, S. L., Peters, C. P., Quaytman, M. S., & Ogden, R. L. (1990). Frequency and correlates of childhood sexual and physical abuse histories in adult female borderline inpatients. *American Journal of Psychiatry, 147,* 214–216.

Shiner, R. L. (2000). Linking childhood personality with adaptation: Evidence for continuity and change across time into late adolescence. *Journal of Personality and Social Psychology, 78,* 310–325.

Shiner, R. L., Masten, A. S., & Tellegen, A. (2002). A developmental perspective on personality in emerging adulthood: Childhood antecedents and concurrent adaptation. *Journal of Personality and Social Psychology, 83,* 1165–1177.

Sinha, B. K., & Watson, D. C. (2001). Personality disorder in university students: A multitrait–multimethod matrix study. *Journal of Personality Disorders, 15,* 235–244.

Sneed, J. R., Balestri, M., & Belfi, B. J. (2003). The use of dialectical behavior therapy strategies in the psychiatric emergency room. *Psychotherapy: Theory, Research, Practice, Training, 40,* 265–277.

Spoth, R. R., Lopez, M., Redmond, C., & Shin, C. (1999). Assessing a public health approach to delay onset and progression of adolescent substance use: Latent transition and log-linear analyses of longitudinal family preventive intervention outcomes. *Journal of Consulting and Clinical Psychology, 67,* 619–630.

Sroufe, L. A., Carlson, E. A., Levy, A. K., & Egeland, B. (1999). Implications of attachment theory for developmental psychopathology. *Development and Psychopathology, 11,* 1–13.

Stein, J. A., Newcomb, M. D., & Bentler, P. M. (1986). Stability and change in personality: A longitudinal study from early adolescence to young adulthood. *Journal of Research in Personality, 20,* 276–291.

Thomas, A., & Chess, S. (1984). Genesis and evolution of behavioral disorders: From infancy to early adult life. *American Journal of Orthopsychiatry, 141,* 1–9.

Tiet, Q. Q., Wasserman, G. A., Loeber, R., McReynolds, L. S., & Miller, L. S. (2001). Developmental and sex differences in types of conduct problems. *Journal of Child and Family Studies, 10,* 181–197.

Torgersen, S., & Alnaes, R. (1989). Localizing DSM-III personality disorders in three-dimensional structural space. *Journal of Personality Disorders, 3,* 18–31.

Torgerson, S., Kringlen, E., & Cramer, V. (2001). The prevalence of personality disorders in a community sample. *Archives of General Psychiatry, 58,* 590–596.

Triandis, H. C. (1996). The psychological measurement of cultural syndromes. *American Psychologist, 51,* 407–415.

Trull, T. J., Useda, J. D., Doan, B. T., Vieth, A. Z., Burr, R. M., Hanks, A. A., & Conforti, K. (1998). Two-year stability of borderline personality measures. *Journal of Personality Disorders, 12,* 187–197.

Turkat, I. D. (1990). *The personality disorders: A psychological approach to clinical management.* New York: Pergamon Press.

Vaglum, P., Friis, S., Karterud, S., Mehlum, L., & Vaglum, S. (1993). Stability of the severe personality disorder diagnosis: A 2- to 5-year prospective study. *Journal of Personality Disorders, 7,* 348–353.

van der Kolk, B. A., Hostetler, A., Herron, N., & Fisler, R. E. (1994). Trauma and the development of borderline personality disorder. *Psychiatric Clinics of North America, 17,* 715–730.

Verhulst, F. C., van der Ende, J., Ferdinand, R. F., & Kasius, M. C. (1997). The prevalence of DSM-III-R diagnoses in a national sample of Dutch adolescents. *Archives of General Psychiatry, 54,* 329–336.

Vetter, P., & Koller, O. (1993). Stability of diagnoses in various psychiatric disorders: A study of long-term course. *Psychopathology, 26,* 173–180.

Watson, D., Clark, L. A., & Harkness, A. R. (1994). Structures of personality and their relevance to psychopathology. *Journal of Abnormal Psychology, 103,* 18–31.

Weaver, T. L., & Clum, G. A. (1993). Early family environments and traumatic experiences associated with borderline personality disorder. *Journal of Consulting and Clinical Psychology, 61,* 1068–1075.

Weissman, M. M. (1993). The epidemiology of personality disorders: A 1990 update. *Journal of Personality Disorders, 7*(Suppl. 1), 44–62.

Westen, D., Ludolph, P., Block, M. J., Wixom, J., & Wiss, F. C. (1990). Developmental history and object relations in psychiatrically disturbed adolescent girls. *American Journal of Psychiatry, 147,* 1061–1068.

Westen, D., Shedler, J., Durrett, C., Glass, S., & Martens, A. (2003). Personality diagnoses in adolescence: DSM-IV Axis II diagnoses and an empirically derived alternative. *American Journal of Psychiatry, 160,* 952–966.

Widiger, T. A. (1998). Four out of five ain't bad. *Archives of General Psychiatry, 55,* 865–866.

Widiger, T. A., Trull, T. J., Clarkin, J. F., Sanderson, C. A., & Costa, P. T., Jr. (2002). A description of the DSM-IV personality disorders with the five-factor model of personality. In P. T. Costa & T. A. Widiger (Eds.), *Personality disorders and the five-factor model of personality* (2nd ed., pp. 89–99). Washington, DC: American Psychological Association Press.

Wiggins, J. S. (1982). Circumplex models of interpersonal behavior in clinical psychology. In P. C. Kendall & J. N. Butcher (Eds.), *Handbook of research methods in clinical psychology* (pp. 183–221). New York: Wiley.

Wolpow, S. (2000). Adapting a dialectical behavior therapy (DBT) group for use in a residential program. *Psychiatric Rehabilitation Journal, 24*(2), 135–142.

Woodberry, K. A., Miller, A. L., Glinski, J., Indik, J., & Mitchell, A. G. (2002). Family therapy and dialectical behavior therapy with adolescents: Part II: A theoretical review. *American Journal of Psychotherapy, 56,* 585–602.

Zaider, T. I., Johnson, J. G., & Cockell, S. J. (2000). Psychiatric comorbidity associated with eating disorder symptomatology among adolescents in the community. *International Journal of Eating Disorders, 28,* 58–67.

Zimmerman, M. (1994). Diagnosing personality disorders: a review of issues and research methods. *Archives of General Psychiatry, 51,* 225–245.

14

Eating Disorders

James Lock
Daniel le Grange

Eating disorders are common psychiatric disorders whose onset is often during adolescence (ages 12–18 years) (Flament, Ledoux, Jeammet, Choquet, & Simon, 1995; Lucas, Beard, & O'Fallon, 1991). The development, maintenance, and treatment of these problematic disorders are understudied, especially as pertains to adolescents (Steiner & Lock, 1998). These disorders share pathological thoughts and behaviors, resulting in physical, social, and psychological deficits (American Psychiatric Association [APA], 1994) Although often conceptualized as developmental disorders, few prospective studies examine normative and pathological phenomena in populations at risk (Lock, Reisel, & Steiner, 2001; Steiner et al., 2003; Steiner, Lock, & Reisel, 1999). This chapter reviews dilemmas in diagnosis, studies of risks for development of eating disorders, their developmental course, and developmentally appropriate treatment considerations for adolescent patients.

DIAGNOSTIC CRITERIA AND NEEDS

The three principal diagnoses used to describe eating disorders are anorexia nervosa (AN), bulimia nervosa (BN), and eating disorder not otherwise specified (EDNOS). Binge eating disorder (BED) is an experimental diagnosis in the *Diagnostic and Statistical Manual of Mental Disorders* (DSM-IV) that has yet to be confirmed as an independent illness for BN (APA, 1994).

According to the DSM-IV, AN is described as a refusal to maintain weight (or gain weight in a period of growth) of 85% of expected weight for height (ideal body weight, or IBW) in the context of an overriding fear of weight gain and a lack of recognition of the physical changes that result from malnutrition (body image distortion or denial of the seriousness of the consequences of malnutrition) (APA, 1994). In postmenarcheal females, these symptoms are accompanied by loss of three consecutive menstrual periods. Patients may purely restrict their intake (restricting subtype), or may engage in binge eating/purging (binge/purge subtype).

BN is defined by DSM-IV as also having both behavioral and psychological components. Behavioral components include severe dieting while maintaining weight in the normal range, episodes of binge eating, and compensatory purgative behaviors (purging, exercise, laxative use, etc.) for a period of 3 months with an intensity of at least two episodes a week on average. These behaviors are accompanied by beliefs and attitudes that overemphasize shape and weight as the sole or major way self-worth and self-esteem are maintained (APA, 1994).

EDNOS, like many of the NOS diagnostic categories in DSM, allows for considerable range of symptoms and attitudes resulting from some form of abnormal eating or dieting practice. What is critical for this diagnosis is that the problem is related to eating, includes both behavioral and psychological components, and is severe enough to cause dysfunction (APA, 1994). Binge eating unaccompanied by compensating behaviors is coded as EDNOS at this time for both adolescents and adults.

DESCRIPTION OF EATING DISORDERS IN ADOLESCENTS

The three major diagnoses used for adolescents with eating disorders are the same as those used with adults, because there is little recognition that adolescents with eating disorders differ from adults with these disorders. Nonetheless, among the diagnostic criteria for AN, there is the suggestion that failure to grow as a result of malnutrition, an event particular to childhood, will substitute for meeting usual weight criteria. In addition, there is the possibility of meeting full criteria without having missed three consecutive menstrual periods if the patient has not previously menstruated, which is more likely for adolescents as well.

However helpful these adjustments might be in making DSM more sensitive to younger persons with AN, there are reasons that the current formulation may not be sufficiently adjusted for adolescents. The weight criteria of 85% IBW or 17.5 kilograms/meters-squared (body mass index, or BMI) is problematic for adolescents because they are often still growing. Calculations used to derive the norms for weight and height are difficult to apply accurately in adolescents who are unusually tall, are male, or have not had onset of menses, leading both to under- and overcalculations of BMI. Menstrual criteria are difficult to apply in younger adolescents who often have not firmly established periodic cycles, again making it difficult to know when three consecutive periods should have taken place in postmenarcheal young women. Moreover, there is no equivalence for amenorrhea in boys with AN, so boys do not have to meet one specified criteria based

on their gender alone. For younger adolescent patients, in our experience, it is sometimes less clear to them what is motivating their restrictive eating, and many report wishes to be healthy rather than a desire to lose weight or a fat phobia per se. We have also found that younger adolescents often do not report body image distortion, but rather more clearly deny, through their actions and sometimes words, the seriousness of their current low weight. These apparent differences between adults and adolescents warrant further study.

For BN, there are few developmental concessions in DSM for adjusting the diagnosis. Perhaps the most important problem with these criteria for adolescents with binge eating and purging behaviors are the requirements of frequency (e.g., an average of twice a week) and duration of symptoms (e.g., for 3 months) elements. These criteria reasonably apply to older, more chronic patients but pose significant problems for the clinician who sees adolescents with binge eating and purging behaviors earlier in their course. Symptoms of these types in adolescents may be intermittent, with varying intensity for briefer periods followed by periods of quiescence.

Many adolescents best fall into the category of EDNOS if one uses strict definitions of DSM. Some studies suggest that up to 40–50% of those with eating disorders would fit this category (Miller, 1998; Ricca et al., 2001; Turner & Bryant-Waugh, 2004). EDNOS may appear to be too imprecise a diagnosis and therefore does not help the clinician to make treatment decisions. However, if one takes a broader view of eating disorders to consider what is common to AN, BN, and EDNOS, an EDNOS perspective may lead to a more comprehensive understanding of eating problems (Fairburn, Cooper, & Shafran, 2003). From this perspective, all persons with eating disorders share the following characteristics: a severely abnormal pattern of eating; an abnormal attitude or set of beliefs about food, weight, and/or shape; a degree of emotional, social, or behavioral dysfunction that results from these behaviors and attitudes (significant problems with school, work, social, or familial functioning); and evidence that these behaviors and attitudes are unlikely to change without intervention. Although such a formulation is controversial in the adult eating disorder literature, child and adolescent practitioners are likely to find this approach conceptually appealing because it better fits an overall developmental perspective (Fairburn et al., in press; Steiner & Lock, 1998).

EPIDEMIOLOGY

The basic understanding of the epidemiology of AN is perhaps best represented by a population-based incidence study conducted in Rochester, Minnesota, over a 50-year span (1935–1984) (Lucas et al., 1991). These authors found the incidence rate of AN for females decreased from 16.6 per 100,000 person-years from 1935 to 1939 to 7 in 1950–1954, and increased to 26.3 in 1980–1984. Importantly, the incidence rates for women over 20 years were constant, while a significant increase for females 15–24 years of age was identified. The overall age-adjusted incidence rate for females was 14.6 and for males, 1.8. Thus the point prevalence is estimated at 0.48% among adolescent females between 15 and 19 years of age (Lucas et al., 1991). These data suggest that there may be a new and larger cohort of young adolescent women developing AN. However, some have suggested that this appearance of increasing incidence may be due simply to improved detection of cases. (Fombonne, 1995; Lucas, Crowson, O'Fallon, & Melton, 1999)

Recent data specific to the epidemiology of BN among adolescents relies on the work of Flament and colleagues (1995), who conducted a two-stage (survey followed up by interviews) screening for the disorder in France among 3,527 unselected secondary school students (Flament et al., 1995). The prevalence rate of BN was estimated to be about 1.1% for girls and 0.2% for boys. BN appears to be somewhat less frequent in this age group than in adult women, where estimates are about 2% (Hoek, 1993). Nonetheless, extreme dieting, binge eating, and purging behaviors all appear to be commonly initiated during adolescence (Stice & Agras, 1998).

The base rates for all eating disorders appears to be greater in females than in males. The rate for AN is 19:2 female to male per 100,000 and 29:1 per 100,000 for BN (Hoek, 1993). Nonetheless, some have identified increased referral rates for males for eating disorders (Braun, Sunday, Huang, & Halmi, 1999). There may be an increased rate of homosexuality among males with eating disorders both among adolescents and adults (Carlat,

Camargo, & Herzog, 1997; French et al., 2001; Lock et al., 2001; Russell & Keel, 2002).

Socioeconomic class has long been a presumed factor in the development of eating disorders. Little evidence supports this claim as pertains to BN; however, limited data do suggest that the majority of patients with AN appear to be from wealthier and more educated groups (le Grange & Lock, 2002; McClelland & Crisp, 2001). Nonetheless, both disorders appear to occur in all ethnic and social groups.

DEVELOPMENTAL COURSE AND OUTCOMES

The course and prognosis of AN and BN appear to differ. Of the two, AN is the most serious in terms of morbidity and mortality. However, BN is often chronic and erodes psychological, social, and vocational development. In addition, there is evidence that many patients transition from AN to BN over time (Bulik, Fear, & Pickering, 1997; Eddy et al., 2002).

Anorexia Nervosa

AN typically develops in early adolescence, though some suggest that there are two particularly vulnerable periods—ages 13–14 and 17–18 (Halmi, Brodland, & Loney, 1973; Lucas et al., 1991). The illness often begins insidiously, with an episode of dieting that gradually leads to life-threatening starvation. At times there can be identifiable precipitating events that begin the dieting process. Examples of these events can include being teased about weight, onset of menses, a friend who begins dieting, transition to a new school or level in school, parental illness, parental dieting, or initiating dating. Patients often report beginning dieting because of a wish to lose weight, eat healthier, or improve performance in a sport. A few adolescents begin consuming less calories in the service of being "good," defined by them as using an ascetic formulation of "the less you consume, the better you are." Regardless of motivation, dieting usually begins informally by cutting out desserts and snacks, but over time, meats and other proteins, fats, and sugars are eliminated (Fairburn, 1997a; Lock, 2002; Lock & le Grange, 2005; Steiner & Lock, 1998).

Once food choices are narrowed, dieting efforts typically are focused on lowering quantities of food consumed even within this limited range of options. Often, detailed calorie counting, exact measuring, and elaborate preparation of foods become the rule. At this point the patient may attempt to remove herself from the company of others while eating, to prepare meals independently of others, and sometimes to cook elaborate meals and desserts for others though not eating anything herself. Alongside this extreme food restriction, a schedule of increased exercise is often used to ensure continued weight loss. At this point, whatever weight goals might have been initially set have typically long been surpassed and the goal of weight loss in itself is firmly established. The patient may also begin to induce vomiting to purge the small portions she does consume or to employ other weight loss strategies including diet pills and laxatives. Eating is often associated with guilt, anxiety, and anger. Paradoxically, with increased weight loss, hunger cues are diminished, making the process of continued food restriction easier. Nonetheless, most patients report extraordinary preoccupation with food. The period over which this cascade of events takes place is variable, but it can be as short as 4–6 weeks or as long as a year or more.

At some point during this process in most postmenarcheal females, menstruation ceases as body fat declines. Interestingly, a subset of females develop amenorrhea very early while others can reach very low weights without losing menstruation, which has led some to suggest the amenorrhea should not be required for the diagnosis (Garfinkel, Lin, & Goering, 1996).

During this process of ever-increasing malnutrition, a variety of medical problems set in. Once malnutrition is present, evidence of physiological compromise is found by lowered body temperature, decreased blood pressure, and decreased heart rate, as well as changes in skin and hair texture and growth. Particularly noteworthy is the development of fine body hair (lanugo). Changes in growth hormone, hypothalamic hypogonadism, bone marrow hypoplasia, structural abnormalities of the brain, cardiac dysfunction, and gastrointestinal difficulties are all common. The most important chronic medical problems for adolescents with AN are the potential for significant growth retardation, pubertal delay or interruption, and peak bone mass reduction (Fisher et al., 1995). Acutely, bradycardia (very slow heart rate), hypothermia (very low body temperature), and dehydration may become life threatening.

The outcome of AN is variable; some patients recover completely, while others develop a fluctuating course of weight gains and losses sometimes leading to BN (Bulik et al., 1997; Eddy et al., 2002; Fairburn, Cooper, Doll, Norman, & O'Connor, 2000). The most unfortunate patients remain at chronically low weights and have a progressively deteriorating course. Studies indicate a mortality rate from 3 to 10%, with half the deaths resulting from suicide (Herzog et al., 2000; Lee, Chan, & Hsu, 2003; Steinhausen, Rauss-Mason, & Seidel, 1991, 1993). It appears that these mortality risks increase at approximately 1% per year for each year of illness (Zipfel, Lowe, Deter, & Herzog, 2000). No other psychiatric illness is so lethal in its chronic form. Although vocational and academic functioning may be good, psychological and social impairment persists even after weight restoration (Deter, Herzog, & Petzold, 1992; Herzog et al., 1999). It appears that a significant subset of up to 30% develops BN as their disordered thoughts and behaviors persist (Bulik et al., 1997; Eddy et al., 2002).

Bulimia Nervosa

Typically binge eating episodes and purging begin in middle adolescence, although full-scale BN appears to develop later, typically around age 18 (Flament et al., 1995; Stice & Agras, 1998). Adolescents with BN often report long histories of weight preoccupation and many with mild to moderate obesity present in childhood. Dissatisfaction with weight and shape is sometimes present for a long period before attempts to change weight begin. Often these adolescents have experimented with a variety of diets for brief periods, only to abandon these efforts. Many report that they develop an urge to binge eat in response to severe dieting and fasting behaviors. Once they have overeaten, they feel guilty and anxious and seek ways to relieve themselves of their fear of gaining weight as a result. This leads to purging in its various forms. Most often purging is through vomiting but can also include the use of laxatives, diuretics, and compensatory exercise (Fairburn et al., 2000).

Adolescents with BN, like their adult counterparts, report a high degree of self-worth being dependent on feeling satisfied with their weight and appearance. Often these adolescents report that they eat very little breakfast or lunch, but when they return to their homes after school, they binge eat. This is a time at which there is usually little parental supervision so that binge eating can occur secretly. Alternately, some adolescents report nighttime binge eating, another time when they are less likely to be observed. Most adolescents, like adults with BN, report intense feelings of shame about these behaviors (Fairburn & Harrison, 2003; le Grange & Lock, 2002; Lock, 2002).

As the disorder becomes more entrenched, adolescents begin to organize their lives around the management of binge eating and the compensatory activities related to it (Lock & le Grange, 2005). They become more irritable and withdraw from friends and families. Often their schoolwork declines. They also report increasingly depressed moods. Once these altered patterns of eating are firmly established and they extend their hold on the adolescent, binge eating and purging become a convenient way to avoid other problems and may be increasingly incorporated into the adolescent's coping strategies. These factors combine to make BN surprisingly resistant to change, even when patients feel motivated to do so. In addition, sometimes adolescents with BN report a history of other impulsive behaviors such as alcohol use and shoplifting.

Although patients with BN experience variations in weight, they rarely approach the low weights associated with AN. Other medical complications, like hypokalemia (low blood levels of potassium), esophageal tears, gastric disturbances, dehydration, and severe changes in blood pressure or heart rate when standing up or sitting down (orthostasis) may require intermittent hospitalization (Fisher, Schneider, Burns, Symons, & Mandel, 2001). Although mortality figures are unknown, death can occur as a result of any of the aforementioned factors.

Without treatment, patients with BN have a variable course, with the majority following a chronic fluctuation of binge–purge behavior (Fairburn et al., 2000; Herzog et al., 1999; Herzog, Keller, Lavori, & Sacks, 1991; Herzog et al., 1993). In treatment studies of adult patients, up to 50% are abstinent at the end of treatment while an additional 20% are improved. At follow-up, most successfully treated patients maintain the gains they have made (Herzog et al., 1993; Wilson & Fairburn, 2002).

ETIOLOGY AND RISKS FOR ADOLESCENT EATING DISORDERS FROM A DEVELOPMENTAL PSYCHOPATHOLOGICAL PERSPECTIVE

It is helpful to view eating disorders from a developmental psychopathological perspective. From this perspective, certain biological vulnerabilities, over time and with exposure to a range of experiences including parenting, abuse, and exposure to media, drive the development of beliefs and behaviors that support classic eating disorders (Lock, le Grange, Agras, & Dare, 2001; Steiner et al., 2003; Steiner & Lock, 1998; Steiner et al., 1999). This confluence of biological, familial, and sociocultural influences apparently reaches a critical threshold for many during adolescence, when most eating disorders begin. Unfortunately, most studies of the development of eating disorders are retrospective or cross-sectional, and therefore implications for the prospective development of an eating disorder are speculative (Steiner et al., 2003; Steiner & Lock, 1998). Nonetheless, the findings of these studies are important in helping to conceptualize a possible etiological and developmental trajectory for eating disorders that we review here.

There are likely biological factors that may underlie vulnerability for the development for eating disorders. For example, there is increasing evidence for the familial clustering of eating disorders and eating attitudes, suggesting a role for heritable causation. However, there are no adequate longitudinal studies controlling shared and nonshared environments (Kendler et al., 1995; Strober & Humphrey, 1987; Strober, Morrell, Burroughs, Salkin, & Jacobs, 1985). These studies suggest there is a 3–10% increase in the prevalence of eating disorders in siblings, 27% in mothers, 16% in fathers, and 29% in first-degree relatives (Strober, Freeman, Lampert, Diamond, & Kaye, 2000). Family history studies show that for AN, greater than 50% of the risk for AN is attributable to additive genetic influences. In addition, there is growing evidence that certain symptoms (e.g., binge eating, self-induced vomiting, dietary restraint, body dissatisfaction, and weight preoccupation) may also be heritable (Bulik, Sullivan, & Kendler, 1998). These findings suggest that there by be a broad phenotype for eating disorders with possible shared genetic predisposition.

The study of the neurobiology of eating disorders has demonstrated impressive hormonal and neurohormonal systems differences in adult and late adolescent patients who are actively ill (Pirke & Platte, 1995). It is not clear whether any of these changes can be generalized to nonchronic adolescent populations, whether they represent specific risk factors, or whether they are brought on by starvation and perpetuate illness, or are simply the result of bodily changes due to starvation and semi-starvation. Most appear to normalize after refeeding. More recent advances using neuroimaging techniques suggest that bulimic patients and anorexic patients differ in serotonin activity; however, the significance of these findings remains unclear. Low levels of the neurotransmitter 5-hydroxytryptamine—serotonin—appear to play a key role in bulimic behavior (Steiger et al., 2001). A study measuring levels of serotonin in women who had recovered from bulimia found persistent serotonergic abnormalities (Kaye, Greeno, et al., 1998; Kaye, Grendall, & Strober, 1998). The deficiency of monoamine activity, even after recovery from the disorder, suggests that neurochemical alterations may contribute to the development of BN.

Early family experiences may also increase developmental risk for eating disorders. Some studies report that families of patients with eating disorders are overly enmeshed, conflict avoidant, and inflexible (Minuchin, Rosman, & Baker, 1978), though these types of familial patterns and interactions are not universally reported (Casper, Hedeker, & McClough, 1992). Other studies suggest that insecure attachment (i.e., dismissive attachment styles) to mothers may contribute to risk for an eating disorder (Ward et al., 2001). According to some studies, families of patients with AN appear more controlling and organized, while families of bulimic patients are more chaotic, conflicted, and critical (Humphrey, 1986, 1987). However, comparisons with families in which there is other psychopathology or to nonclinical families obscure these differences (Casper & Troiani, 2001; Thienemann & Steiner, 1993). Thus, the role of family process, though etiologically implicated in some family therapy approaches, is undetermined (Minuchin et al., 1978; Palazzoli, 1974).

Regardless of any biologically mediated factors or family process variables, there appears to be no clear continuity between eating problems in early childhood (failure to thrive, picky eating, etc.) and those that develop eating disorders during adolescence. Boys are at greater risk of eating disorders in early childhood, while in adolescence girls become more vulnerable. Nonetheless, in one of the few prospective studies of eating problems, Marchi and Cohen (1990) used a lagged design to study two different but overlapping age cohorts (ages 0–10 and 9–18) (Marchi & Cohen, 1990). Subjects were followed for 2.5 years. These authors found that picky eating and digestive problems predate prerestrictive dieting behaviors; pica (eating of non-nutritional substances such as dirt, hair, and clay) and mealtime family fighting were predictive of problems with binge eating and purging. Unfortunately, the total number of subjects was too small to predict true cases of AN or BN.

An early age of onset of weight concerns is considered a risk for later development of AN and BN. It appears, though, that many children express the desire to be thinner (up to 45%) (Maloney, McQuire, & Daniels, 1988). More than a third (37%) try some form of weight loss, while among this latter group, 6.9% score in the pathological range on an adapted version of the Eating Attitude Test (EAT; Maloney, McQuire, & Daniels, 1989; Schur, Sanders, & Steiner, 1999). Girls are more concerned about being thinner, while boys' weight concerns are focused on wishes to be bigger. These observations are consistent with body and weight concerns of adolescents along gender lines and suggest continuity between adolescents and school-age children in this respect.

However, the increased importance of sexual attractiveness and social acceptance and an increased ability to undertake actions related to these concerns independent of parents are also reasons that adolescents are more likely to develop eating disorders. In addition, a somewhat exaggerated focus on weight and shape, as well as dieting, may be normative for many adolescents, leading them to experiment with various weight-loss strategies. This may be due in part to increased focus on bodily appearance, especially in the context of the increased influence of the fashion world during adolescence (Ackard & Peterson, 2001). Rates of dieting and related behaviors increase from middle school years (11–13 years of age) through adolescence with estimates among high school girls approximating 60–70% or higher. This exposes more adolescents to the possibility of extreme or harmful weight-loss strategies that are the most consistently reported associated risks for developing an eating disorder (Patton, Selzer, Coffey, Carlin, & Wolfe, 1999; Steiner et al., 2003). In addition, over time, adolescent girls appear to be less satisfied with their weight and perceive more pressure from the media to decrease weight (McCabe, Ricciardelli, & Finemore, 2001).

These concerns and behaviors are consistent with the developmental stage of adolescence wherein young persons are challenged with increasing personal autonomy that is shaped by their increased capacity for abstract thinking and for personal and sexual intimacy. Attie and Brooks-Gunn (1989) tested the hypothesis that the development of eating problems is related to pubertal onset by prospectively following 193 girls from 7th through 10th grade for 2 years. They found that eating problems emerged in response to pubertal change, especially fat accumulation. In addition, girls who felt most negatively about their bodies at puberty were at highest risk for the development of eating difficulties.

In addition to these pubertal factors, other problems common to adolescence may contribute to the development of an eating disorder. Among these are: teasing by peers (Fabian & Thompson, 1989), discomfort in discussing problems with parents (Larson, 1991), maternal preoccupation with restricting dietary intake (Hill, Weaver, & Blundell, 1990), and acculturation to the Western values in immigrants (Pumariega, 1986). Some studies have reported a high incidence of sexual abuse in women diagnosed with an eating disorder (Perez, Voelz, Pettit, & Joiner, 2002; Wonderlich et al., 2001). However, the nature of the relationship between eating disorders and abuse is difficult to assess because of differences in criteria for evaluating abuse, a high base rate of sexual abuse in the general female population, and a high rate of abuse associated with other psychiatric diagnoses. Unfortunately, the relationship between abuse and eating problems has not been systematically studied in younger patients.

Sociocultural risk factors are also relevant to the development of eating disorders in adolescence. During adolescence, the influence of media, especially the thin ideal of the fashion world, is increasingly salient (Fouts & Burggraf, 1999; McCabe et al., 2001; Pinhaus, Toner, Ali, Garfinkel, & Stuckless, 1999). It is presumed that comparison to these thin ideals leads to increased body dissatisfaction and in some to disordered eating behaviors (Ohring, Graber, & Brooks-Gunn, 2001). A similar hypothesis suggests that for males an increased emphasis on muscularity and lower body fat is leading to increased shape and weight concerns and eating disorders in men (Leit, Pope, & Gray, 2001). It also appears that those who enter Western culture from other regions are at even greater risk (Gowen, Hayward, Killen, Robinson, & Taylor, 1999; Gunewardene, Huon, & Zheng, 2001; Pumariega, 1986). The hypothesis is that these adolescents turn to eating-disordered behaviors in order to increase their acceptance and comfort in their new social environment (Hill & Bhatti, 1995). However, other factors may be related to this apparent increase in vulnerability for developing an eating disorder in these groups, including perfectionism, cultural values, and gender (Davis & Katzman, 1999; Fairburn, Cooper, Doll, & Welch, 1999; McClelland & Crisp, 2001).

ASSESSMENT

Adolescents with eating disorders are often referred by a concerned pediatrician. Families and pediatricians are often reluctant to make these referrals because they are resistant to the idea that changes in eating behaviors are due to an emotional problem. Because dieting and weight concerns are associated with Western culture in general and adolescent young women in particular, it is important to distinguish between these typical and predictable concerns and those that become severe enough to warrant intervention. The clinician should expect that adolescents with eating disorders often deny or minimize symptoms, due in part to a distorted perception of the facts, while others consciously manipulate information to keep clinicians from appreciating the severity of their preoccupations and behaviors. Thus, it is necessary for the clinician to meet with parents to ascertain their perspectives on the referral.

Initially, the clinician should meet with the adolescent to provide a developmentally appropriate entry into the family that respects the adolescent's developing identity. The interviewer should communicate support and warmth, while minimizing presumptions of understanding. Evaluation should include ascertainment of the presence of common triggers such as comments on weight (positive or negative), onset of menses, dating, family conflicts, starting middle school or high school, breakup with a romantic partner, other people beginning dieting in the home or in social circle, and so on. A detailed history about efforts to lose weight should include counting calories, fat restriction, fasting, skipping meals, not drinking, meat and protein restriction, increased exercise, binge eating, purging behaviors (exercise, laxative, diuretics), and use of stimulants and diet pills (both over the counter, health food products, and illegal products).

For patients with AN, there is usually a cascade of restricting activities starting with ridding the diet of fats and sugars, then restricting proteins and meats, and finally restricting amounts. For the patient with BN, restricting periods are less prolonged, often disrupted by binge eating and purging activities in a cycle that leads to increasing frequency of failed restriction, binge eating, and compensatory purgation. A binge may be "objective" (eating significantly more than the average person in a finite period) or "subjective" (eating a normal amount of food, but feeling out of control at the time of eating) (APA, 1994). Both patients with AN and those with BN can have both types of binge eating. However, AN patients are more likely to call a much smaller quantity of food a "binge" than is the typical BN patient. Health consequences of these behaviors should also be evaluated. Patients commonly report dizziness, headaches, fainting spells, weakness, poor concentration, stomach and abdominal pain, and loss of menses. For patients with BN, throat pain, blood in emesis, small dot-like lesions in the schlera of the eyes, and swollen neck glands are also common.

After the interview with the adolescent, parents are interviewed without the patient present. If there are two parents, both need to be present. Parents are asked about the general development of the patient—complications during pregnancy, early feeding, developmental milestones, transitions into preschool and elementary school, aspects of attachment, early temperament and personality traits, family problems during the patient's childhood, and peer and sibling relationships. The clinician may use the information obtained during the interview with the adolescent to compare it to the parents' version of events and explore commonalties as well as differences. Together, these differing perspectives help generate a more comprehensive narrative of the events leading up to and sustaining the current clinical problems.

Because eating disorders affect both mind and body, it is important that a medical and nutritional assessment be conducted. It is also important for clinicians versed in the medical aspects of malnutrition and binge eating and purging behaviors to assess any medical problems that may be present. A basic medical workup for an adolescent with BN would include the following: a complete physical to check for signs of malnutrition (e.g., dehydration, tooth erosion, and lanugo), as well as tests for abnormalities in blood, liver, kidney, and thyroid functioning. These examinations help to assess the degree of illness and its chronicity, as well as to rule out other possible organic reasons for weight loss including infection, diabetes, thyroid disease, or cancers.

Consultation with a dietician with expertise in working with eating disorders is helpful in clarifying the degree of weight loss in AN as well as providing educational advice for the family and patient about the need for proper nutrition for health. This is best done by a nutritionist with experience in the evaluation of patients with eating disorders. For patients with AN, it is often helpful to calculate the BMI—weight (kilograms)/height (meters)^2—in order to determine a reasonable weight range for recovery . For both patients with AN and those with BN, it is important to assess their actual caloric needs compared to their beliefs, which have been distorted by their illness.

Comorbid psychiatric illness in patients with eating disorders is important to assess. Several studies suggest that comorbid psychiatric illness is common for adolescents with eating disorders. For examples, Herzog and colleagues found that 63% of all patients with eating disorders had a lifetime affective disorder (Herzog, Keller, Sacks, Yeh, & Lavori, 1992; Herzog, Nussbaum, & Marmor, 1996). Rastram (1992) found that 35% of patients with chronic AN also had obsessive–compulsive disorder. Although alcohol and drug abuse are commonly diagnosed in adults with eating disorders, particularly among patients with BN, no studies have documented this in younger patients. There is considerable interest in personality problems (e.g., avoidant personality with AN and borderline personality with BN), but it is unclear if these findings are applicable to adolescents or children (Casper et al.,

1992; Herzog, Keller, Lavori, Kenny, & Sacks, 1992). Nonetheless, personality differences have been repeatedly found by multiple methods and from a variety of theoretical backgrounds (temperament, personality, ego psychology), showing anorexic girls to be anxious, inhibited, and controlled, while bulimic patients tend to be more affectively labile and undercontrolled (Casper et al., 1992; Shaw & Steiner, 1997). At the same time, it is possible that the current studies overestimate comorbid illness and eating disorders because many patients with eating disorders who are included in research come from specialized eating disorder clinics and are adults with chronic illness and thereby may overrepresent more seriously compromised individuals.

The assessment of eating disorders remains a complex area of clinical activity, because the disorders present with a mix of disturbances in overlappping domains (e.g., depression, anxiety, obsessionality, and delusions). Patients may appear depressed and unhappy, but this may be specifically related to weight and shape concerns. They may be anxious and obsessed but again exclusively focused on eating and weight loss behaviors. Finally, beliefs and attitudes toward body shape and food or its preparation may be extreme enough in character to suggest delusional thinking. In all these examples, however, the primary problem is the eating disorder and the other symptoms are related to this core problem. In these cases, it is important to focus on the central problem, though attention to other psychiatric disorders if they are truly present is always indicated.

Specific structured interviews (Eating Disorder Examination [EDE]; Binford, le Grange, & Jellar, 2005; Cooper & Fairburn, 1987) are available, as are screening instruments in parent and child versions (Cooper, Cooper, & Fairburn, 1989; Passi, Bryson, & Lock, 2003). However, the adult version of the EDE appears to be feasible for use with most adolescents (Passi et al., 2003). Clinical self-reports are also available: the Eating Disorder Inventory (EDI) has normative data down to age 14 years (Shore & Porter, 1990). The EAT has a version applicable to school-age children (Maloney et al., 1988) and the Kids Eating Disorder Survey (KEDS; Childress, Brewerton, Hodges, & Jarrell, 1993) to middle school children. The utility of these instruments for the clinician resides in the ability to track progress of specific symptoms over time.

TREATMENT FOR ADOLESCENTS WITH EATING DISORDERS

Treatment theories and approaches differ for AN and BN. For AN, there are two main approaches, psychodynamic individual therapy and family therapy. For family therapy, there are a variety of types including psychodynamic family therapy, strategic family therapy, structural family therapy, and specific family-based treatment (i.e., the Maudsley approach). Psychodynamic or cognitive-behavioral therapy are the main individual approaches to AN. For BN, cognitive-behavioral treatment and interpersonal therapies are the main approaches for adults. No treatment has been systematically evaluated for adolescents with BN.

The database for the treatment of eating disorders, at least among adults, has been expanding at a rapid rate over the past 30 years, particularly in the area of cognitive-behavioral treatment for BN. Research in effective treatments for AN has lagged considerably behind that of BN; however, there are some promising leads in terms of family therapy approaches at least for adolescents (Lock, 2001).

Anorexia Nervosa

There are two main approaches to treating adolescents with AN: individual and family approaches. Each approach has strong adherents and a theoretical position to argue its point of view. As already discussed, definitive evidence is lacking on which approach is best, though work with the family seems to have a slight advantage.

In the first half of the 20th century, treatment of AN, like most psychiatric care, was dominated by psychoanalysis with its emphasis on individual treatment. Early psychoanalytic models developed by Waller, Kaufman, and Deutch focused on guilt and oral impregnation fantasies, with weight loss being seen as a defense mechanism (Waller, Kaufman, & Deutch, 1940). These authors proposed that AN resulted from a regression to the oral stage and an abandonment of the genital stage (Thoma, 1967). Later, but still based in the psychoanalytic tradition, Hilda Bruch (1973) suggested that the person with AN is suffering from an inadequate sense of self. To assist with this view, treatment aims at helping to "find a voice" for this deficient self. This deficient self is putatively the result of a mother's failure to support the expression of and need for independence by the adolescent. Thus, by and large, this type of individual treatment focuses on the therapeutic process of developing autonomy and promoting separation from parents, which necessarily limits and to some extent excludes the parents from the treatment process.

An alternative model for the cause of AN was developed by Arthur Crisp, who speculated that AN results from the phobic avoidance of the tasks of adolescence including separation from parents, developing a peer group, and initiation of dating and romantic relationships (Crisp, 1997). In this developmental model, AN is an attempt to cope with anxieties and fears associated with pubertal change and psychosocial maturity. Thus, weight loss that results from excessive dieting and exercise leads to a body shape and hormonal status commensurate with preadolescence. In addition, because of medical and psychological sequelae of these behaviors, and because of parental concerns about them, the patient's role in the family becomes more dependent and like that of a younger child. In these ways, the adolescent thus apparently accomplishes her goal of avoiding adolescent struggles. The initial focus of psychotherapy is on restoration of normal weight so that the adolescent must confront the fears that precipitated the onset of AN. However, the ultimate focus of therapy is on assisting the adolescent to develop mastery over these anxieties through an increased understanding of why she is afraid of taking an adult role. In Crisp's model, treatment is highly focused on supporting the individual adolescent patient but often includes families as a crucial support for both the patient and the therapy itself.

Cognitive-behavioral therapy (CBT) has been used with adult patients with BN and AN. Focus on the cognitive distortions apparent in AN and promoting nutritional health through food logs are two of the main interventions. Studies suggest CBT may be helpful for relapse prevention in adults with AN (e.g., Pike, Walsh, Vitousek, Wilson, & Bauer, 2004). However, the use of CBT in adolescent patients with AN has not been systematically examined.

Family approaches to AN treatment have long been controversial. When Sir William Gull and Charles Leseque independently described AN in the late 19th century, they took somewhat differing views of family involvement (Gull, 1874; Lasègue, 1883). Gull (1874) proposed that families were the worst attendants while Lesèque (1883) viewed family treatment as necessary for recovery. Jean-Martin Charcot appeared to agree with Gull by recommending the suppression of friends and relationships for patients because their presence served to effectively check all progress (Silverman, 1997). Thus, from the outset, a debate about the involvement of family in the treatment of AN was enjoined.

There are several major family approaches to AN treatment based on a range of schools of thought. Traditional family approaches see the patient as developing a problem in response to external factors such as traumas, poor parenting, genetic propensities, and cultural stresses. Family treatment employs the family to counteract the effects of these external causative factors. Thus, family intervention either modifies the problems within the family or, if this fails, separates the child from the family. Systemic family therapy for AN does not see the problem of AN as belonging to the patient but to the family as a whole (Haley, 1973; Selvini Palazzoli, 1974). Specifically within the Milan school of systemic therapy, families of patients with AN are seen as a rigidly organized group that relies on homeostatic mechanisms for maintenance of the status quo that are unusually resistant to change from the outside. Structural family therapy for AN is devised based on observations of psychosomatic families' characteristic transactional patterns that Minuchin described as enmeshed, overprotective, rigid and conflict avoidant (Minuchin et al., 1978). Because the child plays a critical role in the family's overall avoidance of conflict, symptoms are seen as powerfully supported by the family. Structural interventions are designed to alter the family organization by addressing these problematic transactional patterns through challenging alliances between parents and children, encouraging the development of stronger sibling subsystems, and promoting open communication. The result is that the child's emotional involvement with parents is reduced, at the same time improving the effectiveness of the parental dyad. The therapeutic sessions are characterized by direct confrontation by the therapist of parental inadequacies, a strong authoritarian stance on the part of the therapist, and a relatively short focus on the symptoms of AN per se.

Another type of family therapy, devised specifically for AN by Dare and Eisler at the

Maudsley Hospital, incorporates elements of the family therapy schools described previously (Dare & Eisler, 1997; Lock, 2001; Lock, le Grange, et al., 2001). First, this approach takes an agnostic view of the cause of AN consistent with strategic family therapist. It also takes a nonauthoritarian stance while holding the family in positive regard and empowering the family as a resource consistent with Milan approaches to family therapy. It directs the therapist to facilitate parental alignment while forcing siblings into appropriate roles and employing a family meal consistent with structural family therapy. Finally, it places special emphasis on joining the family as a consultant and separating the illness of AN from the patient, which is consistent with post-Milan narrative family approaches. The initial focus of therapy is helping parents to be effective in refeeding their adolescent much in the way an experienced nursing staff on an inpatient service would do. Practitioners of this approach contend that fundamentally AN so distorts normal processes of adolescent development that initial treatment must confront this distortion by paradoxically taking away adolescent autonomy in the service of weight restoration. Once eating and weight are not problematic, treatment focuses on helping the adolescent take control of her eating again under parental guidance and supervision. In the final stages, treatment focuses on dilemmas of adolescence in general (separation from parents, autonomy, social relationships) insofar as they have been affected by AN.

In general, the Maudsley approach views the patient with AN as compromised primarily in terms of her thoughts and preoccupations related to shape weight, dieting, and exercise rather than these symptoms being the result of family problems, inadequate psychological development, or traumatic injury. The principles of the approach are applied consistently regardless of the age of the patient. However, the approach does recognize variations in developmental aspects of the tasks of adolescents; for example, younger adolescents will likely be more preoccupied by the physical changes associated with puberty, while older adolescents are working more on peer relationships and independence. As a result, the particular strategies used to refeed patients are explained to the adolescent and her family in accordance with developmental principles. Whatever the age of the patient, parental control over eating is a temporary intervention with the aim that control over eating will be returned to the adolescent once weight has been restored and eating takes place without struggle.

It is important to point out that in practice family treatments are often combined with individual therapy (Lock, 2002). The main idea is that individual treatment potentially supports autonomy and independence, promotes self-development and confidence, and provides and opportunity for the adolescent to comment on problems and issues without parental involvement (e.g., dating, substance experimentation, and critical evaluations of the parents). Interestingly, in a recent study, Robin and colleagues (1999) compared family treatment similar to the Maudsley approach to an individual psychotherapy that was aimed at enhancing self-efficacy, self-esteem, and self-awareness. It was postulated that those in individual therapy would demonstrate better outcomes on measures of psychological maturity and self-confidence. However, although family treatment restored weight and menses more quickly, there were no differences on outcomes on these psychological variables. Because this study was small (37 total subjects), conclusions based on these findings should be made with caution.

On the other hand, two studies using two variants of the Maudsley approach suggest that seeing the patient independently of her parents may be warranted. Le Grange and colleagues (1992) and Eisler and colleagues (2000) found that, as with schizophrenia and major depression, familial expressed emotion (as expressed by high levels of parental criticism toward the adolescent) may moderate treatment outcome in adolescents with AN (Eisler et al., 2000; le Grange, Eisler, Dare, & Hodes, 1992). Studies from the same group also suggest that high levels of parental criticism are associated with higher treatment dropout and a poorer response to treatment (Szmukler, Eisler, Russell, & Dare, 1985). Specifically, Eisler and colleagues found that in families with high levels of criticism, patients recovered better when the parents were seen separately from the adolescent. From these data, it appears that families that are not highly critical should be seen in whole family therapy (conjointly) in order to maximize the resources available to the patient to recover. On the other hand, when families exhibit high criticism, it may be advisable to prevent the patient from experiencing it so parents are seen separately from their daughter (separated family therapy). While the injunctions and interventions of both conjoint and family therapy are identical and based on the Maudsley approach, the structure of treatment is different.

There is also good reason to consider that individual therapy may have a special role for older adolescents who are more able to intellectually and emotionally utilize insight-oriented psychotherapy in conjunction with family work. According to Russell, Szmukler, Dare, and Eisler (1987), adolescents and adults over the age of 18 appeared to have done better with individual therapy. Developmentally, older adolescents are also more likely to have a need for more privacy around dating, substance use experimentation, and choice of friends, which can be found in the individual therapy situation.

Although AN was identified in the medical literature over 125 years ago, research on the psychological treatments is limited. There are only 13 published outpatient controlled psychotherapy trials for AN (Channon, de Silva, Hemsley, & Perkins, 1989; Crisp et al., 1991; Dare, Eisler, Russell, Treasure, & Dodge, 2001; Eisler et al., 2000; Geist, Heinmaa, Stephens, Davis, & Katzman, 2000; Hall & Crisp, 1987; le Grange, Eisler, Dare, & Russell, 1992; Lock, Agras, Bryson, & Kraemer, 2005; McIntosh et al., 2005; Pike et al., 2005; Robin et al., 1999; Russell et al., 1987; Treasure et al., 1995). These studies were conducted over a 20-year period and employed small sample sizes and variable outcome measures, which render conclusions based on their results problematic. A total of fewer than 600 subjects have been studied in published randomized clinical trials. Nonetheless, among the psychological studies, eight have explored some type of family approach to treatment of the disorder (Crisp et al., 1991; Dare et al., 2001; Eisler et al., 2000; Geist et al., 2000; Hall & Crisp, 1987; le Grange, Eisler, Dare, & Russell, 1992; Lock et al., 2005; Robin et al., 1999; Russell et al., 1987). There have been four trials of adolescents alone, summarized in Table 14.1. These studies suggest that family-based treatment for AN based on the Maudsley approach is effective in 63–94% of cases and appears to be more effective than two forms of individual therapy (supportive and psychodynamic individual therapy), though small cell sizes limit these published studies. In addition, however, preliminary data from a manualized form of the Maudsley approach suggest similar outcomes (Lock & le Grange, 2001).

In addition, although family systemic therapies have not been the subject of any randomized clinical trials, several noncontrolled trials of family therapy suggest that it is efficacious. Minuchin and colleagues (1978) reported good outcomes in 86% of patients in a case series of 53 adolescents with AN treated with structural family therapy. Stierlin and Weber (1989), in another case series of 42 families treated with strategic family therapy, reported that approximately two-thirds had recovered weight and menstruation at follow-up. The therapeutic approaches used in these two studies emphasize the family system as a potential solution for the

TABLE 14.1. Outpatient Psychotherapy Treatment Trials for AN

Study	Type of treatment	n	Age (mean)	Outcomes (Morgan–Russell—good or intermediate)
Russell et al. (1987)	Family therapy and individual therapy	21	15.3	Family therapy = 90%; individual therapy = 18%
le Grange et al. (1992)	Whole family and separated family therapy	18	15.3	68% overall; no differences between groups
Robin et al. (1999)	Family therapy or individual therapy	37	13.9	Family therapy = 94%; individual therapy = 65%; no differences between groups at 1-year follow-up
Eisler et al. (2000)	Family therapy versus separated family therapy	40	15.5	63% overall; no differences between groups
Lock et al. (2005)	Short- versus long-term family therapy	86	15.2	94% overall; no differences between groups

dilemmas of AN in the adolescent patient; however, there is no emphasis on directly changing eating behaviors. Rather, the approach stresses family process, communication, and negotiation of adolescent developmental issues.

Psychopharmacological interventions for AN have been examined in adult samples, but the role of these agents in adolescents is relatively unexplored (Attia, Mayer, & Killory, 2001). During periods of acute medical compromise, psychopharmacological agents are of limited use. Among adults, medications that have been most frequently used include antidepressants and low-dose neuroleptics. Low-dose neuroleptics are used to address severe obsessional thinking, anxiety, and psychotic-like thinking but pose problems with binge induction and little evidence of other benefits compared to controls. Some case reports suggest that some of the newer antipsychotic agents (e.g., olanzapine) may be helpful in reducing severe agitation and thereby increasing toleration of weight gain (Malina et al., 2003). Recent studies suggest that serotonin reuptake inhibitors (SSRIs) are helpful in preventing relapse in adults with AN, but systematic studies are not yet available (Kaye, 1991).

Bulimia Nervosa

There are two main psychological approaches to BN that have developed treatment models: cognitive-behavioral therapy (CBT) and interpersonal psychotherapy (IPT). Both have a research base to support their utility in adults with BN, but little data are available for younger patients. Family approaches to BN in adolescents are understudied, but preliminary data support consideration of family therapy for adolescent patients with BN (le Grange & Lock, 2002; le Grange, Lock, & Dymek, 2003).

The cognitive-behavioral model of BN, developed by Fairburn, assumes that the main factors involved in the maintenance of BN are dysfunctional attitudes toward body shape and weight (Fairburn, Marcus, & Wilson, 1993). Such attitudes lead to an overvaluation of thinness, to bodily dissatisfaction, and to attempts to control shape and weight by excessive dieting. This restrictive pattern then results in both psychological and physiological deprivation often associated with negative mood. As a result of the dietary restriction, hunger is increased, leading to an enhanced probability of binge eating particularly in the presence of negative mood. Because binge eating heightens concerns about weight and shape, it is eventually followed by purging as an attempt to compensate for calories consumed during the binge. The model also suggests that self-esteem, over concern with weight and shape, as well as dietary restraint, are all related constructs, because patients with BN tend to judge their self-worth largely in terms of shape and weight.

IPT for BN as developed by Fairburn is a noninterpretive, nondirective form of individual psychotherapy with little focus on the eating problems accept in the assessment stage. The focus of IPT is on the patient's current relationships. The initial focus is on a detailed analysis of the interpersonal context in which the eating disorder has developed and been maintained. This leads to the formulation of the patient's eating disorder in interpersonal terms and the specification of a limited number of current interpersonal problem areas. Thereafter, the focus of the treatment is on these problem areas, the two most common being interpersonal disputes and difficulty with "role transitions" (e.g., disengaging from parents). Throughout treatment the patient's independent competence is emphasized. At no stage in treatment are there attempts to directly modify the patient's eating habits or attitudes to shape and weight, nor does the treatment contain any of the behavioral or cognitive procedures that specifically characterize CBT for BN. For example, there are no behavioral instructions, nor is there self-monitoring of behavior or cognitions.

Although there are a large number of treatment studies for adult BN, none has specifically included or investigated adolescents with BN. AN and BN are distinct syndromes, but there is considerable overlap in symptomatology. It is reasonable then to consider treatments that have proved to be effective for adolescent AN to be helpful for adolescent patients with BN. There is, however, only scant scientific evidence to support family treatment of adolescents with BN. Eisler and colleagues (2000) found that binge-and-purge type patients with AN did just as well with family therapy as did purely restricting patients with AN, suggesting the binge eating and purging could be managed with the support of parents. In addition, a preliminary case series from the Maudsley group shows that family therapy was helpful for a group of adolescent patients with BN and their families (Dodge, Hodes, Eisler, & Dare, 1995).

Notwithstanding the paucity of systematic data, there are strong clinical reasons to involve the family in the treatment of adolescents with BN. Involving the family provides an opportunity to explore pertinent family issues, behaviors, and attitudes on the part of parents and other family members that can contribute to heightened feelings of shame and guilt, thereby reinforcing symptomatic behavior. Education about BN can be communicated to family members and the impact of the eating disorder on family relationships can be addressed. Many adolescents respond well to parental involvement in meal planning and assisting with efforts to decrease binge eating and purging episodes once the therapist succeeds in assuring them that parental involvement is supportive rather than critical (le Grange & Lock, 2002; le Grange et al., 2003). In fact, family involvement appears to help dilute the feelings of shame and guilt that accompany BN by bringing the problem to light in the family context. At the same time, family involvement helps the therapist to highlight for the parents the medical and psychological problems associated with BN and to elicit their support in helping their child (le Grange, 2002). Such a perspective can help to shift parental attitudes toward the patient and the illness from exasperation and anger to a more productive and sympathetic position.

To date, research in the treatment of BN has focused solely on adults with this disorder, despite the fact that both binge eating and purging often begin during adolescence, and that many cases of BN have their onset in adolescence (Fairburn, Welch, Doll, Davies, & O'Connor, 1997; Stice & Agras, 1998). While significant progress has been made in understanding a range of efficacious treatments for adults with BN, including CBT (Agras, Walsh, Fairburn, Wilson, & Kraemer, 2000; Cooper & Steere, 1995; Fairburn et al., 1991; Fairburn, Kirk, O'Connor, & Cooper, 1986), IPT (Agras et al., 2000; Fairburn, 1997b), and antidepressant medications (Walsh & Devlin, 1995), these treatments have not been studied with an adolescent population.

CBT has been tested in numerous controlled studies and is the most effective psychotherapeutic approach to the treatment of BN, compared to no therapy, nondirective therapy, pill placebo, manualized psychodynamic therapy (supportive–expressive), stress management, or antidepressant treatment. About half of patients with BN recover with CBT, while another 20% are much improved. The only psychotherapeutic treatment that may be as effective as CBT is IPT. A recent multisite study found that CBT was significantly superior to IPT in the number of patients with BN who recovered at the end of treatment (Agras et al., 2000). However, by 8–12 months follow-up, the outcomes for the two treatments were not distinguishable. Hence, because it is slower to exert its effects, IPT should be regarded as a secondary treatment for BN. In the longest follow-up study to date, Fairburn and colleagues (2000) followed bulimic patients treated with CBT for 5 years posttreatment. Nearly 60% of patients studied had no eating disorder and a further 20% had a subclinical disorder at the time of follow-up. The remainder were unrecovered, with a small percentage diagnosed as having AN. Hence, relapse rates for the successfully treated patient are low, and the benefits are long lasting. In the only report available for adolescents with BN treated with CBT, abstinence rates and clinical improvements are similar to those found in adult studies (Lock, in press). However, additional controlled studies of CBT in adolescent populations with bulimia appear to be warranted.

IPT modified for BN has been shown to be an effective therapy for BN (Fairburn, 1997b). As applied to BN, IPT focuses on the interpersonal context within which the eating disorder developed and is maintained with an aim of helping the patient make specific changes in identified problem areas. Little attention is paid to eating habits or attitudes toward weight and shape, nor does the treatment contain any of the specific behavioral or cognitive procedures that characterize CBT, thereby providing a suitable control condition. Three clinical trials and two follow-up studies provide empirical support for the use of IPT to treat BN. Fairburn and colleagues (1986) compared CBT to a short-term focal therapy aimed at identifying and modifying interpersonal problems accompanying BN rather than the eating disorder itself. Patients in both conditions showed improvements that were maintained over a 12-month follow-up period. In a follow-up study designed to replicate and extend these initial findings, 75 patients were randomly assigned to CBT, behavioral therapy (BT), and IPT (Fairburn et al., 1995). End-of-treatment results again indicated that all three treatments had a substantial effect, with results favoring CBT. However, at 12-month follow-up, only CBT and IPT showed consistent improvement.

At 6-year follow-up, patients who received CBT or IPT continued to do well compared to those who received BT. These studies suggest that BN was responsive to IPT as well as CBT, but that the improvements associated with IPT were slower to develop.

Drug therapy has been implemented more often in treatment of BN but has not been found to be as effective as cognitive-behavioral approaches (Agras et al., 1992). Many antidepressants are more effective than placebo in controlled, short-term treatment of binge behavior (Wilson et al., 1999). Medications studied include tricyclic antidepressant, SSRIs, atypical antidepressants (e.g., trazadone and buspuron), and lithium carbonate. The mechanism of action of these medications for BN is unknown, but the aim is to reduce binge-eating episodes and thereby prevent purging. Current treatment suggests that higher dosages of the SSRIs are the medications of choice because of their better safety and side-effect profiles. Longer-term studies have not been conducted. No specific studies of drug therapy for adolescents with BN are available.

CURRENT NEEDS AND FUTURE DIRECTIONS

Although there is abundant clinical wisdom about eating disorders and a developing understanding of how to treat adults with binge eating and purging disorders through CBT, IPT, and medications, we are sorely lacking in clinical trials for treatment of younger cohorts of patients. There are no published systematic treatment trials for adolescents with BN or related disorders employing either psychological or pharmacological therapies. It is apparent that the limited studies of AN provide suggestive evidence that a specific form of family treatment may be helpful (i.e., the Maudsley approach). Definitive treatment trials that compare this treatment to others are lacking. We do not have any medications that appear to be routinely helpful with AN, whether in adults or in adolescents. In addition to these problems, these disorders develop in the context of social, psychological, and physical development, making a developmental perspective on diagnosis and treatment essential. The conceptualization of eating disorders in a developmental context should lead to a clearer understanding of risk factors, treatment approaches, and prevention strategies.

REFERENCES

Ackard, D., & Peterson, D. (2001). Association between puberty and disordered, body image, and other psychological variables. *International Journal of Eating Disorders, 29*, 187–194.

Agras, W. S., Rossiter, E. M., Arnow, B., Schneider, J. A., Telch, C. F., Raeburn, S. D., et al. (1992). Pharmacologic and cognitive-behavioral treatment for bulimia nervosa: A controlled comparison. *American Journal of Psychiatry, 149*(1), 82–87.

Agras, W. S., Walsh, B. T., Fairburn, C. G., Wilson, G. T., & Kraemer, H. C. (2000). A multicenter comparison of cognitive-behavioral therapy and interpersonal psychotherapy for bulimia nervosa. *Archives of General Psychiatry, 57*, 459–466.

American Psychiatric Association. (1994). *Diagnostic and statistical manual of mental disorders* (4th ed.). Washington, DC: Author.

Attia, E., Mayer, L., & Killory, E. (2001). Medication response in the treatment of patients with anorexia nervosa. *Journal of Psychiatric Practice, 7*, 157–162.

Attie, I., & Brooks-Gunn, J. (1989). Development of eating problems in adolescent girls: A longitudinal study. *Developmental Psychology, 25*, 70–79.

Binford, R. B., le Grange, D., & Jellar, C. C. (2005). Eating Disorders Examination versus Eating Disorders Examination—Questionnaire in adolescents with full and partial-syndrome bulimia nervosa and anorexia nervosa. *International Journal of Eating Disorders, 37*, 44–49.

Braun, D., Sunday, S., Huang, A., & Halmi, C. A. (1999). More males seek treatment for eating disorders. *International Journal of Eating Disorders, 25*, 415–424.

Bruch, H. (1973). *Eating disorders: Obesity, anorexia nervosa, and the person within.* New York: Basic Books.

Bulik, C. M., Fear, J., & Pickering, A. (1997). Predictors of the development of bulimia nervosa in women with anorexia nervosa. *Journal of Nervous and Mental Disease, 185*, 704–707.

Bulik, C. M., Sullivan, P. F., & Kendler, K. S. (1998). Heritability of binge eating and broadly defined bulimia nervosa. *Biological Psychiatry, 44*, 1210–1218.

Carlat, D. J., Camargo, C. A., Jr., & Herzog, D. B. (1997). Eating disorders in males: a report on 135 patients. *American Journal of Psychiatry, 154*(8), 1127–1132.

Casper, R., Hedeker, D., & McClough, J. (1992). Personality dimensions in eating disorders and their relevance for subtyping. *Journal of the American Academy of Child and Adolescent Psychiatry, 31*, 830–840.

Casper, R., & Troiani, M. (2001). Family functioning in anorexia by subtype. *International Journal of Eating Disorders, 30*, 338–342.

Channon, S., de Silva, P., Hemsley, D., & Perkins, R. (1989). A controlled trial of cognitive-behavioural and behavioural treatment of anorexia nervosa. *Behaviour Research and Therapy, 27*(5), 529–535.

Childress, A., Brewerton, T., Hodges, E., & Jarrell, M. (1993). The Kids Eating Disorder Survey (KEDS): A study of middle school students. *Journal of the American Academy of Child and Adolescent Psychiatry, 32,* 843–850.

Cooper, P. J., & Steere, J. (1995). A comparison of two psychological treatments for bulimia nervosa: Implications for models of maintenance. *Behaviour Research and Therapy, 33,* 875–885.

Cooper, Z., Cooper, P. J., & Fairburn, C. G. (1989). The validity of the eating disorder examination and its subscales. *British Journal of Psychiatry, 154,* 807–812.

Cooper, Z., & Fairburn, C. G. (1987). The Eating Disorders Examination: A semi-structured interview for the assessment of the specific psychopathology of eating disorders. *International Journal of Eating Disorders, 6,* 1–8.

Crisp, A. H. (1997). Anorexia nervosa as flight from growth: Assessment and treatment based on the model. In D. M. Garner & P. E. Garfinkel (Eds.), *Handbook of treatment for eating disorders* (pp. 248–277). New York: Guilford Press.

Crisp, A. H., Norton, K., Gowers, S., Halek, C., Bowyer, C., Yeldham, D., et al. (1991). A controlled study of the effect of therapies aimed at adolescent and family psychopathology in anorexia nervosa. *British Journal of Psychiatry, 159,* 325–333.

Dare, C., & Eisler, I. (1997). Family therapy for anorexia nervosa. In D. M. Garner & P. E. Garfinkel (Eds.), *Handbook of treatment for eating disorders* (pp. 307–324). New York: Guilford Press.

Dare, C., Eisler, I., Russell, G., Treasure, J. L., & Dodge, E. (2001). Psychological therapies for adults with anorexia nervosa: Randomized controlled trial of outpatient treatments. *British Journal of Psychiatry, 178,* 216–221.

Davis, C., & Katzman, M. (1999). Perfection as acculturation: Psychological correlates of eating problems in Chinese male and female students living in the United States. *International Journal of Eating Disorders, 25,* 65–70.

Deter, J., Herzog, W., & Petzold, E. (1992). The Heidelberg–Mannheim study: Long-term follow-up of anorexia nervosa patients at the University Medical Center—Background and preliminary results. In W. Herzog & W. Vandereycken (Eds.), *The course of eating disorders* (pp. 71–84). Berlin, Germany: Springer-Verlag.

Dodge, E., Hodes, M., Eisler, I., & Dare, C. (1995). Family therapy for bulimia nervosa in adolescents: An exploratory study. *Journal of Family Therapy, 17,* 59–77.

Eddy, K., Keel, P., Dorer, D., Delinsky, S., Franko, D., & Herzog, D. B. (2002). Longitundinal comparison of anorexia nervosa subtypes. *International Journal of Eating Disorders, 31,* 191–202.

Eisler, I., Dare, C., Hodes, M., Russell, G., Dodge, E., &

le Grange, D. (2000). Family therapy for adolescent anorexia nervosa: The results of a controlled comparison of two family interventions. *Journal of Child Psychology and Psychiatry, 41*(6), 727–736.

Fabian, L., & Thompson, J. (1989). Body image and eating disturbances in young females. *International Journal of Eating Disorders, 8,* 63–74.

Fairburn, C. G. (1997a). Eating disorders. In D. Clark & C. G. Fairburn (Eds.), *Cognitive-behavioral therapy: Science and practice* (pp. 160–192). Oxford, UK: Oxford University Press.

Fairburn, C. G. (1997b). Interpersonal psychotherapy for bulimia nervosa. In D. M. Garner & P. E. Garfinkel (Eds.), *Handbook of treatment for eating disorders* (2nd ed., pp. 278–294). New York: Guilford Press.

Fairburn, C. G., Cooper, Z., Doll, H., Norman, P., & O'Connor, M. (2000). The natural course of bulimia nervosa and binge eating disorder in young women. *Archives of General Psychiatry, 57,* 659–665.

Fairburn, C. G., Cooper, Z., Doll, H. A., & Welch, S. L. (1999). Risk factors for anorexia nervosa: Three integrated case-control comparisons. *Archives of General Psychiatry, 56*(5), 468–476.

Fairburn, C. G., Cooper, Z., & Shafran, R. (in press). Cognitive-behavioral therapy for eating disorders: A "transdiagnostic" theory and treatment. *Behaviour Research and Therapy, 41,* 509–528.

Fairburn, C. G., & Harrison, P. J. (2003). Eating Disorders. *The Lancet, 361,* 407–416.

Fairburn, C. G., Jones, R., Peveler, R. C., Carr, S. J., Solomon, R. A., O'Connor, M. E., et al. (1991). Three psychological treatments for bulimia nervosa. A comparative trial. *Archives of General Psychiatry, 48*(5), 463–469.

Fairburn, C. G., Kirk, J., O'Connor, M., & Cooper, P. J. (1986). A comparison of two psychological treatments for bulimia nervosa. *Behaviour Research and Therapy, 24*(6), 629–643.

Fairburn, C. G., Marcus, M. D., & Wilson, G. T. (1993). Cognitive-behavioral therapy for binge eating and bulimia nervosa: A comprehensive treatment manual. In C. G. Fairburn & G. T. Wilson (Eds.), *Binge eating: Nature, assessment, and treatment* (pp. 361–404). New York: Guilford Press.

Fairburn, C. G., Norman, P. A., Welch, S. L., O'Connor, M. E., Doll, H. A., & Peveler, R. C. (1995). A prospective study of outcome in bulimia nervosa and the long-term effects of three psychological treatments. *Archives of General Psychiatry, 52*(4), 304–312.

Fairburn, C. G., Welch, S. L., Doll, H. A., Davies, B. A., & O'Connor, M. E. (1997). Risk factors for bulimia nervosa. A community-based case-control study. *Archives of General Psychiatry, 54*(6), 509–517.

Fisher, M., Golden, N., Katzman, D., Kreipe, R. E., Rees, J., Schebendoch, J., et al. (1995). Eating disorders in adolescents: A background paper. *Journal of Adolescent Health, 16,* 420–437.

Fisher, M., Schneider, M., Burns, J., Symons, H., & Mandel, F. (2001). Differences between adolescents and young adults at presentation to an eating disorder program. *Journal of Adolescent Health, 28,* 222–227.

Flament, M., Ledoux, S., Jeammet, P., Choquet, M., & Simon, Y. (1995). A population study of bulimia nervosa and subclinical eating disorders in adolescence. In H. Steinhausen (Ed.), *Eating disorders in adolescence: Anorexia and bulimia nervosa* (pp. 21–36). New York: Brunner/Mazel.

Fombonne, E. (1995). Anorexia nervosa: No evidence of an increase. *British Journal of Psychiatry, 166,* 462–471.

Fouts, G., & Burggraf, K. (1999). Television situation comedies: Female body images and verval reinforcements. *Sex Roles, 40 ,* 473–481.

French, S., Leffert, N., Story, M., Neumark-Sztainer, D., Hannan, P., & Benson, P. (2001). Adolescents binge/purge and weight loss behaviors: Associations with developmental assets. *Journal of Adolescent Health, 28,* 211–221.

Garfinkel, P., Lin, E., & Goering, P. (1996). Should amenorrhoea be necessary for the diagnosis of anorexia nervosa? Evidence from a Canadian community sample. *British Journal of Psychiatry, 168,* 500–506.

Geist, R., Heinmaa, M., Stephens, D., Davis, R., & Katzman, D. K. (2000). Comparison of family therapy and family group psychoeducation in adolescents with anorexia nervosa. *Canadian Journal of Psychiatry, 45,* 173–178.

Gowen, L., Hayward, C., Killen, J. D., Robinson, J., & Taylor, C. B. (1999). Acculturation and eating disorder symptoms in adolescent girls. *Journal of Research on Adolescence, 9,* 67–83.

Gull, W. (1874). Anorexia nervosa (apepsia hysterica, anorexia hysterica). *Transactions of the Clinical Society of London, 7,* 222–228.

Gunewardene, A., Huon, G., & Zheng, R. (2001). Exposure to westernization and dieting: a cross-cultural study. *International Journal of Eating Disorders, 29,* 289–293.

Haley, J. (1973). *Uncommon therapy: The psychiatric techniques of Milton H. Erickson.* New York: Norton.

Hall, A., & Crisp, A. H. (1987). Brief psychotherapy in the treatment of anorexia nervosa: Outcome at one year. *British Journal of Psychiatry, 151,* 185–191.

Halmi, K., Brodland, G., & Loney, J. (1973). Progress in anorexia nervosa. *Annals of Internal Medicine, 78,* 907–909.

Herzog, D. B., Dorer, D. J., Keel, P. K., Selwyn, S. E., Ekeblad, E. R., Flores, A. T., et al. (1999). Recovery and relapse in anorexia and bulimia nervosa: A 7.5-year follow-up study. *Journal of the American Academy of Child and Adolescent Psychiatry, 38*(7), 829–837.

Herzog, D. B., Greenwood, D. N., Dorer, D. J., Flores, A. T., Ekeblad, E. R., Richards, A., et al. (2000). Mortality in eating disorders: A descriptive study. *International Journal of Eating Disorders, 28,* 20–26.

Herzog, D. B., Keller, M. B., Lavori, P. W., Kenny, G. M., & Sacks, N. R. (1992). The prevalence of personality disorders in 210 women with eating disorders. *Journal of Clinical Psychiatry, 53*(5), 147–152.

Herzog, D. B., Keller, M. B., Lavori, P. W., & Sacks, N. R. (1991). The course and outcome of bulimia nervosa. *Journal of Clinical Psychiatry, 52*(Suppl.), 4–8.

Herzog, D. B., Keller, M. B., Sacks, N. R., Yeh, C. J., & Lavori, P. W. (1992). Psychiatric comorbidity in treatment-seeking anorexics and bulimics. *Journal of the American Academy of Child and Adolescent Psychiatry, 31*(5), 810–818.

Herzog, D. B., Nussbaum, K. M., & Marmor, A. K. (1996). Comorbidity and outcome in eating disorders. *Psychiatric Clinics of North America, 19*(4), 843–859.

Herzog, D. B., Sacks, N. R., Keller, M. B., Lavori, P. W., von Ranson, K. B., & Gray, H. M. (1993). Patterns and predictors of recovery in anorexia nervosa and bulimia nervosa. *Journal of the American Academy of Child and Adolescent Psychiatry, 32*(4), 835–842.

Hill, A., & Bhatti, R. (1995). Body shape perception and dieting in pre-adolescent British Asian girls: Links with eating disorders. *International Journal of Eating Disorders, 17,* 175–183.

Hill, A., Weaver, C., & Blundell, J. (1990). Dieting concerns of 10 year old girls and their mothers. *British Journal of Clinical Psychiatry, 29,* 346–348.

Hoek, H. (1993). Review of epidemiological studies of eating disorders. *International Review of Psychiatry, 5,* 61–74.

Humphrey, L. (1986). Structural analysis of parent–child relationships in eating disorders. *Journal of Abnormal Psychology, 95,* 395–402.

Humphrey, L. (1987). Comparison of bulimic–anorexic and nondistressed families using structural analysis of behavior. *Journal of the American Academy of Child and Adolescent Psychiatry, 26,* 248–255.

Kaye, W. H. (1991). An open trial of fluoxetine in patients with anorexia nervosa. *Journal of Clinical Psychiatry, 52,* 464–471.

Kaye, W. H., Greeno, C. G., Moss, H., Fernstrom, J., Fernstrom, M., Lilenfeld, L. R., et al. (1998). Alterations in serotonin activity and psychiatric symptoms after recovery from bulimia nervosa. *Archives of General Psychiatry, 55,* 927–925.

Kaye, W. H., Grendall, K., & Strober, M. (1998). Serotonin neuronal function and selective serotonin reuptake inhibitor treatment in anorexia nervosa. *Biological Psychiatry, 44,* 825–838.

Kendler, K. S., Walters, E. E., Neale, M. C., Kessler, R. C., Heath, A. C., & Eaves, L. J. (1995). The structure of genetic and environmental risk factors for six major psychiatric disorders in women. *Archives of General Psychiatry, 52,* 374–383.

Larson, C. (1991). Relationship of family communication patterns in Eating Disorder Inventory scores in adolescent girls. *Journal of the American Dietic Association, 91,* 1065–1067.

Lasègue, E. (1883). De l'anorexie hysterique. *Archives Générales de Médecine, 21,* 384–403.

Lee, S., Chan, Y., & Hsu, L. (2003). The intermediate-term outcome of Chinese patients with anorexia nervosa in Hong Kong. *American Journal of Psychiatry, 160,* 967–972.

le Grange, D. (2002). Family therapy in clinical psychology. In *International encyclopedia of the social and behavioral sciences* (Vol. 8, pp. 5401–5406). Oxford, UK: Elsevier.

le Grange, D., Eisler, I., Dare, C., & Hodes, M. (1992). Family criticism and self-starvation: A study of expressed emotion. *Journal of Family Therapy, 14,* 177–192.

le Grange, D., Eisler, I., Dare, C., & Russell, G. (1992). Evaluation of family treatments in adolescent anorexia nervosa: a pilot study. *International Journal of Eating Disorders, 12*(4), 347–357.

le Grange, D., & Lock, J. (2002). Bulimia nervosa in adolescents: Treatment, eating pathology, and comorbidity. *South African Psychiatry Review, 5,* 19–22.

le Grange, D., Lock, J., & Dymek, M. (2003). Family-based therapy for adolescent with bulimia nervosa. *American Journal of Psychotherapy, 57*(2), 237–251.

Leit, R., Pope, H. G., & Gray, J. (2001). Cultural expectations of muscularity in men: The evolution of playgirl centerfolds. *International Journal of Eating Disorders, 29,* 90–93.

Lock, J. (2001). What is the best way to treat adolescents with anorexia nervosa? *Eating Disorders, 9,* 299–302.

Lock, J. (2002). Treating adolescents with eating disorders in the family context: Empirical and theoretical considerations. *Child and Adolescent Psychiatric Clinics of North America, 11,* 331–342.

Lock, J. (in press). Adjusting cognitive-behavioral therapy for adolescents with bulimia nervosa: Results of a case series. *American Journal of Psychotherapy.*

Lock, J., Agras, W. S., Bryson, S., & Kraemer, H. C. (2005). A comparison of short- and long-term family therapy for adolescent anorexia nervosa. *Journal of the American Academy of Child and Adolescent Psychiatry, 44,* 632–639.

Lock, J., & le Grange, D. (2001). Can family-based treatment of anorexia nervosa be manualized? *Journal of Psychotherapy Practice and Research, 10,* 253–261.

Lock, J., & le Grange, D. (2005). *Help your teenager beat an eating disorder.* New York: Guilford Press.

Lock, J., le Grange, D., Agras, W. S., & Dare, C. (2001). *Treatment manual for anorexia nervosa: A family-based approach.* New York: Guilford Press.

Lock, J., Reisel, B., & Steiner, H. (2001). Associated health risks of adolescents with disordered eating: How different are they from their peers? Results from a high school survey. *Child Psychiatry and Human Development, 31,* 249–265.

Lucas, A. R., Beard, C. M., & O'Fallon, W. M. (1991). 50-year trends in the incidence of anorexia nervosa in

Rochester, Minn: A population-based study. *American Journal of Psychiatry, 148,* 917–929.

Lucas, A. R., Crowson, C., O'Fallon, W. M., & Melton, L. (1999). The ups and downs of anorexia nervosa. *International Journal of Eating Disorders, 26,* 397–405.

Malina, A., Gaskill, J., McConaha, C., Guido, F., LaVia, M., Scholar, L., & Kaye, W. H. (2003). Olanzapine treatment of anorexia nervosa: A retrospective study. *International Journal of Eating Disorders, 33,* 234–237.

Maloney, M., McQuire, J., & Daniels, S. (1988). The reliability testing of a children's version of the Eating Attitudes Test. *Journal of the American Academy of Child and Adolescent Psychiatry, 27,* 541–543.

Maloney, M., McQuire, J., & Daniels, S. (1989). Dieting behavior and eating attitudes in children. *Pediatrics, 84,* 482–489.

Marchi, M., & Cohen, P. (1990). Early childhood eating behaviors and adolescent eating disorders. *Journal of the American Academy of Child and Adolescent Psychiatry, 29,* 112–117.

McCabe, M., Ricciardelli, L., & Finemore, J. (2001). The role of puberty, media and popularity with peers on strategies to increase weight, decrease weight and increase muscle tone among adolescent boys and girls. *Journal of Psychosomatic Research, 52,* 145–153.

McClelland, L., & Crisp, A. H. (2001). Anorexia Nervosa and social class. *International Journal of Eating Disorders, 29,* 150–156.

McIntosh, V. V., Jordan, J., Carter, F. A., Luty, S. E., McKenzie, J. M., Bulik, C. M., et al. (2005). Three psychotherapies for anorexia nervosa: A randomized, controlled trial. *American Journal of Psychiatry, 162,* 741–747.

Miller, H. (1998). New eating disorder service. *Psychiatric Bulletin, 22,* 751–754.

Minuchin, S., Rosman, B., & Baker, I. (1978). *Psychosomatic families: Anorexia nervosa in context.* Cambridge, MA: Harvard University Press.

Ohring, R., Graber, J., & Brooks-Gunn, J. (2001). Girls' recurrent and concurrent body dissatisfaction: Correlates and consequences over 8 years. *International Journal of Eating Disorders, 31,* 404–415.

Palazzoli, M. (1974). *Self-starvation: From the intrapsychic to the transpersonal approach to anorexia nervosa.* London: Chaucer.

Passi, V., Bryson, S., & Lock, J. (2003). Assessment of eating disorders in adolescents with anorexia nervosa: Self-report versus interview. *International Journal of Eating Disorders, 33,* 45–54.

Patton, G. C., Selzer, R., Coffey, C., Carlin, J. B., & Wolfe, R. (1999). Onset of adolescent eating disorders: Population based cohort study over 3 years. *British Medical Journal, 318,* 765–768.

Perez, M., Voelz, Z., Pettit, J., & Joiner, T. (2002). The role of acculurative stress and body dissatisfaction in predicting bulimic symptomatology across ethnic groups. *International Journal of Eating Disorders,* 31, 442–454.

Pike, K. M., Walsh, B. T., Vitousek, K., Wilson, G. T., & Bauer, S. (2004). Cognitive behavior therapy in posthospitalization treatment of anorexia nervosa. *American Journal of Psychiatry,* 160, 2046–2049.

Pinhaus, L., Toner, B., Ali, A., Garfinkel, P., & Stuckless, N. (1999). *International Journal of Eating Disorders,* 25, 223–226.

Pirke, M., & Platte, P. (1995). Neurobiology of eating disorders in adolescents. In H. Steinhausen (Ed.), *Eating disorders in adolescence: Anorexia and bulimia nervosa* (pp. 171–179). New York: Aldine de Gruyter.

Pumariega, A. (1986). Acculturation and eating disorders in adolescent girls: A comparative correlational study. *Journal of the American Academy of Child and Adolescent Psychiatry,* 25, 276–279.

Rastram, M. (1992). Anorexia nervosa in 51 Swedish adolescents: Premorbid problems and comorbidity. *Journal of the American Academy of Child and Adolescent Psychiatry,* 31, 819–828.

Ricca, V., Mannucci, E., Mazzani, B., Di Bernardo, M., Zucchi, T., Paionni, A., et al. (2001). Psychopathological and clinical features of outpatients with an eating disorder not otherwise specified. *Eating and Weight Disorders,* 6, 157–165.

Robin, A., Siegal, P., Moye, A., Gilroy, M., Dennis, A., & Sikand, A. (1999). A controlled comparison of family versus individual therapy for adolescents with anorexia nervosa. *Journal of the American Academy of Child and Adolescent Psychiatry,* 38(12), 1482–1489.

Russell, C., & Keel, P. (2002). Homosexuality as a specific risk factor for eating disorders in men. *International Journal of Eating Disorders,* 31, 300–306.

Russell, G. F., Szmukler, G. I., Dare, C., & Eisler, I. (1987). An evaluation of family therapy in anorexia nervosa and bulimia nervosa. *Archives of General Psychiatry,* 44(12), 1047–1056.

Schur, E., Sanders, M., & Steiner, H. (1999). Body dissatisfaction and eating attitudes in young children. *International Journal of Eating Disorders,* 27, 74–82.

Selvini Palazzoli, M. (1974). *Self-starvation: From the intrapsychic to the transpersonal approach.* London: Chaucer.

Shaw, R., & Steiner, H. (1997). Temperament in juvenile eating disorders. *Psychosomatics,* 38, 126–131.

Shore, R., & Porter, J. (1990). Normative and reliability data for 11–18 year olds on the Eating Disorder Inventory. *International Journal of Eating Disorders,* 9, 201–207.

Silverman, J. (1997). Charcot's comments on the therapeutic role of isolation in the treatment of anorexia nervosa. *International Journal of Eating Disorders,* 21, 295–298.

Steiger, H., Gauvin, L., Israel, M., Koerner, N., Ng Ying Kin, N., Paris, J., et al. (2001). Association of serotonin and cortisol indices with childhood abuse in bulimia nervosa. *Archives of General Psychiatry,* 58, 837–843.

Steiner, H., Kwan, W., Walker, S., Miller, S., Sagar, A., & Lock, J. (2003). Risk and protective factors for juvenile eating disorders. *European Child and Adolescent Psychiatry,* 1(12), 38–46.

Steiner, H., & Lock, J. (1998). Anorexia nervosa and bulimia nervosa in children and adolescents: A review of the past 10 years. *Journal of the American Academy of Child and Adolescent Psychiatry,* 37(4), 352–359.

Steiner, H., Lock, J., & Reisel, B. (1999). Apport de l'approche développementale dans la compréhension des troubles des conduites alimentaires. *Prisme,* 30, 52–67.

Steinhausen, H., Rauss-Mason, C., & Seidel, R. (1991). Follow-up studies of anorexia nervosa: A review of four decades of outcome research. *Psychological Medicine,* 21, 447–454.

Steinhausen, H., Rauss-Mason, C., & Seidel, R. (1993). Short-term and intermediate term outcome in adolescent eating disorders. *Acta Psychiatrica Scandinavica,* 88, 169–173.

Stice, E., & Agras, W. S. (1998). Predicting onset and cessation of bulimic behaviors during adolescence. *Behavior Therapy,* 29, 257–276.

Stierlin, H., & Weber, G. (1989). *Unlocking the family door: A systemic approach to the understanding and treatment of anorexia nervosa.* New York: Brunner/Mazel.

Strober, M., Freeman, A., Lampert, C., Diamond, J., & Kaye, W. H. (2000). Controlled family study of anorexia nervosa and bulimia nervosa: evidence of shared liability and transmission of partion syndromes. *American Journal of Psychiatry,* 157, 393–401.

Strober, M., & Humphrey, L. (1987). Family contributions to the etiology and course of anorexia nervosa and bulimia nervosa. *Journal of Consulting and Clinical Psychology,* 55, 654–659.

Strober, M., Morrell, W., Burroughs, J., Salkin, B., & Jacobs, C. (1985). A controlled family study of anorexia nervosa. *Journal of Psychiatric Research,* 19.

Szmukler, G. I., Eisler, I., Russell, G., & Dare, C. (1985). Anorexia nervosa, parental 'expressed emotion' and dropping out of treatment. *British Journal of Psychiatry,* 147, 265–271.

Thienemann, M., & Steiner, H. (1993). Family environment of eating disordered and depressed adolescents. *International Journal of Eating Disorders,* 14, 43–48.

Thoma, H. (1967). *Anorexia nervosa.* New York: International Universities Press.

Treasure, J. L., Todd, G., Brolly, M., Tiller, J., Nehmed, A., & Denman, F. (1995). A pilot study of a randomized trial of cognitive-behavioral analytical therapy vs educational behavioral therapy for adult anorexia nervosa. *Behaviour Research and Therapy, 33*, 363–367.

Turner, H., & Bryant-Waugh, R. (2004). Eating disorder not otherwise specified (EDNOS) profiles of clients presenting at a community eating disorder service. *European Eating Disorders Review, 12*, 18–26.

Waller, J., Kaufman, M., & Deutch, F. (1940). *Evolution of psychosomatic concepts—Anorexia nervosa: A paradigm.* New York: International Universities Press.

Walsh, B. T., & Devlin, M. J. (1995). Pharmacotherapy of bulimia nervosa and binge eating disorder. *Addictive Behaviors, 20*(6), 757–764.

Ward, A., Ramsey, R., Turnbull, S. J., Steele, M., Steele, H., & Treasure, J. L. (2001). Attachment in anorexia nervosa: A transgenerational perspective. *British Journal of Medical Psychology, 74*, 497–505.

Wilson, G. T., & Fairburn, C. G. (2002). Treatments for eating disorders. In P. Nathan & J. Gorman (Eds.), *A guide to treatments that work* (2nd ed., pp. 559–592). New York: Oxford University Press.

Wilson, G. T., Loeb, K. L., Walsh, B. T., Labouvie, E., Petkova, E., Liu, X., & Waternaux, C. (1999). Psychological versus pharmacological treatments of bulimia nervosa: Predictors and process of change. *Journal of Consulting and Clinical Psychology, 67*, 451–459.

Wonderlich, S., Crosby, R., Mitchell, J., Thompson, J., Redlin, J., Demuth, G., et al. (2001). Eating disturbance and sexual trauma in childhood and adulthood. *International Journal of Eating Disorders, 30*, 401–412.

Zipfel, S., Lowe, B., Deter, H. C., & Herzog, W. (2000). Long-term prognosis in anorexia nervosa: Lessons from a 21-year follow-up study. *Lancet, 355*, 721–722.

15

Health and Chronic Illness

Ronald T. Brown
Alexandra Boeving
Angela LaRosa
Laura Arnstein Carpenter

Adolescence is a period of transition with a unique set of developmental challenges. Typically, adolescents experience increasing needs for autonomy within the family system, and peer groups take on greater social significance (Peterson & Leffert, 1995). Peer relationships have been demonstrated to have a significant impact on the psychological adjustment of youth with chronic illnesses (for review, see Schuman & La Greca, 1999; Wolman, Harris, & Blum, 1994). In addition, peer relationships have been demonstrated to be especially critical in disease adaptation as peers may assist adolescents in coping with a chronic illness (Schuman & La Greca, 1999; Wasserstein & La Greca, 1996). Furthermore, as adolescents form beliefs and expectations pertaining to adult roles, health behaviors as well as risk behaviors are formed as well.

This chapter reviews the literature on pertinent health issues as they relate to adolescence. Given the notion that health-related issues encompass both physical health as well as mental health and that psychological adjustment clearly is associated with health outcome

(Brown, Freeman, et al., 2002), the issue of mental health frequently is incorporated under the general area of adolescent health psychology. We incorporate a developmental approach in our discussion of health-related issues, with the underlying framework that adolescence is a period of development in which a number of developmental tasks must be accomplished.

This chapter addresses issues related to chronic illness in adolescence by highlighting key models of adaptation, as well as addressing family systems contributions. We next review developmental demands of adolescence and chronic illness. To accomplish this, we have chosen to review salient issues that adolescents with a chronic illness must negotiate. In our framework, we have chosen four prototypes of chronic disease (i.e., cancer, diabetes, sickle cell disease, and cystic fibrosis) because these are four prevalent chronic diseases among adolescents and present challenging psychosocial issues. We also have outlined particular issues (e.g., adherence to treatment demands, peer relationships, body image, and sexual identity) that adolescents must negotiate in the face of a chronic illness. We next address issues of injury, substance abuse, and sexual activity, given that each of these areas has a profound impact on the health outcome of adolescents. Finally, we present an overview of prevention and intervention efforts that includes promotion of health behaviors in adolescents as well as primary, secondary, and tertiary intervention efforts.

ISSUES RELATED TO CHRONIC ILLNESS IN ADOLESCENCE

Chronic illnesses refer to those medical conditions involving a protracted course that may be fatal or may result in compromised mental or physical functioning and that often are characterized by acute exacerbations that may result in hospitalization or other forms of intensive treatment (Tarnowski & Brown, 2000). Chronically ill adolescents face developmental challenges similar to healthy peers yet also must cope with the illness demands that may frequently be in conflict with the typical developmental tasks of adolescence (Hendry, Shuckswmith, & Philip, 1995). The interface of illness characteristics coupled with the appropriate developmental tasks of adolescence frequently results in distinctive issues that can place significant psychosocial stressors on adolescents with chronic illnesses and their families (Williams, Holmbeck, & Greenley, 2002). Most of these issues are pervasive across illness categories and can be discussed broadly, including adherence to medical regimens, sexuality, body image, and peer group and school concerns, as well as the family systems' contributions to psychosocial adjustment and adaptation to the chronic illness.

Epidemiology

Chronic illness affects approximately 10–20% of adolescents in the United States (Gortmaker, 1985; Newacheck & Halfon, 1975; Thompson & Gustafson, 1996). This figure includes those chronic diseases that are fairly benign and easily managed, such as asthma, as well as those illnesses that have no hope of cure given current state-of-the-art medical science (e.g., sickle cell disease and cystic fibrosis). It must be noted that adolescents have a large number of rare conditions relative to their adult counterparts who evidence a number of small chronic conditions (Thompson & Gustafson, 1996).

Because adolescent chronic conditions are fairly rare, there is significant difficulty in estimating incidence and prevalence of these conditions (Thompson & Gustafson, 1996). A number of studies have revealed asthma to be the most prevalent condition in pediatric populations, while neurological and developmental disabilities and behavior disorders are fairly common. Other chronic conditions at adolescence occur fairly rarely (e.g., chronic renal failure, congenital heart disease, and hemophilia) with prevalence being approximately 1 in 1,000 or even less. While economically disadvantaged adolescents frequently have more severe chronic illnesses, there is little variability in the incidence and prevalence of childhood chronic illnesses across social class and ethnic groups (Thompson & Gustafson, 1996). Variability in specific chronic illnesses across racial or ethnic groups does exist: Chronic diseases such as sickle cell disease affect more African American adolescents, whereas cystic fibrosis affects more individuals who are Caucasian.

Cancer in pediatric populations is slightly albeit steadily increasing according to survey data that have been mounted by the American Cancer Society (Mirro, 2000). Approximately, 19,500 new cases of childhood cancer are diagnosed yearly (occurring with slightly higher frequency in males than females (Centers for Disease Control and Prevention, 1999), with about 11,500 of these cases diagnosed in adolescents. Thus, this incidence rate reflects nearly 14 children per 100,000, with a slightly higher rate in adolescents (Centers for Disease Control and Prevention, 1999). In addition, nearly 151,000 individuals (0.19%) less than 20 years of age have Type I insulin-dependent diabetes mellitus (National Center for Chronic Disease Prevention and Health Promotion, 2000). Approximately 30,000 people in the United States are currently diagnosed with cystic fibrosis (CF), which occurs primarily in individuals of northern European descent (one in 3,200 births). Although far less common, it can be diagnosed in other ethnicities, including African Americans, Native Americans, and Asian Americans (one in 700 births). Approximately 5% of Americans are unaffected carriers of a CF gene, and nearly 2,500 infants are born yearly with CF in the United States. Sickle cell disease occurs in approximately one in every 400 infants born in the United States (approximately 1,000 infants born per year), with the highest incidence rates in peoples of African,

Mediterranean, Turkish, Arabic, and Indian descent (Brown, Mulhern, & Simonian, 2002; Casey & Brown, 2003).

In tandem with these sobering statistics, it should be noted that the significant breakthroughs in medical science have resulted in sustained improvements in the management of many diseases, thereby ensuring survival for many adolescents in this century who in previous years may not have survived their illnesses past childhood. Given the myriad treatment options that are now available for managing chronic diseases during both the pediatric and adult years, appropriate and ongoing management of disease is critical, particularly given the marked increases of life expectancy for many illnesses (William et al., 2002). While concomitant increases in life expectancy have been advanced significantly, concerns pertaining to issues of psychological adjustment and quality of life have become of particular importance at adolescence.

Psychopathology in the Context of Chronic Illness

A plethora of research has been conducted to examine the impact of chronic illness on children's psychosocial functioning. Although there is some discord among findings, the literature broadly reflects little disparity in prevalence of psychopathology between children serving as healthy controls and chronically ill populations (Thompson & Gustafson, 1996). Thompson and Gustafson (1996) have conducted an extensive review of epidemiological studies that have examined the prevalence of psychological adjustment difficulties in children and adolescents with chronic disease. A major problem in attempting to synthesize studies of this type is that different instruments are employed across studies to measure psychological adjustment. However, these studies do indicate that chronically ill children and adolescents are at increased risk for subthreshold symptomatology and behavioral problems across settings (e.g., home and school). Thus, although rates of psychopathology among chronically ill adolescents do not differ markedly from their well peers, there is some evidence to suggest differences in subthreshold symptoms (Thompson & Gustafson, 1996).

In a recent systematic review of children and adolescents diagnosed with cancer, Eiser, Hill, and Vance (2000) found that cancer survivors did not exhibit symptoms of anxiety, depres-

sion, or poor self-esteem relative to matched comparison controls or population norms. In a longitudinal investigation of children and adolescents with sickle cell disease, Thompson and colleagues (2003) prospectively examined behavioral functioning in the context of illness and family functioning variables. Findings revealed that behavior problems were generally within the normative range and did not increase over time but did fluctuate in the context of familial discord. Finally, behavioral problems were more prevalent in those with illness-related complications.

While the prevalence of subthreshold symptomatology is typically higher within chronic illness groups, there is a large degree of individual variation, and it is a minority of ill children who exhibit significant maladjustment (Eiser et al., 2000). As the prevalence of psychopathology is low in this population, it is important to incorporate positive indices of psychosocial outcome (e.g., quality of life) as well as adaptive functional behaviors to determine the adolescent's adaptation to illness. Finally, further attention to the study of individual differences in the process of adjustment is needed to more fully elucidate the risk factors in the development of psychopathology secondary to chronic illness.

MODELS OF ADAPTATION TO CHRONIC ILLNESS

Because adolescents are involved in a number of systems (e.g., families, peer group, and school), it is most reasonable and probably optimal to take a systemic perspective in examining the impact of chronic illness during adolescence. In addition, the challenges of a chronic illness at adolescence and the pathways to successful adjustment and adaptation to a chronic disease occur across biological, psychological, social, educational, and familial domains. For this reason, it is essential to examine adolescent adjustment and adaptation to chronic illness within the context of the adolescents' functioning across a broad array of systems. Several models aim to explain these complex systems and we review them briefly. We devote specific attention to the interpersonal context model (Holmbeck, 2002) as it focuses specifically on adolescence.

The transactional stress and coping model posited by Thompson, Gustafson, Hamlett, and Spock (1992) emphasizes the association between chronic illness and psychological adjustment in the patient as a function of the transactions among biomedical (e.g., severity of disease), developmental (e.g., presence of developmental delays and intellectual functioning), and psychosocial processes (Thompson & Gustafson, 1996). Consistent with the transactional stress and coping model, Wallander and Varni (1995, 1998) have proposed a model that conceptualizes the psychosocial impact of a chronic illness into a risk-and-resistance framework. The most pervasive risk factor associated with any chronic illness includes exposure to stressful events that are both related (e.g., administration of medication, clinic visits, and other daily hassles associated with the disease) and unrelated (major life events, loss of financial resources) to the illness. In an effort to include the role of the family and community systems and subsystems, Patterson (1988) has expanded the stress and coping models reviewed above in the family adjustment and adaptation response (FAAR) model. Specifically, the model differentiates the adjustment of families to the chronic illness based on the demands of the illness, resistance capabilities, and the adaptation of families to endure repeated crises over the course of the chronic illness. An important component of this model is the reciprocal impact of illness on the family and the impact of the family on the illness. Also having its origins in a family systems approach, Rolland (1990) has developed the family systems–illness model for the purpose of guiding the adaptation of individuals with a chronic illness and their families. Specifically, the model posits that a chronic illness results in both threatened and perceived loss for the adolescent who is ill as well as for family members. Although each of these models has been useful in conceptualizing chronic illness for children and adolescents, none of them has been especially useful for adolescent health. For this reason, we focus attention to Holmbeck's model.

Interpersonal Context Model

Specifically with regard to adolescent adaptation and adjustment, Holmbeck and his associates have developed a model that specifically attends to interpersonal contexts as these variables drive developmental outcomes (Holmbeck, 2002). This model provides an excellent exemplar of a systemic focus on adjustment by means of specific attention to the re-

ciprocal relationships among individuals that ultimately create pathways for adjustment. The framework asserts that developmental shifts during the adolescent years have an impact on those individuals who are close to the adolescent, including parents, other caregivers, siblings, and peers, who in turn respond to these developmental changes with specific behaviors that further influence the resolution of the developmental tasks of adolescence (e.g., autonomy, sexuality, and social roles). The model posited by Holmbeck (2002) has particular relevance in the examination of the developmental tasks of adolescence, particularly within the context of a chronic illness. For example, adherence to specific medical regimens may be demanded by the caregivers of an adolescent suffering from a chronic illness, although the adolescent's peer group may negatively sanction or even punish behaviors that are associated with adherence (e.g., restrictions of activities, dietary restrictions, and changes in appearance). Typically, adolescents are developmentally primed to desire autonomy from parental demands and increase peer affiliation. Interventions with adolescents at this developmental stage that require autonomy most appropriately would attempt to balance the social needs of the adolescent coupled with meeting health demands. Meeting the adolescent's need for autonomy from caregivers in one specific arena would be necessary, at the same time increasing the social elements that are attainable by the adolescent in the context of a chronic illness. As Wallander, Eggert, and Gilbert (2003) have astutely observed, most chronic illnesses hinder independence and the adolescent must depend to some extent on either the caregiver or the health care system for the management of his or her illness. Thus, adolescents who suffer from chronic illnesses experience conflict between the desire for autonomy and independence and the need to depend on family members and significant others for illness-related care.

FAMILY SYSTEMS ISSUES

There is now recognition that family systems variables are important predictors for adolescents' adjustment and adaptation to chronic disease (Kazak, Segal-Andrews, & Johnson, 1995). In fact, the models reviewed previously in this chapter (Holmbeck, 2002; Thompson &

Gustafson, 1996) incorporate family functioning as an important domain in the prediction of adolescents' adjustment to a chronic illness. Family relationships can be both a source of support and a stress in the context of a chronic illness, particularly for adolescents. In fact, recent investigations suggest that a primary target of intervention with chronically ill adolescents is the family system whereby positive parenting, reductions of conflict, and conflict resolution may be modeled and taught (Anderson, Brackett, Ho, & Laffel, 2000). In addition, the impact of a chronic illness on an adolescent necessarily influences the adjustment of all family members as well as the entire system. Changes within the family system occur due to the reorganization of family roles, influence on siblings and sibling relationships, and priority shifts in parental attention mandated by the tasks associated with the chronic illness (Anderson & Coyne, 1993; Shannon, 1996). For example, for an adolescent who has just been diagnosed with cancer, the family must reorganize by sharing household chores. Frequently, siblings receive less attention from parents as greater attention is focused on the adolescent with the chronic illness.

The reorganization of the family in response to the stressors associated with an adolescent's chronic illness coupled with the psychological stressors induced by the illness also pose significant stressors on the family system until the system actually reaches a state of homeostasis. In fact, investigations of parental distress in the context of pediatric chronic illness have revealed multiple viable predictors of family stress. Sloper (2000) has provided important data to indicate that for mothers and fathers, appraisal of the strain of the illness together with the reported cohesiveness of the family was an important predictor of distress within the family system. Invasive treatment procedures on the part of the adolescent (Kazak & Barakat, 1997; Kazak, Boyer, et al., 1995), coupled with employment limitations (e.g., not being able to change employment because of a preexisting condition), and financial difficulties resulting from the burden of care (Shannon, 1996; Sloper, 2000) each and collectively contributes to sources of parental distress. Perhaps the most salient parental stressor accompanying a life-threatening adolescent illness is the anxiety and fear associated with the threat of losing one's child (Koocher & O'Malley, 1981).

In summary, family functioning is a vital ingredient to any intervention program with chronically ill adolescents. Intervention with the family and the adolescent must proceed in a developmentally sensitive manner. It is essential to attend to the reciprocity between the adolescent's adjustment and resulting resources for coping as well as those coping resources of the family. Family functioning has consistently been demonstrated to be a strong predictor of the adolescent's psychological adjustment and adaptation to disease (Holden, Chmielewski, Nelson, & Kager, 1997). Moreover, parental coping and adjustment have been demonstrated to have an impact on adolescent coping and adjustment (Frank, Blount, & Brown, 1997; Kupst & Schulman, 1988). Finally, familial functioning also has been associated with adherence to critical treatment regimens as well as appropriate management of disease over the course of time (Miller-Johnson et al., 1994). Specifically, findings across studies have consistently revealed that family cohesion and expressiveness (Varni, Katz, Colegrove, & Dolgin, 1996) reliably predict optimal psychosocial outcomes. Thus these data suggest that chronic illness during adolescence serves as a stressor that clearly has systemic influences in which there are reciprocal effects of parent and child coping and adjustment. The adolescent is a very integral component to this family system and the family influences the adolescent's development in the context of this system.

DEVELOPMENTAL DEMANDS OF ADOLESCENCE AND CHRONIC DISEASE

There is compelling evidence from large-scale epidemiological studies (Cadman, Boyle, Szatmari, & Offord, 1987) and meta-analyses (e.g., Lavigne & Faier-Routman, 1992) to suggest that adolescents who have chronic illnesses are at increased risk for difficulties and problems that have a significant and negative impact on their adjustment (Wallander & Varni, 1998). We next review four chronic illness conditions for the purpose of demonstrating those tasks associated with these various illnesses coupled with the developmental tasks of adolescence. While there are myriad physical diseases from which adolescence may suffer, we have chosen to review four major disease groups (i.e., cancer, Type I insulin-dependent diabetes mellitus, sickle cell disease, and cystic fibrosis) as a prototype because adolescents and their families must negotiate a number of tasks related to these various illnesses, some of which may even impede other general tasks of adolescence. In part, the choice of these diseases for this chapter was based on the data provided by Lavigne and Faier-Routman (1992), in which youth with these chronic illnesses were found to have significant difficulties in adjustment (effect sizes were in the mild to moderate range) relative to healthy controls. In addition, these are the four illness groups for which there is a great deal of research literature pertaining to psychosocial issues and adolescents.

Cancer

Current medical treatments have increased the survival rates of adolescents suffering from various types of cancer (e.g., leukemia, osteosarcoma [cancer of the bone], lymphoma [cancer of the lymph nodes], brain tumors, and other tumors of the central nervous system). Despite the innovative treatments that are now available to manage cancer, these treatments are frequently associated with deleterious adverse side effects, which the medical and psychological communities must address. Along with the obvious physiological impact of the disease, the cancer experience often affects adolescents' emotional functioning (e.g. it causes depression and anxiety), social/educational functioning (frequently inhibited by the adolescent's longterm absence from school), cognitive functioning (frequently impeded when the adolescent is off therapy and begins to suffer from specific nonverbal learning problems as well as attention problems), and family systems functioning.

The adolescent who receives central nervous system (CNS) chemotherapy or radiation therapy (therapies that are frequently administered prophylactically to the brain to prevent cancer cells from infiltrating the CNS) is at less risk for severe cognitive decline than are younger children undergoing similar therapies. Nonetheless, adverse effects of commonly employed CNS chemotherapies and radiation therapy can include impairments in general intellectual and academic functioning (Raymond-Speden, Tripp, Lawrence, & Holdaway, 2000), and specifically in the area of short-term memory, visuomotor coordination, and speed of processing (Cousens, Ungerer, Crawford, & Stevens, 1991; for review, see Brown, Mulhern, & Simonian, 2002; Madan-Swain & Brown, 1991). In addition, childhood cancer survivors frequently sustain cognitive toxicities from the "late effects" of chemotherapy or radiation therapy that sometimes do not appear until adolescence, particularly for females (Brown et al., 1998). Further, for those children or adolescents who have sustained various surgeries for brain tumors, cognitive late effects (defined here as cognitive dysfunction occurring after successful treatment with medical therapy, typically 2 or more years from the time of initial diagnosis) are frequently present and include diminished intellectual functioning, attentional disturbances, and emotional lability. Finally, given the improved prognosis for both children and adolescents who have survived cancer, there is the concern regarding cognitive toxicities, particularly their presence during the late-effects period or after the child or adolescent has been determined to be cured from cancer. When these cognitive toxicities occur at adolescence, there is frequently an interaction with hormones, particularly for adolescent females, thereby designating their cognitive toxicities as clinically significant (Brown et al., 1998). Adolescent females who were diagnosed during early childhood (prior to the age of 4 or 5 years) who have had either chemotherapy or radiation therapy are deemed to be at highest risk for these cognitive late effects (for review, see Brown, Mulhern, & Simonian, 2002).

It should be noted that chronic diseases that also are associated with cognitive impairments pose significant challenges to adolescents' social adjustment and social relationships (for review, see Schuman & La Greca, 1999; Nassau & Drotar, 1997). The reason is attributed to cognitive impairments such as intellectual limitations that may limit social understanding, thereby adversely affecting peer relations. In addition, peer relationships may be limited for adolescents who must attend special programs during the day such as special education classrooms or rehabilitation programs (Schuman & La Greca, 1999).

Further, treatment for various types of cancers that occur at adolescence can often render adverse effects that are of significant concern to the adolescent, such as changes in appearance. It also has been noted that alterations in physical appearance place adolescents with a chronic disease at particular risk for social difficulties (for review, see Schuman & La Greca, 1999). Wasserman, Thompson, Wilimas, and Fairclough (1987) found that nearly one-half of the adolescent and adult survivors of Hodgkin's disease reported unpleasant experiences with classmates, including peer taunting because of their baldness as well as peers avoiding them because of the fear of becoming contagious. For adolescents, who are often acutely sensitive to physical appearance, the social consequences of altered physical appearance due to a chronic illness may be especially acute. In particular, adolescent females with a chronic illness who must endure treatments that result in hair loss, weight gain, or unwelcome facial changes are most apt to resist such therapies thereby making adherence a particular risk factor for this particular population (for review, see Schuman & La Greca, 1999).

The cancer experience may spur social concerns in various areas that may be particularly anxiety producing for adolescents, including peer group response and dating. Adolescents are particularly sensitive to peer group acceptance and rejection, and illness-related variables might contribute greater stressors in these relationships. In addition, as with other chronic diseases that may be present at adolescence (e.g., HIV), dating can be a special challenge at adolescence due to the level of disclosure that adolescents are comfortable with including the specific illness and its associated treatment (Donohoe, 2000).

Sexuality is another salient component of adolescent development in which the impact of the cancer experience and its treatment can be extremely challenging. First, pubertal development can be delayed and ultimately growth curves may taper. Reductions in fertility also can be a concern. Many forms of cancer treatment affect the sex organs as well as the brain in a manner that may result in ovarian failure or low testosterone or sperm production (Crom, Cremer, & Hudson, 2000). It is quite emotionally challenging for an adolescent with developing sexuality to grapple with those concerns of pubertal delay and potential infertility later in life.

Psychosocial interventions should target the emotional sequelae of these treatment effects for adolescents with cancer by means of symptom reduction and coping therapies that emphasize active coping, as well as careful attention to familial functioning as a contributor to adolescent physical and mental health. In addi-

tion, it is of critical importance to attend to the social needs of adolescents with cancer, and for this reason, most pediatric facilities that serve adolescents with cancer have a full array of social and psychological services that are available to the adolescent and the family. In fact, psychological services are considered to be a standard of care in treating children and adolescents during the treatment phase of cancer as well as during the late-effects period. Encouraging social contact with friends is important for the purpose of maintaining peer group continuity for the adolescent. In addition, there has been some research to demonstrate that peer support is critical to adolescent management of the chronic illness (for review, see Schuman & La Greca, 1999). Furthermore, obtaining social support for the adolescent with other youth who are currently in treatment for cancer or who in fact are cancer survivors may be particularly beneficial in terms of increasing hope for survival and having a specific peer group support. Clearly, the impact of peer support for children with cancer needs careful and systematic study. Camps for children and adolescents with cancer often target social support needs as do peer support groups and child life programs that are located in many pediatric cancer centers.

Finally, it also is important for adolescents who are recovering from cancer to develop healthy lifestyle habits. Cancer survivors are at increased risk for developing secondary malignancies and also may suffer from many late effects associated with the cancer experience that also affect physical health (Tyc, 2000). Many health behaviors, including those that are both positive and risky, are introduced and formed during the adolescent years, rendering adolescence a particularly appropriate developmental time for intervention programs that target healthy lifestyles (Williams et al., 2002). Interventions targeting smoking prevention and cessation, skin cancer prevention (sunscreen protection), healthy eating habits, and regular exercise are beneficial to all adolescents but may be especially beneficial to adolescent cancer survivors.

Type I Insulin-Dependent Diabetes Mellitus

As noted throughout this chapter, adolescence poses significant developmental challenges to coping with a chronic illness. These challenges include heightened needs for autonomy, increased motivation to assimilate into peer groups, and biological changes such as hormonal fluctuations (Rovet & Fernandes, 1999). One task associated with many chronic diseases is adherence to treatment regimens. We have chosen Type I insulin-dependent diabetes mellitus to illustrate the issue of adherence because there is an abundance of research on this issue with adolescents. Frequently, diabetes is diagnosed at adolescence, so this poses particular challenges with regard to treatment adherence.

Adherence to treatment demands is of paramount concern for adolescents with Type 1 diabetes (i.e., diabetes that typically has an onset in childhood, is not due to obesity, and must be controlled with insulin). There is no doubt that there are serious ramifications for the adolescent who does not maintain treatment adherence, and a number of secondary medical conditions can result from ongoing poor adherence or poor diabetes control (Johnson, 1995). Diabetes management includes a number of behavioral demands such as special dietary control, a routine exercise program, glucose monitoring, and an ongoing regimen of insulin. These demands typically require modifications in the environments of these youth. Further, peer and family support and involvement are critical in sustaining adequate adherence to diet, exercise, and insulin administration (Pendley et al., 2002). In fact, increasing attention has been devoted to the development of social support because this variable is thought to influence adherence to the diabetes regimen. In addition, greater attention has been devoted to specific assessment of social support for adolescents with diabetes (Bearman & La Greca, 2002), and several studies have been conducted to investigate the impact of social support of the family environment on adherence behaviors (Hanson, Henggeler, Harris, Burghen, & Moore, 1989; Hauser et al., 1990; Johnson, 1995). In fact, family support (i.e., commitment by each of the family members including the adolescent with diabetes) has been demonstrated to be especially predictive of patient adherence (Hauser et al., 1990).

Recent research has also focused on peer support among adolescents with diabetes (Bearman & La Greca, 2002; La Greca & Thompson, 1998; Schuman & La Greca, 1999), indicating that adolescents perceive their friends as providing greater support than their families for "feeling good about diabetes"

(for review, see Schuman & La Greca, 1999). Thus, adolescents with diabetes view their friends as providing significant support for dietary and exercise aspects of diabetes care (La Greca et al., 1995). In fact, findings with ethnic minority youth (Thompson, La Greca, & Shaw, 1997) have provided compelling support to indicate that African American adolescents with diabetes who reported high levels of peer support for dietary adherence, insulin administration, and exercise regimens had significantly better levels of metabolic control than their counterparts without such peer support. Family support for diabetes care among these African American adolescents was unrelated to metabolic control. Bearman and La Greca (2002) also have found friendship support to be associated with adherence for blood glucose testing. Schroff-Pendley and colleagues (2002), in their careful study of both children and adolescents with Type I diabetes, found that adolescents perceived greater diabetes-related peer support than did school-age children. They interpret their findings to suggest a developmental shift in perceptions of peer support.

This review of the literature has indicated that peers also may serve as protective factors for providing support for ongoing disease management. Given the important influences of the peer group on disease adaptation and management, greater research efforts are needed in this area. In addition, peers also may serve as risk factors for poor disease management, particularly for those youth with strong conformity needs who may resist the daily tasks associated with diabetes disease management. As Schuman and La Greca (1999) have noted, what is especially needed is research that goes beyond correlational designs to examine specifically the bidirectional influence of disease on peer relationships and the influence of peers on adolescents' adaptation to disease. Both experimental intervention studies as well as longitudinal designs will be necessary to address this next stage of research.

Of particular concern for adolescent females with Type I diabetes is disordered eating behavior. In fact, some adolescent females use insulin dsyregulation as a means of exerting control on weight, which can result in serious detrimental health outcomes (Williams et al., 2002). Clearly, this is an issue that demonstrates the developmental conflict between the adolescent's striving for peer acceptance and conformity (e.g., consuming the same foods as one's peers) and physical desirability (e.g., maintaining a low weight) and, at the same time, promoting health. Needs for autonomy from the family must be balanced with strict needs for dietary control and administration of insulin, which can be life-threatening if the adolescent fails to adhere to the treatment regimen. In addition, eating disorders are of primary concern for any adolescent female population and should be addressed with females with diabetes due to potential deleterious physiological ramifications.

Intervention and prevention programs for adolescents with Type I diabetes must be developmentally sensitive, particularly when targeting the adolescent age group. Investigators have demonstrated that the initial diagnosis and the beginning intensive treatment for Type I diabetes during early adolescence predicts school dissatisfaction, whereas the initial diagnosis made during later adolescence and its associated management is related to psychological adjustment difficulties (Madsen, Roisman, & Collins, 2002). For this reason, it is imperative that pediatric psychologists attend to developmental concerns when developing treatment goals for managing diabetes.

Sickle Cell Disease

Sickle cell disease is characterized by chronic anemia and significant delays in physical development. The symptoms become more evident as the child grows older, with marked delays in physical development becoming increasingly more pronounced, particularly at adolescence (Brown, Mulhern, & Simonian, 2002; Casey & Brown, 2003). As sickled (malformed) red blood cells begin to obstruct blood vessels and disrupt blood flow, a myriad of medical complications result (for review, see Brown, Mulhern, & Simonian, 2002; Casey & Brown, 2003). Symptoms may include debilitating pain episodes, cerebral vascular accidents (strokes), anemia, vaso-occlusion, major organ failure, leg ulceration, and priapism (the sustained painful erection of the penis). In addition to the physical pain and discomfort associated with priapism, this symptom is often embarrassing and not easily discussed, particularly for adolescent males who are adjusting to their own sexuality. Priapism among adolescent males may contribute to feelings of inadequacy and concerns about sexual dysfunction (Casey & Brown, in press).

Studies of adolescents with sickle cell disease have revealed that they frequently exhibit poor self-esteem and difficulties with body image relative to comparison controls (Morgan & Jackson, 1986). A chronic illness that is present from infancy and persists over the lifespan clearly disrupts social and academic functioning, which in turn impact perceived competence, self-esteem, and body image. Moreover, adolescents with sickle cell disease report less satisfaction with their bodies and spend less time in social activities with peers (for review, see Brown, Mulhern, & Simonian, 2002; Casey & Brown, 2003). These findings in part are attributable to the small body sizes of these youth coupled with their fragility, which clearly limits participation in physical activities including sports.

Females with sickle cell disease have reported greater concerns about sexual development than their male counterparts (Hurtig & Park, 1989), which in turn may be associated with findings of dissatisfaction with body image (for review, see Brown, Doepke, & Kaslow, 1993; Brown, Mulhern, & Simonian, 2002; Casey & Brown, 2003). Thompson, Gil, Burbach, Keith, and Kinney (1993) have noted an increase in disruptive behavior in adolescent boys. These behaviors have been associated as resulting from delayed physical growth. On a related note, Adedoyin (1992) also has found that adolescent males with sickle cell disease exhibit a perceived inability to engage in age appropriate activities, including sports. This may further increase poor competence and feelings of inadequacy. In fact, it has been suggested that school personnel and peers may exclude adolescents from activities in which they are able to participate due to erroneous assumptions about the disease and its physical restrictions (Schuman & La Greca, 1999). Clearly, there is consensus in the literature that adolescents with sickle cell disease relative to healthy controls have greater withdrawal and social skills deficits, some of which may be due to limitations in physical activity that diminish the adolescent's opportunity for peer interaction.

There is some recent evidence that health service utilization among adolescents with sickle cell disease is associated with disease severity as well as parent characteristics (Logan, Radcliffe, & Smith-Whitley, 2002). Logan and associates examined the relationships among parent characteristics (i.e., the parent–adolescent relationship, parents' knowledge of illness, and parents' perceptions of illness-related burden) and the use of routine and urgent health care services among adolescents with sickle cell disease suffering from pain. Findings reveal that after controlling for disease severity and life events, parents' perceptions of more illness-related stress was the most viable predictor of the use of both routine and urgent health care services. In addition, greater knowledge about sickle cell disease also predicted higher frequency of service utilization. Finally, disease severity was strongly associated with urgent service utilization. Based on their data, Logan and colleagues (2002) conclude that enhancing various aspects of parental functioning may aid families in making adaptive decisions regarding health care utilization for pain management in adolescents with sickle cell disease.

Cystic Fibrosis

CF has the highest incidence rate among the autosomal recessive disorders in the Caucasian population (Boat, Welsh, & Beaudet, 1989). CF affects the respiratory and gastrointestinal system. The lungs of these patients develop thick mucous secretions that result in poor airway clearance, frequent lung infections, and chronic inflammation (Quittner, Modi, & Roux, 2003). Adolescents with CF also experience malabsorption, digestive difficulties, and, as a result, poor growth and physical development. Thus, they must consume more calories than their healthy peers. With recent medical advancements, survival rates for this lifelong disease have been steadily increasing so that these individuals have a life expectancy well into early and middle adulthood. This lengthened life expectancy brings up important issues during adolescence that were not apparent in years past due to earlier mortality rates that were associated with cystic fibrosis.

Cystic fibrosis frequently progresses from mild to moderate severity in childhood and becomes much more severe in adolescence and young adulthood (for review, see Quittner et al., 2003). Physical manifestations of the disease become more apparent as the individual ages, and adolescents frequently experience pulmonary exacerbations thereby requiring lengthy and more frequent hospitalizations. Many adolescents begin to view their treatment regimens, which often increase in intensity at adolescence, as interfering with their autonomy

and social activities. Psychological adjustment difficulties tend to increase among adolescents with CF relative to their younger peers. For example, Pearson, Pumariega, and Seilheimer (1991) have provided important data to suggest an increase in symptoms of depression among teenagers with CF relative to their younger counterparts. Similarly, Sawyer, Rosier, Phelan, and Bowes (1998) noted that female adolescents with CF were less well adjusted than their healthy peers. With regard to physical appearance, Zeltzer, Kellerman, Ellenberg, Dash, and Rigler (1980) also found that the adolescent females with CF were especially concerned with the impact of the disease on their physical appearance. However, males have greater concerns with regard to below-average body weight than their female counterparts (Quittner et al., 2003).

D'Auria, Christian, Henderson, and Haynes (2000) interviewed 15 teenagers with CF to understand issues related to peer socialization and found that greater illness severity is associated with placing limits on social activities. In addition, adolescents who had prolonged absences from school felt left out of peer relationships. Friendships have been endorsed by these adolescents as significant sources of emotional support (Graetz, Shute, & Sawyer, 2000). Another issue for adolescents in negotiating the stressors associated with CF includes reluctance to disclose the diagnosis to friends (for review, see Quittner et al., 2003).

Similar to other chronic illnesses in adolescents, peer relationships significantly affect the disease management of adolescents with CF. Christian and D'Auria (1997) have noted that adolescents with cystic fibrosis have reported not adhering to prescribed medication schedules simply because they did not want to be viewed as being different from their peers or risk the loss of a romantic relationship. Qualitative reports have revealed that when going out on dates, adolescents made overt decisions to skip medications or to take several doses of medication upon returning home. Interestingly, those youth who reported friendships characterized by acceptance, validation, and social support also reported a reduction in the need to hide treatment demands associated with their disease (Christian & D'Auria, 1997).

As with other chronic illnesses, family issues also assume prominence for adolescents who suffer from CF. Due to adherence concerns with this population, parents frequently experience difficulties relinquishing medication management to the adolescent (DiGirolamo, Quittner, Ackerman, & Stevens, 1997). Variables that have been demonstrated to be associated with adherence among adolescents with CF include age of the patient, with adherence to dietary recommendations declining as a function of age. Specifically, adolescents with CF have been found to have the lowest rates of adherence (for review, see Quittner et al., 2003).

At adolescence, youth gain greater independence in managing their illness and parental roles in the management of illness demands typically decrease. This transition pertaining to self-management is an especially important issue in young adulthood. Thus, it is important for health care professionals to recognize this transition and begin to work with the family and the adolescent to facilitate the adolescent's self-management of the disease.

Medical and psychological health care providers must attend to important issues of quality of life with regard to sexuality for these youth. A key characteristic of CF is heritability, and thus adolescents must be educated regarding the genetic implications of reproduction as well as safe sex practices (Boylard, 2001). For example, adult women with CF have reported that during puberty they experienced high levels of anxiety with regard to sexuality, delayed pubertal onset, reproduction, and premature death (Johannesson, Carlson, Brucefors, & Hjelte, 1998). Thus, CF is a disease that may impede the typical course of adolescent sexual development.

Unfortunately, few intervention programs for adolescents with CF have been empirically evaluated. A recent multisite clinical trial intervention involving adolescents participating in three arms (i.e., standard medical care, family learning, and behavioral family systems therapy) involving 10 sessions is currently underway and promises to yield important data pertaining to the efficacy of a family-based intervention for adolescents with CF (for review, see Quittner et al., 2003). The promise of such an intervention for adolescents with diabetes and eating disorders (Robin & Siegel, 1999; Wysocki, Harris, & Greco, 2000) suggests its potential in managing some of the family issues associated with adolescents with CF and their families.

In summary, adolescence is a developmental period during which chronic illness poses

unique demands. Salient themes that emerge include needs for autonomy, adherence to complicated treatment demands, issues of sexuality, peer conformity, and the general stressors associated with any chronic illness. Specific demands and developmental conflicts have been highlighted through the various examples of illnesses that we have chosen for the purpose of illustrating the state of the art on research related to issues of adherence, the peer group, family systems issues, autonomy, sexuality, body image, and general psychosocial adjustment.

HEALTH-COMPROMISING BEHAVIORS
Unintentional and Intentional Injuries

Unintentional injury and homicide account for 60% of all deaths among preteens and adolescents and are the leading cause of death among 15- to 19-year-olds. Homicide (considered to be an intentional injury resulting from violence) increased 172% from 1985 to 1994 (Fox, 1996). Firearms have been a major cause in the rise of violence and have recently become the leading cause of death (Murray, Guerra, & Williams, 1997). Specific characteristics of schools have been associated with high delinquency rates that include violence. These characteristics include large school size, absence of individual attention for students, ability grouping and negative labeling, low teacher expectations, lack of structure, and inconsistent treatment by school staff (Dryfoos, 1990). Studies have shown that improvements in school climates are associated with significant decreases in delinquency and violence (for review, see Fuemmeler, 2003).

Unintentional injury also is a pervasive threat to the health of adolescents. Findings have generally suggested that a number of variables associated with unintentional injury are under the control of adolescents and risks for unintentional injury may be diminished by way of increasing skills that promote health-enhancing behaviors (e.g., anger management skills) and reducing health-compromising behaviors (e.g., driving after drinking). Wallander and colleagues (2003) have underscored the notion of schools being involved in prevention efforts for adolescents. Nonetheless, as Wallander and colleagues have concluded, there is a dearth of studies that have effective school-based programs for preventing injury, and this remains an important area for future investigation.

Substance Abuse and Dependence

Teenagers are naturally curious and, for many, substance experimentation is part of the typical adolescent experience. Specifically, tobacco, alcohol, and marijuana are the most commonly used substances among adolescents (Young et al., 2002). However, for a subset of teenagers, adolescent substance experimentation sets the stage for lifelong problems with abuse and dependence. Substance abuse refers to a maladaptive pattern of substance use resulting in clinically significant impairment or distress while substance dependence refers to a maladaptive pattern of use accompanied by symptoms of tolerance or withdrawal. Frequently, the first symptoms of abuse and dependence occur at adolescence. By the age of 18 years, over one-fourth of teenagers meet criteria for abuse and 21.5% meet criteria for dependence of some substance including tobacco, alcohol, marijuana, or other drug substance (Young et al., 2002).

Ongoing alcohol and illicit drug use has been demonstrated to adversely influence many of the vital organ systems in the human body throughout the lifespan, including the brain, stomach, pancreas, and kidneys, and for this reason it has a deleterious impact on health (Wallander et al., 2003). For example, lung cancer from tobacco use is a leading cause of death in this country and also is associated with cardiovascular disease. This is an important area to examine at adolescence because it has been well established that the majority of adult smokers initiated this behavior in adolescence (Chassin, Presson, Sherman, & Edwards, 1990).

The impact of substance abuse on physical health is substantial. Among adults, prolonged drug and alcohol use has been associated with a host of health problems, including cognitive dysfunction, unintentional injury, organ disease, and cancer, to name but just a few. Similar to data regarding adult substance abuse, adolescent substance abuse also has been linked to poor health outcomes. In the short term, among many, these poor outcomes include weigh loss, eczema, headaches, sexually transmitted diseases (STDs), and unintentional injuries. In a 5-year prospective study of adolescents who did and did not receive treatment for substance abuse, Aarons and colleagues (1999) demonstrated that substance abuse severe enough to require treatment resulted in a greater frequency of health problems and that protracted substance abuse was associated with more severe health problems. Further, these investigators demonstrated that early-onset substance abuse is linked to poor health outcomes in late adolescence and early adulthood (Aarons et al., 1999). In addition, the substance abuse can be a risk factor for suicidal behavior in adolescents (Blau & Gullotta, 1996). In fact, of those adolescents who commit suicide, 70% also have been found to abuse alcohol or drugs (Blau & Gullotta, 1996).

Long-term tobacco use has also been associated with very serious health outcomes such as lung cancer and emphysema. The vast majority of smokers first began smoking during adolescence. Although tobacco use among adolescents has been declining since the mid-1990s, a recent study of more than 3,000 adolescents by Young and colleagues (2002) reveals that nearly half of all adolescents have used tobacco. This figure ranges from 8.6% of 12-year-olds to 68% of 17-year-olds. Among 18-year-olds, 16.9% met criteria for nicotine dependence. Interestingly, although many adolescents (and adults) believe that smoking controls weight, in a systematic study of this association among almost 7,000 seventh graders, body mass index (BMI) was positively associated with smoking (Kleges, Robinson, & Zbikowski, 1998). In other words, the smokers had, on average, a higher BMI than the nonsmokers. It is not yet clear whether heavier adolescents are more likely to smoke or whether smoking actually leads to increased BMI.

In addition to creating significant health problems, adolescent substance abuse also impacts morbidity and mortality rates because it is associated with accidental injury, violence, STDs, depression, and suicide (Gruber, Di Clemente, Anderson, & Loidico, 1996). For example, binge drinking during adolescence was associated with more sex partners and less consistent use of condom use at age the age of 21 years (Guo et al., 2002). Similarly, teenagers in substance abuse treatment report a host of sexual risk factors including more partners, less consistent condom use, and more STDs (Tapert, Aarons, Sedlar, & Brown, 2001).

In summary, adolescent substance use and abuse is a serious problem with both short- and long-term health consequences. In the short term, adolescents who abuse substance are more likely to abuse other substances and to suffer adverse health outcomes. In the long term, these adolescents are more likely to become adult substance abusers and to experience associated health risks, occupational problems, and social problems.

Sexual Activity

Sexuality is an integral part of adolescence. Interestingly, teenage sexuality has the conflicted role of being both a normal developmental milestone and a risky, health compromising behavior (Hassan & Creatsas, 2000). The majority of both men and women initiate sexual activity sometime during adolescence. According to the most recent data from the Centers for Disease Control's Youth Risk Behavior Surveillance (Grunbaum et al., 2002), 60% of seniors in high school have reported having had sexual intercourse. Teenagers who become sexually active at a younger age have a greater lifetime number of sexual partners (for review, see Wallander et al., 2003). The health risks of early initiation of sexual activity include STDs, increased risk of cervical cancer, pelvic inflammatory disease, and unplanned pregnancy (for review, see Wallander et al., 2003). The two most obvious health risks of sexual activity are unintended pregnancy and STDs. These two issues are discussed subsequently.

Adolescent Pregnancy

In 1997, the overall teenage pregnancy rate was 91 per 1,000 (Elford & Spence, 2002). Among high school students, almost 5% reported that they had been pregnant or had gotten someone else pregnant (Grunbaum et al., 2002). Compared to women who deliver as adults, women who deliver babies when they are teenagers are more likely to be African American, more likely to be single mothers, and more likely to be diagnosed with an STD (Eure, Lindsay, & Graves, 2002). Teenage pregnancy is associated with significant health risks for both mother and baby. Girls who give birth as teenagers are more likely to experience complications during pregnancy or delivery and to deliver babies with more health problems (Elford & Spence, 2002). Pregnant teenagers frequently do not present for prenatal care until late in pregnancy and as a result receive less prenatal care than do adult mothers

(Elford & Spence, 2002). Younger adolescents who give birth also are at greater risk for complications such as preeclampsia, eclampsia, and preterm delivery (Eure et al., 2002). Moreover, babies born to young adolescent mothers are more likely to be low birthweight (Eure et al., 2002). It also is well documented that low-birthweight babies are at greater risk for developmental problems, including cognitive impairments, developmental delays, and significant health problems.

In addition to medical risks, teenage pregnancy is associated with a host of other difficulties. Among teenagers who give birth, about 90% keep their babies (Elford & Spence, 2002). Being a teenage mother also is associated with social, educational, and economic difficulties. For example, adolescent mothers are more likely to drop out of high school prematurely, to be unmarried, and to be welfare dependent (Elford & Spence, 2002).

Sexually Transmitted Diseases

STD rates tend to be higher among adolescents than among adults, and sexual activity among adolescents puts them at greater risk for pregnancy and STDs. Multiple sexual partners and failure to use condoms are two commonly identified causes for this state of affairs. In addition, certain physiological factors make female adolescents more susceptible to STD infection, including a more prominent exocervix and more frequent retrograde menstruation (Elford & Spence, 2002).

STDs can have serious consequences for reproductive health in teenage girls, including genital cancer, infertility, and ectopic pregnancy (Hassan & Creatsas, 2000). One in ten sexually active females between the ages of 15 and 19 years are believed to be positive for chlamydia (Elford & Spence, 2002). STDs are a health risk to all sexually active teenagers, including males. However, when reproductive health services are available to adolescents they are often available to females only. Although almost three-quarters of adolescent males receive annual physical exams, only 39% receive STD testing or discuss reproductive health with a medical professional (Porter & Ku, 2000). Importantly, the best predictor of an STD infection among adolescents is a past STD infection (Crosby, Leichliter, & Brackbill, 2000). Therefore, programs aimed at prevention among this high-risk group are especially imperative.

Currently, the STD receiving the most media attention is human immunodeficiency virus (HIV). Nationwide, an impressive 89% of students reported being taught in school about acquired immunodeficiency syndrome (AIDS) or HIV infection (Grunbaum et al., 2002). HIV is considered to be a dramatic national public health threat because of the lack of a vaccine or cure and the high risk of eventual death for complications associated with AIDS. Adolescents who are diagnosed with HIV are a particularly high-risk group. In one study, 40% of HIV-positive female adolescents became pregnant after being diagnosed with HIV and over one-third of HIV-positive males and females were later diagnosed with another STD post-HIV diagnosis (Fanburg, Amari, & D'Angelo, 1997). These data clearly indicate that teenagers who acquire HIV may continue to engage in unprotected sexual activity, putting themselves and others at additional risk.

In summary, adolescents are engaging in sexual activity at increasingly early ages. Risky sexual behavior can result in unintended pregnancy and serious health problems. Condom use is the most important tool in STD and pregnancy prevention among sexually active adolescents. However, among sexually active high school students, slightly less than 60% report using a condom during their last sexual experience (Grunbaum et al., 2002). Still, promising data from the Centers for Disease Control's Youth Risk Behavior Surveillance Project suggest that about 85% of teenagers either are not sexually active or are engaging in responsible sexual behavior (i.e., condom use) (Grunbaum et al., 2002). Clearly, adolescent gynecology and obstetrics is associated with a host of legal and psychosocial issues. Therefore, it is important that professionals working with adolescents receive specialty training in pediatric and adolescent gynecology (Creatsas, 1995).

PREVENTION AND INTERVENTION EFFORTS

Promotion of Health Behaviors

Intervention programs for adolescents offer unique opportunities to invest in the health outcomes of adolescents. It should be noted that the most serious and frequent adolescent health problems (i.e., substance abuse, STDs, unintended pregnancy, motor vehicle injuries, and unintentional injuries) are potentially preventable (Brindis, Park, & Ozer, 2002). Early intervention and health promotion activities, including anticipatory guidance, screening, education, counseling, and treatment, may lead to lifelong changes in behavior. Interestingly, it has been suggested that the health of adolescents in this country is more likely to be threatened by social (e.g., homicide and suicide) and behavioral factors (e.g., smoking and eating foods high in fat) than by naturally occurring disease or illness (Fuemmeler, 2003).

Over the last 25 years, the causes of adolescent mortality and morbidity have changed considerably. Previously infectious diseases and cancers led to the majority of deaths in this country (Blum, 1987). In recent years, however, 72% of all deaths among school-age children and adolescents were due to motor vehicle crashes, other intentional injuries, homicide, and suicide, with a large proportion related to alcohol and drug use (Elster & Levenberg, 1997). In recent years, we also are faced with new challenges in adolescent health. More adolescents now than in previous years are involved in behaviors that threaten their health and they engage in multiple health risk behaviors at an earlier age (Gans, Blyth, & Elster, 1990). Finally, despite their socioeconomic status, gender, or race, all adolescents are at risk for involvement in health-risk-taking behaviors that can lead to poor health outcomes (Gans et al., 1990).

Seven categories of risk-taking behaviors account for 70% of adolescent mortality. These include drug and alcohol abuse, unsafe sexual activity, violence, injury-related behavior, tobacco use, inadequate physical activity, and poor dietary habits (Kann, Warren, & Harris, 1998; Park, Mac Donald, & Ozer, 2001). Health promotion targeted at adolescents in order to prevent future risk-taking behaviors can be provided through primary care health care encounters and school and community programs.

Clinic-Based Interventions

To address adolescent risk-taking behaviors in clinical health settings, several national organizations over the last decade have developed practice guidelines to support prevention efforts for adolescents. In 1992, the American Medical Association issued a set of comprehensive recommendations referred to as *Guidelines for Adolescent Preventive Services* (GAPS). The purpose of GAPS is to assist providers and health care administrators to organize the content and administration of preventive services in primary care settings (Elster & Kuznets, 1993). In 1994, the Maternal and Child Health Bureau released *Bright Futures: Guidelines for Health Supervision of Infants, Children and Adolescents* (Green, 1995). *Bright Futures* focuses on family and environmental factors that influence development. These practice guidelines recommend annual preventive visits to primary care providers in order to reinforce health promotion messages, to conduct early screening for the purpose of identifying at-risk adolescents, and to provide counseling and education. Thus far there has been some limited evidence that these guidelines are effective. Winter and Breckenmaker (1991) report that adolescent females who received comprehensive, developmentally appropriate reproductive health counseling improved their adherence to contraceptive regimens. Chan and Witherspoon (1988) demonstrated that initiation of alcohol and cigarette use was less frequent in adolescents who received counseling on these specific topics. Although these studies are promising, more research is needed to better determine the long-term benefits of early clinical intervention services. However, early data suggest that health promotion services administered in clinic settings provide a unique opportunity for personalized interaction, private screening and targeted intervention.

School-Based Interventions

A significant barrier to the effective use of clinic-based early interventions is access to providers by adolescents. Caregivers usually arrange appointments and transportation, and adolescent concerns over confidentiality play a critical role. As a result, the most promising area in which to target the largest number of adolescents for intervention services is through the school system. Nearly all adolescents in this country are enrolled in school (Kann, Warren, Harris & Collins, 1995), and promotion of health in the school setting is accomplished through various means, some of which include the use of intervention in the classroom setting, comprehensive school health education, and school-based health clinics (Reynolds, Paas, & Galvin, 1999).

The Centers for Disease Control and Prevention (CDC) have developed guidelines for comprehensive school health promotion. These guidelines include developing school health policy and environmental changes (i.e., tobacco-free schools), providing health curriculum and education to students, providing teachers and staff with training in health promotion, coordinating efforts with departments of food services and school health clinics, sharing the health promotion messages with families of adolescents and the community, and evaluation of the program. Unfortunately many schools have not met the guidelines addressed by the CDC. For example, although 70% of states, districts and schools require health promotion and physical education, less than 10% of schools provide daily physical activities (Burgeson, Wechsler, & Brener, 2001).

School-based health clinics provide another opportunity to address health promotion for adolescents. School-based health clinics are unique in their accessibility as they are located directly within the school setting. These clinics often provide routine medical care for adolescents, particularly in communities in which adolescents may lack access to health care services in large part due to poor finances and lack of insurance (U.S. Congress Office of Technology Assessment, 1994). Previous research has demonstrated that school-based health clinics can improve academic performance and decrease absentee rates (McCord, Klein, Foy, & Feathergill, 1993) and at the same time decrease emergency room visits for the purpose of seeking primary health care services (Dryfoos, Brindis, & Kaplan, 1996). Despite the positive impact of such programs for providing access to health care, as of yet, there has been little evidence to demonstrate their impact on the reduction of risk-taking behaviors among adolescents.

Community-Based Interventions

Curriculum-based interventions also have included efforts to change community and environmental norms (Flay, Miller, & Hedeker, 1995; Flynn, Worden, Secker-Walker, & Badger, 1992). Community education programs are typically implemented through media campaigns. Although there have been a dearth of studies that have evaluated such community efforts, two investigations focusing on community campaigns for the purpose of reducing tobacco consumption among adolescents (Flynn et al., 1992) and increasing the use of seat belts (Wojitiwicz, Peveler, & Eddy,

1992) have demonstrated efficacy. In addition to the development of health curricula, school-based health services and health-promoting environments include the development of health policy, community partnerships, healthy food services, counseling services, and physical education and also offer health promotion for staff and faculty (Allensworth & Kolbe, 1987). Health promotion for adolescents is a challenge and is typically best accomplished with support from various prevention initiatives. Clinical preventive services through primary care physicians and school-based clinics should complement and reinforce prevention efforts in the schools (i.e., comprehensive school health programs) and communities (i.e., mass media campaigns) (Elster & Levenberg, 1997).

Primary Prevention

The goal of primary prevention is to alter risk factors prior to the onset of disease, thereby preventing disease onset or decreasing the severity of disease burden. Due to the greater emphasis of peer relationships during adolescence and the high percentage of adolescents who attend school, the school environment would seem to be the main site for primary prevention intervention efforts.

Four theoretical approaches have been used to guide the development of school-based curriculum intervention programs. These include the rational, social reinforcement, social norms, and developmental approaches (Rundell & Bruvold, 1998). The rational approach involves the use of factual information in a didactic format, which has been demonstrated to enhance adolescents' knowledge. However, similar to other didactic programs, it has not shown significant change in behaviors (for review, see Fuemmeler, 2003). The social reinforcement approach is based on the use of modeling negative outcomes of the risk-taking behavior and simultaneously role modeling positive outcomes of not engaging in risk-taking behavior. The social norms approach involves creating social groups with desirable social norms or attempting to alter social norms through communication and role modeling. The developmental approach emphasizes improving self-esteem among adolescents, developing plans for achieving future goals, and integrating adolescents into supportive social networks (Braucht, Brakarsh, & Follingstad, 1973). The most successful curriculum-based interventions include theoretically based curricula, engaging social systems (i.e., parents and peers), and/or efforts to change community or environmental norms (Reynolds et al., 1999). These curricula provide activities that disseminate accurate information about the consequences of health-compromising or risk-taking behaviors, attempt to change attitudes, increase self-efficacy, build behavioral skills, set goals, and teach self-monitoring skills (Fuemmeler, 2003).

Primary prevention programs that excel have their roots in developmental theory make use of highly trained personnel, provide factual information about future negative health consequences of specific behaviors and peer norms, and incorporate behavioral strategies and social skills training (Williams et al., 2002). In examining primary prevention research models that allow for empirical evaluation, the gold standard of programs are those that allow for the use of comparison control groups, random assignment to intervention and comparison groups, multiple outcome measures that are characterized by sound psychometric properties, and multiple intervention sites implemented over the course of time (Durlak, 1997).

There are several model school-based primary prevention programs that have targeted a wide range of adolescent health behaviors, including prevention of smoking, alcohol and drug use, early sexual activity, and poor diet and exercise habits, HIV risk reduction and pregnancy. School health clinics also provide primary preventive health care. Researchers have found that school-based health clinics have a positive impact on overall academic achievement, absentee rates, and inappropriate utilization of health care resources (for review, see Fuemmeler, 2003). Three popular targets in primary prevention programs are substance abuse, risky sexual behavior, and cardiovascular risk. The following sections review examples of these programs.

Substance Abuse

Several substance abuse prevention programs have yielded positive results. Perry and associates (Perry, Williams, & Foster, 1993; Perry, Williams, & Veblen-Mortenson, 1996) instituted a 3-year intervention, Project Northland, to prevent or delay the onset of alcohol use by adolescents, as well as to reduce alcohol use among those adolescents who had already started to consume alcohol. It involved a school-based/peer-led curriculum that included parent–child home activities as well as community interventions (e.g., policy changes and enforcement task forces). The program was evaluated in several ways, including student surveys, parent surveys, community leader surveys, alcohol merchant surveys, and the examination of underage purchasing of alcohol. Findings revealed that at the end of the program, students who participated demonstrated a decrease in the use of alcohol and were more likely to perceive that peer drinking was not typical (e.g., less likely to report that peers their age typically consume alcohol on dates). Similarly, the Life Skills Training (LST) Program (Botvin, 1983) is a cognitive-behavioral approach that consists of 12 curriculum units that teach students to resist substance abuse by means of cognitive-behavioral skills, the building of self-esteem, resisting advertising pressure, managing anxiety, communicating effectively, developing personal relationships, and asserting one's rights. The skills are taught using teacher demonstration, behavioral rehearsal, feedback and reinforcement, and assigned homework to be completed out of class. Booster sessions also were provided in the second and third year of the intervention program. In a large 3-year study, pre- and posttest prevention effects were found for cigarette smoking, immoderate alcohol use, and marijuana use (Botvin, Baker, & Dusenbury, 1990). Most important, a follow-up evaluation during the adolescents' senior year in high school also found significant effects for the use of hashish, heroin, PCP, and inhalants.

Risky Sexual Behavior

Primary prevention has been heralded as an important approach for reducing pregnancy and STD at adolescence, but only if it is implemented at preadolescence. Howard and McCabe (1990, 1992) evaluated a program known as Postponing Sexual Involvement, designed to assist middle school students in resisting peer pressure to have sex. Nurses and counselors provided factual information, specific decision-making skills, and information about the proper use of contraceptives over the course of five sessions. The program helped students to develop skills for resisting in sexual activities and to deal assertively with pressure situations (Howard & Mitchell, 1990). Findings revealed that program participants were significantly more likely to postpone sexual in-

volvement than those participants in a comparison condition who only received factual information. Of particular importance is the finding that there was a decreased rate of pregnancy for the intervention group than for those youth in the comparison group. In a similar program focusing specifically on STD risk reduction, Jemmott, Jemmott, and Fong (1998) evaluated an intervention to examine HIV risk reduction among African American sixth- and seventh-grade adolescents. This cognitive-behavioral intervention involved eight 1-hour teaching modules that focused on delaying intercourse or decreasing frequency and safer-sex practices stressing condom use. Dependent measures included self-reports of sexual intercourse, condom use, and unprotected sexual intercourse. Findings revealed that both abstinence and safer-sex interventions were effective in reducing HIV sexual risk behaviors in the short term (i.e., 3-month follow-up). More important, however, safer-sex interventions were especially effective with sexually experienced adolescents over a 1-year period (i.e., 12-month follow-up).

Cardiovascular Risk

In recent years, a number of programs have been developed aimed at changing diet and physical activity for the purpose of reducing risk factors for adult-onset diseases. These programs have addressed tobacco use, dietary habits, and physical fitness among students in fourth through ninth grades (Walter, 1989). Findings from these programs have generally revealed intervention effects for health knowledge, dietary behaviors, blood cholesterol, and obesity (Walter, 1989). One investigation focused on reducing cardiovascular risk by encouraging healthy eating, physical activity, and preventing tobacco use with a large community-based health promotion program (Blackburn et al., 1984). Data revealed that adolescents who received the school-based and community health promotion programs reported healthier food choices and more physical activity, particularly for females, than students who were not involved in the intervention program (Kelder, Perry, Lyle, & Kelp, 1995). Similarly, Baranowski and colleagues (2000) developed an intervention program guided by social cognitive theory that included skills building and behavioral interventions, peer support for healthy eating, and teaching children to ask for more fruits and vegetables at home. The intervention program also included a weekly newsletter, a video with positive role models, and two family nights at a nearby grocery store. Findings were that for those in the intervention group, consumption of vegetables, asking behaviors, and dietary knowledge significantly increased.

Recent research has focused on reviewing successful school-based interventions in order to identify essential components across programs. Those variables that have predicted the success of school-based prevention programs include the structure of the program as well as the intensity of program efforts. For example, programs that have been implemented across school grades and also include booster sessions for maintenance are most successful. It also has been demonstrated that targeting parents and caregivers as well as other family members is important for generalizability and durability of treatment effects (for review, see Wallander et al., 2003). This approach assists in making the curriculum generalizable to settings outside the classroom, thereby increasing ecological validity. Both the independent use of school-based curricula (Perry et al., 1988; Perry, Klepp, & Sillers, 1989) and the inclusion of caregivers and parents in the various programs (Luepker, Perry, & McKinley, 1996; Wojitiwicz et al., 1992) have been demonstrated to be successful. Tobler and Stratton (1997) reviewed 120 programs in a careful meta-analysis and concluded that program content and process are critical variables in assuring efficacy of school-based prevention programs. The programs were classified as being either noninteractive or interactive, whereby noninteractive programs relied exclusively on didactic presentations by a group leader or teacher. Interactive programs emphasized a social process that included adolescent group work, deliberation, and learning. Findings from this meta-analysis revealed that the interactive intervention programs have larger median effect sizes than those programs that were noninteractive. Those programs that were able to change attitudes characteristic of the interactive programs generally produced the most positive effects.

Secondary Prevention

Secondary prevention efforts focus on the early identification and treatment of health problems prior to the progression of significant disease. In addition, secondary prevention efforts at-tempt to thwart negative health behaviors once they have begun (e.g., smoking cessation). Secondary prevention efforts are largely dependent on adequate screening and identification of risk-taking behaviors.

The targets of secondary prevention are guided by statistics for mortality and morbidity. The leading causes of mortality in adolescents are unintentional injuries from motor vehicle accidents and homicides, followed by suicide. Deaths due to cancer, cardiac conditions, and AIDS account for the majority of the remaining mortality among this age group.

Predominant causes of morbidity in adolescents include substance abuse, STDs, teenage pregnancy, and mental health problems. In addition, the early stages of several chronic diseases often begin at adolescence. For example, hypercholesterolemia, hypertension, and obesity, frequently leading to adult coronary artery disease and diabetes, often have their onset at adolescence.

In designing secondary prevention efforts it is important to determine whether disease states are beginning or if adolescents are experimenting as a part of typical development. There is some evidence to suggest that adolescents who experiment with drugs may fare better and be at less risk for later abuse than those who do not experiment with drug substances at adolescence (Shelder & Block, 1990). Current research supports the notion that secondary prevention efforts can reduce the incidence of future health problems (Durlak & Wells, 1998).

Marlatt, Fromme, Coppel, and Williams (1990) studied a secondary prevention intervention for the purpose of addressing alcohol use in college students. The study employed a randomized design for the purpose of assessing the outcomes of a cognitive-behavioral alcohol skills training curriculum, a didactic alcohol program, and a control group. The sample was assessed at 4, 8, and 12 months following the intervention program. Participants were "social" drinkers who wanted to learn more about, or change, their drinking behavior. The goal of the program focused on risk reduction associated with alcohol use, not the promotion of alcohol abstinence. The skills training component was based on social learning principles (Marlatt & George, 1984) and was aimed at the development of coping skills, limit-setting skills, and responsible decision-making skills. The didactic program involved lectures and films on the dangers of alcohol use and was based on a disease model of alcoholism. The control group received no intervention services. At the 1-year follow-up assessment, the students participating in the intervention component noted an overall reduction in self-reported alcohol use, although these findings were not statistically significant. The failure to find significant effects is likely due to the small sample size that largely underpowered the study.

Including a larger cohort of adolescents at higher risk for alcohol abuse than in their previous investigation (Marlatt & George, 1984), in a subsequent investigation Marlatt, Baer, and Kivlakan (1998) assessed an intervention program targeted for students at highest risk for high school drinking patterns. The investigation also included a 2-year follow-up of these students during college. Students at highest risk, based on high school drinking patterns, were targeted for this secondary prevention program. Participants were assigned randomly to an active intervention or a control condition. Treatment in the active intervention involved a brief intervention based on the principles of motivational interviewing (Miller & Rollnick, 1991). In the interview, students' alcohol use was reviewed and feedback was provided on their drinking patterns, risks, and beliefs about the effects of alcohol. In addition, suggestions for risk reduction were outlined. No direct advice was provided, as the goal was to allow the students to take responsibility for change. At the 2-year follow-up assessment, all high-risk students reported fewer alcohol-related problems and drinking less relative to the control group. However, students who received the brief intervention program demonstrated significantly greater declines in alcohol consumption rates and problems over time when compared to the control group. Of note, is the finding that high-risk adolescents in both groups showed a decrease in their alcohol consumption over time. Results from this investigation support the notion that most adolescents go through a developmental period in which those who drink heavily "mature out" of this risk-taking behavior as they transition to employment and family life responsibilities during young adulthood (Gotham, Sherr, & Wood, 1997). It may be that prevention efforts may accelerate this process, thereby sparing some adolescents the negative consequences associated with alcohol. Clearly, additional research efforts in this area are needed.

In a recent investigation designed to provide evidence relevant to a developmentally sensitive intervention and prevention of adolescent psychosocial distress associated with the management of Type I diabetes, Madsen and colleagues (2002) studied 224 adolescents who entered into the Diabetes Control and Complications Trial. Findings revealed that initiation of intensive treatment at early adolescence was associated with increasing school dissatisfaction while initiation of intensive treatment at later adolescence resulted in marginal elevations of psychological distress. These findings are important as they suggest that age at entry into a medical intervention trial designed to enhance disease management moderates the impact of intensive treatment on reported psychosocial distress. Thus, intervention and prevention efforts sensitive to the interaction of developmental tasks with health treatment goals are important for the psychological adjustment and well-being of adolescents with Type I insulin-dependent diabetes mellitus.

Tertiary Prevention Efforts

Tertiary prevention efforts have their focus on any disease or condition that may cause long-term or irreversible damage (e.g., serious injuries, substance dependence, and chronic diseases). Most adolescent tertiary intervention efforts are focused on adherence to medical regimens. The most concrete evidence supporting tertiary intervention efforts with adolescents has been in the area of diabetes. To date, available evidence has shown that in diabetes management, better control of blood glucose levels leads to reductions in long-term diabetes-related complications (Diabetes Control and Complications Research, 1993). For most other chronic conditions, little information is available on specific management guidelines, making specific intervention strategies more difficult to implement and evaluate.

There are few published reports of tertiary prevention studies at adolescence. Quittner, Drotar, and Ievers-Landis (2000) speculate that this may be due to the low prevalence of chronic disorders in adolescents and small number of participants for research. In those studies that have examined tertiary interventions in adolescents with diabetes and asthma, few changes were found in medical adherence or long-term disease outcome, although some positive effects were revealed, particularly in the psychosocial domain. Boardway, Delamater, and Tomakowsky (1993) demonstrated that through the use of stress management training, stress associated with diabetes could be reduced, although no changes in medical adherence or blood glucose control were observed. In an intervention program employing a behavioral family systems approach, Wysocki and colleagues (2000) demonstrated that the family therapy improved parent–adolescent relations, although it did not produce any changes in medical adherence or glucose control. In summary, although tertiary interventions lend some support in enhancing the psychosocial stressors and adjustment associated with chronic illnesses in adolescents, whether such interventions lead to long-term disease outcome and improvements in medical management remain to be demonstrated through future investigation (Williams et al., 2002).

CONCLUSIONS AND FUTURE DIRECTIONS

In this chapter, we have reviewed major health issues as they pertain to adolescence, including chronic illness-related issues specific to this developmental period. We have outlined various theoretical models that have been proposed to predict adaptation and adjustment to the stressors of a chronic illness, as well as the salient issues associated with the adaptation of these stressful diseases. In addition, we have reviewed recent literature related to health-compromising behaviors commonly seen in adolescents, including unintentional and intentional injuries, depression and suicide, substance abuse and dependence, and sexual activity among adolescents. In the interest of promoting a public health model for children and adolescents, we provide a review of literature associated with the promotion of healthy behaviors, including clinical, school, and community-based interventions. Finally, we provide a summary of primary, secondary, and tertiary prevention efforts that have been conducted with adolescents for the purpose of enhancing health.

Theoretical models clearly have been useful in conceptualizing adaptation and stress across a number of chronic illness conditions. Although each of the models that we review underscores specific and unique components of adjustment and adaptation, they all share a number of elements. The most common ele-

ments include the importance of traditional developmental tasks associated with adolescence, issues associated with family functioning (including the adolescent's need for autonomy while negotiating the stressors of a chronic disease), the role of specific environmental stressors (some of which may be associated with chronic illness while others of which are unrelated to the disease), and finally the role of peer and family support in adaptation to disease.

Theoretical models assist with our understanding of the general issues associated with disease and illness and allow for a comparison of various risk and adaptation processes across various illness groups. Future research efforts in this area will need to focus specifically on processes of adaptation for adolescents across chronic illness groups to identify specific risk factors and protective factors as they predict adjustment. This cross-illness theoretical framework would best facilitate broad-based intervention efforts to target youth across chronic disease groups. Notably, there has been a dearth of literature related to the transition to adulthood among adolescents with chronic "childhood" diseases such as CF and sickle cell disease. This is deemed to be an important area of inquiry given that the prognosis for many chronic conditions has improved due to significant medical advancements and technologies. Both correlational studies as well as intervention trials are needed in the evaluation of various theoretical models and to examine their utility in addressing risk and protective factors that are associated with successful adult management and coping in numerous chronic illness groups.

Theoretical model development and research examining adolescents' adaptation to chronic illness to this point has been primarily at a descriptive and correlational level. Although we now are aware of various risk and protective factors that are associated with adolescents' overall adjustment to the stressors of a chronic illness, the next stage of this research will be to validate the correlational models with empirical treatment studies.

Although the percentage of adolescents struggling with chronic illness is relatively low, adolescence is a developmental stage in the lifespan that places youth at specific risk for health-compromising behaviors. These behaviors include both unintentional and intentional injuries, suicide, substance abuse and dependence, and risky sexual activity that may result in adolescent pregnancy and STDs. Clearly, all these health-compromising behaviors that place adolescents at high risk for less than optimal health and even mortality beg for research studies that emphasize both primary and secondary prevention efforts. The literature to date has revealed specific variables that place adolescents at risk for various health-compromising behaviors. In addition, particularly given the high financial impact of these behaviors during adolescence on both the national health care system and private health care industry, there has been increasing interest among the National Institutes of Health in intervention efforts for adolescents that target health risk behaviors. These targets may include the areas of depression and suicide and substance abuse as well as diminishing those risks associated with sexual activity. While such intervention efforts typically have targeted older teens, efforts to employ intervention programs for preadolescents and early adolescents are recommended because of the poor trajectory for teens with early problem onset. The venue of such interventions will be important in order to access those youth most in need of these intervention programs. Therefore, it is essential that the intervention efforts be accessible and affordable.

In particular, school-based interactive intervention programs have demonstrated the most promise, and these efforts with preteenagers also need to be evaluated through controlled clinical trials. In comparison to prevention of substance abuse and risky sexual activity, there have been too few research studies in the area of adolescent unintentional and intentional injuries with perhaps the exception of the study of violence with firearms. Particularly in the area of driving accidents, there has been recent compelling evidence to suggest that psychopathology is a viable risk factor for behaviors that may predispose adolescents to traffic accidents as well as driving casualties (Barkley, Murphy, DuPaul, & Bush, 2000). These studies have been particularly useful in predicting youth who may be at particular risk, and they suggest that it may be possible to specifically target intervention programs for these at-risk adolescents, especially in school settings. The joint efforts of pediatric psychology, law enforcement programs, and the Department of Justice will likely provide fruitful collaboration in future years, particularly as we attempt to mount intervention programs to target those at risk health behaviors that have not been previously examined through systematic and careful investigation.

In an effort to invest in the health promotion of adolescents, there have been significant efforts to develop interventions at the level of the clinic, the school, and the community. The American Academy of Pediatrics, through its primary care guidelines, has long espoused prevention of health problems in children and adolescents by means of assessment and education in the primary care setting. In addition, some of the newer programs including Bright Futures (Jellinek, Patel, & Froehle, 2002) show particular promise in promoting the adaptation of healthy behaviors for all developmental periods including adolescence. For any of these programs to be successful, support will need to be provided by third-party payers in the same manner in which reimbursement for specific diagnostic codes and procedures for chronic disease is currently provided. In addition, careful evaluation of such clinical interventions will be critical in future years, particularly if third-party payers are requested to reimburse these clinical intervention programs.

Although primary care health promotion continues to be an important avenue for intervention, school-based interventions show particular promise in promoting health behaviors during adolescence. Particularly with the increased use of school health clinics, the school can eventually become the venue in which adolescents receive both their health and their mental health care. Although many adolescents rarely see doctors in traditional clinic settings, most adolescents attend school, and as a result, these clinics are accessible to most adolescents and their families. Early detection of health risk behaviors can be accomplished and the promotion of health behaviors may be incorporated with the traditional school curriculum. Health care providers that are employed within the school setting can consult with teachers and other education staff to assist in incorporating important health care routines within the academic curriculum. Further, such health care providers may be perceived as being more familiar and less threatening to the adolescent and may therefore promote honest discussion of sensitive issues regarding sexual behavior and substance use. While school-based interventions have shown some promise, they await empirical support through well-controlled clinical trials.

Finally, community interventions also have the potential to increase health-promoting behaviors and eliminate behaviors that place adolescents at risk for health problems. To accomplish such community efforts, it will be important to have sound partnerships with schools, pediatricians, and law enforcement agencies. Such intervention programs also will require controlled clinical trials.

We have discussed levels of intervention by which clinical, school, and community efforts might take place. Although we expect that such interventions will continue to take place at all levels of the public health spectrum (i.e., primary, secondary, and tertiary prevention), it is anticipated that greater efforts at prevention will emerge, particularly as there is an increased interest in this country in conserving precious health resources. It is recognized that tertiary prevention efforts will continue, particularly for adolescents with chronic health conditions. It is anticipated the secondary prevention efforts will be appropriate when specific risk factors have been identified as designating an adolescent at risk for a chronic illness, disability, or health-compromising behavior. Finally, it is hoped that primary intervention efforts will foster healthy behaviors and mitigate specific risk factors that may later result in chronic disease. Unfortunately, little research has been conducted for most of these efforts. Whether primary, secondary, or tertiary efforts are implemented, each awaits rigorous empirically validated support prior to endorsing them as effective for promoting health among adolescents.

REFERENCES

Aarons, G. A., Brown, S. A., Coe, M. T., Myers, M. G., Garland, A. F., Exxet-Lofstram, R., et al. (1999). Adolescent alcohol and drug abuse and health. *Journal of Adolescent Health, 24,* 412–421.

Adedoyin, M. A. (1992). Psychosocial effects of sickle cell disease among adolescents. *East African Medical Journal, 69,* 370–372.

Allensworth, D., & Kolbe L. (1987). The comprehensive school health program: Exploring an expanded concept. *Journal of School Health. 57,* 409–412.

Anderson, B. J., Brackett, J., Ho, F., & Laffel, L. M. B. (2000). An intervention to promote family teamwork in diabetes management tasks: Relationships among parental involvement, adherence to blood glucose monitoring, and glycemic control in young adolescents with Type I diabetes. In D. Drotar (Ed.), *Pro-* moting adherence to medical treatment in chronic childhood illness: Concepts, methods and interventions (pp. 347–365). Mahwah, NJ: Erlbaum.

Anderson, B. J., & Coyne, J. C. (1993). Family context and compliance behavior in chronically ill children. In N. A. Krasnegor, L. H. Epstein, S. B. Johnson, & S. J. Yaffe (Eds.), *Developmental aspects of health compliance behavior* (pp. 77–89). Hillsdale, NJ: Erlbaum.

Baranowski, T., Davis, M., Resnicow, K., Baranowski, J., Doyle, C., Lin, L. S., et al. (2000). Gimme 5 fruit, juice, and vegetables for fun and health: Outcome evaluation. *Health, Education and Behavior, 27,* 96–111.

Barkley, R. A., Murphy, K. R., DuPaul, G., & Bush, T. (2000). Driving in young adults with attention deficit hyperactivity disorder: Knowledge, performance, adverse outcomes, and the role of executive functioning. *Journal of the International Neuropsychological Society, 8,* 655–672.

Bearman, K., & La Greca, A. (2002). Assessing friend support of adolescents' diabetes care: The Diabetes Social Support Questionnaire—Friend's version. *Journal of Pediatric Psychology, 27*(5), 417–428.

Blackburn, H., Luepker, R. V., Kline, F. G., Bracht, N., Carlaw, R., Jacobs, D., et al. (1984). The Minnesota heart health program: A research demonstration project in cardiovascular disease prevention. In J. D. Matarazzo, J. A. Herd, N. E. Miller, & S. M. Weiss (Eds.), *Behavioral health: A handbook for health enhancement and disease prevention* (pp. 1171–1178). New York: Wiley.

Blau, G. M., & Gullotta, T. P. (1996). *Adolescent dysfunctional behavior.* Thousand Oaks, CA: Sage.

Blum, R. W. (1987). Contemporary threats to adolescent health in the United States. *Journal of the American Medical Association, 257,* 3390–3395.

Boardway, R. H., Delamater, A. M., & Tomakowsky, J. (1993). Stress management training for adolescents with diabetes. *Journal of Pediatric Psychology. 18,* 29–45.

Boat, T. F., Welsh, M. J., & Beaudet, A. L. (1989). Cystic fibrosis. In C. L. Scriver, A. L. Beaudet, W. S. Sly, & D. Valle (Eds.), *The metabolic bases of inherited disease* (pp. 2469–2680). New York: McGraw-Hill.

Botvin, G. J. (1983). *Life skills training: Teachers manual.* New York: Academic Press.

Botvin, G. J., Baker, E., & Dusenbury, L. (1990). Preventing adolescent drug abuse through a multimodal cognitive-behavioral approach: Results of a 3-year study. *Journal of Consulting and Clinical Psychology, 58,* 437–446.

Boylard, D. R. (2001). Sexuality and cystic fibrosis. *American Journal of Maternal Child Nursing, 26*(1), 39–41.

Braucht, G. N., Brakarsh, D., & Follingstad, D. (1973). Deviant drug use in adolescence: A review of psychological correlates. *Psychological Bulletin, 79,* 92–106.

Brindis C., Park, M. J., & Ozer E. M. (2002). Adolescents' access to health services and clinical preventive health care: Crossing the Great Divide. *Pediatric Annals, 31,* 575–581.

Brown, R. T., Doepke, K. J., & Kaslow, N. J. (1993). Risk–resistance–adaptation model for pediatric chronic illness: Sickle cell syndrome as an example. *Clinical Psychology Review, 13,* 119–132.

Brown, R. T., Freeman, W. S., Brown, R. A., Belar, C., Hersch, L., Hornyak, L. M., et al. (2002). The role of psychology in health care delivery. *Professional Psychology: Research and Practice, 33,* 536–546.

Brown, R. T., Madan-Swain, A., Walco, G. A., Cherrick, L., Ievers, C. E., Conte, P. M., et al. (1998). Cognitive and academic late effects among children previously treated for acute lymphocytic leukemia receiving chemotherapy as CNS prophylaxis. *Journal of Pediatric Psychology, 23,* 333–340.

Brown, R. T., Mulhern, R., K., & Simonian, S. (2002). Diseases of the blood and blood-forming organs. In T. J. Boll & S. Bennett Johnson (Eds.), *Handbook of clinical health psychology: Vol. 1. Medical disorders and behavioral applications* (pp. 101–141). Washington, DC: American Psychological Association.

Burgeson, C. R., Wechsler, H., & Brener, N. D. (2001). Physical education and activity: Results from the School Health Policies and Programs Study. *Journal of School Health, 71,* 279–293.

Cadman, D., Boyle, M., Szatmari, P., & Offord, D. R. (1987). Chronic illness, disability, and mental and social well-being: Findings of the Ontario Child Health Study. *Pediatrics, 79,* 805–813.

Casey, R. L., & Brown, R. T. (2003). Psychological aspects of hematologic diseases. *Child and Adolescent Psychiatric Clinics of North America, 12,* 567–584.

Centers for Disease Control and Prevention. (1999). *Youth Risk Behavior Surveillance System.* Retrieved October 20, 2001, from http://cdc.gov/nccdphp/dash/yrbs/.

Chan C., & Witherspoon, J. M. (1988). Health risk appraisal modifies cigarette-smoking behavior among college students. *Journal of General Internal Medicine, 3,* 555–559.

Chassin, L., Presson, C. C., Sherman, S. J., & Edwards, D. A. (1990). The natural history of cigarette smoking: Predicting young-adult smoking outcomes from adolescent smoking patterns. *Health Psychology, 9,* 701–716.

Christian, B. J., & D'Auria, J. P. (1997). The child's eye: Memories of growing up with cystic fibrosis. *Journal of Pediatric Nursing, 12,* 3–12.

Cousens, P., Ungerer, J. A., Crawford, J. A., & Stevens, M. M. (1991). Cognitive effects of childhood leukemia therapy: A case for four specific deficits. *Journal of Pediatric Psychology, 16*(4), 475–488.

Creatsas, G. (1995). Adolescent gynecology and obstetrics. *European Journal of Obstetrics and Gynecology and Reproductive Biology, 58,* 107–109.

Crom, D., Cremer, L., & Hudson, M. M. (2000). The physical aftermath of cancer. In R. G. Steen & J. Mirro (Eds.), *Childhood cancer: A handbook from St. Jude Children's Research Hospital with contributions from St. Jude clinicians and scientists* (pp. 447–459). Cambridge, MA: Perseus.

Crosby, R., Leichliter, J. S., & Brackbill, R. (2000). Longitudinal prediction of sexually transmitted diseases among adolescents: Results of a national study. *American Journal of Preventive Medicine, 18,* 312–317.

D'Auria, J. P., Christian, B. J., Henderson, A. G., & Haynes, B. (2000). The company they keep: The influence of per relationships on adjustment to cystic fibrosis during adolescence. *Journal of Pediatric Nursing, 15*(3), 175–182.

Diabetes Control and Complication Research. (1993). The effect of intensive treatment of diabetes on the development and progression of long-term complications in insulin-dependent diabetes mellitus. *New England Journal of Medicine, 329,* 977–986.

DiGirolamo, A. M., Quittner, A. L., Ackerman, V., & D., & Stevens, J. (1997). Identification and assessment of ongoing stressors in adolescents with a chronic illness: An application of the Behavior Analytic Model. *Journal of Clinical Child Psychology, 26* 53–66.

Donohoe, M. (2000). Social concerns of children with cancer. In R. G. Steen & J. Mirro (Eds.), *Childhood cancer: A handbook from St. Jude Children's Research Hospital with contributions from St. Jude clinicians and scientists* (pp. 471–476). Cambridge, MA: Perseus.

Dryfoos, J. G. (1990). *Adolescents at risk: Prevalence and prevention.* New York: Oxford University Press.

Dryfoos, J. G., Brindis, C., & Kaplan, D. W. (1996). Research and evaluation in school-based health care. *Adolescent Medicine: State of the Art Reviews, 7,* 207–219.

Durlak, J. D. (1997). *Successful prevention programs for children and adolescents.* New York: Plenum Press.

Durlak, J. A., & Wells, A. M. (1998). Evaluation of indicated prevention intervention (secondary prevention) mental health programs for children and adolescents. *American Journal of Community Psychology, 26,* 775–802.

Eiser, C., Hill, J. J., & Vance, Y. H. (2000). Examining the psychological consequences of surviving childhood cancer: Systematic review as a research method in pediatric psychology. *Journal of Pediatric Psychology, 25,* 449–460.

Elford, K. J., & Spence, J. E. H. (2002). The forgotten female: Pediatric and adolescent gynecological concerns and their reproductive consequences. *Journal of Pediatric and Adolescent Gynecology, 15,* 7–77.

Elster, A. B., & Kuznets, N. K. (1993). *AMA guidelines for adolescent preventive services (GAPS): Recommendations and rationale.* Baltimore: Williams & Wilkens.

Elster, A. B., & Levenberg, P. (1997). Integrating comprehensive adolescent preventive services into routine medicine care. *Pediatric Clinics of North America, 44,* 1365–1377.

Eure, C. R., Lindsay, M. K., & Graves, W. L. (2002). Risk of adverse pregnancy outcomes in young adolescent parents in an inner-city hospital. *American Journal of Obstetrics and Gynecology, 186,* 918–920.

Fanburg, J., Amari, S., & D'Angelo, L. (1997). Continued high-risk sexual behavior among known HIV-positive adolescents. *Journal of Adolescent Health, 20,* 149.

Flay, B. R., Miller, T. Q., & Hedeker, D. (1995). The television, school and family smoking prevention and cessation project VIII. Student outcomes and mediating variables. *Preventive Medicine, 24,* 29–40.

Flynn, B. S., Worden, J. K., Secker-Walker, R. H., & Badger, G. J. (1992). Prevention of cigarette smoke through mass media intervention and school programs. *American Journal of Public Health.* 827–834.

Fox, J. A. (1996). *Trends in juvenile violence.* Washington, DC: U.S. Bureau of Justice Statistics.

Frank, N. C., Blount, R. L., & Brown, R. T. (1997). Attributions, coping, and adjustment in children with cancer. *Journal of Pediatric Psychology, 22*(4), 563–576.

Fuemmeler, B. F. (2003). Promotion of health behaviors. In R. T. Brown (Ed.), *Handbook of pediatric psychology in school settings* (pp. 81–98). Mahwah, NJ: Erlbaum.

Gans, J. E., Blyth, D. A., & Elster, A. B. (1990). *America's adolescents: How healthy are they?* Chicago: American Medical Association.

Gortmaker, S. L. (1985). Demography of chronic childhood diseases. In N. Hobbs & J. M. Perrin (Eds.), *Issues in the care of children with chronic illness: A sourcebook on problems, services, and policies* (pp. 135–154). San Francisco: Jossey-Bass.

Gotham, H. J., Sher, K. J., & Wood, P. K. (1997). Predicting stability and change in frequency of intoxication from the college years to beyond: Individual-difference and role transition variables. *Journal of Abnormal Psychology, 106,* 619–629.

Graetz, B. W., Shute, R. H., & Sawyer, M. G. (2000). An Australian study of adolescents with cystic fibrosis: Perceived supportive and nonsupportive behaviors from families and friends and psychological adjustment. *Journal of Adolescent Health, 26,* 64–69.

Green, M. (1995). *Bright futures: Guidelines for health supervision of infants, children and adolescents.* Arlington, VA: National Center for Education in Maternal and Child Health.

Gruber, E., DiClemente, R. J., Anderson, M. M., & Loidico, M. (1996). Early drinking onset and its association with alcohol use and problem behavior in late adolescence. *Preventive Medicine, 25,* 293–300.

Grunbaum, J. A., Kann, L., Kinchen, S. A., Williams, B., Ross, J. G., Lowry, R., & Kolbe, L. (2002). Youth Risk Behavior Surveillance—United States, 2001. *Morbidity and Mortality Weekly Report, 51*(SS04), 1–64.

Guo, J. G., Chung, I., Hill, K. G., Hawkins, J. D.,

Catalano, R. F., & Abbott, R. D. (2002). Developmental relationships between adolescent substance use and risky sexual behavior in young adulthood. *Journal of Adolescent Health, 31,* 254–362.

Hanson, C. L., Henggeler, S. W., Harris, M. A., Burghen, G. A., & Moore, M. (1989). Family system variables and the health status of adolescents with insulin dependent diabetes mellitus. *Health Psychology, 8*(2), 239–253.

Hassan, E. A., & Creatsas, G. C. (2000). Adolescent sexuality: A developmental milestone or sexual risk-taking behavior? The role of health care in the prevention of sexually transmitted diseases. *Journal of Pediatric and Adolescent Gynecology, 13,* 118–124.

Hauser, S., Jacobson, A., Lavori, P., Wolfsdorf, J., Herskowitz, R., Milley, J., et al. (1990). Adherence among children and adolescents with insulin-dependent diabetes mellitus over a four-year longitudinal follow-up: II. Immediate and long-term linkages with the family milieu. *Journal of Pediatric Psychology, 15,* 511–526.

Hendry, L., Schuckswmith, J., & Phillip, K. (1995). *Educating for health: School and community approaches with adolescents.* London: Cassell.

Holden, E. W., Chmielewski, D., Nelson, C. C., & Kager, V. A. (1997). Controlling for general and disease-specific effects in child and family adjustment to chronic childhood illness. *Journal of Pediatric Psychology, 22*(1), 15–27.

Holmbeck, G. (2002). A developmental perspective on adolescent health and illness: An introduction to the special issues. *Journal of Pediatric Psychology, 27*(5), 409–416.

Howard, M., & McCabe, J. A. (1990). Helping teenagers postpone sexual involvement. *Family Planning Perspectives, 22,* 21–26.

Howard, M., & McCabe, J. A. (1992). An information skills approach for younger teens: Postponing sexual involvement program. In B. C. Miller, J. J. Card, R. L. Paikoff, & J. L. Peterson (Eds.), *Preventing adolescent pregnancy* (pp. 83–109). Newbury Park, CA: Sage.

Howard, M., & Mitchell, M. E. (1990). *Postponing sexual involvement: An educational series for preteens.* Atlanta, GA: Grady Memorial Hospital, Emory/Grady Teen Services Program.

Hurtig, A., & Park, K. (1989). Adjustment and coping in children with sickle cell disease. *Annals of the New York Academy of Sciences, 565,* 172–182.

Jellinek, M., Patel, B. P., & Froehle, M. C. (2002). *Bright futures in practice: Practice guide, mental health* (Vol. 1). Arlington, VA: National Center for Education in Maternal and Child Health.

Jemmott, J. B., Jemmott, L. S., & Fong, G. T. (1998). Abstinence and safer sex, HIV risk-reduction interventions for African-American adolescents: A randomized controlled trial. *Journal of the American Medical Association, 279,* 1529–1536.

Johanneson, M., Carlson, M., Brucefors, A. B., & Hjelte, L. (1998). Cystic fibrosis through a female perspective: Psychosocial issues and information concerning puberty and motherhood. *Patient Education and Counseling, 34,* 115–123.

Johnson, S. B. (1995). Managing insulin-dependent diabetes mellitus in adolescence: A developmental perspective. In J. L. Wallander & L. F. Siegel (Eds.), *Adolescent health problems: Behavioral perspectives* (pp. 265–288). New York: Plenum Press.

Kann, L., Warren C., & Harris, W. (1998). *Youth Risk Behavior Survey—United States.* Atlanta, GA: Centers for Disease Control and Prevention.

Kann, L., Warren, C. W., Harris, W. A., & Collins, J. L. (1995). Youth Risk Behavior Surveillance: United States. *Morbidity and Mortality Weekly Report, 44,* 1–55.

Kazak, A. E., & Barakat, L. P. (1997). Brief report: Parenting stress and quality of life during treatment for childhood leukemia predicts child and parent adjustment after treatment ends. *Journal of Pediatric Psychology, 22*(5), 749–758.

Kazak, A. E., Boyer, B., Brophy, P., Johnson, K., Scher, K., Covelman, K., & Scott, S. (1995). Parental perception of procedure related distress and family adaptation in childhood leukemia. *Children's Health Care, 24,* 143–158.

Kazak, A. E., Segal-Andrews, A. M., & Johnson, J. (1995). Pediatric psychology research and practice: A family/systems approach. In M. C. Roberts (Ed.), *Handbook of pediatric psychology* (2nd ed., pp. 84–104). New York: Guilford Press.

Kelder, S., Perry, C. L., Lyle, L. A., & Kelp, K. I. (1995). Community-wide nutrition education: Long-term outcomes of the Minnesota heart health program. *Health Education Research, 10,* 119–131.

Kleges, R. C., Robinson, L. A., & Zbikowsi, S. M. (1998). Is smoking associated with lower body mass in adolescents? A large-scale biracial investigation. *Addictive Behaviors, 23,* 109–113.

Koocher, G. P., & O'Malley, J. E. (1981). *The Damocles syndrome: Psychological consequences of surviving childhood cancer.* New York: McGraw-Hill.

Kupst, M. J., & Schulman, J. L. (1988). Long-term coping with pediatric leukemia: Six-year follow-up study. *Journal of Pediatric Psychology, 13*(1), 7–22.

La Greca, A. M., Auslander, W. F., Greco, P., Spetter, D., Fisher, E. N., & Santiago, J. (1995). I get by with a little help from my family and friends: Adolescents' support for diabetes care. *Journal of Pediatric Psychology, 20,* 449–476.

La Greca, A. M., & Thompson, K. (1998). Family and friend support for adolescents with diabetes. *Analise Psicologica, 16,* 101–113.

Lavigne, J. V., & Faier-Routman, J. (1992). Psychological adjustment to pediatric physical disorders. A meta-analytic review. *Journal of Pediatric Psychology, 17,* 133–157.

Logan, D. E., Radcliffe, J., & Smith-Whitley, K. (2002). Parent factors and adolescent sickle cell disease: Associations with patterns of health service use. *Journal of Pediatric Psychology, 27*(5), 475–484.

Luepker, R. V., Perry, C. L., & McKinley, S. M. (1996). Outcomes of a field trial to improve children's dietary patterns and physical activity: The child and adolescent trial for cardiovascular health (CATCH). *Journal of the American Medical Association, 275,* 768–776.

Madan-Swain, A., & Brown, R. T. (1991). Cognitive and psychosocial sequelae for children with acute lymphocytic leukemia and their families. *Clinical Psychology Review, 11,* 267–294.

Madsen, S. D., Roisman, G. I., & Collins, W. A. (2002). The intersection of adolescent development and intensive intervention: Age-related psychosocial correlates of treatment regimens in the diabetes control and complication trial. *Journal of Pediatric Psychology, 27*(5), 451–459.

Marlatt, G. A., Baer, J. S., & Kivlahan, D. R. (1998). Screening and brief intervention for high-risk college student drinkers: Results from a two-year follow-up assessment. *Journal Consulting and Clinical Psychology, 66,* 604–615.

Marlatt, G. A., Fromme, K., Coppel, D. B., & Williams, E. (1990). Secondary prevention with college drinkers: Evaluation of an alcohol skills training program. *Journal of Consulting and Clinical Psychology, 58,* 805–810.

Marlatt, G. A., & George, W. (1984). Relapse prevention: Introduction and overview of the model. *British Journal of Addiction, 79,* 261–273.

McCord, M. T., Klein, J. D., Foy, J. M., & Feathergill, K. (1993). School-based clinic use and school performance. *Journal of Adolescent Health, 14,* 91–98.

Miller, W. R., & Rollnick, S. (1991). *Motivational interviewing: Preparing people to change addictive behavior.* New York: Guilford Press.

Miller-Johnson, S., Emery, R. E., Marvin, R. S., Clarke, W., Lovinger, R., & Martin, M. (1994). Parent–child relationships and the management of insulin-dependent diabetes mellitus. *Journal of Consulting and Clinical Psychology, 62*(3), 603–610.

Mirro, J. (2000). How common is childhood cancer? In R. G. Steen & J. Mirro (Eds.), *Childhood cancer: A handbook from St. Jude Children's Research Hospital with contributions from St. Jude clinicians and scientists* (pp. 11–18). Cambridge, MA: Perseus.

Morgan, S. A., & Jackson, J. (1986). Psychological and social concomitants of sickle cell anemia in adolescents. *Journal of Pediatric Psychology, 11,* 429–440.

Murray, M. E., Guerra, N. G., & Williams, K. R. (1997). Violence prevention for the 21st century. In R. P. Weisssberg, T. P. Gullotta, R. L. Hampton, B. A. Ryan, & G. R. Adams (Eds.), *Healthy children 1020: Enhancing children's wellness* (pp. 105–128). Thousand Oaks, CA: Sage.

Nassau, J. H., & Drotar, D. (1997). Social competence among children with central nervous system-related chronic health conditions: A review. *Journal of Pediatric Psychology, 22,* 771–793.

National Center for Chronic Disease Prevention and Health Promotion. (2000). *General information and national estimates on diabetes in the United States.* Retrieved June 25, 2003, from www.cdc.gov/diabetes/pubs/factsheet.htm.

Newacheck, P. W., & Halfon, N. (1975). Prevalence and impact of disabling chronic conditions in childhood. *American Journal of Public Health, 88,* 610–617.

Park, M. J., Mac Donald, T. M., & Ozer, E. M. (2001). *Investing in clinical preventive health services for adolescents.* San Francisco: University of California, San Francisco.

Patterson, J. M. (1988). Families Experiencing Stress: I. The family adjustment and adaptation response model. II. Applying the FAAR model to health related issues for intervention and research. *Family Systems Medicine, 6,* 202–237.

Pearson, D. A., Pumariega, A. J., & Seilheimer, D. K. (1991). The development of psychiatric symptomology in patients with cystic fibrosis. *Journal of the American Academy of Child and Adolescent Psychiatry, 30*(2), 290–297.

Pendley, J. S., Kasmen, L. J., Miller, D. L., Donze, J., Swenson, C., & Reeves, G. (2002). Peer and family support in children and adolescents with Type I diabetes. *Journal of Pediatric Psychology, 27*(5), 429–438.

Perry, C. L., Williams, C. L., & Forster, J. L. (1993). Background, conceptualization and design of a community-wide research program on adolescent alcohol use: Project Northland. *Health Education Research, 8,* 125–136.

Perry, C. L., Williams, C. L., & Veblen-Mortenson, S. (1996). Project Northland: Outcomes of a communitywide alcohol use prevention program during early adolescence. *American Journal of Public Health, 86,* 956–965.

Perry, C. L., Luepker, R. V., Murray, D. M., Kurth, C., Mollis, R., Crockett, S., et al. (1988). Parent involvement with children's health promotion: The Minnesota home team. *American Journal of Public Health, 78,* 1156–1160.

Perry, C. L., Klepp, K. I., & Sillers, C. (1989). Community-wide strategies for cardiovascular health: The Minnesota heart health program youth program. *Health Education Research, 4,* 87–101.

Peterson, A. C., & Leffert, N. (1995). What is special about adolescence? In M. Rutter (Ed.), *Psychosocial disturbances in young people: Challenges for prevention* (pp. 3–36). New York: Cambridge University Press.

Porter, L. E., & Ku, L. (2002). Use of reproductive health services among young men, 1995. *Journal of Adolescent Health, 27,* 186–194.

Quittner, A. L., Drotar D., & Ievers-Landis, C. (2000). Adherence to medical treatments in adolescents with cystic fibrosis: The development and evaluation of family-based interventions. In D. Drotar (Ed.), *Promoting adherence to medical treatment in chronic childhood illness: Concepts, methods and interventions* (pp. 383–407). Mahwah, NJ: Erlbaum.

Quittner, A. L., Modi, A. C., & Roux, A. L. (2003). Psychosocial challenges and clinical interventions for children and adolescents with cystic fibrosis: A developmental approach. In R. T. Brown (Ed.), *Handbook of pediatric psychology in school settings.* Mahwah, NJ: Erlbaum.

Raymond-Speden, E., Tripp, G., Lawrence, B., & Holdaway, D. (2000). Intellectual, neuropsychological, and academic functioning in long-term survivors of leukemia. *Journal of Pediatric Psychology, 25*(2), 59–68.

Reynolds, K. D., Pass, M., & Galvin, M. (1999). Schools as a setting for health promotion and disease prevention. In J. M. Raczynski & R. J. DiClemente (Eds.), *Handbook of health promotion and disease prevention.* New York: Kluwer/Plenum Press.

Robin, A. L., & Siegel, P. T. (1999). Family therapy with eating disordered adolescents. In S. W. Russ & T. Ollendick (Eds.), *Handbook of psychotherapies with children and families. Issues in clinical child psychology* (pp. 301–325). New York: Kluwer/Plenum Press.

Rolland, J. S. (1990). The impact of illness on the family. In R. E. Rakel (Ed.), *Textbook of family practice* (4th ed., pp. 80–100). Philadelphia: Saunders.

Rovet, J., & Fernandes, C. (1999). Insulin dependent diabetes mellitus. In R. T. Brown (Ed.), *Cognitive aspects of chronic illness in children* (pp. 142–171). New York: Guilford Press.

Rundell, T. G., & Bruvold, W. H. (1988). A meta-analysis of school-based smoking and alcohol prevention programs. *Health Education Quarterly, 15,* 317–334.

Sawyer, S. M., Rosier, M. J., Phelan, P. D., & Bowes, G. (1998). The self-image of adolescents with cystic fibrosis. *Journal of Adolescent Health, 16,* 204–208.

Schroff-Pendley, J., Kasmen, L. J., Miller, D. L., Donze, J., Swenson, C., & Reeves, G. (2002). Peer and family support in children and adolescents with Type I diabetes. *Journal of Pediatric Psychology, 27,* 429–438.

Schuman, W. B., & La Greca, A. M. (1999). Social correlates of chronic illness. In R. T. Brown (Ed.), *Cognitive aspects of chronic illness in children* (pp. 289–311). New York: Guilford Press.

Shannon, C. (1996). Dealing with stress: Families and chronic illness. In C. L. Cooper (Ed.), *Handbook of stress, medicine, and health* (pp. 321–336). Boca Raton, FL: Circle Press.

Shelder, J., & Block, J. (1990). Adolescent drug use and psychological health: A longitudinal inquiry. *American Psychologist, 45,* 612–630.

Sloper, P. (2000). Predictors of distress in parents of children with cancer: A prospective study. *Journal of Pediatric Psychology, 25*(2), 79–91.

Tapert, S. F., Aaarons, G. A., Sedlar, G. R., & Brown, S. A. (2001). Adolescent substance use and sexual risk-taking behaviors. *Journal of Adolescent Health, 28,* 181–189.

Tarnowski, K. J., & Brown, R. T. (2000). Psychological

aspects of pediatric disorders. In M. Hersen & R. T. Ammerman (Eds.), *Advanced abnormal child psychology* (2nd ed., pp. 131–150). Mahwah, NJ: Erlbaum.

Thompson, K. M., LaGreca, A. M., & Shaw, K. H. (1997). *Ethnic differences in family and friend support adolescents with diabetes.* Unpublished manuscript, University of Miami, Coral Gables, FL.

Thompson, R. J., Armstrong, F. D., Link, C. L., Pegelow, C. H., Moser, F., & Wan, W. C. (2003). A prospective study of the relationship over time of behavior problems, intellectual functioning, and family functioning in children with sickle cell disease: A report from the Cooperative Study of Sickle Cell Disease. *Journal of Pediatric Psychology, 28,* 59–65.

Thompson, R. J., Jr., Gil, K. M., Burbach, D. J., Keith, B. R., & Kinney, T. R. (1993). Psychological adjustment of mothers of children and adolescents with sickle cell disease: The role of stress, coping methods, and family functioning. *Journal of Pediatric Psychology, 18,* 549–559.

Thompson, R. J., & Gustafson, K. (1996). *Adaptation to chronic childhood illness.* Washington, DC: American Psychological Association.

Thompson, R. J., Gustafson, K. E., Hamlett, K. W., & Spock, A. (1992). Psychological adjustment of children with cystic fibrosis: The role of child cognitive processes and psychiatrically referred and nonreferred children. *Journal of Pediatric Psychology, 15,* 745–759.

Tobler, N. S., & Stratton, H. H. (1997). Effectiveness of school-based drug prevention programs: A meta-analysis of the research. *Journal of Primary Prevention, 18,* 71–128.

Tyc, V. (2000). Practicing a healthy lifestyle after cancer therapy. In R. G. Steen & J. Mirro (Eds.), *Childhood cancer: A handbook from St. Jude Children's Research Hospital with contributions from St. Jude clinicians and scientists* (pp. 527–534). Cambridge, MA: Perseus.

U.S. Congress Office of Technology Assessment. (1994). *Health care reform, school-based health centers can promote access to care* (GAO/HEEHS-94–66). Washington, DC: U.S. Government Printing Office.

Varni, J. W., Katz, E. R., Colegrove, R., Jr., & Dolgin, M. (1996). Family functioning predictors of adjustment in children with newly diagnosed cancer: A prospective analysis. *Journal of Child Psychology and Psychiatry, 3,* 321–328.

Wallander, J. L., Eggert, K. M., & Gilbert, K. K. (2003). Adolescent health related issues. In R. T. Brown (Ed.), *Handbook of pediatric psychology in school settings* (pp. 503–520). Mahwah, NJ: Erlbaum.

Wallander, J. L., & Varni, J. W. (1995). Appraisal, coping, and adjustment in adolescents with a physical disability. In J. L. Wallander & L. J. Siegel (Eds.), *Adolescent health problems: Behavioral perspectives* (pp. 209–231). New York: Guilford Press.

Wallander, J. L., & Varni, J. W. (1998). Effects of pediatric chronic physical disorders on child and family adjustment. *Journal of Child Psychology and Psychiatry, 39,* 29–46.

Walter, H. J. (1989). Primary prevention of chronic disease among children: The school based "Know your body" intervention trials. *Health Education Quarterly, 16,* 201–214.

Wasserman, A. L., Thompson, E. L., Wilimas, J. A., & Fairclough, D. L. (1987). The psychological status of survivors of childhood/adolescent Hodgkin's disease. *American Journal of Diseases of Children, 141,* 626–631.

Wasserstein, S., & La Greca, A. M. (1996). Can peer support buffer against behavioral consequences of parental discord? *Journal of Clinical Child Psychology, 25,* 177–182.

Williams, G. W., Holmbeck, G. N., & Greenley, R. N. (2002). Adolescent health psychology. *Journal of Consulting and Clinical Psychology, 70,* 828–842.

Winter, L., & Breckenmaker, L. C. (1991). Tailoring family planning services to the special needs of adolescents. *Family Planning Perspective, 21,* 203–214.

Wojitiwics, G. C., Peveler, L. A., & Eddy, J. M. (1992). The Midfield highs school safety belt incentive program. *Journal of School Health, 52,* 407–410.

Wolman, C., Resnick, M. D., Harris, L. J., & Blum, R. W. (1994). Emotional well-being among adolescents with and without chronic conditions. *Journal of Adolescent Health, 15,* 199–204.

Wysocki, T., Harris, M. A., & Greco, P. (2000). Randomized control trial behavior therapy for families of adolescents with insulin-dependent diabetes mellitus. *Journal of Pediatric Psychology, 25,* 23–33.

Young, S. E., Corley, R. P., Stallings, M. C., Rhee, S. H., Crowley, T. J., & Hewitt, J. K. (2002). Substance use, abuse, and dependence in adolescence: Prevalence, symptom profiles and correlates. *Drug and Alcohol Dependence, 68,* 309–322.

Zeltzer, L., Kellerman, J., Ellenberg, L., Dash, J., & Rigler, D. (1980). Psychologic effects of illness in adolescence II: Impact of illness in adolescents—Crucial issues and coping styles. *Journal of Pediatrics, 97*(1) 132–138.

VI

GENDER IDENTITY
AND SEXUAL DISORDERS

16

Gender Identity Disorder

Kenneth J. Zucker

In this chapter, I provide an overview of the clinical and research literature on gender identity disorder (GID) during adolescence, borrowing from the literature on both children and adults when appropriate. I also give some consideration to another psychosexual disorder, transvestic fetishism (TF), which can occur during adolescence as some TF youth also struggle with gender identity issues. It should be noted that GID occurs in both males and females, although TF (with or without co-occurring GID) occurs only in males.

Some readers of this volume are probably aware that GID is currently very popular in the media. On television, episodes of *Chicago Hope*, *ER*, *Law & Order*, and *Party of Five* have all had storylines on the topic. Two critically acclaimed films, *Ma Vie en Rose* (My Life in Pink) in 1997 (Kline, 1998) and *Boys Don't Cry* in 1999, have also focused an artistic gaze on the subject. Indeed, in the latter film, Hilary Swank won an Academy Award for her role as Brandon Teena. Teena (born Teena Brandon), a female-to-male transsexual from Nebraska, was raped and subsequently murdered in 1993 at the age of 21 after two of his male friends discovered that he was "really" a woman (Sloop, 2000; Willox, 2003). And, finally, the print media have given attention to GID, including articles in *Time* (Cloud, 2000), *Satur-*

day Night (Bauer, 2002), and *Today's Parent* (Hoffman, 2003). Thus, it is timely to provide an updated review on youth who experience distress about their gender identity.

TERMINOLOGY

Several terms are used throughout this chapter, so it is useful to provide a brief definition of each. These are (1) sex, (2) gender, (3) gender identity, (4) gender role (masculinity–femininity), (5) sexual orientation, and (6) sexual identity.

Sex

The term "sex" refers to attributes that collectively, and usually harmoniously, characterize biological maleness and femaleness. In humans, the most well-known attributes that constitute biological sex include the sex-determining genes, the sex chromosomes, the H–Y antigen, the gonads, sex hormones, the internal reproductive structures, and the external genitalia (Grumbach, Hughes, & Conte, 2003; Migeon & Wisniewski, 1998; Money & Ehrhardt, 1972; Vilain, 2000). Over the past couple of decades, there has, of course, also been great interest in the possibility that the human brain has certain sex-dimorphic neuroanatomic structures which, perhaps, emerge during the course of prenatal physical sex differentiation (see, e.g., Arnold, 2003; Chung, De Vries, & Swaab, 2002; Swaab, Chung, Kruijver, Hofman, & Hestiantoro, 2003).

Our understanding about biological sex has been a gradual, cumulative process. From historical studies, it is clear that knowledge about it has included many false and flawed notions (Laqueur, 1992). In modern times, the common "person on the street" likely can identify the sex chromosomes as constituting an important component of biological sex; yet, it should be remembered that it was only in the 1950s that reliable techniques were developed to karyotype the sex chromosomes (Moore & Barr, 1955).

In the 1990s, there were substantial developments in understanding aspects of biological sex that had been speculated about for several decades. For example, although it had long been surmised that the presence of the Y chromosome was necessary for the gonads to differentiate along male lines (i.e., testicular differentiation), it was only in 1990 that the "testis-determining factor" (TDF) was identified (Vilain & McCabe, 1998). As described by Haqq and Donahoe (1998), the TDF is located on the short arm of the Y chromosome, with subsequent identification of SRY (the sex-determining gene region of the Y chromosome) (Donahoe & Schnitzer, 1996). In addition, Mullerian inhibiting substance is another protein involved in the temporal sequence of events that leads to male sex differentiation, as it results in the regression of the Mullerian duct, the anlagen of the uterus, fallopian tubes, and the upper vagina.

Gender

"Gender" is a term that is often used to refer to psychological or behavioral characteristics associated with males and females (Ruble & Martin, 1998). From a historical perspective, it is of interest to note that gender as a technical term is much younger than the technical term "sex." Indeed, as late as the mid-1950s, the term "gender" was not even part of the professional lexicon that purported to study psychological similarities and differences between males and females (see Haig, 2004). In fact, the first term introduced to the literature was "gender role" (not gender), which Money (1955)

defined as "all those things that a person says or does to disclose himself or herself as having the status of boy or man, girl or woman, respectively. It includes, but is not restricted to, sexuality in the sense of eroticism" (p. 254).

Over the past four-plus decades, three major developments have occurred with regard to the usage of the terms "sex" and "gender." First, as some scholars have noted, there has been a tendency, at least in some quarters, to conflate the use of the two terms, so that it is not always clear if one is referring to biological or psychological characteristics that distinguish males from females (Gentile, 1993; Haig, 2004). As noted by Unger and Crawford (1993), a good example of this is the title of a scholarly journal, *Sex Roles*, which began publishing in 1975. Because this journal typically publishes articles pertaining to psychological and behavioral characteristics associated with males and females, it might be more aptly titled *Gender Roles*.

Second, scholars have argued that the use of the terms "sex" and "gender" are related to assumptions about causality, in that the former is used to refer exclusively to biological processes and the latter is used to refer exclusively to psychological or sociological processes (for critiques of this division, see Maccoby, 1988; Money, 1985; Unger, 1979; for an exchange on this point, see Deaux, 1993; Gentile, 1993; Unger & Crawford, 1993; see also Laner, 2000). As a result, some researchers who study humans employ such terms as "sex-typical," "sex-dimorphic," and "sex-typed" to characterize sex differences in behavior, as they are descriptively more neutral with regard to putative etiology.

The third development, as noted by Zucker and Bradley (1995), is that Money's original use of the term "gender role" has been decomposed into three conceptually distinct component parts that are identified by the terms "gender identity," "gender role," and "sexual orientation."

Gender Identity

As a term, "gender identity" was introduced into the literature by Hooker and Stoller, almost simultaneously in the early 1960s (see Money, 1985). For example, Stoller (1964) used the slightly different term "core gender identity" to describe a young child's developing "fundamental sense of belonging to one sex"

(p. 453). This term was adopted by cognitive-developmental psychologists, such as Kohlberg (1966), who defined gender identity in relation to the child's ability to accurately discriminate males from females and then to identify his or her own gender status correctly—a task considered by some to be the first "stage" in "gender constancy" development, whose end state is the knowledge of gender invariance (Kohlberg, 1966; Martin, Ruble, & Szkrybalo, 2002).

Gender Role

The term "gender role" has been used extensively by developmental psychologists to refer to behaviors, attitudes, and personality traits that a society, in a given culture and historical period, designates as masculine or feminine—that is, more "appropriate" to or typical of the male or female social role (Ruble & Martin, 1998). It should be recalled, however, that defining gender roles in this way assumes that they are completely arbitrary and social in origin, a view not universally shared by researchers in the field. From a descriptive point of view, the measurement of gender role behavior in children has included several easily observable phenomena, including affiliative preference for same-sex versus opposite-sex peers, fantasy roles, toy interests, dress-up play, and interest in rough-and-tumble play. In adolescents, less attention has been given to the measurement of gender role behaviors, but some parameters that have been studied include personality attributes with stereotypical masculine or feminine connotations (e.g., Cate & Sugawara, 1986; Keyes, 1984; Massad, 1981), body gestures (Rekers, Sanders, & Strauss, 1981), activity interests (Berenbaum, 1999), and occupational aspirations (Brown, 1982; Mussen, 1962).

Sexual Orientation

The term "sexual orientation" is defined by a person's relative responsiveness to sexual stimuli. The most salient dimension of sexual orientation is probably the sex of the person to whom one is attracted sexually. This stimulus class is obviously how one defines a person's sexual orientation as heterosexual, bisexual, or homosexual. In contemporary sexological research, sexual orientation is often assessed by psychophysiological techniques, such as penile plethysmography and vaginal photoplethys-mography (Chivers, Rieger, Latty, & Bailey, 2004; Rosen & Beck, 1988), although structured interview assessments or self-report questionnaires have become increasingly common, particularly when respondents do not have a compelling reason to conceal their sexual orientation.

The paraphilias (*para*: akin to, faulty, abnormal; *philia*: abnormal appetite or liking for) also need to be considered in relation to the concept of sexual orientation (see Money, 1984, 1986). For example, the stimulus class of age is of importance in determining whether a person's sexual orientation is complicated by an age-atypical sexual preference, as in the cases of pedophilia (prepubertal children) and hebephilia (pubescent children, usually around 11–14 years), regardless of whether the superordinate sexual orientation is heterosexual or homosexual (e.g., Freund, Watson, & Rienzo, 1989). TF is one of the paraphilias and it often is first manifested during adolescence.

Sexual Identity

It is important to uncouple the construct of sexual orientation from the construct of *sexual identity*. A person may, for example, be predominantly aroused by homosexual stimuli yet not regard him- or herself as "a homosexual" (see, e.g., Ross, 1983). Indeed, there is a substantial body of evidence indicating disjunctions among various operational definitions of homosexuality, such as behavioral experience, attraction, and identity (for a detailed analysis, see Laumann, Gagnon, Michael, & Michaels, 1994).

Sociologists, particularly those of the "social scripting" and "social constructionist" schools, have articulated the sexual orientation–sexual identity disjunction most forcefully, arguing that the incorporation of sexual orientation into one's sense of identity is a relatively recent phenomenon, culturally variable, and the result of a complex interplay of sociohistorical events (Gagnon, 1990; Weeks, 1991). Nowadays, in postmodern Western culture, individuals with a minority sexual orientation frequently choose from a multiplicity of labels in characterizing their sexual identity (gay, pomo homo [postmodern homosexual] queer, questioning, etc.). Indeed, Rust (1999) reported no less than 21 different sexual identity labels that were generated by women who had had bisexual sexual experiences!

HISTORICAL CONTEXT

In the 19th-century European literature in sexology, there were several accounts of adults who struggled with a sense of profound discomfort about what we now term their gender identity (Hoenig, 1985). Subsequently, Hirschfeld (1923) coined the term "transsexual," which was popularized by Benjamin (1966), an endocrinologist who played a pivotal role in humanizing the modern clinical care of adults with gender dysphoria (Memorial for Harry Benjamin, 1988; for a comprehensive review of these developments, see Meyerowitz, 1998, 2002). The term "gender dysphoria" has been defined as a sense of awkwardness or discomfort in the anatomically congruent gender role and the desire to possess the body of the opposite sex, together with the negative affect associated with these ideas (Fisk, 1973). Clinically, it has been used to refer to the whole gamut of individuals who, at one time or another, experience sufficient discomfort with their biological sex to form the wish for sex reassignment.

A turning point in the recognition of transsexualism as a clinical phenomenon was the publication of the Christine Jorgensen case (a male-to-female transsexual) by the Danish endocrinologist, Hamburger (1953), which helped crystalize the notion that adults' discontent with their gender identity might impel them to seek radical physical transformations. For various reasons, transsexualism in adult males was more commonly described than in adult females, but in recent decades considerably more work has appeared on gender dysphoria in females (e.g., Cromwell, 1999; Devor, 1997; Halberstam, 1998; Lothstein, 1983; Prosser, 1998), strengthening the view that intense gender dysphoria occurred in both sexes.

Several summary accounts have made the case that the wish to become a member of the opposite sex is not a novelty of 20th-century social life in the West (reviewed in Zucker & Bradley, 1995). What is new, however, is the availability of hormonal and surgical techniques for transforming aspects of biological sex to conform to the felt psychological state (Hausman, 1992). This development is particularly relevant to biological females, in that although cross-sex hormones have been available for both sexes for decades, surgical advances and refinements in phalloplasty (surgical creation of a penis) have lagged behind vaginoplasty (surgical creation of a neovagina) because of greater technical problems (Hage, 1996).

The relevance of the adult syndrome of transsexualism to the study of both children and adolescents became apparent from life history interviews, which indicated that the patient's gender dysphoria, or discontent, often originated in childhood. As was the case for adults, the early reports on apparent GID in children focused predominantly, if not exclusively, on boys (Green & Money, 1960). Much less of the early work focused on adolescents; however, with the establishment of specialized gender identity clinics for children and adolescents, it became apparent that girls could also struggle quite intensely with gender identity issues.

A DEVELOPMENTAL PSYCHOPATHOLOGY FRAMEWORK

Sroufe (1990) has argued that adaptational failure must be defined with respect to normative developmental tasks. Thus, if one seeks to understand why some adolescents develop a sense of substantial distress regarding their gender identity, it is of great importance to understand how the vast majority of youth develop a more positive sense of being male or female. In many respects, the study of sex differences in psychosexual differentiation (e.g., with regard to gender identity, gender role behavior [masculinity–femininity], and sexual orientation) shares some clear similarities with the model that links developmental psychology and psychopathology. In the general population of males and females, these behavioral components show, on average, very strong sex differences: Most females have a female gender identity and most males have a male gender identity; most females have a feminine gender role behavioral pattern and most males have a masculine gender role pattern; and most females are erotically attracted to males and most males are erotically attracted to females (Collaer & Hines, 1995).

Although no one has attempted to formally document the extent of these behavioral differences by meta-analysis and the effect size metric (Cohen, 1988), I have little doubt that the effects would be quite large. Thus, there is a great deal of room to study the source of these differences, which can include both biological and psychosocial mechanisms. It could be argued, therefore, that understanding the mechanisms that underlie psychosexual differentiation in typical youth might inform us about similar mechanisms in atypical youth.

DESCRIPTION OF THE DISORDER IN ADOLESCENTS

Core Symptoms

Adolescents diagnosed with GID show a strong psychological identification with the opposite sex. More important, they also verbalize a strong desire to become a member of the opposite sex and indicate an extreme unhappiness about being male or female. The subjective experience of such youth can be characterized by the term "gender dysphoria." In its full form, the clinical picture includes several characteristics: (1) a frequently stated desire to be a member of the opposite sex; (2) verbal or behavioral expressions of anatomic dysphoria (e.g., in girls, stating a desire to have a penis; to masculinize their bodies via contrasex hormones; and to have bilateral mastectomy; for sophisticated adolescents, they will also express the desire for both a hysterectomy and oophorectomy; in boys, stating a desire to have their penis and testes removed and to have the surgical creation of a neovagina and clitoris; to feminize their bodies via contrasex hormones, electrolysis, and reduction in size of the Adam's apple); and (3) a strong desire to pass socially as a member of the opposite sex, which is often attempted via modification of phenotypical social markers of gender, such as hair and clothing style and the adoption of a stereotypical name associated with the opposite sex. To illustrate the core phenomenology, I offer two clinical vignettes.

Case 1

Samantha (IQ = 100), who had adopted the name of Sam, is a 17-year-old biological female. She requested an assessment after informing her mother that she was a "transsexual" and not a lesbian, as she had previously thought. Sam lived with her mother and her mother's common-law partner, who had functioned as a father figure for her since middle childhood. Sam's biological parents separated when she was 3, following several years of pa-

ternal spousal abuse. The reconstituted family was of a lower-middle-class socioeconomic background. As a child, Sam was considered by her family to be a "tomboy." She preferred to play with boys, enjoyed stereotypical masculine activities (e.g., playing with racing cars), and often enacted male roles during pretend play (e.g., a police officer). Although her hairstyle was conventionally feminine, Sam had a strong aversion to wearing stereotypical feminine clothing, such as dresses, although she would reluctantly wear them to special occasions, such as church attendance or grade school graduation. During childhood, Sam did not verbalize a desire to be a boy. Because Sam never seemed to express an overt unhappiness about being a girl, her parents, retrospectively, said that they never had considered that she might be struggling with her feeling about being a girl: "We just thought that she was a tomboy who would grow out of it." Upon entry into high school, Sam began to experience more social ostracism from other girls. For example, she was often teased for her masculine style of dress. In grade 9, Sam became aware of her sexual attraction to females, but it was only in grade 10 that she tentatively disclosed to her mother that she thought that she was a lesbian. In grade 9, Sam cut her hair very short, so, along with her style of dress, she was perceived by naive observers to be a boy. At this time, she began a sexual relationship with another girl who claimed to be bisexual. Because of Sam's phenotypical physical appearance, her girlfriend's parents thought that she was a boy, but when they learned that she was, in fact, a biological female, they forbade their daughter to continue the relationship with Sam. At the time of assessment, Sam recalled that she had found the transition to puberty extremely distressing. She was horrified when she began to menstruate and when she started to develop breasts. Accordingly, she began to wear several layers of t-shirts to conceal her breast development. Sam reported that looking at her feminized body was extremely difficult. As an example, Sam noted that when she showered she was compelled to look "straight ahead" and to count backward from 100. As these feelings intensified, Sam reported a deepening sense of despair and acknowledged several episodes of cutting herself. When asked about suicidal feelings, Sam sobbed, stating that she had thought of killing herself on numerous occasions: "I can't take it anymore." She indicated a desire to have a sex change operation, which would include taking hormones to masculinize her physical appearance (e.g., facial hair and voice deepening), wanted her breasts removed, and wanted to have an operation that would give her a "dick." She indicated that she saw herself as "one of the guys" and that her sexual attraction to girls was experienced as heterosexual; indeed, she reported that the earlier thought that she might be a lesbian nauseated her: "Doc, to be honest, lesbians make me sick. No offense. I got nothin' against lesbians. It's just not for me. I want to be normal."

Case 2

Christopher (IQ = 89), who had adopted the name of Chrissy, is a 15-year-old biological male. He requested an assessment after informing his mother that he was intending on living as a girl upon the completion of grade 9. When seen several months later for an assessment, Chrissy was dressed in feminine attire and would be perceived as an adolescent girl by a naive observer. For the assessment, Chrissy was dressed in flared jeans, suede boots with heels, a bra stuffed with water balloons (to simulate breasts), and a velvet tank top, along with a variety of jewelry. His hair was shoulder length and dyed platinum blonde. Chrissy lived with his mother. The parents had separated when Chrissy was 6, following the father's disclosure that he was no longer in love with his wife and was having an affair. The family was of a lower-middle-class socioeconomic background. As a child, Chrissy showed a variety of extreme cross-gender behaviors. He preferred to play with girls, enacted female roles in fantasy play, enjoyed playing with Barbie dolls, and cross-dressed frequently. He found rough-and-tumble play frightening and other stereotypical masculine activities aversive. He was often teased by other children and was frequently called "girly, sissy, and fag." He frequently told his mother that he wanted to be a girl, but his mother reported that she figured he would "grow out of it." Chrissy never did well in school academically. Upon entry into high school, Chrissy felt very isolated from his same-age peers and stopped going to school for weeks at a time. He spent a lot of time at home with his mother, who suffered from periodic agoraphobia and thus was often at home herself. In grade 9, Sam became aware of his sexual attraction to males but never considered himself to be gay: "I'm a girl who likes boys." He had not had, however, any sexual experiences with same-age peers although mother and Chrissy did report that he had been subjected to sexual abuse by an older boy when he was around the age of 8 and that this had lasted for several years, stopping only when he disclosed what was happening to his mother. At the time of assessment, Chrissy indicated that the transition to puberty was unpleasant. He found the deepening of his voice and the beginning of hair growth on his face, arms, and legs very unpleasant. Accordingly, Chrissy frequently shaved the hair off of his body and applied makeup to conceal any signs of facial hair. Chrissy indicated that he found penile erection "gross" and indicated that he never looked at or touched his genitals. Chrissy indicated a desire to have a sex change operation, which would include taking hormones to feminize his physical appearance, wanted to take contrasex hormones to induce breast development, and wanted his penis and testicles removed: "now, today." He also reported a strong desire to be pregnant and was surprised to learn that a sex change operation would not result in the capacity to bear a child.

DIAGNOSTIC CRITERIA

Table 16.1 shows the DSM-IV-TR (American Psychiatric Association, 2000) diagnostic criteria for GID, as they apply to adolescents. In the development of the diagnostic criteria for GID in DSM-IV (American Psychiatric Association, 1994), the Subcommittee on Gender Identity Disorders (Bradley et al., 1991) had recommended that the two DSM-III and DSM-III-R diagnoses of gender identity disorder of childhood and transsexualism (which was to be used for both adolescents and adults) be collapsed into one overarching diagnosis, gender identity disorder, with the diagnostic criteria reflecting age-related, developmental differences in clinical presentation. Because the presenting indicators of GID in adolescence were thought to be more closely related to the indicators seen in adults, it was for this reason that the criteria were differentiated from those provided for children.

It can be seen in Table 16.1 that the Point A criteria contain four possible indicators of a "strong and persistent cross-gender identification": (1) a stated desire to be the other sex, (2)

TABLE 16.1. DSM-IV-TR Criteria for Gender Identity Disorder

A. A strong and persistent cross-gender identification (not merely a desire for any perceived cultural advantages of being the other sex).

In adolescents . . . the disturbance is manifested by symptoms such as a stated desire to be the other sex, frequent passing as the other sex, desire to live or be treated as the other sex, or the conviction that he or she has the typical feelings and reactions of the other sex. . . .

B. Persistent discomfort with his or her sex or sense of inappropriateness in the gender role of that sex.

In adolescents . . . the disturbance is manifested by symptoms of such as preoccupation with getting rid of primary and secondary sex characteristics (e.g., request for hormones, surgery, or other procedures to physically alter sexual characteristics to simulate the other sex) or belief that he or she was born the wrong sex.

C. The disturbance is not concurrent with a physical intersex condition.

D. The disturbance causes clinically significant distress or impairment in social, occupational, or other important areas of functioning.

Specify if (for sexually mature individuals):
    Sexually Attracted to Males
    Sexually Attracted to Females
    Sexually Attracted to Both
    Sexually Attracted to Neither

Note. From American Psychiatric Association (2000). Copyright 2000 by the American Psychiatric Association. Reprinted by permission. Only criteria for adolescents are listed.

frequent passing as the other sex, (3) desire to live or be treated as the other sex, and (4) the conviction that he or she has the typical feelings and reactions of the other sex. The Point B criteria contain two possible indicators of a "persistent discomfort with [one's sex] or sense of inappropriateness in the gender role of that sex": (1) preoccupation with getting rid of primary and secondary sex characteristics; or (2) the belief that one was born the wrong sex.

Reliability and Validity

What is known about the reliability and validity of the DSM criteria for GID as they apply to adolescents? Unfortunately, we actually know very little as there have been no formal studies.

Indeed, the empirical state of affairs differs dramatically when compared to research on children with GID, for which there has been a substantial body of work documenting the validity of the DSM criteria (see, e.g., Johnson et al., 2004; Zucker, 1992; Zucker & Bradley, 1995). In part, this reflects the general relative lack of empirical research on adolescents when compared to their child counterparts with GID.

From a front-line clinical perspective, one could argue that, in practice, the application of the diagnostic criteria is not particularly difficult, because it is relatively uncommon, at least in specialized child and adolescent gender identity clinics, to encounter an adolescent who has only very mild gender dysphoria. But this may well not be the case in general clinical practice (see, e.g., Rosenberg, 2003). Thus, it is important to keep in mind that the indicators of GID are meant to capture a "strong and persistent cross-gender identification" (Point A) and a "persistent discomfort" with one's gender (Point B), not transient feelings.

Unfortunately, the DSM criteria are somewhat vague in helping the front-line clinician make this distinction. Consider two examples from the Point A criteria. Note, for example, that the first indicator of the Point A criterion refers to a "stated desire" to be the other sex and that the third indicator refers to a "desire to live or be treated as the other sex." It is unlikely that these indicators were intended to reflect merely an episodic desire to be of the other sex or to live as the other sex, but, for some reason, neither indicator included a specific reference to persistence or intensity. On this point, revisions to the criteria appear warranted.

From a practical point of view, it could be argued that the odds of making a misdiagnosis of GID are probably not that high, primarily because normative data suggest that the frequent wish to be of the opposite sex in both referred and nonreferred samples appears to be extremely low. For example, in the standardization of the Child Behavior Checklist (CBCL), a commonly used parent-report measure of behavior problems in children and adolescents, the percentage of adolescent boys and girls (ages 12–16) whose parents endorsed the item "Wishes to be of opposite sex" was extremely low; indeed, for some sex × age cells, the percentage was 0 (see Achenbach & Edelbrock, 1983, p. 33). Thus, against base rates, even a periodic desire to become a member of the opposite sex is quite atypical.

The DSM-IV criterion with regard to the "preoccupation" with one's primary and secondary sex characteristics (Point B-2) reflects well the adolescent expression of gender dysphoria as it pertains to discomfort with somatic sex, as the distress over physical sex markers is so pervasive. Nonetheless, even here, one has to exert some caution in making the diagnosis. For example, a study by Lee (2001) found that there was a great deal of overlap in feelings of "anatomic dysphoria" among female-to-male transsexual women and self-identified "butch" lesbians. Similarly, the recently described phenomenon of "tranny boys" among young lesbian women (see, e.g., McCarthy, 2003; Theobald, 2003), in which, for example, there appears to be a desire for "partial" sex reassignment (e.g., mastectomy, but not masculinizing hormone treatment), calls for caution in differential diagnosis.

Special Diagnostic Considerations

In DSM, the clinician can specify for "sexually mature individuals" information about sexual attraction (orientation) to males, females, both, or neither (see Table 16.1). In the clinical sexology literature on adults with GID, these categories have been termed, in relation to the patient's *birth sex*, heterosexual, homosexual, bisexual, or asexual (Blanchard, Clemmensen, & Steiner, 1987).

There are at least two reasons why it is important to consider the sexual orientation of an adolescent with GID: theoretical reasons (see the section "Etiology") and clinical reasons. Most adolescents with GID who have an early onset (i.e., starting in childhood; see the section "Age of Onset") are sexually attracted to members of their birth sex, and this is also the case with adults with GID (Blanchard et al., 1987). Thus, as noted earlier, Sam was attracted sexually to biological females and Chrissy was attracted sexually to biological males. In contrast, most adolescents with GID who have a late onset (i.e., starting in adolescence), as is the case with youth with TF, are sexually attracted to the opposite sex.

From an assessment perspective, it is important to understand how the adolescent conceptualizes his or her emerging sexual attractions. For example, as noted earlier, Sam appeared to initially self-label herself as a lesbian when she became aware of her sexual attraction to girls, but, as her gender dysphoria intensified, she re-jected that label and considered her sexual identity to be heterosexual because she felt like a boy who was attracted to girls. Thus, although she was sexually attracted to females, she did not experience this attraction as homosexual. As discussed in more detail in the section "Treatment," it is common clinical practice to explore with GID adolescents the psychological interface between their gender identity and sexual orientation.

EPIDEMIOLOGY

Prevalence

The prevalence of GID in adolescents has not been formally studied by epidemiological methods. Nevertheless, Meyer-Bahlburg's (1985) characterization of GID as a rare phenomenon is not unreasonable. For example, Bakker, van Kesteren, Gooren, and Bezemer (1993) inferred the prevalence of GID in adults in The Netherlands—1 in 30,400 women and 1 in 11,000 men—from the number who received "cross-gender" hormonal treatment at the main adult gender identity clinic in that country.

This approach suffers, however, from at least two limitations: First, it relies on the number of patients who attend specialty clinics serving as gateways for hormonal and surgical sex reassignment, which may not see all gender-dysphoric adults. In some countries in which health insurance covers the costs of sex-reassignment surgery (SRS), it is mandatory to receive a recommendation for sex reassignment from a specialized gender clinic team; however, for adults who are able to afford the cost of sex reassignment, they are less likely to be seen in a specialized gender clinic and thus would not contribute to estimates of prevalence, as in the study by Bakker and colleagues (1993) (see, e.g., Lawrence, 2003). In North America, this may be even more true nowadays as the number of university or hospital-based gender identity clinics has dwindled (Petersen & Dickey, 1995), and there has been a concomitant increase of paraprofessional support and search for care within sexual and gender minority communities (Broad, 2002; Feldman & Bockting, 2003). Second, the assumption that GID in adolescence will persist into adulthood is not necessarily true (see the section "Developmental Course and Outcomes"). Thus, gauging the prevalence of GID in adolescence from prevalence data on adults should be done with caution.

Sex Differences in Referral Rates

Among children between the ages of 3 and 12, it has been found that boys are referred more often than girls for concerns regarding gender identity. In our own clinic, we found a sex ratio of 5.75:1 ($n = 358$) of boys to girls based on consecutive referrals from 1975 to 2000 (Cohen-Kettenis, Owen, Kaijser, Bradley, & Zucker, 2003). In the Cohen-Kettenis and colleagues (2003) study, comparative data were available on children evaluated at the sole gender identity clinic for children in Utrecht, The Netherlands. Although the sex ratio was significantly smaller at 2.93:1 ($n = 130$), it still favored referral of boys over girls. Among adolescents between the ages of 13 and 20, however, the sex ratio in our clinic narrowed considerably, at 1.32:1 ($n = 72$) of males to females (Zucker, Owen, Bradley, & Ameeriar, 2002). This ratio is remarkably similar to the 1.20:1 ($n = 133$) ratio of male-to-female adolescents reported by Cohen-Kettenis and Pfäfflin (2003, p. 166) in the Netherlands. Thus, across both clinics, there was a sex-related skew in referrals during childhood, which lessened considerably during adolescence.

How might this developmental disparity in the sex ratio be best understood? One possibility is that it reflects accurately the change in prevalence of GID in males and females between childhood and adolescence, but because prevalence data from the general population are lacking, this remains a matter of conjecture. Another possibility is that social factors play a role. For example, in childhood, it is well established that parents, teachers, and peers are less tolerant of cross-gender behavior in boys than in girls (Fagot, 1985; Sandnabba & Ahlberg, 1999; Zucker, Wilson-Smith, Kurita, & Stern, 1995), which might result in a sex differential in clinical referral (for review, see Zucker & Bradley, 1995).

Zucker, Bradley, and Sanikhani (1997) and Cohen-Kettenis and colleagues (2003) provided data that supported this prediction, in which it was shown that girls may need to display more cross-gender behavior than boys before a referral is initiated. This higher threshold for referral appeared consistent with the fact that, in both the Toronto and Utrecht clinics, girls were referred, on average, about 10 months later than were boys (mean age = 8.1 years vs. 7.3 years, respectively), a significant difference, despite the fact that the girls showed, on average, higher levels of cross-gender behavior than the boys. However, it is important to note that the sexes did not differ in the percentage who met the complete DSM criteria for GID; thus, there was no gross evidence for a sex difference in false-positive referrals.

Another factor that could affect sex differences in referral rates pertains to the relative salience of cross-gender behavior in boys versus girls. For example, it has been long observed that the sexes differ in the extent to which they display sex-typical behaviors; when there is significant between-sex variation, it is almost always the case that girls are more likely to engage in masculine behaviors than boys are likely to engage in feminine behaviors (e.g., Cole, Zucker, & Bradley, 1982; Sandberg, Meyer-Bahlburg, & Yager, 1993). Thus, the base rates for cross-gender behavior, at least within the range of normative variation, may well differ between the sexes.

In adolescence, the picture may change considerably in that extreme cross-gender behavior is subject to more equivalent social pressures across sex and thus there is a lowering in the bias toward a greater referral of boys. Along similar lines, it is possible that gender dysphoria in adolescent girls is more difficult to ignore than it is during childhood, as the intensification of concerns with regard to physical sex transformation becomes more salient to parents and other adults involved in the life of the adolescent (e.g., teachers) (see, e.g., Cohen-Kettenis & Everaerd, 1986; Streitmatter, 1985); however, in a community sample of adolescents, Young and Sweeting (2004) found that, like in childhood, cross-gender behavior was reacted to more harshly in boys than in girls.

Social Class, Ethnicity, and Culture

The association of GID with demographic variables, such as social class and ethnicity, and with culture, has been examined to varying degree. In our clinic, children with GID are represented in all socioeconomic groups, as defined by Hollingshead's (1975) Four-Factor Index of Social Status, and this was also the case in the child sample from The Netherlands reported by Cohen-Kettenis and colleagues (2003). In a study in which we compared our child and adolescent patients (Zucker et al., 2002), we found that the child patients were significantly more likely to come from a higher social class background than were the adolescent patients. We also found that the child patients were more likely to be Caucasian than were the adolescent patients (83.0% vs. 65.3%). The child patients were also more likely to speak English as their first language and to be born in Canada than were the adolescent patients. Unfortunately, we do not know if these child–adolescent differences in demographics are unique to youngsters with GID or would be characteristic of clinic-referred youngsters in general who are seen from the same catchment area (cf. Swanson et al., 2003).

There is certainly a considerable amount of evidence that GID occurs in both Western and non-Western cultures, although there has been much more written about the apparent similarity in phenomenology with regard to adults than to children and adolescents (Herdt, 1994; Kulick, 1998; Newman, 2002; Poasa, Blanchard, & Zucker, 2004; Tucker & Keil, 2001). It is less clear, however, whether or not the surface similarity in behavior reflects an underlying common etiology or is an example of equifinality (i.e., different starting points leading to the same outcome) (Cicchetti & Rogosch, 1996).

Age of Onset

At the time of assessment, parents sometimes remark that their adolescent had behaved in a cross-gendered manner "since day one." Upon questioning, what parents usually mean is that cross-gender behaviors were apparent once the child was old enough to engage in specific sex-dimorphic activities (e.g., toy play and dress-up play). Most typically, this is during the toddler and preschool years (2–4 years), which corresponds to the developmental period in which normative behavioral sex differences pertaining to gender identity and gender role first emerge (Martin et al., 2002; Ruble & Martin, 1998). Indeed, in one retrospective chart study, Zucker and Bradley (1995) showed that the vast majority of adolescents with GID showed multiple indicators of cross-gender behavior, including the wish to be of the opposite sex, in childhood.

In general, then, the clinical presentation of an adolescent who meets DSM criteria for GID includes a long history of pervasive cross-gender behavior. There are two main exceptions to this pattern. One exception concerns

adolescents with both TF and gender dysphoria (Zucker & Blanchard, 1997). Such youth typically do not have a childhood history of cross-gender behavior (Zucker & Bradley, 1995) but develop the strong fantasy of being a girl as part of a sexual arousal pattern termed "autogynephilia." This pattern is defined, for example, as a male's propensity to be sexually aroused by the thought or image of himself as a female (Blanchard, 1989). The other exception pertains to a relatively small subgroup of adolescents who appear to develop an obsession with gender identity in the context of either a preexisting obsessive–compulsive disorder or Asperger's disorder. In both disorders, the general tendency for obsessional and ruminative thinking switches from one content domain to another (e.g., food, religion, sex→gender), but there is no childhood history of cross-gender behavior.

Case 3

David (IQ = 114) is a 14-year-old boy with a diagnosis of Asperger's disorder who was referred because of a preoccupation with gender identity and co-occurring sex-transformation fantasies. Around a year prior to our assessment, David, in the course of ordinary "surfing" on the Internet, came across a website titled *WonderBreast* (www.wonderbreast.com), which pertains to breast enhancement. Over the next 12 months, he became deeply preoccupied with, and thinking about, a sex change operation. He asked his parents to buy him "pills" (i.e., hormone tablets) for a "sex change." At different points during this period, he shaved his legs, eyebrows, and underarms, and, on one occasion, put on his mother's nail polish. Shortly before the assessment, David wrote a letter (to himself):

> I want to be a girl and I'm struggling more and more with it. It's on my mind 24/7 [24 hours/7 days per week] and I can't concentrate because of it. My parents don't understand and they don't know what to do or how to deal with it. I don't completely know why I want to be female, but I do vaguely know some reasons: My preference would be to be the girl in a boy–girl relationship because I want to be the caregiver. . . . I want to be the mother figure. . . . There are more options as the girlfriend. Another reasons is because I want fashion, clothing, and looks . . . matter to me more. Girls have all that . . . I want to go [to the assessment] because I'm getting to the point where

it's hard to function because of [this]. I need to know whether it's an actual problem or if it's just me (in my head). If I was able to get it done, I would want specific things. I would want to have a beautiful face, with freckles. . . . I would have nice, full lips. I would want to have nice curves on my body (big boobs/butt). . . . I would want to be beautiful all around. . . . Then, I'd go shopping. . . . After I get it done, I'm going to get my name changed.

There was no childhood history of gender identity problems or pervasive behavioral femininity. Childhood gender-typed play was stereotypically masculine and peer affiliation preferences were for male playmates. Based on clinical history and interview data, there was no evidence for TF or autogynephilia or other paraphilias (e.g., exhibitionism, sadism, masochism, and simple fetishism). David's sexual orientation in fantasy was exclusively heterosexual. He had not yet had any interpersonal sexual experiences. He was "disgusted" at the thought of homosexuality. One aspect of David's history that appeared to be of particular relevance was that he had had a long fascination with a particular type of toy, Animorphs (scholastic.com/animorphs/index.htm), which allowed for "identity transformations." David proudly told the interviewer that he owned all 54 books on them. He was also interested in the Calvin and Hobbes comic strip "Transmorgified." There was about a 2-month lag between referral and assessment. During this period, three events occurred that appeared to affect the natural history of the gender preoccupation. First, the consultant psychiatrist who referred David told his parents that he could not possibly have GID because he had not shown any signs of the disorder as a child. This information was then conveyed to David by his parents. Second, David was started on both Luvox (150 milligrams at bedtime) and Risperdal (0.25 milligrams at 8:00 P.M.). Third, David was informed that he was now on a waiting list to be seen in our clinic. By the time we saw him, David indicated that his desire to become a woman and to have a sex change had remitted. This was supported by the social worker involved in the patient's care and the parents. When asked why he had changed his mind, David commented that "I realized that most likely I would not like what I would be . . . I would most likely end up living alone and miserable," but he was unable to state why it took so long to have this "realization." He went on to state that the idea of cross-dressing was now "really weird . . . the clothes don't make the person . . . it can only slightly change your looks." He said that, at present, nothing made him feel feminine and "growing a beard . . . makes me feel masculine."

ASSOCIATED BEHAVIOR AND EMOTIONAL PROBLEMS

The assessment of associated behavior and emotional problems in adolescents with GID has relied on several measurement approaches, including standardized parent-report questionnaires, personality tests, self-report questionnaires of emotional disturbance, and projective tests. Understanding the extent to which adolescents with GID have other psychological and psychiatric difficulties is important, not only for theoretical reasons but also for the delivery of clinical care.

In our clinic, we have used the parent and teacher versions of the CBCL to assess general behavior problems. In the original standardization of the CBCL, factor analysis was performed on six sex-by-age groupings (4–5 years, 6–11 years, and 12–16 years). Two broad-band factors were identified, termed Internalizing and Externalizing, respectively. Across the six groupings, there were both common and unique narrow-band factors (see Achenbach & Edelbrock, 1983).

CBCL Data on Adolescents with Gender Identity Disorder

Table 16.2 presents parent-report data for 46 gender-referred adolescents for five CBCL indices of disturbance.[1] For comparative purposes, we show data from 343 gender-referred children and standardization data from the CBCL for referred and nonreferred adolescents.

On all five indices, the gender-referred adolescents had significantly higher levels of behavioral disturbance than did the gender-referred children (all p's < .001). Because the two age groups of GID patients differed on several demographic variables, it was necessary to see if the CBCL differences remained significant after controlling for these differences in demographics. Four of the five comparisons remained statistically significant (p's ranged from < .003 to < .001). The difference for the Exter-

TABLE 16.2. Ratings of Behavioral Disturbance on the Child Behavior Checklist

Measures	Gender-dysphoric adolescents (n = 46)		Gender-dysphoric children (n = 343)		Referred adolescents (n = 500)		Nonreferred adolescents (n = 500)	
	M	SD	M	SD	M	SD	M	SD
No. of elevated narrow-band scales[a]	4.35	6.22	1.95	2.43	—	—	—	—
No. of items[b]	49.83	18.35	34.65	17.92	—	—	—	—
Sum of items[c]	70.04	29.43	44.03	26.67	57.40	25.20	19.15	14.50
Internalizing T	69.15	8.47	60.75	11.03	65.00	8.65	50.50	8.55
Externalizing T	66.17	8.83	59.67	11.85	66.10	8.65	50.20	8.45

Note. Data on gender-dysphoric children and adolescents from Zucker et al. (2002). Nonreferred and referred samples consist of boys and girls ages 12–16, from Achenbach and Edelbrock (1983, Appendix D). For the probands, all CBCL items pertaining to gender identity scored 1 or 2 were set to 0 to avoid artificial inflation of general behavior problems.
[a]Absolute range, 0–9.
[b]Absolute range, 0–118.
[c]Absolute range, 0–236.

nalizing T-score was reduced to a trend level of significance ($p = .069$). More important, it can be seen in Table 16.2 that the GID adolescents had, on average, levels of behavioral disturbance comparable to the standardization sample of referred adolescents and considerably higher levels of behavioral disturbance when compared to the nonreferred adolescents. For the three measures for which there were comparative data on the nonreferred adolescents (sum of items, Internalizing and Externalizing T-scores), the effect sizes, using Cohen's d, were large: 3.50, 2.18, and 1.88, respectively. Using cutoff scores provided by Achenbach and Edelbrock (1983, Table 7-6, p. 63), 47.4% of the child GID sample and 84.7% of the adolescent GID sample had a sum score that was in the clinical range (> 90th percentile).

Taken together, the CBCL data suggest that adolescents with GID are as likely to have as many behavior problems as are other referred adolescents and to have considerably more behavioral disturbance than nonreferred adolescents. Given the increased degree of behavior problems in our adolescent sample, compared to the child sample, the data suggest that the persistence of GID is a risk factor for the intensification of general behavior problems.

Case 4

William, a First Nations 15-year-old boy (Verbal IQ = 60; Performance IQ = 94; Full Scale IQ = 75), was referred because of an intense desire to be a girl. When seen for assessment, he was noted to be quite thin with a poor complexion. He was wearing a tight pair of jeans and a snug top, as well as high heels. Although William would likely be perceived as a teenage girl by a naive observer, his presentation was not entirely unambiguous due to the presence of facial hair and a deep voice. At the time of assessment, he was living in a group home. He had not attended school on a regular basis since grade 5. His family history was characterized by a variety of child abuse parameters such that he was moved to a foster family, where, unfortunately, the stepfather sexually abused him for many years. His gender identity conflict co-occurred with a variety of other behavioral and psychiatric difficulties, including depression, impulsivity, suicide attempts, and self-mutilation. William would often insert sharp metal objects into his rectum and he would tell his therapist that the goal was "to kill myself from the inside out." His first response to Card I of the Rorschach reflected the trauma of his earlier sexual abuse: "A pig getting stabbed in the rear end." The CBCL was completed by William's placement supervisor who identified 81 items as characteristic of his behavior, which summed to 132. Both the Internalizing and Externalizing T-scores fell well within the clinical range, and of the nine narrow-band scales, eight were elevated. Peak narrow-band factors were Hostile–Withdrawn (T = 86), Hyperactive (T = 84), and Somatic Complaints (T = 83). Despite his very low Verbal IQ, William was a gifted artist and his drawings reflected, in remarkable detail, the multiple parameters of his distressed state: His drawings were characterized by mutilations, split-off body parts, massive anger at the world (one drawing was entitled "FUCK-OFF!!!"), and idealized and highly sexualized representations of himself as a girl.

Only one other study has utilized the CBCL in the assessment of behavior problems in GID adolescents. Cohen-Kettenis and van Goozen (2002) reported data on 29 adolescents with GID (11 males, 18 females). Collapsed across sex, the Internalizing T-score (mean = 64.02) was intermediate between the means for my child and adolescent samples, as was the Externalizing T-score (mean = 61.05). Nine (31%) of the 29 patients had a sum score in the clinical range. Unfortunately, their sample included only 39.7% of their series of 73 patients, which threatens the internal validity of the study. This is an important point because, in our comparative study of children in Toronto and The Netherlands (Cohen-Kettenis et al., 2003), in which CBCL data were available on almost all the patients, there were no significant clinic differences in degree of behavior problems.

Other Measures of Psychopathology

Several other studies on the psychological and psychiatric functioning of Dutch adolescents referred for gender identity concerns have also been reported. For example, Smith, van Goozen, and Cohen-Kettenis (2001) compared 20 adolescents (mean age = 16.6 years) who later received both hormone treatment and SRS with 14 adolescents (mean age = 17.3 years) for whom the request for sex reassignment was rejected. The "rejected" group consisted of adolescents who were not "transsexuals despite the fact that some did have gender identity problems" (p. 473). Unfortunately, Smith and colleagues did not indicate if this meant that the "rejected" group did not meet DSM criteria for GID because the parameter used to diagnosis "transsexualism" was not reported.

At the time of initial assessment, Smith and colleagues (2001) reported that both the treated and untreated groups had, on average, elevated scores on the Dutch version of the Symptom Checklist-90 (Derogatis, 1983). At follow-up, the treated group (mean age = 21.0 years) (i.e., those who underwent sex reassignment) showed a greater diminution in SCL-90 symptomatology than did the untreated group

(mean age = 21.6 years). Smith et al. also reported that more than half of the untreated group had, at the time of initial assessment, at least one clinician-diagnosed DSM disorder; unfortunately, comparable psychiatric diagnostic data on the treated group were not provided. Importantly, the treated group showed a substantial reduction in mean scores on the Utrecht Gender Dysphoria Scale (UGDS; Cohen-Kettenis & van Goozen, 1997) whereas the untreated group showed a much more modest reduction on the UGDS and remained significantly higher than the mean score of a standardization referent group.

In another study, Cohen, de Ruiter, Ringelberg, and Cohen-Kettenis (1997) evaluated the presence of psychological disturbance using the Rorschach Comprehensive System. Adolescents with GID were found to be intermediate between clinic-referred adolescents and nonpatients on an index of perceptual inaccuracy but did not differ from nonpatients with regard to thought disturbance or negative self-image (see also Smith, Cohen, & Cohen-Kettenis, 2002). Two methodological aspects of the Cohen and colleagues (1997) study deserve comment: First, only a subgroup of the GID patients were administered the Rorschach, and this subgroup was likely better functioning than the subgroup that was excluded (see Smith et al., 2001); second, the clinical controls included youth for whom a Rorschach protocol was available, raising the possibility that such youth were more disturbed than referred youth in general because a clinical decision had been made to administer a projective test. Taken together, then, the method of subject recruitment for the study may have led to an underestimation of psychological disturbance in the GID group and an overestimation of psychological disturbance in the clinical controls.

Summary

Adolescents with GID appear to show, on average, about as many behavioral difficulties as other referred youth and more than nonreferred youth. It is likely that multiple factors contribute to their difficulties, including risk factors common to many referred youth (Zucker et al., 2002). But, it is also likely that adolescents with GID have risk factors specific to their unique minority status (i.e., a markedly atypical gender identity) and, in this regard, likely share the same risk factors that have been identified in gay and lesbian adolescents, including stigmatization, rejection by the peer group, and discrimination (see, e.g., D'Augelli, 2002; Lombardi, Wilchins, Priesing, & Malouf, 2001; Mathy, 2002, Meyer, 2003; Sadowsky & Gaffney, 1998; Savin-Williams & Ream, 2003).

DEVELOPMENTAL COURSE AND OUTCOME

Information on the persistence and desistance of GID is of great importance, both theoretically and clinically. Regarding psychosexual differentiation, three outcomes have been identified: (1) persistence of GID, with a co-occuring homosexual sexual orientation; (2) desistance of GID, with a co-occurring homosexual sexual orientation; and (3) desistance of GID, with a co-occurring heterosexual sexual orientation. Regarding prospective follow-up studies of children, mainly boys, the second of these three outcomes has proved to be the most common (i.e., a desistance of GID with a co-occurring homosexual sexual orientation) (Green, 1987; Zucker, 2003b; Zucker & Bradley, 1995). From a developmental perspective, this suggests that gender identity, at least among children with GID, is malleable and likely influenced by psychosocial experiences, such as therapeutic interventions.

Unfortunately, we do not know a great deal about the long-term outcome among adolescents who have been evaluated for gender identity concerns. For example, the case report literature is very small and little confidence can be drawn from it in making general conclusions (see, e.g., Davenport & Harrison, 1977; Dulcan & Lee, 1984; Kronberg, Tyano, Apter, & Wijsenbeek, 1981; Meyenburg, 1999; Newman, 1970; Philippopoulos, 1964; Wren, 2002).

To date, the best data on long-term outcome on adolescents come from the Dutch group in Utrecht. Cohen-Kettenis and van Goozen (1997) reported that 22 (66.6%) of 33 adolescents went on to receive SRS. At initial assessment, the mean age of the 22 adolescents who received SRS was 17.5 years (range, 15–20). Of the 11 who did not receive SRS, 8 were not recommended for it because they were not diagnosed with transsexualism (presumably the DSM-IV diagnosis of GID); the 3 remaining patients were given a diagnosis of transsexualism but the "real-life test" (i.e., living for a

time as the opposite sex prior to the institution of contrasex hormonal treatment and surgery) was postponed because of severe comorbid psychopathology and/or adverse social circumstances.

These data suggest a very high rate of persistence of GID, which is eventually treated by SRS. It should be noted that the persistence rate could be even higher than 66% because Cohen-Kettenis and van Goozen (1997) did not provide follow-up information on the 11 patients who were not recommended to proceed with the real-life test or were unable to implement it.

In another study, Smith and colleagues (2001) reported that 20 (48.7%) of 41 other adolescent patients went on to receive SRS. At initial assessment, the mean age of the 20 adolescents who received SRS was 16.6 years (range, 15–19). Of the 21 who did not receive SRS (mean age = 17.3 years; range, 13–20), the reasons were similar to that reported in the earlier study. Data from Smith and colleagues suggest that a substantial number of the patients who did not receive SRS were still gender dysphoric at the time of a follow-up assessment that occurred, on average, 4.3 years later.

Data from our own clinic are relatively consistent with the findings from the Dutch group. Zucker and Bradley (1995) reported that 19 (43.2%) of 44 GID adolescents had been referred for assessment to the adult gender identity clinic in our hospital because of a continued wish for SRS. Of these cases, three patients had received both hormone treatment and SRS; a number of the others have been placed on cross-sex hormonal treatment but had not yet been approved for surgery. Many of the remaining adolescents continued with a chronic gender dysphoria, being unable or unwilling to comply with the real-life test requirements for SRS.

Case 5

Stella, a 16-year-old female, was referred by her youth group therapist when she revealed that she felt she was a boy and was interested in SRS. She had begun treatment with the referring therapist following several minor suicide attempts. The history revealed moderate cross-gender interests, a preference for boys as playmates, and a role as protector when socializing with girls. Intense interest in SRS began to emerge around age 13 after watching a TV show about it. She began to feel that surgery would make her feel "complete the way she is and feels" and would make her physically acceptable. Around this same time, Stella changed her appearance to look very "punk" and began to ask that she be called "Spike." Subsequently, she referred to herself as "Sid" after Sid Vicious, a punk-rock musician. She became involved in the drug culture and was sexually involved with a girl, to whom she introduced herself as a male with a congenitally absent penis. She liked to be identified as male and would get upset when her maleness was challenged. Reaction to puberty had been very negative, with Stella refusing to wear a bra. She had been concealing her breasts and using feminine napkins to simulate male genitals. At the time of assessment, she maintained that she still had not begun her periods, a concern that was only later revealed to have been a deception. She refused to use the girl's washroom, maintaining that she didn't urinate at school. The parents were disapproving of both her sexual orientation and thoughts about SRS, although her father felt he could accept her as a lesbian. Stella was very negative about her mother whom she perceived as "wimpish." When Stella informed her parents that she desired SRS, her mother declared her "dead" and withdrew from her emotionally. Interestingly, during psychotherapy, Stella noted that her mother was quite despondent when she was conceived and attempted to induce a miscarriage via rigorous exercise. Stella had more positive feelings about her father, with whom she shared an interest in repairing cars.

It was felt that Stella's gender dysphoria had remained relatively mild in childhood, but, for reasons that were not entirely clear during the assessment (aside from her hearing of SRS on TV), it had intensified amid the psychosexual demands of early adolescence. Although Stella did not clearly state that she wished to pursue SRS, her behavior and manner of relating suggested significant cross-gender identification. She was followed in supportive psychotherapy and gradually clarified a more appropriate (less antisocial) male identity and went on to SRS. At follow-up, she has been functioning well and is attending university.

When one compares the rates of persistence between patients first seen in childhood versus adolescence for GID, the data appear to show a higher rate in the latter group (Zucker, 2003b). This suggests, therefore, that there is a consid-erable narrowing, with age, of plasticity with regard to long-term gender identity differentiation. There are, of course, alternative interpretations. One possibility is that there is a high rate of "false positives" within child samples (i.e., youngsters who are not "truly" GID and therefore not really at risk for persistence); however, this does not appear to be the case in the sense that the vast majority of child patients met the DSM criteria for GID, if not at the time of assessment, then earlier (see Cohen-Kettenis et al., 2003). Thus, understanding variation in natural history of GID appears to be a legitimate empirical question for which there are, at present, few answers. Like other aspects of the self, however, gender identity appears to become more fixed with development and it is this consolidation that likely contributes to the reason one sees such a high rate of persistence among adolescents.

ETIOLOGY

Biological and psychosocial theories (and, more narrowly, hypotheses) have been developed to account for both between- and within-sex variations in psychosexual differentiation. In this section, I provide a selective overview of these theories and a summary of the empirical database.

Biological Mechanisms

For over 40 years now, the most prominent biological hypothesis that has guided research on psychosexual differentiation pertains to the role of prenatal sex hormones (and, in some lower animals, perinatal sex hormones). The classic version of the theory posits that prenatal exposure to androgens (a male-typical hormone) both masculinizes and defeminizes postnatal sex-dimorphic behavior (Collaer & Hines, 1995; Ellis & Ames, 1987; Meyer-Bahlburg, 1984; Mustanski, Chivers, & Bailey, 2002; Rahman & Wilson, 2003). The theory has guided literally thousands of experimental studies of lower animals in which the effects of the manipulation of the prenatal and perinatal hormonal milieu are evaluated with regard to species-specific sex-dimorphic behaviors (for reviews, see Dixson, 1998; Wallen, 1996; Wallen & Baum, 2002). If the theory has plausibility for the human situation, then variations in postnatal sex-dimorphic behavior should be related to variations in exposure to prenatal sex hormones.

Female and male fetuses differ significantly in their exposure to prenatal androgen (Grumbach et al., 2003). In turn, this affects the sex-dimorphic differentiation of the external genitalia and, so the theory goes, sex-sensitive structures in the brain. It is argued that these neural effects account, in part, for the large sex differences with regard to gender identity, gender role, and sexual orientation (Collaer & Hines, 1995; Hines, 2004). The theory also posits that within-sex variation in exposure to prenatal sex hormones might also explain within-sex variation in postnatal sex-dimorphic behaviors (see, e.g., Bailey & Zucker, 1995).

In some respects, GID is an ideal test of the model. In males, there are three indicators of marked behavioral feminization (female gender identity, feminine gender role preference, and sexual attraction to males) and in females the same three indicators show marked behavioral masculinization (male gender identity, masculine gender role preference, and sexual attraction to females). For many years, however, a fundamental problem with the model has been noted: For the vast majority of individuals with GID, the differentiation of the external genitalia is invariably *normal*, which would appear to rule out the presence of a grossly sex-atypical prenatal hormonal milieu (leading to under-masculinization of the external genitalia in males and masculinization of the external genitalia in females) (Meyer-Bahlburg, 1984). Over the past couple of decades, however, new research on lower animals has shown that it is possible to manipulate the prenatal hormonal environment and cause sex-dimorphic behavioral effects but leave the structure of the external genitalia intact.

In female rhesus macaques (*Macaca mulatta*), for example, Goy, Bercovitch, and McBrair (1988) induced behavioral masculinization in the absence of genital masculinization by varying the timing of exogenous injections of testosterone propionate during the pregnancy. From an interpretive point of view, this methodology is of interest because it eliminates a possible confound—that the masculinized behavior is, in part, a function of how the social group reacts to the anomalous genitalia of the female offspring. Goy and colleagues found that early-exposed females, who were genitally masculinized, showed increased rates of maternal and peer mounting (male-typical

behaviors) and lowered rates of grooming of their own mothers (a female-typical behavior) compared to normal females but did not differ from normal females in their rates of rough play. In contrast, late-exposed females, who were not genitally masculinized, showed increased rates of rough play and peer mounting but did not differ from normal females in their rates of maternal mounting. The mothers of the early-exposed females were more likely to inspect their genitalia than were the mothers of normal females, but the mothers of the late-exposed females were not. Goy and colleagues concluded that "the individual behavior traits that are components of the juvenile male role are independently regulated by the organizing actions of androgen and have separable critical periods" (p. 552). The association between prenatal androgen exposure and increased rates of some male-typical behaviors, despite the absence of genital masculinization, suggests that there can be a *dissociation* of morphological and behavioral effects in nonhuman primates.

Thus, this crucial finding leaves open the possibility that similar mechanisms operate in humans. As a result, researchers have sought to identify sex-dimorphic behavioral markers that might be affected by more subtle variations in the prenatal hormonal milieu—that is, variations that do not affect the configuration of the external genitalia (for recent reviews of the model with regard to sexual orientation in individual without GID, see Lippa, 2003; Mustanski et al., 2002; Rahman & Wilson, 2003; for recent reviews of the model with regard to individuals with physical intersex conditions, largely without GID, see Zucker, 1999).

At present, the empirical evidence has yielded a mixed picture with regard to sex-dimorphic behavioral effects that might have a biological basis in GID. For example, on sex-dimorphic tests of verbal and spatial ability, the evidence is inconsistent for the presence of sex-atypical patterns in both male and female adults with GID (Cohen-Kettenis, van Goozen, Doorn, & Gooren, 1998; Haarldsen, Opjordsmoen, Egeland, & Finset, 2003; van Goozen, Slabbekoorn, Gooren, Sanders, & Cohen-Kettenis, 2002). A similar inconsistency has been reported in two studies of sex-dimorphic fingerprint patterns (Green & Young, 2000; Slabbekoorn, van Goozen, Sanders, Gooren, & Cohen-Kettenis, 2000).

An increased rate of left- or mixed-handedness has been consistently reported in adult females with GID (Green & Young, 2001; Herman-Jeglinska, Dulko, & Grabowska, 1997; Slabbekoorn et al., 2000) compared to same-sex controls, but the corresponding findings in adult males has been inconsistent; however, Zucker, Beaulieu, Bradley, Grimshaw, and Wilcox (2001) reported an elevated rate of left-handedness in boys with GID compared to same-sex clinical controls. The increased rate of left-handedness in females with GID is consistent with a prenatal masculinization hypothesis (summarized in Lalumière, Blanchard, & Zucker, 2000), but the increased rate of left-handedness in boys with GID is paradoxical, which has led to alternative interpretations of the effect, including the role of prenatal developmental instability (Lalumière et al., 2000).

Males with GID have an excess of brothers to sisters (sibling sex ratio) and a later birth order (Blanchard & Sheridan, 1992; Blanchard, Zucker, Bradley, & Hume, 1995; Blanchard, Zucker, Cohen-Kettenis, Gooren, & Bailey, 1996; Green, 2000; Zucker, Green, et al., 1997). Additional evidence shows that males with GID are born later primarily in relation to the number of older brothers, but not sisters. In the Blanchard et al. (1995) study, for example, clinical control boys showed no evidence for an altered sibling sex ratio or a late birth order. One biological explanation to account for these results pertains to maternal immune reactions during pregnancy. The male fetus is experienced by the mother as more "foreign" (antigenic) than the female fetus. Based on studies with lower animals, it has been suggested that one consequence of this is that the mother produces antibodies that have the consequence of demasculinizing or feminizing the male fetus but no corresponding masculinizing or defeminizing of the female fetus (Blanchard & Klassen 1997). This model would predict that males born later in a sibline might be more affected, because the mother's antigenicity increases with each successive male pregnancy, which is consistent with the empirical evidence on sibling sex ratio and birth order among GID probands. At present, however, this proposed mechanism has not been formally tested in humans.

An ideal test of the prenatal hormone hypothesis would be to have measurements on known sex-dimorphic neuroanatomical structures. Unfortunately, postmortem access to brain material is usually required for this, which, as can be imagined, is difficult to come by. One study used MRI to visualize the corpus callosum, but there were no differences in size or shape of the splenium between adults with GID and controls (Emory, Williams, Cole, Amparo, & Meyer, 1991). Interpretation of the null finding is difficult because Emory et al. did not find sex differences in controls and there is a more general controversy over whether there are reliable normative sex differences in the structure of the corpus callosum (Bishop & Wahlsten, 1997).

Zhou, Hofman, Gooren, and Swaab (1995) reported that, in six adult males with GID, the size of the central division of the bed nucleus of the stria terminalis (BSTc) was in the range of unaffected genetic females. Subsequently, Kruijver and colleagues (2000) reported that the number of neurons in the BSTc of the GID males was similar to that of unaffected genetic females. In contrast, the neuron number of one adult female with GID was found to be in the range similar to that of unaffected genetic males.

Given the small number of patients for whom these rich postmortem neuroanatomical data were available, the results need to be interpreted with the usual caution. Three other issues make the matter even more complex. First, Chung and colleagues (2002) subsequently reported that the sex-dimorphic aspect of the BSTc in unaffected males and females could not be shown until *adulthood*, thus raising the possibility that the effect is caused by circulating sex hormones, and not sex differences in prenatal hormonal exposure. Second, if this is the case, the sex-atypical findings for patients with GID might be attributed to administration of contrasex hormones in adulthood. Finally, there is some evidence, at least in rats, that neural structures can be affected by variations in the social environment and experiences, including sexual behavior (see, e.g., Breedlove, 1995, 1997; Juraska, 1998), thus reversing the more traditional direction-of-effect interpretations typically given to these kinds of findings. Accordingly, the etiological significance of the BSTc findings is uncertain.

Psychosocial Mechanisms

Psychosocial factors can be considered with regard to predisposing, precipitating, and perpetuating (or maintaining) factors. To merit causal status, psychosocial factors would need to influence the onset of cross-gender behaviors and feelings (Zucker & Bradley, 1995). A multifactorial model of causality can, however, also entertain perpetuating factors, which can exacerbate any type of predisposing factor, including biological influences.

Given the early behavioral onset of GID, psychosocial mechanisms that are operative during adolescence are most likely perpetuating or maintaining factors. As one example, it was noted earlier that for some adolescents, the emerging awareness of homoerotic attractions appeared to intensify the cross-gender identification. It is very unlikely, however, that a discomfort with homoerotic feelings can induce gender dysphoria on its own. It is more likely that there is already a significant vulnerability in the adolescent's sense of self as a male or a female, which is further compounded by having to address sexual orientation issues.

Many parents of adolescents with GID will report a period during childhood in which the cross-gender behavior was tolerated or encouraged, often being viewed as "only a phase." Thus, during the preschool years, when gender identity is in a phase of consolidation (Martin et al., 2002), many adolescents with GID appear to grow up in an environment that enhances their cross-gender fantasies. It has been my experience that very few adolescents seen for a GID evaluation have had therapy to help them with their gender identity issues as children (Zucker & Bradley, 1995). For children seen for a GID evaluation, it is possible that the subsequent therapeutic exposure that many of these youngsters receive may interrupt the natural history, thus lessening the likelihood of persistence. On this point, however, systematic evidence is lacking.

Another factor that may serve as a perpetuating variable concerns the degree of family psychopathology. Many clinicians have noted that families that are stressed or burdened by psychiatric difficulties are less able to address the therapeutic needs of children, whatever they may be. Thus, one could hypothesize that adolescents with GID come from families that have more stress and more parental psychopathology than do children with GID. Although it appears that parents of children with GID have, on average, higher rates of psychopathology than do the parents of nonreferred control children (Zucker & Bradley, 1995), a comparison of families with children versus ad-

olescents with GID has not been carried out. Thus, it is not established that there are greater family problems and psychiatric difficulties in adolescent than in child patients with GID.

Finally, it might be argued that adolescents with GID are already burdened by considerably more general behavioral difficulties than are their child counterparts (Zucker et al., 2002). Along with other factors, these more general difficulties may make it harder for adolescents to address their gender identity problem. In fact, for many adolescents, the desire to change sex is seen as a way of solving many of their other problems in living, which is unrealistic.

ASSESSMENT

As noted earlier, the prevalence of GID is quite uncommon. Thus, some of the boundary problems that are often encountered in diagnostic assessment are much less likely to be an issue in the evaluation of youth who are referred for gender identity concerns.

In contrast to the empirical state of affairs for children, the development of reliable and valid assessment techniques for adolescents has lagged behind (for a review of child assessment techniques for GID, see Johnson et al., 2004; Zucker, 1992; Zucker & Bradley, 1995). Nonetheless, there are several assessment tools that can be used in the assessment of adolescents with gender identity issues, which can complement a clinical interview that confirms the presence of the DSM criteria for GID. Table 16.3 lists these measurement instruments. They can be used to establish the degree of current gender dysphoria, the extent of both current and childhood cross-behavior, and characterize the adolescent's sexual orientation, both in fantasy (e.g., crushes, dreams, and masturbation) and in behavior.

Table 16.4 shows data from the Recalled Childhood Gender Identity/Gender Role Questionnaire (Zucker, Mitchell, Bradley, Tkachuk, & Allin, 2004). This is a 23-item questionnaire designed to measure recalled sex-typed behavior during childhood. Factor analysis identified a two-factor solution: Factor 1 contains 18 items pertaining to childhood gender role and gender identity. Factor 2 contains 3 items pertaining to parent–child relations (e.g., relative closeness to mother vs. father). It can be seen in Table 16.4 that both male and female adoles-

TABLE 16.3. Methods of Assessment

Variable	Measure	References
Gender identity	Draw-a-Person test	Jolles (1952)
	Utrecht Gender Dysphoria Scale	Cohen-Kettenis & van Goozen (1997)
	Gender Identity Questionnaire (Adolescent Version)	Zucker et al. (2005)
Gender role	Gender Identity/Role Questionnaire (parental report)	Zucker & Bradley (unpublished)
	Recalled Childhood Gender Identity/ Role Scale (self-report)	Zucker, Mitchell, Bradley, Tkachuk, & Allin (2004)
	Rorschach (Sex-Typed Coding Manual)	Zucker et al. (1992)
Sexual orientation	Erotic Response and Sexual Orientation Scale	Storms (1980)
	Modified Zuckerman Heterosexual and Homosexual Experiences Scale	Zucker et al. (1996)
	Kinsey Interview Ratings	Kinsey et al. (1948)

cents with GID recalled significantly more cross-gender behavior during childhood than did the adolescents with TF (Factor 1). On Factor 2, the female adolescents with GID felt closer to their mothers than did the male GID and TF adolescents to their fathers; in addition, the adolescents with TF felt closer to their fathers than did the male adolescents with GID.

Figure 16.1 lists the items on a new Gender Identity Questionnaire (GIQ) that can be used with adolescents (and adults) (Zucker et al., 2005). It was designed to complement a previously developed Gender Identity Interview for Children (Zucker et al., 1993) by capturing a range of developmentally sensitive markers indicative of cross-gender identification and gender dysphoria. The GIQ was completed by 462 adolescents and young adults. Factor analysis identified one common factor in which all 27 items had a factor loading $\geq .30$ (median, .86; range, .34–.96), accounting for 61.3% of the variance. In Zucker and colleagues (2005), gender identity patients reported significantly more gender dysphoria than did the heterosexual and homosexual participants. Using a cut-point of 3.00, specificity was 99.7% and sensitivity was 90.4%.

In Table 16.5, illustrative mean scores from 12 clinic-referred adolescents are shown: three were referred for concerns about their sexual orientation, two were referred because of TF, and seven were referred because of GID. It is clear that there is a clear separation between those referred for current gender identity concerns versus those who did not have such issues.

TABLE 16.4. Factor Scores on the Recalled Childhood Gender Identity/Gender Role Questionnaire of Adolescents with Gender Identity Disorder and Transvestic Fetishism

Group	GID males (*n* = 29)	GID females (*n* = 25)	TF (*n* = 33)
Factor 1[a]			
M	2.60	2.15	3.97
SD	0.92	0.58	0.75
Factor 2[b]			
M	0.86	2.23	1.43
SD	0.94	1.06	1.25

Note. Data from Zucker et al. (2004).
[a]Absolute range, 1.00–5.00.
[b]Absolute range, –0.66–4.33.

TREATMENT

Ethical Considerations

Any contemporary child clinician responsible for the therapeutic care of children and adolescents with GID will quickly be introduced to complex social and ethical issues pertaining to the politics of sex and gender in postmodern Western culture and have to think them through carefully. Is GID really a disorder or

Time Frame: Past 12 Months

Instructions: Girls may vary a lot in how they think and feel about themselves in terms of gender, ranging from feeling totally comfortable in being a girl to uncertainty through pursuing a change into a boy. Thus, we are not talking about reactions to some social disadvantages of girls in our society, but about the basic sense of being a girl. You will be reading some questions about how you have been thinking and feeling in this regard about yourself during the past 12 months. Please answer each of the questions with one of the five answers of *Always, Often, Sometimes, Rarely,* or *Never.* Use the Comments section after each question to record any specific things that you want to add to your answer.

01. In the past 12 months, have you felt satisfied being a girl?

ALWAYS___ OFTEN___ SOMETIMES___ RARELY___ NEVER___ [12 months]

Comments:

02. In the past 12 months, have you felt uncertain about your gender, that is, feeling somewhere in between a girl and a boy?
03. In the past 12 months, have you felt pressured by others to be a girl, although you don't really feel like one?
04. In the past 12 months, have you felt, unlike most girls, that you have to work at being a girl?
05. In the past 12 months, have you felt that you were not a real girl?
06. In the past 12 months, have you felt, given who you really are (e.g., what you like to do, how you act with other people), that it would be better for you to live as a boy rather than as a girl?
07. In the past 12 months, have you had dreams?

YES ____   NO ____

If NO, skip to Question 8.

If YES, Have *you* been in your dreams?

YES ____   NO ____

If NO, skip to Question 8.
If YES, In the past 12 months, have you had dreams in which you were a boy?

08. In the past 12 months, have you felt unhappy about being a girl?
09. In the past 12 months, have you felt uncertain about yourself, at times feeling more like a boy and at times feeling more like a girl?
10. In the past 12 months, have you felt more like a boy than like a girl?
11. In the past 12 months, have you felt that you did not have anything in common with either boys or girls?
12. In the past 12 months, have you been bothered by seeing yourself identified as female or having to check the box "F" for female on official forms (e.g., employment applications, driver's license, passport)?
13. In the past 12 months, have you felt comfortable when using girls's restrooms in public places?
14. In the past 12 months, have strangers treated you as a boy?
15. In the past 12 months, at home, have people you know, such as friends or relatives, treated you as a boy?
16. In the past 12 months, have you had the wish or desire to be a boy?
17. In the past 12 months, at home, have you dressed and acted as a boy?
18. In the past 12 months, at parties or at other social gatherings, have you presented yourself as a boy?
19. In the past 12 months, at work or at school, have you presented yourself as a boy?
20. In the past 12 months, have you disliked your body because it is female (e.g., having breasts or having a vagina)?
21. In the past 12 months, have you wished to have hormone treatment to change your body into a boy's?
22. In the past 12 months, have you wished to have an operation to change your body into a boy's (e.g., to have your breasts removed or to have a penis made)?
23. In the past 12 months, have you made an effort to change your legal sex (e.g., on a driver's license or credit card)?
24. In the past 12 months, have you thought of yourself as a "hermaphrodite" or an "intersex" rather than as a boy or girl?
25. In the past 12 months, have you thought of yourself as a "transgendered person"?
26. In the past 12 months, have you thought of yourself as a boy?
27. In the past 12 months, have you thought of yourself as a girl?

FIGURE 16.1. Gender Identity Questionnaire for Adolescents (Female Version). The version for males is comparable in form, with appropriate change in pronouns and content (Questions 12–13, 22). Responses are scored on a 1-5 point scale, with a higher score indicating more gender dysphoria. Reverse scoring is required for Questions 1, 13, and 27. An interviewer-led format is also available (e.g., for adolescents who cannot read). The questionnaire also includes a "lifetime" version.

TABLE 16.5. Mean Score on the Gender Identity Questionnaire for Adolescents (Examples)

Case	Sex	Age at assessment (years)	Diagnosis	Mean score[a]
01	F	13	Homosexual	1.07
02	M	13	Homosexual	1.07
03	M	18	Homosexual	1.33
04	M	14	TF	1.37
05	M	16	TF	1.92
06	F	13	GID	3.92
07	F	13	GID	3.96
08	M	14	?GID[b]	1.61
09	F	16	GID	3.92
10	F	17	GID	3.33
11	M	19	GID	3.18
12	M	19	GID	3.18

[a]Absolute range, 1–5.
[b]Case 3 in the text.

just a "normal" variant of gendered behavior (see, e.g., Bartlett, Vasey, & Bukowski, 2000; Bradley & Zucker, 2003; Danforth & Schlozman, 2003; Pickstone-Taylor, 2003; Pleak, 1999; Rosenberg, 2002, 2003; Zucker, 2003a)? Is marked cross-gender behavior inherently harmful or is it simply harmful because of social factors? How does the clinician deal with an adolescent who states that she wants to have a sex-change operation because she is attracted sexually to girls and her religion tells her that homosexuality is wrong, so the only way she can be "normal" and have sex with a girl is by becoming a boy? If a teenager requests immediate cross-sex hormonal and surgical intervention as a therapeutic for gender dysphoria, should the clinician comply? These and other questions force the clinician to think long and hard about theoretical, ethical, and treatment issues.

Developmental Considerations

As noted earlier, the empirical literature suggests that there are important developmental considerations to bear in mind, in that there is some evidence to suggest that GID is less responsive to psychosocial interventions during adolescence (and, certainly by young adulthood) than it is during childhood. Thus, the lessening of malleability and plasticity over time in gender identity differentiation is an important clinical consideration.

Therapeutic Approaches

If GID in adolescence is not responsive to psychosocial treatment, should the clinician recommend the same kinds of physical interventions that are used with adults (Harry Benjamin Standards of Care for Gender Identity Disorders, 1998)? Prior to such a recommendation, most clinicians will encourage adolescents with GID to consider alternatives to this invasive and expensive treatment. One area of inquiry can, therefore, explore the meaning behind the adolescent's desire for SRS and if there are viable alternative lifestyle adaptations. In this regard, the most common area of exploration pertains to the patient's sexual orientation. Almost all adolescents with GID recall that they always felt uncomfortable growing up as boys or as girls; however, for some adolescents the idea of a "sex change" did not begin to crystalize until they became aware of homoerotic attractions. For some of these youngsters, the idea that they might be gay or homosexual is abhorrent. For some such adolescents, psychoeducational work can explore their attitudes and feelings about homosexuality. Group therapy, in which such youngsters have the opportunity to meet gay adolescents, can be a useful adjunct in such cases. In some cases, the gender dysphoria will resolve and a homosexual adaptation ensues (Zucker & Bradley, 1995). For others, however, a homosexual adaptation is not possible and the gender dysphoria does not abate.

Case 6

Carlos (IQ = 122) is a 14-year-old boy from a Spanish-speaking, working-class family from South America, that had immigrated to Canada prior to the patient's birth. His parents had a long history of marital discord up until the father's death, which had been preceded by a chronic illness, when the patient was 12. Carlos had been very effeminate during childhood, with periodic thoughts about wanting to be a girl. During the year prior to the assessment, he began to cross-dress publicly and expressed to his mother and siblings that he wanted to be a girl. The intensification of the wish to be a girl appeared to coincide with his emerging awareness of sexual attractions to other males. Carlos stated that he did not want to be "gay" because a homosexual identity was viewed with disdain in his country of origin. He went on to say that if he could be a female, then he would be "normal" (i.e., his attraction to males would then be considered heterosexual). Carlos was seen for 2 years in individual psychotherapy. During this period, we helped Carlos to transfer to an alternative school that catered to bright adolescents who had trouble coping (or were not stimulated enough) in the traditional high school setting. He began attending this school in the female social role, introducing himself as Lucia. Although Lucia enjoyed a class that talked about gay issues and he participated in a community group for gay, lesbian, bisexual, transgender, and questioning youth, Lucia did not see living her life as a gay person an alternative adaptation. After 2 years in therapy, contrasex hormonal treatment was instituted.

For adolescents in which the gender dysphoria appears chronic, the clinician can consider two main options: (1) management until the adolescent turns 18 and can be referred to an adult gender identity clinic or (2) "early" institution of contrasex hormonal treatment. Regarding the latter, Gooren and Delemarre-van de Waal (1996) recommended that one option with gender-dysphoric adolescents is to prescribe puberty-blocking luteinizing hormone-release agonists (e.g., depot leuprolide or depot triptorelin) that facilitate more successful passing as the opposite sex (see also Cohen-Kettenis & van Goozen, 1998; Wren, 2000). Thus, for example, in male adolescents, such medication can suppress the development of secondary sex characteristics, such as facial hair growth and voice deepening, which makes it more difficult to pass in the female social role. Cohen-Kettenis and van Goozen (1997, 1998) reported that early cross-sex hormone treatment for adolescents under the age of 18 years, judged free of gross psychiatric comorbidity, facilitated the complex psychosexual and psychosocial transition to living as a member of the opposite sex and results in a lessening of the gender dysphoria (see also Smith et al., 2001).

Although such early hormonal treatment is controversial (Cohen-Kettenis, 1994, 1995; Meyenburg, 1994), it may well be the treatment of choice once the clinician is confident that other options have been exhausted. One issue that is not yet resolved concerns who the best candidates are for early hormonal treatments. Cohen-Kettenis and van Goozen (1997) have suggested that the least risky subgroup of adolescents with GID comprises those who show little evidence of psychiatric impairment. In my own clinic, the vast majority of adolescents with GID would not qualify on this basis (Zucker et al., 2002); however, by adolescence, the issue is a tricky one because it is not clear to what extent the psychiatric impairment is a consequence of the chronic gender dysphoria (Newman, 1970).

FUTURE DIRECTIONS

In this chapter, I have provided an overview of the literature on GID in adolescence. Since GID first appeared in DSM-III in 1980, considerable advances have been made in some areas. For example, the phenomenology of GID is now well-described and extant assessment procedures are available to conduct a thorough and competent diagnostic evaluation; however, there has been less work in this area for adolescents than there has been for children. Like other psychiatric disorders that affect adolescents, it is apparent that complexity, not simplicity, is the guiding rule of thumb in any effort to make sense of the origins of GID.

It appears that both biological and psychosocial factors contribute to the disorder's genesis and maintenance, and we are making some progress in identifying specific markers of both processes; however, very little work has utilized adolescent as opposed to both child and adult samples. We are only beginning to obtain data on the "natural history" of adolescents with GID, particularly when carried out from a prospective standpoint, and almost nothing in the way of empirical research has been carried out with regard to psychological interventions. Indeed, the current state of the art suggests a rather poor prognosis for the resolution of GID if it persists into adolescence. Unfortunately, research on adolescents with GID has lagged behind research on their child counterparts, but it is hoped that this chapter will contribute to a more comprehensive understanding of those adolescents who struggle so intensely with their feelings about being male or female.

NOTE

1. Two items on the CBCL specifically pertain to cross-gender behavior (Item 5: "behaves like opposite sex" and Item 110: "wishes to be of opposite sex."). It has been our experience that certain other items on the CBCL are endorsed in a manner that reflect the adolescent's cross-gender-identification. For example, a parent might endorse Item 84 ("strange behavior") and then provide an example such as "thinks she's a boy." For all the analyses reported here, these items were scored as 0's to avoid any artificial inflation of the disturbance indices.

REFERENCES

Achenbach, T. M., & Edelbrock, C. (1983). *Manual for the Child Behavior Checklist and Revised Child Behavior Profile*. Burlington: University of Vermont, Department of Psychiatry.

American Psychiatric Association. (1994). *Diagnostic and statistical manual of mental disorders* (4th ed.). Washington, DC: Author.

American Psychiatric Association. (2000). *Diagnostic and statistical manual of mental disorders* (4th ed., Text rev.). Washington, DC: Author.

Arnold, A. P. (2003). The gender of the voice within: The neural origin of sex differences in the brain. *Current Opinion in Neurobiology, 13,* 759–764.

Bailey, J. M., & Zucker, K. J. (1995). Childhood sex-typed behavior and sexual orientation: A conceptual analysis and quantitative review. *Developmental Psychology, 31,* 43–55.

Bakker, A., van Kesteren, P. J. M., Gooren, L. J. G., & Bezemer, P. D. (1993). The prevalence of transsexualism in the Netherlands. *Acta Psychiatrica Scandinavica, 87,* 237–238.

Bartlett, N. H., Vasey, P. L., & Bukowski, W. M. (2000). Is gender identity disorder in children a mental disorder? *Sex Roles, 43,* 753–785.

Bauer, G. (2002, November). Gender bender. *Saturday Night, 117*(6), 60–62, 64.

Benjamin, H. (1966). *The transsexual phenomenon.* New York: Julian Press.

Berenbaum, S. A. (1999). Effects of early androgens on sex-typed activities and interests in adolescents with congenital adrenal hyperplasia. *Hormones and Behavior, 35,* 102–110.

Bishop, K. M., & Wahlsten, D. (1997). Sex differences in the human corpus callosum: Myth or reality? *Neuroscience and Biobehavioral Reviews, 21,* 581–601.

Blanchard, R. (1989). The concept of autogynephilia and the typology of male gender dysphoria. *Journal of Nervous and Mental Disease, 177,* 616–623.

Blanchard, R., Clemmensen, L. H., & Steiner, B. W. (1987). Heterosexual and homosexual gender dysphoria. *Archives of Sexual Behavior, 16,* 139–152.

Blanchard, R., & Klassen, P. (1997). H–Y antigen and homosexuality in men. *Journal of Theoretical Biology, 185,* 373–378.

Blanchard, R., & Sheridan, P. M. (1992). Sibship size, sibling sex ratio, birth order, and parental age in homosexual and nonhomosexual gender dysphorics. *Journal of Nervous and Mental Disease, 180,* 40–47.

Blanchard, R., Zucker, K. J., Bradley, S. J., & Hume, C. S. (1995). Birth order and sibling sex ratio in homosexual male adolescents and probably prehomosexual feminine boys. *Developmental Psychology, 31,* 22–30.

Blanchard, R., Zucker, K. J., Cohen-Kettenis, P. T., Gooren, L. J. G., & Bailey, J. M. (1996). Birth order and sibling sex ratio in two samples of Dutch gender-dysphoric homosexual males. *Archives of Sexual Behavior, 25,* 495–514.

Bradley, S. J., Blanchard, R., Coates, S., Green, R., Levine, S. B., Meyer-Bahlburg, H. F. L., et al. (1991). Interim report of the DSM-IV subcommittee on gender identity disorders. *Archives of Sexual Behavior, 20,* 333–343.

Bradley, S. J., & Zucker, K. J. (2003). [Reply to Pickstone-Taylor]. *Journal of the American Academy of Child and Adolescent Psychiatry, 42,* 266–267.

Breedlove, S. M. (1995). Another important organ. *Nature, 378,* 15–16.

Breedlove, S. M. (1997). Sex on the brain. *Nature, 389,* 801.

Broad, K. L. (2002). GLB + T?: Gender/sexuality movements and transgender collective (de)constructions. *International Journal of Sexuality and Gender Studies, 7,* 241–264.

Brown, C. A. (1982). Sex typing in occupational preferences of high school boys and girls. In I. Gross, J. Downing, & A. d'Heurle (Eds.), *Sex role attitudes and cultural change* (pp. 81–88). Dordrecht, The Netherlands: D. Reidel.

Cate, R., & Sugawara, A. I. (1986). Sex role orientation and dimensions of self-esteem among middle adolescents. *Sex Roles, 15,* 145–158.

Chivers, M. L., Rieger, G., Latty, E., & Bailey, J. M. (2004). A sex difference in the specificity of sexual arousal. *Psychological Science, 15,* 736–744.

Chung, W. C. J., De Vries, G. J., & Swaab, D. F. (2002). Sexual differentiation of the bed nucleus of the stria terminalis in humans may extend into adulthood. *Journal of Neuroscience, 22,* 1022–1033.

Cicchetti, D., & Rogosch, F. A. (1996). Equifinality and multifinality in developmental psychopathology. *Development and Psychopathology, 8,* 597–600.

Cloud, J. (2000, September 25). His name is Aurora. *Time,* pp. 90–91.

Cohen, J. (1988). *Statistical power analysis for the social sciences* (2nd ed.). Hillsdale, NJ: Erlbaum.

Cohen, L., de Ruiter, C., Ringelberg, H., & Cohen-Kettenis, P. T. (1997). Psychological functioning of adolescent transsexuals: Personality and psychopathology. *Journal of Clinical Psychology, 53,* 187–196.

Cohen-Kettenis, P. T. (1994). Die Behandlung von Kindern und Jugendlichen mit Geschlechtsidentitäts-störungen an der Universität Utrecht [Clinical management of children and adolescents with gender identity disorders at the University of Utrecht]. *Zeitschrift für Sexualforschung, 7,* 231–239.

Cohen-Kettenis, P. T. (1995). Replik auf Bernd Meyenburg's "Kritik der hormonellen Behandlung Judendlicher mit Geschlechtsidentitätsstörungen" [Rejoinder to Bernd Meyenburg's "Criticism of hormone treatment for adolescents with gender identity disorders"]. *Zeitschrift für Sexualforschung, 8,* 165–167.

Cohen-Kettenis, P. T., & Everaerd, W. (1986). Gender role problems in adolescence. *Advances in Adolescent Mental Health, 1*(Pt. B), 1–28.

Cohen-Kettenis, P. T., Owen, A., Kaijser, V. G., Bradley, S. J., & Zucker, K. J. (2003). Demographic characteristics, social competence, and behavior problems in children with gender identity disorder: A cross-national, cross-clinic comparative analysis. *Journal of Abnormal Child Psychology, 31,* 41–53.

Cohen-Kettenis, P. T., & Pfäfflin, F. (2003). *Transgenderism and intersexuality in childhood and adolescence: Making choices.* Thousand Oaks, CA: Sage.

Cohen-Kettenis, P. T., & van Goozen, S. H. M. (1997). Sex reassignment of adolescent transsexuals: A follow-up study. *Journal of the American Academy of Child and Adolescent Psychiatry, 36,* 263–271.

Cohen-Kettenis, P. T., & van Goozen, S. H. M. (1998). Pubertal delay as an aid in diagnosis and treatment of a transsexual adolescent. *European Child and Adolescent Psychiatry, 7,* 246–248.

Cohen-Kettenis, P. T., & van Goozen, S. H. M. (2002). Adolescents who are eligible for sex reassignment surgery: Parental reports of emotional and behavioural problems. *Clinical Child Psychology and Psychiatry, 7,* 412–422.

Cohen-Kettenis, P. T., van Goozen, S. H. M., Doorn, C. D., & Gooren, L. J. G. (1998). Cognitive ability and cerebral lateralization in transsexuals. *Psychoneuroendocrinology, 23,* 631–641.

Cole, H. J., Zucker, K. J., & Bradley, S. J. (1982). Patterns of gender-role behaviour in children attending traditional and non-traditional day-care centres. *Canadian Journal of Psychiatry, 27,* 410–414.

Collaer, M. L., & Hines, M. (1995). Human behavioral sex difference: A role for gonadal hormones during early development? *Psychological Bulletin, 118,* 55–107.

Cromwell, J. (1999). *Transmen and FTMs: Identities, bodies, genders, and sexualities.* Urbana, IL: University of Illinois Press.

Danforth, N., & Schlozman, S. C. (2003). Our offices: Safe and tolerant places. *Journal of the American Academy of Child and Adolescent Psychiatry, 42,* 1522–1523.

D'Augelli, A. R. (2002). Mental health problems among lesbian, gay, and bisexual youths ages 14 to 21. *Clinical Child Psychology and Psychiatry, 7,* 433–456.

Davenport, C. W., & Harrison, S. I. (1977). Gender identity change in a female adolescent transsexual. *Archives of Sexual Behavior, 6,* 327–341.

Deaux, K. (1993). Sorry, wrong number—A reply to Gentile's call. *Psychological Science, 4,* 125–126.

Derogatis, L. (1983). *SCL-90: Administration, scoring and procedures manual for the revised version.* Baltimore: Clinical Psychometric Research.

Devor, H. (1997). *FTM: Female-to-male transsexuals in society.* Bloomington: Indiana University Press.

Dixson, A. F. (1998). *Primate sexuality: Comparative studies of the prosimians, monkeys, apes, and human beings.* Oxford, UK: Oxford University Press.

Donahoe, P. K., & Schnitzer, J. J. (1996). Evaluation of the infant who has ambiguous genitalia, and principles of operative management. *Seminars in Pediatric Surgery, 5,* 30–40.

Dulcan, M. K., & Lee, P. A. (1984). Transsexualism in the adolescent girl. *Journal of the American Academy of Child Psychiatry, 23,* 354–361.

Ellis, L., & Ames, M. A. (1987). Neurohormonal functioning and sexual orientation: A theory of homosexuality-heterosexuality. *Psychological Bulletin, 101,* 233–258.

Emory, L. E., Williams, D. H., Cole, C. M., Amparo, E. G., & Meyer, W. J. (1991). Anatomic variation of the corpus callosum in persons with gender dysphoria. *Archives of Sexual Behavior, 20,* 409–417.

Fagot, B. I. (1985). Beyond the reinforcement principle: Another step toward understanding sex role development. *Developmental Psychology, 21,* 1097–1104.

Feldman, J., & Bockting, W. (2003). Transgender health. *Minnesota Medicine, 86*(7), 25–32.

Fisk, N. (1973). Gender dysphoria syndrome (the how, what, and why of a disease). In D. Laub & P. Gandy (Eds.), *Proceedings of the Second Interdisciplinary Symposium on Gender Dysphoria Syndrome* (pp. 7–14). Palo Alto, CA: Stanford University Press.

Freund, K., Watson, R., & Rienzo, D. (1989). Heterosexuality, homosexuality, and erotic age preference. *Journal of Sex Research, 26,* 107–117.

Gagnon, J. H. (1990). The explicit and implicit use of the scripting perspective in sex research. *Annual Review of Sex Research, 1,* 1–43.

Gentile, D. A. (1993). Just what are sex and gender, anyway? A call for a new terminological standard. *Psychological Science, 4,* 120–122.

Gooren, L., & Delemarre-van de Waal, H. (1996). The feasibility of endocrine interventions in juvenile transsexuals. *Journal of Psychology and Human Sexuality, 8*(4), 69–84.

Goy, R. W., Bercovitch, F. B., & McBrair, M. C. (1988). Behavioral masculinization is independent of genital masculinization in prenatally androgenized female rhesus macaques. *Hormones and Behavior, 22,* 552–571.

Green, R. (1987). *The "sissy boy syndrome" and the development of homosexuality.* New Haven, CT: Yale University Press.

Green, R. (2000). Birth order and ratio of brothers to

sisters in transsexuals. *Psychological Medicine, 30,* 789–795.

Green, R., & Money, J. (1960). Incongruous gender role: Nongenital manifestations in prepubertal boys. *Journal of Nervous and Mental Disease, 131,* 160–168.

Green, R., & Young, R. (2000). Fingerprint asymmetry in male and female transsexuals. *Personality and Individual Differences, 29,* 933–942.

Green, R., & Young, R. (2001). Hand preference, sexual preference, and transsexualism. *Archives of Sexual Behavior, 30,* 565–574.

Grumbach, M. M., Hughes, I. A., & Conte, F. A. (2003). Disorders of sex differentiation. In P. R. Larsen, H. M. Kronenberg, S. Melmed, & K. S. Polonsky (Eds.), *Williams textbook of endocrinology* (10th ed., pp. 842–1002). Philadelphia: Saunders.

Hage, J. J. (1996). Metaidioplasty: An alternative phalloplasty technique in transsexuals. *Plastic and Reconstructive Surgery, 97,* 161–167.

Haig, D. (2004). The inexorable rise of gender and the decline of sex: Social change in academic titles. *Archives of Sexual Behavior, 33,* 87–96.

Halberstam, J. (1998). *Female masculinity.* Durham, NC: Duke University Press.

Hamburger, C. (1953). The desire for change of sex as shown by personal letters from 465 men and women. *Acta Endocrinologica, 14,* 361–375.

Haraldsen, I. R., Opjordsmoen, S., Egeland, T., & Finset, A. (2003). Sex-sensitive cognitive performance in untreated patients with early onset gender identity disorder. *Psychoneuroendocrinology, 28,* 906–915.

Harry Benjamin International Gender Dysphoria Association. (1998). *The standards of care for gender identity disorders,* Fifth version. Düsseldorf, Germany: Symposian Publishing.

Hausman, B. L. (1992). Demanding subjectivity: Transsexualism, medicine, and the technologies of gender. *Journal of the History of Sexuality, 3,* 270–302.

Haqq, C. M., & Donahoe, P. K. (1998). Regulation of sexual dimorphism in mammals. *Physiological Reviews, 78,* 1–33.

Herdt, G. (Ed.). (1994). *Third sex, third gender: Beyond sexual dimorphism in culture and history.* New York: Zone Books.

Herman-Jeglinska, A., Dulko, S., & Grabowska, A. M. (1997). Transsexuality and adextrality: Do they share a common origin? In L. Ellis & L. Ebertz (Eds.), *Sexual orientation: Toward biological understanding* (pp. 163–180). Westport, CT: Praeger.

Hines, M. (2004). *Brain gender.* New York: Oxford University Press.

Hirschfeld, M. (1923). Die intersexuelle konstitution. *Jahrbuch für Sexuelle Zwischenstufen, 23,* 3–27.

Hoenig, J. (1985). The origin of gender identity. In B. W. Steiner (Ed.), *Gender dysphoria: Development, research, management* (pp. 11–32). New York: Plenum Press.

Hoffman, J. (2003, August). Boys will be . . . girls. *Today's Parent, 20*(7), 109–116.

Hollingshead, A. B. (1975). *Four factor index of social status.* Unpublished manuscript, Department of Sociology, Yale University, New Haven, CT.

Johnson, L. L., Bradley, S. J., Birkenfeld-Adams, A. S., Radzins Kuksis, M. A., Maing, D. M., Mitchell, J. N., & Zucker, K. J. (2004). A parent-report Gender Identity Questionnaire for children. *Archives of Sexual Behavior, 33,* 105–116.

Jolles, I. (1952). A study of validity of some hypotheses for the qualitative interpretation of the H–T–P for children of elementary school age; I. Sexual identification. *Journal of Clinical Psychology, 8,* 113–118.

Juraska, J. M. (1998). Neural plasticity and the development of sex differences. *Annual Review of Sex Research, 9,* 20–38.

Keyes, S. (1984). Gender stereotypes and personal adjustment: Employing the PAQ, TSBI and GHQ with samples of British adolescents. *British Journal of Social Psychology, 23,* 173–180.

Kinsey, A. C., Pomeroy, W. B., & Martin, C. E. (1948). *Sexual behavior in the human male.* Philadelphia: Saunders.

Kline, T. J. (1998). Alain Berliner's *Ma Vie en Rose* (1997): Crossing dress, crossing boundaries. *Gender and Psychoanalysis, 3,* 435–449.

Kohlberg, L. (1966). A cognitive-developmental analysis of children's sex-role concepts and attitudes. In E. E. Maccoby (Ed.), *The development of sex differences* (pp. 82–173). Stanford, CA: Stanford University Press.

Kronberg, J., Tyano, S., Apter, A., & Wijsenbeek, H. (1981). Treatment of transsexualism in adolescence. *Journal of Adolescence, 4,* 177–185.

Kruiver, F. P. M., Zhou, J.-N., Pool, C. W., Hofman, M. A., Gooren, L. J. G., & Swaab, D. F. (2000). Male-to-female transsexuals have female neuron numbers in a limbic nucleus. *Journal of Clinical Endocrinology and Metabolism, 85,* 2034–2041.

Kulick, D. (1998). *Travesti: Sex, gender, and culture among Brazilian transgendered prostitutes.* Chicago: University of Chicago Press.

Lalumière, M. L., Blanchard, R., & Zucker, K. J. (2000). Sexual orientation and handedness in men and women: A meta-analysis. *Psychological Bulletin, 126,* 575–592.

Laner, M. R. (2000). "Sex" versus "gender": A renewed plea. *Sociological Inquiry, 70,* 462–474.

Laqueur, T. (1992). *Making sex: Body and gender from the Greeks to Freud.* Cambridge, MA: Harvard University Press.

Laumann, E. O., Gagnon, J. H., Michael, R. T., & Michaels, S. (1994). *The social organization of sexuality: Sexual practices in the United States.* Chicago: University of Chicago Press.

Lawrence, A. A. (2003). Factors associated with satisfaction or regret following male-to-female sex reassignment surgery. *Archives of Sexual Behavior, 32,* 299–315.

Lee, T. (2001). Trans(re)lations: Lesbian and female to male transsexual accounts of identity. *Women's Studies International Forum, 24,* 347–357.

Lippa, R. A. (2003). Are 2D:4D finger-length ratios related to sexual orientation? Yes for men, no for women. *Journal of Personality and Social Psychology, 85,* 179–188.

Lombardi, E. L., Wilchins, R. A., Priesing, D., & Malouf, D. (2001). Gender violence: Transgender experiences with violence and discrimination. *Journal of Homosexuality, 42,* 89–101.

Lothstein, L. M. (1983). *Female-to-male transsexualism: Historical, clinical, and theoretical issues.* Boston: Routledge & Kegan Paul.

Maccoby, E. E. (1988). Gender as a social category. *Developmental Psychology, 24,* 755–765.

Martin, C. L., Ruble, D. N., & Szkrybalo, J. (2002). Cognitive theories of early gender development. *Psychological Bulletin, 128,* 903–933.

Massad, C. M. (1981). Sex role identity and adjustment during adolescence. *Child Development, 52,* 1290–1298.

Mathy, R. M. (2002). Transgender identity and suicidality in a nonclinical sample: Sexual orientation, psychiatric history, and compulsive behaviors. *Journal of Psychology and Human Sexuality, 14(4),* 47–65.

McCarthy, L. (2003). *Off that spectrum entirely: A study of female-bodied transgender-identified individuals.* Unpublished doctoral dissertation, University of Massachusetts, Amherst.

Memorial for Harry Benjamin. (1988). *Archives of Sexual Behavior, 17,* 1–31.

Meyenburg, B. (1994). Kritik der hormonellen Behandlung Judendlicher mit Geschlechtsidentitätsstörungen [Criticisms of hormone treatment for adolescents with gender identity disorders]. *Zeitschrift für Sexualforschung, 7,* 343–349.

Meyenburg, B. (1999). Gender identity disorder in adolescence: Outcomes of psychotherapy. *Adolescence, 34,* 305–313.

Meyer, I. H. (2003). Prejudice, social stress, and mental health issues in lesbian, gay, and bisexual populations: Conceptual issues and research evidence. *Psychological Bulletin, 129,* 674–697.

Meyer-Bahlburg, H. F. L. (1984). Psychoendocrine research on sexual orientation: Current status and future options. *Progress in Brain Research, 61,* 375–398.

Meyer-Bahlburg, H. F. L. (1985). Gender identity disorder of childhood: Introduction. *Journal of the American Academy of Child Psychiatry, 24,* 681–683.

Meyerowitz, J. (1998). Sex change and the popular press: Historical notes on transsexuality in the United States, 1930–1955. *GLQ, 4,* 159–187.

Meyerowitz, J. (2002). *How sex changed: A history of transsexuality in the United States.* Cambridge, MA: Harvard University Press.

Migeon, C. J., & Wisniewski, A. B. (1998). Sexual differentiation: From genes to gender. *Hormone Research, 50,* 245–251.

Money, J. (1955). Hermaphroditism, gender and precocity in hyperadrenocorticism: Psychologic findings. *Bulletin of the Johns Hopkins Hospital, 96,* 253–264.

Money, J. (1984). Paraphilias: Phenomenology and classification. *American Journal of Psychotherapy, 38,* 164–179.

Money, J. (1985). The conceptual neutering of gender and the criminalization of sex. *Archives of Sexual Behavior, 14,* 279–290.

Money, J. (1986). *Lovemaps: Clinical concepts of sexual/erotic health and pathology, paraphilia, and gender transposition in childhood, adolescence, and maturity.* New York: Irvington.

Money, J., & Ehrhardt, A. A. (1972). *Man and woman, boy and girl: The differentiation and dimorphism of gender identity from conception to maturity.* Baltimore: Johns Hopkins Press.

Moore, K. L., & Barr, M. L. (1955). Smears from the oral mucosa in the detection of chromosomal sex. *Lancet, 2,* 57–58.

Mussen, P. H. (1962). Long-term consequences of masculinity of interests in adolescence. *Journal of Consulting Psychology, 26,* 435–440.

Mustanski, B. S., Chivers, M. L., & Bailey, J. M. (2002). A critical review of recent biological research on human sexual orientation. *Annual Review of Sex Research, 13,* 89–140.

Newman, L. E. (1970). Transsexualism in adolescence: Problems in evaluation and treatment. *Archives of General Psychiatry, 23,* 112–121.

Newman, L. K. (2002). Sex, gender and culture: Issues in the definition, assessment and treatment of gender identity disorder. *Clinical Child Psychology and Psychiatry, 7,* 352–359.

Petersen, M. E., & Dickey, R. (1995). Surgical sex reassignment: A comparative survey of international centers. *Archives of Sexual Behavior, 24,* 135–156.

Philippopoulos, G. S. (1964). A case of transvestism in a 17-year-old girl: Psychopathology–psychodynamics. *Acta Psychotherapeutica, 12,* 29–37.

Pickstone-Taylor, S. D. (2003). Children with gender nonconformity [Letter]. *Journal of the American Academy of Child and Adolescent Psychiatry, 42,* 266.

Pleak, R. R. (1999). Ethical issues in diagnosing and treating gender-dysphoric children and adolescents. In M. Rottnek (Ed.), *Sissies and tomboys: Gender nonconformity and homosexual childhood* (pp. 34–51). New York: New York University Press.

Poasa, K. H., Blanchard, R., & Zucker, K. J. (2004). Birth order in transgendered males from Polynesia: A quantitative study of Samoan fa'afafine. *Journal of Sex and Marital Therapy, 30,* 13–23.

Prosser, J. (1998). *Second skins: The body narratives of transsexuality.* New York: Columbia University Press.

Rahman, Q., & Wilson, G. D. (2003). Born gay? The

psychobiology of human sexual orientation. *Personality and Individual Differences, 34,* 1337–1382.

Rekers, G. A., Sanders, J. A., & Strauss, C. C. (1981). Developmental differentiation of adolescent body gestures. *Journal of Genetic Psychology, 138,* 123–131.

Rosen, R. C., & Beck, J. G. (1988). *Patterns of sexual arousal: Psychophysiological processes and clinical applications.* New York: Guilford Press.

Rosenberg, M. (2002). Children with gender identity issues and their parents in individual and group treatment. *Journal of the American Academy of Child and Adolescent Psychiatry, 41,* 619–621.

Rosenberg, M. (2003). Recognizing gay, lesbian, and transgender teens in a child and adolescent psychiatry practice. *Journal of the American Academy of Child and Adolescent Psychiatry, 42,*1517–1521.

Ross, M. W. (1983). *The married homosexual man: A psychological study.* Boston: Routledge & Kegan Paul.

Ruble, D. N., & Martin, C. L. (1998). Gender development. In W. Damon (Series Ed.) & N. Eisenberg (Vol. Ed.), *The handbook of child psychology. Vol. 3: Social, emotional, and personality development* (5th ed., pp. 933–1016). New York: Wiley.

Rust, P. C. (1999, June). *Lesbianism and bisexuality: Cultural categories and the distortion of human sexual experience.* Paper presented at the meeting of the International Academy of Sex Research, Stony Brook, NY.

Sadowski, H., & Gaffney, N. (1998). Gender identity disorder, depression, and suicidal risk. In D. Di Ceglie (Ed.), *A stranger in my own body: Atypical gender identity development and mental health* (pp. 126–136). London: Karnac Books.

Sandberg, D. E., Meyer-Bahlburg, H. F. L., & Yager, T. J. (1993). Feminine gender role behavior and academic achievement: Their relation in a community sample of middle childhood boys. *Sex Roles, 29,* 125–140.

Sandnabba, N. K., & Ahlberg, C. (1999). Parents' attitudes and expectations about children's cross-gender behavior. *Sex Roles, 40,* 249–263.

Savin-Williams, R. C., & Ream, G. L. (2003). Suicide attempts among sexual-minority male youth. *Journal of Clinical Child and Adolescent Psychology, 32,* 509–522.

Slabbekoorn, D., van Goozen, S. H. M., Sanders, G., Gooren, L. J. G., & Cohen-Kettenis, P. T. (2000). The dermatoglyphic characteristics of transsexuals: Is there evidence for an organizing effect of sex hormones? *Psychoneuroendocrinology, 25,* 365–375.

Sloop, J. M. (2000). Disciplining the transgendered: Brandon Teena, public representation, and normativity. *Western Journal of Communication, 64,* 165–189.

Smith, Y. L. S., Cohen, L., & Cohen-Kettenis, P. T. (2002). Postoperative psychological functioning of adolescent transsexuals: A Rorschach study. *Archives of Sexual Behavior, 31,* 255–261.

Smith, Y. L. S., van Goozen, S. H. M., & Cohen-Kettenis, P. T. (2001). Adolescents with gender identity disorder who were accepted or rejected for sex reassignment surgery: A prospective follow-up study. *Journal of the American Academy of Child and Adolescent Psychiatry, 40,* 472–481.

Sroufe, L. A. (1990). Considering normal and abnormal together: The essence of developmental psychopathology. *Development and Psychopathology, 2,* 335–347.

Stoller, R. J. (1964). The hermaphroditic identity of hermaphrodites. *Journal of Nervous and Mental Disease, 139,* 453–457.

Storms, M. D. (1980). Theories of sexual orientation. *Journal of Personality and Social Psychology, 38,* 783–792.

Streitmatter, J. L. (1985). Cross-sectional investigations of adolescent perception of gender roles. *Journal of Adolescence, 8,* 183–193.

Swaab, D. F., Chung, W. C. J., Kruijver, F. P. M., Hofman, M. A., & Hestiantoro, A. (2003). Sex difference in the hypothalamus in the different stages of human life. *Neurobiology of Aging, 24,* S1–S6.

Swanson, D. P., Spencer, M. B., Harpalani, V., Dupree, D., Noll, E, Ginzburg, S., & Seaton, G. (2003). Psychosocial development in racially and ethnically diverse youth: Conceptual and methodological challenges in the 21st century. *Development and Psychopathology, 15,* 743–771.

Theobald, S. (2003, May 2). I'm a girl–just call me "he." *The Guardian.*

Tucker, J. B., & Keil, H. H. J. (2001). Can cultural beliefs cause a gender identity disorder? *Journal of Psychology and Human Sexuality, 13*(2), 21–30.

Unger, R. K. (1979). Toward a redefinition of sex and gender. *American Psychologist, 34,* 1085–1094.

Unger, R. K., & Crawford, M. (1993). The troubled relationship between terms and concepts. *Psychological Science, 4,* 122–124.

van Goozen, Slabbekoorn, D., Gooren, L. J. G., Sanders, G., & Cohen-Kettenis, P. T. (2002). Organizing and activating effects of sex hormones in homosexual transsexuals. *Behavioral Neuroscience, 116,* 982–988.

Vilain, E. (2000). Genetics of sexual development. *Annual Review of Sex Research, 11,* 1–25.

Vilain, E., & McCabe, E. R. B. (1998). Mammalian sex determination: From gonads to brain. *Molecular Genetics and Metabolism, 65,* 74–84.

Wallen, K. (1996). Nature needs nurture: The interaction of hormonal and social influences on the development of behavioral sex differences in rhesus monkeys. *Hormones and Behavior, 30,* 364–378.

Wallen, K., & Baum, M. J. (2002). Masculinization and defeminization in altricial and precocial mammals: Comparative aspects of steroid hormone action. *Hormones, Brain and Behavior, 4,* 385–423.

Weeks, J. (1991). *Against nature: Essays on history, sexuality, and identity.* London: Rivers Oram Press.

Willox, A. (2003). Branding Teena: (Mis)representations in the media. *Sexualities, 6*, 407–425.

Wren, B. (2000). Early physical intervention for young people with atypical gender identity development. *Clinical Child Psychology and Psychiatry, 5*, 220–231.

Wren, B. (2002). "I can accept my child is transsexual but if I ever see him in a dress I'll hit him": Dilemmas in parenting a transgendered adolescent. *Clinical Child Psychology and Psychiatry, 7*, 377–397.

Young, R., & Sweeting, H. (2004). Adolescent bullying, relationships, psychological well-being, and gender atypical behavior: A gender diagnosticity approach. *Sex Roles, 50*, 525–537.

Zhou, J.-N., Hofman, M. A., Gooren, L. J., & Swaab, D. F. (1995). A sex difference in the human brain and its relation to transsexuality. *Nature, 378*, 68–70.

Zucker, K. J. (1992). Gender identity disorder. In S. R. Hooper, G. W. Hynd, & R. E. Mattison (Eds.), *Child psychopathology: Diagnostic criteria and clinical assessment* (pp. 305–342). Hillsdale, NJ: Erlbaum.

Zucker, K. J. (1999). Intersexuality and gender identity differentiation. *Annual Review of Sex Research, 10*, 1–69.

Zucker, K. J. (2003a, September). *Debating DSM.* Paper presented at the meeting of the Harry Benjamin International Gender Dysphoria Association, Gent, Belgium.

Zucker, K. J. (2003b, September). *Persistence and desistance of gender identity disorder in children.* Paper presented at the meeting of the Harry Benjamin International Gender Dysphoria Association, Gent, Belgium.

Zucker, K. J., Beaulieu, N., Bradley, S. J., Grimshaw, G. M., & Wilcox, A. (2001). Handedness in boys with gender identity disorder. *Journal of Child Psychology and Psychiatry, 42*, 767–776.

Zucker, K. J., & Blanchard, R. (1997). Transvestic fetishism: Psychopathology and theory. In D. R. Laws & W. O'Donohue (Eds.), *Sexual deviance: Theory, assessment, and treatment* (pp. 253–279). New York: Guilford Press.

Zucker, K. J., & Bradley, S. J. (1995). *Gender identity disorder and psychosexual problems in children and adolescents.* New York: Guilford Press.

Zucker, K. J., Bradley, S. J., Oliver, G., Blake, J., Fleming, S., & Hood, J. (1996). Psychosexual development of women with congenital adrenal hyperplasia. *Hormones and Behavior, 30*, 300–318.

Zucker, K. J., Bradley, S. J., Lowry Sullivan, C. B., Kuksis, M., Birkenfeld-Adams, A., & Mitchell, J. N. (1993). A gender identity interview for children. *Journal of Personality Assessment, 61*, 443–456.

Zucker, K. J., Bradley, S. J., & Sanikhani, M. (1997). Sex differences in referral rates of children with gender identity disorder: Some hypotheses. *Journal of Abnormal Child Psychology, 25*, 217–227.

Zucker, K. J., Deogracias, J. J., Johnson, L. L., Meyer-Bahlburg, H. F. L., Kessler, S. J., & Schober, J. M. (2005, July). *The Gender Identity Questionnaire for Adults and the Recalled Childhood Gender Questionnaire—Revised: Final analyses.* Poster session presented at the meeting of the International Academy of Sex Research, Ottawa, ON, Canada.

Zucker, K. J., Green, R., Coates, S., Zuger, B., Cohen-Kettenis, P. T., Zecca, G. M., et al. (1997). Sibling sex ratio of boys with gender identity disorder. *Journal of Child Psychology and Psychiatry, 38*, 543–551.

Zucker, K. J., Lozinski, J. A., Bradley, S. J., & Doering, R. W. (1992). Sex-typed responses in the Rorschach protocols of children with gender identity disorder. *Journal of Personality Assessment, 58*, 295–310.

Zucker, K. J., Mitchell, J. N., Bradley, S. J., Tkachuk, J., & Allin, S. (2004). *The Recalled Childhood Gender Identity/Gender Role Questionnaire: Psychometric properties.* Manuscript submitted for publication.

Zucker, K. J., Owen, A., Bradley, S. J., & Ameeriar, L. (2002). Gender-dysphoric children and adolescents: A comparative analysis of demographic characteristics and behavioral problems. *Clinical Child Psychology and Psychiatry, 7*, 398–411.

Zucker, K. J., Wilson-Smith, D. N., Kurita, J. A., & Stern, A. (1995). Children's appraisals of sex-typed behavior in their peers. *Sex Roles, 33*, 703–725.

17

Sexual Risk Behavior

Beth A. Kotchick
Lisa Armistead
Rex L. Forehand

With the tragic consequences of the world AIDS epidemic continuing to mount, the need for comprehensive and effective prevention strategies is critical. Researchers and clinicians alike are carefully considering the range of factors that predispose the world's most vulnerable populations to exposure to the disease. Unlike many other devastating diseases, AIDS uniquely lends itself to potential control and prevention through behavioral change. Sexual contact with a person infected with HIV, the virus known to cause AIDS, is a primary avenue for new infections, especially for young persons between the ages of 13 and 25 (Centers for Disease Control and Prevention [CDC], 2001). As such, professional and public attention has increasingly been directed to the numerous health risks of unsafe sexual behavior among adolescents, and to the examination of the psychosocial context in which sexual initiation and sexual risk-taking behavior occur (see Kotchick, Shaffer, Forehand, & Miller, 2001).

This chapter examines adolescent sexual risk behavior, its associated risks to health and well-being, and the factors identified in the clinical and public health literature related to the promotion of sexual risk-taking and risk-reduction practices. It is written with the scholarly practitioner in mind; all those who work with adolescents in a clinical or community setting must acknowledge that sexuality is a part of the typical adolescent experience and thus is worthy of exploration and understanding as case conceptualizations are being formed. While relatively few adolescents may be specifically referred for treatment as a result of concern over their sexual risk behavior or its consequences, sexual risk taking may be an important piece of the larger clinical picture. For example, sexual risk taking may be part of a constellation of problem behaviors in need of clinical intervention (e.g., among youth with conduct disorder or antisocial disorder), or it may be a contributing factor to psychological or emotional distress (e.g., depression and anxiety). And certainly, the biological and social impact of puberty and its associated physical changes during adolescence is large enough to warrant some attention from clinical providers no matter what is identified as the presenting problem.

However, a recent review of empirically supported treatments for adolescent mental health problems revealed that most treatment studies do not address physical or sexual development in either their evaluation of treatment effects or the development of interventions themselves (Weisz & Hawley, 2002). Likewise, it is unclear whether treatment providers make a common practice of considering sexual development or sexual behavior in their assessment, conceptualization, or treatment of their adolescent clients.

Thus, this chapter provides a context within which adolescent sexual behavior may be considered by identifying factors across multiple systems that may promote risk or interfere with healthy sexual development. In doing so, we strive to present the available research on adolescent sexual risk behavior and its prevention from a multisystemic perspective. Such a view holds that adolescent sexual risk behavior is shaped by factors falling into several nested levels of influence, including the self, the family, and the social context.

We begin by summarizing the available data on the prevalence of sexual risk behavior among adolescents. Next, we discuss adolescent sexual development and consider the social and political forces that shape the definition of appropriate and inappropriate sexual expression during adolescence. Third, we provide information pertaining to the health and psychosocial risks associated with sexual risk behavior among youth, including AIDS, other sexually transmitted diseases, and teenage pregnancy. Fourth, we describe what is currently understood about the psychosocial factors that have been associated with adolescent sexual risk behavior. Fifth, we offer a discussion of the theoretical underpinnings of prevention efforts designed to reduce adolescent sexual risk behavior, as well as a review of the empirically evaluated prevention programs currently available. Finally, we offer some thoughts regarding what is needed to enhance our understanding of adolescent sexual risk behavior and its prevention.

ADOLESCENT SEXUAL RISK: BEHAVIORAL TRENDS

Adolescent Sexual Activity

Consistent data across a number of national surveys indicate that American adolescents are initiating sexual activity at earlier ages, and that a considerable number of adolescents are currently sexually active. According to the 2003 Youth Risk Behavior Surveillance (YRBS) data, just over 45% of students in grades 9–12 have engaged in sexual intercourse (Grunbaum et al., 2004). This figure represents a decline in youth reporting sexual activity from previous YRBS reports when 49.9% of sampled students indicated they were sexually experienced (Kann et al., 1998). However, a substantial number of young persons in the Unites States continue to report that they have engaged in sexual intercourse at least once. Rates of sexual activity appear to be higher for males, ethnic minority adolescents, and adolescents of lower socioeconomic status (Grunbaum et al., 2004; Leigh, Morrison, Trocki, & Temple, 1994; Seidman & Reider, 1994).

National survey data published during the past 5 years also reveal that a considerable proportion of teenagers are initiating sexual activity by early or middle adolescence, with estimates ranging from nearly 7% to 17% of teens reporting sexual initiation prior to age 13 or grade 9 (Grunbaum et al., 2004; Resnick et al., 1997). Early initiation of sexual activity appears to be more prevalent among ethnic minority adolescents: black and Hispanic teens tend to report higher rates of sexual involvement at younger ages than their Caucasian peers (Grunbaum et al., 2004; Leigh et al., 1994; Romer et al., 1994; Seidman & Reider, 1994; Stanton et al., 1994). These differences are most likely due to socioeconomic and community factors. For example, a study of African American high school students identified as being a high risk for school dropout found that 77% of sexually active females experienced sexual intercourse for the first time between ages 13 and 14, and 73% of sexually active males became sexually experienced between the ages of 12 and 13 (Ramirez-Valles, Zimmerman, & Juarez, 2002).

Noncoital sexual behaviors, such as mutual masturbation and oral sex, are also of significant concern. These sexual behaviors are associated with the risk of contracting sexually transmitted diseases and are often viewed as precursors, and thus predictors, of sexual intercourse. However, the prevalence of noncoital behaviors is difficult to ascertain. Many surveys of adolescent sexual behavior either limit their assessment to penile–vaginal sexual intercourse or fail to explicitly define what is meant by sexual intercourse in their measures. In addition, real and perceived difficulties in obtaining parental consent for surveys about sexual activity among adolescents, as well as reluctance on the part of federal funding agencies to sponsor such research, have hampered behavioral scientists' efforts to document the prevalence of noncoital behaviors among the nation's youth (see Remez, 2000, for discussion).

Nevertheless, the studies that do exist suggest that sexual activity other than penile–vaginal intercourse is quite common among adolescents. For example, data collected in the 1980s indicates that roughly 20% of 13–18-year-olds report having ever had oral sex (Coles & Stokes, 1985), while another survey of junior high school students in 1982 indicated that 53% of males and 42% of females had experienced oral sex (Newcomer & Udry, 1985). A more recent study found that approximately 20% of 12–15-year-old adolescents receiving general health examinations in the Washington, DC, area reported having experienced oral sex (Boekeloo & Howard, 2002). Recent media reports appearing in such publications as the *New York Times*, *Washington Post*, *Talk* magazine, and *Seventeen* magazine provide further support that noncoital behavior is prevalent, particularly among younger teens who have not yet experienced penile–vaginal intercourse (Remez, 2000). Most important, these reports indicate that youth who are engaging in these behaviors do not see them as risky, or even intimate; rather, oral sex is viewed as a safe alternative to sexual intercourse for those who wish to remain abstinent, and as casual as a good-night kiss (e.g., Jarrell, 2000).

Adolescent Sexual Risk Behavior

Considering the rate of sexual activity among adolescents, it is of significant concern that many sexually active teenagers engage in behaviors that are considered risky or unsafe and that may expose them to HIV/AIDS, other sexually transmitted diseases (STDs), or unintended pregnancy. For example, recent national data indicate that 25.6% of sexually active students used alcohol or drugs at the time of their most recent sexual experience (Grunbaum et al., 2004). Regarding condom use, only half of sexually active adolescents report using a condom during their most recent sexual encounter (Grunbaum et al., 2004), and only a small proportion (i.e., approximately 10–20%) of sexually active adolescents report using condoms consistently (DiClemente et al., 1992; Kann et al., 1995; Seidman & Rieder, 1994). When assessed, the use of condoms or other barrier methods of protection (e.g., dental dams) during oral sex appears to be extremely low (Boekeloo & Howard, 2002).

Sexual risk may also be measured by the number of sexual partners reported by adolescents. Because adolescents tend to engage in sexual activities in the context of serial monogamous sexual relationships that are of short duration, their exposure to multiple sexual partners and, subsequently, their risk of HIV infection and other negative consequences of sexual risk-taking behavior is increased (Overby & Kegeles, 1994). The most recent data from the CDC and the YRBS system indicate that approximately 14% of high school students nationwide report having had at least four sexual partners in their lifetime, with male students being more likely than female students to report having had four or more lifetime sexual partners (Grunbaum et al., 2004).

Gender and Ethnicity

Although sexual activities appear to vary by adolescent gender and race, male and female adolescents across all studied ethnic groups engage in some sexual practices that place them at risk for HIV, STDs, or pregnancy (Luster & Small, 1994; Tubman, Windle, & Windle, 1996). For example, boys report higher rates of sexual activity and more sexual partners than do girls (Grunbaum et al., 2004; Tubman et al., 1996), but girls tend to report less consistent use of condoms with their sexual partners than do boys (Romer et al., 1994; Shrier, Emans, Woods, & DuRant, 1996).

In terms of ethnicity, earlier national surveys have found higher rates of sexual activity and less consistent use of condoms among ethnic minority youth as compared to white adolescents (Airhihenbuwa, DiClemente, Wingood, & Lowe, 1992; Brown, DiClemente, & Park, 1992); however, more recent studies have found that both male and female black high school students were more likely to report using a condom the last time they had sexual intercourse than were their white or Hispanic peers (Grunbaum et al., 2004). In one of the only studies of adolescent sexual risk behavior to include Asian adolescents, Hou and Basen-Engquist (1997) found that Asian Pacific Islander youth were more likely to have multiple sexual partners but less likely to report having used alcohol or drugs prior to sexual intercourse than their white peers. Clearly, studies examining racial and gender differences in sexual behavior and risk-reduction strategies yield inconsistent results, with the findings depending on the racial groups being compared and the sexual behaviors being considered.

SOCIAL AND DEVELOPMENTAL PERSPECTIVES

The confluence of biological, cognitive, and psychosocial changes occurring during the period of adolescence results in a developmental stage characterized by growth and transition. At the same time, adolescents find themselves in many situations that provide ample opportunity for young persons to make decisions about engaging in behaviors such as sexual risk behavior that have important implications for health and safety (Millstein, Petersen, & Nightingale, 1993). Several different perspectives have been offered to account for the propensity of adolescents to act in ways that could potentially compromise their physical and emotional well-being. Some authors suggest that adolescents engage in risk behaviors to mark their transition to adulthood (e.g., Jessor, Costa, Jessor, & Donovan, 1983). This is the central premise of problem behavior theory, which posits that sexual risk behavior is linked with other problem or risk behaviors, such as substance use and delinquent activity, and represents a general tendency toward nonconformity and a desire to identify oneself as mature and independent (Jessor et al., 1983; Jessor & Jessor, 1977).

Critics of problem behavior theory would argue that applying a label of "problematic" or "deviant" to adolescent sexual behavior ignores the developmental processes occurring during this period, including the process by which a child becomes a physically mature, and thus sexually mature, adult. Puberty is accompanied by numerous physical, hormonal, emotional, and social changes, with the end result being a fully physically mature person who now has the capacity to conceive and bear children. Puberty also brings with it an increased awareness of one's own sexuality and a natural interest in romantic and sexual relationships. Research concerning pubertal development has highlighted that both boys and girls are maturing at earlier ages than in the past. For example, the average age of menarche among American girls is currently 12–13 years, down from age 16 approximately 150 years ago (Hamburg, 1992).

The downward trend in the age at which youth become physically mature has been identified as one potential explanation for the increase in adolescent sexual activity seen over the past several decades (Chapin, 2000). Sexual experimentation in adolescence has become, to many developmentalists, a normative event in modern society (Ensminger, 1987). Certainly, when nearly half of high school students report being sexually experienced, one can no longer classify that event as being atypical (Grunbaum et al., 2004). However, although their bodies may have matured to the point of being sexual "equals" with adults, physically mature adolescents are still undergoing substantial growth in other areas that directly affect how they handle and respond to sexual situations.

Perhaps most important, the cognitive development occurring during adolescence is critical to understanding risk behavior. It is during adolescence that individuals develop the ability to engage in abstract thinking and to anticipate the potential consequences of their actions. Adolescents do not yet have the ability to engage in the hypothetical reasoning necessary to realistically evaluate the probability that behavior in the present may have negative consequences in the future (Cothran & White, 2002), which leads to a sense of personal invulnerability or optimistic bias (Elkind, 1967). Thus, the "normative" physical development that often characterizes early to middle adolescence does not necessarily equate with the cognitive maturity needed to safely engage in sexual behavior with minimal risk of adverse health consequences.

HEALTH RISKS ASSOCIATED WITH ADOLESCENT SEXUAL BEHAVIOR

Concern over adolescents' ability to consider the health consequences of risky sexual behavior is certainly well warranted. Sexual risk-taking behavior, such as inconsistent condom use and sex with multiple partners, has already had devastating effects on the health of American adolescents. Recent surveillance data indicate that over 4,200 cases of AIDS have been diagnosed in the United States among persons between 13 and 19 years of age, with another 2,532 cases of HIV infection within this age bracket being reported from states with confidential HIV infection reporting (CDC, 2001). However, these figures likely represent a gross underestimate of the number of individuals who become infected during adolescence. The most recent surveillance data indicate that another 32,700 cases of HIV have been identified among adults ages 20–29 (CDC, 2001). Because HIV has a median incubation period of approximately 10 years, a large proportion of adults diagnosed with AIDS in their 20s are thought to have become infected with HIV during their adolescence (Chesney, 1994; Joseph, 1991; Rosenberg, Biggar, & Goedert, 1994). As such, many more adolescents may be unknowingly infected with HIV than the current surveillance data reports.

National data also reveal that 15–19-year-old adolescents have the highest rates of gonorrhea and chlamydia in the United States (CDC, 2000; Department of Health and Human Services, 1997), and infections appear to be on the rise (CDC, 2000). For example, the rates of gonorrhea among adolescents increased 13% between 1997 and 1999 (CDC, 2000). In addition, a national survey conducted between 1970 and 1990 indicated that new herpes infections increased most dramatically among Caucasian teens between the ages of 12 and 19 (Fleming et al., 1997).

The United States also has one of the highest teenage pregnancy rates among Western industrialized countries (see Kirby et al., 1994). Recent data suggest that nearly 4 in 10 young women become pregnant at least once before they reach the age of 20, with 80% of these pregnancies being unintended and 79% among unmarried teens (Henshaw, 1998; Martin, Hamilton, Ventura, Menacher, & Park, 2002). The annual financial cost of teen pregnancy for the United States totals approximately $7 billion, and the social costs are great for the adolescent: Teen mothers are less likely to complete high school and often end up on welfare (National Campaign to Prevent Teen Pregnancy, 2002).

Statistics such as these underscore the fact that the consequences of adolescent sexual risk-taking behavior are of grave concern and are in immediate need of efforts to prevent their occurrence. To do so effectively, we need to identify and understand the factors that contribute to sexual risk behavior among American adolescents. This includes a better understanding of the psychosocial context surrounding the initiation of sexual activity, as well as the factors influencing adolescents' decisions to engage in behaviors (e.g., sex with multiple partners and unprotected sexual intercourse) considered to be sexually "risky" because of potential exposure to HIV/AIDS, other STDs, or pregnancy.

CONTRIBUTING FACTORS: A MULTISYSTEMIC PERSPECTIVE

Sexual risk behavior, like many other problematic behaviors of youth, has been studied for quite some time (see Brooks-Gunn & Furstenberg; 1989; Goodson, Evans, & Edmundson, 1997; Miller & Moore, 1990, for earlier reviews). However, the research that has accumulated thus far still leaves two important issues to be addressed. First, most existing literature on adolescent sexuality has framed *all* sexual behavior among youth as being problematic, resulting in little empirical attention having been devoted to the typical developmental processes involved in becoming a sexually healthy adult. Second, until fairly recently, empirical studies of adolescent sexual behavior have made little effort to integrate the literature into a conceptual framework that simultaneously considers multiple systems of influence and the complexity of their combined effects on adolescent behavior (see Miller, Forehand, & Kotchick, 2000; Resnick et al., 1997; Small & Luster, 1994, for exceptions).

In this chapter, we briefly summarize the literature on adolescent sexual risk behavior from a multisystemic perspective (Figure 17.1). Such an approach is guided by Bronfrenbrenner's (1979, 1989) ecological systems theory, which emphasizes the reciprocal relations among multiple systems of influence on a person's behavior. According to this perspective, an accurate and comprehensive understanding of adolescent sexual risk behavior must necessarily include some knowledge of both the personal and the environmental factors that may contribute to the decision to become sexually active and, subsequently, the decision to engage in risk-promoting or risk-reducing sexual behaviors.

Our approach is similar to that adopted by other leading researchers in the area of adolescent risk behavior, most notably ecodevelopmental theory proposed by Szapocznik and Coatsworth (1999). Like our multisystemic perspective, ecodevelopmental theory suggests

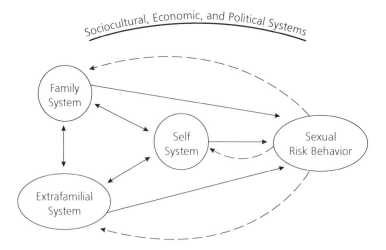

FIGURE 17.1. A multisystemic perspective on adolescent sexual risk behavior.

that understanding the risk and protective factors that contribute to adolescent behavior requires consideration of the multiple social systems (e.g., family, peers, school, and neighborhood) that provide a context within which those factors occur (see Perrino, Gonzalez-Soldevilla, Pantin, & Szapocznik, 2000; Szapocznik & Coatsworth, 1999). What these perspectives share is an approach to organizing knowledge about adolescent sexual risk behavior into a framework that considers the breadth and complexity of the adolescent sexual experience, and a commitment to applying this framework to the development of the most comprehensive intervention and prevention efforts.

To this end, we focus our attention on three "systems" of influence believed to be the primary contributors to adolescent sexual behavior: the self, family, and extrafamilial systems (see Figure 17.1). Interventions designed to reduce or prevent sexual risk behavior may target each system independently, though perhaps the most effective approach is to simultaneously address all three systems and their interaction.

The Self System: Biological, Psychological, and Behavioral Variables

The most proximal set of factors related to sexual risk behavior is contained within the adolescent him- or herself. Many studies have sought to identify the biological, psychological, and behavioral variables that are related to sexual risk behavior with varying success.

Biological Factors

Adolescent age, pubertal timing, and physical development, as well as gender and ethnicity, represent the self-system variables that may be considered biologically determined and that have been shown to relate to adolescent sexual risk behavior.

Not surprisingly, older adolescents report more sexual activity and having more partners than do younger teens (e.g., Grunbaum et al., 2004; Harvey & Spigner, 1995; Miller et al., 2000). In addition, older age has been associated with less consistent condom use in both minority and mixed-race samples (Anderson et al., 1990; Pendergrast, DuRant, & Gaillard, 1992; Reitman et al., 1996; Shrier et al., 1996). This latter finding is most likely due to the context surrounding sexual relationships among older adolescents; older adolescents are more likely than their younger peers to be involved in stable, monogamous romantic relationships in which sexual intercourse is a sign of intimacy and attachment (Feiring, 1996). In such relationships, contraceptive use is geared more toward pregnancy prevention than disease prevention, and the use of barrier methods, such as condoms, is less frequently endorsed.

A variable inherently confounded with age is pubertal development. Early pubertal development has been found to relate to an earlier age of sexual debut for both males and females (Capaldi, Crosby, & Stoolmiller, 1996; Miller, Norton, Curtis, Hil, Schvaneveldt, & Young, 1997; Miller, Norton, Fan, & Christopherson,

1998). In addition, self-report of appearing older or more mature than peers has been found to relate to earlier sexual involvement in a nationally representative sample (Resnick et al., 1997). Earlier age at menarche has also been found to correlate with riskier sexual practices, most likely by increasing the risk of early-maturing girls affiliating with older boyfriends, which, in turn, increases the chance of engaging in sexual risk behavior (Mezzich et al., 1997). In addition, Baumeister, Flores, and Marin (1995) found that, among Latina adolescents, later age at menarche was associated with *not* becoming pregnant in adolescence.

As noted earlier, adolescent age, gender, and race have all been correlated with various measures of sexual risk behavior. However, the findings are often inconsistent, with the results varying by the sexual risk behaviors being examined. Inconsistencies in rates of sexual risk behavior across age, gender and racial groups may also be explained by the psychosocial factors that are so inherently tied with those categorical variables. For example, adolescent age is often confounded with physical development, which has an impact not only on the adolescent but also on the way he or she is perceived by others. Likewise, both race and gender have multiple psychosocial correlates that may account for the differences found with respect to adolescent sexual behavior, including socioeconomic status (SES), education, access to health care and family planning services, experience of sexual coercion, and cultural expectations for male and female sexual behavior (e.g., Biglan, Noell, Ochs, Smolkowski, & Metzler, 1995). A review of all the literature pertaining to adolescent age, gender, and race and their relation to sexual risk behavior is well beyond the scope of this chapter; the reader is referred to Kotchick and colleagues (2001) for a more comprehensive examination of these issues.

Psychological Factors

Several cognitive and emotional factors have been identified as important predictors of sexual risk. In terms of cognitive factors, better academic performance has been associated with decreased sexual risk in a number of studies (e.g., East, 1998; Jessor, Van Den Bos, Vanderryn, Costa, & Turbin, 1995; Perkins, Luster, Villarruel, & Small, 1998; Small & Luster, 1994). For example, adolescents who

became pregnant had lower grade point averages (GPAs) (Hardy, Astone, Brooks-Gunn, Shapiro, & Miller, 1998), while higher grades have been associated with sexual abstinence, fewer sexual partners, and more condom use among youth (Luster & Small, 1994). In the only prospective study in this area, Scaramella, Conger, Simons, and Whitbeck (1998) found that eighth-grade GPA was a significant predictor of whether an adolescent reported experiencing a pregnancy by the 12th grade.

What teens know about sex and its risks has received considerable attention as a predictor of sexual risk behavior. However, there does not appear to be a clear association between knowledge of sexuality or sexual risk and adolescent sexual risk-taking practices. Some studies indicate that greater knowledge about sexual risk practices and prevention was significantly associated with more consistent condom use (e.g., Reitman et al., 1996; Stanton et al., 1994), contraception use in general (Jemmott & Jemmott, 1990), or fewer sexual partners (Zimet et al, 1992), while others have found no association between knowledge and sexual risk practices (e.g., Brown et al., 1992; Romer et al., 1994). The lack of consensus regarding the relation between accurate knowledge of sexuality and sexual risk practices is consistent with the observation of many researchers in the area of sexual risk behavior prevention that knowledge alone does not necessarily translate to behavior or behavior change (e.g., Baldwin, Whitely, & Baldwin, 1990; St. Lawrence, Jefferson, Alleyne, & Brasfield, 1995).

Other cognitive processes, such as perception of personal risk or attitudes toward sex in general, may provide the missing link between sexual knowledge and sexual behavior. Unfortunately, the findings pertaining to these factors have not been much clearer. Some studies have found that youth who perceived themselves to be more vulnerable to potential negative sexual health outcomes were more likely to engage in risk-reduction strategies such as condom use (Pendergrast et al., 1992; Zimet et al., 1992) or to have fewer sexual partners (Miller et al., 2000), while others found that increased perception of risk was associated with greater levels of sexual risk-taking behavior (Langer & Tubman, 1997; Millstein & Moscicki, 1995). Still others found no association between risk perception and sexual risk behavior (Orr, Beiter, & Ingersoll, 1991; Shafer & Boyer,

1991). These inconsistencies are most likely due to the exclusive use of concurrent analyses to evaluate the relationship between risk perception and risk behavior, thus making it impossible to determine the direction and nature of the relationship between these two variables (Millstein & Moscicki, 1995).

Attitudes concerning the morality of sex and toward risk-reduction practices themselves have been more consistently associated with sexual risk behaviors. For example, more liberal attitudes about teenage sexuality have been found to relate to higher levels of sexual risk-taking behavior (Jemmott & Jemmott, 1990). Several researchers also have documented the finding that adolescent attitudes toward risk-reduction strategies, like condom use, are associated with their use; adolescents with more positive attitudes toward condoms tend to report greater use of condoms (e.g., Jemmott & Jemmott, 1990; Reitman et al., 1996).

Similarly, adolescents who report higher levels of religiosity are less likely to engage in sexual intercourse (Bingham & Crockett, 1996; Levinson, Jaccard, & Beamer, 1995; Neumark-Sztainer, Story, French, & Resnick, 1997) and more likely to use a condom during sex than their less religious peers (Jemmott & Jemmott, 1992). However, in several of these studies, the relationship between religiosity and sexual risk behavior was of only marginal significance, particularly once family structure, SES, and age were considered (e.g., Jemmott & Jemmott, 1992). A more recent study found no relation between religiosity and adolescent sexual behavior among minority youth (Miller et al., 2000).

Self-efficacy, or the belief that one has the ability to perform a particular action effectively (Bandura, 1977), has been a central concept in social-cognitive theories of HIV prevention in general (see Herlocher, Hoff, & DeCarlo, 1995, for a review of HIV prevention theories). However, relatively little research examines the role of self-efficacy in promoting safer sexual practices among adolescents. Reitman and colleagues (1996) found that adolescents who believed they could take precautionary measures to avoid HIV had fewer sexual partners and reported more condom use than their peers who had lower self-efficacy scores. Likewise, general and AIDS-specific self-efficacy were related to more condom use within a sample of high-risk female minority adolescents (Overby & Kegeles, 1994).

Various indicators of psychosocial or emotional distress (e.g., depressive symptoms, anxiety, and poor self-esteem) have been found to relate to adolescent sexual activity, with higher levels of distress being associated with greater sexual activity (e.g., Harvey & Spigner, 1995; Luster & Small, 1994; Orr et al., 1991; Tubman et al., 1996). In terms of sexual risk behavior itself, Luster and Small (1994) found that adolescent males who engaged in high-risk sexual behaviors reported more suicidal ideation than those who engaged in low risk-taking sexual behaviors. Low self-esteem also has been associated with inconsistent use of contraceptives among adolescent girls (Miller et al., 2000).

Related to psychological distress, several researchers have found that a history of victimization is associated with sexual risk-taking behaviors. Sexual abuse, in particular, has been related to outcomes of risky sexual behavior, such as teenage pregnancy (Roosa, Tein, Reinholtz, & Angelini, 1997). Among a sample of adolescent females, Biglan and colleagues (1995) found that 41.7% reported at least one experience of sexual coercion, described as the use of aversive behavior to force someone into sexual intercourse. Compared to those who did not report a history of sexually coercive experiences, those who did were more likely to engage in various sexual risk behaviors, including having sex under the influence of drugs or alcohol and having sex with an unknown partner, and were more likely to experience negative outcomes of such behaviors. In another study, a history of childhood sexual abuse was related to earlier pregnancy among African American adolescents (Fiscella, Kitzman, Cole, Sidora, & Olds, 1998).

Behavioral Factors

Sexual risk-taking behaviors are correlated with a number of other behaviors, including delinquency, substance use, and other indices of sexual activity in general. Problem behavior theory (Jessor & Jessor, 1977) postulates that problem behaviors cluster together such that a subset of adolescents are engaging in multiple risk behaviors across several areas. For example, the boys and girls who engage in more delinquent behavior (e.g., skipping school and stealing) during adolescence also report having a greater number of sexual partners (Devine, Long, & Forehand, 1993). Similarly, fighting and other measures of delinquency (e.g., school suspension or expulsion and drug use) emerged as significant predictors of rapid repeated pregnancies among a sample of adolescent mothers (Gillmore, Lewis, Lohr, Spencer, & White, 1997). Adolescents who report higher rates of aggressive or delinquent behavior also experience a higher incidence of teenage pregnancy or parenthood (e.g., Scaramella et al., 1998; Stouthamer-Loeber & Wei, 1998).

A number of other studies have documented the relationship between substance use and sexual risk practices. The national YRBS data indicate that high-risk sexual behaviors (e.g., multiple sexual partners and no condom use at last intercourse) were most prevalent among adolescents who had used illicit substances during the past year (Lowry, Holtzman, Truman, Kann, Collins, & Kolbe, 1994). Others have found that a history of alcohol and/or drug use correlated with inconsistent condom use (Brown et al., 1992; Cooper, Pierce, & Huselid, 1994; Fullilove et al., 1993; Keller et al., 1991; Luster & Small, 1994; Miller et al., 2000; Millstein & Moscicki, 1995; Shrier et al., 1996) and having multiple sexual partners (Devine et al., 1993; Duncan, Strycker, & Duncan, 1999; Fullilove et al., 1993; Koniak-Griffin & Brecht, 1995; Tubman et al., 1996).

Use of alcohol or drugs immediately prior to or during sexual encounters is also related to decreased condom use (Bagnall, Plant, & Warwick, 1990; Fullilove et al., 1993; Jemmott & Jemmott, 1993; Strunin & Hingson, 1992). For example, among inner-city black male adolescents, those who report a higher frequency of having had sex while "high" are more likely to have unprotected sexual intercourse, a greater number of sexual partners, and a greater number of "risky" sexual partners (Jemmott & Jemmott, 1993). Similarly, adolescents who frequently combine alcohol consumption and sexual behavior are seven times less likely to use a condom (Bagnall et al., 1990). Dermen, Cooper, and Agocha (1998) conducted a test of expectancy theories and found that those adolescents who expected that alcohol consumption would decrease sexual inhibitions were more likely to have sex under the influence of alcohol, as well as engage in other risk behaviors, such as unprotected sex.

The robust relationship between adolescent sexual risk-taking behavior and other risk behaviors, such as drug use or engagement in delinquent activities, may be explained, in part, by personality characteristics, including a tendency toward sensation seeking or impulsivity. Indeed, some research has found that higher levels of sexual risk-taking behavior are reported among youth who also score higher on measures of sensation seeking (Brown et al., 1992; Neumark-Sztainer et al., 1997) and who perceive themselves as having little behavioral control (Mezzich et al., 1997; Millstein & Moscicki, 1995).

In addition, problem behavior theory (Jessor & Jessor, 1977) has attempted to explain the strong co-occurrence of risky sex with other potentially harmful behaviors by considering all adolescent risk behavior as similar in purpose and development. In a longitudinal study employing latent growth curve modeling, Duncan and colleagues (1999) found strong support for problem behavior theory, as the development of three types of substance use (alcohol, cigarettes, and other drugs) covaried with the development of risky sexual behaviors. In addition, a study of female adolescents with and without substance abuse disorders found that substance use problems and risky sexual behavior were strongly related and shared many of the same risk factors (e.g., behavioral dysregulation and childhood victimization) (Mezzich et al., 1997).

Not only do other risk behaviors (e.g., drug use) correlate with sexual risk taking among sexually active youth, but so do other aspects of sexual behavior. In essence, risk builds on risk, such that adolescents at risk for exposure to HIV, STDs, or pregnancy because of their sexual risk practices are likely to be engaging in multiple behaviors considered to be sexually risky. For example, early sexual debut is related to multiple aspects of risky sexual behavior (Crockett, Bingham, Chopak, & Vicary, 1996); adolescents who were younger at the initiation of sexual activity report less condom use at first intercourse (Melchert & Burnett, 1990; St. Lawrence & Scott, 1996) and in subsequent sexual encounters (Melchert & Burnett, 1990; Smith, 1997) as well as have higher rates of pregnancy than do their peers who were older at sexual initiation (Roosa et al., 1997; Smith, 1997). Others have found that the number of sexual partners is inversely related to condom use (DiClemente et al., 1992), and that number of years that an adolescent has been sexually active is positively correlated to a variety of sexual risk behaviors (Gillmore, Butler, Lohr, & Gilchrist, 1992).

The Family System: Family Structure and Family Process

Familial influences on adolescent sexual activity can be divided into two primary categories: family structure variables and family process variables. In general, the latter category of variables has received more attention than the former category. However, there is evidence that structural factors, such as single parenting, SES, and parental education, should not be ignored.

Structural Factors

Several studies have shown that living in two-parent family is often a protective factor against risky sexual behavior and its outcomes, such as pregnancy (e.g., Baumeister et al., 1995; Jemmott & Jemmott, 1992; Metzler, Noell, Biglan, Ary, & Smolkowski, 1994; Santelli, Lowry, Brener, & Robin, 2000). Whether this protection stems from the greater socioeconomic resources often enjoyed by intact or two-parent families or whether differences in family processes related to family structure account for the increased risk is unclear.

In terms of SES, teens living in poverty have been identified as being at greater risk for early pregnancy than their higher-income peers (Gordon, 1996; Roosa et al., 1997). However, it is important to note that one recent study (Miller, Forehand, & Kotchick, 1999) examined several aspects of adolescent sexual risk behaviors (e.g., number of sex partners and consistency of condom use) and failed to find any relationship between family structural variables (i.e., parental education, marital status, and family income) and these risk outcomes. Unfortunately, further conclusions regarding family structure variables such as these are difficult to draw, as these particular variables are often statistically controlled in data analyses due to their covariance with other variables.

Family Process Factors

The most widely studied family process variable in the adolescent sexual risk behavior literature is parenting. Research concerning the role parents play in the sexual socialization of their children has generally focused on three aspects of parenting: parental monitoring, the quality of the parent–adolescent relationship, and parent–adolescent communication about sex.

Parental monitoring or supervision of adolescents' social activities has been associated with less risky sexual behavior among youth, including less frequent sexual behavior (Romer et al, 1994), fewer sexual partners (e.g., Miller et al., 2000; Rodgers, 1999), and more consistent use of contraception (e.g., Luster & Small, 1994; Rodgers, 1999). Related to parental monitoring, adolescents' ratings of parental strictness have also been shown to be significantly associated with lower levels of sexual risk behavior. In a survey of African American adolescent males, Jemmott and Jemmott (1992) noted that perceived parental strictness related to different aspects of sexual risk for each parent—having a strict mother was related to fewer sexual partners, while having a strict father was related to more consistent condom use.

Parental monitoring may also be protective for adolescents by limiting their involvement in other risk behaviors that have been associated with sexual risk practices. Indeed, better parental monitoring has been associated with lower levels of problem behavior and drug abuse among adolescents (e.g., Barber, Olsen, & Shagle, 1994; Steinberg, 1987). In a more recent study, low levels of perceived parental monitoring were associated with participation in several health risk behaviors, including sexual risk behavior, substance use, drug trafficking, school truancy, and violent behaviors (Li, Feigelman, & Stanton, 2000).

However, there is evidence that suggests that the relationship between parental monitoring and adolescent sexual risk may be protective only to a certain point. Indeed, excessive control by parents that denies adolescents adequate autonomy is associated with a higher probability that adolescents will engage in sexual risk-taking behavior (Rodgers, 1999). This finding is consistent with research demonstrating that either too much or too little parental control is associated with increased problem behaviors among adolescents (Mason, Cauce, Gonzales, & Hiraga, 1996).

The quality of an adolescent's relationship with her or his parents, including how the adolescent perceives this relationship, is an important aspect of the family system that appears to affect sexual risk behaviors. Parental support and involvement have been associated with decreased sexual risk behaviors and reduced risk of pregnancy (e.g., Jaccard & Dittus, 2000; Jaccard, Dittus, & Gordon, 1996; Luster & Small, 1994; Scaramella et al., 1998). In fact, Jaccard and his colleagues have found that a single item assessing adolescents' satisfaction with their relationship with their mothers was the best predictor of adolescent sexual behavior: Higher relationship satisfaction is related to a lower probability of sexual intercourse and pregnancy, and a higher probability of birth control use (e.g., Jaccard et al., 1996; Jaccard & Dittus, 2000).

Although other studies provide partial support for these findings, most of them have not documented such a clear or uniform association between parent–adolescent relationships and sexual risk behaviors. For example, data from a national longitudinal study of adolescents in grades 7–12 found that parent–child connectedness was the key family factor in the development of a variety of general (i.e., nonsexual) risky behaviors, even after controlling for demographic characteristics. However, a lower probability of involvement in pregnancy by the 12th grade was not among the outcomes predicted by family connectedness (Resnick et al., 1997).

The quality of the parent–adolescent relationship is also reflected in the frequency and quality of parent–adolescent communication, and communication between adolescents and parents is particularly important for the transmission of information regarding sexuality, HIV/AIDS, and appropriate risk-reduction strategies for adolescents. Family communication about sex and its potential risks has been found to relate to more correct knowledge about sexuality and AIDS among adolescents (e.g., Pick & Palos, 1995; Sigelman, Derenowski, Mullaney, & Siders, 1993). More important, parent–adolescent communication about sex is associated with several measures of decreased sexual risk-taking behavior among adolescents (e.g., Baumeister et al., 1995; Kotchick, Dorsey, Miller, & Forehand, 1999; Luster & Small, 1994; Miller et al., 1999; Miller, Kotchick, Dorsey, Forehand, & Ham, 1998). Parent–adolescent communication about sex and condom use has also been found to moderate the relationship between peer sexual behavior and adolescent sexual behavior, such that peer norms were more strongly related to adolescent sexual behavior among adolescents who had not discussed sex

or condoms with their parents (Whitaker & Miller, 2000). Although there is clear evidence suggesting that parents have a positive impact on their adolescent children's sexual decision making, many parents do not discuss sexuality or sexual risk with their children (e.g., Miller, Kotchick, et al., 1998), citing discomfort, lack of knowledge, or fear that their openness may encourage adolescent sexual behavior.

Although many researchers have shown that parental communication about sex is related to decreased sexual risk behavior among adolescents, most of this research has only examined whether or not the communication occurred, rather than the particular characteristics of how, why, or when the communication happened. However, recent research by Miller and her colleagues have noted that several aspects of parent–child sexual communication, including the timing of the discussions (Miller, Levin, Whitaker & Xu, 1998), the content or topics discussed (Dutra, Miller, & Forehand, 1999; Miller, Kotchick, et al., 1998), and the process of the communication itself (Dutra et al., 1999) all contribute uniquely to the relation between parental communication and adolescent sexual behavior. For example, research with high-risk minority adolescents has demonstrated that parent–adolescent discussions about sex have their greatest impact on sexual risk behavior when they occur prior to the first sexual encounter (Miller, Levin, et al., 1998). Likewise, when youth perceive their parents as being positive and supportive during discussions about sex, they report having fewer sexual partners and more consistent condom use than their peers who perceive communication with their parents to be less positive (Miller et al., 2000).

In addition to providing structure (in the form of parental monitoring), support (through a positive parent–child relationship), and information (by communicating about sexual topics), parents communicate their values and expectations about sexuality via their own behavior (Metzler et al., 1994). For example, there is a documented increase in the risk of teenage pregnancy among the adolescent children of teenage mothers (Hardy et al., 1998). However, research concerning the relationship between current parental sexual behavior and adolescent sexual risk practices is less available. One study of ethnic minority families found that maternal sexual risk behavior was predictive of adolescent sexual risk behavior, although the significance of maternal sexual behavior was reduced once maternal attitudes about adolescent sexual activity and mother–adolescent communication about sex were added to the model (Kotchick et al., 1999).

In addition to direct modeling effects, adolescent sexual behavior may also be indirectly modeled through transmission of parental attitudes toward sex and sexual risk taking. There is clear evidence that perceived parental disapproval of risky sexual behavior is a predictor of more consistent contraceptive use (Jaccard et al., 1996; Jaccard & Dittus, 2000; Stanton et al., 1994), as well as less sexual activity in general. However, adolescent perceptions of maternal approval of birth control has been associated with an increased likelihood of sexual initiation during a 1-year follow-up period, suggesting that some adolescents may misinterpret parental messages about safer sexual practices as being supportive of sexual activity in general (Jaccard & Dittus, 2000). Still, the findings of that study were deemed "fragile" by the authors, and the results clearly linked perceived maternal approval of birth control with increased use of protection during intercourse (Jaccard & Dittus, 2000). More research is needed to understand the complex relationship between the perceptions that teens hold concerning their parents' attitudes about sex and risk reduction and adolescent sexual behavior.

The Extrafamilial System: Peers, Neighborhood, and Schools

For adolescents who are in the midst of developing their own identities and establishing more complex social networks, the point of reference by which they guide their behavior naturally shifts from the family to the social environment (Forehand & Wierson, 1993). Peers, neighborhoods, and other community factors all relate in important, though poorly understood, ways to adolescent sexual risk behavior.

Peers

Relative to the relationships between family variables and sexual behavior during adolescence, associations between peer factors and sexual behaviors have received less attention in the literature. The studies examining the latter issue indicate that as peers become an important source of reinforcement, modeling, and support during adolescence (Forehand & Wierson, 1993), adolescents whose peers are

sexually active are more likely to be sexually active themselves (e.g., Miller et al., 2000; Romer et al., 1994). In addition, indicators of sexual risk-taking behavior among adolescents' peer groups (e.g., pregnancy and inconsistent condom use) have been shown to relate to increased adolescent sexual risk (Gillmore et al., 1997; Millstein & Moscicki, 1995). More subjectively, adolescents' perceptions of their peers' behaviors have also been found to relate to sexual risk taking, as several researchers have found that consistent condom use is associated with the perception of condom use among friends (e.g., Romer et al., 1994; Stanton et al., 1994).

Beyond peer sexual behavior, other characteristics of an adolescent's peer group appear to be related to adolescent sexual risk behavior. Research has repeatedly indicated that association with a deviant peer group, such as one that is involved with alcohol and drug use or delinquency, has been related to participation in high-risk sexual practices (e.g., Brewster, 1994; Miller et al., 2000). A prospective study by Scaramella and colleagues (1998) found that deviant peer affiliations in the 8th grade was significantly related to sexual risk behavior in the 12th grade.

Neighborhood/Community

On the broadest level of the extrafamilial system, the neighborhood or community in which the adolescent lives also appears to influence the types of risk behaviors in which he or she may be involved. The community provides myriad levels of social support, through schools, jobs, social contacts, and other resources. The community can also serve to hinder an adolescent's development or place the adolescent at greater risk, through a lack of future opportunities, insufficient monitoring, or socioeconomic disadvantage or instability. For example, lower neighborhood SES, increased levels of female employment, and higher divorce rates within the community were all associated with greater sexual risk taking among African American adolescent girls (Brewster, 1994), and neighborhood poverty was associated with earlier ages of sexual debut among African American males (Ramirez-Valles et al., 2002). The degree of social support garnered from extrafamilial sources is also likely to be important, as less social support has been found to relate to more frequent engagement in sexual risk behaviors among African American adolescents (St. Lawrence et al., 1994).

Schools

An important aspect of an adolescent's community is the school environment. Simply being in school, versus having dropped out, serves as a protective role in terms of adolescent sexual risk behavior. Youth who have dropped out of school are more likely to initiate sex at earlier ages, fail to use contraception, or become involved in a pregnancy than students who remain in school (Brewster, Cooksey, Guilkey, & Rindfuss, 1998; Darroch, Landry, & Oslak, 1999; Manlove, 1998). Greater attachment to school is also associated with less sexual risk behavior (e.g., Brewster et al., 1998; Lammers, Ireland, Resnick, & Blum, 2000; Manlove, 1998), as are plans to attend college (Blum, Buehring, & Rinehart, 2000; Halpern, Joyner, Udry, & Suchindran, 2000). Schools also provide the context in which the majority of formal sexuality education and prevention messages are delivered (see Kirby, 2002). Pendergrast and colleagues (1992) have noted that increased exposure to sexual education in the schools, particularly on the avoidance of STDs, is related to increased condom use.

A Multisystemic Model of Adolescent Sexual Risk Behavior

Much has been learned about the variables that are related to adolescent sexual risk behavior, and factors at the individual, family, and extrafamilial levels have been identified as potential targets for preventive interventions. Based on this research, social and political attention have been devoted to the larger contextual variables and environmental conditions that appear to promote sexual risk taking by adolescents, and public policies dedicated to empowering youth and their families have been implemented (e.g., Children Now & Kaiser Family Foundation, 1999).

A multisystemic perspective would suggest that the relations among these systems are as important as the individual risk factors falling within each system in terms of their impact on adolescent sexual behavior. Although some research has begun to address the influence of factors from across multiple systems on sexual risk among adolescents (e.g., Luster & Small, 1994), very few studies have addressed the ef-

fects of each system as a whole and/or their interaction on behavior.

As an example of the kind of research now sorely needed to evaluate more comprehensive models of adolescent sexual risk behavior, Miller and colleagues (2000) examined self, family, and extrafamilial factors and their association with sexual risk taking among ethnic minority adolescents. Their findings indicated that factors from all three systems emerged as predictors of four different measures of sexual risk behavior. In addition, there was a linear relationship between the number of systems identified as being "at risk" based on scores on significant predictors and several indicators of adolescent sexual risk behavior.

Studies such as this are needed to identify how factors from multiple systems of influence interact or combine with each other to shape behavior. A multisystemic perspective suggests that the relationships among various systems of influence are transactional and interactional, such that risks or resources from one may serve to either potentiate or buffer against the effects of others, and that each system influences other systems, as well as sexual behavior itself. In addition, sexual behavior itself may also exert some influence on the self, family, and extrafamilial systems in a feedback mechanism that continually shapes and reshapes the relations among the systems (see Kotchick et al., 2001; Szapocznik & Coatsworth, 1999). However, few studies have been undertaken to examine adolescent sexual risk behavior at such a comprehensive level.

Nevertheless, the literature that does exist provides a solid foundation on which prevention efforts may be built. Available preventive interventions designed to delay onset of sexual activity or reduce sexual risk behavior vary in the extent to which they have addressed factors within each of the three levels we have discussed: self, family, and extrafamilial. While the earliest generation of HIV/STD/pregnancy prevention programs most often targeted individual level variables, and typically only one individual level component (i.e., knowledge), more recently developed programs attempt to address factors at two or even all three levels. As the research into the correlates and predictors of adolescent sexual risk behavior advances and becomes more comprehensive, it is expected that prevention efforts will also expand beyond their current boundaries.

PREVENTION INTERVENTIONS

Well over 100 prevention programs designed either to reduce sexual risk behavior or to delay sexual intercourse among adolescents have been developed. Some, but not all, have been empirically evaluated, though many are currently in place in schools, youth centers, churches, and other community organizations around the country. Of those empirically tested, only a handful has demonstrated rigorous support for their efficacy. The purpose of this section of the chapter is to assist researchers and practitioners in understanding the essential components of effective interventions and in identifying programs with the most evidence-based promise of success.

Essential Components of Successful Interventions

Kirby (2001) has proposed a number of qualities necessary for sex and HIV education programs to be successful in reducing sexual risk behavior, and thus the incidence of HIV, other STDs, and pregnancy, among youth. The qualities include those specific to the development, content, and delivery of an intervention.

With respect to intervention development, Kirby (2001) emphasized the importance of relying on a theoretical framework with demonstrated influence on health behavior. Theories are not always explicitly considered in intervention development; however, when they are, four theories or models of behavior change are most commonly used to develop preventive interventions targeting teen sexual behavior: social learning theory; cognitive-behavioral theory; social influence or inoculation model; and information–motivation–behavioral skills model (for a more detailed discussion of these theories, please see Armistead, Kotchick, & Forehand, 2004). All the interventions discussed subsequently are grounded in one or more theoretical approaches.

Turning to content, Kirby (2001) illuminated the importance of presenting a clear message with respect to abstinence and/or condom use. In fact, message clarity and consistency appear to be the most important qualities distinguishing ineffective and effective interventions. In addition, provision of accurate information about the risks of sexual behavior, strategies for avoiding intercourse, and successful condom use is essential. Kirby also indicated that

specific sexual behaviors should be targeted and the social pressures that influence those behaviors discussed.

With regard to content delivery, there are five important considerations, according to Kirby (2001). First, an intervention must last a sufficient length of time (i.e., more than a few hours). Brief interventions are rarely successful with respect to sustained behavior change. Second, it is important to provide youth with relevant examples and to offer opportunities to practice skills, perhaps through role plays. Examples might include role playing refusal to engage in intercourse. Third, instruction methods must include active engagement from participants, rather than being simply didactic in nature. Through active engagement, participants will have the opportunity to transform the information so that it is most relevant for their lives. Fourth, it is critical that information, as well as teaching methods and materials, be culturally and developmentally appropriate for the target youth. For example, an intervention designed for African American youth might use African proverbs and/or feature African American youth in visual materials (e.g., posters or videos). Finally, the intervention facilitators should be adequately trained and enthusiastic about the program and must believe that it is likely to be effective.

Empirically Supported Prevention Interventions

As previously mentioned, more than 100 prevention programs targeting HIV, STD, and teen pregnancy have been utilized with adolescents. We employed the following guidelines in determining which programs to include in the subsequent discussion of prevention programs. First, we included only interventions with empirical evidence of effectiveness as determined either by the CDC (1999) or The National Campaign to Prevent Teen Pregnancy (Kirby, 2001). Second, we included only studies conducted in the United States or Canada that targeted adolescents between the ages of 12 and 18. Third, certain methodological standards must have been met in order for the programs to be discussed in this review. These standards include the use of an experimental or quasi-experimental design, a sample size of at least 100, and measurement of the intervention's impact on sexual or contraceptive behavior, pregnancy, or childbearing outcomes (see Kirby,

2001). Finally, we have chosen to focus only on studies published in the last decade (1992–2002) because they represent the most advanced knowledge of proven prevention strategies.

We begin our discussion by reviewing those interventions focused on altering sexual risk behavior itself, subsequently termed sexual risk reduction programs, which are the most commonly employed type of intervention. Table 17.1 provides a summary of the 10 empirically supported programs reviewed in this chapter and includes information about program characteristics and the major program components.

A review of program characteristics reveals that many programs were conducted with ethnically and economically diverse high school youth. When study samples were not ethnically or economically diverse, they consisted only of ethnic minority participants and/or those from the lower socioeconomic bracket. The focus on ethnic minority youth and those from the lower socioeconomic bracket reflects the higher rates of teen pregnancy, HIV, and other STDs occurring among these youth relative to middle- and upper-class Caucasian youth (Kotchick et al., 2001). In addition, all but two of the studies targeted high school age youth. Unfortunately, waiting until youth are in high school to discuss sexual risk reduction is common and reflects the cultural proscriptions against providing comprehensive sexuality education to youth at younger ages. However, as previously mentioned, it is ideal to intervene with youth around sexual behavior *before* they begin engaging in it. Thus, some of the newer, although still uncompleted, interventions discussed later include younger youth.

Turning to program format, all interventions listed in Table 17.1 were implemented via multiple group-based sessions, ranging in number from 4 to 20. Of note, although some interventions adhered to the more traditional weekly session format, two spread the intervention across multiple years. For example, Draw the Line involved a total of 20 sessions, implemented across the sixth through eighth grades. Decisions regarding the scheduling of sessions depend, at least in part, on practical considerations such as the intervention site. For example, it is more feasible to spread an intervention across multiple years in a school setting than in a community setting.

All interventions were designed to increase the likelihood of maximum impact by presenting the information in a dynamic and interactive format. For example, Street Smart, an intervention for runaway youth, included a component where teens created soap opera dramatizations in order to practice the skills taught in the intervention. In addition, in a unique and potentially powerful attempt to influence the behavior of youth, Becoming a Responsible Teen also included a component that involved discussion groups held with HIV-infected youth. This component was included in an attempt to promote accurate perceptions of vulnerability to HIV infection.

In terms of program components, the majority of the interventions focused exclusively on the individual factors involved in risky sexual behavior (e.g., knowledge, attitudes, and skills) rather than on family or extrafamilial factors. In particular, it is important to note that the majority of sexual risk reduction interventions rely on a "single-target" approach to intervention, as opposed to focusing on youth in the context of dating or romantic relationships. While negotiation skills are often covered, participants' romantic relationships (e.g., role of intimacy and companionship) are not often directly addressed. However, a few interventions did target change in family or peer systems. For example, Safer Choices was unique in that these investigators targeted individual variables, familial variables, and extrafamilial variables. Specifically, the investigators attempted to incorporate parents into the intervention through homework and parent newsletters. In addition, some students were trained to be peer educators who would reinforce safer sex messages in the school environment (e.g., at assemblies).

Participants in all interventions received information about the risks of unprotected sex and methods for protecting oneself (e.g., abstinence and condom use). Moreover, two intervention programs (i.e., Safer Choices and AIDS Prevention for Adolescents in School) also attempted to change youths' perceptions of the frequency with which their peers were engaging in sexual behavior. These interventions used group discussions about the rate of youth sexual behavior in an attempt to debunk the misperception that "everyone is doing it" (Coyle, Kirby, Marin, Gomez, & Gregorich, 2000).

Values clarification was also a part of several of the interventions (i.e., Focus on Kids, AIDS Prevention for Adolescents in School, Becoming a Responsible Teen, and Healthy Oakland

TABLE 17.1. Empirically Supported Sexual Risk Reduction Interventions

Program title (author[s], publication date)	Sample description		Study	
	SES (sample size)	Age/grade/gender/ethnicity	Program delivery	Program content
Draw the Line/Respect the Line (Coyle et al., 2000)	Mixed SES (n = 2,829)	Mean age = 11.5 years; 50% female; mixed ethnicity	20 sessions delivered in middle schools across 3 years; teachers trained as interventionists	Information about the consequences of sex; limit setting with refusal skills
Reducing the Risk (Hubbard, Giese, & Rainey, 1998)	Mixed SES (n = 212)	9–12th grades; 52% female; 85% white	16 sessions delivered in health-ed classes in schools; teachers trained as interventionists	AIDS education; refusal skills
AIDS Prevention for Adolescents in School (Walter & Vaughn, 1993)	Low SES (n = 867)	9th and 11th grades; 58% female; mixed ethnicity	6 sessions delivered in classes at schools; teachers trained as interventionists	AIDS education; cognitive skills for risk appraisal; norms of teen sexual behavior; values clarification; skills to delay intercourse or use condoms
Safer Choices (Coyle et al., 2001)	Mixed SES (n = 3,058)	High school; 52% female; mixed ethnicity	20 sessions delivered in the 9th and 10th grades (10 each year); teachers trained as interventionists plus parent education, school health protection council, and school–community linkages	Information about the consequences of sex; norms of teen sexual behavior; skills for avoiding sex or using condoms
Get Real About AIDS (Main et al., 1994)	SES not reported (n = 979)	9th–12th grades; 49% female; mostly white and Hispanic	15 sessions delivered in classes at schools; teachers trained as interventionists plus posters in the schools	AIDS education; norms of teen sexual behavior; condom use skills; skills for identifying and avoiding risk
Becoming a Responsible Teen (St. Lawrence, Brasfield, et al., 1995)	Low SES (n = 225)	Mean age = 15.3 years; 72% female; 100% black	8 sessions delivered in a community setting	AIDS education; sexual decisions and pressures; condom use skills; social skills and risk avoidance
Be Proud, Be Responsible (Jemmott, Jemmott, & Fong, 1998)	Low income (n = 659)	Mean age = 11.8 years; 53% female; 100% black	8 1-hour modules delivered on school campuses over two Saturdays; trained adult or peer interventionists	Small-group discussions; informational videos and games; skill-building exercises
Healthy Oakland Teens (Ekstrand et al., 1996)	Low income (n = 250)	Mean age = 13 years; 52% female; mostly black	5 sessions delivered in classes at schools; trained adult or peer interventionists	Information on sexuality, substance abuse, HIV, and STDs; risk perception; values clarification; norms of teen sexual behavior; refusal skills and condom skills
Intensive AIDS Education in Jail (Magura, Kang, & Shapiro, 1994)	SES not reported (n = 157)	Mean age = 18 years; 100% male; 65% black, 33% Hispanic	4 sessions delivered in a juvenile correctional facility; trained project staff were interventionists	Small-group discussions; AIDS education; decision-making skills
Focus on Kids (Stanton, Li, Galbraith, Feigelman, & Kaljee, 1996)	Low income (n = 383)	Mean age = 11 years; 44% female; 100% black	8 sessions delivered in recreational centers; trained project staff were interventionists	AIDS education; values clarification; community projects

Teens). For example, Becoming a Responsible Teen devoted a discussion session to sexual decisions and values. Subsequent to viewing a video, the participants continued this discussion with an emphasis on support from friends and family around one's sex-related personal values.

With respect to behavioral outcomes of the interventions, all programs collected follow-up data (at least 3 months and typically 12 months) and demonstrated efficacy at reducing risky behaviors. The outcomes measured included initiation of sexual behavior for sexually inexperienced youth and, among sexually active youth, condom use, intercourse frequency, and number of partners. Although some studies did not demonstrate a positive effect for delay of sexual intercourse (but did affect other risky behaviors, such as unprotected intercourse), it is important to note that in no case did an intervention hasten the onset of intercourse. This finding refutes the argument that the discussion of adolescent sexual behavior, its consequences, and means of protection that occurs in sex education programs will lead to an increase in adolescent sexual behavior. These study findings indicate that interventions targeting the sexual risk behavior that can lead to HIV, STDs, and teen pregnancy can be, but are not always, effective. Perhaps the most exciting results offered are that in the majority of these studies, teen protective behaviors persisted at follow-up assessments occurring at least 12 months after the intervention. Moreover, one intervention sustained its effect on condom use and number of partners at a 31-month follow-up. These findings are very important given that the potential negative effects of risky sexual behaviors loom well beyond the early adolescent years. Thus, interventions must be powerful enough to have an enduring impact.

Missing from our review are those prevention programs that exclusively promote abstinence as a method of sexual risk reduction. The reason these politically popular programs were not included is that they did not meet the criteria of having been empirically demonstrated to significantly reduce sexual risk behavior among youth. Thus, we chose not to include them in our review of empirically supported prevention programs. The interested reader is referred to Kirby (2001) for more information concerning the effectiveness of abstinence-only interventions.

Promising and Innovative Family-Based Prevention Programs

Several prevention programs are currently being evaluated and appear to offer promise with respect to their impact on youth sexual behavior. These new programs set themselves apart from existing prevention efforts by incorporating families and targeting children younger than those reached by the programs reviewed previously (e.g., CHAMP Family Program, McKay & Williams, 2002; Parents Matter! Program, Kotchick et al., 2002). For example, the Parents Matter! Program is a group intervention for African American parents of fourth- and fifth-grade students. Parents participating in the treatment groups of this intervention learn about the numerous health and sexual risks facing youth as they transition into adolescence and are taught general parenting skills, such as monitoring and relationship building, that are known to be protective for youth. Following this foundation, the intervention emphasizes the importance of parent–child communication about sexual health and provides training in specific communication skills that parents can use to initiate discussions or respond to their children's questions about sexuality (Kotchick et al., 2002).

Nontraditional Prevention Programs

Research indicates that improving females' educational and employment opportunities reduces their pregnancy rates (Kirby, 2001). In addition, male and female youth most at risk for HIV and other STDs are those with relatively poor educational and career opportunities (e.g., Airhihenbuwa et al., 1992; Brown et al., 1992). Thus, some professionals working with youth have targeted the improvement of educational and career opportunities, rather than or in addition to sexual behavior per se, as the intervention focus. These interventions, known as youth development programs, have aims broader than simply a reduction in youth sexual risk behavior. Specifically, they focused on enhancing factors such as involvement with other adults, attachment to school, employment opportunities, and educational goals (Kirby, 2001).

There are four youth development programs that met the methodological and other criteria discussed above. Table 17.2 presents the program name and investigators of these in-

TABLE 17.2. Empirically Supported Youth Development Programs

Program title	Reference
Teen Outreach Program	Philliber & Allen (1992)
Abecedarian Project	Campbell (1999)
Seattle Social Development Project	Hawkins, Catalano, Kosterman, Abbott, & Hill (1999)
Carrera Program	Philliber, Kaye, Herring, & West (2000)

terventions. Unlike the interventions focused exclusively on sexual behavior, the youth development programs are generally more different than they are similar. Next, we discuss interesting features of these interventions with respect to methodology, program format, and content, as well as behavioral outcomes.

As with the sexual risk-reduction programs, the youth development projects focus primarily on youth demographically at risk for negative outcomes. However, there is a much broader age range represented in the youth development interventions, compared to those focused exclusively on the reduction of sexual risk behavior.

As one would expect, the format and content of the programs varied considerably depending on the age of the youth. However, unlike most of the sexually specific interventions, the youth development programs are consistent in their incorporation of multiple systems in their interventions, with components focusing on the individual, family, and extrafamilial factors that are related to sexual risk behavior among youth.

The most distinctly different program is the Abecedarian program that included a preschool and elementary school component and lasted up to 8 years. The preschool component consisted of enriched full-day child care year round from infancy to kindergarten. The elementary school intervention involved a teacher devoted to the home–school connection (e.g., increasing parental involvement in the child's learning and enhancing parent–school communication).

The interventions focused on teens were implemented in schools and community settings. The format included small groups, and the content focused on values, decision making, com-

munication skills, and parenting. These interventions were also service learning programs, and treatment youth participated in an average of 46 hours of service in the school or community.

Though different in their methodology, format, and content, each of the four youth development programs had a positive impact on the same outcome: Participants in the treatment groups in all four intervention studies evidenced lower pregnancy or birth rates than did control group participants. Most interesting, three of the programs followed youth into young adulthood and demonstrated a positive impact with respect to unintended pregnancy.

CURRENT NEEDS AND FUTURE DIRECTIONS

If the recent decline in the proportion of high school students who report being sexually active is indicative of a true behavioral trend (Grunbaum et al., 2004), then it may be surmised that the plethora of prevention programs and media attention currently devoted to the need to reduce adolescent sexual risk behavior are having some positive effects. However, the development of effective prevention programs is wholly dependent on the study of adolescent sexual risk behavior and its predictors or correlates. Thus, we would like to conclude this chapter by offering our thoughts on the unmet needs, unanswered questions, promising directions, and lingering challenges that face researchers and practitioners with regard to adolescent sexual risk behavior.

Challenges for Research

Before addressing specific methodological challenges facing researchers in the area of adolescent sexual risk behavior, we first want to acknowledge that such work is conducted in an often politically, and certainly morally, charged climate. One cannot consume or conduct research concerning adolescent sexual behavior without being acutely aware of the impact of social and political forces on the research questions asked or the methods used to address them. For example, most research on the topic of adolescent sexuality and its prevention is conducted with high school students, despite evidence suggesting that sexual risk behaviors are becoming increasingly prevalent among younger adolescents and even among preteens (e.g., Grunbaum et al., 2004). The cultural prohibition against measuring sexual behavior, thoughts, or attitudes among younger adolescents or preadolescents has resulted in few studies of sexual behavior in these younger cohorts, and has even culminated in the withdrawing of grant funding to projects that sought to collect such sorely needed data (see Lilienfeld, 2002). Likewise, the ongoing debate over whether "abstinence only" or comprehensive sexuality education should be the central curriculum in federally and state funded programs clearly indicates that the issue of prevention is susceptible to moral, political, and emotional biases (Levesque, 2000). It is hoped that the efficacy trials of some of the newer-generation prevention efforts that target youth in this younger age range through the more socially acceptable avenue of their parents will highlight the need for greater attention to the growing numbers of sexually mature and sexually active youth.

Political climate aside, substantial improvements in research design and focus are needed to answer the questions raised by the available literature: What are the factors that contribute to the developmental pathways ending with sexual initiation, and are they the same factors that guide decision making about engaging in risk behavior? What is the chronological sequence of events that influence sexual risk-taking behavior? How are all the factors identified as correlates of adolescent sexual risk behavior related, and in what manner do they exert direct and indirect effects on each other and on sexual behavior? How do adolescent gender, ethnicity, and social class interact with these factors to differentially place certain youth at increased risk of the adverse consequences of sexually risky behavior?

These questions reflect the need to move beyond simply identifying when, how, and why risky sexual practices develop, and to begin to integrate our knowledge and efforts into understanding the whole picture. Thus, more attention must be given to the development of comprehensive models that take into account factors from multiple systems of influence and their combined effects on adolescent sexual risk-taking behavior. Recent advances in statistical methodology and measurement strategies (e.g., structural equation modeling) now offer researchers the tools they need to address the multiple systems of influence noted in this review and to move our knowledge and understanding of adolescent sexuality to a more comprehensive level.

With respect to the variables identified for study, the most extensively studied factors so far are those from the self system. Future research should focus more attention on familial and extrafamilial factors that may contribute to adolescent sexual risk behavior. In particular, the specific factors within these contexts that are predictive of sexual risk behavior must be better defined before they will be useful additions to prevention efforts. Furthermore, many of the self system variables found to be related to sexual risk behavior are not amenable to change (e.g., age, gender, and race) and may merely serve as proxies for the familial or extrafamilial conditions or factors associated that truly influence behavior. Again, understanding how these systems and variables interact and intersect to exert influence on adolescent behavior should be a top priority for future research efforts.

As summarized in a review by Kotchick and colleagues (2001), there are several other methodological limitations that pose challenges to researchers interested in assessing adolescent sexual risk behavior. For example, the measurement of events as private and sensitive as sexual behavior results in an exclusive reliance on self-report measures of the outcome variables (Jemmott & Jemmott, 1994). However, there are many concerns about the reliability of such data (McFarlane & St. Lawrence, 1999), and several studies have demonstrated that adolescents tend to be poor reporters of sexual behavior (e.g., Capaldi, 1996). Most self-report methods rely on recall of sexual behaviors during some specified time frame, such as the past 3 weeks or within the last 6 months. Alternatively, adolescents may be asked about lifetime rates of behavior or number of sexual partners. Either way, adolescents tend to be inconsistent in their reporting over time (e.g., Capaldi, 1996), and the reliability of recalled sexual behaviors appears to decrease as the length of the recall period increases (McFarlane & St. Lawrence, 1999).

Recall of sexual events is affected not only by the length of the recall period but also by the method of data collection. Data collected by interviews, particularly face-to-face interviews, introduce social desirability and situational demand characteristics, such as the age, gender, or race of the interviewer, which may influence responding, and little is known about the reliability of interview methods for assessing sexual behavior. The good news is that innovative methods have recently been developed that appear to enhance the validity of self-report measures of adolescent sexual behavior. For example, both automated sexual behavior diaries and audio computer-assisted self-interviewing methods result in greater reporting of sensitive behavior than traditional face-to-face interviews or paper-and-pencil self-administered questionnaires (e.g., Des Jarlais et al., 1999; Minnis & Padian, 2001; Turner et al., 1998).

In terms of research design, with very few exceptions, studies of adolescent sexual risk behavior have employed cross-sectional designs (see Devine et al., 1993; Scaramella et al., 1998, for exceptions). Such studies allow for the identification of variables related to sexual behavior but not for the specification of the direction of those relationships. There is a substantial need for longitudinal or prospective studies that can elucidate these bidirectional relationships to identify the true "influencing" factors that may be the active ingredients in effective intervention efforts.

Finally, the variables identified as correlates or predictors of adolescent sexual risk behavior are not always defined as accurately, precisely, or consistently as they could be. This lack of specificity may result in the misinterpretation of significant associations between predictors and outcomes or prevent meaningful relationships from being detected at all. The review of findings that document an unclear relationship between sexual knowledge and sexual risk behavior illustrates this point well. One likely reason for the lack of agreement among researchers is the inconsistency of measures used to assess sexual knowledge. The majority of studies assessing sexual knowledge created their own questionnaire for the purposes of the study, and without validation or replication (e.g., DiClemente et al., 1992; Langer & Tubman, 1997; Melchert & Burnett, 1990). Although the content of the various measures across studies had some elements in common, it is impossible to conduct viable comparisons across studies without consistency in methods. Clearly, this research would benefit from the establishment of a validated and consistently implemented measure of sexual knowledge, in order to specify the construct as well as its relationship to sexual risk behavior.

As a second example of the importance of specificity in measures, Miller, Levin, and colleagues (1998) recently found that the timing of parental discussions about condoms was important in influencing adolescent use of condoms: discussions that occurred prior to adolescent sexual debut were particularly important in promoting condom use. This finding underscores the importance of "fine tuning" measures rather than examining a broadly conceived variable such as "parent–child communication" or even "discussions about sex or condoms."

In the same manner, it is difficult to compare the results of studies that define sexual risk taking differently. For example, the consistent use of contraceptives has been defined as "contraceptive use during last sexual encounter" (e.g., Fullilove et al., 1993; Hou & Basen-Engquist, 1997), "frequency of contraceptive use during past six months" (e.g., Miller, Clark, & Wendell, 1997; Neumark-Sztainer et al., 1997), and "use of contraceptives at sexual initiation" (e.g., Melchert & Burnett, 1990; St. Lawrence & Scott, 1996). Each measures a slightly different, albeit related, aspect of contraceptive use.

CHALLENGES FOR PREVENTION

As reviewed earlier, a number of effective programs have been developed that provide youth with the knowledge, skills, and resources to manage their transition to sexual adulthood more safely. Nevertheless, there is room for improvement and advancement with respect to prevention program development. First, more attention must be given to programs that successively intervene across multiple contexts. Extrafamilial contexts, such as school and neighborhood conditions, offer particular promise for inclusion as both targets and resources in prevention programs designed to reduce STD infection, pregnancy, and the transmission of HIV among youth.

Second, prevention programs typically start too late. Early-intervention efforts that take place prior to the initiation of sexual activity are the most effective, and with the rates of sexual activity in younger cohorts increasing, it is imperative that prevention specialists reach youth sooner. As exemplified in some promising new interventions (e.g., Kotchick et al., 2002), the family represents a very powerful socializing force in the lives of children and adolescents, and one that is more politically amenable to early intervention. Parents are in a unique and powerful position to shape young people's attitudes and behaviors and to socialize them to become sexually healthy adults. They can do this, in part, by providing accurate information about sex and its risks, consequences, and responsibilities and by imparting skills to make responsible decisions about health. However, the strength of parents as interventionists stems from their unique ability to engage their children in dialogues about sexual development and decision making that occur early and are continuous (i.e., not one-time events), sequential (i.e., building on each other as the child's cognitive, emotional, physical, and social development and experiences change), and time-sensitive (i.e., information is immediately responsive to the child's questions and anticipated needs rather than programmed to a curriculum).

Finally, the literature suggests that targets for intervention should include competencies specific to both sexual behavior and more general areas of psychosocial or family functioning. For adolescents, knowledge, attitudes, and sexual self-efficacy represent specific competencies known to be related to reduced sexual risk taking. For parents, specific targets for intervention include knowledge of adolescent sexual behavior, monitoring of dating behavior, and skills to communicate with their adolescent children about sex. However, broader indices of functioning, such as depression and anxiety, self-esteem, school involvement, and parent–child relationship quality, are all appropriate targets for interventions seeking to promote well-being and reduce sexual risk behavior among adolescents. In this sense, we would encourage prevention and intervention efforts that have as their ultimate goal the development of healthy and well-adjusted youth. Risk reduction would be part, but only a part, of such programs, and the result would be teens and families that value and foster sexual health and safety as part of overall well-being.

ACKNOWLEDGMENTS

The writing of this chapter was supported, in part, by the Centers for Disease Control and Prevention, the William T. Grant Foundation, and the University of Georgia's Institute for Behavioral Research. Parts of this chapter are based on our earlier writings, including Armistead, Kotchick, and Forehand (2004).

REFERENCES

Airhihenbuwa, C. O., DiClemente, R. J., Wingood, G. M., & Lowe, A. (1992). Perspective: HIV/AIDS education and prevention among African-Americans: A focus on culture. *AIDS Education and Prevention, 4*, 267–276.

Anderson, J. E., Kann, L., Holtzman, D., Arday, S., Truman, B., & Kolbe, L. (1990). HIV/AIDS knowledge and sexual behavior among high school students. *Family Planning Perspectives, 22*, 252–255.

Armistead, L., Kotchick, B. A., & Forehand, R. (2004). Teenage pregnancy, sexually transmitted diseases, and HIV/AIDS. In L. A. Rapp-Paglicci, C. N. Dulmas, & J. S. Wodarski (Eds.), *Handbook of preventive interventions for children and adolescents* (pp. 227–254). Hoboken, NJ: Wiley.

Bagnall, G., Plant, M., & Warwick, W. (1990). Alcohol, drugs and AIDS-related risks: results from a prospective study. *AIDS Care, 2*, 309–317.

Baldwin, J. I., Whitely, S., & Baldwin, J. D. (1990). Changing AIDS and fertility-related behavior. The effectiveness of AIDS education. *Journal of Sex Research, 27*, 245–262.

Bandura, A. (1977). *Social learning theory.* Englewood Cliffs, NJ: Prentice-Hall.

Barber, B. K., Olsen, J. E., & Shagle, S. C. (1994). Associations between parental psychological and behavioral control and youth internalized and externalized behaviors. *Child Development, 65*, 1120–1136.

Baumeister, L. M., Flores, E., & Marin, B. (1995). Sex information given to Latina adolescents by parents. *Health Education Research, 10*, 233–239.

Biglan, A., Noell, J., Ochs, L., Smolkowski, K., & Metzler, C. (1995). Does sexual coercion play a role in the high-risk sexual behavior of adolescent and young adult women? *Journal of Behavioral Medicine, 18*, 549–568.

Bingham, C. R., & Crockett, L. J. (1996). Longitudinal adjustment patterns of boys and girls experiencing early, middle, and late sexual intercourse. *Developmental Psychology, 32*, 647–658.

Blum, R. W., Beuhring, T., & Rinehart, P. M. (2000). *Protecting teens: Beyond race, income, and family structure.* Minneapolis: Center for Adolescent Health, University of Minnesota.

Boekeloo, B. O., & Howard, D. E. (2002). Oral sexual experiences among young adolescents receiving general health examinations. *American Journal of Health Behavior, 26*, 306–314.

Brewster, K. L. (1994). Neighborhood context and the transition to sexual activity among young Black women. *Demography, 31*, 603–614.

Brewster, K. L., Cooksey, E. C., Guilkey, D. K., & Rindfuss, R. R. (1998). The changing impact of religion on the sexual and contraceptive behavior of adolescent women in the United States. *Journal of Marriage and the Family, 60*, 493–504.

Brooks-Gunn, J., & Furstenberg, F. F. (1989). Adolescent sexual behavior. *American Psychologist, 44,* 249–257.

Bronfenbrenner, U. (1979). *The ecology of human development.* Cambridge, MA: Harvard University Press.

Bronfenbrenner, U. (1989). Ecological systems theory. *Annals of Child Development, 6,* 187–249.

Brown, L. K., DiClemente, R. J., & Park, T. (1992) Predictors of condom use in sexually active adolescents. *Journal of Adolescent Health, 13,* 651–657.

Campbell, F. A. (1999, April). Long-term outcomes from the Abecedarian study. In F. A. Campbell (Chair), *How high-quality early childhood programs enhance long-term development: Comparison of findings and models.* Symposium presented at the biennial meeting of the Society for Research in Child Development, Albuquerque, NM.

Capaldi, D. M. (1996). The reliability of retrospective report for timing of first sexual intercourse for adolescent males. *Journal of Adolescent Research, 11,* 375–387.

Capaldi, D. M., Crosby, L., & Stoolmiller, M.(1996). Predicting the timing of first sexual intercourse for at-risk adolescent males. *Child Development, 67,* 344–359.

Centers for Disease Control and Prevention. (1999). *HIV/AIDS Prevention Research Synthesis Project: Compendium of HIV prevention interventions with evidence of effectiveness.* Atlanta, GA: Author.

Centers for Disease Control and Prevention. (2000). *Tracking the hidden epidemics: Trends in STDs in the United States.* Retrieved July 15, 2002, from www.cdc.gov

Centers for Disease Control and Prevention. (2001). *HIV/AIDS Surveillance Report, 13*(1).

Chapin, J. R. (2000). Adolescent sex and mass media: A developmental approach. *Adolescence, 35,* 799–811.

Chesney, M. A. (1994). Prevention of HIV and STD infections. *Preventive Medicine, 23,* 655–660.

Children Now & Kaiser Family Foundation. (1999). *Talking with kids about tough issues.* Retrieved August 17, 1999, from www.talkingwithkids.org

Coles, R., & Stokes, G. (1985*). Sex and the American teenager.* New York: Harper & Row.

Cooper, M. L., Peirce, R. S., & Huselid, R. F. (1994). Substance use and sexual risk taking among black adolescents and white adolescents. *Health Psychology, 13,* 251–262.

Cothran, M. M., & White, J. P. (2002). Adolescent behavior and sexually transmitted diseases: The dilemma of human papillomavirus. *Health Care for Women International, 23,* 306–319.

Coyle, K. K., Basen-Enquist, K. M., Kriby, D. B., Parcel, G. S., Banspach, S. W., & Collins, J. L. (2001). Safer Choices: Long-term impact of a multi-component school-based HIV, STD, and pregnancy prevention program. *Public Health Reports, 116,* 82–93.

Coyle, K. K., Kirby, D., Marin, B., Gomez, C., & Gregorich, S. (2000). *Effect of Draw the Line/Respect the Line on sexual behavior in middle schools.*

Unpublished manuscript, ETR Associates, Santa Cruz.

Crockett, L. J., Bingham, C. R., Chopak, J. S., & Vicary, J. R. (1996). Timing of first sexual intercourse: The role of social control, social learning, and problem behavior. *Journal of Youth and Adolescence, 25,* 89–111.

Darroch, J. E., Landry, D. J., & Oslak, S. (1999). Age differences between sexual partners in the United States. *Family Planning Perspectives, 31,* 160–167.

Department of Health and Human Services. (1997). *Sexually Transmitted Disease Surveillance—1996.* Retrieved September 29, 1998, from wonder.cdc.gov/wonder/STD/STDD016.PCW.html

Dermen, K. H., Cooper, M. L., & Agocha, V. B. (1998). Sex-related alcohol expectancies as moderators of the relationship between alcohol use and risky sex in adolescents. *Journal of Studies on Alcohol, 59,* 71–77.

Des Jarlais D. C., Paone, D., Milliken, J. Turner, C. F., Miller, H., Gribble, J., et al. (1999). Audio-computer interviewing to measure risk behaviour for HIV among injecting drug users: a quasi-randomised trial. *Lancet, 353,* 1657–1661.

Devine, D., Long, P., & Forehand, R. (1993). A prospective study of adolescent sexual activity: Description, correlates, and predictors. *Advances in Behaviour Research and Therapy, 15,* 185–209.

DiClemente, R. J., Durbin, M., Siegel, D., Krasnovsky, F., Lazarus, N., & Comacho, T. (1992). Determinants of condom use among junior high school students in a minority, inner-city school district. *Pediatrics, 89,* 197–202.

Duncan, S. C., Strycker, L. A., & Duncan, T. A. (1999). Exploring associations in developmental trends of adolescent substance use and risky sexual behavior in a high-risk population. *Journal of Behavioral Medicine, 22,* 21–34.

Dutra, R., Miller, K. S., & Forehand, R. (1999). The process and content of sexual communication with adolescents in two-parent families: Associations with sexual risk-taking behavior. *AIDS and Behavior, 3,* 59–66.

East, P. L. (1998). Racial and ethnic differences in girls' sexual, marital, and birth expectations. *Journal of Marriage and the Family, 60,* 150–162.

Ekstrand, M. L., Siegel, D. S., Nido, V., Faigeles, B., Cummings, G. A., Battle, R., et al. (1996, July). *Peer-led AIDS prevention delays onset of sexual activity and changes peer norms among urban junior high school students.* Paper presented at the XI International Conference on AIDS, Vancouver, BC, Canada.

Elkind, D. (1967). Egocentrism in adolescence. *Child Development, 38,* 1024–1038.

Feiring, C. (1996). Concept of romance in 15 year-old adolescents. *Journal of Research on Adolescence, 6,* 181–200.

Fiscella, K., Kitzman, H. J., Cole, R. E., Sidora, K. J., & Olds, D. (1998). Does child abuse predict adolescent pregnancy? *Pediatrics, 101,* 620–624.

Fisher, W. A., Williams, S. S. Fisher, J. D., & Malloy, T.

E. (1999). Understanding AIDS risk behavior among sexually active urban adolescents: An empirical test of the information–motivation–behavioral skills model. *AIDS and Behavior, 3*, 13–23.

Fleming, D. T., McQuillian, G. M., Johnson, R. E., Nahmias, A. J, Aral, S. O., Lee, F. K., & St. Louis, M. E. (1997). Herpes simplex virus type 2 in the United States, 1976–1994. *New England Journal of Medicine, 337*, 1105–1111.

Forehand, R., & Wierson, M. (1993). The role of developmental factors in planning behavioral interventions for children: Disruptive behavior as an example. *Behavior Therapy, 24*, 117–141.

Fullilove, M. T., Golden, E., Fullilove, R. E., Lennon, R., Porterfield, D., Schwarcz, S., & Bolan, G. (1993). Crack cocaine use and high-risk behaviors among sexually active black adolescents. *Journal of Adolescent Health, 14*, 295–300.

Gillmore, M. R., Butler, S. S., Lohr, M. J., & Gilchrist, L. (1992). Substance use and other factors associated with risky sexual behavior among pregnant adolescents. *Family Planning Perspectives, 24*, 255–261, 268.

Gillmore, M. R., Lewis, S. M., Lohr, M. J., Spencer, M. S., & White, R. D. (1997). Repeat pregnancies among adolescent mothers. *Journal of Marriage and the Family, 59*, 536–550.

Goodson, P., Evans, A., & Edmundson, E. (1997). Female adolescents and onset of sexual intercourse: A theory-based review of research from 1984 to 1994. *Journal of Adolescent Health, 21*, 147–156.

Gordon, C. P. (1996). Adolescent decision making: A broadly based theory and its applications to the prevention of early pregnancy. *Adolescence, 31*, 561–584.

Grunbaum, J., Kann, L., Kinchen, S. A., Ross, J. G., Hawkins, J., Lowry, R., et al. (2004). Youth Risk Behavior Surveillance—United States, 2003. *Morbidity and Mortality Weekly Report, 53*(SS-2), 2–29.

Halpern, C. T., Joyner, K., Udry, J. R., & Suchindran, C. (2000). Smart teens don't have sex (or kiss much either). *Journal of Adolescent Health, 26*, 213–225.

Hamburg, D. (1992). *Today's children: Creating a future for a generation in crisis.* New York: Times Books.

Hardy, J. B., Astone, N. M., Brooks-Gunn, J., Shapiro, S., & Miller, T. L. (1998). Like mother, like child: Intergenerational patterns of age at first birth and associations with childhood and adolescent characteristics and adult outcomes in the second generation. *Developmental Psychology, 34*, 1220–1232.

Harvey, S. M., & Spigner, C. (1995). Factors associated with sexual behavior among adolescents: A multivariate analysis. *Adolescence, 30*, 253–264.

Hawkins, J. D., Catalano, R. F., Kosterman, R., Abbott, R., & Hill, K. G. (1999). Preventing adolescent health-risk behaviors by strengthening protection during childhood. *Archives of Pediatrics and Adolescent Medicine, 153*, 226–234.

Henshaw, S. K. (1998). Unintended pregnancy in the United States. *Family Planning Perspectives, 1*, 24–29.

Herlocher, T., Hoff, C., & DeCarlo, P. (1995). *Can theory help in HIV prevention?* [HIV Prevention Fact Sheet]. San Francisco: University of California.

Hou, S., & Basen-Engquist, K. (1997). Human immunodeficiency virus risk behavior among White and Asian/Pacific Islander high school students in the United States: Does culture make a difference? *Journal of Adolescent Health, 20*, 68–74.

Hubbard, B. M., Giese, M., II, & Rainey, J. (1998). A replication of Reducing the Risk, a theory-based sexuality curriculum for adolescents. *Journal of School Health, 68*, 243–247.

Jaccard, J., & Dittus, P. J. (2000). Adolescent perceptions of maternal approval of birth control and sexual risk behavior. *American Journal of Public Health, 90*, 1426–1430.

Jaccard, J., Dittus, P. J., & Gordon, V. V. (1996). Maternal correlates of adolescent sexual and contraceptive behavior. *Family Planning Perspectives, 28*, 159–165.

Jarrell, A. E. (2000, April 2). The face of teenage sex grows younger. *New York Times.* Retrieved April 5, 2000, from search.nytimes.com

Jemmott, J. B., & Jemmott, L. S. (1993). Alcohol and drug use during sexual activity: Predicting the HIV-risk-related behaviors of inner-city black male adolescents. *Journal of Adolescent Research, 8*, 41–57.

Jemmott, J. B., & Jemmott, L. S. (1994). Interventions for adolescents in community settings. In R. J. DiClemente & J. L. Peterson (Eds.), *Preventing AIDS: Theories and methods of behavioral interventions* (pp. 141–174). New York: Plenum Press.

Jemmott, J. B., III, Jemmott, L. S., & Fong, G. T. (1998). Abstinence and safer sex: A randomized trial of HIV sexual risk-reduction interventions for young African American adolescents. *Journal of the American Medical Association, 279*, 1529–1536.

Jemmott, L. S., & Jemmott, J. B. (1990). Sexual knowledge, attitudes, and risky sexual behavior among inner-city Black male adolescents. *Journal of Adolescent Research, 5*, 346–369.

Jemmott, L. S., & Jemmott, J. B. (1992). Family structure, parental strictness, and sexual behavior among inner-city black male adolescents. *Journal of Adolescent Research, 7*, 192–207.

Jessor, R., Costa, F., Jessor, L., & Donovan, J. E. (1983). Time of first intercourse: A prospective study. *Journal of Personality and Social Psychology, 44*, 608–626.

Jessor, R., & Jessor, S. L. (1977). *Problem behavior and psychosocial development.* New York: Academic Press.

Jessor, R., Van Den Bos, J., Vanderryn, J., Costa, F. M., & Turbin, M. S. (1995). Protective factors in adolescent problem behavior: Moderator effects and developmental change. *Developmental Psychology, 31*, 923–933.

Joseph, S. C. (1991). AIDS and adolescence: A challenge

to both treatment and prevention. *Journal of Adolescent Health, 12,* 614–618.

Kann, L., Kinchen, S. A., Williams, B. I., Ross, J. G., Lowry, R., Hill, C., et al. (1998). Youth Risk Behavior Surveillance—United States, 1997. *Morbidity and Mortality Weekly Report, 47*(SS-3), 1–89.

Kann, L., Warren, C. W., Harris, W. A., Collins, J. L., Douglas, K. A., Collins, M. E., et al.. (1995). Youth Risk Behavior Surveillance—United States, 1993. *Morbidity and Mortality Weekly Report, 44,* 1–57.

Keller, S. E., Bartlett, J. A., Schleifer, S. J., Johnson, R. L., Pinner, E., & Delaney, B. (1991). HIV-relevant sexual behavior among a healthy inner-city heterosexual adolescent population in an endemic area of HIV. *Journal of Adolescent Health, 12,* 44–48.

Kirby, D. (2001). *Emerging answers: Research findings on programs to reduce teen pregnancy.* Washington, DC: National Campaign to Prevent Teen Pregnancy.

Kirby, D. (2002). The impact of schools and school programs upon adolescent sexual behavior. *Journal of Sex Research, 39,* 27–33.

Kirby, D., Short, L., Collins, J., Rugg, D., Kolbe, L., Howard, M., et al. (1994). School-based programs to reduce sexual risk behaviors: A review of effectiveness *Public Health Reports, 109,* 339–360.

Koniak-Griffin, D., & Brecht, M. (1995). Linkages between sexual risk taking, substance use, and AIDS knowledge among pregnant adolescents and young mothers. *Nursing Research, 44,* 340–346.

Kotchick, B. A., Armistead, L., Forehand, R., Long, N., Miller, K., Kelly, A., et al. (2002, November). *The Parents Matter! Program: A preliminary report.* Paper presented at the annual meeting of the Association for the Advancement of Behavior Therapy, Reno, NV.

Kotchick, B. A., Dorsey, S., Miller, K. S., & Forehand, R. (1999). Adolescent sexual risk-taking behavior in single-parent ethnic minority families. *Journal of Family Psychology, 13,* 93–102.

Kotchick, B. A., Shaffer, A., Forehand, R., & Miller, K. (2001). Adolescent sexual risk behavior: A multi-system perspective. *Clinical Psychology Review, 21,* 493–519.

Lammers, C., Ireland, M., Resnick, M., & Blum, R. (2000). Influences on adolescents' decisions to postpone onset of sexual intercourse: A survival analysis of virginity among youths aged 13–18 years. *Journal of Adolescent Health, 26,* 42–48.

Langer, L. M., & Tubman, J. G. (1997). Risky sexual behavior among substance-abusing adolescents: Psychosocial and contextual factors. *American Journal of Orthopsychiatry, 67,* 315–322.

Leigh, B. C., Morrison, D. M., Trocki, K., & Temple, M. T. (1994). Sexual behavior of American adolescents: Results from a U.S. national survey. *Journal of Adolescent Health, 15,* 117–125.

Levesque, R. J. (2000). Sexuality education: What adolescents' educational rights require. *Psychology, Public Policy, and Law, 6,* 953–988.

Levinson, R. A., Jaccard, J., & Beamer, L. (1995). Older adolescents' engagement in casual sex: Impact of risk perception and psychosocial motivation. *Journal of Youth and Adolescence, 24,* 349–364.

Li, X., Feigelman, S., & Stanton, B. (2000). Perceived parental monitoring and health risk behaviors among urban low-income African American children and adolescents. *Journal of Adolescent Health, 27,* 43–48.

Lilienfeld, S. O. (2002). When worlds collide: Social sciences, politics, and the Rind et al. (1998) child sexual abuse meta-analysis. *American Psychologist, 57,* 176–188.

Lowry, R., Holtzman, D., Truman, B. I., Kann, L., Collins, J. L., & Kolbe, L. J. (1994). Substance use and HIV-related sexual behaviors among U.S. high school students: Are they related? *American Journal of Public Health, 84,* 1116–1120.

Luster, T., & Small, S. A. (1994). Factors associated with sexual risk-taking behaviors among adolescents. *Journal of Marriage and the Family, 56,* 622–632.

Magura, S., Kang, S., & Shapiro, J. L. (1994). Outcomes of intensive AIDS education for male adolescent drug users in jail. *Journal of Adolescent Health, 15,* 457–463.

Main, D. S., Iverson, D. C., McGloin, J., Banspach, S. W., Collins, K., Rugg, D., & Kolbe, L. J. (1994). Preventing HIV infection among adolescents: Evaluation of a school-based education program. *Preventive Medicine, 23,* 409–417.

Manlove, J. (1998). The influence of high school dropout and school disengagement on the risk of school-age pregnancy. *Journal of Research on Adolescence, 8,* 187–220.

Martin, J. A., Hamilton, B. E., Ventura, S. J., Menacher, F., & Park, M. M. (2002). Births. *National Vital Statistics Reports, 50*(5).

Mason, C. A., Cauce, A. M., Gonzales, N., & Hiraga, Y. (1996). Neither too sweet nor too sour: Problem peers, maternal control, and problem behavior in African American adolescents. *Child Development, 67,* 2115–2130.

McFarlane, M., & St. Lawrence, J. S. (1999). Adolescents' recall of sexual behavior: Consistency of self-report and effect of variations in recall duration. *Journal of Adolescent Health, 25,* 199–206.

McKay, M., & Williams, J. (July, 2002). *The CHAMPS (Collaborative HIV Prevention and Adolescent Mental Health Project) family program.* Workshop conducted at the annual NIMH conference on the Role of Families in Preventing and Adapting to HIV/AIDS, Miami, FL.

Melchert, T., & Burnett, K. F. (1990). Attitudes, knowledge, and sexual behavior of high-risk adolescents: Implications for counseling and sexuality education. *Journal of Counseling and Development, 68,* 293–298.

Metzler, C. W., Noell, J. Biglan, A., Ary, D., & Smolkowski, K. (1994). The social context for risky sexual behavior among adolescents. *Journal of Behavioral Medicine, 17,* 419–438.

Mezzich, A. C., Tarter, R. E., Giancola, P. R., Lu, S., Kirisci, L., & Parks, S. (1997). Substance use and risky sexual behavior in female adolescents. *Drug and Alcohol Dependence, 44*, 157–166.

Miller, B. C., & Moore, K. A. (1990). Adolescent sexual behavior, pregnancy, and parenting: Research through the 1980s. *Journal of Marriage and the Family, 52*, 1025–1044.

Miller, B. C., Norton, M. C., Curtis, T., Hill, E. J., Schvaneveldt, P., & Young, M. H. (1997). The timing of sexual intercourse among adolescents: family, peer, and other antecedents. *Youth and Society, 29*, 54–83.

Miller, B. C., Norton, M. C., Fan, X., & Christopherson, C. R. (1998). Pubertal development, parental communication, and sexual values in relation to adolescent sexual behaviors. *Journal of Early Adolescence, 18*, 27–52.

Miller, K. S., Clark, L. F., & Wendell, D. A. (1997). Adolescent heterosexual experience: A new typology. *Journal of Adolescent Health, 20*, 179–186.

Miller, K. S., Forehand, R., & Kotchick, B. A. (1999). Adolescent sexual behavior in two ethnic minority samples: The role of family variables. *Journal of Marriage and the Family, 61*, 85–98.

Miller, K. S., Forehand, R., & Kotchick, B. A. (2000). Adolescent sexual behavior in two ethnic minority groups: A multi-system perspective. *Adolescence, 35*, 313–333.

Miller, K. S., Kotchick, B. A., Dorsey, S., Forehand, R., & Ham, A. Y. (1998). Family communication about sex: What are parents saying and are their adolescents listening? *Family Planning Perspectives, 30*, 218–222 & 235.

Miller, K. S., Levin, M. L., Xu, X., & Whitaker, D. J. (1998). Patterns of condom use among adolescents: The impact of maternal–adolescent communication. *American Journal of Public Health, 88*, 1542–1544.

Millstein, S. G., & Moscicki, A. (1995). Sexually-transmitted disease in female adolescents: Effects of psychosocial factors and high risk behaviors. *Journal of Adolescent Health, 17*, 83–90.

Millstein, S. G., Petersen, A. C., & Nightingale, E. O. (1993). *Promoting the health of adolescents: New directions for the twenty-first century.* Oxford: Oxford University Press.

Minnis, A. M., & Padian, N. S. (2001). Reliability of adolescents' self-reported sexual behavior: A comparison of two diary methodologies. *Journal of Adolescent Health, 28*, 394–403.

National Campaign to Prevent Teen Pregnancy. (2002). *Research, resources, and information.* Retrieved July 15, 2002, from www.teenpregnancy.org

Neumark-Sztainer, D., Story, M., French, S. A., & Resnick, M. D. (1997). Psychosocial correlates of health compromising behaviors among adolescents. *Health Education Research: Theory and Practice, 12*, 37–52.

Newcomer, S. F., & Udry, J. R. (1985). Oral sex in an adolescent population. *Archives of Sexual Behavior, 14*, 41–46.

Orr, D. P., Beiter, M., & Ingersoll, G. (1991) Premature sexual activity as an indicator of psychosocial risk. *Pediatrics, 87*, 141–147.

Overby, K. J., & Kegeles, S. M. (1994). The impact of AIDS on an urban population of high-risk female minority adolescents: Implications for intervention. *Journal of Adolescent Health, 15*, 216–227.

Pendergrast, R. A., DuRant, R. H., & Gaillard, G. L. (1992). Attitudinal and behavioral correlates of condom use in urban adolescent males. *Journal of Adolescent Health, 13*, 133–139.

Perkins, D. F., Luster, T., Villarruel, F. A., & Small, S. (1998). An ecological, risk-factor examination of adolescents' sexual activity in three ethnic groups. *Journal of Marriage and the Family, 60*, 660–673.

Perrino, T., Gonzalez-Soldevilla, A., Pantin, H., & Szapocznik, J. (2000). The role of families in adolescent HIV prevention: A review. *Clinical Child and Family Psychology Review, 3*, 81–96.

Philliber, S., & Allen, J. P. (1992). Life options and community service: Teen Outreach Program. In B. C. Miller, J. J. Card, R. L. Paikoff, & J. L. Peterson (Eds.), *Preventing adolescent pregnancy* (pp. 139–155). Newbury Park, CA: Sage.

Philliber, S., Kaye, J. W., Herring, S., & West, E. (2000). *Preventing teen pregnancy: An evaluation of the Children's Aid Society Carrera Program.* Accord, NY: Philliber Research Associates.

Pick, S., & Palos, P. A. (1995). Impact of the family on the sex lives of adolescents. *Adolescence, 30*, 667–675.

Ramirez-Valles, J., Zimmerman, M. A., & Juarez, L. (2002). Gender differences of neighborhood and social control processes: A study of the timing of first intercourse among low-achieving, urban, African American youth. *Youth and Society, 33*, 418–441.

Reitman, D., St. Lawrence, J. S., Jefferson, K. W., Alleyne, E., Brasfield, T. L., & Shirley, A. (1996). Predictors of African American adolescents' condom use and HIV risk behavior. *AIDS Education and Prevention, 8*, 499–515.

Remez, L. (2000). Oral sex among adolescents: Is it sex or is it abstinence? *Family Planning Perspectives, 32*, 298–304.

Resnick, M. D., Bearman, P. S., Blum, R. W., Bauman, K. R., Harris, K. M., Jones, J., et al. (1997). Protecting adolescents from harm. *Journal of the American Medical Association, 278*, 823–832.

Rodgers, K. B. (1999). Parenting processes related to sexual risk-taking behaviors of adolescent males and females. *Journal of Marriage and the Family, 61*, 99–109.

Romer, D., Black, M. Ricardo, I., Feigelman, S., Kaljee, L., Galbraith, J., et al. (1994). Social influences on the sexual behavior of youth at risk for HIV exposure. *American Journal of Public Health, 84*, 977–985.

Roosa, M. W., Tein, J. Y., Reinholtz, C., & Angelini, P. J. (1997). The relationship of childhood sexual abuse to teenage pregnancy. *Journal of Marriage and the Family, 59*, 119–130.

Rosenberg, P. S., Biggar R. J., & Goedert J. J. (1994). Declining age at HIV infection in the United States. *New England Journal of Medicine, 330,* 789–90.

Santelli, J. S., Lowry, R., Brener, N. D., & Robin, L. (2000). The association of sexual behaviors with socioeconomic status, family structure, and race/ethnicity among US adolescents. *American Journal of Public Health, 90,* 1582–1588.

Scaramella, L. V., Conger, R. D., Simons, R. L., & Whitbeck, L. B. (1998). Predicting risk for pregnancy by late adolescence: A social contextual perspective. *Developmental Psychology, 34,* 1233–1245.

Seidman, S. N., & Reider, R. O. (1994). A review of sexual behavior in the United States. *American Journal of Psychiatry, 151,* 330–341.

Shafer, M. A., & Boyer, C. B. (1991). Psychosocial and behavioral factors associated with risk of sexually transmitted diseases, including human immunodeficiency virus, among urban high school students. *Journal of Pediatrics, 119,* 826–833.

Shrier, L. A., Emans, S. J., Woods, E. R., & DuRant, R. H. (1996). The association of sexual risk behaviors and problem drug behaviors in high school students. *Journal of Adolescent Health, 20,* 377–383.

Siegelman, C. K., Derenowski, E. B. Mullaney, H. A., & Siders, A. T. (1993). Parents' contributions to knowledge and attitudes regarding AIDS. *Journal of Pediatric Psychology, 18,* 221–235.

Small, S. A., & Luster, T. (1994). Adolescent sexual activity: An ecological, risk-factor approach. *Journal of Marriage and the Family, 56,* 181–192.

Smith, C. A. (1997). Factors associated with early sexual activity among urban adolescents. *Social Work, 42,* 334–346.

St. Lawrence, J. S., Brasfeld, T. L., Jefferson, K. W., Alleyne, E., O'Bannon, R. E., III, & Shirley, A. (1995). Cognitive-behavioral intervention to reduce African American adolescents' risk for HIV infection. *Journal of Consulting and Clinical Psychology, 63,* 221–237.

St. Lawrence, J. S., Jefferson, K. W., Alleyne, E., & Brasfield, T. L. (1995). Comparison of education vs. behavioral skills training interventions in lowering sexual HIV-risk behavior of substance-dependent adolescents. *Journal of Consulting and Clinical Psychology, 63,* 154–157.

St. Lawrence, J. S., Jefferson, K. W., Banks, P. G., Clince, T. R., Alleyne, E., & Brasfield, T. L. (1994). Cognitive-behavioral group intervention to assist substance-dependent adolescents in lowering HIV infection risk. *AIDS Education and Prevention, 6,* 424–435.

St. Lawrence, J. S., & Scott, C. P. (1996). Examination of the relationship between African American adolescents' condom use at sexual onset and later sexual behavior: Implications for condom distribu-

tion programs. *AIDS Prevention and Education, 8,* 258–266.

Stanton, B., Li, X., Black, M., Ricardo, I., Galbraith, J., Kalijee, L., & Feigelman, S. (1994). Sexual practices and intentions among preadolescent and early adolescent low-income urban African-Americans. *Pediatrics, 93,* 966–973.

Stanton, B. F., Li, X., Galbraith, J., Feigelman, S., & Kaljee, L. (1996). Sexually transmitted diseases, human immunodeficiency virus, and pregnancy prevention: Combined contraceptive practices among urban African-American early adolescents. *Archives of Pediatrics and Adolescent Medicine, 150,* 17–24.

Steinberg, L. (1987). Familial factors in delinquency: A developmental perspective. *Journal of Adolescent Research, 2,* 255–268.

Stouthamer-Loeber, M., & Wei, E. H. (1998). The precursors of young fatherhood and its effect on delinquency of teenage males. *Journal of Adolescent Health, 22,* 56–65.

Strunin, L., & Hingson, R. (1992). Alcohol, drugs, and adolescent sexual behavior. *International Journal of the Addictions, 27,* 129–146.

Szapocznik, J., & Coatsworth, J. D. (1999). An ecodevelopmental framework for organizing the influences on drug abuse: A developmental model for risk and prevention. In M. Glantz & C. R. Hartel (Eds.), *Drug abuse: Origins and interventions* (pp. 331–366). Washington, DC: American Psychological Association.

Tubman, J. G., Windle, M., & Windle, R. C. (1996). Cumulative sexual intercourse patterns among middle adolescents: Problem behavior precursors and concurrent health risk behaviors. *Journal of Adolescent Health, 18,* 182–191.

Turner, C. F., Ku, L., Rogers, S. M., Lindberg, L. D., Pleck, J. H., & Sonenstein, F. L. (1998). Adolescent sexual behavior, drug use, and violence: Increased reporting with computer survey technology. *Science, 280,* 867–873.

Walter, H. J., & Vaughn, R. D. (1993). AIDS risk reduction among a multi-ethnic sample of urban high school students. *Journal of the American Medical Association, 270,* 725–730.

Weisz, J. R., & Hawley, K. M. (2002). Developmental factors in the treatment of adolescents. *Journal of Clinical and Consulting Psychology, 70,* 21–43.

Whitaker, D. J., & Miller, K. S. (2000). Parent–adolescent discussions about sex and condoms: Impact on peer influences of sexual risk behavior. *Journal of Adolescent Research, 15,* 251–273.

Zimet, G. D., Bunch, D. B., Anglin, T. M., Lazebnik, R., Williams, P., & Krowchuk, D. P. (1992). Relationship of AIDS-related attitudes to sexual behavior changes in adolescents. *Journal of Adolescent Health, 13,* 493–498.

18

Deviant Sexual Behavior

Howard E. Barbaree
Calvin M. Langton

This chapter focuses on deviant sexual behavior in adolescents. As an introduction to the chapter, deviant sexual behavior is discussed in terms of (1) the statistical prevalence of particular sexual behaviors in a specific population, (2) moral and religious condemnation of unusual sexual behaviors, (3) potential harmful effects of sexual behaviors, and (4) criminal sanctions. The purpose of the introduction is to compare and contrast three related concepts: sexual deviance, sexual abuse, and sexual crime.

At the outset and throughout the chapter, we make a distinction between sexual deviance and issues relating to other sexual behaviors or conditions evident in adolescence, namely, sexual orientation and homosexuality, gender identity and dysphoria, and gender-atypical behavior. These topics are beyond the scope of the present discussion and are addressed in a separate chapter in this book (see Zucker, Chapter 16, this volume).

DEVIANT SEXUAL BEHAVIOR

"Deviance" is a statistical term, denoting the tendency in a distribution of scores of any quantifiable variable for the values of individual observations to disperse from the average value or midpoint. Accordingly, sexual behavior is said to be deviant when it is outside the "norm" for a particular population of individuals. We can determine whether or not a sexual behavior is deviant if we know the group membership of the individual who has engaged in the behavior and what sexual practices are usual for that group. For example, an unmarried 18-year-old girl engaging in sexual intercourse would be considered normative in modern Western society because such behavior is not unusual in her peer group (Leitenberg & Saltzman, 2000, 2003). However, such behavior would be considered deviant in many parts of the world where such behavior is unusual in the local population.

DEVIANT SEXUAL BEHAVIOR IN CHILDREN AND ADOLESCENTS

High-quality scientific studies of sexual behavior in adolescents are few in number. The result is that we have very little objective information about the normal developmental course of sexual behavior. There have been many explanations offered to account for this lack of basic and fundamental knowledge. For example, it has been suggested that research on children's sexuality is discouraged by legal and ethical considerations where the mere act of observing or inquiring about sexual behavior in children could lay the experimenter open to charges of sexual abuse (Bancroft, 1989). And the development of sexual modesty and embarrassment from childhood to adolescence has frustrated the accumulation of reliable and accurate information on sexual behaviors in children and adolescents. Friedrich, Grambsch, Broughton, Kuiper, and Beilke (1991) surveyed mothers of 880 2–12-year-olds using a behavior checklist that included a number of sexual behaviors. These overt sexual behaviors decreased with age in this sample in both sexes. Money and Ehrhardt (1972) observed this same decline and suggested that as children get older they seek to conceal their sexual behavior in order to conform to society's rules on modesty and manners.

Even when studies have been done, the observations made have led to widely different interpretations depending on culture and social climate (Vizard, Monck, & Misch, 1995). In Norway, for example, Gundersen, Melas, and Skar (1981) conducted individual interviews with 60 preschool teachers concerning their observations of sexual behavior of their pupils. Many of the teachers reported seeing children exploring their own bodies, manipulating their own genitals, exhibiting an interest in their fellow students' genitals, and engaging in behaviors they described as "coitus training." In the United States, Cantwell (1988) described the same behaviors in very young children but judged these preschool and school-age children as "perpetrators" of inappropriate sexual behavior and recommended an educational program of prevention (Vizard et al., 1995).

We do know that adolescents engage in many of the deviant sexual behaviors exhibited by adults, including child molestation, paraphilia, and fetishism (Zolondek, Abel, Northey, & Jordan, 2001). Perhaps ironically, we may know more about deviant than normative sexual behavior in these age groups. Whereas research into normative sexual behavior of children and adolescents has been difficult and frustrating, research into deviant sexual behavior has become widespread. Upon disclosure, these sexual behaviors become the subject of intense investigation and scrutiny by the school authorities, child protective agencies, the police, the courts, and correctional authorities. These cases are often referred to clinical practitioners for evaluation and intervention. As a consequence, a large clinical and scientific literature now exists on deviant sexual behavior in adolescents. Because our scientific knowledge is based almost entirely on research with clinical cases, it likely suffers from what has been called external validity bias (Rind, Tromovitch, & Bauserman, 2001).

When considering whether or not a sexual behavior is deviant, the issue is complicated during adolescence by the fact that normative sexual behavior changes over age and between developmental stages. In the normal course of development from childhood through adolescence, sexual behavior becomes more frequent, extensive, and complex, following a developmental sequence from hugging and kissing in the earliest stages to fondling and touching of the breasts and genitals in later stages to more intimate interactions involving oral–genital contact and penetrative intercourse in the final stage (Smith & Udry, 1985). When the sexual behavior of an adolescent is consistent with sexual behavior exhibited by his or her peers in their own age group, such sexual behavior is considered to be normative.

However, when children engage in sexual behaviors that are unusual for their current age group, these behaviors are considered deviant even though these same behaviors may be normative later in development. Again, sexual intercourse in young girls provides an illustrative example. Leitenberg and Saltzman (2000) conducted a statewide survey of a representative sample of adolescent girls in 8th–12th grades (n = 4,201) in Vermont. Participants were asked to report their age at first experience of consensual sexual intercourse. Prior to age 14, only 5% of surveyed girls reported that they had engaged in sexual intercourse. Therefore, to this stage in development, sexual intercourse is rare or unusual in the peer group and such behavior might be said to be deviant. However, by the time these girls were 18 years of age, 51% of them reported that they had engaged in sexual intercourse. At this level of prevalence, sexual intercourse would be considered a normative behavior. From a developmental perspective, when a sexual behavior appears earlier in the development sequence than usual in the population, we regard such sexual behavior as deviant.

If we restrict ourselves to the statistical definition of deviance, no value judgment of the sexual behavior is made or conveyed. But deviant sexual behaviors have been characterized in negative terms in a number of ways, including (1) as immoral as a result of religious or moral condemnation, (2) as pathological by diagnosis as a mental disorder, (3) by association as a correlate with negative outcomes, (4) as abusive when the deviant sexual behavior involves nonconsenting partners or children, and (5) as criminal when the behavior violates the criminal law.

RELIGIOUS OR MORAL CONDEMNATION OF DEVIANT SEXUAL BEHAVIOR

In colloquial usage, the term "sexual deviance" has acquired a pejorative connotation and conveys at least a tone of moral disapproval, more often outright condemnation. It seems a prominent human trait and a pervasive aspect of human society that religious and moral judgments are readily made about all forms of sexual behavior, but particularly when the sexual behavior is unusual. For the obvious example, the world's religions have condemned homosexual behavior throughout history. But religious disapproval has not been restricted to less prevalent sexual behavior. Leaders in the early Christian church expressed disapproval of sexual intercourse between a husband and his wife even when performed for the purposes of procreation (Tannahill, 1992, pp. 138–141). In this chapter, we resist the human tendency to condemn sexual behaviors on moral or religious grounds, except, of course, as explained later, in the case of sexual abuse, on the basis of its harmful effects on victims.

Resisting the general temptation to make moral judgments of deviant sexual behaviors is especially important when considering such behavior in children and adolescents. Young children may not yet have an ability to appreciate that particular sexual behaviors are considered to be morally wrong, socially inappropriate, harmful, or illegal (Pithers & Gray, 1998). In addition, according to many authorities in this field, and as discussed below, deviant sexual behaviors in adolescents are often the result of abusive experiences they have endured as a child (e.g., Craissati, McClurg, & Browne, 2002), in which case moral or religious condemnation is akin to blaming the victim.

DIAGNOSIS AS A MENTAL DISORDER

Sexual deviation is often used as a synonym for "sexual perversion" or "paraphilia" (Travin & Protter, 1993). When the object of sexual desire is unusual, an underlying pathology of sexual interest is inferred and a mental health professional will make a diagnosis of paraphilia according to criteria set out in DSM-IV (American Psychiatric Association, 1994). For example, when the objects of desire are children, women's undergarments, or animals, diagnoses of pedophilia, fetishism, and zoophilia would be made, respectively. Paraphilias are discussed later in more detail in relation to diagnosis and assessment.

DEVIANT SEXUAL BEHAVIOR AND ASSOCIATED NEGATIVE OUTCOMES

Deviant sexual behaviors may come to be viewed as undesirable because they are associated with less desirable circumstances or outcomes. We continue with the previous example of girls engaging in consenting sexual intercourse at an early age. Such girls exhibit more behavior problems than similar-age girls who are not yet sexually active (Irwin & Millstein, 1992; Jessor & Jessor, 1977), and these behavior problems include suicide, alcohol use, drug use, truancy, and pregnancy (Leitenberg & Saltzman, 2000). Later, in adulthood, these girls are more likely to endorse symptoms of psychological distress (Leitenberg & Saltzman, 2003). Girls who engage in sexual intercourse early in adolescence experience greater family conflict and exhibit less positive affect (McBride, Paikoff, & Holmbeck, 2003), are more likely to come from a single-parent family (Wyatt, Durvasula, Guthrie, LeFranc, & Forge, 1999), and are less likely to achieve their educational goals (Hayes, 1987). There are reasons to believe that the younger the girl is when she first has intercourse, the more likely she is to have had a much older partner. For example, Elo, King, and Furstenberg (1999) found that 45% of women who first had intercourse when they were 14 years of age or younger had partners 4 or more years older than themselves compared to 18% who first had intercourse between ages 15 and 17. Lindberg, Sonenstein, Ku, and Martinez (1997) found that the youngest teenage mothers in their sample were the most likely to have had substantially older partners. These findings suggest that when a girl experiences first intercourse at a very young age, she may have been subject to the undue influence of a much older partner, even though she described the interaction as consenting

It is not known whether early sexual intercourse causes these less desirable outcomes or if early sexual intercourse is a result of these undesirable circumstances. Of course, early intercourse together with these outcomes may be a result of some other unknown determining factor (Billy, Lindale, Grady, & Zimmerle, 1988; Bingham & Crockett, 1996; Costa, Jessor, Donovan, & Fortenberry, 1995).

SEXUAL ABUSE

A significant subset of deviant sexual behaviors is referred to as sexually abusive. To properly define sexual abuse, we must first define consent to sexual relations. Movies, television, and other popular media often portray the pleasurable aspects of sexual activity but place much less emphasis on the significant risks to participants. There are well-known health risks of sexual intercourse, including the acquisition of sexually transmitted diseases and HIV, with the potential for serious negative health outcomes. Girls have their own specific set of risks. Pregnancy and the subsequent birth of a child will present the teenage mother with difficult choices between abortion, giving the child up for adoption, or raising the child in very difficult circumstances. Parenthood leads to serious long-term lifestyle changes and financial challenges. Sexual relationships, particularly during adolescence, are associated with negative emotional states including jealousy, rejection, and abandonment. Of course, sex can have a number of benefits as well, including increased psychological well-being, the solidification of human partnerships, the formation of family units, and procreation. Considering the potential risks and rewards of sexual relations, the decision to engage in sexual activity can be a critically important decision with long-term consequences for the individual.

There is now widespread recognition that adults have the right to make autonomous decisions concerning their participation in sexual relations (United Nations General Assembly, 1994) by weighing for themselves the balance between the potential risks and rewards of any sexual relationship. This recognition is the result of the long history of the emancipation of women and more recent feminist scholarship and activism (Brownmiller, 1975). The absolute right of women to refuse sexual relations has been articulated in the slogan "no-means-no" used in campaigns on college campuses over the past 15 years to raise consciousness of this important principle (Monson, Langhinrichsen-Rohling, & Binderup, 2000). Perhaps the ultimate recognition of women's right to refuse sexual relations is contained in laws against rape in marriage that have been enacted over the past several years in many Western jurisdictions. While the right to refuse sexual relations has been won largely by women for women, the resulting principle that consent is required to be obtained before sexual relations begin is now a benefit afforded to all persons

When sexual interactions are forced against a nonconsenting person, the sexual interactions are, by definition, abusive. In these circumstances, the person (adult or adolescent) who forces sex is referred to as the perpetrator or as a sexual abuser while the nonconsenting person is recognized as a victim of sexual abuse. Though it has been argued that prevalence rates of sexual abuse are high (e.g., Koss, Gidycz, & Wisniewski, 1987), there is general agreement that sexual abuse is outside the norm in our society. Therefore, sexual abuse is a subset of deviant sexual behavior; not all deviant sexual behaviors are abusive, but all abusive sexual behaviors are considered deviant.

Considering the relationship between sexual abuse and consent to sexual relations, it follows that sex between an adult (or older adolescent) and a child is inherently abusive because children are unable to provide true consent (Finkelhor, 1979). Finkelhor articulated two preconditions to true consent: (1) full knowledge regarding what is being consented to, and (2) absolute freedom to accept or decline. Young children have not yet developed the capacity to give consent to sexual relations because (1) they have not yet developed the intellectual ability or the knowledge to properly weigh the risks and rewards of sexual relations, and (2) children are susceptible to influence by adults, who, by virtue of their maturity and greater experience easily exert control over children (Ondersma et al., 2001). In short, children are neither knowledgeable nor autonomous beings and as a consequence they are not able or free to make their own decisions regarding sexual relations. Over the past 25 years, the influence of the child protection, victim's rights, and woman's movements have combined with emerging scientific research regarding the harmful effects of child sexual abuse (CSA) leading to a dramatic shift in public awareness and concern. Children have come to be viewed as potential victims of sexual exploitation by adults or adolescents, and as such, they deserve and require what protection society can provide (Ondersma et al., 2001; Myers, Diedrich, Lee, Fincher, & Stern, 1999).

An important distinction is to be made here between "willingness" and "consent." A child may be "willing" to engage in sexual interactions. They may express a desire for sexual interactions and they may even seem to initiate sexual interactions. However willing they may be, according to the foregoing argument, they do not have the psychological capacity to give consent. Therefore, all sexual interactions between an adult and a child are, by definition, abusive to the child. CSA has been used in the psychological literature to describe virtually all sexual interactions between children or adolescents and significantly older persons, as well as between same-age children or adolescents when coercion or a power imbalance is involved (Rind, Tromovitch, & Bauserman, 1998).

SEXUAL CRIME

In all jurisdictions in modern Western society, criminal laws against sexual assault have been enacted to protect the individual's right to autonomy and self-determination in sexual relations. Although these laws contain language that varies from jurisdiction to jurisdiction, they all prohibit all forms of sexual behavior, including touching, kissing, and intercourse when the prospective sexual partner does not give consent. Forcing another person of any age to engage in sexual relations of any kind is against the law in every modern Western society.

In addition, in every jurisdiction in modern Western society, criminal laws specifically protect children from sexual victimization by adults and/or adolescents. When a child is unwilling and sexual interactions are forced on them, the sexual crime is referred to as child rape, or simply as sexual assault. When the child is willing and agrees to sexual interactions with an adult, the sexual crime is sometimes referred to as statutory rape (Leitenberg & Saltzman, 2000, 2003; Oberman, 1994).

Laws against CSA require the establishment of an age below which the individual is considered to be unable to provide consent to sexual relations. This is often referred to as the age of consent. According to Leitenberg and Saltzman (2003), in the United States, 15 states have established 18 years, 6 states have set 17 years, and 28 states have chosen 16 years as their age of consent. Only one American state has established age 14 as the age of consent (Donovan, 1997). In Europe, one-half of the separate legal jurisdictions use 14 as the age of consent, whereas most of the remainder has set 15 or 16 as the age of consent (Graupner, 2000). In Canada, the age of consent is 14 years (Rodrigues, 2004).

The intent of these laws is to protect children from sexual victimization and exploitation by adults. In the same vein, very young children require protection from older children or adolescents who might take advantage of a very young child. However, it was not the original intent of these laws to criminalize sexual interactions between adolescent peers when such interactions are a normal part of adolescent development. Unfortunately, such criminalization does occur.

THE ADOLESCENT MALE SEXUAL PARTNER: BOYFRIEND OR SEXUAL ABUSER?

Imagine the situation when two 13-year-old neighbors, one male and the other female, engage in sexual intercourse while their parents are at work. Because these two adolescents are of equal age and maturity, it would be inappropriate to label such interactions "abusive." At 13 years of age, the law would state that neither one of them has the psychological capacity to consent to sexual activity. But, because their interactions did not involve any force or violence or threats of violence, and there is no power imbalance between them, according to the definition of sexual abuse provided previously, we would not be able to determine which of these individuals is the abuser and which the victim. If we agree that there has been no abuse in this situation, we should also agree that it would be inappropriate to subject either of these adolescents to criminal prosecution.

Now consider that these two adolescents are separated by several years in age. In this circumstance we have to consider that the relationship was abusive, and that the older of the two was the "abuser." The question then arises: How much of an age difference is required before we regard this situation as either (1) abusive, and/or (2) criminal? It seems reasonable to suggest that when an older individual has sex with a child who is below the age of consent, it should not be considered abusive or criminal when the older individual's age is close to the age of the younger. In the research literature, CSA is said to occur when there is at least a 5-year difference between partners (Finkelhor, 1984). For the purposes of this chapter, we define CSA as sexual interactions between a child under the age of 14 years with a person more than 5 years older than the child.

According to Leitenberg and Saltzman (2003), in the United States, four states require a minimum of a 5-year age difference between partners in order for the sexual interaction to qualify as a statutory rape offense (Donovan, 1997). However, 29 states do not require any age discrepancy for these laws to be prosecuted. Among these states, some require more severe penalties based on the magnitude of the age discrepancy, the absolute age of the defendant (e.g., 20 and over), and whether or not he is a repeat offender. However, in these states, when the "alleged (usually female) victim" is at all younger than the age of consent, her (usually male) sexual partner of any age can be charged with a criminal sexual offense (statutory rape; Leitenberg & Saltzman, 2003). With respect to the aforementioned example of the male and female 13-year-olds, the male partner could be prosecuted and convicted of sexual assault in many U.S. states.

In the study described earlier by Leitenberg and Saltzman (2000), young girls were asked to report the age at which they first experienced sexual intercourse, and, in addition, they were asked to report the age of their partner during their first experience. For 11- to 12-year-old girls, only 37% reported that their partners were of similar age. Twenty-nine percent and 34% reported that their partners were 2–4.5 years older and more than 5 years older, respectively. For 13- to 15-year-olds, 45%, 43%, and 12% reported that their partners were of similar age, 2–4.5 years older, and more than 5 years older, respectively. This study confirmed

the concern about the welfare of very young girls having much older partners. For girls who first had intercourse in early adolescence (11–12 years of age), much older partners (+5 years) were associated with more suicide attempts, more alcohol and drug abuse, and a higher incidence of pregnancy. For older girls (13+ years), much older partners (+5 years) did not lead to significantly more problems, except for truancy. Therefore, a large number of male adolescents not much older than their female partners have consensual sex with girls below the age of consent and would be subject to criminal proceedings in many states in the United States.

The following discussion illustrates how peer-to-peer sexual relations in adolescence have been accommodated in Canadian law (Rodrigues, 2004). When sexual relations involve a person under the age of consent (12–13 years of age) with a person who is peer-age or only marginally older (12–15 years of age) and who has no other relationship with the underage person that would make the relationship a nonpeer relationship (teacher, coach, etc.), then the sexual relations would be viewed as an example of peer-to-peer relations. In this circumstance, the older adolescent would be allowed to offer the defense at trial that the alleged victim consented to sexual activity. In this case, the older adolescent would perhaps not be subject to successful criminal prosecution in Canada. However, when the alleged victim is below the age of consent, the alleged perpetrator cannot use the defense that the alleged victim consented to sexual activity when the alleged victim is less than 12 years of age, or when the alleged perpetrator is over the age of 16.

The Canadian law also takes age into account in determining criminal sanctions in cases of sexual assault. As in most Western jurisdictions, youthful offenders are provided with a criminal justice system that is separate from the adult system, where the penalties are less severe and the emphasis is on rehabilitation rather than punishment. It is interesting to note here the different ways in which the law treats immaturity in the victim as compared immaturity in the perpetrator. For the victim below the age of consent, the law regards the individual to be "incapacitated" by their immaturity, lacking the psychological resources to make autonomous decisions regarding sexual behavior. In contrast, the perpetrator of the same age is not viewed as being incapacitated. They are held to be fully responsible for their criminal sexual behavior. In Canada, when the perpetrator is older than 12 but below the age of consent (14), the law regards the individual to be capable to make decisions regarding sexual behavior and therefore fully responsible for criminal sexual behavior, though deserving of less severe punishment on account of their immaturity. Under the age of 12, in Canada, as in most Western jurisdictions, the alleged perpetrator is "exempt" from prosecution, and this may be a recognition that below this age, the individual does not have the "capacity" to appreciate the fact that the behavior was illegal.

THE NATURE OF DEVIANT SEXUAL BEHAVIOR

This section of the chapter deals with the nature of deviant sexual behavior in adolescence. It is divided into three sections, following a developmental sequence. In the first section, we examine the effect of CSA on the development of deviant sexual behavior in adolescence. In the second section, we consider the role of the family and environmental context within which deviant sexual behavior arises. In the third section, we describe the characteristics known to be associated with adolescent sexual abusers.

The Effects of Child Sexual Abuse

The effect of CSA is considered more broadly in a separate chapter in this book (see Chapter 20, this volume). Therefore, in this chapter, the effect of CSA is subject to a more focused discussion, with the emphasis on the specific effects on later deviant sexual behavior.

Using a large (n = 4,023) nationwide (U.S.) probability sample of adolescents ages 12–17, Kilpatrick and his colleagues (Kilpatrick et al., 2000, 2003) surveyed symptoms of posttraumatic stress disorder (PTSD), major depression, and substance abuse/dependence. A significant minority of this representative sample of adolescents (15.5% of boys and 19.3% of girls) met diagnostic criteria for at least one of these DSM-IV diagnoses. Adolescents who reported experiencing sexual assault were 2.4 times more likely to have comorbid PTSD and a major depressive episode, 6.73 times more likely to have comorbid PTSD and substance abuse/dependence, and 4.43 times more likely

to have comorbid major depressive episode and substance abuse/dependence (Kilpatrick et al., 2003). Similarly, adolescents who reported being victims of sexual assault were 2.4 times more likely to abuse alcohol or to be alcohol dependent, and over two and a half times more likely to abuse hard drugs (Kilpatrick et al., 2000).

Numerous nonclinical studies of high school students have reported that CSA is associated with a wide variety of high-risk behaviors (Dallam et al., 2001), including antisocial behavior, conduct disorders, self-destructive behavior, substance abuse, younger age at first coitus, more frequent and risky sexual activity, not using condoms or birth control, sexually transmitted diseases, increased HIV risk, and teen pregnancy (Bensley, Spieker, Van Eenwyk, & Schoder, 1999; Bensley, Van Eenwyk, Spieker, & Schoder, 1999; Fiscella, Kitzman, Cole, Sidora, & Olds, 1998; Harrison, Fulkerson, & Beebe, 1997; Hibbard, Brack, Rauch, & Orr, 1988; Hibbard, Ingersoll, & Orr, 1990; Nagy, DiClemente, & Adcock, 1995; Stock, Bell, Boyer, & Connell, 1997). Moreover, studies of high school students have reported that sexual abuse has a particularly negative impact on the behavior of adolescent males (e.g., Chandy, Blum, & Resnick, 1996; Garnefski & Arends, 1998; Hibbard et al., 1990). Chandy and colleagues (1996) examined gender-specific outcomes for 370 abused boys and 2,681 abused girls who were identified in a study of over 36,000 students in grades 7 to 12. Compared with their female counterparts, male adolescents who acknowledged experiencing CSA were at significantly higher risk for poor school performance, delinquent activities, sexual risk taking, and dropping out of high school.

A long-standing and prevalent clinical assumption regarding adolescent sex offenders has been that many have been sexually abused as children and, therefore, that sexually deviant behavior somehow stems from early sexual victimization (e.g., Breer, 1987; McCormack, Rokous, Hazelwood, & Burgess, 1992; Muster, 1992). By 1990, numerous authorities in the field had reported that a significant minority (19–49%) of youthful sex offenders had experienced CSA (Becker, Cunningham-Rathner, & Kaplan, 1986; Becker, Kaplan, Cunningham-Rathner, & Kavoussi, 1986; Fehrenbach, Smith, Monastersky, & Deisher, 1986; Longo, 1982; Pierce & Pierce, 1987). Before 1990, clinical experience suggested that even higher rates were to be found in specific subgroups of sex offenders (e.g., male adolescents who molest younger boys; Davis & Leitenberg, 1987). Some specific samples had been reported to have rates of CSA of as high as 75% (a sample of incarcerated child molesters who had offended against boys, Robertson, 1990; a sample of children younger than age 6 who had engaged in sexual abuse, Johnson, 1988).

Johnson (1988), studying 47 boys between the ages of 4 and 13 who had engaged in sexually abusive behaviors, found an inverse relationship between the children's own sexual victimization and the age at which their sexual behavior problems began. Of the children who began their sexually abusive behavior when they were age 6 or younger, 72% reported having been sexually abused themselves, while 42% of the children who began their sexually abusive behaviors between the ages of 7 and 11 were victims of sexual abuse. In children who began sexually abusing between ages 11 and 12, only 35% acknowledged having been sexually abused. Friedrich and Luecke (1988) studied a group of school-age children (4–11 years, mean = 7.3 years) who had engaged in genital contact involving coercion and found that the sexual abuse experience had been more severe than reported for a sample of sexually abused children.

By the mid-1990s, research on CSA in adolescent sex offenders was becoming more systematic. Worling (1995) reviewed the extant literature on CSA in adolescent sex offenders and reported that of the 1,268 adolescent male sex offenders in these samples, 31% reported some form of sexual abuse, approximately triple the rate typically reported in studies of men in the general population (Peters, Wyatt, & Finkelhor, 1986). While the rates of CSA varied widely in these studies (19–55%), Worling reported that the rates were different comparing studies that had been based on data collected at pretreatment (22%) compared with the rates reported in studies that collected data after substantial treatment had been completed (52%). Worling speculated that this result was a reflection of the clinical reports that many adolescent sex offenders only acknowledge sexual victimization after they have formed a trusting relationship with a therapist (Becker, 1988; Kahn & Lafond, 1988). These data would argue that the reported rates of CSA experienced in sex offenders may be underestimates because

most studies have recorded data at pretreatment, or in circumstances in which there was no treatment involvement.

An alternative perspective is that at least some offenders claim to have been sexually abused as children in order to mitigate their responsibility for abusive behavior, perhaps once they recognize that CSA represents a clinical focus of treatment. The use of polygraph testing examining sexual offenders' self-reported history of personal victimization indicates that overreporting does occur (Hindman & Peters, 2001). Clearly, overreliance on self-reported data would place methodological limitations on our current understanding of the etiological role of CSA in later sexual offending behavior.

Nevertheless, from the data that have been reported, the rates of CSA seems to vary across groups of adolescent sex offenders subdivided according to characteristics of their offense history. For example, more adolescent sex offenders against children report a history of CSA compared with adolescent offenders against peers or adults (Awad & Saunders, 1991; O'Brien, 1991), and offenders who assault a male child are more likely to report sexual victimization than those who offended exclusively against female children (Hanson & Slater, 1988). However, Worling (1995) has pointed out that in these studies, age and gender of victim were confounded. While youthful sex offenders victimize females of all ages, they do not offend against adult males. Therefore, when the research findings suggest that CSA rates are higher among offenders against children, it may be that this finding is entirely due to the fact that all male victims are children.

Benoit and Kennedy (1992) examined institution records of adolescent offenders who assaulted only children, thereby eliminating the confound. Offenders who assaulted both male and female children were combined with those who assaulted only male children and it was found that 36% of adolescents who assaulted even one male child disclosed a history of sexual abuse. Conversely, only 16% of those who offended against female children reported sexual victimization.

Worling (1995) presented data from 87 adolescent male sex offenders between the ages of 12 and 19 years. Initial victimization and offending histories were collected by therapists during regular clinical interactions with the adolescents, which ranged in duration from 2 to 50 months with a mean of 13 months. Sexual victimization was recorded and corroborated by reports from child welfare or probation agencies. The sample of subjects was divided into four groups: offenders against female adolescents and adults ($n = 27$); offenders against female children ($n = 29$); offenders against only male children ($n = 12$); and offenders against both male and female children ($n = 19$). Overall, 43% of the participants reported sexual victimization. Comparing the four groups in terms of the frequency of sexual victimization, the four groups were significantly different, and the overall statistical significance was attributable to the finding that 75% of adolescents who had ever assaulted a male child disclosed a history of childhood sexual abuse, in comparison to only 25% who had only assaulted females of any age.

In summary, the literature indicates that most adolescent offenders who assault even one male child report a history of sexual abuse. This finding corroborates clinical observations (Breer, 1987; Davis & Leitenberg, 1987) and is similar to the results with adult offenders against children (Hanson & Slater, 1988). According to Worling (1995), there are a number of possible explanations for these results: The first is based on a learning or conditioning process where physiological arousal is seen as a component of the experience of victimization. Sexual abuse often involves sexual stimulation of the victim (Breer, 1987; Wheeler & Berliner, 1988). If some boys subsequently masturbate to fantasies of their early sexual experience— the abuse of a young boy—they may be conditioning their sexual arousal to cues of young boys (Becker & Stein, 1991; Laws & Marshall, 1990; McGuire, Carlysle, & Young, 1965). The second possible explanation is that sexual victimization may raise questions of sexual orientation for a male child; in particular, a male victim may wonder whether he is homosexual because of sexual arousal experienced during the assault (Gilgun & Reiser, 1990). The adolescent offenders' subsequent sexual offenses against male children may represent some form of "recapitulation" of the victimization incident, whereby the offender attempts to regain a sense of control and mastery over homosexual conflicts (Breer, 1987; Watkins & Bentovim, 1992). Perhaps the most parsimonious explanation is based on social learning principles. Quite simply, it is possible that some male child victims will model the behavior of their offender (Laws & Marshall, 1990).

The following two studies provide support for the conditioning and modeling theories of CSA's role in the development of deviant sexual behavior. Veneziano, Veneziano, and LeGrande (2000) studied 74 consecutive adolescent male sex abusers who had been referred or court-ordered to a residential treatment facility. Of the 74 subjects, 92% had been sexually abused, as documented by the family, the criminal justice system, or the referral source. After eliminating those subjects who had no experience of CSA, data analysis indicated that the subjects who were themselves first sexually abused when they were younger than the age of 5 were twice as likely to victimize someone younger than the age of 5. Similarly, they were twice as likely to have sexually abused males if they had been so abused by males. If they were victimized by a relative, they were one and a half times more likely to victimize a relative. The boys who had been subjected to anal intercourse were 15 times more likely to abuse their victims in this fashion. If they had been fondled, they were seven times more likely to fondle their victims, and if their sexual abuse had involved fellatio, they were twice as likely to have engaged in fellatio with their victims.

In a similar study, Burton (2003) studied a sample of 179 adolescent males incarcerated in youth residential facilities, 46% of whom had been convicted of sexual offenses, and the remainder for other violent offenses from armed robbery to murder. These participants had been specifically selected for the study: In an anonymous survey, these youth reported that they had been sexually abused, and they admitted to committing a sexual offense. Results indicated that these youth tended to abuse the same type of person who abused them. A youth who was abused by a relative was 2.95 times more likely to abuse a relative than a youth who was abused by a nonrelative. Similarly, a youth who was abused by a stranger was 2.87 times more likely to abuse a stranger than a youth who was abused by a nonstranger. A youth who was abused by a friend or neighbor was 4.54 times more likely to abuse a friend or neighbor than a youth who was not sexually abused by a friend or neighbor. These youth were more likely to abuse the same gender of person who abused them; a youth who was abused by a male was 6.05 times more likely to abuse a male, and a youth who was abused by a female was 3.89 times more likely to abuse a female. Youth were more likely to use the *modus operandi* of the person who had abused them; a youth who was sexually abused with favors, games, or babysitting was 9.22 times more likely to use these same methods than a youth who was not so abused. Similarly, a youth who was abused with threats against him was 3.88 times more likely to use threats himself. Finally, youth who were sexually penetrated as part of the victimization experience were 4.13 times more likely to penetrate their own victims. This suggests that sexual abuse of children by some adolescent sex offenders may be a reenactment of their own sexual abuse or a learned behavior pattern (Burton, 2003; Longo, 1982; McCormack et al., 1992; Ryan, Miyoshi, Metzner, Krugman, & Fryer, 1996).

The following study also provides support for the conditioning model. Lambie, Seymour, Lee, and Adams (2002) examined the moderating factors that may prevent a victim of male sexual abuse from entering the "victim–offender cycle." Two groups were interviewed as part of the study: a resilient group (*n* = 47) that had experience with sexual victimization but no history of perpetration, and a victim–offender group (*n* = 41). Compared with the offender group, the resilient group was less likely to have fantasized and masturbated about the abuse, less likely to report deriving pleasure from the abuse, more likely to have had frequent social contact with adolescent peers, and more likely to have had more family and nonfamily support during childhood.

Although these findings provide general support for the role of CSA in the development of deviant sexual behavior, it is important and worthwhile to note that CSA is neither necessary nor sufficient for later deviant sexual behavior. Most male victims of sexual abuse do not become sex offenders (Finkelhor, 1986), and 25% of the offenders against male children in Worling's (1995) study did not report a history of sexual abuse.

Family and Environmental Context

It is important at this point to describe the experiential and environmental contexts within which deviant sexual behaviors arise. Deviant sexual behavior in adolescents is strongly influenced by the youngster's family environment, their early sexual experiences, particularly the experience of CSA, and their early sexual behavior. Of course, not all adolescents who display deviant sexual behavior have experienced CSA, nor have they all grown up in families that allow or promote the development of these behaviors. But, as will be seen, empirical data confirm the clinical impressions of professionals in the field that family context, early sexual behavior, and the experience of CSA are critically important factors in the development of deviant sexual behavior.

As has been reported for the adult sex offender (Barbaree, Hudson, & Seto, 1993), the families of adolescent sexual abusers are characterized by frequent violence, family instability, and disorganization (Awad, Saunders, & Levene, 1984; Deisher, Wenet, Paperny, Clarke, & Fehrenbach, 1982; Fehrenbach et al., 1986; Lewis, Shankok, & Pincus, 1979; Longo, 1982; Smith, 1988). Although these same family characteristics and backgrounds may be said to apply to persons who later exhibit a wide variety of dysfunctional behaviors (e.g., criminal behavior and substance abuse), the families that particularly seem to produce sexual deviance are characterized by (1) instability and lack of resources, (2) the failure to promote or establish strong emotional bonds particularly between parent and child, (3) early exposure to sexual material and behavior, (4) an environment in which the child is at high risk for sexual abuse or sexual exploitation by an adult, and (5) lack of resources to cope with the effects of CSA.

Further, the more serious and harmful adolescent sex offenders more often report having engaged in problematic sexual behavior prior to the age of 12 (Burton, 2000). Children naturally engage in a wide range of sexual behaviors (Friedrich et al., 1991). However, sexually abused children exhibit a higher frequency of sexual behaviors than do nonabused children (Berliner, 1991; Gale, Thompson, Moran, & Sack, 1988). In a review of the literature on the effects of childhood maltreatment, Kendall-Tackett, Williams, and Finkelhor (1993) found that 13 of 45 studies examining these effects reported the occurrence of sexual behaviors earlier in development than expected. Twenty-eight percent of 1,353 maltreated children had engaged in sexual behaviors, but these studies showed a large range in the proportion of children showing premature sexual behaviors (i.e., 7–90%). Although most maltreated children may not exhibit highly sexualized behaviors, the available data suggest that sexual behaviors may occur earlier than expected in development in approximately one-quarter of all maltreated children. These premature sexual behaviors are some of the most distinguishing consequences of childhood sexual victimization (Pithers & Gray, 1998).

The Child Sexual Behavior Inventory (CSBI) is a 36-item checklist completed by the child's caregiver who rates behaviors manifested over the previous 6 months along a scale from 0–4 reflecting the frequency of problematic sexual behaviors (Freidrich, Grambsch, Damon, & Hewitt, 1985). The CSBI was developed on sexually abused and abuse-free children ages 2–12. The inventory has shown discriminant validity in the sense that it shows significant differences in the frequency of sexual behaviors between children referred to clinical services subsequent to their experience of CSA and nonreferred children. Problematic sexual behavior exhibited by the children who had experienced CSA include touching the sex parts of another child, touching animals' sex parts, asking others to engage in sex, rubbing sex parts against other people, inserting objects in vagina or rectum, and trying to undress other children. These problem sexual behaviors were extremely rare in the nonreferred sample.

Gray, Busconi, Houchens, and Pithers (1997) reported on a sample of children with sexual behavior problems. This sample was composed of 65% boys and 35% girls. Mental health practitioners, child protective agencies, and the courts referred these children for treatment after they had been identified as a result of their own victimization. Gray and colleagues defined children with sexual behavior problems as 6–12-year-olds who had engaged in sexual behaviors that were (1) repetitive; (2) unresponsive to adult intervention and supervision; (3) equivalent to a criminal violation, if performed by an adult; (4) pervasive, occurring across time and situations; or (5) a diverse array of sexual acts.

Although the sample of children with sexual behavior problems had experienced all recognized forms of child maltreatment, sexual abuse predominated. Sexual abuse occurred in 95% of the 66 children for whom data could be collected. All the females in this study had been sexually abused, as were 93% of the males. Physical abuse was the second most common type of victimization, experienced by 48% of the entire sample, with 52% of the males and 42% of the females being affected. One-third of all the children had been emotionally abused. More than half the children with

sexual behavior problems were victims of multiple forms of abuse with the most frequent combination being sexual and physical abuse. Considering all forms of abuse, the average number of victimizers per child was 2.5. Most of the children's abusers were male (73.2%). Other children and adolescents were responsible for nearly 40% of abuse to these children, with 16.7% of the perpetrating children being 5–10 years old and 22.7% being 11–18 years old. Young adults, ages 19–25, represented 6.1% of the children's abusers, and older adults accounted for 33% of their abusers. The average age of these children at the time of their own maltreatment was 3.4 years.

It is important to recognize, particularly in the context of this chapter on deviant sexual behavior in adolescents, that sexual behavior problems in childhood are precursors to deviant sexual behavior in adolescence. Burton (2000) compared three groups of incarcerated adolescents who admitted to sexual offending in an anonymous survey project on measures of trauma, sexual offending, and the relationship between trauma and sexual offending. Burton divided his sample into those who admitted to offending before the age of 12 only, those who admitted to offending after the age of 12 only, and those who offended before and after the age of 12. Approximately half of the total sample who reported any sexually aggressive behavior reported having begun their aggressive behavior prior to the age of 12. Further, the severity and complexity of the sexual aggression was greater for those individuals for adolescents who reported continuous sexual aggression (both before and after the age of 12).

Families of children with sexual behavior problems are characterized as being unstable with few resources. In a study of children with sexual behavior problems, Gray and colleagues (1997) found that half of the caregivers were single parents. Although most caregivers in this sample had completed high school, their annual family incomes were low, with 38% of these families falling below the U.S. federal poverty level. Poverty has been shown to be highly associated with all forms of child maltreatment (Coulton, Korbin, Su, & Chow, 1995; Garbarino & Sherman, 1980; Gelles, 1992; Tzeng & Schwarzin, 1990; Zuravin, 1989). The Third National Incidence Study of Child Abuse and Neglect (Sedlak & Broadhurst, 1996) compared families with incomes over $30,000 with families with incomes under $15,000. The poorer families had 12–16 times the incidence of physical abuse and 18 times the incidence of CSA (Sedlack & Broadhurst, 1996).

Second, these families fail to establish strong emotional bonds (Blaske, Borduin, Henggeler, & Mann, 1989). In recent years, the etiological significance of insecure childhood attachment among sexual offenders has received theoretical consideration (Marshall, 1989; Ward, Hudson, Marshall, & Siegert, 1995) and tentative empirical support (Smallbone & Dadds, 1998, 2000; Ward, Hudson, & Marshall, 1996). Childhood attachment insecurity among sexual offenders has been proposed to lead to disruptions in empathy and to the failure to achieve intimacy in adolescence and adulthood (Marshall, 1989; Ward et al., 1995), contributing to sexually abusive behaviors (Smallbone & McCabe, 2003).

Three specific aspects of the parent–child relationship have been found to be associated with the development of early-onset behavioral problems (Loeber & Stouthamer-Loeber, 1987; Reiss et al., 1995): parent–child conflict, inadequate parental monitoring of children, and lack of positive involvement between parent and child. Parents of children with conduct disorder are more likely to fight with their child, administer harsh punishment, and dislike their child; they are less likely to create an emotionally supportive home, to express concern for their child's welfare, or to foster intellectual stimulation and provide emotional support. At least one study has found that these three dimensions of the parent–child relationship contribute independently to child conduct problems, with the presence of each factor separately contributing to the development and maintenance of problematic childhood behaviors. Wasserman, Miller, Pinner, and Jaramillo (1996) have noted that the combination of a difficult child (e.g., impulsive and irritable) and an adverse family context (e.g., incompetent parenting) leads to a persistent pattern of oppositional and aggressive behavior

In the families of children with sexual behavior problems, all three of these parent–child conditions were found (Pithers & Gray, 1998). Parents of children with sexual behavior problems indicated that they had difficulty fulfilling their parental role as a result of qualities of their children that they found undesirable or disappointing (Pithers & Gray, 1998). They

considered their children to be overreactive to changes in routine, difficult to calm when upset, and excessively demanding. The parents regarded interactions with their children as generally unrewarding. Further, parents of children with sexual behavior problems reported feeling emotionally distant from their children, suggesting an impaired parent–child attachment (Pithers & Gray, 1998).

Third, these families promote or allow early exposure to sexual material and behavior. Friedrich and colleagues (1991) surveyed mothers of 880 2–12-year-olds using a behavior checklist that included a number of sexual behaviors. These authors report that increased overt sexual behavior in children was positively related to family nudity and general behavior problems. Ford and Linney (1995) compared adolescent sex offenders, violent nonsexual offenders, and nonviolent offenders. The content of early childhood memories and exposure to pornographic material differed among the groups. Forty-two percent of the sex offenders reported exposure to hard-core sex magazines, compared to 29% of the violent and nonviolent offenders. *Post hoc* comparisons indicated that the sex offenders were exposed to pornographic magazines at the youngest ages, between 5 and 8 years old, with child molesters being the most frequently exposed.

Fourth, these families allow an environment to exist in which the child is at high risk for both sexual and physical abuse (Awad & Saunders, 1989; Becker, Cunningham-Rathner, & Kaplan, 1986; Becker, Kaplan, et al., 1986; Fehrenbach et al., 1986; Lewis et al., 1979; Longo, 1982; Robertson, 1990; Smith, 1988; Van Ness, 1984). In the Ford and Linney (1995) study cited earlier, adolescent child molesters were found to have experienced more physical and sexual abuse than violent nonsexual and nonviolent offender groups. Some of these families include an adult perpetrator of CSA. In families of children with sexual behavior problems, Gray and colleagues (1997) found that excluding the sexual abuse perpetrated by the child who had been referred for sexual behavior problems, 62% of the families contained at least one additional person who had performed a sexually abusive act. In the 72 families involved in the study, there was a total of 87 additional perpetrators, an average of 1.3 additional sexual abusers per family. Further, sexual abuse perpetrators within the family tended to act against other family members, with 94% of the victims being within the extended family and 84.8% of the abuse occurred with the abuser's or victim's own home.

But, even when the family does not contain another perpetrator of CSA, some of these families fail their children by allowing the child to be sexually abused, through neglect, ignorance, or incompetence. Hummel, Thomke, Oldenburger, and Specht (2000) compared adolescent child molesters with (*n* = 16) and without (*n* = 20) a history of sexual abuse. Adolescent child molesters who had a history of sexual abuse reported more frequent absence of the parent from the family home.

Finally, these families do not have the resources required to cope effectively with the effects of CSA once it has occurred. Friedrich and Luecke (1988) observed that after CSA, appropriate parenting is the exception, rather than the rule, and this further exacerbated the trauma of sexual abuse. While highly skilled, nurturing parents may assist children to overcome difficulties early in life, a rejecting parental response will worsen behavior problems (Henggeler, 1989; McCord, 1979; Patterson & Stouthamer-Loeber, 1984). Parental incompetence and parents' relative detachment from their children predispose their child to maltreatment but also reduce the moderating effect of the parental relationship on subsequent behavior problems (Pithers & Gray, 1998). The fact that these families fail to cope effectively with the effects of CSA makes it even more

likely that the child victim will engage later in aggressive and/or deviant sexual behavior (Pithers & Gray, 1998).

Characteristics of Adolescent Sexual Abusers

Adolescent Male Sexual Abusers

Adolescent male offenders show all the same variations of sexually abusive behaviors as do older offenders. Zolondek and colleagues (2001) used a standardized self-report questionnaire to survey 485 boys between the ages of 11 and 17 who were seeking evaluation or treatment for possible sexually deviant behavior. Table 18.1 presents the percent of this sample endorsing each of 13 sexually deviant behaviors, with the age of onset, number of victims, and estimated number of acts associated with each behavior. The most prevalent deviant sexual behavior was child molestation (60.8%), with use of pornography (31.6%) and fetishism (24.6%) endorsed less frequently. Sadism (2.1%) and masochism (1.9%) were the least frequently endorsed behaviors.

Fehrenbach and colleagues (1986) examined 305 offenders 18 years of age or younger. Within the 279 male offenders, the most common offense was fondling (59%), then rape (23%), exhibitionism (11%), and other noncontact offenses (7%). Wasserman and Kappel (1985) examined the sexual behaviors in the offenses of

TABLE 18.1. Percentage of Juvenile Sexual Offenders Engaging in Behaviors, Mean Age of Onset, Mean Number of Victims, and Average Number of Acts

Behavior	Percentage reporting	Age of onset (years)	Number of victims	Number of acts
Exhibitionism	11.5	11.4	6.0	11.1
Fetishism	26.4	10.8	NA	46.0
Voyeurism	17.0	11.0	8.8	16.9
Zoophilia	5.0	10.8	Unknown	11.6
Obscene phone calls	16.4	12.3	10.0	Unknown
Masochism	1.9	9.7	NA	40.9
Child molestation	60.8	11.9	4.2	11.1
Unwanted rubbing/touching	17.0	11.7	9.1	15.4
Sadism	2.1	11.0	2.4	11.2
Transvestism	4.6	11.5	NA	9.4[a]
Phone sex	15.4	12.4	Unknown	11.7
Pornography	31.6	11.4	NA	22.9
Transsexualism	3.3	10.1	NA	NA

Note. From Zolondek, Abel, Northey, and Jordan (2001). Copyright 2001 by Sage Publications. Reprinted by permission.
[a]Mean number of times per month.

161 (149 male) under 19-year-old or younger offenders. Some form of penetration was involved in 59% of offenses, while 31% involved intercourse, 12% oral–genital contact, and 16% genital fondling; 12% were judged to be noncontact offenses.

Intercourse becomes more common as the age of both offender and victim increases. Awad and Saunders's (1989) sample of 11- to 16-year-old child molesters had mainly fondled their victims, whereas Smith, Monastersky, and Deisher's (1987) older sample of 262 adolescent sex offenders (mean age = 15.3 years) had raped, or attempted to rape, in 77.5% of cases. When the victims were children who were younger than the adolescent offender, rape occurred in 21–24% of instances compared to 67% of offenses involving same-age or older victims (Groth, 1977; Wasserman & Kappel, 1985).

Adolescent offenders seem to use less force than adult offenders (McDermott & Hindelang, 1981). In the case of rape, a victim of an adolescent offender is one-third as likely to have had a weapon used against her and one-half as likely to be physically injured compared to a similar assault by an adult. Nevertheless, physical injury results from one-third of offenses perpetrated by adolescents (McDermott & Hindelang, 1981). Both Wasserman and Kappel (1985) and Fehrenbach and colleagues (1986) found a low rate of weapon usage (4–8%) among adolescent offenders, but in approximately half of their cases some form of threat was used. The level of reported coercion varies with the age of the victim. Victims report higher levels of coercion than offenders, and younger victims seem to be subject to less force (Davis & Leitenberg, 1987). Groth (1977) reported that 43% of offenses against a peer or older victim involved a weapon, whereas when the victim was a much younger child, no weapons were involved.

Miranda and Corcoran (2000) compared the characteristics of sexually abusive behavior between adolescent and adult sex offenders and found that the adolescents were more likely than adults to commit incest offenses, and they were more likely to use force in the commission of their offenses than the adults. However, the adults were more likely to penetrate the victim vaginally, anally, or orally than the adolescents, and the adolescents were more likely to engage in digital penetration. Adult offenders perpetrated a higher number of abusive acts than ad-

olescents and maintained their abusive relationships with victims over a longer period of time than adolescents.

The Victims of Male Adolescent Sexual Abusers. Typically the victims of assaults by adolescent sex offenders are younger children. Fehrenbach and colleagues (1986) found that 62% of the victims of their sample of abusers were less than 12 years of age, with 44% less than 6. In both, Deisher and colleagues' (1982) and Wasserman and Kappel's (1985) samples, 50–66% were less than 10, and only a quarter were older than 20 years of age. Incarcerated adolescent offenders, who are typically older than a nonincarcerated group (Groth, 1977; Longo, 1982; Van Ness, 1984), had older victims, but these victims were still usually younger than the offenders themselves. The only exception to this general rule seems to be when noncontact offenses such as exhibitionism and obscene telephone calls are involved; in these instances peer-age and adult females were more frequent targets (Fehrenbach et al., 1986). In studies in which adolescent child molesters are defined on the basis of being 4–5 years older than the victim, the majority of these victims are even younger than this age-defined discrepancy. Indeed, the victims are typically only 6–9 years of age, with male victims younger than female victims (Awad & Saunders, 1989; Becker, Cunningham-Rathner, & Kaplan, 1986; Pierce & Pierce, 1987).

The majority (69–84%) of the victims of sexual assaults by adolescents are female (Awad et al., 1984; Fehrenbach et al., 1986; Groth, 1977; Longo, 1982; Van Ness, 1984; Wasserman & Kappel, 1985), and this is especially true in noncontact offenses (Fehrenbach et al., 1986). However, as the age of the victim decreases, the victim is more likely to be male, as 45–63% of the child victims of adolescent perpetrators are male (Awad & Saunders, 1989; Shoor, Speed, & Bartlett, 1966; Van Ness, 1984).

Most of the victims of adolescents are known to the offender and are usually friends or relatives. Relatives constitute between 6% and 40% of victims (Fehrenbach et al., 1986; Groth, 1977; Wasserman & Kappel, 1985) while friends were victims in 41–51% of cases reported (Fehrenbach et al., 1986; Groth, 1977). Strangers were victims in 17–48% of cases (Fehrenbach et al., 1986; Groth, 1977; Van Ness, 1984). There is an increasing tendency toward victimizing strangers in rape compared with child molestation. For example, in a sample of adolescent rapists, Vinogradov, Dishotsky, Doty, and Tinklenberg (1988) found that only one-third knew their victim before the rape took place. In contrast, almost all of Awad and Saunders's (1989) child molesters knew their victims, either as relatives, children of friends of the parents, or children the offenders had been babysitting.

Incidence and Prevalence of Sexual Abuse by Male Adolescents. Ageton (1983) estimated that 2–4% of adolescent males have reported committing sexually assaultive behavior. While the prevalence of sexual assault among adolescents may be low, a substantial proportion of all sexual offenses can be attributed to adolescents. The best available estimates suggest that approximately 20% of all rapes and between 30 and 50% of child molestations are perpetrated by adolescent males (Becker, Kaplan, et al., 1986; Brown, Flanagan, & McLeod, 1984; Deisher et al., 1982; Groth, Longo, & McFadin, 1982). Table 18.2 presents data from the *Uniform Crime Report* for 2002 (Federal Bureau of Investigation, 2002) for four violent crimes: murder, forcible rape, aggravated assault, and other sexual offenses. Persons under the age of 18 account for 16.7% of all forcible rapes and 20.61% of other sexual offenses, and these percentages are consistent with figures from 10 years ago (1993). Nevertheless, there have been substantial reductions in the numbers of persons arrested for violent crimes over this same 10-year period, a decrease that is matched by reductions in child sexual victimization, a phenomenon that is at present not completely understood or explained (Finkelhor & Jones, 2004). Lalumière, Quinsey, Harris, and Rice (2005) have listed the many speculations to explain this decrease, including an increase in the number of incarcerated men, an increase in policing resources, a smaller relative number of young men, changes in the laws on abortion, a proliferation in the number of prevention programs, and a decrease in the tolerance for risk-taking behavior. Although these authors favor the latter, there are no convincing data supporting one of these explanations over another.

Age of Onset. Groth and colleagues (1982) reported the modal age for first offense in 83 rapists as 16 years (range 9–47), whereas the 54 child molesters showed a bimodal distribution, peaking in early adolescence around 14 years of age, and again in the early 30s. Longo (1982) found 14.3 years was the mean age of first sexual assault among adult offenders. Whereas a first sexual assault seems to occur most often in early adolescence, Lewis and colleagues (1979) found that most adolescent sex offenders had committed deviant sexual acts by 6 years of age.

Role of Antisocial History, Attitudes, Behavior, and Peer Group. A history of delinquency is common in adolescent sex offenders (Saunders, Awad, & White, 1986). Among adolescent sex offenders, a history of prior nonsexual crime was found in 28–50% of cases (Becker, Cunningham-Rathner, & Kaplan, 1986; Becker, Kaplan, et al., 1986; Fehrenbach et al., 1986); a prior sexual offense in 46–90% of cases (Awad et al., 1984; Becker, Kaplan, et al., 1986; Pierce & Pierce, 1987); aggressive acts and other antisocial behavior in 50–86% of cases (Awad & Saunders, 1989; Shoor et al., 1966; Van Ness, 1984); and arrests and incarceration in 33% of child molesters (Shoor et al., 1966) and 50% of adolescent incest offend-

TABLE 18.2. FBI Uniform Crime Report: Ten-Year Arrest Trends in the United States, 1993 to 2002

Offenses charged	Total persons, 2002	% of total persons arrested under 18 years of age		% change total persons, 1993–2002
		1993	2002	
Murder and non-negligent manslaughter	8,933	26.42	9.90	−64.3
Forcible rape	17,394	16.70	16.59	−26.5
Aggravated assault	299,286	15.41	12.72	−23.0
Sex offenses (except forcible rape and prostitution)	59,193	19.38	20.61	−8.9

ers (Becker, Cunningham-Rathner, & Kaplan, 1986).

Jacobs, Kennedy, and Meyer (1997) presented a comprehensive descriptive study of incarcerated adolescent offenders with an analysis of group differences between sexual and nonsexual offenders. The study used a relatively large sample ($n = 156$) with standardized psychometric measures and substantial institutional and therapeutic record reviews. The groups were described and compared on measures of delinquent history, intelligence, academic achievement, and psychopathology. Whereas the goal of the research was to identify characteristics unique to sexual offenders that could lead to theories as to why adolescent offenders act out as they do, the results did not reveal a meaningful pattern of differences between the groups on the variables measured. The data supported the conclusion that sexual offending by incarcerated adolescents is likely to be but one expression of antisocial, violent behavior by these adolescents.

Sexual Experience and Knowledge. Between 59% and 86% of adolescent sex offenders report having experienced previous consensual intercourse (Becker, Cunningham-Rathner, & Kaplan, 1986; Groth, 1977; Longo, 1982). However, while comparing four groups of young men (17–20-year-old college students, 16–20-year-old sex offenders, 16–20-year-old non-sex offenders, and 10–15-year-old sex offenders), Daleiden, Kaufman, Hilliker, and O'Neil (1998) reported that youthful sex offenders reported fewer consenting sexual experiences and more involvement in nonconsenting and paraphilic behaviors than both incarcerated nonsexual offenders and college males.

Comorbid Mental Disorders. Awad and colleagues (1984) and Lewis and colleagues (1979) found an equally high prevalence of psychiatric symptoms in both adolescent non-sex offenders and adolescent sex offenders. Psychiatric problems have been found in between 70–87% of adolescent offenders (Awad & Saunders, 1989; Awad et al., 1984; Lewis et al., 1979); prior psychiatric treatment in 33% of young offenders (Awad & Saunders, 1989); conduct disorder in 48% of young offenders, with rapists (75%) being more likely than child molesters (38%) to receive this diagnosis (Kavoussi, Kaplan, & Becker, 1988); and sub-stance abuse in over 10% of these adolescents (Kavoussi et al., 1988). Similar to adult sex offenders, adolescent offenders have exhibited high rates of emotional problems (Deisher et al., 1982; Groth, 1977; Shoor et al., 1966; Van Ness, 1984).

Baumbach (2002) points out that prenatal alcohol exposure can seriously harm the fetus, resulting in a wide range of physical and central nervous system abnormalities. A follow-up study of persons prenatally exposed to alcohol found that 49% of adolescents and adults had repeatedly displayed inappropriate sexual behavior. Although these persons are likely to present to sexual offender treatment programs, they are unlikely to be recognized as neurologically impaired because the sequelae of prenatal alcohol exposure are subtle and are seldom accurately identified by clinicians. Nevertheless, persistent impairments in response inhibition, memory, and executive functions are common in this group.

Several studies have noted a frequent presence of long-standing "learning problems" and other neuropsychological impairments in sexual offender populations (Lewis et al., 1979; Ryan, 1991, 1998; Tarter, Hegedus, Alterman, & Katzgaar, 1983). In addition, a few investigators have published data that implicitly suggested that attention-deficit/hyperactivity disorder (ADHD) may be more prevalent in adolescent sex offenders (Kavoussi et al., 1988; Ryan, 1991) and adult (Kafka & Prentky, 1998) sex offender populations. The findings from these studies are consistent with other research that has demonstrated that (1) children and adolescents with ADHD frequently display comorbid antisocial-spectrum disorders (Loney, 1987; Lynam, 1996), exceeding 50–60% in many samples (Biederman, Newcorn, & Sprich, 1991) and (2) ADHD is, by itself, a strong predictor of delinquency and conduct disorders in adolescence and adulthood (Klein & Manuzza, 1991).

Fago (2003) studied 72 children between 6 and 17 years of age, all of whom were referred for sexually aggressive behavior and were evaluated in an outpatient treatment center. These evaluations were consistent with multimodal assessment protocols that have been recommended in the literature on behaviorally disruptive children (Achenbach, 1985, 1993; Breen & Altpeter, 1990; Conners, 1994; Hinshaw, Simmel, & Heller, 1995), including a cognitive assessment using the Wechsler scales.

Two index scales (freedom from distractibility/working memory and processing speed), composed of 4 of 11 subscales on these instruments (arithmetic, digit span, symbol search, digit symbol coding) have been found to be particularly sensitive to attention and related executive function/cognitive-processing deficits (Biederman et al., 1991, 1993; Kaufman & Lichtenberger, 1999).

Results from this survey indicated that 59 (82%) were identified as having a diagnosis of ADHD or other neurodevelopmental disorder with deficits in executive function. This prevalence is approximately 20 times greater than the 3–5% prevalence figure for ADHD that is estimated to occur in the general population (American Psychiatric Association, 1994; Anderson, Williams, McGee, & Silva, 1987; Sandburg, Weiselberg, & Shaffer, 1980), and it is also significantly greater than the 17% base rate for ADHD diagnosis in all children evaluated at the study site during the period of the investigation. In addition, there was a modest trend toward younger sexually aggressive children having a more probable diagnosis of ADHD/neurodevelopmental disorders, in that 89% of the study subjects who were age 13 or younger were diagnosed with neurodevelopmental disorders, whereas only 77% of the 15–17-year-olds received these diagnoses.

Recidivism. There is a strong belief among professionals in the area that recidivism risk of adolescent sex offenders is low, and lower than that of adults. For example, Trivits and Reppucci (2002) provide an incomplete narrative review of studies reporting recidivism rates in adolescent and adult sex offenders and conclude that although recidivism rates of both groups were not nearly as high as popular opinion would suggest, recidivism rates for youth (generally 8–12%) were lower that those for adults (generally 20–40%). However, making conclusive comparisons between groups in recidivism rates is a complex and difficult task. Important confounding variables that confuse the comparison include length of follow-up (the average interval of time from the offender's release from custody to the date on which the recidivism data were recorded), outcome measures (criminal charges vs. criminal convictions), and level of risk for the samples being compared (Hanson & Bussiére, 1998).

Worling and Långström (2006) have conducted an exhaustive review and found 20 studies of recidivism of adolescent sex offenders. They report a wide range in recidivism percentages of between 0 and 75%, with a mean recidivism rate of 15% (SD = 15.99). These studies had a mean follow-up interval of 4.4 years (range = 0.5 years to 9.58 years). Hanson and Bussiére (1998) conducted a meta-analysis of the world's literature on sex offender recidivism, including 61 separate studies providing recidivism data on a total of 28,972 offenders. Of the samples included in the study, 52 were samples of adult offenders, 6 were samples of adolescent offenders only, and 3 were samples of both adult and adolescent offenders. These authors report an overall recidivism rate of 13.4% over an average follow-up period between 4 and 5 years. Taken together, these studies support the conclusion that there is no evidence for lower rates of recidivism for adolescent or adolescent sex offenders compared with the larger population of sex offenders (both adult and adolescent combined).

Adolescent Female Sexual Abusers

There has been some controversy as to what extent females are represented among adolescent sex offenders. An early study (Roberts, McBee, & Bettis, 1969) examined adolescent sex offenders (less than 16 years of age) and reported that 43% of their sample was female, compared to only 20% in a comparison group of non-sex offender adolescents. However, more recent data suggest that while females account for 18% of all under-18-year-old arrests, they constitute only 7% of all sex offenders and only 2% of rapists (Brown et al., 1984). Early prejudicial attitudes regarding what was appropriate sexual behavior for males compared with females complicate our interpretation of these statistics. For example, in Markey's (1950) report on 25 male and 25 female adolescent offenders, the predominant offense for females was simply "having intercourse"; at least two of these female "sex delinquents" would be seen more recently to be the victims of an incestuous sexual assault. At any rate, there is general agreement that females make up only a small minority of adolescent sex offenders.

Fehrenbach and Monastersky (1988) presented descriptive data on a group of 28 female adolescent sex offenders seen in an outpatient clinic. The sexual offenses for which the subjects were referred were either rape (mean = 15;

53.6%), or indecent liberties (mean = 13; 46.4%). Rape involved oral, anal, or vaginal intercourse with the victim or penetration of the victim with either an object or a finger. Indecent liberties involved a variety of sexual touching of the victim by the offender or having the victim touch the offender, all short of penetration. Unlike adult female sex offenders described in the previous literature, all adolescent offenders committed their offenses independently, without accomplices or co-offenders.

With one exception, the victims were all children 12 years of age or younger. Excluding that one victim, the mean age of victims was 5.2 years. Typically the victims of assaults by adolescent female sex offenders are younger children. Fehrenbach and colleagues (1986) found that 62% of the victims of their sample of male abusers were less than 12 years of age, with 44% less than 6. However, in the Fehrenbach and Monastersky (1988) sample of female offenders, the victims of the female perpetrators were all less than 6 years old. Ten of the offenders (35.7%) had assaulted males and 16 (57.1%) committed offenses against females. Two offenders (7.1%) had assaulted both male and female victims. The offenders were not strangers to any of their victims, three victims were offenders' siblings (10.7%), one was a step-sibling (3.6%), four were foster siblings (14.3%), and four were otherwise related (14.3%). Sixteen (57.1%) of the victims were acquaintances of the offender. Nineteen of the offenses (67.9%) took place while the subject was babysitting the victim. Four (14.3%) of the subjects were found to have committed more than one sexual offense. None of the subjects was found to have committed any other violent or interpersonal offense like assault. Only four (14.3%) had committed a delinquent act not directly involving another person, such as theft. Six (21.4%) of the subjects reported a history of being physically abused. Fourteen (50%) reported having been sexually abused.

Matthews, Hunter, and Buz (1997) studied 67 adolescent female sexual offenders who had been referred for either community-based or residential treatment following a documented history of sexual perpetration. These young girls were compared to a group of 70 adolescent male sex offenders across three parameters: developmental and psychiatric characteristics, history of maltreatment, and sexual perpetration characteristics. Compared with the adolescent males, the females reported even more extensive and pervasive childhood maltreatment. In addition, females were also exposed to the modeling of interpersonal aggression by females as well as males. Finally, the majority of these adolescent female sex offenders demonstrated repetitive patterns of sexual offending with multiple victims, suggesting psychosexual disturbances equivalent in severity to the comparison group of males.

ASSESSMENT

In this section, the focus is on two aspects of assessment of deviant sexual behavior in adolescents: the assessment of deviant sexual interests and the evaluation of risk for reoffense.

Assessment of Deviant Sexual Interests

Historically, the concept of deviant sexuality has been invoked as a construct to explain deviant sexual behavior. The construct has been variously referred to as paraphilia, deviant sexual preferences, deviant sexual arousal, and deviant sexual interest. In adults, deviant sexual arousal was identified early on as an important motivator for sexual assaults, particularly against children (Abel, Blanchard, & Jackson, 1974; Freund, 1967). Self-reported deviant arousal is related to recidivism in adolescent sex offenders (Schram, Milloy, & Rowe, 1991; Worling & Curwen, 2000).

Diagnosis

One method of assessing and specifying deviant sexual interest is through the diagnosis of a paraphilia, specifically a deviant (para) attraction (philia). There are various forms of paraphilias, depending on the target of the attraction, and these targets can include (1) nonhuman objects (as in fetishism), (2) the suffering or humiliation of oneself or one's partner (masochism and sadism, respectively), and (3) children or other nonconsenting persons. Common paraphilias seen among adolescents include pedophilia (sexual activity with a prepubescent child or children [must be 16 years of age and at least 5 years older than the child or children involved]), exhibitionism (exposure of one's genitals to an unsuspecting stranger), fetishism (use of nonliving objects [e.g., female undergarments]), frotteurism (touching or rubbing against a nonconsenting person), and transvestic fetishism (cross-dressing). These are listed and described further in DSM-IV (American Psychiatric Association, 1994). All paraphilias involve recurrent, intense, sexually arousing fantasies, sexual urges, or behaviors involving a deviant sexual activity or deviant choice of partner. To meet DSM criteria for paraphilia, these fantasies, urges, and behaviors must be experienced over at least a 6-month period, and they must cause clinically significant distress or impairment in social, occupational, or other important areas of functioning.

While diagnosis of paraphilia can be informative and descriptive of the sexual interests of some individual cases, there are a number of disadvantages of diagnosis as an assessment methodology, especially in the situation in which it is the only source of assessment information: (1) diagnoses of paraphilia have not been assessed for their reliability or validity, and (2) these diagnoses involve the use of vague diagnostic criteria that include constructs that are not operationally defined and for which there are no valid measures (O'Donohue, Regev, & Hagstrom, 2000).

In addition, the validity of diagnoses often depend on the validity of the self-report by the subject being assessed. Self-report has an extreme lack of credibility among professionals in this area. It is universally accepted that, perhaps not surprisingly, sex offenders of all ages often lie about their true sexual preferences or interests. Consequently, the field has sought to develop assessment methodologies that have the ability to determine sexual interests in a way that is not susceptible to manipulation by the person being assessed.

These assessments can be accomplished in a number of ways, but the methods currently available for adolescents that have the best empirical support are phallometric assessment, visual reaction time, and the criminal history of sexually deviant behavior.

Phallometric Assessment

Phallometric assessment involves the measurement of erectile responses through direct calibration of changes in circumference or volume of the penis during presentations of sexual stimuli depicting children and adults. Phallometric testing of adolescents who have committed sexual offenses against children has received less empirical attention compared to adult sex offenders, partly because there have been ethical and practical objections to its use. However, what empirical data there are supports the use of phallometry with adolescent sex offenders.

For example, Seto, Lalumière, and Blanchard (2000) used phallometric assessment to compare three groups of subjects: 40 adolescent (ages 14–17) sex offenders against children, 75 young adult (ages 18–21) sex offenders against children, and 39 young adult comparison subjects. The responses of adolescents with female victims were not different from the responses of comparison subjects. Young adult offenders, regardless of victim sex, had larger relative responses to child stimuli than comparison subjects. Using a cut score of 0 (indicating equal or greater arousal to children than to adults), sensitivity was 42% for adolescents with any male victim, and specificity was 92% for the comparison subjects. These results suggest that phallometric testing can identify pedophilic interests among adolescent sex offenders.

Past research has revealed that greater sexual interest in children compared to adults is more likely to be observed among adult child molesters when their sexual offense histories include male victims, more than one victim, younger victims, and extrafamilial victims (e.g., Freund & Blanchard, 1989; Freund & Watson, 1991; Seto, Lalumière, & Kuban, 1999). This finding has been replicated in adolescent offenders. Hunter, Goodwin, and Becker (1994) found that those offenders who abused only male children showed greater arousal to children during phallometric testing than those offenders who had abused female children or both male and female children. There is additional strong evidence that a history of CSA combines with choice of victim gender to determine strength of deviant arousal. Becker, Hunter, Stein, and Kaplan (1989) found that adolescent offenders with a history of sexual victimization and a history of offending against male children were more likely to show deviant arousal to audiotaped cues. Murphy, DiLillo, Haynes, and Steere (2001) found that the gender of the victim was the best predictor of deviant arousal, but these authors also found an important interaction: Those individuals who had male victims and who had been sexually abused themselves showed significantly greater responding to deviant cues than did other groups.

Visual Reaction Time

An alternative to plethysmographic assessment has been proposed by Osborn, Abel, and Warberg (1995) using visual reaction time or the amount of time an individual looks at a stimulus. The visual reaction time, first investigated by Rosenzweig (1942), is now used in a variety of frameworks (Abel, Rouleau, Lawry, Barrett, & Camp, 1990; Wright & Adams, 1994). More recently, visual reaction time was successfully compared to plythysmography in the assessment of sexual interest of adult child molesters (Abel, Huffman, Warberg, & Holland, 1998).

Abel and colleagues (2004) have extended the application of visual reaction time to the assessment of adolescent sex offenders. These authors compared visual reaction times to pictorial representations of children and adults of both genders. Participants were male adolescents (n = 1,704) undergoing treatment for paraphilias. This large group of participants was subdivided into two groups: child molesters (n = 1,170) and nonmolesters (n = 534). The former group admitted to molesting a child who was at leasts 5 years younger than themselves. The visual stimuli presented were pictorial representation of clothed individuals of both genders in four age groups: 2–4-year-olds, 8–10-year-olds, 14–17-year-olds, and adults over the age of 21. Participants were seated in front of a computer that was linked to a slide projector and shown how to advance the slides by pressing a key on the computer keyboard. Participants were asked to rate their own sexual arousal to each picture. The computer measured the length of time each participant took to rate each picture. Results indicated that the amount of time male adolescent child molesters viewed slides of children was significantly longer than nonmolesters. In addition, viewing time of slides of children for male adolescent child molesters was significantly correlated with their number of victims and the number of times they carried out acts of child molestation. These findings support the use of visual reaction time as a measure of sexual interest in adolescent sex offenders.

History of Deviant Sexual Behavior

Another potential assessment methodology to assess deviant sexual interests in adolescents is a scale based on offense history information developed by Michael Seto and his associates (Screening Scale for Pedophilic Interests [SSPI]; Seto & Lalumière, 2001). Among child molesters, phallometrically measured sexual interest in children is associated with having male victims, multiple victims, younger victims, and extrafamilial victims. These sexual offense history variables are also associated with risk for sexual recidivism (Hanson, 1997). The items for the SSPI were scored from information about the child molester's sexual offense histories. Each item was initially coded as present or absent: any male victims; more than one victim; any prepubescent victim (a child under the age of 12); and any extrafamilial victims (a child who was not the offender's son or daughter, stepson or stepdaughter, or a member of his extended family).

A study of 1,113 adult child molesters was conducted to determine if these sexual offense history variables were related to phallometrically determined sexual interest in children. Using a cutoff score that classified 90% of a sample of 206 non-child molesters as not having pedophilic interests, SSPI scores identified pedophilic interests among child molesters significantly better than chance. Individuals with the highest SSPI score were more than five times as likely to be show pedophilic interests in phallometric testing than individuals receiving the lowest score. The Receiver Operating Characteristic (ROC) area under the curve for the SSPI was .70 (SE = .02), indicating diagnostic accuracy that is significantly better than chance.

Seto, Murphy, Page, and Ennis (2003) extended the development of the SSPI in a study of three samples of adolescent sex offenders who underwent phallometric testing for pedophilic interests. Scores on the SSPI were positively correlated with a phallometric index of relative sexual arousal to children in all three samples. Specifically, scores on the SSPI had a correlation of .56 with phallometrically measured sexual interest in children among 40 adolescent sex offenders with child victims. The positive relationship between SSPI scores and pedophilic responding held up despite the use of different penile measures, stimulus sets, procedures, and scoring methods across the three samples. These authors suggest that if replicated in an independent and larger sample, the SSPI could be used as an alternative measure for adolescent sex offenders with child victims when phallometric data are unavailable.

Assessment of Risk for Recidivism

Scientific research has consistently shown that actuarial methods of risk assessment are more accurate than clinical judgments alone in predicting future reoffense among sex offenders released into the community (e.g., Barbaree, Seto, Langton, & Peacock, 2001). Unfortunately, at the present time, there is not yet enough follow-up research to establish and validate an actuarial tool for adolescents (Worling & Långström, 2006). At best, with adolescents, we are able to inform clinical decisions with what Hanson (2000) has called *empirically guided clinical judgment*. Unlike actuarial scales, there is no link between a total score and a specific probability of a reoffense. But, the advantage of empirically guided clinical judgment in comparison to unstructured clinical judgment is that there is the promise of higher accuracy given the scientific evidence in favor of the risk factors. Two such instruments in use in North America have been described as promising (Doren, 2002; Leversee & Pearson, 2001). These are the Juvenile Sex Offender Assessment Protocol (J-SOAP; Prentky & Righthand, 2001) and the Estimate of Risk of Adolescent Sexual Offense Recidivism (ERASOR; Worling & Curwen, 2001). Both tools have the advantage of offering explicit scoring instructions for a fixed number of risk factors, and both are designed to assist clinicians to estimate the risk of a sexual reoffense for individuals ages 12–18.

The original version of the J-SOAP had scoring criteria for 23 factors in four risk domains: (1) Sexual Drive/Sexual Preoccupation, (2) Impulsive, Antisocial Behavior, (3) Clinical/Treatment, and (4) Community Adjustment. The instrument has undergone two revisions based on empirical analysis of estimates of reliability and validity. The present 28-item J-SOAP is available free of charge at www.csom.org.

The ERASOR was modeled after the Sexual Violence Risk scale (SVR-20; Boer, Hart, Kropp, & Webster, 1997). The 25 risk factors included in the ERASOR (Version 2.0; Worling & Curwen, 2001) fall into 5 categories: (1) Sexual Interests, Attitudes, and Behaviors, (2) Historical Sexual Assaults, (3) Psychosocial Functioning, (4) Family/Environmental Functioning, and (5) Treatment. A coding manual is available from the author (Worling). Research is currently underway in various locations around the world but preliminary findings reported, while indicating good reliability (Worling, 2002), have not yet demonstrated the predictive validity of the instrument (Morton, 2003).

TREATMENT

If treatment is effective in reducing deviant behaviors among adolescent offenders, then treatment of the adolescent could go a long way toward reducing the impact of sexual assault in our society. Treatments currently in use for the adolescent sexual offender have not been developed specifically for this population based on the scientific analysis of their own unique treatment needs. Rather, treatments have been developed for use with other populations and adapted for use with this population, specifically sex-offender-specific cognitive-behavioral treatment with emphasis on relapse prevention (adult sex offenders), and multisystemic therapy (antisocial youth).

Cognitive-behavioral therapy has been used widely with adult sex offenders targeting cognitions and behaviors that contribute to offending (e.g., Abel, Mittleman, & Becker, 1985). Relapse prevention strategies, developed originally for use with addictions (Marlatt & Gordon, 1985), have been adapted and used with adult sex offenders (Laws, 1989). Modern or current programs for the treatment of adult sex offenders most often combine the cognitive-behavioral treatment with relapse prevention (e.g., Marques, Day, Nelson, & West, 1994). Typical programs would attempt to prevent future offending through (1) the reduction of distorted cognitions supportive of sexual assault including the offender's denial and/or minimization of his role in previous assaults and an increase in empathy for the victims of sexual assault and greater awareness of victim harm in sexual assault through cognitive restructuring, (2) reductions in deviant sexual arousal and fantasy through verbal satiation and covert sensitization, (3) sex education and values clarification, (4) acquisition of knowledge about offense cycles or behavioral chains leading to their own offending, and (5) the development of strategies for the offender's use to avoid or escape from situations in which the offender is at high risk to reoffend.

These programs for adult sex offenders (e.g., Abel et al., 1985) have been adapted for use with the youthful sex offender. The best known of these was developed by Judith Becker and her associates (Becker, 1990; Becker, Kaplan, & Kavoussi, 1988; Hunter & Santos, 1990). Use of this model of therapy with this population is an endorsement of the view that adolescent sex offenders can be effectively treated as younger versions of the adult sex offender.

More recently, programs reflecting both theoretical and empirical advances in the field have been developed (see Marshall, Fernandez, Hudson, & Ward, 1998), and treatment interventions designed specifically for adolescent sex offenders have appeared (e.g., Rich, 1998). These initiatives are consistent with findings in the wider criminological literature indicating that effective treatment programs should be delivered in a format designed to accommodate characteristics of the offender that influence his or her response to the intervention (e.g., intelligence, communication ability, and emotionality; see Andrews & Bonta, 2003). These specialized interventions are an endorsement of the view that adolescent sex offenders present with specific treatment needs at least some of which are distinct from those found among adult sex offenders.

Multisystemic therapy (MST; Henggeler & Lee, 2003) is an intensive family-based treatment that addresses the known determinants of serious antisocial behavior in adolescents and their families. MST treats those factors in the youth's environment that are contributing to his or her behavior problems. Such factors might pertain to individual characteristics of the youth (e.g., poor problem-solving skills), family relations (e.g., inept discipline), peer relations (e.g., association with delinquent peers), and school performance (e.g., academic difficulties). On a highly individualized basis, treatment goals are developed in collaboration with the family, and family strengths are used as levers for therapeutic change. Specific interventions used in MST are based on the best of the empirically supported treatment approaches such as cognitive-behavioral therapy and the pragmatic family therapies. The primary goals of MST are to reduce rates of antisocial behavior in the adolescent, reduce out-of-home placements, and empower families to resolve future difficulties. Use of this form of therapy with adolescent sex offenders is an endorsement of the view that the sexual aggression is one form of antisocial behavior in youth.

The randomized controlled trial (RCT) is the preferred method for establishing the efficacy of any psychological or medical treatment (McConaghy, 1999; Shadish & Ragsdale, 1996). Borduin, Henggeler, Blaske, and Stein (1990) used an RCT to evaluate the efficacy of MST as a treatment for adolescent sex offenders. These authors report that MST was effective in reducing recidivism in the treated sample compared with a comparison group during the follow-up period. It is interesting to note here that MST is not a treatment that specifically targets sexual behavior. However, it does target factors in the offender's environment that might contribute to sexual offending, including many family variables. Given the importance of family environment to the development of deviant sexual behaviors in adolescents, it is perhaps not surprising that an intervention targeting family variables is effective.

In 1997, a small group of members of the Association for the Treatment of Sexual Abusers launched the Collaborative Outcome Data Project. The project team included some of the most well-respected authorities in the area, from both sides of the debate. Hanson and colleagues (2002) reported the first set of conclusions as a result of a meta-analysis of 43 studies of both adult and adolescent sexual offender recidivism (combined n = 9,454). Hanson and colleagues coded treatment studies as to the adequacy of their research designs to control for potentially confounding variables as described earlier. Combining experimental with quasi-experimental designs, Hanson and colleagues found a significant treatment effect. Among current psychological treatments (those programs initiated after 1980 or those initiated before 1980 but still in operation), the authors report a significant effect in reducing rates of both sexual and general recidivism by approximately 40%. Current treatments were described as cognitive-behavioral therapies (or MST with adolescents), most often with an emphasis on relapse prevention. Older forms of treatment (prior to 1980) were found to have little effect. Importantly, the treatment effect remained significant when considering only studies in which dropouts were explicitly included with the treatment group. On the face of it, this study encourages the conclusion that sexual offender treatment can be effective in reducing recidivism among sexual offenders.

SUMMARY AND CONCLUSIONS

This chapter has defined deviant sexual behavior in adolescents by distinguishing it from normative or usual sexual behavior in the reference or local population of adolescents. In addition, deviant sexual behavior among adolescents was defined by contrast with related but similar terms, including, sexual perversion, sexual abuse, and sexual crime. This chapter highlighted the important contribution of CSA to the development of deviant sexuality in adolescence, along with the important contribution of family context. Family context was shown to provide the occasion or setting in which children suffer sexual victimization, but also in which parental incompetence and neglect fail to provide the ameliorating effects parental and family support might otherwise provide the victim of CSA. This chapter also identified sexual behavior problems in childhood as precursors to deviant sexuality in adolescence. We described the characteristics of adolescent sex offenders, both male and female, their offending behavior, their victims, comorbid mental disorders, and the age at onset of their deviant sexual behaviors, along with the incidence and prevalence of deviant sexual behavior among adolescents. Recidivism rates among adolescent sex offenders were compared with those of adult offenders. The chapter described two important aspects of clinical assessment of adolescent sex offenders: assessment of their deviant sexual interests and assessment of their risk for reoffense or recidivism. Finally, the chapter described various approaches to effective treatment of the adolescent sex offender.

REFERENCES

Abel, G. G., Blanchard, E. B., & Jackson, M. (1974). The role of fantasy in the treatment of sexual deviation. *Archives of General Psychiatry, 30,* 467–475.

Abel, G. G., Huffman, J., Warberg, B., & Holland, C. L. (1998). Visual reaction time and plethysmography as measures of sexual interest in child molesters. *Sexual Abuse: A Journal of Research and Treatment, 10,* 81–95.

Abel, G. G., Jordan, A., Rouleau, J. L., Emerick, R., Barboza-Whitehead, S., & Osborn, C. (2004). The use of visual reaction time to assess male adolescents who molest children. *Sexual Abuse: A Journal of Research and Treatment, 16,* 255–265.

Abel, G. G., Mittelman, M. S., & Becker, J. V. (1985). Sex offenders: Results of assessment and recommendations for treatment. In M. H. Ben-Aron, S. J. Hucker, & C. D. Webster (Eds.), *Clinical criminology: The assessment and treatment of criminal behavior* (pp. 207–220). Toronto, ON, Canada: M&M Graphics.

Abel, G. G., Rouleau, J. L., Lawry, S. S. Barrett, D. H., & Camp, N. L. (1990). *A non-invasive, physiologic measure of adult sexual preference.* Paper presented at the 16th annual meeting of the International Academy of Sex Research, Sigtuna, Sweden.

Achenbach, T. M. (1985). *Assessment and taxonomy of child and adolescent psychopathology.* Beverly Hills, CA: Sage.

Achenbach, T. M. (1993). Taxonomy and comorbidity of conduct problems: Evidence from empirically based approaches. *Development and Psychopathology, 5,* 51–64.

Ageton, S. (1983). *Sexual assault among adolescents.* Lexington, MA: Lexington Books.

Anderson, J., Williams, S., McGee, R., & Silva, P. (1987). DSM-III disorders in preadolescent children. *Archives of General Psychiatry, 44,* 69–76.

Andrews, D. A., & Bonta, J. L. (2003). *The psychology of criminal conduct* (3rd ed.). Cincinnati, OH: Anderson.

American Psychiatric Association. (1994). *Diagnostic and statistical manual of mental disorders* (4th ed.). Washington, DC: Author.

Awad, G. A., & Saunders, E. (1989). Adolescent child molesters: Clinical observations. *Child Psychiatry and Human Development, 19,* 195–206.

Awad, G. A., & Saunders, E. (1991). Male adolescent sexual assaulters: Clinical observations. *Journal of Interpersonal Violence, 6,* 446–460.

Awad, G. A., Saunders, E., & Levene, J. (1984). A clinical study of male adolescent sex offenders. *International Journal of Offender Therapy and Comparative Criminology, 28,* 105–116.

Bancroft, J. (1989). *Human sexuality and its problems.* Churchill, UK: Livingstone.

Barbaree, H. E., Hudson, S. M, & Seto, M. C. (1993). Sexual assault in society: The role of the juvenile offender. In H. E. Barbaree, W. L. Marshall, & S. M. Hudson (Eds.), *The juvenile sex offender* (pp. 1–24). New York: Guilford Press.

Barbaree, H. E., Seto, M. C., Langton, C. M., & Peacock, E. J. (2001). Evaluating the predictive accuracy of six risk assessment instruments for adult sex offenders. *Criminal Justice and Behavior, 28,* 490–521.

Baumbach, J. (2002). Some implications of prenatal alcohol exposure for the treatment of adolescents with sexual offending behaviors. *Sexual Abuse: A Journal of Research and Treatment, 14,* 313–327.

Becker, J. V. (1988). The effects of child sexual abuse on adolescent sexual offenders. In G. E. Wyatt & G. J. Powell (Eds.), *Lasting effects of child sexual abuse* (pp. 193–207). Newbury Park, CA: Sage.

Becker, J. V. (1990). Treating adolescent sexual offenders. *Professional Psychology: Research and Practice, 21,* 362–365

Becker, J. V., Cunningham-Rathner, J., & Kaplan, M. S. (1986). Adolescent sexual offenders: Demographics, criminal and sexual histories, and recommendations for reducing future offenses. Special Issue: The prediction and control of violent behavior: II. *Journal of Interpersonal Violence, 1,* 431–445.

Becker, J. V., Hunter, J., Stein, R., & Kaplan, M. S. (1989). Factors associated with erectile response in adolescent sex offenders. *Journal of Psychopathology and Behavioral Assessment, 11,* 353–362.

Becker, J. V., Kaplan, M. S., Cunningham-Rathner, J., & Kavoussi, R. J. (1986). Characteristics of adolescent incest sexual perpetrators: Preliminary findings. *Journal of Family Violence, 1,* 85–97.

Becker, J. V., Kaplan, M., & Kavoussi, R. (1988). Measuring the effectiveness of treatment for the aggressive adolescent sex offender. *Annals of the New York Academy of Science, 528,* 215–222.

Becker, J. V., & Stein, M. (1991). Is sexual erotica associated with sexual deviance in adolescent males? *International Journal of Law and Psychiatry, 14,* 85–95.

Benoit, J. L., & Kennedy, W. A. (1992). The abuse of male adolescent sex offenders. *Journal of Interpersonal Violence, 7,* 543–548.

Bensley, L. S., Spieker, S. J., Van Eenwyk, J., & Schoder, J. (1999). Self-reported abuse history and adolescent problem behaviors: II Alcohol and drug use. *Journal of Adolescent Health, 24,* 173–180.

Bensley, L. S., Van Eenwyk, J., Spieker, S. J., & Schoder, J. (1999). Self-reported abuse history and adolescent problem behaviors: I. Anti-social and suicidal behaviors. *Journal of Adolescent Health, 24,* 163–172.

Berliner, L. (1991, June). Effects of sexual abuse on children. *Violence Update, 1,* 10–11.

Biederman, J., Faraone, S. J., Spencer, T., Wilens, T., Norman, D., Lapey, K. A., et al. (1993). Patterns of psychiatric comorbidity, cognition, and psychosocial functioning in adults with attention-deficit disorder. *American Journal of Psychiatry, 150,* 1792–1798.

Biederman, J., Newcorn, J., & Sprich, S. (1991). Comorbidity of attention deficit hyperactivity with conduct, depressive, anxiety and other disorders. *American Journal of Psychiatry, 148,* 564–577.

Billy, J. O., Lindale, N. S., Grady, W. R., & Zimmerle, D. M. (1988). Effects of sexual activity on adolescent social and psychological development. *Social Psychology Quarterly, 51,* 190–212.

Bingham, C. R., & Crockett, L. J. (1996). Longitudinal adjustment of boys and girls experiencing early, middle, and late sexual intercourse. *Deviant Psychology, 32,* 647–658.

Blaske, D. M., Borduin, C. M., Henggeler, S. W., & Mann, B. J. (1989). Individual, family, and peer characteristics of adolescent sex offenders and assaultive offenders. *Developmental Psychology, 25,* 846–855.

Boer, D. P., Hart, S. D., Kropp, P. R., & Webster, C. D. (1997). *Manual for the Sexual Violence Risk-20.* Burnaby, BC, Canada: The Mental Health, Law, & Policy Institute, Simon Fraser University.

Borduin, C. M., Henggeler, S. W., Blaske, D. M., & Stein, R. J. (1990). Multisystemic treatment of adolescent sexual offenders. *International Journal of Offender Therapy and Comparative Criminology, 34,* 105–113.

Breen, M. J., & Altepeter, T. S. (1990). *Disruptive behavior disorders in children: Treatment-focused assessment.* New York: Guilford Press.

Breer, W. (1987). *The adolescent molester.* Springfield, IL: Charles C. Thomas.

Brown, E. J., Flanagan, T. J., & McLeod, M. (Eds.). (1984). *Sourcebook of criminal justice statistics—1983.* Washington, DC: Bureau of Justice Statistics.

Brownmiller, S. (1975). *Against our will: Men, women and rape.* New York: Simon & Schuster.

Burton, D. L. (2000). Were adolescent sexual offenders children with sexual behavior problems? *Sexual Abuse: A Journal of Research and Treatment, 12,* 37–48.

Burton, D. L. (2003). Male adolescents: Sexual victimization and subsequent sexual abuse. *Child and Adolescent Social Work Journal, 20,* 277–296.

Cantwell, H. B. (1988). Child sexual abuse: Very young perpetrators. *Child Abuse and Neglect, 13,* 65–75.

Chandy, J. M., Blum, R. W., & Resnick, M. D. (1996). Gender-specific outcomes for sexually abused adolescents. *Child Abuse and Neglect, 20,* 1219–1231.

Conners, C. K. (1994). *Attention deficit hyperactivity disorder: Assessment and treatment for children and adolescents.* Toronto, ON, Canada: Multi-Health Systems.

Costa, F. M., Jessor, R., Donovan, J. F., & Fortenberry, J. D. (1995). Early initiation to sexual intercourse: The influence of psychosocial unconventionality. *Journal of Research on Adolescence, 5,* 93–121.

Coulton, C., Korbin, J., Su, M., & Chow, J. (1995). Community level factors and child maltreatment rates. *Child Development, 66,* 1262–1276.

Craissati, J., McClurg, G., & Browne, K. (2002). Characteristics of perpetrators of child sexual abuse who have been sexually victimized as children. *Sexual Abuse: A Journal of Research and Treatment, 14,* 225–239.

Daleiden, E. L., Kaufman, K. L., Hilliker, D. R., & O'Neil, J. N. (1998). The sexual histories of youthful males: A comparison of sexual offending, nonsexual offending and nonoffending groups. *Sexual Abuse: A Journal of Research and Treatment, 10,* 195–209.

Dallam, S. J., Gleaves, D. H., Cepeda-Benito, A., Silberg, J. L., Kaemer, H. C., & Spiegel, D. (2001). The effects of child abuse: Comment on Rind, Tromovitch, and Bauserman (1998). *Psychological Bulletin 2001, 127,* 715–733.

Davis, G. E., & Leitenberg, H. (1987). Adolescent sex offenders. *Psychological Bulletin, 101,* 417–427.

Deisher, R. W., Wenet, G. A., Paperny, D. M., Clark, T. F., & Fehrenbach, P. A. (1982). Adolescent sexual offense behavior: The role of the physician. *Journal of Adolescent Health Care, 2,* 279–286.

Donovan, P. (1997). Can statutory rape laws be effective in preventing adolescent pregnancy? *Family Planning Perspectives, 29,* 30–34.

Doren, D. M. (2004). Stability of the interpretive risk percentages for the RRASOR and Static-99. *Sexual Abuse: A Journal of Research and Treatment, 16,* 25–36.

Elo, I. T., King, R. B., & Furstenberg, F. F. (1999). Adolescent females: Their sexual partners and the fathers of their children. *Journal of Marriage and the Family, 61,* 74–84.

Fago, D. P. (2003). Evaluation and treatment of neurodevelopmental deficits in sexually aggressive children and adolescents. *Professional Psychology: Research and Practice, 34,* 248–257.

Federal Bureau of Investigation. (2002). *Uniform Crime Report.* Washington, DC: Author.

Fehrenbach, P. A., & Monastersky, C. (1988). Characteristics of female adolescent sexual offenders. *American Journal of Orthopsychiatry, 53,* 148–151.

Fehrenbach, P. A., Smith, W., Monastersky, C., & Deisher, R. W. (1986). Adolescent sexual offenders: Offender and offense characteristics. *American Journal of Orthopsychiatry, 56,* 225–233.

Finkelhor, D. (1979). What's wrong with sex between adults and children? Ethics and the problem of sexual abuse. *American Journal of Orthopsychiatry, 49,* 692–697.

Finkelhor, D. (1984). *Child sexual abuse: New theory and research.* New York: Free Press.

Finkelhor, D. (1986). Abusers: Special topics. In D. Finkelhor (Ed.), *A sourcebook on child sexual abuse* (pp. 119–142). Newbury Park, CA: Sage.

Finkelhor, D., & Jones, L. M. (2004, January). Explanations for the decline in child sexual abuse cases. *Juvenile Justice Bulletin,* pp. 1–12.

Fiscella, K., Kitzman, H. J., Cole, R. E., Sidora, K. J., & Olds, D. (1998). Does child abuse predict adolescent pregnancy? *Pediatrics, 101*(4, Pt. 1), 620–624.

Ford, M. E., & Linney, J. A. (1995). Comparative analysis of juvenile sex offenders, violent nonsexual offenders, and status offenders. *Journal of Interpersonal Violence, 10,* 56–70.

Freund, K. (1967). Erotic preference in pedophilia. *Behavior Research and Therapy, 5,* 339–348.

Freund, K., & Blanchard, R. (1989). Phallometric diagnosis of pedophilia. *Journal of Consulting and Clinical Psychology, 57,* 100–105.

Freund, K., & Watson, R. J. (1991). Assessment of the sensitivity and specificity of a phallometric test: An update of phallometric diagnosis of pedophilia. *Psychological Assessment, 3,* 254–260.

Friedrich, W. N., Grambsch, P., Broughton, D., Kuiper, J., & Beilke, R. J. (1991). Normative sexual behavior in children. *Pediatrics, 88,* 456–464.

Friedrich, W. N., Grambsch, P., Damon, L., & Hewitt, S. (1985). Child Sexual Behavior Inventory: Normative and clinical comparisons. *Psychological Assessment, 4,* 303–311.

Friedrich, W. N., & Luecke, W. J. (1988). Young school-age sexually aggressive children. *Professional Psychology Research and Practice, 19,* 155–164

Gale, J., Thompson, R. J., Moran, T., & Sack, W. H. (1988). Sexual abuse in young children. *Journal of Pediatric Psychology, 11,* 47–57.

Garbarino, J., & Sherman, D. (1980). High-risk neighborhoods and high-risk families: The human ecology of child maltreatment. *Child Development, 51,* 188–198.

Garnefski, N., & Arends, E. (1998). Sexual abuse and adolescent maladjustment: Differences between male and female victims. *Journal of Adolescence, 21,* 99–107.

Gelles, R. (1992). Poverty and violence towards children. *American Behavioral Scientist, 35,* 258–274.

Gilgun, J. F., & Reiser, E. (1990). The development of sexual identity among men sexually abused as children. *Families in Society: The Journal of Contemporary Human Services, 71,* 515–523.

Graupner, H. (2000). Sexual consent: The criminal law in Europe and overseas. *Archives of Sexual Behavior, 29,* 415–461.

Gray, A., Busconi, A., Houchens, P., & Pithers, W. D. (1997). Children with sexual behavior problems and their caregivers: Demographics, functioning, and clinical patterns. *Sexual Abuse: A Journal of Research and Treatment, 9,* 267–290.

Groth, A. N. (1977). The adolescent sexual offender and his prey. *International Journal of Offender Therapy and Comparative Criminology, 21,* 249–254.

Groth, A., Longo, R. E., & McFadin, J. (1982). Undetected recidivism among rapists and child molesters. *Crime and Delinquency, 28,* 450–458.

Gundersen, B. H., Melas, P. S., & Skar, J. E. (1981). Sexual behavior of pre-school children: Teachers' observations. In L. L. Constantine & F. M. Martinson (Eds.), *Children and sex: New findings, new perspectives* (pp. 45–61). Boston: Little, Brown.

Hanson, R. K. (1997). *The development of a brief actuarial risk scale for sexual offense recidivism* (User Report 1997-04). Ottawa, ON, Canada: Department of the Solicitor General of Canada.

Hanson, R. K. (2000). *Risk assessment.* Beaverton, OR: Association for the Treatment of Sexual Abusers.

Hanson, R. K., & Bussiére, M. T. (1998). Predicting relapse: A meta-analysis of sexual offender recidivism studies. *Journal of Consulting and Clinical Psychology, 66,* 348–362.

Hanson, R. K., Gordon, A., Harris, A. J. R., Marques, J. K., Murphy, W., Quinsey, V. L., & Seto, M. C. (2002). First report of the collaborative outcome data project on the effectiveness of psychological treatment for sex offenders. *Sexual Abuse: A Journal of Research and Treatment, 14,* 169–194.

Hanson, R. K., & Slater, S. (1988). Reactions to motivational accounts of child molesters. *Journal of Child Sexual Abuse, 2,* 43–59.

Harrison, P. A., Fulkerson, J. A., & Beebe, T. J. (1997).

Multiple substance use among adolescent physical and sexual abuse victims. *Child Abuse and Neglect, 21,* 529–539.

Hays, C. H. (1987). *Risking the future: Adolescent sexuality, pregnancy, and childbearing.* Washington, DC: National Academy Press.

Henggeler, S. (1989). *Delinquency in adolescence.* Newbury Park, CA: Sage.

Henggeler, S. W., & Lee, T. (2003). Multisystemic treatment of serious clinical problems. In A. E. Kazdin & J. R. Weisz (Eds.), *Evidence-based psychotherapies for children and adolescents* (pp. 301–322). New York: Guilford Press.

Hibbard, R. A., Brack, C. J., Rauch, S., & Orr, D. P. (1988). Abuse, feelings, and health behaviors in a student population. *American Journal of Diseases of Childhood, 142,* 326–330.

Hibbard, R. A., Ingersoll, G. M., & Orr, D. P. (1990). Behavioral risk, emotional risk, and child abuse among adolescents in a nonclinical setting. *Pediatrics, 86,* 896–901.

Hindman, J., & Peters, J. M. (2001). Polygraph testing leads to better understanding adult and juvenile sex offenders. *Federal Probation, 65,* 8–15.

Hinshaw, S. P., Simmel, C., & Heller, T. L. (1995). Multimethod assessment of covert antisocial behavior in children: Laboratory observations, adult ratings, and child self-report. *Psychological Assessment, 7,* 209–219.

Hummel, P., Thomke, V., Oldenburger, H. A., & Specht, F. (2000). Male adolescent sex offenders against children: Similarities and differences between those offenders with and those without a history of sexual abuse. *Journal of Adolescence, 23,* 305–317.

Hunter, J. A., Goodwin, D. W., & Becker, J. V. (1994). The relationship between phallometrically measured deviant sexual arousal and clinical characteristics in juvenile sexual offenders. *Behavior Research and Therapy, 32,* 533–538.

Hunter, J. A., & Santos, D. (1990). The use of specialized cognitive-behavioral therapies in the treatment of juvenile sexual offenders. *International Journal of Offender Therapy and Comparative Criminology, 34,* 239–248.

Irwin, C. E., & Millstein, S. G. (1992). Risk-taking behaviors and biopsychological development during adolescence. In E. J. Sussman, T. V. Feagans, & W. J. Ray (Eds.), *Emotion, cognition, health and development in children and adolescents* (pp. 95–102). Hillsdale, NJ: Erlbaum.

Jacobs, W. L., Kennedy, W. A., & Meyer, J. B. (1997). Juvenile delinquents: A between group comparison study of sexual and nonsexual offenders. *Sexual Abuse: A Journal of Research and Treatment, 9,* 201–217.

Jessor, R., & Jessor, S. L. (1977). *Problem behavior and psychological development: A longitudinal study of youth.* New York: Academic Press.

Johnson, T. C. (1988). Child perpetrators: Children who molest other children: Preliminary findings. *Child Abuse and Neglect, 12,* 219–229.

Kafka, M. P., & Prentky, R. A. (1998). Attention-deficit/hyperactivity disorder in males with paraphilias and paraphilia-related disorders: A comorbidity study. *Journal of Clinical Psychiatry, 59,* 388–396.

Kahn, T. J., & Lafond, M. A. (1988). Treatment of adolescent sexual offenders. *Child and Adolescent Social Work, 5,* 135–148.

Kaufman, A. S., & Lichtenberger, E. O. (1999). *Essentials of WAIS-III assessment.* New York: Wiley.

Kavoussi, R. J., Kaplan, M., & Becker, J. V. (1988). Psychiatric diagnoses in adolescent sex offenders. *Journal of the American Academy of Child and Adolescent Psychiatry, 27,* 241–243.

Kendall-Tackett, K. A., Williams, L. M., & Finkelhor, D., (1993). Impact of sexual abuse on children: A review and synthesis of recent empirical studies. *Psychological Bulletin, 113,* 164–180.

Kilpatrick, D. G., Acierno, R., Schnurr, P. P., Saunders, B., Resnick, H. S., & Best, C. L. (2000). Risk factors for adolescent substance abuse and dependence: Data from a national sample. *Journal of Consulting and Clinical Psychology, 68,* 19–30.

Kilpatrick, D. G., Ruggiero, K. J., Acierno, R., Saunders, B. E., Resnick, H. S., & Best, C. L. (2003). Violence and risk of PTSD, major depression, substance abuse/dependence, and comorbidity: Results from the national survey of adolescents. *Journal of Consulting and Clinical Psychology, 71,* 692–700.

Klein, S., & Manuzza, S. (1991). Long-term outcome of hyperactive children: A review. *Journal of the American Academy of Child and Adolescent Psychiatry, 30,* 1120–1134.

Koss, M. P., Gidycz, C. A., & Wisniewski, N. (1987). The scope of rape: Incidence and prevalence of sexual aggression and victimization in a national sample of higher education students. *Journal of Consulting and Clinical Psychology, 55,* 162–170.

Lalumière, M. L., Quinsey, V. L., Harris, G. H., & Rice, M. E. (2005). *The causes of rape: Understanding individual differences in the male propensity for sexual aggression.* Washington, DC: American Psychological Association.

Lambie, I., Seymour, F., Lee, A., & Adams, P. (2002). Resiliency in victim–offender cycle in male sexual abuse. *Sexual Abuse: A Journal of Research and Treatment, 14,* 31–48.

Laws, D. R. (1989). *Relapse prevention with sex offenders.* New York: Guilford Press.

Laws, D. R., & Marshall, W. L. (1990). A conditioning theory of the etiology and maintenance of deviant sexual preferences and behavior. In W. L. Marshall, D. R. Laws, & H. E. Barbaree (Eds.), *Handbook of sexual assault: Issues, theories, and treatment of the offender* (pp. 209–229). New York: Plenum Press.

Leitenberg, H., & Saltzman, H. (2000). A statewide survey of age at first intercourse for adolescent females and age of their male partners: Relation to other risk behaviors and statutory rape implications. *Archives of Sexual Behavior, 29,* 203–215.

Leitenberg, H., & Saltzman, H. (2003). College women who had sexual intercourse when they were underage minors (13–15): Age of their male partners, relation to current adjustment, and statutory rape implications. *Sexual Abuse: A Journal of Research and Treatment, 15,* 135–147.

Leversee, T., & Pearson, C. (2001). Eliminating the pendulum effect: A balanced approach to the assessment, treatment, and management of sexually abusive youth. *Journal of the Center for Families, Children and the Courts, 3,* 45–57.

Lewis, D. O., Shankok, S. S., & Pincus, J. H. (1979). Juvenile male sexual assaulters. *American Journal of Psychiatry, 136,* 1194–1196.

Lindberg, L. D., Sonenstein, F. L., Ku, L., & Martinez, G. (1997). Age differences between minors who give birth and their adult partners. *Family Planning Perspectives, 29,* 61–66.

Loeber, R., & Stouthamer-Loeber, M. (1987). Prediction. In H. C. Quay (Ed.), *Handbook of juvenile delinquency* (pp. 325—382). New York: Wiley.

Loney, J. (1987). Hyperactivity and aggression in the diagnosis of attention deficit disorder. In B. B. Lahey & A. E. Kazdin (Eds.), *Advances in clinical child psychology* (Vol. 10, pp. 99–135). New York: Plenum Press.

Longo, R. E. (1982). Sexual learning and experience among adolescent sexual offenders. *International Journal of Offender Therapy and Comparative Criminology, 26,* 235–241.

Lynam, D. R. (1996). Early identification of chronic offenders: Who is the fledgling psychopath? *Psychological Bulletin, 120,* 209–234.

Marlatt, G. A., & Gordon, J. R. (1985). *Relapse prevention: Maintenance strategies in the treatment of addictive behaviors.* New York: Guilford Press.

Markey, O. B. (1950). A study of aggressive sex misbehavior in adolescents brought to juvenile court. *American Journal of Orthopsychiatry, 20,* 719–731.

Marques, J. K., Day, D. M., Nelson, C., & West, M. A. (1994). Effects of cognitive-behavioral treatment on sex offender recidivism: Preliminary results of a longitudinal study. *Criminal Justice and Behavior, 21,* 28–54.

Marshall, W. L. (1989). Intimacy, loneliness, and sexual offenders. *Behavior Research and Therapy, 27,* 491–503.

Marshall, W. L., Fernandez, Y. M., Hudson, S. M., & Ward, T. (Eds.). (1998). *Sourcebook of treatment programs for sex offenders.* New York: Plenum Press.

Matthews, R., Hunter, J. A., & Buz, J. (1997). Juvenile female sexual offenders: Clinical characteristics and treatment issues. *Sexual Abuse: A Journal of Research and Treatment, 9,* 187–199.

McBride, C. K., Paikoff, R. L., & Holmbeck, G. N. (2003). Individual and familial influences on the onset of sexual intercourse among urban African American adolescents. *Journal of Consulting and Clinical Psychology, 71,* 159–167.

McConaghy, N. (1999). Methodological issues concerning evaluation of treatment for sexual offenders: Randomization, treatment dropouts, untreated controls, and within-treatment studies. *Sexual Abuse: A Journal of Research and Treatment, 11,* 183–193.

McCord, J. (1979). Some child-rearing antecedents of criminal behavior in adult men. *Journal of Personality and Social Psychology, 8,* 1477–1486.

McCormack, A., Rokous, F. E., Hazelwood, R. R., & Burgess, A. W. (1992). An exploration of incest in the childhood development of serial rapists. *Journal of Family Violence, 7,* 219–228.

McDermott, M. J., & Hindelang, M. J., (1981). *Juvenile criminal behavior in the United States: Its trends and patterns* (Analysis of National Crime Victimization Survey Data to Study Serious Delinquent Behavior, Monograph No. 1). Washington, DC: Office of Juvenile Justice and Delinquency Prevention.

McGuire, R., Carlysle, J., & Young, B. (1965). Sexual deviation as conditioned behavior: A hypothesis. *Behavior Research and Therapy, 2,* 185–190.

Miranda, A. O., & Corcoran, C. L. (2000). Comparison of perpetration characteristics between male juvenile and adult sexual offenders: Preliminary results. *Sexual Abuse: A Journal of Research and Treatment, 12,* 179–188.

Money, J., & Ehrhardt, A. (1972). *Man and woman: Boy and girl.* Baltimore: Johns Hopkins University Press.

Monson, C. M., Langhinrichsen-Rohling, J., & Binderup, T. (2000). Does "no" really mean "no" after you say "yes." *Journal of Interpersonal Violence, 15,* 1156–1175.

Morton, K. E. (2003). *Psychometric properties of four risk assessment measures with male adolescent sexual offenders.* Unpublished master's dissertation. Carleton University.

Murphy, W. D., DiLillo, D., Haynes, M. R., & Steere, E. (2001). An exploration of factors related to deviant sexual arousal among juvenile sex offenders. *Sexual Abuse, 13,* 91–103.

Muster, N. J. (1992). Treating the adolescent victim-turned-offender. *Adolescence, 27,* 441–450.

Myers, J. E. B., Diedrich, S., Lee, D., Fincher, K. M., & Stern, R. (1999). Professional writing on child sexual abuse from 1900 to 1975: Dominant themes and impact on prosecution. *Child Maltreatment, 4,* 201–216.

Nagy, S., DiClemente, R., & Adcock, A. G. (1995). Adverse factors associated with forced sex among southern adolescent girls. *Pediatrics, 96*(5, Pt. 1), 944–946.

Oberman, M. (1994). Turning girls into women: Reevaluating modern statutory rape law. *Journal of Criminal Law and Criminology, 85,* 15–79.

O'Brien, M. J. (1991). Taking sibling incest seriously. In

M. Q. Patton (Ed.), *Family sexual abuse: Frontline research and evaluation* (pp. 75–92). Newbury Park, CA: Sage.

O'Donahue, W., Regev, L. G., & Hagstrom, A. (2000). Problems with the DSM-IV diagnosis of pedophilia. *Sexual Abuse: A Journal of Research and Treatment, 12,* 95–105.

Ondersma, S. J., Chaffin, M., Berliner, L., Cordon, I., Goodman, G. S., & Barnett, D. (2001). Sex with children is abuse: Comment on Rind, Tromovitch, and Bauserman (1998). *Psychological Bulletin 2001, 127,* 707–714.

Patterson, G. R., & Stouthamer-Loeber, M. (1984). The correlation of family management practices and delinquency. *Child Development, 55,* 1299–1307.

Peters, S. D., Wyatt, G. E., & Finkelhor, D. (1986). Prevalence. In D. Fineklhor (Ed.), *A sourcebook on child sexual abuse* (pp. 15–59). Newbury Park, CA: Sage.

Pierce, J. H., & Pierce, R. L. (1987). Incestuous victimization by juvenile sex offenders. *Journal of Family Violence, 2,* 351–364.

Pithers, W. D., & Gray, A. (1998). The other half of the story: Children with sexual behavior problems. *Psychology, Public Policy, and Law, 4,* 200–217.

Prentky, R. A., & Righthand, S. C. (2001). *Juvenile sex offender assessment protocol: Manual* [Online]. Unpublished document. Retrieved 2003 from www.csom.org

Reiss, D., Hetherington, E. M., Plomin, R., Howe, G. W., Simmens, S. J., Henderson, S. H., O'Connor, T. J., et al. (1995). Genetic questions for environmental studies: Differential parenting and psychopathology in adolescence. *Archives of General Psychiatry, 52,* 925–936.

Rich, S. D. (1998). A developmental approach to the treatment of adolescent sexual offenders. *The Irish Journal of Psychology, 19,* 102–118.

Rind, B., Tromovitch, P., & Bauserman, R. (1998). A meta-analytic examination of assumed properties of child sexual abuse using college samples. *Psychological Bulletin 1998, 124,* 22–53.

Rind, B., Tromovitch, P., & Bauserman, R. (2001). The validity and appropriateness of methods, analyses, and conclusions in Rind et al. (1998): A rebuttal of victimological critique from Odersma et al. (2001) and Dallam et al. (2001). *Psychological Bulletin, 127,* 734–758.

Roberts, R. E., McBee, G. W., & Bettis, M. C. (1969). Youthful sex offenders: An epidemiological comparison of types. *Journal of Sex Research, 5,* 29–40.

Robertson, J. M. (1990). Group counseling and the high risk offender. *Federal Probation, 54,* 48–51.

Rodrigues, G. P. (2004). *Pocket criminal code.* Toronto, ON, Canada: Thomson Carswell.

Rosenzweig, S. (1942). The photoscope as an objective device for evaluating sexual interest. *Psychosomatic Medicine, 4,* 150–157.

Ryan, G. (1991). Incidence and prevalence of sexual offenses committed by juveniles. In G. Ryan & S. Lane (Eds.), *Juvenile sexual offending: Causes, consequences, correction* (pp. 9–19). Boston: Lexington Books.

Ryan, G. (1998). The relevance of early life experience to the behavior of sexually abusive youth. *The Irish Journal of Psychology, 19,* 32–48.

Ryan, G., Miyoshi, T. J., Metzner, J. L., Krugman, R. D., & Fryer, G. E. (1996). Trends in a national sample of sexually abusive youths. *Journal of the American Academy of Child and Adolescent Psychiatry, 33,* 17–25.

Sandburg, S., Weiselberg, M., & Shaffer, D. (1980). Hyperkinetic and conduct problem children in primary school population: Some epidemiological considerations. *Journal of Child Psychology and Psychiatry, 21,* 293–311.

Saunders, E. B., Awad, G. A., & White, G. (1986). Male adolescent sexual offenders: The offender and the offense. *Canadian Journal of Psychiatry, 31,* 542–549.

Schram, D. D., Milloy, C. D., & Rowe, W. D. (1991). *Juvenile sex offenders: A follow-up study of reoffense behavior.* Olympia: Washington State Institute for Public Policy.

Sedlak, A. J., & Broadhurst, D. D. (1996). *Executive summary: Third National Incidence Study of Child Abuse and Neglect.* Washington, DC: Department of Health and Human Services.

Seto, M. C., & Lalumière, M. L. (2001). A brief screening scale to identify pedophilic interests among child molesters. *Sexual Abuse, 13,* 15–25.

Seto, M. C., Lalumière, M. L., & Blanchard, R. (2000). The discriminative validity of a phallometric test for pedophlic interests among adolescent sex offenders against children. *Psychological Assessment, 12,* 319–327.

Seto, M. C., Lalumière, M. L., & Kuban, M. (1999). The sexual preferences of incest offenders. *Journal of Abnormal Psychology, 108,* 267–272.

Seto, M. C., Murphy, W. D., Page, J., & Ennis, L. (2003). Detecting anomalous sexual interests in juvenile sex offenders. In R. A. Prentky, E. S. Janus, & M. C. Seto (Eds.), *Sexually coercive behavior: Understanding and management.* New York: Annals of the New York Academy of Sciences Press.

Shadish, W. R., & Ragsdale, K. (1996). Random versus nonrandom assignment in controlled experiments: Do you get the same answer? *Journal of Consulting and Clinical Psychology, 64,* 1290–1305.

Shoor, M., Speed, M. H., & Bartlet, C. (1966). Syndrome of the adolescent child molester. *American Journal of Psychiatry, 122,* 783–789.

Smallborne, S. W., & Dadds, M. R. (1998). Childhood attachment and adult attachment in incarcerated adult male sex offenders. *Journal of Interpersonal Violence, 13,* 555–573.

Smallborne, S. W., & Dadds, M. R. (2000). Attachment and coercive sexual behavior. *Sexual Abuse: A Journal of Research and Treatment, 12,* 3–15.

Smallborne, S. W., & McCabe, B. (2003) Childhood attachment, childhood sexual abuse, and onset of masturbation among adult sexual offenders. *Sexual Abuse: a Journal of Research and Treatment, 15*, 1–9.

Smith, W. R. (1988). Delinquency and abuse among juvenile sexual offenders. *Journal of Interpersonal Violence, 3*, 400–413.

Smith, W. R, Monastersky, C., & Deisher, R. W. (1987). MMPI-based personality types among juvenile sexual offenders. *Journal of Clinical Psychology, 43*, 422–430.

Smith, E. A., & Udry, J. R. (1985). Coutal and non-coital sexual behaviours of white and black adolescents. *American Journal of Public Health, 75*, 1200–1203.

Stock, J. L., Bell, M. A., Boyer, D. K., & Connell, F. A. (1997). Adolescent pregnancy and sexual risk-taking among sexually abused girls. *Family Planning Perspective, 29*, 200–203, 227.

Tannahill, R. (1992). *Sex in history*. Chelsea, MI: Scarborough House.

Tarter, R. E., Hegedus, A. M., Alterman, A. L., & Katzgaar, L. (1983). Cognitive capacities of juvenile violent, nonviolent, and sexual offenders. *Journal of Nervous and Mental Disease, 171*, 564–567.

Travin, S., & Protter, B. (1993). *Sexual perversion: Integrative treatment approaches for the clinician*. New York: Plenum Press.

Trivits, L. C., & Reppucci, N. D. (2002). Application of Megan's Law to juveniles. *American Psychologist, 57*, 690–704.

Tzeng, O., & Schwarzin, H. (1990). Gender and race differences in child sexual abuse correlates. *International Journal of Intercultural Relations, 14*, 135–161.

United Nations General Assembly. (1994). *Declaration on the elimination of violence against women*. Geneva, Switzerland: Office of the United Nations High Commissioner for Human Rights.

Van Ness, S. R. (1984). Rape as instrumental violence: A study of youth offenders. Special Issue: Gender issues, sex offenses, and criminal justice: Current trends. *Journal of Offender Counseling, Services and Rehabilitation, 9*, 161–170.

Veneziano, C., Veneziano, L., & LeGrande, S. (2000). The relationship between adolescent sex offender behaviors and victim characteristics with prior victimization. *Journal of Interpersonal Violence, 15*, 363–374.

Vinogradov, S., Dishotsky, N. I., Doty, A. K., & Tinklenberg, J. R. (1988). Patterns of behavior in adolescent rape. *American Journal of Orthopsychiatry, 58*, 179–187.

Vizard, E., Monck, E., & Misch, P. (1995). Child and adolescent sex abuse perpetrators: A review of the research literature. *Journal of Child Psychology and Psychiatry, 56*, 731–756.

Ward, T., Hudson, S. M., & Marshall, W. L. (1996). Attachment style in sex offenders: A preliminary study. *Journal of Sex Research, 33*, 17–26.

Ward, T., Hudson, S. M., & Marshall, W. L., & Siegert, R. J. (1995). Attachment style and intimacy deficits in sexual offenders: A theoretical framework. *Sexual Abuse: A Journal of Research and Treatment, 7*, 317–335.

Wasserman, J., & Kappel, S. (1985). *Adolescent sex offenders in Vermont*. Burlington: Vermont Department of Health.

Watkins, B., & Bentovim, A. (1992). The sexual abuse of male children and adolescents: A review of current research. *Journal of Child Psychology and Psychiatry, 33*, 197–248.

Wheeler, J. R., & Berliner, L. (1988). Treating the effects of sexual abuse on children. In G. E. Wyatt & G. J. Powell (Eds.), *Lasting effects of child sexual abuse* (pp. 227–247). Newbury Park, CA: Sage.

Worling, J. R. (1995). Sexual abuse histories of adolescent male sex offenders: Differences on the basis of the age and gender of their victims. *Journal of Abnormal Psychology, 104*, 610–613.

Worling, J. R. (2002, October). *Risk assessment with adolescents: Current research and practice*. Invited address at 21st Annual Research and Treatment Conference, Association for the Treatment of Sexual Abusers, Montreal.

Worling, J. R., & Curwen, T. (2000). Adolescent sexual offender recidivism: Success of specialized treatment and implications for risk prediction. *Child Abuse and Neglect, 24*, 965–982.

Worling, J. R., & Curwen, T. (2001). Estimate of Risk of Adolescent Sexual Offense Recidivism (the ERASOR: Version 2.0). In M. C. Calder (Ed.), *Juveniles and children who sexually abuse: Frameworks for assessment* (pp. 372–397). Lyme Regis, Dorset, UK: Russell House. (Available by contacting author at jworling@ican.net)

Worling, J. R., & Långström, N. (2006). Risk of sexual recidivism in adolescents who offend sexually: Correlates and assessment. In H. E. Barbaree & W. L. Marshall (Eds.), *The juvenile sex offender* (2nd ed., pp. 219–247). New York: Guilford Press.

Wright, L. W., & Adams, H. E. (1994). Assessment of sexual preference using a choice reaction time task. *Journal of Psychopathology and Behavioral Assessment, 16*, 221–231.

Wyatt. G., Durvasula, R. S., Guthrie, D., LeFranc, E., & Forge, N. (1999). Correlates of first intercourse among women in Jamaica. *Archives of Sexual Behavior, 28*, 139–157.

Zolondek, S. C., Abel, G. G., Northey, W. F., & Jordan, A. D. (2001). The self-reported behaviors of juvenile sexual offenders. *Journal of Interpersonal Violence, 16*, 73–85.

Zuravin, S. (1989). The ecology of child abuse and neglect: Review of the literature and presentation of data. *Victims and Violence, 4*, 101–120.

VII

MALTREATMENT AND TRAUMA

19

Relationship Violence

Ernest N. Jouriles
David A. Wolfe
Edward Garrido
Anna McCarthy

For many adolescents, the early- to mid-teenage years are a period in which romantic relationships begin to emerge. These relationships often occupy a significant portion of adolescents' time (Richards, Crowe, Larson, & Swarr, 1998; Thompson, 1994) and serve many positive functions (Connolly & Johnson, 1996; Feiring, 1996, 1999; Gray & Steinberg, 1999). Unfortunately, a surprisingly large number of adolescent romantic relationships are marked by physical, psychological, and sexual violence, and the consequences of such violence can be devastating.

Research on violence in adolescent romantic relationships has a short history. The groundbreaking efforts of a few research teams (e.g., Henton, Cate, Koval, Lloyd, & Christopher, 1983; Makepeace, 1981) made it clear that physical violence occurred in dating relationships and among adolescent couples. Although systematic research on adolescent relationship violence is still sparse, significant progress has been made in our understanding of this phenomenon. For example, early efforts directed at understanding dating violence were often de-

void of theory or discussed/applied theory in a very general manner. Recently, however, comprehensive and integrative theoretical frameworks exclusive to adolescent dating violence have been devised and empirically tested (e.g., O'Leary & Slep, 2003; Wolfe, Wekerle, Scott, Straatman, & Grasley, 2004). The early assessment of adolescent dating violence typically involved measures originally developed for use with adult populations; that is, measures designed to assess adult relationship violence were simply applied to adolescent samples. Recent developments have yielded new measures that more fully capture the behaviors and attitudes of adolescents (e.g., Wolfe, Scott, Reitzel-Jaffe, et al., 2001). In addition, until recently, intervention programs addressing adolescent dating violence were practically unheard of. Investigators now are beginning to develop and carefully evaluate such interventions, although the number of empirically validated interventions is still very small (Wekerle & Wolfe, 1999).

This chapter begins by describing different types of relationship violence, followed by a brief review of epidemiological findings. We then provide an overview of the course, precursors, and outcomes of relationship violence and several of the theories used to explain its development. Next, we discuss issues associated with the assessment of dating violence and provide an overview and critique of intervention/prevention programs that have been developed to deal with this phenomenon. We conclude with a brief discussion of future directions.

DEFINING ADOLESCENT DATING VIOLENCE

Dating during adolescence is difficult to define, in part, because dating patterns and behaviors change dramatically during the course of adolescence. For example, in early adolescence dating typically occurs in the context of small groups of mixed-sex friends; that is, friends meet, go out, and do things together as a group (Connolly, Craig, Goldberg, & Pepler, 1999). Romantic interest may be expressed in the context of these groups, but romantic activity rarely occurs (Connolly et al., 1999). From these group experiences, adolescents progress toward going out with/dating a single individual (in addition to going out with groups). These initial "single-dating" experiences are typically casual and short term, progressing to more serious, exclusive relationships in mid to late adolescence (Feiring, 1996; Furman & Buhrmester, 1992).

Researchers in the area of adolescent dating violence have approached the task of defining dating in several different ways. Some researchers provide an explicit definition of *date* or *dating* for their adolescent participants. Foshee, Bauman, and Linder (1999), for example, asked adolescents if they had ever been on a date, defined as "very informal activities, such as meeting at a mall, sporting event, or park, as well as more formal activities" (p. 324). Others leave it to the adolescents to determine what is meant by *date* or *dating*. However, what appears to be most common in this literature is for researchers to ask adolescents to report on violence occurring in the context of a relationship (e.g., between the adolescent participant and a "boyfriend" or "girlfriend"). It might be argued that there are important differences between violence occurring in the context of a boyfriend/girlfriend relationship and violence occurring on a date (e.g., the former being more restrictive), but the implications of defin-

ing adolescent violence in these different contexts is not known.

Violence typically is defined as the occurrence of one or more specific acts of violence (on a date or between a boyfriend or girlfriend). As a result, the definition of violence is synonymous with the specific items naming or describing violent acts on measures that assess violence. Multiple types of violence occur in the context of adolescent dating relationships, including physical, psychological, and sexual violence. Thus, it is useful to consider definitions for each of these different types of violence.

Physical violence often is defined in terms similar to that of adults, and has often been measured by items (or slight modifications of items) from Straus's (1979) Conflict Tactics Scales. For example, physical violence may be defined by any of the following acts: *threw something at partner; physically restrained partner; pushed, grabbed, or shoved partner; slapped partner; kicked, bit, or hit partner with fist; choked partner; beat up partner; threatened partner with a knife or gun.* Typically, the occurrence of one or more of these acts over a specified period of time (e.g., the last 4 months or the entire length of the dating partners' relationship) is used to signify the occurrence of physical relationship violence.

Psychological violence has also been defined with items from Straus's (1979) Conflict Tactics Scales, including *insulted or swore at partner; sulked or refused to talk; stomped out of room or house; cried; done/said something in spite; threatened to hit or throw something; threw, hit, or kicked something.* Adolescent-focused measures have begun to emerge, which address some of the more unique behaviors shown among this age group. For example, O'Leary and Slep (2003) and Wolfe, Scott, Reitzel-Jaffe, and colleagues (2001) recently assessed additional classes of behavior that might be conceptualized as psychological violence. These include efforts directed at damaging relationships between the partner and his or her peers (e.g., "I spread rumors about him or her"; "I tried to turn his or her friends against him or her"), control tactics (e.g., "I tried to keep my boyfriend/girlfriend from seeing or talking to his or her family"; "I monitored my partner's time and made him or her account for his or her whereabouts"), and jealous tactics (e.g., "I was jealous and suspicious of my boyfriend's/girlfriend's friends"; "I accused my boyfriend/girlfriend of seeing another girl/boy"). Again, the occurrence of one or more of these acts over a specified period of time is used to signify the occurrence of psychological violence.

Sexual violence includes forced or coerced sexual activity. Examples of such items from the Sexual Experiences Survey (Koss & Oros, 1982) include kissing or petting through the use of physical force, intercourse through the use of physical force, intercourse because he threatened to end the relationship, intercourse because pressured by his continual arguments (female respondents are asked if these acts occurred). Examples of such items from the Conflict in Adolescent Dating Relationship Inventory (Wolfe, Scott, Reitzel-Jaffe, et al., 2001) include (again, from the female's point of view) "He touched me sexually when I didn't want him to"; "He kissed me when I didn't want him to"; "He threatened me in an attempt to have sex with me"; "He forced me to have sex with him when I didn't want to." As with physical and psychological violence, the occurrence of one or more of these acts over a specified period of time is used to indicate sexual violence.

Although the definition of adolescent dating violence (physical, psychological, and sexual) may, in some ways, appear straightforward (i.e., in the context of a relationship or on a date and the occurrence of a specific act or behavior deemed to be violent), it is complicated by a number of issues. For example, researchers who have asked questions to assess how specific acts of violence were intended or perceived have found that many adolescents downplay the occurrence of physical and psychological violence; that is, these acts are often rationalized as occurring in the context of "joking" or "flirting" or as a means of gaining attention (e.g., Molidor & Tolman, 1998). There also are differences in the ways males and females perceive acts of violence, with respect to their meaning and consequences (Molidor & Tolman, 1998; Watson, Cascardi, Avery-Leaf, & O'Leary, 2001). For example, Molidor and Tolman found that females were more likely than males to report that the relationship worsened or ended as a consequence of the violence (more examples are provided in the section on outcomes). Such research highlights the importance of considering the context of the violent acts when defining and studying relationship violence. Another issue to consider is the developmental level of the ado-

lescent and the fact that different types of violence may be more relevant for adolescents of different ages. For example, Wolfe, Scott, Reitzel-Jaffe, and colleagues (2001) found relational violence (i.e., efforts directed at damaging relationships between the partner and his or her peers) to be more common among younger than older teens. This finding may reflect younger adolescents' relative immaturity in the areas of negotiating intimacy and handling relationship conflict.

EPIDEMIOLOGY

According to national survey data collected in the United States, 9.5% of students (grades 9–12) have been hit, slapped, or physically hurt on purpose by a boyfriend or girlfriend during a 12-month period (Centers for Disease Control [CDC], 2002). This estimate is based on a scientifically drawn sample, but the survey measure only included a single question about dating violence and the question was asked at only one time point. Other estimates of the prevalence of physical dating violence tend to be much higher, with most ranging from about 20% to over 50% (e.g., Cascardi, Avery-Leaf, O'Leary, & Slep, 1999; Jezl, Molidor, & Wright, 1996; Molidor & Tolman, 1998). Although these other estimates are not based on national samples, they are based on samples representative of specific high schools and include a much more extensive assessment of physical dating violence.

Comparable national data on the prevalence of psychological and sexual violence occurring in the context of dating relationships are not available for high school students (e.g., the CDC survey does not report on psychological violence or sexual violence occurring *in the context of a dating relationship*). However, estimates from other samples suggest that rates for psychological violence, in general, tend to be higher than those reported for physical violence, and rates for sexual violence vary (sometimes they are higher than those reported for physical violence and sometimes they are lower) depending on the specific criteria used for sexual violence. For example, Wolfe, Scott, Reitzel-Jaffe, and colleagues (2001) found in a large sample of high school students ($n = 1,019$) that the prevalence rates for self-reports of the perpetration of specific acts of psychological violence ranged from 25.6% ("I ridiculed or made fun of him or her in front of others") to 54% ("I spoke to him or her in a hostile or mean tone of voice"). On the other hand, the prevalence rates for self-reports of the perpetration of acts of physical violence ranged from 7% ("I slapped him or her or pulled his or her hair") to 11% ("I kicked, hit, or punched him or her"). The prevalence rates for self-reports of sexual violence ranged from 2.2 to 2.5% for items that involve forced sexual activity ("I forced him or her to have sex when he or she didn't want to"; "I threatened him or her in an attempt to have sex with him or her"). However, prevalence rates for unwanted kissing and touching were much higher—15.2–20.6% ("I kissed him or her when she did not want me to"; "I touched him or her sexually when he or she did not want me to").

It is also important to consider the co-occurrence of different forms of relationship violence. Physical violence most often occurs in relationships in which psychological violence has occurred (e.g., Jezl et al., 1996; Murphy & O'Leary, 1989). Similarly, it appears that sexual violence, defined as forced sexual activity, typically occurs in relationships in which physical violence has also occurred (Buzy et al., 2004; Silverman, Raj, Mucci, & Hathaway, 2001).

Age of Onset

The age of onset for adolescent dating violence is difficult to pinpoint, but it is most likely close to the onset of dating, which varies tremendously across individuals (Connolly & Johnson, 1996; Feiring, 1996). Most of our knowledge on the incidence of dating violence is with adolescents who are at least high school age (over 14 years of age), and it is clear that 14-year-olds (ninth graders) report both perpetrating and experiencing violence in the context of boyfriend/girlfriend relationships (e.g., Howard & Wang, 2003). Although research on violence experienced by middle school children is practically nonexistent, it appears that relationship violence does commence during the middle school years for at least some children/adolescents (see Avery-Leaf & Cascardi, 2002, for a review). In fact, to the extent that cross-sex teasing or harassment might be considered a form of psychological violence, it might be argued that certain forms of relationship violence are evident in the early school years.

Teasing and harassment initially emerge in the context of same-sex relationships. This can include malicious whispering, name calling, and note passing; it can also include, or be based on, the romantic interests and choices of an individual (McMaster, Connolly, Pepler, & Craig, 2002). Between grades 6 and 8, cross-sex teasing and harassment become increasingly more common, with pubertal maturation and mixed-sex socialization both associated with increased cross-sex harassment (McMaster et al., 2002). Although same-sex teasing and harassment *sometimes* have a sexual component, cross-sex harassment *often* entails behaviors that might be construed as sexual advances. Examples of these behaviors include making sexual comments or gestures, rating sexual parts of someone's body, pulling at someone's clothes in a sexual way (e.g. pulling up a shirt and pulling down pants), or brushing up against someone in a sexual way on purpose. Although younger teens have some concept of the various forms of teasing and harassment and why they are wrong, such behaviors among peers or friends are usually discounted as "just joking" (Berman, Izumi, & Arnold, 2002). This minimizing view continues throughout midadolescence, and becomes a familiar excuse for dating violence and/or a misperception of care and commitment from a partner. At the same time these teasing behaviors are also sometimes thought to be ways adolescents express romantic interest, which is why it is difficult for teens and adults alike to differentiate the more harmful behaviors.

Sexual teasing and harassment of others may be a warning sign of a developmental pattern of interpersonal aggression and a precursor for hostile interactions with dating partners (Connolly, Pepler, Craig, & Taradash, 2000; McMaster, Connolly, Pepler, & Craig, 2002). In one of the few studies to track relationship aggression from childhood to adolescence, children who perpetrated the most same- and cross-sex teasing and harassment were substantially more likely to report perpetrating aggression in their dating relationships (Pepler, Craig, Connolly, & Henderson, 2002).

Gender and the Prevalence of Relationship Violence

Adolescent females report engaging in physical violence toward dating partners at rates that are comparable to or higher than those reported by adolescent males (e.g., Cascardi et al., 1999; Chase, Treboux, & O'Leary, 2002; Molidor & Tolman, 1998; O'Keefe, 1997). Adolescent females also report engaging in more psychological violence than adolescent males (Cascardi et al., 1999; Wolfe, Scott, Reitzel-Jaffe, et al., 2001). In contrast, adolescent males are more likely than females to report sexual violence and coercion (e.g., Bennett & Fineran, 1998; Molidor & Tolman, 1998; O'Keefe, 1997; Swan & Snow, 2002; Wolfe, Scott, Reitzel-Jaffe, et al., 2001), but this depends on how sexual violence is defined. For example, it appears that females are more likely to engage in certain forms of sexual intrusiveness (e.g., kissing against victim's will and fondling), whereas males are more likely to commit arguably much more severe acts, such as attempted and forced intercourse (Poitras & Lavoie, 1995).

There are a number of complications in comparing and interpreting prevalence rates for relationship violence for males and females, and these complications arise, in part, from the definitions of violence typically employed. That is, if the occurrence of specific acts of violence is used to determine the prevalence of violence, then females appear as violent, if not more violent, than males; however, if acts of violence that result in injuries are used, then males come across as being more violent than females (e.g., Arias, Samios, & O'Leary, 1987; Bookwala, Frieze, Smith, & Ryan, 1992; Makepeace, 1986; Molidor & Tolman, 1998; Riggs, 1993). Thus, it could be argued from a health perspective that males' violence toward females is clearly a larger problem than females' violence toward males, even though prevalence rates for specific acts of violence tell a different story. Differential consequences of males' and females' relationship violence are covered in the next section.

Ethnic/Cultural and Socioeconomic Differences in Adolescent Dating Violence

Research on ethnic and cultural differences in the experience of adolescent dating violence has been somewhat limited due to a reliance on predominantly Anglo, middle-class samples (Jackson, 1999; Sugarman & Hotaling, 1989). Results of those studies that have examined race or ethnicity generally indicate higher rates for African Americans compared to Anglos (Foshee, Linder, MacDougall, & Bangdiwala, 2001; Howard & Wang, 2003; Malik,

Sorenson, & Aneshensel, 1997; O'Keefe, 1997). For example, an examination of female responses to the Youth Risk Behavior Survey revealed that African-American girls were twice as likely as their Anglo counterparts to report being the victim of physical violence (Howard & Wang, 2003). Moreover, Foshee and colleagues (2001) found that adolescent girls' ethnicity (i.e., being nonwhite) was a significant, longitudinal predictor of becoming a perpetrator of mild and severe forms of dating violence. Less consistent findings have been reported for Latino and Asian American samples, with some studies reporting slightly higher rates of dating violence perpetration/victimization (relative to Anglos) among Latino adolescents (O'Keefe, 1997) and slightly lower rates among Asian American adolescents (Malik et al., 1997).

An important consideration when interpreting the effects of ethnic/cultural differences on adolescent dating violence is the role of socioeconomic status (SES) as a potential confounding variable. Indeed, when factors associated with SES are controlled for (e.g., parent's income and occupation), the contribution of race/ethnicity is often rendered nonsignificant (O'Keefe, 1997). One potential explanation might be that lower SES adolescents encounter more stress at home due to problems that often go hand-in-hand with diminished resources (e.g., poverty and unemployment of parents). This increased amount of stress may, in turn, lead to a greater likelihood of experiencing/witnessing marital and family violence, a potential precursor to relationship violence (O'Keefe & Sela-Amit, 1997; Stets & Henderson, 1991). Accordingly, although Malik and colleagues (1997) found that African American adolescents were significantly more likely to perpetrate dating violence, the finding was no longer statistically significant after accounting for exposure to family violence.

DEVELOPMENTAL COURSE AND OUTCOMES

There has been some speculation that the prevalence of physical relationship violence increases with age during adolescence and on into early adulthood. That is, on the basis of a review of cross-sectional studies conducted with different age groups, O'Leary (1999) speculated that between the ages of 15 and 25, prevalence rates for physical relationship violence increase dramatically. However, there is also evidence to the contrary. Specifically, in one of the few prospective studies on the topic of dating violence, women's rates for experiencing violence were higher during high school than during the college years (Humphrey & White, 2000; Smith, White, & Holland, 2003).

Results from several cross-sectional studies of dating violence among high school students suggest that the prevalence of physical relationship violence may increase over the course of high school. For example, an analysis of the 1999 national Youth Risk Behavior Survey indicated that 9th-grade females reported the lowest prevalence rates for experiencing dating violence (8.02%), whereas 12th-grade females reported the highest prevalence rates (10.88%), but differences in prevalence across the four grades were not statistically significant (Howard & Wang, 2003). Similarly, in a large survey of adolescents, Malik and colleagues (1997) found adolescent age to be an important correlate of involvement in dating violence; older adolescents generally were more likely to be involved in dating violence than younger adolescents, but this association was not completely linear.

Regarding the course of adolescent dating violence, there is some evidence that during the high school years, physical relationship violence remains stable over time. In other words, when violence occurs in the context of an adolescent dating relationship, it often reoccurs. This is true when the dating relationship remains intact; that is, male and female adolescents have been found to be violent toward the *same* partner over time (O'Leary & Slep, 2003). This is also true across partners or relationships. That is, when males and females have been violent in one relationship, they tend to be violent in subsequent relationships as well (Cano, Avery-Leaf, Cascardi, & O'Leary, 1998; Chase, Treboux, O'Leary, & Strasberg, 1998). It is also noteworthy that experiencing dating violence in high school increases the risk for experiencing dating violence in college (Humphrey & White, 2000; Smith et al., 2003). Similarly, violence during the year prior to marriage predicts violence during the early years of marriage (O'Leary et al., 1989).

A number of variables appear to play a key role in the development of relationship violence. Among these are exposure to violence during childhood/adolescence, beliefs and attitudes that view male aggression against females as justifiable, antisocial behavior in childhood and adolescence, trauma symptoms, peer influences, and verbal conflict within the relationship. We review some of the evidence implicating each of these variables below. We also review findings on more immediate precursors to relationship violence (i.e., situational factors that appear to predict relationship violence) and then discuss outcomes.

Exposure to Violence

Exposure to violence during childhood/adolescence consistently is found to correlate with the perpetration of dating violence, and there is evidence that it correlates with victimization as well (e.g., Jankowski, Leitenberg, Henning, & Coffey, 1999; O'Keefe, 1998; Smith et al., 2003; Wolfe, Wekerle, Reitzel-Jaffe, & Lefebvre, 1998). Much of this literature focuses on exposure to "family" violence (i.e., witnessing interparent violence or experiencing child abuse). Both the witnessing of interparent violence and the experiencing of child abuse have been found to be associated with dating violence, but findings are not consistent across studies. That is, some investigators have found the witnessing of interparent violence and not the experiencing of child abuse to be associated with dating violence (e.g., Wolf & Foshee, 2003, for females only). Others have found the experiencing of child abuse and not the witnessing of interparent violence to be associated with dating violence (e.g., Brendgen, Vitaro, Tremblay, & Wanner, 2002; Wolf & Foshee, 2003, for males only).

The vast majority of research on exposure to violence during childhood/adolescence is cross-sectional, with the exposure to violence variable measured retrospectively and then correlated with current or recent incidents of relationship violence. Prospective research on dating violence is beginning to emerge, however, and the findings from these studies are consistent with those from cross-sectional studies. For example, Smith and colleagues (2003) collected data on childhood victimization experiences retrospectively, but they collected data on victimization experiences during college prospectively. These investigators found women who reported childhood victimization experiences (coercive sexual acts, parental physical abuse, or interparent physical abuse prior to the age of 14) to be at increased risk for experiencing violence from a romantic partner during college.

Several investigators also have found exposure to other types of violence, in addition to family violence, to be important in the prediction of partner violence. For example, Malik and colleagues (1997) found exposure to community violence to relate to involvement in dating violence, independent of exposure to family violence. These investigators also found that many of the relations between demographic characteristics (e.g., ethnicity) and involvement in dating violence are accounted for by exposure to violence. In addition, exposure to friends' aggression or violent behavior has been found to predict partner violence in several longitudinal investigations (e.g., Brendgen et al., 2002; Capaldi, Dishion, Stoolmiller, & Yoerger, 2001; Jouriles, McDonald, Swank, Norwood, & Buzy, 2002).

Beliefs and Attitudes

Adolescent beliefs and attitudes about dating violence consistently relate to self-reports of the perpetration of relationship violence, particularly among males (e.g., O'Keefe, 1997; Riggs & O'Leary, 1996; Slep, Cascardi, Avery-Leaf, & O'Leary, 2001). There are also data consistent with the idea that beliefs and attitudes justifying the use of violence against dating partners mediate the relation between exposure to violence and the perpetration of dating violence. For example, Foshee, Bauman, and Linder (1999) found that violence in adolescent males' family of origin predicted more positive outcome expectations for using dating violence and more acceptance of dating violence as a means of dealing with potential relationship conflict. These attitudes, in turn, were associated with the perpetration of dating violence and were found to mediate the association between exposure to violence and the perpetration of dating violence. Similarly, Grych, Kinsfogel, Hart, Klockkow, and Robbins (2003) found evidence that attitudes justifying the use of relationship violence mediate the association between exposure to family aggression and the perpetration of dating violence.

A close inspection of this literature, however, suggests the need for a couple of caveats when interpreting findings about beliefs and attitudes. First, it is important to recognize that many different types of beliefs and attitudes about dating violence exist. Specifically, beliefs and attitudes about dating violence include those indicating that (1) relationship violence, in general, is justified (e.g., "It's okay for a boy to hit his girlfriend"), (2) relationship violence is justified in particular contexts (e.g., "It's okay for a boy to hit his girlfriend if she insults him"), (3) positive and negative expectations about the consequences of dating violence (e.g., "If I hit a dating partner, my friends would think I was cool") and (4) the perceived prevalence or normalcy of dating violence (e.g., "Most boys hit their girlfriends"), among others. Although many of these different beliefs and attitudes have been associated with the perpetration of dating violence, there is some evidence for differential associations as well. For example, Foo and Margolin (1995) investigated beliefs justifying dating violence in two different contexts—after being humiliated by the partner and in self-defense. Justification of relationship violence after being humiliated contributed unique variance in both males' and females' dating violence. On the other hand, justification of relationship violence performed in self-defense did not contribute unique variance in dating violence. These findings highlight the need for more attention to potentially important distinctions between different types of beliefs and attitudes about dating violence.

Second, the cross-sectional nature of most of the research on this topic leaves open the possibility that certain beliefs and attitudes about dating violence are a product of one's dating experiences rather than a precursor or cause. Consistent with this notion, Foshee and colleagues (2001) found several measures of attitudes and beliefs about dating violence (e.g., negative expectations of the consequences of dating violence and perceived prevalence or normalcy of dating violence) to be associated with the perpetration of dating violence cross-sectionally but not longitudinally. Similar findings are reported by Wolfe and colleagues (2004). On the other hand, there is longitudinal research indicating that certain attitudes and beliefs about violence predict future dating violence. For example, Foshee and colleagues did find that males who reported a greater amount of acceptance of gender-based dating violence (e.g., "Sometimes boys have to hit their girlfriends to get them back under control") were more likely to engage in dating violence a year and a half later. This relation emerged even after accounting for other predictors of dating violence (e.g., violence in the family of origin and other problem behaviors). Similarly, Brengden and colleagues (2002) found males' general beliefs about fighting (e.g., "Winning a fight is the best fun there is" and "A person who won't fight is just no good") assessed at age 12 predicted violence directed at a dating partner at ages 16 and 17. Again, these findings highlight the importance of distinguishing between different types of attitudes, but they also indicate that at least some attitudes and beliefs about violence are precursors to dating violence and not just outcomes or justifications for violent behavior.

Violent and Antisocial Behavior

In a comprehensive review of the adult literature on male batterers, Holtzworth-Munroe and Stuart (1994) estimated that a substantial portion of all batterers (25–50%) act violently toward individuals other than their partners. Research on the co-occurrence of partner violence and other forms of violence/antisocial behavior is sparse among adolescents, although there is some evidence for significant overlap (e.g. Brendgen et al., 2002; Capaldi & Clark, 1998). That is, many of the adolescents who engage in partner violence also engage in acts of violence and antisocial behavior targeted at individuals other than their partners. For example, a study of 5,500 male and female high school students in South Carolina indicated that severe dating violence (victim/perpetrator combined) was significantly related to physical fighting, drug use (illegal drugs, anabolic steroids, tobacco or alcohol), and high-risk sexual behavior (Coker et al., 2000). In short, the results of survey studies suggest that involvement in dating violence is associated with a wide range of antisocial behavior.

Moreover, there is a growing body of longitudinal evidence indicating that antisocial behavior during childhood and adolescence is a precursor to partner violence in late adolescence and early adulthood. For example, in a large New Zealand sample, a composite measure of childhood/adolescent problem behavior (which included juvenile police contacts, conduct problems, aggressive delinquency, and substance abuse) predicted men's partner violence at age 21 (Magdol, Moffitt, Caspi, &

Silva, 1998). In a sample of rural families, a construct labeled "antisocial behavioral trait," defined by a variety of deviant acts including fighting, traffic violations, lying, gambling, and arrests occurring during childhood and adolescence, was associated with frequent and persistent partner violence in adulthood (Simons, Wu, Johnson, & Conger, 1995). In a sample of males at risk for delinquency, a broad measure of antisocial behavior obtained at grade 12 predicted men's physical and psychological aggression toward female partners during early adulthood (Capaldi et al., 2001). In a modified probability sample of adolescents living in a midwestern city, a broad measure of delinquent behavior over a 12-month period predicted involvement in relationship violence 10 years later (Giordano, Millhollin, Cernkovich, Pugh, & Rudolph, 1999). In short, there is consistent evidence that antisocial behavior in childhood and adolescence predicts later partner violence.

It is also important to highlight that victims of dating violence, as well as the perpetrators of such violence, appear to engage in antisocial behavior. For example, Howard and Wang (2003) found that females who reported being victims of dating violence during the previous 12 months were four times more likely to have engaged in binge drinking, 10 times more likely to have used cocaine or inhalants, 7 times more likely to have had multiple sex partners, and 5 times more likely to have had sex without a condom relative to females without a history of dating violence. Silverman and colleagues (2001) also found adolescent females who reported experiencing physical dating violence to have problems with substance use and high-risk sexual behavior. These investigators also found victims of dating violence to report using unhealthy weight control techniques (such as taking diet pill or laxatives) and suicidality. Buzy and colleagues (2004) documented both a cross-sectional and longitudinal association between general alcohol use and victimization among adolescent females. Thompson, Wonderlich, Crosby, and Mitchell (2001) found that dating violence and sexual victimization were predictors of both purging and diet pill consumption among adolescent females. It is not clear if these other problem behaviors precede or follow victimization. However, it does seem to be clear that victims of dating violence often experience other difficul-

ties and/or exhibit unhealthy or problem behaviors.

Trauma Symptoms

Developmental traumatology (DeBellis &
Putnam, 1994) posits trauma-related symptoms as a key mediator of maltreatment history
and subsequent maladaptive outcomes, via
stress-induced changes in developing neurobiology. Given both the discrete maltreatment
events and chronic family stressors that often
accompany these events (e.g., substance abuse,
multiple home and partner changes, chaotic
routines, and neglect-related accidents;
Wekerle & Wall, 2002), the biological stress
system response is chronically mobilized,
which can lead to permanent structural and
functional changes to the brain (DeBellis,
2001). Affected children have some degree of
ongoing trauma symptoms, with greater episodic activation following acute maltreatment-
related cue exposure.

Elevated trauma symptoms have been consistently found among victims of sexual abuse
(Briere, 1992), physical abuse, and neglect
(Widom, 1999) and witnesses of parental conflict and violence (Kitzmann, Gaylord, Holt, &
Kenny, 2003). Applied to dating violence, trauma symptoms may interfere with acknowledging when "rough and tumble play" crosses the
line to abusive behavior, due to the confusing
positive affect in the earlier stages and the potentially heightened tolerance of abuse among
maltreatment victims (Capaldi & Gorman-
Smith, 2003). Furthermore, playful grabbing
or restraining by a dating partner may trigger
activation of maltreatment-related memories,
increasing the risk of escalating aggressive responses (Meiser-Stedman, 2002). Such trauma-
related symptoms are especially elevated
among females with maltreatment backgrounds in both community (Wolfe et al.,
2001) and child protection samples (Wekerle,
Scott, Wekerle, & Pittman, 2001). Thus, the
dating context poses new challenges, especially
for maltreated youth, whereby strong feelings,
physical proximity, and sexual involvement
may contribute to a resurgence of trauma
symptoms owing to similar cues to the original
abusive event(s) (Wekerle & Wolfe, 2003).

Wolfe and colleagues (2004) examined in a
community sample of adolescents how a history of child maltreatment, including mild to
moderate forms of abuse and neglect, may relate to the later emergence of dating violence.
Three risk constructs (i.e., trauma symptoms,
attitudes justifying dating violence, and empathy and self-efficacy in dating relationships)
were identified as important factors that may
partially explain this connection. Using cross-
lagged analyses to control for correlational relationships, the only construct that predicted
change in dating violence over 1 year was trauma-related symptoms, for both boys and girls.
Teens' attitudes about the use of abusive methods with dating partners, as well as their self-
reported empathy and self-efficacy, were not
significant predictors of dating violence over
time, despite being correlated with dating violence at both time periods. The role of trauma
symptoms on dating violence also has been
documented among girls and women with
known maltreatment experiences (Messman-
Moore & Long, 2000; Wekerle et al., 2001).
Thus, findings from several studies underscore
the importance of trauma symptoms in understanding the association between childhood
maltreatment and dating violence.

Peer Influences

Systematic research evaluating the contribution
of peer influences on dating violence is sparse,
but there have been several longitudinal studies
pointing to the potential importance of peer influences. For example, Capaldi and colleagues
(2001) examined the longitudinal influence of
adolescent males' peer networks in the perpetration of dating violence by hypothesizing and
testing a path model. Deviant peer association
during midadolescence (13–16 years of age)
predicted degree of observed hostile talk about
females during late adolescence (17–18 years of
age), which, in turn, predicted levels of aggression toward a dating partner during young
adulthood (ages 20–23). Brendgen and colleagues (2002) found that the aggression levels
of males' friends (assessed at age 12) predicted
both concurrent acceptance of dating violence
among participants and their later likelihood of
engaging in dating violence in mid to late adolescence (age 16–17). Jouriles and colleagues
(2002) found that affiliation with peers who
engage in violent behavior predicted partner violence 3 years later. There is also some indication that peers may influence the likelihood of
victimization. For example, Howard, Qiu, and

Boekeloo (2003) found that adolescents who reported being exposed to peer-drinking activities (e.g., "Hanging out with friends who drank") were two to four times more likely to report being the victim of dating violence during the previous 3 months.

Relationship Conflict

Several different dimensions of relationship conflict have been examined as correlates of dating violence. For example, Riggs, O'Leary, and Breslin (1990) queried a sample of undergraduate students who were in a dating relationship about problems that had recently caused difficulties in their relationship. They found a positive association between number of problems reported and the perpetration of physical violence for both males and females. Similarly, Riggs and O'Leary (1996) found higher rates of physical violence for those undergraduate students who reported more frequent episodes of relationship conflict. In another study involving an undergraduate student sample, Riggs (1993) found higher rates of both perpetrating dating violence and being the victim of such violence among students who judged their relationship's conflict to be more severe. Thus, the frequency and severity of relationship conflict have been documented as correlates of dating violence.

Results from studies examining general relationship satisfaction as a correlate of dating violence have been more mixed than those that have examined relationship conflict. For example, Gaertner and Foshee (1999) found that decreased levels of relationship satisfaction were associated with an increased probability of having utilized violence. O'Keefe (1997), however, found that degree of relationship satisfaction did not predict perpetration of physical aggression for males or females. Similarly, Arias, Samios, and O'Leary (1987) found no association for males between their reported levels of aggression and their degree of liking or loving their partner. Studies examining particular aspects of relationship satisfaction are less common. Ronfeldt, Kimerling, and Arias (1998) found that undergraduate males who were less satisfied with the decision-making responsibilities (i.e., power) in their relationships were more likely to report having perpetrated physical aggression. Related to these findings, O'Leary and colleagues (1989) found that couples reported higher levels of relationship vio-

lence during the year prior to marriage, when relationship satisfaction was at a peak, as compared to when the couples were married. These findings, as a group, suggest that relationship dissatisfaction may not be a consistent precursor to relationship violence; indeed, it appears that a lot of dating violence occurs in "happy" or "satisfied" relationships.

Immediate Precursors

More immediate precursors to the perpetration of relationship violence may include feelings of jealousy, anger, emotional hurt, and acts of violence perpetrated by one's partner (Follingstad, Wright, Lloyd, & Sebastian, 1991; Molidor & Tolman, 1998; O'Keefe, 1997; O'Keefe & Treister, 1998). In addition, sex differences appear to exist in the motives behind such feelings. Adolescent females, for example, are more likely to report using violence to express anger or emotional hurt for unwanted sexual advances or for being verbally/psychologically abused, whereas adolescent males are more likely to use violence as retaliation for being hit first (Follingstad et al., 1991; Molidor & Tolman, 1998; Scott, Wekerle, & Wolfe, 1997). It has also been hypothesized that adolescent males use physical violence as a means of expressing anger for being rejected sexually (i.e., having sexual advances turned down) (O'Keefe & Treister, 1998), or for gaining control over a partner (Foshee et al., 2001; O'Keefe, 1997; Ronfeldt et al., 1998).

Outcomes

As indicated previously in the section "Epidemiology," there appear to be sex differences in response to relationship violence. In general, female victims are more likely than male victims to experience fear and hurt and to express a desire to leave the situation for self-protection (Follingstad et al., 1991; Jackson, Cram, & Seymour, 2000; O'Keefe & Treister, 1998). Molidor and Tolman (1998) found sex differences in reactions to the "worst" incident of violence. Males frequently reported that they "laughed" as their reaction to the worst incident, whereas females frequently reported that they "cried" or had to fight back in self-defense. Not surprisingly, after instances of dating violence, females are also more likely to report damaging physical and psychological consequences (e.g., bruises and depression)

(Bookwala et al., 1992; O'Keefe, 1997) and that the violence posed a threat to the status of the relationship (Molidor & Tolman, 1998). Males, particularly those with a history of aggression in their relationships, are less likely to report the potential for negative relationship consequences (e.g., breakup) as a result of dating violence (Riggs & Caulfield, 1997), in some instances indicating that the relationship would stay the same or improve as a result of the aggression (Molidor & Tolman, 1998).

THEORIES

Many researchers have used principles derived from broad and widely applied theories, such as social learning theory (Bandura, 1973, 1977) and attachment theory (Bowlby, 1969, 1972, 1980), in their attempts to understand and explain the perpetration of adolescent dating violence. Other researchers have developed models specific to adolescent relationship violence, often including principles and variables suggested by these broad theories into their models. Examples of such models include the contextual–situational model (Riggs & O'Leary, 1989), the dyadic longitudinal model (O'Leary & Slep, 2003), the relationship sensitivity model (Downey & Feldman, 1996), and the male peer support model (DeKeseredy, 1988, 1990; DeKeseredy & Schwartz, 1993). In the section that follows, we focus on models specific to the etiology of dating violence among adolescents. We describe the models and comment on some of the empirical findings consistent with these models' predictions.

Riggs and O'Leary (1989) developed the "background–situational" model for courtship aggression, which was initially developed for college dating relationships but has been used to guide research on adolescent dating violence (e.g., O'Keefe, 1997). The model includes two general categories of variables: (1) contextual or background variables, which predict aggressive behavior in general, and (2) situational variables, which predict incidents of aggression directed at a romantic partner (i.e., when and in what situations dating violence is likely to occur). Background variables in this model include exposure to violence in the family of origin, attitudes justifying the use of aggression, aggressive/impulsive personality characteristics, psychopathology, and difficulties effectively regulating emotion. These variables are hypothesized to lead to aggressive behavior across situations (i.e., increase aggressive behavior in general). Situational variables include expectations of a positive outcome to violence, stress, the use of alcohol, partners' use of aggression, and relationship conflict. Each of these variables are hypothesized to contribute to an increased likelihood of violence in a particular situation or directed at a particular partner.

Riggs and O'Leary (1989) rely heavily on social learning theory to explain the links among many of the background variables, situational variables, and relationship violence. For example, Riggs and O'Leary maintain that aggression is learned, often via observation/modeling processes, and parents are one of the main sources of early learning. Similarly, exposure to violence contributes to the learning of beliefs and attitudes accepting of aggression and expectations associated with the use of aggression toward a partner in particular situations.

Empirical support for Riggs and O'Leary's (1989) framework has come primarily from studies examining individual components as correlates or predictors of dating violence, and, as indicated above in the "Developmental Course and Outcomes" section, there are data indicating a relation between many of the variables in the background–situational model and dating violence. Several investigators have also attempted to examine the model more broadly. O'Keefe (1997), for example, examined the predictive ability of various background and situational components of the model in explaining dating violence among an ethnically diverse sample of over 1,000 high school students. She found that the variables specified in the Riggs and O'Leary model accounted for 55% of the variance in the dating violence reports of both males and females, with contextual variables explaining more of the variance for males and situational variables more of the variance for females.

More recently, O'Leary and Slep (2003) proposed the dyadic longitudinal model of adolescent dating aggression. What is new to this model is the emphasis on dyadic influences in the prediction of physical violence. That is, an adolescent female's use of psychological aggression is hypothesized to predict her male partner's use of physical aggression, and vice versa. This model is based, in part, on research and data suggesting the importance of relationship conflict and communication problems in the prediction of violence among young couples. This model is also based on the notion that dyadic influences may be much more important in adolescent romantic relationships than in adult relationships because of the fluid nature of most adolescent relationships. Although research on dyadic influences in adolescent romantic relationships is sparse, O'Leary and Slep found evidence consistent with their hypotheses. Specifically, both males' and females' psychological aggression predict their partner's use of physical aggression, concurrently and prospectively.

Downey and colleagues (e.g., Downey, Bonica, & Rincon, 1999; Downey & Feldman, 1996; Downey, Lebolt, Rincon, & Freitas, 1998) draw upon attachment theory in their development of the rejection sensitivity model for intimate relationships. The core construct of this model is rejection sensitivity—a disposition to expect, perceive, and overreact to rejection experiences. This disposition is hypothesized to result from early childhood experiences of rejection from parents. That is, children's expectations regarding the availability, reliability, and responsivity of caretakers form the basis for their behavior and expectations in future romantic relationships, including those engaged in during adolescence (Hazan & Shaver, 1987, 1994). For example, the formation of a secure attachment style in childhood is the result of consistent and responsive childrearing and is found in adolescence and adulthood to be associated with positive relationship outcomes (e.g., trust, relationship satisfaction, longer relationships). An insecure attachment style, on the other hand, stems from childrearing that is inconsistent, unresponsive, or aversive (i.e., violent) and is often associated with relationship difficulties, such as a lack of trust in a partner, difficulties with separation, and greater interpersonal sensitivity (Crittenden & Ainsworth, 1989).

Adolescents and adults high in rejection sensitivity have developed the expectation that when they seek acceptance and support from significant others, they will probably be rejected. These individuals place a high value on avoiding rejection. They often experience anticipatory anxiety when expressing needs and vulnerabilities to relationship partners, and when they encounter rejection cues, no matter how minimal or ambiguous, they readily perceive intentional rejection, which can lead to hostility and violence. Although this theory has

not received much empirical attention in the dating violence literature, at least two investigative teams have found measures of rejection sensitivity to relate to dating violence among adolescent males (e.g., Brendgen et al., 2002; Downey, Feldman, & Ayduk, 2000), with Brendgen and colleagues (2002) documenting a prospective relation between rejection sensitivity at age 12 and dating violence at ages 16 and 17.

DeKeseredy's (1988, 1990; DeKeseredy & Schwartz, 1993) male peer support model draws upon feminist theory, which hypothesizes that aggression against women is a product of the socialization of males to be in control of situations and relationships. Feminist theory stresses that socialization processes encouraging male dominance and female subservience are part of societal expectations regarding status and power. Males, according to this view, are socialized to be aggressive, dominant, and repressive in the expression of emotions such as fear and concern; in contrast, females are encouraged to be passive, compliant, and repressive in the expression of anger (Miedzian, 1995; Serbin, Powlishta, & Gulko, 1993). Moreover, the power imbalance suggested by these beliefs is thought to often lead to the acceptance of male entitlement, wherein the female may feel obligated to cater to the needs of her partner as caregiver, sex provider, and so forth (Dutton, 1995).

As implied by the model's name, DeKeseredy's model focuses on the presumed effects of the male peer support group on dating violence. The argument is made that involvement in certain male peer groups is associated with beliefs and attitudes that justify violence toward women or sexually objectify women. Moreover, the strong sense of cohesion that exists in these groups is thought to provide a supportive environment (i.e., one free of deterrence) for the perpetration of dating violence.

The male peer support model has been evaluated primarily in undergraduate samples. Humphrey and Kahn (2000) assessed the potential risk for violence toward women by members of certain fraternities and athletic teams, which were judged to be high risk for promoting violence toward women in ratings by undergraduate students. Results indicated that members of the perceived high-risk organizations scored significantly higher than members of the perceived low-risk organizations on measures of sexual aggression, hostility toward women, and peer support for sexual assault. Schwartz, DeKeseredy, Tait, and Alvi (2001) examined the impact of peer-provided, pro-abuse advice on undergraduate males' propensity for engaging in sexual violence. Degree of proabuse advice was assessed by asking participants if any of their male friends had told them things like: "It is all right for a man to hit his date or girlfriend in certain situations" and "Your dates or girlfriends should have sex with you when you want." Results indicated that males who reported two or more friends had provided them with proabuse advice had significantly higher rates of sexual coercion, attempted rape, and forced rape, relative to men with no such friends.

Results consistent with the male peer support model have also been observed in a sample of male adolescents at risk for antisocial behavior. Specifically, Capaldi and colleagues (2001) measured hostile talk about women by male peers by instructing their participants to "talk about what they liked and disliked about the girls they knew" (p. 64). The content of these videotaped, 5-minute interactions was coded for degree of hostility and was found to be a prospective predictor of males perpetrating psychological and physical aggression toward a female partner in young adulthood.

ASSESSMENT AND TREATMENT

Assessment

Adolescent dating violence typically is assessed via adolescent self-report. Specifically adolescents report on their own violent behavior or use of violence, their victimization experiences, or both. Although it is not uncommon in the research literature to see single-question assessments of dating violence, it is most commonly assessed through the use of a multi-item questionnaire, and as indicated in the section on defining adolescent dating violence, a number of questionnaires have been used to assess violence in adolescent dating relationships. Examples include the Conflict Tactics Scales (Straus, 1979), the Conflict in Adolescent Dating Relationship Inventory (Wolfe, Scott, Reitzel-Jaffe, et al., 2001), and the Sexual Experiences Survey (Koss & Oros, 1982). These measures ask adolescents to report on whether specific violent acts occurred during a specified time period (e.g., 6 months). Typically, these measures are administered to adolescents in a paper-and-

pencil format, and adolescents complete these measures anonymously and independently (although the measures are often completed in a classroom setting). Depending on the purpose of the assessment, each of these measures can be used (or modified to be used) to assess the perpetration of violence, victimization experiences, or both.

One of the key issues in terms of assessing adolescent dating violence is the field's heavy reliance on self-reports. Self-reports are potentially very valuable for the collection of private, sensitive, and potentially stigmatizing information. However, the possibility of participants giving socially desirable responses, in lieu of those that are more honest, becomes a prime concern. This appears to be particularly the case when considering reports of perpetration. Riggs, Murphy, and O'Leary (1989), for example, asked undergraduates the likelihood of their reporting the occurrence of both socially undesirable (e.g., physical dating violence) and socially desirable (e.g., reasoning) conflict-oriented behaviors for themselves and their partner on an anonymous questionnaire. Not surprisingly, results indicated that participants were significantly more likely to say that they would report both their own and their partner's socially desirable, rather than undesirable, behaviors. However, when asked the likelihood of their reporting negative behavior, participants were more likely to say they would report their partner's behavior than their own, particularly when asked about more severe forms of dating aggression.

Another inherent difficulty with relying on self-report data is the possibility of memory failures occurring, particularly when the recall period asked of participants is an extremely long one (e.g., 1 year). In one study, for example, adolescents were asked, across three separate time points, to give estimates of the number of cumulative instances of physical and sexual aggression occurring during the previous month, 6 months, and year. Results indicated that adolescents provided estimates of the reported rates that were not significantly different from one another (Hilton, Harris, & Rice, 1998).

Considering the difficulties already discussed involving self-reports (e.g., social desirability and memory failures), it is not surprising that interpartner agreement regarding the frequency of relationship violence among adults tends to be fairly low (e.g., Jouriles & O'Leary, 1985;

O'Leary, Vivian, & Malone, 1992). This is particularly true when considering partner agreement on specific questions of violence (Moffitt et al., 1997). One solution is to aggregate questions that assess dating violence. Moffit and colleagues (1997), for example, found that interpartner agreement regarding the incidence of dating violence was much improved when items were aggregated into scales.

In addition to relying predominantly on self-reports, researchers have tended to confine their assessments of dating violence to one partner. Considering that dating violence is an interpersonal phenomenon, assessments involving only one partner will provide researchers with only "half the picture." Indeed, the majority of research examining potential predictors of dating violence has involved intrapersonal factors, such as witnessing or experiencing familial violence, alcohol or drug use, and attachment styles. Conversely, relatively little research has involved potential interpersonal predictors, such as communication styles, problem-solving skills, and relationship satisfaction.

Intervention and Prevention Efforts

It is generally agreed that the period of adolescence provides fertile ground for those interested in affecting the attitudes and beliefs teens may have regarding dating relationships (Wekerle & Wolfe, 1998). To begin with, about half of all adolescents report having had some dating experience by the age of 14 or 15 (Connolly & Johnson, 1996; Feiring, 1996), with the percentage increasing to over 80% by the age of 16 (Dickinson, 1975; Hansen, 1977). Although these dating experiences typically are brief in nature, lasting an average of 4 months (Feiring, 1996), they nevertheless require adolescents to acquire and modify important relationship skills, such as strategies for dealing with and resolving interpersonal conflict. This natural development on the part of adolescents, of a relationship-oriented knowledge base, may provide those interested in implementing an intervention with an opportunity to reinforce nonviolent conflict resolution strategies as well as other "healthy" relationship behaviors.

Moreover, adolescents are likely motivated to avoid teasing from their peers that, during this period, generally concerns the lack of interest in establishing heterosexual romantic rela-

tionships (Shapiro, Baumeister, & Kessler, 1991). Thus, to meet the expectations of their peers, adolescents may place great importance in initiating and developing dating relationships. As a result, adolescents may be highly motivated to acquire information about healthy relationships, an important predictor of the successful modification of "risk behaviors" (Fisher & Fisher, 1992).

Despite the potential advantages of implementing an intervention aimed at affecting the dating attitudes and skills of adolescents, there has been a noticeable lack of such efforts (Wekerle & Wolfe, 1999). Wekerle and Wolfe (1999), for example, discovered in their review of the published literature covering the past 20 years the existence of only six adolescent relationship violence prevention/intervention programs. Furthermore, most of the prevention/intervention programs that have been evaluated suffer from a variety of methodological limitations, clouding the interpretation of their findings. For example, very few evaluations employ a true experimental design of random assignment of participants to intervention and control conditions (see Wolfe et al., 2003, for an exception). Most choose, instead, to adopt a quasi-experimental design of assigning classes or schools randomly to intervention or regular curriculum conditions. Additionally, most evaluations of programs do not measure changes in abusive behavior (see Foshee et al., 1998, for an exception). Rather, the assessment of change is typically limited to attitudes that justify the use of abusive behavior within a romantic relationship (Wekerle & Wolfe, 1999). Attitude change is important in and of itself; indeed, according to some theories, it is a prerequisite to behavior change. However, the global assessment of attitudes is unlikely to predict specific change in abusive behavior (Deaux & Wrightsman, 1984). Finally, few studies conduct longitudinal assessments of outcome (i.e., pretreatment, posttreatment, and follow-up).

Intervention programs that have been implemented generally assume that all teens can benefit from greater awareness of issues pertaining to violence because acts of violence and abuse in adolescent dating relationships are relatively commonplace and developmentally relevant. Therefore, intervention strategies are often based on a public health perspective of risk and protective health factors, rather than individual psychopathology (Wolfe, Wekerle, & Scott, 1997). A public health approach implies a focus on prevention and early intervention, with additional services available for targeted groups (e.g., high-risk youth), or to address the harmful consequences of victimization. Emerging prevention programs challenge inappropriate attitudes and behaviors and offer positive alternatives. They may also include resilience-promoting activities, such as skill-building, recognition of early warning signs, awareness of forms of violence, and help-seeking strategies. Below are several considerations in addressing dating violence from a broad, prevention standpoint.

Gender Considerations

There is some indication that intervention efforts must be careful to avoid the adoption of a theoretical model focusing exclusively on male perpetration. Boys, in particular, are seldom willing to engage in discussion of relationship violence and personal responsibility that does not acknowledge, at some level, the reality of girls' aggression. Such programs are at a heightened risk of creating a backlash among male participants if the intervention is viewed as an attack on males in general (Hilton, Harris, Rice, Krans, & Lavigne, 1998). Jaffe, Sudermann, Reitzel, and Killip (1992), for example, conducted a 1-day intervention involving presentations made by members of the community (e.g., police officers and domestic violence personnel) aimed specifically at addressing issues related to wife assault. Although overall results indicated improvements in adolescents' attitudes and behavioral intentions, for some males, the intervention was actually found to have effects opposite of those intended (e.g., a greater acceptance of violence and attitudes justifying rape). Finally, girls may need to be made aware that relational and other forms of nonphysical aggression are inappropriate, regardless of their male partner's apparent lack of injury or indifference (Odgers & Moretti, 2002).

Program Delivery

The majority of interventions identified by Wekerle and Wolfe (1999) were school-based and were typically administered as part of existing health classes. These programs often involve activities aimed at increasing awareness and dispelling myths about relationship violence and sexual assault. Most often such activities include school auditorium presentations involving videotapes, plays, professional theater groups, or a speech from a survivor; classroom discussion facilitated by teachers or service providers; or specific programs and curricula that encourage students to examine attitudes and behaviors that promote or tolerate violence. These curricula have primarily used didactic approaches to orient students to the different ways in which abuse and violence may be expressed, and examining their own attitudes and gender role stereotypes (Avery-Leaf, Cascardi, O'Leary, & Cano, 1997; Lavoie, Vezina, Piche, & Boivin, 1995).

The practical benefits of carrying out a school-based intervention include being able to disseminate the curriculum to a large number of adolescents at once, having access to students' records, and the presence of staff (e.g., teachers, counselors) familiar with students. Additionally, the classroom setting provides a "natural" context for adolescents and thus addresses potential issues of participant reactivity and attrition. These interventions are not, however, free of challenges and potential obstacles. For example, as Hammond, Yung, and Kadis (1990) have pointed out, because involvement in such programs is contingent upon school attendance, school dropouts and adolescents prone to truancy are excluded. Additionally, interventions should consider culturally relevant information and differences among participants and avoid a "one size fits all" approach (Heppner, Neville, Smith, Kivlighan, & Gershuny, 1999). A classroom setting may also make it difficult for adolescents to contribute to group discussions of sensitive and potentially embarrassing situations and topics. This is particularly the case when program facilitators do not discourage ridicule of peer responses or the reassurance of confidentiality. Additionally, because of a heightened awareness and sensitivity to issues of relationship violence, there may be a resulting increase in adolescents' reports of such instances. Thus, the training of school staff to meet these demands needs to be established in advance (Wekerle & Wolfe, 1999). Finally, designers of interventions need to determine the best "dosage" of information and training (i.e., some programs are delivered in one session, whereas most are extended over 10–20 lesson plans), as well as the possible role of booster sessions that would expand the curriculum in accordance with developmental changes.

One such school-based program that has been evaluated is "Safe Dates" (Foshee, 1996; Foshee et al., 2000). Over 1,500 eighth- and ninth-grade students participated in 10 classroom sessions and related activities, such as a poster contest. This project is one of the few studied that has included a follow-up assessment to explore long-term prevention effects. Although some of the positive behavioral changes had disappeared at a 1-year follow-up, some of the critical changes in variables that mediate dating violence (e.g., dating violence norms, conflict management skills, and awareness of community services for dating violence) were maintained.

Community-based interventions (typically conducted in small coed groups) provide their own unique advantages. For example, as a result of the comparatively smaller group sizes, a community-based program may find it easier to conduct interactive, role-playing exercises that include all of the adolescents. These types of exercises are thought to be vital to intervention efforts because they provide opportunities for individualized feedback about performance, which has been found to be one of the most effective ways to improve behavioral acquisition (Foshee et al., 1996). Additionally, community-based programs allow for a more homogenous group of adolescents (i.e., teens with similar backgrounds, needs, strengths) to interact with one another, and in so doing, provide a more comfortable atmosphere for the exchange of opinions and experiences.

As an example of a community-based program, Wolfe and colleagues (2003) developed the Youth Relationships Project (YRP) to assist adults in empowering youth to end violence in relationships through education, skill development, and social competence. This program reflects an incremental strategy aimed at self-awareness and social change (i.e., examining oneself first, and moving on to one's peers, school environment, social institutions, and cultural influences), and is delivered through an 18-session program in community settings. The program targets not only abusive behaviors but also the social factors underlying discriminatory attitudes and assumptions, such as sexism, racism, and other forms of discrimination that make girls and minorities particularly susceptible to violence or oppression. Two-year follow-up results involving random assignment to an intervention or control condition suggest this approach is effective in reducing physical and emotional abuse perpetration toward dating partners, for both girls and boys.

FUTURE DIRECTIONS

As indicated at the beginning of this chapter, research on violence in adolescent romantic relationships has a short history. As a result, there is much more to learn about violence in adolescent dating relationships than many of the other adolescent problems and disorders covered in this volume. It is clear that violence in adolescent dating relationships is a problem, with potentially serious consequences. It is also clear that much more needs to be learned about how relationship violence develops, the course of relationship violence, and how best to reduce/prevent occurrences of such violence.

To advance this field, there is a strong need to improve the assessment of adolescent dating violence. As noted, the assessment of adolescent dating violence typically involves self-reports using paper-and-pencil surveys. Strides have been made in the assessment of relationship violence via surveys, and many of the recently developed surveys are quite sophisticated. However, sole reliance on paper-and-pencil surveys, almost without exception across studies, to assess this phenomenon might be considered a serious limitation. In fact, sole reliance on any single method to assess a complex construct might be considered a limitation.

There is also a need for theoretical formulations for teen dating violence that specifically take into account the developmental period of adolescence and the process of romantic relationship development. Studies that have examined theoretically derived pathways and constructs have accounted for some of the variance in violence in relationships, such as child maltreatment and other forms of trauma. However, because abusive behavior is multiply determined, other important risk and protective factors have likely received inadequate attention. These include, for example, the influence of early attachment experiences, early and contemporary peer relationships, and underlying interpersonal skills that likely play a role in the formation of healthy versus abusive behavior toward romantic partners.

There is also a critical need for longitudinal

investigations of gender-specific developmental pathways to adolescent dating violence, similar to the findings that low-level teasing or aggression by pre- and early-adolescent girls increases their risk of later victimization by male partners (McMaster et al., 2002). Longitudinal research on the impact of dating violence may clarify sex differences in initiation and response to more and less severe verbal and physical tactics commonly used in adolescent dating relationships. The dynamic that is evolving between girls and boys in their early experiences at forming intimate relationships is fundamentally different than the patterned forms of aggression seen among adult partners, requiring a more developmentally guided approach to these issues. Similarly, the study of partnerships and dating violence could be advanced by examining the stability of violence across different relationships, the age differential of partners, the level of substance use in the partnership, and the overall quality of relationships.

As noted herein, the current limited state of knowledge on the predictors of abusive behavior requires caution in how the findings are applied to prevention and intervention initiatives. For example, school-based prevention programs for adolescent dating violence and related risk factors have derived from cognitive-behavioral models of intervention, and as such tend to focus on altering adolescents' knowledge and attitudes about dating violence (Wekerle & Wolfe, 1999). Although these programs are likely helpful for changing norms, a broader scope is needed. In particular, the association between affective states (especially anger) suggests that efforts to address dating violence might successfully target co-occurring risk behaviors that may have an underlying affective component, such as delinquency, substance abuse, and unsafe sexual behavior (Silverman, Raj, Mucci, & Hathaway, 2001). Given that youths' early involvement in dating violence is an indicator of future risk, developmentally informed early interventions that specifically address affective and behavioral skill components of conflict resolution are needed to promote positive youth development (Wolfe et al., 2003). Adolescence is an important transitional period in this regard, because it offers opportunities to strengthen healthy choices and replace negative patterns carried forward from previous relationships with more adaptive ones.

REFERENCES

Arias, I., Samios, M., & O'Leary, K. D. (1987). Prevalence and correlates of physical aggression during courtship. *Journal of Interpersonal Violence, 2,* 82–90.

Avery-Leaf, S., & Cascardi, M. (2002). Dating violence education: Prevention and early intervention strategies. In P. A. Schewe (Ed.), *Preventing violence in relationships: Interventions across the life span* (pp. 79–105). Washington, DC: American Psychological Association.

Avery-Leaf, S., Cascardi, M., O'Leary, K. D., & Cano, A. (1997). Efficacy of a dating violence prevention program on attitudes justifying aggression. *Journal of Adolescent Health, 21,* 11–17.

Bandura, A. (1973). *Aggression: A social learning analysis.* Englewood Cliffs, NJ: Prentice-Hall.

Bandura, A. (1977). *Social learning theory.* Englewood Cliffs, NJ: Prentice-Hall.

Bennett, L., & Fineran, S. (1998). Sexual and severe physical violence among high school students. *American Journal of Orthopsychiatry, 68,* 645–652.

Berman, H., Izumi, J., & Arnold, C. T. (2002). Sexual harassment and the developing sense of self among adolescent girls. *Canadian Journal of Counseling, 36,* 265–280.

Bookwala, J., Frieze, I. H., Smith, C., & Ryan, K. (1992). Predictors of dating violence: A multivariate analysis. *Violence and Victims, 7,* 297–311.

Bowlby, J. (1969). *Attachment and loss: Vol. 1. Attachment.* New York: Basic Books.

Bowlby, J. (1972). *Attachment and loss: Vol. 2. Separation, anxiety, and anger.* New York: Basic Books.

Bowlby, J. (1980). *Attachment and loss: Vol. 3. Loss, sadness, and depression.* New York: Basic Books.

Brendgen, M., Vitaro, F., Tremblay, R. E., & Wanner, B. (2002). Parent and peer effects on delinquency-related violence and dating violence: A test of two mediational models. *Social Development, 11,* 225–244.

Briere, J. (1992). *Child abuse trauma: Theory and treatment of the lasting effects.* Newbury Park, CA: Sage.

Buzy, W. M., McDonald, R., Jouriles, E. N., Swank, P., Rosenfield, D., Shimek, J., & Corbitt-Shindler, D. (2004). Adolescent girls' alcohol use as a risk factor for relationship violence. *Journal of Research on Adolescence, 14,* 449–470.

Cano, A., Avery-Leaf, S., Cascardi, M., & O'Leary, K. D. (1998). Dating violence in two high school samples: Discriminating variables. *Journal of Primary Prevention, 18,* 431–446.

Capaldi, D. M., & Clark, S. (1998). Prospective family predictors of aggression towards female partners for at-risk young men. *Developmental Psychology, 34,* 1175–1188.

Capaldi, D. M., Dishion, T. J., Stoolmiller, M., & Yoerger, K. (2001). Aggression toward female partners by at-risk young men: The contribution of male adolescent friendships. *Developmental Psychology, 37,* 61–73.

Capaldi, D. M., & Gorman-Smith, D. (2003). The development of aggression in young male/female couples. In P. Florsheim (Ed.), *Adolescent romantic relations and sexual behavior: Theory, research, and practical implications* (pp. 243–278). Mahwah, NJ: Erlbaum.

Cascardi, M., Avery-Leaf, S., O'Leary, K. D., & Smith-Slep, A. M. (1999). Factor structure and convergent validity of the conflict tactics scale in high school students. *Psychological Assessment, 11,* 546–555.

Centers for Disease Control and Prevention. (2002). Surveillance Summaries, June 28, 2002. *Morbidity and Mortality Weekly Report, 51*(No. SS-4).

Chase, K. A., Treboux, D., & O' Leary, K. D. (2002). Characteristics of high-risk adolescents' dating violence. *Journal of Interpersonal Violence, 17,* 33–49.

Chase, K. A., Treboux, D., O'Leary, K. D., & Strasberg, Z. (1998). Specificity of dating aggression and its justification among high-risk adolescents. *Journal of Abnormal Child Psychology, 26,* 467–473.

Coker, A. L., McKeown, R. E., Sanderson, M., Davis, K. E., Valois, R. F., & Huebner, E. S. (2000). Severe dating violence and quality of life among South Carolina high school students. *American Journal of Preventive Medicine, 19,* 220–227.

Connolly, J. A., Craig, W., Goldberg, A., & Pepler, D. (1999). Conceptions of cross-sex friendships and romantic relationships in early adolescence. *Journal of Youth and Adolescence, 28,* 481–494.

Connolly, J. A., & Johnson, A. M. (1996). Adolescents' romantic relationships and the structure and quality of their close interpersonal ties. *Personal Relationships, 3,* 185–195.

Connolly, J. A., Pepler, D., Craig, W., & Taradash, A. (2000). Dating experiences of bullies in early adolescence. *Child Maltreatment, 5,* 297–308.

Crittenden, P., & Ainsworth, M. (1989). Attachment and child abuse. In D. Cicchetti & V. Carlson (Eds.), *Child maltreatment: Theory and research on the causes and consequences of child abuse and neglect* (pp. 432–463). New York: Cambridge University Press.

Deaux, K., & Wrightsman, L. S. (1984). *Social psychology in the 80s.* Monterey, CA: Brooks-Cole.

DeBellis, M. D. (2001). Developmental traumatology: The psychobiological development of maltreated children and its implications for research, treatment, and policy. *Development and Psychopathology, 13,* 539–564.

DeBellis, M. D., & Putnam, F. W. (1994). The psychobiology of childhood maltreatment. *Child and Adolescent Psychiatric Clinics of North America, 3,* 663–678

DeKeseredy, W. S. (1988). *Woman abuse in dating relationships: The role of male peer support.* Toronto: Canadian Scholar's Press.

DeKeseredy, W. S. (1990). Woman abuse in dating relationships: The contribution of male peer support. *Sociological Inquiry, 60,* 236–243.

DeKeseredy, W. S., & Schwartz, M. D. (1993). Male peer support and woman abuse: An expansion of DeKeseredy's model. *Sociological Spectrum, 13,* 393–413.

Dickinson, G. E. (1975). Dating behavior of Black and White adolescents before and after desegregation. *Journal of Marriage and the Family, 37,* 602–608.

Downey, G., Bonica, C., & Rincón, C. (1999). Rejection sensitivity and adolescent romantic relationships. In W. Furman, B. B. Brown, & C. Feiring (Eds.), *The development of romantic relationships in adolescence* (pp. 148–174). New York: Cambridge University Press.

Downey, G., & Feldman, S. I. (1996). Implications of rejection sensitivity for intimate relationships. *Journal of Personality and Social Psychology, 70,* 1327–1343.

Downey, G., Feldman, S. I., & Ayduk, O. (2000). Rejection sensitivity and male violence in romantic relationships. *Personal Relationships, 7,* 45–61.

Downey, G., Lebolt, A., Rincón, C., & Freitas, A. L. (1998). Rejection sensitivity and children's interpersonal difficulties. *Child Development, 69,* 1074–1091.

Dutton, D. G. (1995). *The domestic assault of women: Psychological and criminal justice perspectives* (2nd ed.). Vancouver: University of British Columbia Press.

Feiring, C. (1996). Concepts of romance in 15-year-old adolescents. *Journal of Research on Adolescence, 6*(2), 181–200.

Feiring, C. (1999). Gender identity and the development of romantic relationships in adolescence. In W. Furman, B. B. Brown, & C. Fering (Eds.), *The development of romantic relationships in adolescence* (pp. 211–232). New York: Cambridge University Press.

Fisher, J. D., & Fisher, W. A. (1992). Changing AIDS risk behavior. *Psychological Bulletin, 111,* 455–474.

Follingstad, D. R., Wright, S., Lloyd, S., & Sebastian, J. A. (1991). Sex differences in motivations and effects in dating violence. *Family Relations: Journal of Applied Family and Child Studies, 40,* 51–57.

Foo, L., & Margolin, G. (1995). A multivariate investigation of dating aggression. *Journal of Family Violence, 10,* 351–377.

Foshee, V. A. (1996). Gender differences in adolescent dating abuse prevalence, types and injuries. *Health Education Research, 11,* 275–286.

Foshee, V. A., Bauman, K. E., Greene, W. F., Koch, G. G., Linder, G. F., & MacDougall, J. E. (2000). The Safe Dates Program: 1-year follow-up results. *American Journal of Public Health, 90,* 1619–1622.

Foshee, V. A., Bauman, K. E., & Linder, F. (1999). Family violence and the perpetration of adolescent dating violence: Examining social learning and social control processes. *Journal of Marriage and the Family, 61,* 331–343.

Foshee, V. A., Linder, F., Bauman, K. E., Langwick, S. A., Arriaga, X. B., Heath, J. L., et al. (1998). The Safe Dates Project: Theoretical basis, evaluation design, and selected baseline findings. *American Journal of Preventive Medicine, 12*, 39–47.

Foshee, V. A., Linder, F., MacDougall, J. E., & Bangdiwala, S. (2001). Gender differences in the longitudinal predictors of adolescent dating violence. *Preventive Medicine: An International Journal Devoted to Practice and Theory, 32*, 128–141.

Furman, W., & Buhrmester, D. (1992). Age and sex differences in perceptions of networks of personal relationships. *Child Development, 63*, 103–115.

Gaertner, L., & Foshee, V. A. (1999). Commitment and the perpetration of relationship violence. *Personal Relationships, 6*, 227–239.

Giordano, P. C., Millhollin, T. J., Cernkovich, S. A., Pugh, M. D., & Rudolph, J. L. (1999). Delinquency, identity, and women's involvement in relationship violence. *Criminology, 27*, 17–40.

Gray, M. R., & Steinberg, L. (1999). Adolescent romance and the parent-child relationship: A contextual perspective. In W. Furman, B. B. Brown, & C. Fering (Eds.), *The development of romantic relationships in adolescence* (pp. 235–262). New York: Cambridge University Press.

Grych, J. H., Kinsfogel, K., Hart, N., Klockow, L. L., & Robbins, D. (2003, April). *Investigating links between family relationships and abuse in adolescent dating relationships: Cognitive, affective, and attachment processes*. Paper presented at the meeting of the Society for Research in Child Development, Tampa, FL.

Hammond, W. R., Yung, B. R., & Kadis, P. (1990). *Positive Adolescent Choices Training (PACT)*. ERIC Clearinghouse on Higher Education, AASCU ERIC Model Programs Inventory Project.

Hansen, S. L. (1977). Dating choices of high school students. *The Family Coordinator, 26*, 133–138.

Hazan, C., & Shaver, P. (1987). Romantic love conceptualized as an attachment process. *Journal of Personality and Social Psychology, 52*, 511–524.

Hazan, C., & Shaver, P. (1994). Attachment as an organizational framework for research on close relationships. *Psychological Inquiry, 5*, 1–22.

Henton, J. M., Cate, R. M., Koval, J., Lloyd, S., & Christopher, F. S. (1983). Romance and violence in dating relationships. *Journal of Family Issues, 4*, 467–482.

Heppner, M. J., Neville, H. A., Smith, K., Kivlighan, D. M., & Gershuny, B. S. (1999). Examining immediate and long-term efficacy of rape prevention programming with racially diverse college men. *Journal of Counseling Psychology, 46*, 16–26.

Hilton, N. Z., Harris, G. T., & Rice, M. E. (1998). On the validity of self-reported rates of interpersonal violence. *Journal of Interpersonal Violence, 13*, 58–72.

Hilton, N. Z., Harris, G. T., Rice, M. E., Krans, T. S., & Lavigne, S. E. (1998). Antiviolence education in high schools: Implementation and evaluation. *Journal of Interpersonal Violence, 13*, 726–742.

Holtzworth-Munroe, A., & Stuart, G. (1994). Typologies of male batterers: Three subtypes and the differences among them. *Psychological Bulletin, 116*, 476–497.

Howard, D. E., Qiu, Y., & Boekeloo, B. (2003). Personal and social contextual correlates of adolescent dating violence. *Journal of Adolescent Health, 33*, 9–17.

Howard, D. E., & Wang, M. Q. (2003). Risk profiles of adolescent girls who were victims of dating violence. *Adolescence, 38*, 1–14.

Humphrey, J. A., & White, J. W. (2000). Women's vulnerability to sexual assault from adolescence to young adulthood. *Journal of Adolescent Health, 27*, 419–424.

Humphrey, S. E., & Kahn, A. S. (2000). Fraternities, athletic teams, and rape. *Journal of Interpersonal Violence, 15*, 1313–1322.

Jackson, S. M. (1999). Issues in the dating violence research: A review of the literature. *Aggression and Violent Behavior, 4*, 233–247.

Jackson, S. M., Cram, F., & Seymour, F. W. (2000). Violence and sexual coercion in high school students' dating relationships. *Journal of Family Violence, 15*, 23–36.

Jaffe, P. G., Sudermann, M., Reitzel, D., & Killip, S. M. (1992). An evaluation of a secondary school prevention program on violence in intimate relationships. *Violence and Victims, 7*, 129–146.

Jankowski, M. K., Leitenberg, H., Henning, K., & Coffey, P. (1999). Intergenerational transmission of dating aggression as a function of witnessing only same sex parents vs. opposite sex parents vs. both parents as perpetrators of domestic violence. *Journal of Family Violence, 14*, 267–279.

Jezl, D. R., Molidor, C. E., & Wright, T. L. (1996). Physical, sexual, and psychological abuse in high school dating relationships: Prevalence rates and self-esteem issues. *Child and Adolescent Social Work Journal, 13*, 69–87.

Jouriles, E. N., McDonald, R., Swank, P. R., Norwood, W. D., & Buzy, W. M. (2002). *Men's domestic violence and other forms of deviant behavior* (Final Report). Washington, DC: National Institute of Justice. Retrieved November 12, 2003, from http://www.ncjrs.org/pdffiles1/nij/grants/197206.pdf

Jouriles, E. N., & O'Leary, K. D. (1985). Interspousal reliability of reports of marital violence. *Journal of Consulting and Clinical Psychology, 53*, 419–421.

Kitzmann, K. M., Gaylord, N. K., Holt, A. R., Kenny, E. D. (2003). Child witnesses to domestic violence: A meta-analytic review. *Journal of Consulting and Clinical Psychology, 71*, 339–352

Koss, M. P., & Oros, C. J. (1982). Sexual Experiences Survey: A research instrument investigating sexual aggression and victimization. *Journal of Consulting and Clinical Psychology, 50*, 455–457.

Lavoie, F., Vezina, L., Piche, C., & Boivin, M. (1995). Evaluation of a prevention program for violence in teen dating relationships. *Journal of Interpersonal Violence, 10*, 516–524.

Magdol, L., Moffitt, T. E., Caspi, A., & Silva, P. A. (1998). Developmental antecedents of partner abuse: A prospective-longitudinal study. *Journal of Abnormal Psychology, 107*, 375–389.

Makepeace, J. M. (1981). Courtship violence among college students. *Family Relations, 30,* 97–102.

Makepeace, J. M. (1986). Gender differences in courtship violence victimization. *Family Relations, 35,* 383–388.

Malik, S., Sorenson, S., & Aneshensel, C. (1997). Community and dating violence among adolescents: Perpetration and victimization. *Journal of Adolescent Health, 21,* 291–302.

McMaster, L. E., Connolly, J., Pepler, D., & Craig, W. M. (2002). Peer to peer sexual harassment in early adolescence: A developmental perspective. *Development and Psychopathology, 14,* 91–105.

Meiser-Stedman, R. (2002). Towards a cognitive-behavioral model of PTSD in children and adolescents. *Clinical Child and Family Psychology Review, 5,* 217–232.

Messman-Moore, T. L., & Long, P. J. (2000). Child sexual abuse and revictimization in the form of adult sexual abuse, adult physical abuse, and adult psychological maltreatment. *Journal of Interpersonal Violence, 15,* 489–502.

Miedzian, M. (1995). Learning to be violent. In E. Peled, P. G. Jaffe, & J. L. Edelson (Eds.), *Ending the cycle of violence: Community responses to children of battered women* (pp. 10–24). Thousand Oaks, CA: Sage.

Moffitt, T. E., Caspi, A., Krueger, R. F., Magdol, L., Margolin, G., Silva, P. A., & Sydney, R. (1997). Do partners agree about abuse in their relationship? A psychometric evaluation of interpartner agreement. *Psychological Assessment, 9,* 47–56.

Molidor, C., & Tolman, R. M. (1998). Gender and contextual factors in adolescent dating violence. *Violence against Women, 4,* 180–194.

Murphy, C. M., & O'Leary, K. D. (1989). Psychological aggression predicts physical aggression in early marriage. *Journal of Consulting and Clinical Psychology, 57,* 579–582.

Odgers, C. L., & Moretti, M. M. (2002). Aggressive and antisocial girls: Research update and challenges. *International Journal of Forensic Mental Health Services, 1,* 103–119.

O'Keefe, M. (1997). Predictors of dating violence among high school students. *Journal of Interpersonal Violence, 12,* 546–568.

O'Keefe, M. (1998). Factors mediating the link between witnessing interparental violence and dating violence. *Journal of Family Violence, 13,* 39–57.

O'Keefe, M., & Sela-Amit, M. (1997). An examination of the effects of race/ethnicity and social class on adolescent's exposure to violence. *Journal of Social Service Research, 22,* 53–71.

O'Keefe, M., & Treister, L. (1998). Victims of dating violence among high school students: Are the predictors different for males and females? *Violence against Women, 4,* 195–223.

O'Leary, K. D. (1999). Developmental and affective issues in assessing and treating partner aggression. *Clinical Psychology: Science and Practice, 6,* 400–414.

O'Leary, K. D., Barling, J., Arias, I., Rosenbaum, A., Malone, J., & Tyree, A. (1989). Prevalence and stability of physical aggression between spouses: A longitudinal analysis. *Journal of Consulting and Clinical Psychology, 57,* 263–268.

O'Leary, K. D., & Slep, A. M. (2003). A dyadic longitudinal model of adolescent dating aggression. *Journal of Clinical Child and Adolescent Psychology, 32,* 314–327.

O'Leary, K. D., Vivian, D., & Malone, J. (1992). Assessment of physical aggression against women in marriage: The need for multimodal assessment. *Behavioral Assessment, 14,* 5–14.

Pepler, D. J., Craig, W. M., Connolly, J., & Henderson, K. (2002). Bullying, sexual harassment, dating violence, and substance use among adolescents. In C. Wekerle & A. M. Wall (Eds.), *Violence and addiction equation: Theoretical and clinical issues in substance abuse and relationship violence* (pp. 153–168). New York: Brunner-Routledge.

Poitras, M., & Lavoie, F. (1995). A study of the prevalence of sexual coercion in adolescent heterosexual dating relationships in a Quebec sample. *Violence and Victims, 10,* 299–313.

Richards, M. H., Crowe, P. A., Larson, R., & Swarr, A. (1998). Developmental patterns and gender differences in the experience of peer companionship during adolescence. *Child Development, 69,* 154–163.

Riggs, D. S. (1993). Relationship problems and dating aggression: A potential treatment target. *Journal of Interpersonal Violence, 8,* 18–35.

Riggs, D. S., & Caulfield, M. B. (1997). Expected consequences of male violence against their female dating partners. *Journal of Interpersonal Violence, 12,* 229–240.

Riggs, D. S., Murphy, C. M., & O'Leary, K. D. (1989). Intentional falsification in reports of interpartner aggression. *Journal of Interpersonal Violence, 4,* 220–232.

Riggs, D. S., & O'Leary, K. D. (1989). A theoretical model of courtship aggression. In M.A. Pirog-Good & J. E. Stets (Eds.), *Violence in dating relationships: Emerging social issues* (pp. 53–71). New York: Praeger.

Riggs, D. S., & O'Leary, K. D. (1996). Aggression between heterosexual dating partners: An examination of a causal model of courtship aggression. *Journal of Interpersonal Violence, 11,* 519–540.

Riggs, D. S., O'Leary, K. D., & Breslin, F. (1990). Multiple predictors of physical aggression in dating couples. *Journal of Interpersonal Violence, 5,* 61–73.

Ronfeldt, H. M., Kimerling, R., & Arias, I. (1998). Satisfaction with relationship power and the perpetration of dating violence. *Journal of Marriage and the Family, 60,* 70–78.

Schwartz, M. D., DeKeseredy, W. S., Tait, D., & Alvi, S. (2001). Male peer support and a feminist routine activities theory: Understanding sexual assault on the college campus. *Justice Quarterly, 18,* 623–649.

Scott, K. L., Wekerle, C., & Wolfe, D. A. (1997, April). *Considered sex differences in youth self-reports of vi-*

olence and their implications for the development of violent relationships. Poster presented at the biennial meeting of the Society for Research in Child Development, Washington, DC.

Serbin, L. A., Powlishta, K. K., & Gulko, J. (1993). The development of sex typing in middle childhood. *Monographs of the Society for Research in Child Development, 58* (Serial No. 232).

Shapiro, J. P., Baumeister, R. F., & Kessler, J. W. (1991). A three-component model of children's teasing: Aggression, humor, and ambiguity. *Journal of Social and Clinical Psychology, 10,* 459–472.

Simons, R. L., Wu, C.-I., Johnson, C., & Conger, R. D. (1995). A test of various perspectives on the intergenerational transmission of domestic violence. *Criminology, 33,* 141–172.

Silverman, J. G., Raj, A., Mucci, L. A., & Hathaway, J. E. (2001). Dating violence against adolescent girls and associated substance use, unhealthy weight control, sexual risk behavior, pregnancy, and suicidality. *Journal of the American Medical Association, 286,* 572–579.

Slep, A. M. S., Cascardi, M. Avery-Leaf, S., & O'Leary, K. D. (2001). Two new measures of attitudes about the acceptability of teen dating aggression. *Psychological Assessment, 13,* 306–318.

Smith, P. H., White, J. W., & Holland, L. J. (2003). A longitudinal perspective on dating violence among adolescent and college-age women. *American Journal of Public Health, 93,* 1104–1109.

Stets, J. E., & Henderson, D. A. (1991). Contextual factors surrounding conflict resolution while dating: Results from a national study. *Family Relations: Journal of Applied Family Studies, 40,* 29–36.

Straus, M. A. (1979). Measuring intrafamily conflict and violence: The Conflict Tactics (CT) scales. *Journal of Marriage and the Family, 41,* 75–88.

Sugarman, D. B., & Hotaling, G. T. (1989). Dating violence: Prevalence, context, and risk markers. In M. A. Pirog-Good & J. E. Stets (Eds.), *Violence in dating relationships: Emerging social issues* (pp. 3–32). New York: Praeger.

Swan, S. C., & Snow, D. L. (2002). A typology of women's use of violence in intimate relationships. *Violence Against Women, 8,* 286–319.

Thompson, K. M., Wonderlich, S. A., Crosby, R. D., & Mitchell, J. E. (2001). Sexual violence and weight control techniques among adolescent girls. *International Journal of Eating Disorders, 29,* 166–176.

Thompson, S. (1994). Changing lives, changing genres: Teenage girls' narratives about sex and romance, 1978–1986. In A. S. Rossi (Ed.), *Sexuality across the life course* (pp. 209–232). Chicago: University of Chicago Press.

Watson, J. M., Cascardi, M., Avery-Leaf, S., & O'Leary, K. D. (2001). High school students' responses to dating aggression. *Violence and Victims, 16,* 339–348.

Wekerle, C., & Wall, A. (2002). *The violence and addiction equation: Theoretical and clinical issues in substance abuse and relationship violence.* New York: Brunner-Routledge.

Wekerle, C., & Wolfe, D. A. (1998). Prevention of physical abuse and neglect: Windows of opportunity. In P. K. Trickett & C. Schellenbach (Eds.), *Violence against children in the family and the community* (pp. 339–370). New York: APA Books.

Wekerle, C., & Wolfe, D. A. (1999). Dating violence in mid-adolescence: Theory, significance, and emerging prevention initiatives. *Clinical Psychology Review, 19,* 435–456.

Wekerle, C., & Wolfe, D. A. (2003). Child maltreatment. In E. J. Mash & R. A. Barkley (Eds.), *Child psychopathology* (pp. 632–684). New York: Guilford Press.

Wekerle, C., Wolfe, D. A., Hawkins, D. L., Pittman, A., Glickman, A., & Lovald, B. E. (2001). Childhood maltreatment, posttraumatic stress symptomatology, and adolescent dating violence: Considering the value of adolescent perceptions of abuse and a trauma mediational model. *Development and Psychopathology, 13,* 847–871.

Widom, C. S. (1999). Posttraumatic stress disorder in abused and neglected children grown up. *American Journal of Psychiatry, 156,* 1223–1229.

Wolf, K. A., & Foshee, V. A. (2003). Family violence, anger expression styles, and adolescent dating violence. *Journal of Family Violence, 18,* 309–316.

Wolfe, D. A., Scott, K., Reitzel-Jaffe, D., Wekerle, C., Grasley, C., & Straatman, A. (2001). Development and validation of the conflict in adolescent dating relationships inventory. *Psychological Assessment, 13,* 277–293.

Wolfe, D. A., Scott, K., Wekerle, C., & Pittman, A. (2001). Child maltreatment: Risk of adjustment problems and dating violence in adolescence. *Journal of the American Academy of Child and Adolescent Psychiatry, 40,* 282–298.

Wolfe, D. A., Wekerle, C., Reitzel-Jaffe, D., & Lefebvre, L. (1998). Factors associated with abusive relationships among maltreated and non-maltreated youth. *Development and Psychopathology, 10,* 61–85.

Wolfe, D. A., Wekerle, C., & Scott, K. (1997). *Alternatives to violence: Empowering youth to develop healthy relationships.* Thousand Oaks, CA: Sage.

Wolfe, D. A., Wekerle, C., Scott, K., Straatman, A., & Grasley, C. (2004). Predicting abuse in adolescent dating relationships over 1 year: The role of child maltreatment and trauma. *Journal of Abnormal Psychology, 113,* 406–415.

Wolfe, D. A., Wekerle, C., Scott, K., Straatman, A., Grasley, C., & Reitzel-Jaffe, D. (2003). Dating violence prevention with at-risk youth: A controlled outcome evaluation. *Journal of Consulting and Clinical Psychology, 71,* 279–291.

20

Abuse and Trauma

David A. Wolfe
Jennine S. Rawana
Debbie Chiodo

The World Health Organization (2002) recently published the first world report on violence and health, declaring that violence is a leading worldwide public health problem. While noting that the effects of trauma, particularly abuse, are harmful for all age groups, the report underscores the need to address the unique issues of abuse and trauma affecting adolescents in particular. Adolescence is considered a time of particularly high vulnerability to traumatic events. For example, 11% of youth had experienced a traumatic event by age 11, which rose to 43% by age 18 (Giaconia, Reinherz, Silverman, & Pakiz, 1994). In addition to violence in the home, adolescents are exposed to a variety of risky situations that may result in traumatic experiences as they become increasingly independent from their families and influenced by peers, such as sexual assault and gang- or community-related violence.

Physical and sexual abuse are two types of traumatic experiences that are particularly relevant to adolescents. Not only do traumatic experiences occur frequently in this population, but they also can take the form of interpersonal violence, such as physical or sexual abuse, which seem to increase the risk of developing posttraumatic stress disorder (PTSD) and other psychopathologies, compared with other forms of traumatic experiences such as disasters (Brown, Cohen, Johnson, & Smailes, 1999; Kessler, Sonnega, Bromet, Hughes, & Nelson, 1995). In a 17-year longitudinal study with a normative sample, 11% of participants reported experiencing physical or sexual abuse before age 18 (Silverman, Reinherz, & Giaconia, 1996). Even higher rates were found in a community sample of 665 youth (ages 9–17 years), with nearly 26% of the sample reporting a history of physical abuse (Flisher et al., 1997).

The focus of this chapter is to examine how abuse and trauma occurring prior to or during adolescence affect ongoing development and psychopathology. A discussion of abuse and trauma during adolescence must take into careful consideration the ongoing developmental processes that interact with such events, including biological, cognitive, social, and behavioral changes. We consider abuse and trauma to be life-course problems, associated with a broad range of symptoms that may shift significantly over the course of development. Symptoms related to the impact of abuse and trauma are often enmeshed with problem behaviors that obtain more prominence, such as suicide, aggression, or substance abuse, disguising the underlying factors. Rather than a disorder per se, acute or chronic exposure to abuse or trauma disrupts normal developmental progress in an unpredictable fashion and may be a contributing factor to many other emotional and behavioral disorders.

There is some ambiguity associated with the term "trauma" that merits clarification. Sometimes the term is used to describe a traumatic event, and at other times it refers to psychological reactions to that event and to the longer-term impact of such reactions on psychological adjustment. The term is used herein to refer to "an event far beyond usual human experience that overwhelms the senses and ability to cope with the event at that time" (UNICEF, 1998, p. 6). Rather than focusing on the types of abuse and trauma, this chapter examines research pertaining to the effects of various forms of human-made trauma on adolescent development and adjustment. The three most prominent forms of abuse and trauma affecting adolescents include being the target of direct *physical violence and intimidation* by caregivers or peers; being the target of direct *sexual violence* such as incest and sexual assault, either by peers or adults; and being *exposed to violence* targeted toward others at home, including exposure to domestic violence, or in the community. This chapter also presents some information on bullying, an area of increasing importance in adolescent peer relationships. Interested readers are referred to recent work by Yule, Stuvland, Baingana, and Smith (2003) for a detailed discussion of children and youth in war-related trauma.

The impact of trauma on adolescent development varies considerably according to the nature of the relationship of the offender to the adolescent (e.g., parent, person of trust, peer, and stranger); the context of the traumatic events (e.g., abusive or violent acts among peers, in the home, or in the community); and the severity, duration, and chronicity of the events. Although these events all have different aspects, they share important elements. Abuse and traumatic events create fear and apprehension in the victim, and a sense of helplessness; many of these acts also pose a threat to one's sense of safety and well-being or have a delayed impact leading to subsequent feelings of self-blame or betrayal.

Central to this definition is the notion that acts of abuse and trauma involve the inappropriate use of power and authority, which has the potential to harm children's ongoing development and future well-being (Wolfe, Jaffe, Jette, & Poisson, 2003), regardless of setting. Such acts may also include a failure to protect the child from harm or meet minimal standards of care, similar to established definitions of child neglect. Furthermore, regardless of setting and perpetrator, abuse is seldom a single event but rather a process with multiple implications. That is, the nature and impact of abuse change over time and in relation to previous abuse and typically involve a chronic situation in which there is differing intensity during different phases of the individual's involvement (Cicchetti, Toth, & Maughan, 2000). This important transactional process underlies much of the following discussion of harm stemming from abuse and trauma that occurred either before or during adolescence.

In brief, this chapter focuses on the underlying common elements associated with the impact of trauma on adolescents, taking into account the unique dynamics of different forms of abuse and trauma when research indicates their particular relevance. Much of the research in this area has involved adolescent outcomes of earlier physical and sexual abuse, so this literature forms a large basis for the organization and findings throughout. Because abuse and trauma are not disorders but, rather, represent causal agents affecting developmental psychopathology, in the section on theories and etiology we identify abuse-related factors that contribute to harmful outcomes and dimensions of harm associated with such acts. Assessment and intervention approaches are discussed in relation to empirically supported approaches.

A DEVELOPMENTAL PSYCHOPATHOLOGY PERSPECTIVE ON ABUSE AND TRAUMA IN ADOLESCENTS

Due to differences in developmental stages, adolescents understand and react to similar traumatic events differently than do children. Zubenko (2002) lists a number of ways in which responses to loss and crises may differ. For example, while preschoolers may cry and throw temper tantrums and school-age children may exhibit somatic and sleep complaints, adolescents may seek isolation and become less communicative. Or, while younger children may display irritability, aggression, or revert back to "magical" thinking, adolescents may exhibit hopelessness or increase risk-taking behaviors, such as substance abuse or risky sexual activity. As children become adolescents, their trauma reactions become more similar to those of adults, being more likely to exhibit symptoms of numbing, withdrawal, and hyperarousal (Lubit, Rovine, DeFrancisci, & Eth, 2003). Thus, it is important to identify not only the differences in how children and adolescents experience trauma but also in how they react to it, which may look very different from how younger children and adults cope with trauma.

Along with increased physical development, adolescence is also a time when childhood patterns of thinking, feeling, and behaving crystalize, and it is a period of greater expression of interpersonal violence (Eckenrode, Powers, & Garbarino, 1997). Some adolescents are violently assaulted by peers in the community; however, as the Task Force on Adolescent Assault Victim Needs (1996) has pointed out, no best-practice guidelines exist that address the specific needs and vulnerabilities of adolescents who suffer violent injury (although there are such guidelines for adolescents with suicidal behaviors [Shaffer & Pfeffer, 2001] and adolescents who sexually abuse others [Shaw, 1999]). Thus, violently injured teens are usually treated like other *un*intentionally injured children (in children facilities), or other unintentionally or violently injured adults (in adult facilities).

Adolescence is a crucial time to develop a healthy sexual identity. At an age when adolescents typically begin to explore and learn to manage sexual feelings, violation of one's body may exert especially harmful consequences for development. Adolescent victims of sexual abuse may be more likely to exhibit posttraumatic symptomatology than child sexual abuse victims (Wolfe, Sas, & Wekerle, 1994), and that may display higher levels of depressive symptoms, lower self-worth, less social support, and more negative reactions from others (Feiring, Taska, & Lewis, 1999). One explanation for these developmental differences may be that children are often seen as "less responsible" for abuse than adolescents, which affects perceived support and negative reactions by

others, and thus attributions of causal responsibility developed by adolescent victim (Feiring et al., 1999).

Characteristics of the sexual abuse itself that are more prominent in adolescents as compared to children include a parental perpetrator, a higher likelihood of having experienced force, and having been abused at least 10 times (Feiring et al., 1999). The developmental tasks of adolescence may put sexual abuse victims at increased risk for psychological distress in that the stresses of abuse combined with the discovery of the abuse process and the normative stresses of adolescence make abuse victims within this developmental period particularly vulnerable to experiencing psychological problems related to affect regulation (e.g., depression) and self-evaluation.

A number of factors need to be considered with adolescent (and child) trauma victims that are less of a factor with adult victims. Family support and environment play essential roles in mitigating between trauma exposure and the subsequent development of problems (Cyr et al., 2003; Schetky, 2003; Spencer, Dupree, Cunningham, Harpalani, & Munoz-Miller, 2003; Youngstrom, Weist, & Albus, 2003). Although family support and self-concept may not moderate exposure to violence, they moderate the *effects* of that violence on internalizing and externalizing problems for adolescents (Youngstrom et al., 2003). *Ipso facto*, family conflict is a risk factor for the development of depression and distress in addition to abuse (Meyerson, Long, Miranda, & Marx, 2002). Physically abused female and male adolescents and sexually abused females perceive their home environments as more conflictual than do nonabused youth (sexually abused males did not differ from nonsexually abused males; Meyerson et al., 2002).

In addition to parental response to trauma, other added dimensions in youth trauma are the impact of trauma on the adolescent's development, the possibility of delayed onset of PTSD symptoms, and the fact that child PTSD symptoms may not resemble adult PTSD symptomatology (Schetky, 2003). Thus, in addition to developmental status, a number of extraneous factors can have a great impact on the effects of trauma on adolescent functioning more so than with adult victims; that is, trauma symptoms are not solely attributable to violence exposure (Spencer et al., 2003).

DESCRIPTION OF ABUSE AND TRAUMA IN ADOLESCENTS

Because many studies on the effect of trauma on children also involve adolescents, we can draw some limited conclusion as to how the findings apply to adolescent victims. Finkelhor (1995) has identified the need to differentiate between localized and developmental effects when looking at the developmental aspects of victimization. He defines localized effects as the common PTSD symptoms, such as avoidance and fearfulness, which are frequently found in traumatized children and may subside over time and with proper treatment. The main concern in this section is with developmental effects, which are more general and pervasive and interfere with important age-appropriate tasks such as the development of self-esteem and emotional regulation (Finkelhor, 1995).

Core Symptoms

Traumatic and stressful life events occurring in childhood may lead to a diverse spectrum of psychopathological manifestations for adolescents. Given the same traumatic event, some adolescents will be more likely to develop PTSD than others, and there is some evidence to suggest that an individual's cognitive style can influence the severity of posttraumatic and other symptoms (Bolger & Patterson, 2001; Moran & Eckenrode, 1992). For example, Moran and Eckenrode (1992) found that in a sample of maltreated adolescent girls, those with a more internal locus of control were less depressed on average than those with a more external locus of control. Moreover, the trauma response is related to the degree of exposure. That is, there is a dose–response relationship between the extent of childhood trauma and rates of psychiatric disorders in childhood (Sadowski et al., 2003). The extent of the psychological impact of trauma on the primary victims depends on many factors: the age when the trauma occurs, how long the abuse lasts, who does it, the form of the abuse, and the response of significant others (Gladstone et al., 2004).

Enduring a traumatic event or a series of traumatic events in childhood can predispose some adolescents to developing a variety of symptoms consistent with a diagnosis of PTSD (American Psychiatric Association [APA], 1994). It is broadly estimated that there is a lifetime prevalence for PTSD of 1–14% in the general population (APA, 1994). Such symptoms may include responses of intense fear, helplessness, or horror; an enduring avoidance of any stimuli associated with the trauma; chronic symptoms of hyperarousal; and impaired overall functioning. Among those who have been exposed to a traumatic stressor, estimates of those who will go on to develop PTSD vary between 9% and 25% (Breslau et al., 1998; Green, 1994; Kessler et al., 1995). Based on data from the National Survey of Adolescents (NSA; $n = 4\,023$), Kilpatrick and colleagues (2003) reported that the 6-month prevalence of PTSD was 3.7% for male adolescents and 6.3% for female adolescents (ages 12–17). Overall, the literature suggests that of children exposed to abuse, approximately one-third will develop PTSD (Ackerman, Newton, McPherson, Jones, & Dykman, 1998; Famularo, Fenton, Augustyn, & Zuckerman, 1996).

Associated Characteristics

Importantly, core symptoms related to PTSD may transform in adolescence into associated characteristics that may no longer resemble acute trauma symptoms. The impact of trauma may remain clinically and/or diagnostically significant yet not warrant the diagnosis of PTSD (Amsel & Marshall, 2003). For example, Kiser, Heston, Millsap, and Pruitt (1991) investigated a population of physically and/or sexually abused children and adolescents and found that those who did not develop PTSD symptoms exhibited more anxiety, depression, and externalizing behaviors than those diagnosed with PTSD. Many of the children and adolescents who did not meet PTSD criteria were still adversely affected by their exposure to the trauma and were still experiencing significant responses to the trauma. These results further suggest that the diagnosis of PTSD does not necessarily identify children most affected by the trauma.

There is empirical support for multiple domains of adolescent functioning in which consequences of traumatic exposure may emerge. These domains include, for example, fear, depression, dissociative complaints, behavioral problems, school problems, and sexual problems (McNally, 1996b). Also, some adolescents develop a negative self-image, which may express itself in low appreciation, a negative self-concept, a negative body image, or an eating disorder (Ackard & Neumark-Sztainer, 2003; Finkelhor, 1990). Lipschitz, Winegar, Hartnick, Foote, and Southwick (1999) reported that eating disorders and somatization disorders were diagnosed in 25% and 34% of adolescents (respectively) exposed to childhood trauma and diagnosed with PTSD.

Adolescents with a history of sexual abuse reported more fear, more depressive complaints, more posttraumatic symptoms, more dissociate complaints, more anger, and more sexual problems than those who had experienced a different stressful event, such as a serious accident, a disaster, or the death of someone close to them (Bal, Crombez, Van Oost, & De Bourdeaudhuji, 2003). These findings were similar for boys and girls. Moreover, these adolescents reported a more negative self-image and more negative emotions compared to either a control group of adolescents who experienced no traumatic experiences or a traumatic experience other than sexual abuse.

Studies of the long-term effects of trauma often do not differentiate between the social and contextual factors that may have an impact on both the risk of being exposed to trauma and the risk of developing psychopathology. To address such limitations, Fergusson, Horwood, and Lynskey (1997) studied a birth cohort of children up to the age of 18 with regular assessments of family, social, and related circumstances throughout childhood. At the age of 18, cohort members were then asked to provide retrospective accounts of childhood exposure to physical maltreatment, and a series of measures of personal adjustment were obtained. Increasing exposure to physical punishment in childhood was associated with significant increases in psychiatric disorder, suicide attempts, substance abuse/dependence, criminal offending, and rates of victimization. Adolescents who reported that they had been exposed to frequent, severe punishment or harsh and abusive treatment during their childhood had rates of these outcomes that were 1.5 to 3.9 times higher than those rates for young people who had reported that their parents had never used physical punishment. While the associations between reported physical punishment or maltreatment and adjustment outcomes at age 18 were slightly reduced after adjusting for family and social circumstances, those reporting abuse continued to be at increased risk of involvement in self-inflicted or interpersonal violence and were more prone to alcohol dependence.

Special Diagnostic Considerations with Adolescents

Exposure to childhood traumas of the type noted in this chapter may mean a whole host of physical, behavioral, and emotional problems for youth, both in the short and long term. The specificity of adolescent response to previous trauma is difficult to predict precisely because the presentation of symptoms appears to be a commonality of psychological responses that may differ according to the type and severity of trauma, the age of onset, and the duration of exposure. Because the symptoms of PTSD often overlap with those of other disorders, there may be instances in which the underlying PTSD syndrome is missed or not considered in the assessment or treatment of the traumatized adolescent. For example, the hyperactivity, distractibility, and interpersonal problems that often accompany PTSD in youth may be misrepresented as a diagnosis of attention-deficit/hyperactivity disorder (ADHD).

Child abuse and PTSD are very much underrecognized and untreated in adolescents (Cohen, 1998). Professionals working with youth must look beyond the presenting "acting out," "self-harming," or "depressive behaviors" of the adolescent and assess for early victimization and trauma. This practice entails moving beyond the individual and focusing on the social and psychological contexts in which the behaviors may arise. It is also likely that the adolescent may suffer from both PTSD and an associated disorder or that the associated disorder is a reaction to PTSD through mediating life circumstances. Nevertheless, careful attention to the differential diagnosis leads to appropriate and efficient treatment planning.

Much is still unknown as to why some children exposed to abuse and trauma but not others develop PTSD and other disorders. In a study examining the prevalence of trauma outcomes in children and adolescents who had experienced physical abuse only, sexual abuse only, or both, those who had experienced both were most likely to experience PTSD and other disorders (Ackerman et al., 1998). Kessler and colleagues (1995) found that the traumas that were most often linked to PTSD were rape, physical abuse, and neglect. Similarly, Reinherz, Giaconia, Lefkowitz, and Pakiz (1993) report that of adolescents with PTSD, the most common type of trauma experienced was sexual or physical assault. Other common diagnoses of abused children are oppositional defiant disorder (ODD), conduct disorder (CD), ADHD, and phobic disorder (Ackerman et al., 1998). Multiple factors contribute to one's risk of developing PTSD and other psychopathology, such as level of exposure, extent of disruption in social support, and psychopathology existing before trauma (Pine & Cohen, 2002).

An important practical and clinical question is whether adolescents who meet full diagnostic criteria for PTSD are different in some significant way from those who meet partial PTSD criteria. Ruchkin, Schwab-Stone, Koposov, Vermeiren, and Steiner (2002) found in their sample of Russian male juvenile delinquents that adolescents who met diagnostic criteria for partial PTSD had rates of psychopathology similar to those in the no-PTSD group and had similar numbers of comorbid diagnoses (one or two). The adolescent group diagnosed with full PTSD, however, revealed a wide range of comorbid diagnoses (generally more than three) and differed not only from the no-PTSD group but also from the partial PTSD group in most diagnoses and self-reported behaviors. These findings underscore the special attention required in understanding the distinction between full and partial PTSD for appropriate treatment planning and intervention.

EPIDEMIOLOGY

Prevalence estimates for adolescent exposure to traumatic events vary a lot depending on the factors mentioned later (e.g., the scope of the definition of trauma and how questions are asked). Within community samples looking at exposure to general stressful events, approximately 42–72% of adolescents (11–19 years) have experienced a major stressful event, which may include abuse, the death or serious illness of a family member, and a natural disaster, among others (Bal, Crombez, et al., 2003; Bal, Van Oost, De Bourdeaudhuji, & Crombez, 2003). Another community survey found that 25% of youth have experienced a high-magni-

tude stressor event (e.g., abuse, physical violence, serious accident, and natural disaster) by the age of 16 years, and that 6% of youth had experienced such an event in the past 3 months (Costello, Erkanli, Fairbank, & Angold, 2002).

Physical and Sexual Violence

The number of adolescents who endorse experiencing an unwanted sexual experience and/or dating violence varies tremendously between surveys, likely due in large part to the nature of the question(s) asked (Hanson, 2002). Even the definition of what constitutes an "assault" may vary tremendously between studies, from verbal aggression to physical harm. Almost half of adolescent females report having experienced sexual aggression (Maxwell, Robinson, & Post, 2003), and by the age of 18 years, 40% of females and 16% of males have had an unwanted sexual experience (Kellogg & Hoffman, 1995). However, other community studies have reported lower levels of sexual violence. Ackard and Neumark-Sztainer (2002) found that 9% of high-school girls and 6% of boys had ever experienced dating violence and/or date rape.

A survey of Canadian child protective service agency investigations of child abuse revealed that 40% of physical abuse cases involved adolescents between the ages of 12 and 15 years, with most of these cases being isolated incidents involving older children and injuries (Trocmé et al., 2001). In the United States, at least one-quarter of all incidents reported to child protective service agencies involve youth ages 12–15 years old, and according to the Second National Incidence Study of Child Abuse and Neglect in 1988, approximately 44% of all cases of maltreatment known to professionals involved adolescents (Garbarino, Eckenrode, & Powers, 1997). According to the Third National Incidence Study in 1996, approximately 20% of all cases of maltreatment reported by Child Protection Services involved adolescents (King, Trocmé, & Thatte, 2003). It is important to note that many instances of assault or abuse are likely to go unreported for a variety of reasons. Adolescents might fear that they will not be believed, or that there will be negative consequences for disclosing information. Boney-McCoy and Finkelor (1995) conducted a phone survey of 2,000 youth and found that of those who reported having experienced an assault of any kind, 26% had not disclosed this information to anyone prior to the study. Similarly, of adolescents who were victims of sexual assault, only two-thirds were found to have reported the incident to anyone (Hanson et al., 2003). These findings suggest that in all likelihood, estimates of both adolescent physical and sexual abuse are quite conservative.

Exposure to Domestic Violence

Margolin and Gordis (2000) report that it is difficult to determine the prevalence rate of children and adolescents exposed to domestic violence because it is not usually formally recorded by the police or child protection agencies. Researchers have cited that at least 3.3 million children and adolescents are exposed to domestic violence, although this figure may be an underestimation, as the data were collected about 20 years ago and did not include divorced parents or children under age 3 (Osofsky, 2003). Community studies report that approximately 20% of children and adolescents are exposed to domestic violence (McClosky, Figueredo, & Koss, 1995; McCloskey & Walker, 2000). Approximately half of the children and adolescents who are maltreated also experience exposure to domestic violence (Kellogg & Menard, 2003).

Community Violence

Many studies have examined the rates at which adolescents experience violence in their communities. While the term "community violence" has not been consistently defined across the literature, resulting in researchers using different definitions across studies, most research converges on the findings that children and adolescents are being exposed to incidents of community violence at exceedingly high rates. Guterman, Hahm, and Cameron (2002) reported that 20% of high school students have experienced serious violent victimization (e.g., assault with a weapon and getting "jumped") in the past year. Between the years of 1976 and 2002, the rate of violent victimization among adolescents between the ages of 12 and 19 was higher than that of all other age groups (Klaus & Rennison, 2002). Using both cross-sectional and longitudinal data, a large community sample of adolescents found that one-third of junior and high school students witness violence

in their communities (Schwab-Stone et al., 1999). Results from the National Longitudinal Study of Adolescent Health indicated that in a sample of 17,036 adolescents, risk factors for engaging in violent behaviors (e.g., taking part in a group fight and pulling a knife/gun on someone) were witnessing and being the target of violence, carrying a weapon to school, and emotional problems. Protective factors were being older, good academic performance, and expecting to finish high school, although these results varied for males and females.

Other factors that predict adolescent exposure to community violence have also been studied, such as geographical residence, ethnicity, and family income. For example, Stein, Jaycox, Kataoka, Rhodes, and Vestal (2003) reviewed the literature on adolescent exposure to community violence, including prevalence rates, as well as the different types and predictors of community violence. Rates of witnessing community violence were consistently higher than rates of actual victimization, and predictors of exposure to community violence (excluding sexual assault and rape) included being male, older, and residing in an urban, low-income, minority community. Similarly, only 12% of inner-city children report that they had *not* witnessed any violence (Mazza & Reynolds, 1999). In a sample of urban resident adolescents residing in New York City, 87% reported having witnessed some form of violence in their lifetime (Pastore, Fisher, & Friedman, 1996). According to the NSA study mentioned earlier, prevalence rates of witnessing violence (e.g., having seen someone actually or threatened to be shot, stabbed, sexually assaulted, and mugged) decreases as family income increases (Crouch, Hanson, Saunders, Kilpatrick, & Rensick, 2000). This relationship held true for Caucasian youth (34.4% witnessed violence) but not for African American youth (57.2% witnessed violence), whose increased income level was not a protective factor for decreased violence exposure. In a cross-cultural study of a Belgium community sample of 1,624 adolescents, 27% had been chased by gangs or individuals, 45% had been beaten up or mugged, and 20% had been threatened with serious physical harm (Vermeiren, Ruchkin, Leckman, Deboutte, & Schwab-Stone, 2002). These rates are reportedly lower compared to American rates but still highlight the problem of child and adolescent violence exposure in European communities.

Bullying

Although bullying is a common problem across countries, direct comparison of prevalence and outcomes has not always been possible because of methodological variation across studies. Most researchers generally define bullying as aggressive behaviors characterized by repetition and an imbalance of power (Smith & Brain, 2000). Specifically, "Bullying is a form of aggression that is hostile and proactive, and involves both direct and indirect behaviors that are repeatedly targeted at an individual or group perceived as weaker" (Elinoff, Chafouleas, & Sassu, 2004, p. 888). The Health Behavior in School-aged Children (HBSC) study is one of the few studies to examine bullying across countries in nationally representative samples by standard measures and methods (Nansel et al., 2004). Nansel and colleagues (2004) examined prevalence data on bullying across 25 countries, including the United States, Canada, and Europe. Students between the ages of 11 and 15 were provided with a standard definition of bullying and asked to report how frequently they had been the victim of bullying at school during the current school term and how frequently they had been the perpetrators of bullying at school. Involvement in bullying at school—as bully, victim, or both—ranged from 9 to 54%. Children classified as being victims ranged from 5 to 20%, with an average across countries of 11%. With respect to bullying others, rates ranged from 3 to 20%, with an overall average of 10%. For those children classified as both bullies and victims, prevalence rates ranged from 1 to 20%, with the countries averaging 6% overall.

Nansel and colleagues (2001) reported that in the first nationally representative sample of American youth, 30% reported moderate or frequent involvement in bullying, as a bully (13%), one who was bullied (11%), or both (6%). This overall rate is similar to another multidistrict study that found that 24% of early adolescent children report being bullied (Seals & Young, 2003). These authors also reported that males were more likely than females to be both perpetrators and targets of bullying. These sex differences, however, may be related to age and type of bullying. Regarding age, many researchers have found that bullying is less common in adolescents compared to middle school children (Borg, 1999; O'Moore & Smith, 1997; Whitney & Smith,

1993). As well, a meta-analysis of 35 child and adolescent studies by Scheitauer (as cited in Smith, 2004) found that females under the age of 7 and over the age of 12 tend to use more relational aggression (i.e., damage to one's peer relationships) than same-age males, and both males and females equally use relational aggression between the ages of 8 and 12. Generally, males tend to engage in more physical bullying.

Many researchers have studied the psychological impact of bullying on adolescents. Depression, suicidal thoughts and behaviors, and referrals to psychiatric services are more common in adolescents who have been bullied compared to those who have not (Mills, Guerin, Lynch, Daly, & Fitzpatrick, 2004). James, Sofroniou, and Lawlor (2003) examined adolescent reactions to bullying and found that victims reported feelings of anger and frustrations regardless of the frequency of bullying, while feelings of sadness and anxiety increased with the frequency of bullying. Adolescents who had had rumors spread about them experienced more sadness and anxiety compared to those who did not, and adolescents who had been excluded from peers experienced more sadness than those who were not; 21% of this group reported feeling suicidal.

Gender-identity issues may also contribute to the short- and long-term impact of bullying. Young and Sweeting (2004) reported that adolescent males who exhibit gender-atypical behaviors reported more victimization, more loneliness, fewer male friends, and greater distress than did gender-typical peers. Rivers (2004) studied gay, lesbian, or bisexual adults about their experiences of bullying in childhood and adolescence and found that 17% of the adults reported more posttraumatic symptoms and depression compared to controls; a small number of participants used drugs and alcohol to help them cope with bullying memories. They also did not report these bullying incidents to their parents or teachers. On a more positive note, these adults still had a positive attitude toward their sexual orientation and did not have low-self esteem compared to controls (Rivers, 2001).

Internet harassment is emerging as a significant and psychological issue for young people (Finkelhor, Mitchell, & Wolak, 2000). Though studies related to Internet harassment are few, research indicates that 6% of youth who use the Internet have been harassed in the past year

(Finkelhor et al., 2000). Based on data from the United Kingdom (British Broadcasting Corporation, 2002), lifetime estimates for youth harassed via email are 4%, and 7% of youth in the same study reported being the target of harassment in Internet chat rooms. Using the largest U.S. sample of youth Internet users to date, Ybarra and Mitchell (2004) reported that 15% of youth were identified as Internet harassers ($n = 219$) and 7% were identified as being harassed online in the past year. Adolescent males with depression symptoms were three times more likely to report an Internet harassment experience during the past year than youth with mild or absent symptoms (Ybarra, 2004). It was interesting to note that this relationship was not evident in adolescent females, implying that there may be gender differences in the impact of Internet harassment.

Age of Onset

The younger a child is when physical or sexual abuse begins the greater number of mental health diagnoses he or she is likely to have (Ackerman et al., 1998). Similarly, earlier age of onset of PTSD (by age 14) increases one's risk of having multiple disorders by age 18 (Giaconia et al., 1994). The age of onset of PTSD has also been found to be related to associated impairments. Adolescents with early-onset PTSD were more likely to have interpersonal problems and those with late-onset PTSD were more likely to have poor academic performance (Giaconia et al., 1994). In the Detroit Area Survey of Trauma, the prevalence of traumatic events was found to peak between the ages of 16 and 20 years (Breslau et al., 1998). Similarly, in a longitudinal study following children from kindergarten to age 18, the peak age of developing PTSD was between 16 and 17 years of age, with a median of 16 years; however, one-third of the youth with PTSD had developed this disorder by age 14 (Giaconia et al., 1994).

Sex Differences

Although sex differences in experiencing physical abuse are minimal (e.g., Silverman et al., 1996), it is largely established that girls are more likely than boys to experience sexual abuse (Ackerman et al., 1998; Silverman et al., 1996). In their phone survey, Boney-McCoy and Finkelor (1995) found that 15% of girls

and 6% of boys had been the victims of one or more incidents of sexual assault. Sexual abuse of females is more likely to be reported than that of males (Chandy, Blum, & Resnick, 1996; Shaw, 2000), and thus the difference in the rates of sexual abuse for boys and girls may not be as great as the numbers suggest. Finally, girls are more likely than boys to experience sexual abuse by a parental figure, whereas boys are more likely to be abused by a person outside the family (Feiring et. al., 1999).

Sex differences are also apparent in outcomes of abuse and trauma for adolescents. In general, girls are more likely to internalize their experiences while boys tend to externalize. Specifically, girls are more likely to have mood or anxiety symptoms after experiencing a traumatic stress, whereas boys are more likely to show behavioral symptoms (Pine & Cohen, 2002). For example, Ackerman and colleagues (1998) found that abused boys were more likely to display symptoms of ADHD, ODD, and CD, whereas girls were more likely to have separation anxiety and phobic disorder. Pertaining to sexual abuse, girls show more intrusive thoughts and greater hyperarousal than boys, both of which are PTSD symptoms (Feiring et al., 1999). Furthermore, girls are more likely to use a ruminative response style and to report feelings of shame for the abuse (Feiring et al., 1999). Boys, on the other hand, tend to report more eroticism and less sexual anxiety.

With these findings in mind, it is not surprising that girls are at least twice as likely as boys to develop PTSD (Kessler et al., 1995; Kilpatrick et al., 2003). Kilpatrick and colleagues (2003) found that the 6-month prevalence for PTSD in adolescents between the ages of 12 and 17 was 6.3% for females but only 3.7% for males. However, this is not to suggest that there are not other negative effects of trauma on boys. Boys who have been exposed to trauma may be more likely than girls to have substance abuse problems, aggressive behavior, and suicidal thoughts (Garnefski & Arends, 1998). Furthermore, at least one study suggests that of children and adolescents who do develop PTSD, boys are more vulnerable than girls to adverse brain development (DeBellis et al., 2002).

In studies of adolescent dating violence, gender emerges as a significant issue. Estimates of physical victimization among girls range from 8 to 57% and 6 to 38% for boys; estimates of sexual victimization range from 14 to 43% for girls and 0.3 to 36% for boys (Hickman, Jaycox, & Aronoff (2004). O'Keefe (1997) reported that boys and girls reported anger as their primary reason for violence, although girls were more likely to report using violence as self-defense, whereas boys used violence to exert control over their dating partner.

Social Class, Ethnicity, and Culture

There is limited evidence as to the influence of social class on exposure to abuse and trauma and trauma outcomes in adolescents. In a German sample of adolescents between the ages of 14 and 24, Perkonigg, Kessler, Storz, and Wittchen (2000) found that low social class membership increased one's risk of both experiencing traumatic events and developing PTSD. Similarly, adolescents who had parents with less than a college education were significantly more likely than those with higher-educated parents to have experienced multiple traumas (Turner & Butler, 2003), although Kessler and colleagues (1995) did not find this relationship. Nonetheless, after having experienced traumatic events, those with higher education and income were less vulnerable to developing PTSD.

Some cultural differences with regard to trauma and trauma outcomes have been reported, although studies in this area are limited. For example, African American children are overrepresented as victims of physical but not sexual abuse (Ackerman et al., 1998). Hispanic children are more likely than African American or European American children to be abused by a parent figure, to be living with the perpetrator at the time of abuse, and to suffer more chronic abuse (Feiring, Coates, & Taska, 2001). Recently, with a sample of 649 college students, Turner and Butler (2003) reported that nonwhites had significantly more traumatic experiences in childhood and adolescence than did whites. Almost half of the nonwhite participants reported having experienced seven or more traumatic events in their lifetime, whereas only a quarter of white participants had such experiences.

No racial differences were found with regard to diagnosis of PTSD or other psychopathologies for adolescents who were victims of abuse (Kessler et al., 1995). PTSD diagnoses in a sample of Cambodian refugee youth were quite similar to those previously found in North American samples of Caucasian and African Americans (Sack, Seeley, & Clarke, 1997). Similarly, demographics such as age and gender were more important than race or ethnicity in predicting outcomes of adolescents who had experienced traumatic events (Kilpatrick et al., 2003). Given the lack of consistency in the findings regarding racial and ethnic differences, it is likely that many experiences of trauma transcend cultural boundaries (Mennen, 1995).

DEVELOPMENTAL COURSE AND OUTCOMES

The impact of trauma in adolescence is greatly influenced by the youth's developmental stage. Because adolescents are still struggling with issues of separation and individuation and the evolving definition of the self, the long-term effects of exposure to trauma on the developing adolescent are far ranging. Thus, traumatic experiences may affect not only their short-term responses but also how they adapt in the future. Here we examine the burgeoning research on this issue in terms of social-cognitive impairments, emotional and behavioral disorders, and adult outcomes.

Social-Cognitive Impairments

Experiencing abuse prior to or during adolescence may affect the types of coping strategies the adolescent learns to use for all new stressful situations into adulthood, as well as subsequent psychosocial development (Shapiro & Levendosky, 1999). Children and adolescents may learn to "turn off" feelings of pain and distress during abuse, thereby learning to avoid dealing with painful situations (Weems, Saltzman, Reiss, & Carrion, 2003). Poor coping strategies learned in childhood or adolescence may reemerge when faced with new stressors in later adolescence or adulthood, particularly if these new stressors provoke similar feelings of shame and helplessness (Gibson & Leitenberg, 2001).

The role of coping style has recently received considerable attention as a possible mediator between experiencing a traumatic event and adjustment difficulties. For example, poor adjustment following child sexual abuse was mediated by avoidant coping strategies, whereas active coping mediated the relationship between sexual trauma and the occurrence of anger (Bal, Van Oost, et al., 2003). In a study of female adolescents (14–16 years) with a history of sexual abuse, avoidant coping strategies mediated the relationship between childhood sexual or physical abuse and current interpersonal conflict (Shapiro & Levendosky, 1999). In addition, attachment style mediated between the childhood abuse or neglect and coping strategy, suggesting an intricate and complicated pathway between maltreatment and current adolescent difficulties. In a recent study of Palestinian adolescents living in a residential training school, maltreatment was associated with a greater reliance on avoidant or "emotion-focused" coping strategies, which in turn was associated with higher levels of emotional difficulties (Thabet, Tischler, & Vostanis, 2004). Emotion-focused coping strategies referred to ways of regulating or minimized the accompanying distress in stressful situations.

Traumatic experiences before age 16 were assessed in a study of undergraduate women (mean age = 18.6 years), including sexual abuse, physical abuse, and witnessing domestic violence (Leitenberg, Gibson, & Novy, 2004). The greater the history of child or adolescent abuse, the greater the reliance of these women on disengagement methods of coping, such as wishful thinking, problem avoidance, social withdrawal, and self-criticism. Interestingly, they did not find a corresponding decrease in the use of engagement coping methods (e.g., problem solving and social support) as a function of child abuse or stressor histories (Leitenberg et al., 2004).

Emotional and Behavioral Disorders

Adolescence is the time at which many youth are exposed to a number of risky situations for the first time, such as substance use, dating, sexual activity, and unhappiness with body image, particularly with the onset of puberty, and delinquency (Wolfe, Jaffe, & Crooks, in press). Adolescents learn to negotiate and regulate these types of activities, and if development is disrupted during this time by a traumatic experience, the acquisition of the skills needed to develop healthy responses to these situations may be hampered. These activities may also be used as outlets for coping with the overwhelming stress of trauma upon an immature emotional coping system. Following is a summary of the associated characteristics that may occur during adolescence for youth with a history of

traumatic exposure. While some of these characteristics may be comorbid with PTSD, others may develop as coping mechanisms leading to lifelong impairment.

Substance Use

Research has established a causal link that adolescents with a history of adverse childhood experiences have an enhanced risk of alcohol and substance abuse disorders, compared with nontraumatized populations (Harrison, Fulkerson, & Beebe, 1997; Lipschitz et al., 2003), with the highest rates of multiple substance use among victims of both physical and sexual abuse (Harrison et al., 1997; Moran, Vuchinich, & Hall, 2004). Seventy percent of 212 adolescents participating in a long-term residential drug program reported lifetime trauma exposure, and 29% of the trauma-exposed met criteria for current PTSD (Jaycox, Ebener, Damesek, & Becker, 2004). For girls and boys in early adolescence, sexual abuse is associated with extreme substance use, increasing the likelihood more than fourfold (Bergen, Martin, Richardson, Allison, & Roeger, 2004). Adolescents with trauma exposure initiate the use of substances at an earlier age than do their peers (Harrison et al., 1997), and for 80% of girls with both PTSD and a substance use disorder (SUD), the age of onset for PTSD preceded or developed concurrently with the SUD (Lipschitz et al., 2003). Male adolescents with a history of sexual abuse report more extreme and frequent use of marijuana, and more extreme alcohol use, while sexually abused females report more frequent alcohol use (Chandy et al., 1996). Rheingold, Smith, Ruggiero, Saunders, Kilpatrick, and Resnick (2004) reported that adolescents who experience the death of a close friend have increased PTSD, depression, and substance abuse symptoms.

Much of the research on trauma and SUD has assessed the prevalence of trauma in adolescents receiving treatment for SUDs. For adolescents in SUD treatment, higher levels of trauma symptoms are associated with higher levels of substance use, mental health and physical problems, and HIV risk behaviors (Stevens, Murphy, & McKnight, 2003). Grella and Joshi (2003) found that 59% of girls and 39% of boys in SUD treatment had a history of physical and/or sexual abuse, and that those adolescents had greater service needs upon treatment admission. Those adolescents with a history of physical abuse had a lower likelihood of remaining abstinent after treatment. In their sample of adolescents receiving long-term residential SUD treatment, 71% reported exposure to trauma at some point in their lifetime, which also included witnessing or community violence in addition to maltreatment (Jaycox at al., 2004). Those adolescents who had experienced trauma (but without PTSD symptoms) left treatment sooner than those who did not have a history of trauma exposure. Findings such as these emphasize the need to consider the effects of traumatic exposure in adolescents with substance use problems, because treatment may be less successful if trauma experiences are not addressed and resolved.

Although these findings are significant, the mechanisms whereby childhood traumatization can increase the likelihood of substance abuse in adolescence remain unclear. Some authors have argued that it is not simply exposure to childhood trauma that is a risk factor for later substance abuse in adolescence but the subsequent ability of the traumatized child to regulate his or her affect in adolescence and later adulthood (Deykin & Buka, 1997; Hilarski, 2004).

Depression and Anxiety

Higher rates of depression are a very common finding in the maltreatment literature. Adolescent girls with a history of sexual abuse in either pre- or early adolescence, show more depression (e.g., Johnson, 2001), with a longer duration of the abuse predicting a greater severity of depressive symptoms and lower levels of self-esteem (Cecil & Matson, 2001). Family functioning—in particular, a lack of family cohesion—also predicts internalizing problems in sexually abused adolescents (Bal, De Bourdeaudhuji, Crombez, & Van Oost, 2004).

Adolescents with a history of early childhood trauma also have an increased risk of developing anxiety-related disorders and fears, in addition to core symptoms of PTSD noted previously (Fergusson et al., 1997; Swanston, Plunkett, O'Toole, Shrimpton, Parkinson, & Oates, 2003; Tebbutt, Swanston, Oates, & O'Toole, 1997). By adolescence, often the core symptoms of PTSD, such as sleeplessness or intense fear, are masked such that a child who had been traumatized years before may suffer the onset of dissociation, disorganization,

depression, aggression, suicidal behavior, hypersexual behavior, and anxiety. Pettigrew and Burcham (1997) suggested that there may be specificity between childhood sexual abuse and anxiety disorders, such as PTSD, which can be very long lasting. While the traditional symptoms of PTSD will progressively lesson over time, the full impact of early trauma may not be experienced until the youth reaches adulthood and engages in adult relationships and responsibilities (Yehuda, Spertus, & Golier, 2001). For example, poor adaptation following trauma experiences may be expressed as relational difficulties with others, such as lack of closeness, trust, and intimacy. Furthermore, PTSD symptoms may reemerge following a subsequent trauma related or unrelated to the original trauma, a life stressor, or by a cue of the original trauma.

Risky Sexual Behaviors

The acquisition of healthy sexual practices and attitudes is another important skill in adolescence, and interference can have long-lasting implications both emotionally and physically. Female adolescents with a history of sexual abuse and/or sexual assault, for example, are more likely to initiate consensual sexual activity at an earlier age, to have had multiple sexual partners, to engage in unprotected sex, and/or to have a history of sexually transmitted diseases (Buzi et al., 2003; Fergusson et. al., 1997; Johnson, 2001). Female victims of sexual abuse prior to age 16 are also at increased risk of sexual assault in later adolescence and young adulthood (Fergusson et al., 1997). Male adolescents with a history of sexual abuse have a greater risk for sexual risk taking (Chandy et al., 1996). Experiences of physical abuse from a parent or parental figure or witnessing interparental violence also significantly increases the odds of engaging in risky sexual practices (Elliott, Avery, Fishman, & Hoshiko, 2002).

Dating Violence

Research supports the link between adolescent dating violence and early childhood trauma (see Jouriles, Wolfe, Garrido, & McCarthy, Chapter 19, this volume). For example, youth with histories of maltreatment have increased risk for relationship-based difficulties (Bank & Burraston, 2001; Wekerle & Avougoustis,

2003) and have more than a three and a half times greater risk of involvement in adult domestic violence (Coid et al., 2001). In a school-based sample of high school students, childhood experiences of abuse and trauma was associated with violence toward a dating partner in high school; dating violence remained stable for those individuals with maltreatment backgrounds over 1 year and was associated with other adjustment problems such as trauma-related symptoms (Wolfe, Wekerle, Scott, Straatman, & Grasley, 2004). Adolescents who carry forward their posttraumatic stress-related problems, moreover, have difficulty distinguishing when "rough-and-tumble play" crosses the line to become abusive behavior (Capaldi & Gorman-Smith, 2003). Especially for maltreated youth, dating relationships may pose new challenges whereby strong feelings and sexual involvement may contribute to a resurgence of trauma symptoms due to similar cues signaling the original abusive event or events (Wekerle & Wolfe, 2003).

Eating-Disordered Behaviors

A history of sexual abuse increases the risk for a variety of eating-disordered behaviors in both female and male adolescents, increasing the odds up to 29 times for specific behaviors (Ackard & Neumark-Sztainer, 2003), especially for girls (Chandy et al., 1996). Dating violence and date rape are both associated with higher rates of eating-disordered behaviors, with over half of those adolescents reporting both dating violence and eating disorders also reporting suicide attempts (Ackard & Neumark-Sztainer, 2002). Both physical and sexual abuse are related to binge and purge behaviors in 5th–12th graders, with the strongest associations with those who have experienced both types of abuse (Ackard, Neumark-Sztainer, Hanna, French, & Story, 2001). Moreover, sexual victimization is associated with weight regulation practices, with stronger relationships with more extreme weight regulatory behaviors, independent of physical abuse or dating violence (Thompson, Wonderlich, Crosby, & Mitchell, 2001). The latter researchers also reported that sexual victimization increases the probability of purging behaviors by 18%. Interestingly, abused youth who have discussed their experiences of abuse report less binge and purging behaviors than those who have not (Ackard et al., 2001).

Delinquency and Violence

Delinquent and violent behaviors are particularly of concern during adolescence, and are also linked to histories of abuse and trauma. The National Youth Survey has reported that violent adolescent victimization by both family and nonfamily members has an immediate and sustained impact on juvenile offending (Fagan, 2003), especially for boys (Chandy et al., 1996). Incarcerated juvenile delinquents report higher levels of exposure to sexual and community violence and PTSD symptoms, particularly for those youth who commit more violent crimes (Wood, Foy, Layne, Pynoos, & James, 2002). A study of Russian male juvenile delinquents found that two-thirds of their sample met criteria for partial or full PTSD criteria, with the experience or witnessing of violence victimization as the most common reported traumas (Ruchkin et al., 2002). These researchers suggested that the PTSD symptoms may be associated with the difficulties with behavior inhibition and poor coping often seen in youth with conduct problems, in addition to an association with the prior violence exposure and temperamental behavior activation. More violent adolescents use more maladaptive coping strategies, have been exposed to higher levels of violence, and exhibit greater levels of trauma symptoms relative to both less violent and nonviolent peers (Flannery, Singer, & Wester, 2003).

Suicidality

Although suicidal cognitions may be present in children, these symptoms may be more common in adolescents who have the means and knowledge to attempt suicide. A community survey of Italian adolescents revealed that over half the sample who had been victimized at school in the past 12 months had experienced suicidal cognitions, while approximately one-third of those youth who had been victimized at home and 20% who had witnessed violence in the home also experienced suicidal ideations (Baldry & Winkel, 2003). After controlling for witnessing violence, direct victimization by the father predicted suicidal cognitions for boys, while direct victimization by both parents predicted suicidal cognitions for girls (Baldry & Winkel, 2003).

Adolescents who have experienced sexual abuse have at least a threefold risk of suicidal thoughts and/or attempts; similarly, adolescents who have experienced dating violence or date rape also show a higher risk for suicidal thoughts and/or attempts (Ackard & Neumark-Sztainer, 2002), especially for girls (Chandy et al., 1996). In their community study of Australian eighth graders, Martin, Bergen, Richardson, Roeger, and Allison (2004) found that 55% of sexually abused boys and 29% of sexually abused girls had attempted suicide. For boys, sexual abuse was strongly and independently associated with suicidal thoughts, plans, threats, deliberate self-injury, and suicide attempts, after controlling for current levels of depression, hopelessness, and family dysfunction (Martin et al., 2004). Compared to nonabused boys, sexually abused boys who reported a high level of current distress about the abuse had a 10-fold increased risk for suicidal plans and threats, and a 15-fold risk for suicidal attempts.

Conduct Problems

Greenwald (2002) has suggested that trauma exposure plays a key role in the development and persistence of conduct problems in adolescents, arguing that the effects of trauma can help to account for a number of core features of CD such as a lack of empathy, impulsivity, anger, acting out, and resistance to treatment. Witnessing or experiencing community violence were significant risk factors for conduct problems over a 1-year period in early adolescence (approximately 10–14 years of age; Pearce, Jones, Schwab-Stone, & Ruchkin, 2003). These associations, however, were moderated by level of religiousness and parental involvement with their children. Sexual abuse has also been found to be a significant predictor of antisocial behaviors for adolescents, at least doubling the odds of exhibiting antisocial behaviors, even after controlling for level of family dysfunction and depressive symptoms (Bergen, Martin, Richardson, & Allison, & Roeger, 2004). Findings from earlier years of the National Youth Survey demonstrated that victimization in the previous year accounted for 26% of conduct problems in 11-year-olds (Hilarski, 2004).

In sum, adolescents who have experienced abuse and trauma often show a wide range of problem behaviors other than PTSD, suggesting that these experiences have a generalized effect on adjustment and development. In general, girls are more likely to develop internalizing problems, while boys show more externalizing problems. Compared to boys, girls are more likely to develop PTSD symptoms after exposure to a traumatic event (Elklit, 2002), sexual abuse (Feiring et al., 1999), or witnessing of or exposure to community violence (Foster, Kuperminc, & Price, 2004). Interestingly, Foster and colleagues (2004) found that although girls are equally likely to develop PTSD symptoms whether witnessing or experiencing community violence, boys are more distressed by the experience of violence. Feiring and her colleagues (1999) theorize that sexually abused girls are more likely than boys to develop internalizing and PTSD symptoms because they feel more shame, experience more fears related to a heightened sense of vulnerability and sense of the world as a dangerous place, have higher levels of hyperarousal and intrusive thoughts, and in general have a greater ruminative response style.

Adult Outcomes

As adulthood approaches, developmental impairments stemming from previous trauma and abuse can lead to more pervasive and chronic psychiatric disorders, including anxiety and panic disorders, depression, eating disorders, sexual problems, and personality disturbances (Brown et al., 1999; Kendler et al., 2000). Researchers associated with the Centers for Disease Control and Prevention have retrospectively studied the co-occurrence of multiple forms of adverse childhood experiences (ACEs) in adults (Felitti et al., 1998). Ten types of ACEs were investigated: childhood abuse (emotional, physical, and sexual), neglect (emotional and physical), and household dysfunction (growing up in domestic violence, parental marital discord, and substance-abusing, mentally ill, or criminal household members) that the participant had reported experiencing prior to 18 years of age. Strong cumulative relationships were found between experiencing ACEs and health-related problems in adulthood such as smoking, adult alcohol problems, drug abuse, unintended pregnancies, male involvement in teen pregnancy, sexually transmitted infections, suicide attempts, and common chronic diseases. For example, persons who had experienced four or more categories of childhood exposure, compared to those who had experienced none, had a 4- to 12-fold greater health risk for alcoholism, drug abuse, depression, and suicide attempt (Felitti et al., 1998). With respect to types of trauma experiences, of individuals who reported physical abuse, 98% reported more than one ACE, 90% reported more than two ACEs, and 42% reported more than five ACEs. Other researchers have also found sex differences in the distribution of cumulative traumas, with a larger proportion of males experiencing seven-plus traumatic experiences and a smaller proportion experiencing zero to two traumas (Turner & Butler, 2003). These findings underscore the importance of assessing different areas of trauma.

Traumatic experiences in adolescence relating to sexual activity or dating relationships appear to have a particularly large impact on adult functioning in these areas, likely because adolescence is the time when skills are developed that provide a template for all future relationships. For example, being the victim of dating violence in adolescence was a better predictor of being a dating violence victim as a college student than was childhood sexual or physical abuse, or the witnessing of interparental violence (Smith, White, & Holland, 2003). Males who were physically punished, were sexually abused, or witnessed domestic violence in childhood had a greater risk for sexually coercive behavior in adolescence and young adulthood (White & Smith, 2004). This study provides evidence for the importance of providing dating-violence intervention programs for youth who have engaged in coercive dating behaviors, as these youth may continue to perpetrate these behaviors in adulthood.

The psychological functioning of men (*n* = 76) who had been the victim of multiple and severe incidents of sexual, physical, and/or emotional abuse during childhood placement in a religiously affiliated institution was recently examined (Wolfe, Francis, & Straatman, in press). The abuse was perpetrated by several adults in positions of authority and trust at the institution. DSM-IV criteria were met for current PTSD (42%), alcohol (21%), and mood-related disorders (25%). Over one-third suffered chronic sexual problems, and over one-half had a history of criminal behavior. The researchers found that the importance of the institution, the role of the perpetrator(s) within the setting, and the community's response to allegations of abuse affected the long-term adjustment of these men, in addition to postabuse events such as arrest, denial, or punishment of the offender.

THEORIES AND ETIOLOGY CONCERNING THE IMPACT OF ABUSE AND TRAUMA IN ADOLESCENTS

Theoretical explanations for the harmful effects of abuse and trauma take into account developmental processes and how they might interact with the particular pattern and trauma of maltreatment, including the setting (e.g., familial or nonfamilial) and the child's relationship to the offender. Finkelhor and Browne's (1985) early conceptualization of harm resulting from child abuse has guided the field, especially in terms of looking beyond symptom expression to the underlying psychological dynamics that form the core of the psychological injury (i.e., traumatic sexualization, betrayal, stigmatization, and powerlessness). Powerlessness, for example, refers to the situation whereby the child's will, desire, and sense of self-efficacy are thwarted and rebuked, and it is often linked to fears, worries, and depression. Such feelings may not be identified until years later, once the individual reaches an age whereby he or she can recognize this betrayal dynamic as the source of feelings of self-blame, guilt, and powerlessness (Williams, 1988). Clinically, these dynamics contribute to the trauma-related outcomes most commonly reported in the literature on the long-term effects of sexual and physical abuse: PTSD, depression, suicide, sexual promiscuity, susceptibility to repeat abusive acts, attempts to gain power over others, and poor academic performance (Briere, 1992; Brown et al., 1999; Lange et al., 1999; Tyler, 2002).

Developmental traumatology has also emerged as an important theoretical perspective on the effects of trauma across the lifespan. This perspective involves the study of the interactions among the complex factors of genetic constitution, psychosocial environment, and critical periods of vulnerability and resiliency in individuals experiencing abuse or trauma, with the view toward disentangling the effect of trauma on neurobiological development (DeBellis, 2001; DeBellis & Putnam, 1994). To illustrate, Perry (2001) points out that when a child lives in a persistent state of fear, the primary areas of the brain that are processing information may be very different from the primary brain areas functioning in a child living in a safe environment. Under chronic stress, there is more of a selective development of *nonverbal* cognitive capacities when the youth is constantly hypervigilant for danger cues: He or she will overinterpret nonverbal cues at the expense of verbal cues. Due to their traumatic experiences, these youth have learned that picking up on nonverbal cues (e.g., facial expressions) is more important than verbal information; thus, chronically traumatized children are less efficient at processing and storing information (Perry, 2001). Due to this overreliance on nonverbal cues, cognition becomes dominated by subcortical and limbic areas. Compared to a nontraumatized child living in a safe environment, the traumatized child has different parts of the brain controlling his or her cognitive functioning. Due to chronic experiences of danger, the traumatized youth has a foreshortened sense of the future, placing too much emphasis on immediate reward (Perry, 2001), and thus impeding the normal cognitive development in adolescence of the effects of his or her actions on the future.

More generally, developmental psychopathology considers that abusive or traumatic acts can affect children's development diversely and progressively over time (Cicchetti & Lynch, 1995). This explanation places children's experiences in a broader context that includes their perception of the emotional climate of their families or caregivers, their previous experiences with conflict and abuse, their interpretations of violence and maltreatment, and their available coping abilities and resources to countermand stress and inadequate caregiving. Related to this developmental viewpoint are the effects of two independent dimensions of *life threat* and *social betrayal* associated with trauma experiences. Life-threatening situations may lead to symptoms of fear, anxiety, hyperarousal, and intrusive memories, whereas social betrayal is associated with symptoms of dissociation, amnesia, numbing, and abusive relationships (Freyd, 1997; Wekerle & Wolfe, 2003).

Recently, Wolfe and colleagues (2003) proposed a framework for understanding the dynamics of abuse in relation to familial and nonfamilial settings. The two central features of the framework—contributors to harm and dimensions of harm—were intended to identify patterns and constructs for further empirical development. The factors contributing to harm

include aspects of the youth's environment that further influence adjustment difficulties over the life course. Four factors contributing to harm include the significance and role of the setting (e.g., school, family, and religion); the role of the perpetrator within the setting (e.g., parent, religious leader, teacher, or other trusted adult); the degree and nature of child or youth involvement with the institution or organization (the extent to which an offender has the opportunity to take advantage of the youth's commitment, desire to participate, etc.); and abuse and postabuse events (e.g., the use of power structure, rules, or belief system to gain trust or maintain silence). This latter factor also includes an institution's response to allegations of abuse by individuals within their organization, which can prolong the impact of the trauma.

Dimensions of harm have been identified on the basis of both familial and nonfamilial forms of abuse and trauma, similar to Finkelhor and Browne's (1985) model. These are termed "betrayal" and "diminished trust," which has a profound effect on the following factors: interpersonal relationships and their willingness to trust persons in their community; shame, guilt, and humiliation, in which the victim feels that he or she was somehow responsible for the abuse, or misattributes such acts to his or her personal faults or weaknesses; fear of/disrespect for authority, in which the youth may fear individuals in positions of authority or may lose respect for them as a result of their abuse of power (others may feel powerless to stop the abuse, resulting in symptoms of depression, anxiety, and PTSD); avoidance of reminders, which may trigger painful flashbacks and often disrupts or impedes their daily life; and injury and vicarious trauma, ranging from self-abuse to suicidal attempts. Supportive evidence for these dimensions emerges throughout the following discussion of biological and developmental influences.

Biological Influences

The developing brain is extremely sensitive to stress, which contributes to functional deficits and vulnerability to future stressors. Neural systems that are activated repetitively may permanently alter the number of synaptic connections, microarchitecture, dendritic density, and the expression of a host of important structural and functional cellular constituents, such as enzymes and neurotransmitter receptors (Lubit et al., 2003). The two distinct response systems in reaction to trauma and abuse are hyperarousal and dissociation (Perry, 2001). Hyperarousal represents the "alarm" stage following traumatic events, in which arousal, anxiety, and modulation of limbic and cortical processing is activated by the reticular activating system (RAS). Under acute stress, activity is increased in related brain areas of the locus coeruleus and the ventral tegmental nucleus, triggering an increase in the release of norephinephrine (NE) that is projected to all major areas of the brain. NE, in turn, plays a critical role in regulating arousal, vigilance, affect, behavioral irritability, locomotion, attention, response to stress, sleep, and the startle response.

The hyperarousal response also affects the hippocampus, which is a key center for memory and learning. There is a surge in the release of cortisol associated with chronic or repeated stress, which alters hippocampal structure and volume and increases the risk of functional memory and learning problems. This explanation was supported in a study of inpatient adolescents, whereby greater severity of trauma experiences was associated with reduced autobiographical memory of childhood (de Decker, Hermans, Raes, & Eelen, 2003). Similarly, chronic activation of the hypothalamic–pituitary–adrenal axis as a result of abuse or trauma is very taxing and can result in profound cognitive distortions due to being constantly on alert for danger in the environment.

While hyperarousal involves the overuse of some systems, dissociation is related to the *disuse* of the early alarm response, or defeat (Perry, 2001). There are major differences in the central nervous system activation between the hyperarousal and dissociation systems. Although there is also an increase in the circulation of NE in a dissociative episode, vagal tone also increases dramatically, thereby *decreasing* blood pressure and heart rate, in contrast to hyperarousal. Because dopaminergic systems are active, modulation of mood and emotions and mediation of pain are diminished.

A younger age at the time of trauma exposure is a risk factor for more severe trauma sequelae because of the developmental vulnerabilities inherent in several of the brain structures involved in the processing of trauma. This finding applies even in late adolescence. For example, Maercker and Karl (2003) examined two groups of adult men who had been trau-matized by political imprisonment, either in their late adolescent years (17–22 years) or in middle adulthood. Those men who had been traumatized in late adolescence had a higher rate of autonomic arousal than did the men who had been traumatized in middle adulthood, even years after their imprisonment.

Developmental Influences

Abuse and trauma influence the major developmental tasks of adolescence, which include separation and emancipation, intimacy, identity, and vocation and mastery (Task Force on Adolescent Assault Victim Needs, 1996). Consequently, the effects of experiencing trauma may vary depending on the adolescent's stage of development. In early adolescence victimization can delay the separation and individuation process by causing the adolescent to regress to overdependency on parents and less on peers. Younger adolescents may also possess feelings of invincibility and lack experience, maturity, and decision-making abilities that reduce exposure to danger. In middle adolescence, normal experiences include risk taking and conflicts with adults over responsibility and independence. However, those who experience trauma or abuse during this developmental stage may be at especially high risk for injury due to peer influences. The need to prove oneself and to experiment, in tandem with inexperience, limited decision-making skills, and increasing autonomy greatly increase access to high-risk situations. Finally, abuse or trauma during late adolescence can temporarily or permanently interrupt the ability to solidify progress into becoming a self-sufficient and independent young adult (Task Force on Adolescent Assault Victim Needs, 1996).

Adolescents increasingly acquire the abilities needed to think abstractly and logically, to consider the future more, to take on the perspective of the third person, and to place greater importance on their roles in life (Zubenko, 2002). Accordingly, they are better able than a few years prior to infer the motives behind others' actions and/or maltreatment, although they may still not be able to fully comprehend the reasons. The full impact of prior or contemporary abuse may not be appreciated until the individual further develops and engages in more mature relationships and responsibilities and develops more sophisticated cognitive capabilities (Lubit et al., 2003). Essentially, abuse and trauma, including neglect, exacerbate the potential stressfulness of developmental changes, such as the onset of puberty, more difficult classes, or changing from one school to another, resulting in a greater likelihood of cognitive deficits (Kendall-Tackett & Eckenrode, 1996).

Importantly, situational influences can increase or decrease one's risk of poor adjustment outcomes following trauma. Persons who were exposed to childhood sexual abuse but did not go on to develop adjustment difficulties were characterized by positive family factors, such as parental care and parental attachment, and more positive peer affiliations in adolescence (Lynskey & Fergusson, 1997). Similar studies have found intrapersonal, interpersonal, and contextual factors that support the ability to recover from the impact of abuse and trauma, such as family cohesion, social support, and the presence of caring relationships in the family, at school, and in the community (Resnick et al., 1997).

ASSESSMENT

Assessment of trauma-related symptoms should include comprehensive clinical interviews with the youth and his or her parents/guardians. The adolescent should be encouraged to talk about the details of the traumatic event in order for the clinician to identify current stressors and psychological symptoms related to the trauma, the types of coping skills used, and the impact of the trauma on overall functioning. The symptoms of reexperiencing, avoidance, and hyperarousal should be queried, as they comprise the main PTSD diagnostic criteria. Researchers have also emphasized the need for assessment instruments that measure PTSD across different areas of functioning, such as school and home (Kratochwill, 1996; McNally, 1996a). Several assessment scales are available to clinicians and researchers to assess PTSD symptoms, which should be accompanied by a comprehensive clinical interview.

In general, assessment measures range from structured interviews administered by clinicians to self-report scales completed by clients. Although there are no structured interviews available to specifically assess for the presence of PTSD symptoms, there are other general standardized interviews for children and adolescents that contain modules that assess PTSD

symptoms. Some of these include the Diagnostic Interview for Children and Adolescents—Revised (DICA-R; Reich, 1997), the Diagnostic Interview Schedule for Children—Version IV (DISC-IV; Shaffer, Fisher, Lucas, Dulcan, & Schwab-Stone, 2000), and the Schedule for Affective Disorders and Schizophrenia for School-Age Children—Present and Lifetime Version (K-SADS-PL; Kaufman, Birmaher, Brent, & Rao, 2000). There are also scales available to assess traumatic sequelae in adolescents. Because these are relatively new measures that have been developed over the past few decades, the psychometric properties of these measures have yet to be fully established. Many of these scales are based on adult measures that have been changed to meet the developmental needs of adolescents and children and, unfortunately, have few adolescent norms. The following is an overview of some of the more promising measures to assess trauma, violence exposure, dissociative symptoms, and bullying with adequate psychometric properties; the reader is referred to Ohan, Myers, and Collett (2002) for a comprehensive review of trauma-related scales.

The Children's Post-Traumatic Stress Reaction Index (CPTS-RI; Frederick, Pynoos, & Nader, 1992; Pynoos et al., 1987) is a 20-item measure that is the children's version of the Posttraumatic Stress Reduction Index used with adults. It can be used both as a clinician administered scale and a self-report measure for children and youth ages 8–18 years old. As well as assessing the symptoms of PTSD, the measure classifies symptoms into three clusters: Numbing/Avoiding, Reexperiencing, and Hyperarousal. The CPTS-RI can be used with youth of diverse cultural backgrounds and traumatic experiences based on its use in extensive trauma research (e.g., Allwood, Bell-Dolan, & Husain, 2002; Gordon, Staples, Blyta, & Bytyqi, 2004).

The Children's PTSD Inventory (CPTSDI, Saigh, 2002; Saigh et al., 2000) is a clinician-administered scale for youth ages 7–18. The items are based on developmental modifications of the PTSD DSM-IV criteria (Ohan et al., 2002). This measure has five subscales: Situational reactivity, Reexperiencing, Avoidance and Numbing, Increased Arousal, and Significant Impairment. The Child PTSD Symptom Scale (CPSS) is used with children and youth ages 8–15 years old, and has age-appropriate norms. The CPSS is the child version of the Posttraumatic Diagnostic Scale for Adults (Foa, Johnson, Feeny & Treadwell, 2001) and has developmentally appropriate wording to assess PTSD symptoms. The three main subscales are Reexperiencing, Avoidance, and Arousal, as well as Functional Impairment. It has been used with different cultural groups (e.g., Kataoka et al., 2003) and to measure treatment improvement (e.g., Stein, Jaycox, Kataoka, Wong, et al., 2003).

The Children's Impact of Events Scale—13 (CRIES-13; Children and War Foundation, 1998) is based on the revised Impact of Event Scale (Weiss & Marmar, 1997), and it is used with individuals ages 8 and older. This self-report measure has 13 items measuring PTSD symptoms over the past 14 days and provides information on levels of intrusion, avoidance, and arousal in children and adolescents. It has been used in research with children from different cultural backgrounds (e.g., those who have experienced conflict in Bosnia) (Smith, Perrin, Dyregrov, & Yule, 2002). Ohan and colleagues (2002) suggest that this measure and the CPTS-RI are the best measures to use to assess post-traumatic symptoms in different cultural populations.

The Trauma Symptom Checklist for Children (TSCC; Briere, 1996) is a 54-item measure (ages 7–16) that is used to assess distress and related symptoms after an acute or chronic trauma, not PTSD diagnostic symptoms per se. There are also 44- and 40-item versions that do not contain sexual trauma symptoms, known as the TSCC-Alternative Form (Zlotnick, Shea, Begin, & Pearlstein, 1996). The TSCC has six subscales: Anxiety, Depression, Anger, Posttraumatic Stress, Dissociation, and Sexual Concerns, and two validity scales to detect underreporting. An advantage of this measure is that is has a large normative base and can be useful to examine symptom profiles and symptom course following trauma (Ohan et al., 2002).

The Clinician-Administered PTSD Scale for Children (CAPS-C; Nader et al., 2002) is used to assess the frequency and intensity of symptoms associated with PTSD, as well as the impact of those symptoms on personal functioning such as overall distress, coping skills, and impairment. This measure is used to assess children and adolescents ages 8–18 and is based on the CAPS, developed for use with adults (Blake et al., 1995). Although the psychometric data on the CAPS-C is limited, it has been used

widely as a measure of coping strategies in youth following a trauma (Stallard, Velleman, Langsford, & Baldwin, 2001) and treatment changes (March, Amaya-Jackson, Murray, & Schulte, 1998; Seedat, Lockhat, Kaminer, Zungu-Dirwayi, & Stein, 2001).

Scales to measure more specific exposure to abuse and trauma also exist, such as exposure to violence in the home (e.g., Childhood Trauma Questionnaire [CTQ]; Bernstein & Finkelhor, 1998) and in the community (e.g., Children's Report of Exposure to Violence [CREV]; Cooley-Quille, Turner, & Beidel, 1995). The CTQ retrospectively measures the frequency of emotional, physical, and sexual abuse, as well as emotional and physical neglect during childhood and adolescents in individuals 12 years old and older. It has a range of clinical (e.g., to facilitate dialogue with a youth about abuse experiences) and research (e.g., quick, easy to complete, good preliminary psychometric research) uses. The CREV is a 29-item scale that can be used with children and adolescents ages 8–18, which assesses children's exposure to violence through the media as reported by others, directly witnessed, and directly experienced. It also includes three categories of victims: Self, Strangers, and Familiar Persons. Researchers have also used a modified version of the Life Events Scale (Singer, Anglin, Song, & Lunghofer, 1995), a 34-item measure that assesses the frequency of several types of community violence (e.g., threats, beatings, knife attacks, and shootings) in multiple locations over the past year and lifetime (Kataoka et al., 2003. This measure has been shown to have acceptable reliability in elementary, middle school, and high schools in multicultural inner-city populations (Singer et al., 1995).

Appropriate measures to assess bullying experiences in adolescents include the Peer Relations Questionnaire (PRQ; Rigby & Slee, 1993), the Peer Relations Assessment Questionnaire (PRAQ; Rigby 1997), and the Revised Bully/Victim Questionnaire (R-BVQ; Olweus, 1996). The first two measures can be used with children and adolescents ages 8–18, and the latter one for adolescents ages 11–16. All measures have large normative samples (the PRQ and PRAQ are normed in Australia, and the R-BVQ is normed in Norway) and good psychometric properties (Griffin & Gross, 2004).

With respect to dissociative symptoms, the Adolescent Dissociative Experiences Schedule

(A-DES; Armstrong, Putnam, Carlson, Libero, & Smith, 1997) is an adolescent version of the Dissociative Experiences Schedule (Bernstein & Putnam, 1986; van IJzendoorn & Schuengel, 1996). It is a self-report measure for use with adolescents ages 11–17 years old and is comprised of four subscales: Dissociative Amnesia, Absorption and Imaginative Involvement, Passive Influence, and Depersonalization/Derealization.

TREATMENT AND PREVENTION

In general, few studies have examined the treatment of PTSD in children and adolescents, resulting in a reliance on the adult literature (Foa & Meadows, 1997). Nonetheless, individual interventions with a trauma-focused cognitive-behavioral framework have received the most support with children and adolescents (Cohen, Berliner, & Mannarino, 2000, 2003; Cohen, Deblinger, Mannarino, & Steer, 2004; Davis & Siegel, 2000; Pfferbaum, 1997). There is also a lot of research supporting empirically derived school-based programs to treat and prevent trauma symptoms in adolescents and, to a lesser extent, residential-based programs. These issues are discussed next.

Trauma-Focused Cognitive-Behavioral Therapy

Over the past 10 years the majority of research has focused on treating children and youth who have been sexually abused (Saywitz, Mannarino, Berliner, & Cohen, 2000). Pine and Cohen (2002) reviewed six randomized controlled trails that used trauma-focused cognitive-behavioral therapy (TF-CBT) to treat PTSD and anxiety symptoms in children who have been sexually abused, and they concluded that there is relatively strong evidence of the efficacy of CBT. These studies also reported a decrease in PTSD symptoms, and the inclusion of parents produced significantly more improvements in externalizing and depressive symptoms. Most studies have involved preadolescents, with only one including older adolescents (i.e., King et al., 2000; ages 5–17 years old). Cohen, Berliner, and Mannarino (2000) also concluded that no single treatment approach will likely be applicable for all traumatized children as this population presents with a diversity of emotional and behavioral difficulties. Although there has been a lot of empirical support for TF-CBT, the mechanisms by which children and adolescent's improve are beginning to be explored. Another recent review has outlined the empirical support for the four major components of TF-CBT for children and adolescents, again relying on adult PTSD literature: exposure, cognitive processing and reframing, stress management, and parental treatment (see Cohen, Mannarino, Berliner, & Deblinger, 2000, for a discussion of these components).

School-Based Intervention Programs

Many researchers have developed school-based trauma intervention programs (Glodich, Allen, & Arnold, 2001; March et al., 1998; Saltzman, Pynoos, Layne, Steinberg, & Aisenberg, 2001; Saltzman, Steinberg, Layne, Aisenberg, & Pynoos, 2001). These programs are useful in that they can target a large number of students who may have been exposed to a community trauma or share other similar traumatic experiences. School-based programs can also be useful to treat children and adolescents who live in underserviced areas, such as rural communities. March and colleagues (1998) used a school-based group CBT program to treat children and adolescents who experienced PTSD symptoms after a single-incident stressor. The authors used multimodality trauma treatment (MMTT), which is a manualized CBT treatment that is based on social and biological theories underlying PTSD and incorporates anxiety-management training, relaxation training, a problem-solving approach to anger control, and a stimulus hierarchy. The results indicated that children and adolescents treated with MMTT showed significant improvement on PTDS, depression, and anxiety. This treatment modality provided evidence that gradual exposure to anxiety-provoking material resulted in symptom reductions. Unfortunately, the study did not use a control group, and the average age included school-age children (age 12) and not adolescents. Hickman and colleagues (2004) completed a review of dating violence treatment and prevention programs, most of which were school based. They concluded that the evaluation literature related to these projects is limited and has many methodological problems (e.g., no comparison groups and brief follow-up periods). Promising findings for a community-based intervention program, the

Youth Relationships Project, were discussed in relation to early intervention for at-risk youth from abusive or traumatic backgrounds (Wolfe et al., 2003).

School-based programs have also been effective at reducing bullying, although decreases in the rates of victimization before and after implementing the programs vary across studies. Smith (2004) presented information on more than 12 multischool intervention programs implemented in various countries. Many of the programs are based on a seminal antibullying initiative in Norway, the Bullying Prevention Program (Kallestad & Olweus, 2003). The goal of the program is to facilitate schools being safe and positive learning environments by reducing existing bullying problems, preventing future bullying problems, and achieving better peer relations at school. This is accomplished by a whole-school approach that is underlined by redirecting bullying into more prosocial behaviors. The whole-school approach involves giving information to all school administrators, teachers, and staff, as well as parents, about bullies and victims (e.g., common myths and causes) and intervention and prevention guidelines. The program resulted in substantial reductions (50% or more) in students' reports of bullying and victimization, general antisocial behaviors, and improvements in school climate (e.g., improved order and discipline in classrooms and more positive attitude toward schoolwork and the school; Kallestad & Olweus, 2003). Other programs based on this model in other countries typically report a range of 5–20% decrease in victimization (Smith, 2004). Despite the success of Olweus's program, the actual mechanisms of improvement have yet to be determined. Kallestad and Olweus (2003) report evidence that the successful implementation of the program was not related to the degree of implementation of a specific component of the program but instead by variables related to teachers. For instance, teachers who recognized or suspected bullying in their classrooms, and who saw themselves, their colleagues, and their schools as important agents of changes, were more likely to implement the program. As well, schools with higher levels of open communication implemented more of the program.

Other factors that affect the success of bullying programs include the extent to which schools take ownership of the antibullying program and the importance of a sustained period of intervention, as opposed to a "one-time" effort. Antibullying programs should focus on broader school climate issues and relationships in schools, as opposed to focusing on bullying alone (Roland & Galloway, 2002). As well, programs in which implementation was systematically monitored were more effective than programs without any monitoring (Smith, Schneider, Smith, & Ananiadou, 2004).

Other researchers have developed programs that target trauma experiences in different cultural groups, which are often underserviced. Kataoka and colleagues (2003) completed an 8-week group TF-CBT program for Latino immigrant students who had been exposed to community violence and their families. Many (69%) of the children had been exposed to weapon-related violence involving a knife or gun. This school-based program was a collaborative venture between school clinicians, educators, and researchers. The program compared 152 children who completed the intervention program to 46 wait-list controls. There was a significant decrease in PTSD symptoms in the intervention group, although this decrease was only significant for depression scores, not PTSD scores, compared to the wait-list control. De Arellano and colleagues (2005) present a description of a community-based program that provided in-home and in-school evidenced-based treatment services for children and adolescents who have been abused and exposed to or victimized by crime. These authors provide a practical guide to the challenges of engaging these families and implementing the interventions across various settings, particularly in the family home. Outcome data on the effectiveness of the program have yet to be published, although the authors point out that it incorporates behavioral and cognitive-behavioral principles that are effective in treating posttraumatic symptoms in children and adolescents (de Arellano et al., 2005).

Residential-Based Intervention Program

Rivard and colleagues (Rivard et al., 2003, 2004) have published preliminary information on an intervention program aimed at youth with histories of maltreatment and exposure to family and community violence. Their program is based on the sanctuary model (Bloom, 1997), which was developed to treat adults with traumatic histories. A main tenet of the model is strengthening the therapeutic environment (i.e., modeling healthy relationships) in order to empower youth in positive ways. It also teaches youth effective adaptive and coping skills within a cognitive-behavioral framework. Preliminary data from the focus groups highlight the challenges of changing the organizational culture of the residence and improving staff and youth communication among each other and with community partners.

Pharmacotherapy

Although there is some evidence that psychotropic medications such as selective serotonin reuptake inhibitors (SSRIs) are efficacious in decreasing PTSD symptoms in adults (e.g., Hagh-Shenas, Goldstein, & Yule, 1999) and children (e.g., Seedat & Stein, 2001; Seedat et al., 2001; for review, see Schoenfeld, Marmar, & Neylan, 2004), only one randomized controlled pilot study has compared the efficacy of pharmacological treatment of trauma-related symptoms among children and adolescents (Robert, Blackeney, Villarreal, Rosenberg, & Meyer, 1999). As well, other researchers (Seedat et al., 2001; Wheatley, Plant, Reader, Brown, & Cahill, 2004) have reported beneficial effects of the SSRI citalopram in adolescents in open trials. Thus, although there is some support for pharmacological treatment of trauma symptoms in adolescents, it is too early to draw conclusions.

In sum, research on treating trauma in adolescents can be divided into individual or small-group programs and large-scale school-based programs. With respect to individual programs, interventions that are based on TF-CBT have the most empirical support. However, the majority of this research consists of treating abuse in younger children and may not translate into large treatment effects for adolescents, despite the evidence showing its effectiveness with adults. There is a need to have randomized controlled trials of TF-CBT with adolescents with a variety of traumatic experiences to incorporate developmental modifications that may be necessary. There are numerous examples of school-based programs being used to treat and prevent trauma in adolescents. Many of them show promising preliminary results (e.g., MMTT; March et al., 1998) or more established results (e.g., the Bullying Prevention Program; Olweus, 1995). The benefit of these school-based programs is that they can address the larger contextual and social factors that are important in preventing trauma in youth, such as the role of teachers, geographical location, school climate, interpersonal relationships, and culture.

REFERENCES

Ackard, D. M., & Neumark-Sztainer, D. (2002). Date violence and date rape among adolescents: associations with disordered eating behaviors and psychological health. *Child Abuse and Neglect, 26,* 455–473.

Ackard, D. M., & Neumark-Sztainer, D. (2003). Multiple sexual victimizations among adolescent boys and girls: prevalence and associations with eating behaviors and psychological health. *Journal of Child Sexual Abuse, 12,* 17–37.

Ackard, D. M., Neumark-Sztainer, D., Hanna, P. J., French, S., & Story, M. (2001). Binge and purge behavior among adolescents: associations with sexual and physical abuse in a nationally representative sample: The Commonwealth Fund survey. *Child Abuse and Neglect, 25,* 771–785.

Ackerman, P. T., Newton, J. E. O., McPherson, W. B., Jones, J. G., & Dykman, R. A. (1998). Prevalence of posttraumatic stress disorder and other psychiatric diagnoses in three groups of abused children (sexual, physical, and both). *Child Abuse and Neglect, 22,* 759–774.

Allwood, M. A., Bell-Dolan, D., & Husain, S. A. (2002). Children's trauma and adjustment reactions to violent and nonviolent war experiences. *Journal of the American Academy of Child and Adolescent Psychiatry, 41,* 450–457.

American Psychiatric Association (1994). *Diagnostic and statistical manual of mental disorders* (4th ed.). Washington, DC: Author.

Amsel, L., & Marshall, R. D. (2003). Clinical management of subsyndromal psychological sequelae of the 9/11 terror attacks. In S. W. Coates, J. L. Rosenthal, & D. S. Schechter (Eds.), *September 11: Trauma and human bonds* (pp. 75–97). Hillsdale, NJ: Analytic Press.

Armstrong, J. G., Putnam, F. W., Carlson, E. B., Libero, D. Z., & Smith, S. R. (1997). Development and validation of a measure of adolescent dissociation. The Adolescent Dissociative Experiences Scale. *Journal of Nervous and Mental Disease, 185,* 491–497.

Bal, S., Crombez, G., Van Oost, P., & De Bourdeaudhuji, I. (2003). The role of social support in well-being and coping with self-reported stressful events in adolescents. *Child Abuse and Neglect, 27,* 1377–1395.

Bal, S., De Bourdeaudhuji, I., Crombez, G., & Van Oost, P. (2004). Differences in trauma symptoms and family functioning in intra- and extra familial sexually abused adolescents. *Journal of Interpersonal Violence, 19,* 108–123.

Bal, S., Van Oost, P., De Bourdeaudhuji, I., & Crombez, G. (2003). Avoidant coping as a mediator between self-reported sexual abuse and stress-related symptoms in adolescents. *Child Abuse and Neglect, 27,* 883–897.

Baldry, A. C., & Winkel, F. W. (2003). Direct and vicarious victimization at school and at home as risk factors for suicidal cognition among Italian adolescents. *Journal of Adolescence, 26,* 703–716.

Bank, L., & Burraston, B. (2001). Abusive home environments as predictors of poor adjustment during adolescence and early childhood. *Journal of Community Psychology, 29,* 195–217.

Bergen, H. A., Martin G., Richardson, A. S., Allison, S., & Roeger, L. (2004). Sexual abuse, antisocial behavior and substance use: Gender differences in young community adolescents. *Australian and New Zealand Journal of Psychiatry, 38,* 34–41.

Bernstein, D., & Finkelhor, L. (1998). *Childhood Trauma Questionnaire: A retrospective self-report.* San Antonio, TX: Psychological Corporation.

Bernstein, E. M., & Putnam, F. W. (1986). Development, reliability, and validity of a dissociation scale. *Journal of Nervous and Mental Disease, 174,* 727–735.

Blake, D. D., Weathers, F. W., Nagy, L. M., Kaloupek, D. G., Gusman, F. D., Charney, D. S., & Keane, T. M. (1995). The development of a Clinician-Administered PTSD Scale. *Journal of Traumatic Stress, 8,* 75–90.

Bloom, S. (1997). *Creating sanctuary: Toward the evolution of sane societies.* New York: Routledge.

Bolger, K. E., & Patterson, C. J. (2001). Pathways from child maltreatment to internalizing problems: Perceptions of control as mediators and moderators. *Development and Psychopathology, 13,* 913–940.

Boney-McCoy, S., & Finkelhor, D. (1995). Prior victimization: A risk factor for child sexual abuse and for PTSD-related symptomatology among sexually abused youth. *Child Abuse and Neglect, 19,* 1401–1421.

Borg, M. G. (1999). The extent and nature of bullying among primary and secondary schoolchildren. *Educational Research, 41,* 137–153.

Breslau, N., Kessler, R. C., Chilcoat, H. D., Schultz, L. R., Davis, G. C., & Andreski, P. (1998). Trauma and posttraumatic stress disorder in the community: The 1996 Detroit area survey of trauma. *Archives of General Psychiatry, 55,* 626–632.

Briere, J. N. (1992). *Child abuse trauma: Theory and treatment of the lasting effects.* Thousand Oaks, CA: Sage.

Briere, J. (1996). *Trauma Symptom Checklist for Children (TSCC): Professional manual.* Lutz, FL: Psychological Assessment Resources.

British Broadcasting Corporation. (2002). *Youngsters targeted by digital bullies* [Online]. Available: news.bbc.co.uk/hi/english/uk/newsid_1929000/1929944.stm

Brown, J., Cohen, P., Johnson, J. G., & Smailes, E. M. (1999). Childhood abuse and neglect: Specificity and effects on adolescent and young adult depression and suicidality. *Journal of the American Academy of Child and Adolescent Psychiatry, 38,* 1490–1496.

Buzi, R. S., Tortolero, S. R., Roberts, R. E., Ross, M. W., Addy, R. C., & Markham, C. M. (2003). The impact of a history of sexual abuse on high-risk sexual behaviors among females attending alternative schools. *Adolescence, 38,* 595–605.

Capaldi, D. M., & Gorman-Smith, D. (2003). The development of aggression in young male–female couples. In P. Florsheim (Ed.), *Adolescent romantic relations and sexual behavior: Theory, research, and practical implications* (pp. 243–278). Mahwah, NJ: Erlbaum.

Cecil H., & Matson, S. C. (2001). Psychological functioning and family discord among African-American adolescent females with and without a history of childhood sexual abuse. *Child Abuse and Neglect, 25,* 983–988.

Chandy, J. M., Blum, R. W., & Resnick, M. D. (1996). Gender-specific outcomes for sexually abused adolescents. *Child Abuse and Neglect, 20,* 1219–1231.

Children and War Foundation. (1998). *The Children's Impact of Event's Scale (13) CRIES-13* [Online]. Available: www.childrenandwar.org/CRIES-13.doc

Cicchetti, D., & Lynch, M. (1995). Failures in the expectable environment and their impact on individual development: The case of child maltreatment. In D. Cicchetti & D. J. Cohen (Eds.), *Developmental psychopathology: Vol. 2. Risk, disorder, and adaptation.* (pp. 32–71). Oxford, UK: Wiley.

Cicchetti, D., Toth, S. L., & Maughan, A. (2000). An ecological-transactional model of child maltreatment. In A. Sameroff, M. Lewis, & S. Miller (Eds.), *Handbook of developmental psychopathology* (2nd ed., pp. 689–722). New York: Kluwer/Plenum Press.

Cohen, J. (1998). Practice parameters for the assessment and treatment of children and adolescents with posttraumatic stress disorder. *Journal of the American Academy of Child and Adolescent Psychiatry, 37*(Suppl. 10), 4S-26S.

Cohen, J. A., Berliner, L., & Mannarino, A. P. (2000). Treating traumatized children: A research review and synthesis. *Trauma Violence and Abuse, 1,* 29–46.

Cohen, J. A., Berliner, L., & Mannarino, A. P. (2003). Psychosocial and pharmacological interventions for child crime victims. *Journal of Traumatic Stress, 16,* 175–186.

Cohen, J. A., Deblinger, E., Mannarino, A. P., & Steer, R. A. (2004). A multi-site, randomized controlled trial for children with sexual abuse-related PTSD symptoms. *Journal of the American Academy of Child and Adolescent Psychiatry, 43,* 393–402.

Cohen, J. A., Mannarino, A. P., Berliner, L., & Deblinger, E. (2000). Trauma-focused cognitive behavioral therapy for children and adolescents: An empirical update. *Journal of Interpersonal Violence, 15,* 1202–1223.

Coid, J., Petruckevitch, A., Feder, G., Chung, W., Richardson, J., & Moorey, S. (2001). Relation between childhood sexual and physical abuse and risk of revitimization in women: A cross-sectional survey. *The Lancet, 358,* 450–454.

Cooley-Quille, M. R., Turner, S. M., & Beidel, D. C. (1995). Emotional impact of children's exposure to community violence: A preliminary study. *Journal of the American Academy of Child and Adolescent Psychiatry, 34,* 1362–1368.

Costello, E. J., Erkanli, A., Fairbank, J. A., & Angold, A. (2002). The prevalence of potentially traumatic events in childhood and adolescence. *Journal of Traumatic Stress, 15,* 99–112.

Crouch, J. L., Hanson, R. F., Saunders, B. E., Kilpatrick, D. G., & Resnick, H. S. (2000). Income, race/ethnicity, and exposure to violence in youth: Results from the national survey of adolescents. *Journal of Community Psychology, 28,* 625–641.

Cyr, M., Wright, J., Toupin, J., Oxman-Martinez, J., McDuff, P., & Theriault, C. (2003). Predictors of maternal support: The point of view of adolescent victims of sexual abuse and their mothers. *Journal of Child Sexual Abuse, 12,* 39–65.

Davis, L., & Siegel, L. J. (2000). Posttraumatic stress disorder in children and adolescents: A review and analysis. *Clinical Child and Family Psychology Review, 3,* 135–154.

de Arellano, M. A., Waldrop, A. E., Deblinger, E., Cohen, J. A., Danielson, C. K., & Mannarino, A. R. (2005). Community outreach program for child victims of traumatic events: A community-based project for underserved populations. *Behavior Modification Special, Beyond Exposure for Posttraumatic Stress Disorder Symptoms: Broad-Spectrum PTSD Treatment Strategies, 29,* 130–155.

DeBellis, M. D. (2001). Developmental traumatology: The psychobiological development of maltreated children and its implications for research, treatment, and policy. *Development and Psychopathology Special, Stress and Development: Biological and Psychological Consequences, 13,* 539–564.

DeBellis, M. D., Keshavan, M. S., Frustaci, K., Shifflett, H., Iyengar, S., & Beers, S. R., & Hall, J. (2002). Superior temporal gyrus volumes in maltreated children and adolescents with PTSD. *Biological Psychiatry, 51,* 544–552.

DeBellis, M. D., & Putnam, F. W. (1994). The psychology of childhood maltreatment. *Child and Adolescent Psychiatric Clinics of North America, 3,* 663–678.

de Decker, A., Hermans, D., Raes, F., & Eelen, P. (2003). Autobiographical memory specificity and trauma in inpatient adolescents. *Journal of Clinical Child and Adolescent Psychology, 32,* 22–31.

Deykin, E. Y., & Buka, S. L. (1997). Prevalence and risk factors for posttraumatic stress disorder among chemically dependent adolescents. *American Journal of Psychiatry, 154,* 752–757.

Eckenrode, J., Powers, J. L., & Garbarino, J. (1997). Youth in trouble are youth who have been hurt. In J. Garbarino & J. Eckenrode (Eds.), *Understanding abusive families: An ecological approach to theory and practice* (pp.166–193). San Francisco: Jossey-Bass.

Elinoff, M. J., Chafouleas, S. M., & Sassu, K. A. (2004). Bullying: considering for defining and intervening in school settings. *Psychology in the Schools Special, Differentiation of Emotional Disturbance and Social Maladjustment, 41,* 887–897.

Elklit, A. (2002). Victimization and PTSD in a Danish national youth probability sample. *Journal of the American Academy of Child and Adolescent Psychiatry, 41,* 174–181.

Elliott, G. C., Avery, R., Fishman, E., & Hoshiko, B. (2002). The encounter with family violence and risky sexual activity among young adolescent females. *Violence and Victims, 17,* 569–592.

Fagan, A. A. (2003). The short- and long-term effects of adolescent violent victimization experienced within the family and community. *Violence and Victims, 18,* 445–459.

Famularo, R., Fenton, T., Augustyn, M., & Zuckerman, B. (1996). Persistence of pediatric posttraumatic stress disorder after 2 years. *Child Abuse and Neglect, 20,* 1245–1248.

Feiring, C., Coates, D. L., & Taska, L. S. (2001). Ethnic status, stigmatization, support, and symptoms development following sexual abuse. *Journal of Interpersonal Violence, 16,* 1307–1329.

Feiring, C., Taska, L., & Lewis, M. (1999). Age and gender differences in children's and adolescents' adaptation to sexual abuse. *Child Abuse and Neglect, 23,* 115–128.

Felitti, V. J., Anda, R. F., Nordenberg, D., Williamson, D. F., Spitz, A. M., & Edwards, V., et al. (1998). Relationship of childhood abuse and household dysfunction to many of the leading causes of death in adults: The adverse childhood experiences (ACE) study. *American Journal of Preventive Medicine, 14,* 245–258.

Fergusson, D. M., Horwood, L. J., & Lynskey, M. T. (1997). Childhood sexual abuse, adolescent sexual behaviors and sexual revictimization. *Child Abuse and Neglect, 21,* 789–803.

Finkelhor, D. (1990). Early and long-term effects of child sexual abuse: An update. *Professional Psychology: Research and Practice, 21,* 325–330.

Finkelhor, D. (1995). The victimization of children: A developmental perspective. *American Journal of Orthopsychiatry, 65,* 177–193.

Finkelhor, D., & Browne, A. (1985). The traumatic impact of child sexual abuse: A conceptualization. *American Journal of Orthopsychiatry, 55,* 530–541.

Finkelhor, D., Mitchell, K., & Wolak, J. (2000). *Online victimization: A report on the nation's youth* [Online]. National Centre for Missing and Exploited Children. Available: www.unh.edu/ccrc/Youth_ Internet_info_page.html

Flannery, D. J., Singer, M. I., & Wester, K. L. (2003). Violence, coping, and mental health in a community sample of adolescents. *Violence and Victims, 18,* 403–418.

Flisher, A. J., Kramer, R. A., Grosser, R. C., Alegria, M., Bird, H. R., & Bourdon, K. H. et al. (1997). Correlates of unmet need for mental health services by children and adolescents. *Psychological Medicine, 27,* 1145–1154.

Foa, E., Johnson, K., Feeny, N., & Treadwell, K. R. (2001). The child PTSD symptom scale: A preliminary examination of its psychometric properties. *Journal of Clinical Child Psychology, 30,* 376–384.

Foa, E. B., & Meadows, E. A. (1997). Psychosocial treatments for posttraumatic stress disorder: A critical review. *Annual Review of Psychology, 48,* 449–480.

Foster, J. D., Kuperminc, G. P., & Price, A. W. (2004). Gender differences in posttraumatic stress and related symptoms among inner-city minority youth exposed to community violence. *Journal of Youth and Adolescence, 33,* 59–69.

Frederick, C. Pynoos, R., & Nader, K. (1992). *Reactor Index to Psychic Trauma Form C (child).* Unpublished manuscript, University of California at Los Angeles.

Freyd, J. J. (1997). Violations of power, adaptive blindness and betrayal trauma theory. *Feminism and Psychology, 7,* 22–32.

Garbarino, J., Eckenrode, J., & Powers, J. L. (1997). The maltreatment of youth. In J. Garbarino & J. Eckenrode (Eds.), *Understanding abusive families: An ecological approach to theory and practice* (pp.145–165). San Francisco: Jossey-Bass.

Garnefski, N., & Arends, E. (1998). Sexual abuse and adolescent maladjustment: Differences between male and female victims. *Journal of Adolescence, 21,* 99–107.

Giaconia, R. M., Reinherz, H. Z., Silverman, A. B., & Pakiz, B. (1994). Ages of onset of psychiatric disorders in a community population of older adolescents. *Journal of the American Academy of Child and Adolescent Psychiatry, 33,* 706–717.

Gibson, L. E., & Leitenberg, H. (2001). The impact of child sexual abuse and stigma on methods of coping with sexual assault among undergraduate women. *Child Abuse and Neglect, 25,* 1343–1361.

Gladstone, G., Parker, G., Mitchell, P., Malhi, G., Wilhelm, K., & Austin, M.P. (2004). Implications of childhood trauma for depressed women: An analysis of pathways from childhood sexual abuse to deliberate self-harm and revitalization. *American Journal of Psychiatry, 161,* 1417–1425.

Glodich, A., Allen, J. G., & Arnold, L. (2001). Protocol for a trauma-based psychoeducational group intervention to decrease risk-taking, reenactment, and further violence exposure: Application to the public high school setting. *Journal of Child and Adolescent Group Therapy, 11,* 87–107.

Gordon, J. S., Staples, J. K., Blyta, A., & Bytyqi, M. (2004). Treatment of posttraumatic stress disorder in postwar Kosovo high school students using mind–body skills groups: A pilot study. *Journal of Traumatic Stress, 17,* 143–147.

Green, B. L. (1994). Psychosocial research in traumatic stress: An update. *Journal of Traumatic Stress, 7,* 341–362.

Greenwald, R. (2002). The role of trauma in conduct disorder. *Journal of Aggression, Maltreatment, and Trauma, 6,* 5–23.

Grella, C. E., & Joshi, V. (2003). Treatment processes and outcomes among adolescents with a history of abuse who are in drug treatment. *Child Maltreatment, 8,* 7–18.

Griffin, R. S., & Gross, A. M. (2004). Childhood bullying: Current empirical findings and future directions for research. *Aggression and Violent Behavior, 9,* 379–400.

Guterman, N. B., Hahm, H. C., & Cameron, M. (2002). Adolescent victimization and subsequent use of mental health counseling services. *Journal of Adolescent Health, 30,* 336–345.

Hagh-Shenas, H., Goldstein, L., & Yule, W. (1999). Psychobiology of post-traumatic stress disorder. In W. Yule (Ed.), *Post-traumatic stress disorders: concepts and therapy* (pp. 139–160). New York: Wiley.

Hanson, R. F. (2002). Adolescent dating violence: Prevalence and psychological outcomes. *Child Abuse and Neglect, 26,* 447–451.

Hanson, R., Kievit, L., Saunders, B., Smith, D., Kilpatrick, D., Resnick, H., & Ruggiero, K (2003). Correlates of Adolescent Reports of Sexual Assault: Findings from the national survey of adolescents. *Child Maltreatment: Journal of the American Professional Society on the Abuse of Children, 8,* 261–272.

Harrison, P. A., Fulkerson, J. A., & Beebe, T. J. (1997). Multiple substance use among adolescent physical and sexual abuse victims. *Child Abuse and Neglect, 21,* 529–539.

Hickman, L. J., Jaycox, L. H., & Aronoff, J. (2004). Dating violence among adolescents: Prevalence, gender distribution, and prevention program effectiveness. *Trauma Violence and Abuse, 5,* 123–142.

Hilarski, C. (2004). Victimization history as a risk factor for conduct disorder behaviors: Exploring connections in a national sample of youth. *Stress, Trauma, and Crisis: An International Journal, 7,* 47–59.

James, D. J., Sofroniou, N., & Lawlor, M. (2003). The response of Irish adolescents to bullying. *Irish Journal of Psychology, 24,* 22–34.

Jaycox, L. H., Ebener, P., Damesek, L., & Becker, K. (2004). Trauma exposure and retention in adolescent substance abuse treatment. *Journal of Traumatic Stress, 17,* 113–121.

Johnson, P. (2001). In their own voices: Report of a study on the later effects of child sexual abuse. *Journal of Sexual Aggression, 7,* 41–56.

Kallestad, J. H., & Olweus, D. (2003). Predicting teachers' and schools' implementation of the Olweus bullying prevention program: A multilevel study [Online]. *Prevention and Treatment, 6.* Available: http://journals.apa.org/prevention/volume6/pre0060021a.html

Kataoka, S. H., Stein, B. D., Jaycox, L. H., Wong, M., Escudero, P., & Tu, W. et al. (2003). A school-based mental health program for traumatized Latino immigrant children. *Journal of the American Academy of Child and Adolescent Psychiatry, 42,* 311–318.

Kaufman, J., Birmaher, B., Brent, D., & Rao, U. (2000). Kiddi-SADS-Present and Lifetime Version. *Journal of the American Academy of Child and Adolescent Psychiatry, 39,* 1208.

Kellogg, N. D., & Hoffman, T. J. (1995). Unwanted and illegal sexual experiences in childhood and adolescence. *Child Abuse and Neglect, 19,* 1457–1468.

Kellogg, N. D., & Menard, S. W. (2003). Violence among family members of children and adolescents evaluated for sexual abuse. *Child Abuse and Neglect, 27,* 1367–1376.

Kendall-Tackett, K. A., & Eckenrode, J. (1996). The effects of neglect on academic achievement and disciplinary problems: A developmental perspective. *Child Abuse and Neglect, 20,* 161–169.

Kendler, K. S., Bulik, C. M., Silberg, J., Hettema, J. M., Myers, J., & Prescott, C. A. (2000). Childhood sexual abuse and adult psychiatric and substance use disorders in women: An epidemiological and co-twin control analysis. *Archives of General Psychiatry, 57,* 953–959.

Kessler, R. C., Sonnega, A., Bromet, E., Hughes, M., & Nelson, C. B. (1995). Posttraumatic stress disorder in the national comorbidity survey. *Archives of General Psychiatry, 52,* 1048–1060.

Kilpatrick, D. G., Ruggiero, K. J., Acierno, R., Saunders, B. E., Resnick, H. S., & Best, C. L. (2003). Violence and risk of PTSD, major depression, substance abuse/dependence, and comorbidity: results from the national survey of adolescents. *Journal of Consulting and Clinical Psychology, 71,* 692–700.

King, G., Trocmé, N., & Thatte, N. (2003). Substantiation as a multi-tier process: The results of a NIS-3 analysis. *Child Maltreatment: Journal of the American Professional Society on the Abuse of Children, 8,* 173–182.

King, N. J., Tonge, B. J., Mullen, P., Myerson, N., Heyne, D., & Rollings, S. (2000). Treating sexually abused children with posttraumatic stress symptoms: A randomized clinical trial. *Journal of the American Academy of Child and Adolescent Psychiatry, 39,* 1347–1355.

Kiser, L. J., Heston, J., Millsap, P. A., & Pruitt, D. B. (1991). Physical and sexual abuse in childhood: Relationship with post-traumatic stress disorder. *Journal of the American Academy of Child and Adolescent Psychiatry, 30,* 776–783.

Klaus, P., & Rennison, C. M. (2002). *Age patterns in violent victimization, 1976–2002* (NCJ 190104). Washington, DC: U.S. Department of Justice, Office of Justice Programs, Bureau of Justice Statistics.

Kratochwill, T. R. (1996). Posttraumatic stress disorder in children and adolescents: commentary and recommendations. *Journal of School Psychology: Special Posttraumatic Stress Disorder, 34,* 185–188.

Lange, A., de Beurs, E., Dolan, C., Lachnit, T., Sjollema, S., & Hanewald, G. (1999). Long-term effects of childhood sexual abuse: Objective and subjective characteristics of the abuse and psychopathology in later life. *Journal of Nervous and Mental Disease, 187,* 150–158.

Leitenberg, H., Gibson, L. E., & Novy, P. L. (2004). Individual differences among undergraduate women in methods of coping with stressful events: The impact of cumulative childhood stressors and abuse. *Child Abuse and Neglect, 28,* 181–192.

Lipschitz, D. S., Rasmusson, A. M., Anyan, W., Gueorguieva, R., Billingslea, E. M., Cromwell, P. F., & Southwick, S. M. (2003). Posttraumatic stress disorder and substance use in inner-city adolescent girls. *Journal of Nervous and Mental Disease, 191,* 714–721.

Lipschitz, D., Winegar, R., Hartnick, E., Foote, B., & Southwick, S. (1999). Posttraumatic stress disorder in hospitalized adolescents: psychiatric comorbidity and clinical correlates. *Journal of the American Academy of Child and Adolescent Psychiatry, 38,* 385–392.

Lubit, R., Rovine, D., DeFrancisci, L., & Eth, S. (2003). Impact of trauma on children. *Journal of Psychiatric Practice, 9,* 128–138.

Lynskey, M. T., & Fergusson, D. M. (1997). Factors protecting against the development of adjustment difficulties in young adults exposed to childhood sexual abuse. *Child Abuse and Neglect, 21,* 1177–1190.

Maercker, A., & Karl, A. (2003). Lifespan-development differences in physiologic reactivity to loud tones in trauma victims: A pilot study. *Psychological Reports, 93,* 941–948.

March, J. S., Amaya-Jackson, L., Murray, M. C., & Schulte, A. (1998). Cognitive-behavioral psychotherapy for children and adolescents with posttraumatic stress disorder after a single-incident stressor. *Journal of the American Academy of Child and Adolescent Psychiatry, 37,* 585–593.

Margolin, G., & Gordis, E. B. (2000). The effects of family and community violence on children. *Annual Review of Psychology, 51,* 445–479.

Martin, G., Bergen, H. A., Richardson, A. S., Roeger, L., & Allison, S. (2004). Sexual abuse and suicidality: Gender differences in a large community sample of adolescents. *Child Abuse and Neglect, 28,* 491–503.

Maxwell, C. D., Robinson, A. L., & Post, L. A. (2003). The nature and predictors of sexual victimization and offending among adolescents. *Journal of Youth and Adolescence, 32,* 465–477.

Mazza, J. J., & Reynolds, W. M. (1999). Exposure to violence in younger inner-city adolescents: Relationships with suicidal ideation, depression and PTSD symptomology. *Journal of Abnormal Child Psychology, 27,* 203–213.

McCloskey, L. A., Figueredo, A. J., & Koss, M. P. (1995). The effects of systemic family violence on children's mental health. *Child Development, 66,* 1239–1261.

McCloskey, L. A., & Walker, M. (2000). Posttraumatic

stress in children exposed to family violence and single-event trauma. *Journal of the American Academy of Child and Adolescent Psychiatry, 39,* 108–115.

McNally, R. J. (1996a). Assessment of posttraumatic stress disorder in children and adolescents. *Journal of School Psychology, 34,* 147–161.

McNally, R. J. (1996b). Cognitive bias in the anxiety disorders. In D. A. Hope (Ed.), *Perspectives on anxiety, panic, and fear: Current theory and research in motivation* (Vol. 43, pp. 211–250). Lincoln: University of Nebraska Press.

Mennen, F. E. (1995). The relationship of race/ethnicity to symptoms in childhood sexual abuse. *Child Abuse and Neglect, 19,* 115–124.

Meyerson, L. A., Long, P. J., Miranda Jr., R., & Marx, B. P. (2002). The influence of childhood sexual abuse, physical abuse, family environment, and gender on the psychological adjustment of adolescents. *Child Abuse and Neglect, 26,* 387–405.

Mills, C., Guerin, S., Lynch, F., Daly, I., & Fitzpatrick, C. (2004). The relationship between bullying, depression and suicidal thoughts/behaviour in Irish adolescents. *Irish Journal of Psychological Medicine, 21,* 112–116.

Moran, P. B., & Eckenrode, J. (1992). Protective personality characteristics among adolescent victims of maltreatment. *Child Abuse and Neglect, 16,* 743–754.

Moran, P. B., Vuchinich, S., & Hall, N. K. (2004). Associations between types of maltreatment and substance use during adolescence. *Child Abuse and Neglect, 28,* 565–574.

Nader, K. O., Kriegler, J., Blake, D., Pynoos, R., Newman, E., & Weather, F. (2002). *The Clinician-Administered PTSD Scale, Child and Adolescent Version (CAPS-CA).* White River Junction, VT: National Center for PTSD.

Nansel, T., Craig, W., Overpeck, M., Saluja, G., Ruan, J., and Health Behaviour in School-aged Children Bullying Analyses Working Group. (2004). Cross-national consistency in the relationship between bullying behaviours and psychosocial adjustment. *Archives of Pediatric and Adolescent Medicine, 158,* 730–736.

Nansel, T. R., Overpeck, M., Pilla, R. S., Ruan, W. J., Simons-Morton, B., & Scheidt, P. (2001). Bullying behaviors among US youth: Prevalence and association with psychosocial adjustment. *Journal of the American Medical Association, 285,* 2094–2100.

Ohan, J. L., Myers, K., & Collett, B. R. (2002). Ten-year review of rating scales. IV: Scales assessing trauma and its effects. *Journal of the American Academy of Child and Adolescent Psychiatry, 41,* 1401–1422.

O'Keefe, M. (1997). Predictors of dating violence among high school students. *Journal of Interpersonal Violence, 12,* 546–568.

Olweus, D. (1995). Bullying or peer abuse at school: Facts and interventions. *Current Directions in Psychological Science, 4,* 196–200.

Olweus, D. (1996). *The revised Olweus Bully/Victim Questionnaire.* Bergen, Norway: Research Center for Health Promotion (HEMIL Center), University of Bergen.

O'Moore, A. M., & Smith, P. K. (1997). Bullying behaviour in Irish schools: A nationwide study. *Irish Journal of Psychology, 18,* 141–169.

Osofsky, J. D. (2003). Prevalence of children's exposure to domestic violence and child maltreatment: Implications for prevention and intervention. *Clinical Child and Family Psychology Review, 6,* 161–170.

Pastore, D. R., Fisher, M., & Friedman, S. B. (1996). Violence and mental health problems among urban high school students. *Journal of Adolescent Health, 18,* 320–324.

Pearce, M. J., Jones, S. M., Schwab-Stone, M. E., & Ruchkin, V. (2003). The protective effects of religiousness and parent involvement on the development of conduct problems among youth exposed to violence. *Child Development, 74,* 1682–1696.

Perkonigg, A., Kessler, R. C., Storz, S., & Wittchen, H. (2000). Traumatic events and post-traumatic stress disorder in the community: Prevalence, risk factors and comorbidity. *Acta Psychiatrica Scandinavica, 101,* 46–59.

Perry, B. D. (2001). The neurodevelopmental impact of violence in childhood. In D. Schetky & E. P. Benedek (Eds.), *Textbook of child and adolescent forensic psychiatry* (pp. 221–238). Washington, DC: American Psychiatric Press.

Pettigrew, J., & Burcham, J. (1997). Effects of childhood sexual abuse in adult female psychiatric patients. *Australian and New Zealand Journal of Psychiatry, 31,* 208–213.

Pfferbaum, B. (1997). Posttraumatic stress disorder in children: A review of the past 10 years. *Journal of the American Academy of Child and Adolescent Psychiatry, 36,* 1503–1511.

Pine, D. S., & Cohen, J. A. (2002). Trauma in children and adolescents: risk and treatment of psychiatric sequelae. *Biological Psychiatry, 51,* 519–531.

Pynoos, R., Frederick, C., Nader, K., Arroyo, W., Steinberg, A., Eth, S., et al. (1987). Life threat and posttraumatic stress in school-age children. *Archives of General Psychiatry, 44,* 1057–1063.

Reich W. (1997). *Diagnostic Interview for Children and Adolescents: Revised DSM-IV version.* Toronto, ON, Canada: Multi-Health Systems.

Reinherz, H. Z., Giaconia, R. M., Lefkowitz, E. S., & Pakiz, B. (1993). Prevalence of psychiatric disorders in a community population of older adolescents. *Journal of the American Academy of Child and Adolescent Psychiatry, 32,* 369–377.

Resnick, M. D., Bearman, P. S., Blum, R. W., Bauman, K. E., Harris, K. M., & Jones, J. et al. (1997). Protecting adolescents from harm: findings from the national longitudinal study on adolescent health. *Journal of the American Medical Association, 278,* 823–832.

Rheingold, A. A., Smith, D. W., Ruggiero, K. J., Saunders, B. E., Kilpatrick, D. G., & Resnick, H. S.

(2004). Loss, trauma exposure, and mental health in a representative sample of 12–17-year-old youth: Data from the national survey of adolescents. *Journal of Loss and Trauma Special: Risk and Resiliency Following Trauma and Traumatic Loss, 9*, 1–19.

Rigby, K. (1997). *The Peer Relations Assessment Questionnaire*. Point Lonsdale, Victoria, Australia: Professional Reading Guide.

Rigby, K., & Slee, P. T. (1993). *The Peer Relations Questionnaire*. Point Lonsdale, Victoria, Australia: Professional Reading Guide.

Rivard, J. C., Bloom, S. L., Abramovitz, R., Pasquale, L. E., Duncan, M., & McCorkle, D., Gelman, A. (2003). Assessing the implementation and effects of a trauma-focused intervention for youths in residential treatment. *Psychiatric Quarterly, 74*, 137–154.

Rivard, J. C., McCorkle, D., Duncan, M. E., Pasquale, L. E., Bloom, S. L., & Abramovitz, R. (2004). Implementing a trauma recovery framework for youths in residential treatment. *Child and Adolescent Social Work Journal, 21*, 529–550.

Rivers, I. (2001). The bullying of sexual minorities at school: its nature and long-term correlates. *Educational and Child Psychology, 18*, 32–46.

Rivers, I. (2004). Recollections of bullying at school and their long-term implications for lesbians, gay men, and bisexuals. *Crisis, 25*, 169–175.

Robert, R., Blackeney, P. E., Villarreal, C., Rosenberg, L., & Meyer, W. J. (1999). Imipramine treatment in pediatric burn patients with symptoms of acute stress disorder: A pilot study. *Journal of the American Academy of Child and Adolescent Psychiatry, 38*, 873–882.

Roland, E., & Galloway, D. (2002). Classroom influences on bullying. *Educational Research, 44*, 299–312.

Ruchkin, V. V., Schwab-Stone, M., Koposov, R., Vermeiren, R., & Steiner, H. (2002). Violence exposure, posttraumatic stress, and personality in juvenile delinquents. *Journal of the American Academy of Child and Adolescent Psychiatry, 41*, 322–329.

Sack, W. H., Seeley, J. R., & Clarke, G. N. (1997). Does PTSD transcend cultural barriers? A study from the Khmer adolescent refugee project. *Journal of the American Academy of Child and Adolescent Psychiatry, 36*, 49–54.

Sadowski, H., Trowell, J., Kolvin, I., Weeramanthri, T., Berelowitz, M., & Gilbert, L. H. (2003). Sexually abused girls: Patterns of psychopathology and exploration of risk factors. *European Child and Adolescent Psychiatry, 12*, 221–230.

Saigh, P. A. (2002). *The Children's Post Traumatic Stress Disorder—Inventory* (CPTSD-I). New York: Author.

Saigh, P. A., Yasik, A., Oberfield, R., Green, B., Halamandaris, P., Rubenstein, H., et al. (2000). The Children's PTSD Inventory: Development and reliability. *Journal of Traumatic Stress, 13*, 369–380

Saltzman, W. R., Pynoos, R. S., Layne, C. M., Steinberg, A. M., & Aisenberg, E. (2001). Trauma- and grief-fo-

cused intervention for adolescents exposed to community violence: Results of a school-based screening and group treatment protocol. *Group Dynamics Special Issue: Group-Based Interventions for Trauma Survivors, 5*, 291–303.

Saltzman, W. R., Steinberg, A. M., Layne, C. M., Aisenberg, E., & Pynoos, R. S. (2001). A developmental approach to school-based treatment of adolescents exposed to trauma and traumatic loss. *Journal of Child and Adolescent Group Therapy, 11*, 43–56.

Saywitz, K. J., Mannarino, A. P., Berliner, L., & Cohen, J. A. (2000). Treatment of sexually abused children and adolescents. *American Psychologist, 55*, 1040–1049.

Schetky, D. H. (2003). PTSD in children and adolescents: An overview with guidelines for forensic assessment. In R. I. Simon (Ed.), *Posttraumatic stress disorder in litigation: Guidelines for forensic assessment* (pp. 91–118). Washington, DC: American Psychiatric Association.

Schoenfeld, F. B., Marmar, C. R., & Neylan, T. C. (2004). Current concepts in pharmacotherapy for posttraumatic stress disorder. *Psychiatric Services, 55*, 519–531.

Schwab-Stone, M., Chen, C., Greenberger, E., Silver, D., Lichtman, J., & Voyce, C. (1999). No safe haven II: The effects of violence exposure on urban youth. *Journal of the American Academy of Child and Adolescent Psychiatry, 38*, 359–367.

Seals, D., & Young, J. (2003). Bullying and victimization: Prevalence and relationship to gender, grade level, ethnicity, self-esteem, and depression. *Adolescence, 38*, 735–747.

Seedat, S., & Stein, D. J. (2001). Biological treatment of PTSD in children and adolescents. In S. Eth (Ed.), *PTSD in children and adolescents: Review of psychiatry* (Vol. 20, pp. 87–116). Washington, DC: American Psychiatric Association.

Seedat, S., Lockhat, R., Kaminer, D., Zungu-Dirwayi, N., & Stein, D. J. (2001). An open trial of citalopram in adolescents with post-traumatic stress disorder. *International Clinical Psychopharmacology, 16*, 21–25.

Shaffer, D., Fisher, P., Lucas, C., Dulcan, M., & Schwab-Stone, M. (2000). NIMH Diagnostic Interview Schedule for Children version IV (NIMH DISC-IV): Description, differences from previous versions, and reliability of some common diagnoses. *Journal of the American Academy of Child and Adolescent Psychiatry 39*, 28–38.

Shaffer, D., & Pfeffer, C. R. (2001). Practice parameters for the assessment and treatment of children and adolescents with suicidal behavior. *Journal of the American Academy of Child and Adolescent Psychiatry, 40*(Suppl. 7), 4S–23S.

Shapiro, D. L., & Levendosky, A. A. (1999). Adolescent survivors of childhood sexual abuse: The mediating role of attachment style and coping in psychological and interpersonal functioning. *Child Abuse and Neglect, 23*, 1175–1191.

Shaw, J. (2000). Children, adolescents and trauma. *Psychiatric Quarterly, 71*, 227–243.

Shaw, J. A. (1999). Practice parameters for the assessment and treatment of children and adolescents who are sexually abusive of others. *Journal of the American Academy of Child and Adolescent Psychiatry, 38*(Suppl. 12), 55S-76S.

Silverman, A. B., Reinherz, H. Z., & Giaconia, R. M. (1996). The long-term sequelae of child and adolescent abuse: A longitudinal community study. *Child Abuse and Neglect, 20*, 709–723.

Singer, M. I., Anglin, T. M., Song, L. Y., & Lunghofer, L. (1995). Adolescents' exposure to violence and associated symptoms of psychological trauma. *Journal of the American Medical Association, 273*, 477–482.

Smith, J. D., Schneider, B. H., Smith, P. K., & Ananiadou, K. (2004). The effectiveness of whole-school antibullying programs: A synthesis of evaluation research. *School Psychology Review, 33*, 547–560.

Smith, P. K. (2004). Bullying: Recent developments. *Child and Adolescent Mental Health, 9*, 98–103.

Smith, P. K., & Brain, P. (2000). Bullying in schools: Lessons from two decades of research. *Aggressive Behavior Special: Bullying in the Schools, 26*, 1–9.

Smith, P., Perrin, S., Dyregrov, A., & Yule, W. (2002). Principle components analysis of the Impact of Events Scale with children of war. *Personality and Individual Differences, 34*, 315–332.

Smith, P. H., White, J. W., & Holland, L. J. (2003). A longitudinal perspective on dating violence among adolescent and college-age women. *American Journal of Public Health, 93*, 1104–1109.

Spencer, M. B., Dupree, D., Cunningham, M., Harpalani, V., & Munoz-Miller, M. (2003). Vulnerability to violence: A contextually-sensitive, developmental perspective on African-American adolescents. *Journal of Social Issues, 59*, 33–49.

Stallard, P., Velleman, R., Langsford, J., & Baldwin, S. (2001). Coping and psychological distress in children involved in road traffic accidents. *British Journal of Clinical Psychology, 40*, 197–208.

Stein, B. D., Jaycox, L. H., Kataoka, S., Rhodes, H. J., & Vestal, K. D. (2003). Prevalence of child and adolescent exposure to community violence. *Clinical Child and Family Psychology Review, 6*, 247–264.

Stein, B. D., Jaycox, L. H., Kataoka, S. H., Wong, M., Tu, W., & Elliott, M. N., & Fink, A. (2003). A mental health intervention for schoolchildren exposed to violence: A randomized controlled trial. *JAMA: Journal of the American Medical Association, 290*, 603–611.

Stevens, S. J., Murphy, B. S., & McKnight, K. (2003). Traumatic stress and gender differences in relationship to substance abuse, mental health, physical health, and HIV risk behavior in a sample of adolescents enrolled in drug treatment. *Child Maltreatment, 8*, 46–57.

Swanston, H., Plunkett, A., O'Toole, B., Shrimpton, S., Parkinson, P., & Oates, K. (2003). Nine years after child sexual abuse. *Child Abuse and Neglect, 27*, 967–984.

Task Force on Adolescent Assault Victim Needs. (1996). Adolescent assault victim needs: A review of issues and a model protocol. *Pediatrics, 98*, 991–1001.

Tebbutt, J., Swanston, H., Oates, R. K., & O'Toole, B. (1997). 5 years after child sexual abuse: Persisting dysfunction and problems of prediction. *Journal of the American Academy of Child and Adolescent Psychiatry, 36*, 330–339.

Thabet, A. A. M., Tischler, V., & Vostanis, P. (2004). Maltreatment and coping strategies among male adolescents living in the Gaza Strip. *Child Abuse and Neglect, 28*, 77–91.

Thompson, K. M., Wonderlich, S. A., Crosby, R. D., & Mitchell, J. E. (2001). Sexual victimization and adolescent weight regulation practices: A test across community based samples. *Child Abuse and Neglect, 25*, 291–305.

Trocmé, N., MacLaurin, B., Fallon, B., Daciuk, J., Billingsley, D., Tourigny, M., et al. (2001). *Canadian Incidence Study of Reported Child Abuse and Neglect: Final report.* Ottawa, ON, Canada: Minister of Public Works and Government Services Canada.

Turner, H. A., & Butler, M. J. (2003). Direct and indirect effects of childhood adversity on depressive symptoms in young adults. *Journal of Youth and Adolescence, 32*, 89–103.

Tyler, K. A. (2002). Social and emotional outcomes of childhood sexual abuse: A review of recent research. *Aggression and Violent Behavior, 7*, 567–589.

UNICEF. (1998). *Report of programme workshop in the area of psychosocial care and protection.* Nyeri, Kenya: Author.

van IJzendoorn, M. H., & Schuengel, C. (1996). The measurement of dissociation in normal and clinical populations: Meta-analytic validation of the dissociative experiences scale (DES). *Clinical Psychology Review, 16*, 365–382.

Vermeiren, R., Ruchkin, V., Leckman, P. E., Deboutte, D., & Schwab-Stone, M. (2002). Exposure to violence and suicide risk in adolescents: A community study. *Journal of Abnormal Child Psychology, 30*, 529–537.

Weems, C. F., Saltzman, K. M., Reiss, A. L., & Carrion, V. G. (2003). A prospective test of the association between hyperarousal and emotional numbing in youth with a history of traumatic stress. *Journal of Clinical Child and Adolescent Psychology, 32*, 166–171.

Weiss, D. S., & Marmar, C. R. (1997). The Impact of Event Scale—Revised. In J. P. Wilson & T. M. Keane (Eds.), *Assessing psychological trauma and PTSD* (pp. 399–411). New York: Guilford Press.

Wekerle, C., & Avgoustis, E. (2003). Child maltreatment, adolescent dating, and adolescent dating violence. In P. Florsheim (Ed.), *Adolescent romantic relations and sexual behavior* (pp. 213–242). Mahwah, NJ: Erlbaum.

Wekerle, C., & Wolfe, D. A. (2003). Child maltreatment. In E. J. Mash & R. A. Barkley (Eds.), *Child psychopathology* (2nd ed., pp. 632–684). New York: Guilford Press.

Wheatley, M., Plant, J., Reader, H., Brown, G., & Cahill, C. (2004). Clozapine treatment of adolescents with posttraumatic stress disorder and psychotic symptoms. *Journal of Clinical Psychopharmacology, 24,* 167–173.

White, J. W., & Smith, P. H. (2004). Sexual assault perpetration and reperpetration: From adolescence to young adulthood. *Criminal Justice and Behavior, 31,* 182–202.

Whitney, I., & Smith, P. K. (1993). A survey of the nature and extent of bullying in junior/middle and secondary schools. *Educational Research, 34,* 3–25.

Williams, G. (1988). Sexual abuse of children. In G. Albee, J. Joffe, & L. D. Dusenbury (Eds.), *Prevention, powerlessness, and politics: A book of readings on social change* (pp. 141–160). Newbury Park, CA: Sage.

Wolfe, D. A., Francis, K. J., & Straatman, A. (in press). Child abuse in religiously-affiliated institutions: Long-term impact on men's mental health. *Child Abuse and Neglect.*

Wolfe, D. A., Jaffe, P., & Crooks, C. (in press). *Sex, drugs, and violence in adolescence: Engaging youth in education and prevention.* New Haven, CT: Yale University Press.

Wolfe, D. A., Jaffe, P., Jette, J., & Poisson, S. (2003). The impact of child abuse in community institutions and organizations: Advancing professional and scientific understanding. *Clinical Psychology: Science and Practice, 10,* 179–191.

Wolfe, D. A., Wekerle, C., Scott, K., Straatman, A. L., & Grasley, C. (2004). Predicting abuse in adolescent dating relationships over 1 year: The role of child maltreatment and trauma. *Journal of Abnormal Psychology, 113,* 406–415.

Wolfe, D. A., Sas, L., & Wekerle, C. (1994). Factors associated with the development of post-traumatic stress disorder among child victims of sexual abuse. *Child Abuse and Neglect, 18,* 37–50.

Wood, J., Foy, D. W., Layne, C., Pynoos, R., & James, C. B. (2002). An examination of the relationships between violence exposure, posttraumatic stress symp-

tomatology, and delinquent activity: An "ecopathological" model of delinquent behavior among incarcerated adolescents. *Journal of Aggression, Maltreatment and Trauma, 6,* 127–147.

World Health Organization. (2002). *World Report on violence and health: Summary.* Geneva: Author.

Ybarra, M. L. (2004). Linkages between depressive symptomatology and Internet harassment among young regular Internet users. *CyberPsychology and Behavior, 7,* 247–257.

Ybarra, M., & Mitchell, K. (2004). Youth engaging in online harassment: Associations with caregiver–child relationships, Internet use, and personal characteristics. *Journal of Adolescence, 27,* 319–336.

Yehuda, R., Spertus, I. L., & Golier, J. A. (2001). Relationship between childhood traumatic experiences and PTSD in adults. In S. Eth (Ed.), *PTSD in children and adolescents* (pp. 117–158). Washington, DC: American Psychiatric Association.

Young, R., & Sweeting, H. (2004). Adolescent bullying, relationships, psychological well-being, and gender-atypical behavior: A gender diagnosticity approach. *Sex Roles, 50,* 525–537.

Youngstrom, E., Weist, M. D., & Albus, K. E. (2003). Exploring violence exposure, stress, protective factors and behavioral problems among inner-city youth. *American Journal of Community Psychology, 32,* 115–129.

Yule, W., Stuvland, R., Baingana, F. K., & Smith, P. (2003). Children in armed conflict. In B. L. Green, M. J. Friedman, J. de Jong, S. D. Solomon, T. M. Keane, J. A. Fairbank, et al. (Eds.), *Trauma interventions in war and peace: Prevention, practice, and policy* (pp. 217–242). New York: Kluwer.

Zlotnick, C., Shea, M. T., Begin, A., & Pearlstein, T. (1996). The validation of the Trauma Symptom Checklist—40 (TSC-40) in a sample of inpatients. *Child Abuse and Neglect, 20,* 503–510.

Zubenko, W. N. (2002). Developmental issues in stress and crisis. In W. N. Zubenko & J. A. Capozzoli (Eds.), *Children and disasters: A practical guide to healing and recovery* (pp. 85–100). New York: Oxford University Press.

Author Index

Subject Index

Page numbers followed by *f* indicate figure; *t*, table.